Nutrition and Metabolism in the Surgical Patient

Nutrition and Metabolism in the Surgical Patient

Second Edition

Edited by

Josef E. Fischer, M.D.
Christian R. Holmes Professor and Chairman of Surgery
University of Cincinnati College of Medicine
Cincinnati

Surgeon-in-Chief
University Hospital, Christian R. Holmes Hospital, and
University of Cincinnati Medical Center
Cincinnati

Little, Brown and Company
Boston New York Toronto London

Second Edition

Library of Congress Cataloging-in-Publication Data

Nutrition and metabolism in the surgical patient / edited by Josef E. Fischer.—2nd ed.
p. cm.
Rev. ed. of: Surgical nutrition. c1983.
Includes bibliographical references and index.
ISBN 0-316-28390-8
1. Surgery—Nutritional aspects. 2. Metabolic manifestations of general diseases. I. Fischer, Josef E., 1937– . II. Surgical nutrition.
[DNLM: 1. Postoperative Care. 2. Nutritional Support—methods. 3. Metabolism—physiology. WO 183 N976 1996]
RD52.N88S868 1996
617—dc20
DNLM/DLC
for Library of Congress 95-31028
CIP

Printed in the United States of America
MV-NY

Editorial: Nancy E. Chorpenning
Production Editor: Katharine S. Mascaro
Indexer: Jill Jordan of AlphaByte & Co.
Production Supervisor: Michael A. Granger
Cover Designer: Ethan W. Thomas

Dedication

In the summer of 1966, a new intern appeared on the pediatric surgical service of the Massachusetts General Hospital, a service on which I was chief resident. He had graduated from the University of Pennsylvania, where he had worked in the Harrison Department of Surgical Research. In the next laboratory there was a resident by the name of Stanley Dudrick who was doing some very interesting experiments in Dr. Jonathan Rhoads' laboratory. Ron Abel, the new intern, carefully observed what Dr. Dudrick had accomplished, namely the nutritional support of animals purely by vein. When Ron Abel came to the Massachusetts General Hospital, he quickly told the chief resident on the pediatric surgical service about this astounding development. I was that chief resident on the pediatric surgical service. Although skeptical at first, we invited Dr. Dudrick to the Massachusetts General Hospital to tell us about his discoveries, and, with Dr. William Abbott, set up our own hyperalimentation unit in 1968. My own interest, and the Hyperalimentation Unit at the Massachusetts General Hospital, was born. It was Ron Abel who brought that information to us and originally provided the spark.

Dr. Abel subsequently pursued a career in cardiac surgery. Some of his original work on starvation and cardiac function and on renal failure still stands as classic—work which included the use of essential amino acids and hypertonic dextrose in the treatment of patients with acute renal failure. A loyal friend who was at the same time brilliant, unpredictable, at times impossible to deal with, but always inquisitive and continually striving for excellence, Ron Abel was a pioneer in the field of nutritional support.

Ron Abel was tragically killed in an automobile accident in November 1993. This volume is dedicated to his memory.

Contents

Preface

Over 10 years have passed since the publication of the first edition of *Surgical Nutrition.* At that time, the book signaled the end of perhaps the second phase of nutritional support. During the first phase—the establishment of in-hospital nutritional support—the field was one of unbridled enthusiasm, with widespread application of newer techniques prior to the requirement for proof of efficacy. By the time *Surgical Nutrition,* from which this volume has grown, first appeared in 1983, the field had developed to the point where proof of efficacy was being demanded. Enthusiasm had given way to prospective trials and cost-consciousness—characteristics which stand us in good stead even today in our cost-conscious era.

Once again, the field of nutrition is in transition. This new, completely revised edition of *Nutrition and Metabolism in the Surgical Patient* is a snapshot, as it were, of changes in our understanding of metabolism, mediators, and mechanisms in an effort to formulate the best ways to support patients who may be critically ill. By comparison with the first book, it is easy to understand the need for completely rethinking the goals and content in our revised edition.

The field has evolved considerably. Whereas the emphasis was initially on parenteral nutrition, the focus is now on the gut. Investigations are proceeding apace as to what specific advantage the gut brings to nutritional support. Parenteral nutrition is used only if enteral support is not possible. Nutritional pharmacology (the term originally proposed by J. Wesley Alexander), in which such naturally-occurring components as arginine, glutamine, omega-3 fatty acids, and other components documented in this volume are given in supranormal amounts, has come into its own as a discrete field. The study of total parenteral nutrition has also evolved into examination of the mechanisms and mediators by which changes in metabolism occur in illness. Extensive and important chapters in *Nutrition and Metabolism of the Surgical Patient* are devoted to the study of such metabolism and mediators. To comprehend metabolism and the changes in illness is to understand how to intervene.

This volume is intended hopefully to be used by a variety of individuals with skills varying from the least sophisticated to the most knowledgeable of physicians, nurses, dietitians, and pharmacists dealing with nutritional support. We have tried to make this book a mixture of the theoretical; the background for what we do and why we do it; as well as some of the basics of intermediary metabolism; the causation and pathophysiology of cytokines and mediators; and the practical aspects of how we care for patients, what the complications are, and how they may be prevented. To the extent that these attempts are successful, and they are difficult to encompass in a single volume, I owe it all to the excellent group of contributors, to the editors at Little, Brown and Company, and especially to Nancy Chorpenning, with whom I have enjoyed a wonderful professional relationship for many years. This book would not have been possible without the excellent editorial assistance of Steve Wiesner. My loyal and efficient office staff—Judy Braun, Gilda Young, Mary Wiesman, and Joann Trodahl—protect me from myself. And to my family, who have endured my working on this volume for more Saturday and Sunday mornings and evenings than I care to remember, my profound thanks for what is seemingly an endless amount of support.

I hope that this volume, as it captures the current field of nutritional support in the mid-1990's, will accomplish at least several of the goals that we have set for it.

J.E.F.

Contributing Authors

Steve F. Abcouwer, Ph.D.
Instructor in Surgery, Harvard Medical School; Assistant Biochemist, Department of Surgical Oncology, Massachusetts General Hospital, Boston
12. Glutamine as a Metabolic Intermediate

Naji N. Abumrad, M.D.
Professor and Chairman, Department of Surgery; Dean, School of Medicine, State University of New York at Stony Brook, Stony Brook, New York
4. Energy Metabolism

J. Wesley Alexander, M.D., Sc.D.
Professor of Surgery, University of Cincinnati College of Medicine; Director, Transplantation Division, University Hospital, Cincinnati
17. Translocation as It Applies to Metabolism

Adrian Barbul, M.D.
Associate Professor of Surgery, Johns Hopkins Medical Institutions; Assistant Surgeon-in-Chief, Sinai Hospital of Baltimore, Baltimore
14. Arginine

R. Daniel Beauchamp, M.D.
Associate Professor of Surgery and Cell Biology, Vanderbilt University School of Medicine; Associate Clinical Director, Vanderbilt Cancer Center, Vanderbilt University Medical Center, Nashville, Tennessee
5. Growth Factors

Scott M. Berry, M.D.
Chief Resident and Nutrition Support Fellow, Department of Surgery, University of Cincinnati Medical Center, Cincinnati
28. Parenteral Nutrition, 29. Enteral Nutrition, 30. Critical Evaluation of Results: Cost and Benefit of Nutrition Support

Palmer Q. Bessey, M.D.
Professor of Surgery, University of Rochester School of Medicine; Director of Trauma and Critical Care, Co-Director of Burn Center, and Attending Surgeon, Strong Memorial Hospital, Rochester, New York
21. Metabolic Response to Trauma and Infection

Timothy R. Billiar, M.D.
Associate Professor of Surgery, University of Pittsburgh School of Medicine; Attending Surgeon, Presbyterian University Hospital, Pittsburgh
16. Nitric Oxide

Barrie P. Bode, Ph.D.
Instructor in Surgery, Harvard Medical School; Assistant Biochemist, Department of Surgical Oncology, Massachusetts General Hospital, Boston
12. Glutamine as a Metabolic Intermediate

Robert H. Bower, M.D.
Professor of Surgery, University of Cincinnati College of Medicine; Chief, Surgery Service, Cincinnati Veterans Affairs Medical Center, Cincinnati
29. Enteral Nutrition

Timothy E. Bowling, M.D.
Honorary Research Fellow, Department of Gastroenterology and Nutrition, Central Middlesex Hospital, NHS Trust; Senior Registrar, Department of Gastroenterology, The Middlesex Hospital, UCLH NHS Trust, London
2. Intestinal Digestion and Absorption of Nutrients

Robert A. Burns, Ph.D.
Associate Director, Nutrition Research, Mead Johnson and Company, Evansville, Indiana
9. Vitamins

Simon Bursztein, M.D.
Full Professor, Faculty of Medicine, Technion-Israel Institute of Technology, Bat-Galim; Director, Department of General Intensive Care, Rambam Medical Center, Haifa, Israel
4. Energy Metabolism

Gordon P. Buzby, M.D.
Associate Professor of Surgery, University of Pennsylvania School of Medicine; Attending Surgeon, Hospital of the University of Pennsylvania, Philadelphia
23. Changes in Immunologic Function

Yvon A. Carpentier, M.D.
Professor of Surgery and Director, L. Deloyers Laboratory for Experimental Surgery, Clinique de Nutrition, Free University of Brussels; Director, One Day Clinic, Hôpital Erasne, Brussels, Belgium
8. Plasma Lipoproteins and Intravenous Lipid Emulsions

Alex C. Cech, M.D.
Resident, Department of Surgery, University of Pennsylvania School of Medicine, Philadelphia
22. Nutrition and Neoplasia

Tsueng H. Chang, Ph.D.
Assistant Professor of Surgery, Albert Einstein College of Medicine of Yeshiva University; Assistant Professor of Surgery, Montefiore Medical Center, Bronx, New York
20. Starvation: Metabolic and Physiologic Responses

Wei-Kuen Cheong, M.B., B.S., M.R.C.P.
Physican, Internal Medicine, Medicine II, Singapore General Hospital, Singapore
10. Essential Trace Metals: Deficiencies and Requirements

John M. Daly, M.D.
Lewis Atterbury Stimson Professor and Chairman of Surgery, Cornell University Medical College; Surgeon-in-Chief, New York Hospital, New York
22. Nutrition and Neoplasia

Richard J. Deckelbaum, M.D., C.M.
Robert R. Williams Professor of Nutrition and Director, Institute of Human Nutrition, College of Physicians and Surgeons of Columbia University; Director, Division of Gastroenterology and Nutrition, Department of Pediatrics, Babies Hospital, New York
8. Plasma Lipoproteins and Intravenous Lipid Emulsions

Denis Y. Dubois, M.D.
Scientific Collaborator, L. Deloyers Laboratory for Experimental Surgery, Clinique de Nutrition, Free University of Brussels, Brussels, Belgium
8. Plasma Lipoproteins and Intravenous Lipid Emulsions

Josef E. Fischer, M.D.
Christian R. Holmes Professor and Chairman of Surgery, University of Cincinnati College of Medicine; Surgeon-in-Chief, University Hospital, Christian R. Holmes Hospital, and University of Cincinnati Medical Center, Cincinnati
24. Nutritional Support in Hepatic Failure, 25. Nutritional Management in Acute Renal Failure

Herbert R. Freund, M.D.
Professor of Surgery, Hebrew University-Hadassah Medical School; Chief of Surgery, Hadassah University Hospital, Mount Scopus, Jerusalem
26. Nutrition of Heart and Lung

Roberto Gennari, M.D.
Research Fellow, Transplantation Division, Department of Surgery, University of Cincinnati College of Medicine, Cincinnati
17. Translocation as It Applies to Metabolism

Harry L. Greene, M.D.
Clinical Professor, Indiana School of Medicine; Senior Director, Nutritional Sciences, Mead Johnson Nutrition Group, Evansville, Indiana
9. Vitamins

George K. Grimble, B.Sc., Ph.D.
Reader in Clinical Nutrition, Roehampton Institute of London, Whitelands College; Honorary Senior Lecturer, Department of Clinical Biochemistry, Kings College School of Medicine and Dentistry, London
2. Intestinal Digestion and Absorption of Nutrients

Per-Olof Hasselgren, M.D., Ph.D.
Professor of Surgery, University of Cincinnati College of Medicine; Attending Surgeon, University of Cincinnati Medical Center, Cincinnati
3. Mediators, Hormones, and Control of Metabolism: Regulation of Protein, Carbohydrate, and Lipid Metabolism in Critical Illness

Graham L. Hill, M.D., Ch.M.
Professor of Surgery, Faculty of Medicine, The University of Auckland School of Medicine; Consultant in Colon and Rectal Surgery and Director, Surgical Nutrition and Metabolism Laboratory, Auckland Hospital, Auckland, New Zealand
19. Nutritional Assessment: The Assessment of the Nutritional and Metabolic Status of Surgical Patients

Harriet Williams Hopf, M.D.
Assistant Professor of Anesthesia and Surgery, University of California, San Francisco, School of Medicine; Anesthesiologist, University of California Medical Center and Hospitals, San Francisco
15. Nutrition in Wound Healing

Thomas K. Hunt, M.D.
Professor and Vice Chair, Department of Surgery, University of California, San Francisco, School of Medicine; Surgeon, University of California Medical Center and Hospitals, San Francisco
15. Nutrition in Wound Healing

Obi J. Imegwu, M.D.
National Institute of General Medicine Research Fellow, Department of Surgery, Albert Einstein College of Medicine of Yeshiva University; Resident in Surgery, Montefiore Medical Center, Bronx, New York
20. Starvation: Metabolic and Physiologic Responses

Danny O. Jacobs, M.D., M.P.H.
Associate Professor of Surgery, Harvard Medical School; Associate Surgeon, Brigham and Women's Hospital, Boston
1. Body Composition

Khursheed N. Jeejeebhoy, M.B., B.S., Ph.D.
Professor of Medicine, Nutrition and Physiology, University of Toronto, Toronto
10. Essential Trace Metals: Deficiencies and Requirements

John C. Kucharczuk, M.D.
Postdoctoral Research Fellow, Harrison Department of Surgical Research, University of Pennsylvania School of Medicine; Surgical Resident, Hospital of the University of Pennsylvania, Philadelphia
23. Changes in Immunologic Function

Joseph A. Lacy, M.S., R.D.
Nutritionist, Department of Parenteral and Enteral Nutrition, University of Cincinnati Medical Center, Cincinnati
30. Critical Evaluation of Results: Cost and Benefit of Nutrition Support

Stanley M. Levenson, M.D.
University Professor Emeritus, Department of Surgery, Albert Einstein College of Medicine of Yeshiva University; Director, Surgical Intensive Care—Burn Unit, Department of Surgery, Jacobi Medical Center, Bronx, New York
20. Starvation: Metabolic and Physiologic Responses

John I. Lew, A.B.
Research Fellow, Harrison Department of Surgical Research, University of Pennsylvania School of Medicine; Medical Student, Department of Surgery, Hospital of the University of Pennsylvania, Philadelphia
13. Intestinal Fuels: Implications for Improvement of Intestinal Growth and Function

Michael A. Lieberman, Ph.D.
Professor of Molecular Genetics, University of Cincinnati College of Medicine, Cincinnati
7. Carbohydrates

Tory A. Meyer, M.D.
Surgical Resident and Research Fellow, Department of Surgery, University of Cincinnati College of Medicine, Cincinnati
25. Nutritional Management in Acute Renal Failure

Patricia Molina, M.D., Ph.D.
Assistant Professor of Surgery, State University of New York at Stony Brook, Stony Brook, New York
4. Energy Metabolism

Francis D. Moore, M.D.
Moseley Professor of Surgery Emeritus, Harvard Medical School; Surgeon-in-Chief Emeritus, Peter Bent Brigham Hospital, Boston
11. Two Dozen Syndromes: Pattern Recognition in Diagnosis and Treatment of Fluid and Electrolyte Disorders

Michael S. Nussbaum, M.D.
Assistant Professor of Surgery, University of Cincinnati College of Medicine; Attending Surgeon and Director of Surgical Endoscopy, University of Cincinnati Medical Center, Cincinnati
28. Parenteral Nutrition

Michael D. Peck, M.D., Sc.D.
Associate Professor of Surgery, University of Miami School of Medicine; Assistant Director, University of Miami/Jackson Memorial Burn Center, Miami
18. Omega-3 and Other Polyunsaturated Fatty Acids: Modulation of the Inflammatory Response

Gary W. Raff, M.D.
Chief Resident in Surgery, University Hospital, University of Medicine and Dentistry of New Jersey, Newark, New Jersey
25. Nutritional Management in Acute Renal Failure

Malcolm K. Robinson, M.D.
Clinical Fellow in Surgery, Harvard Medical School; Assistant to the Surgeon-in-Chief, Department of Surgery, Brigham and Women's Hospital, Boston
1. Body Composition

John L. Rombeau, M.D.
Professor of Surgery, University of Pennsylvania School of Medicine; Attending Surgeon, Hospital of the University of Pennsylvania, Philadelphia
13. Intestinal Fuels: Implications for Improvement of Intestinal Growth and Function

David B. A. Silk, M.D.
Co-Director and Consultant Physician, Department of Gastroenterology and Nutrition, Central Middlesex Hospital, NHS Trust, London
2. Intestinal Digestion and Absorption of Nutrients

Richard L. Simmons, M.D.
Professor of Surgery, University of Pittsburgh School of Medicine; Chief of Surgery and Attending Surgeon, Presbyterian University Hospital, Pittsburgh
16. Nitric Oxide

Wiley W. Souba, M.D., Sc.D.
Professor of Surgery, Harvard Medical School; Chief of Surgical Oncology and Director, Nutrition Support Unit, Massachusetts General Hospital, Boston
12. Glutamine as a Metabolic Intermediate

E. Aubrey Thompson, Ph.D.
Professor and Vice Chairman, Department of Human Biological Chemistry and Genetics, University of Texas Medical Branch, University of Texas Medical School at Galveston, Galveston, Texas
5. Growth Factors

Gregory M. Tiao, M.D.
Surgical Resident and Research Fellow, University of Cincinnati College of Medicine, Cincinnati
24. Nutritional Support in Hepatic Failure

John W. Vester, M.D.
Professor of Medicine and Biochemistry Emeritus and Associate Dean Emeritus, University of Cincinnati College of Medicine; Director of Research and Chairman Emeritus, Endocrine Section, Good Samaritan Hospital; Attending Staff Emeritus, Internal Medicine, University Hospital, Cincinnati
7. Carbohydrates

Brad W. Warner, M.D.
Assistant Professor of Surgery, University of Cincinnati College of Medicine; Attending Surgeon, Division of Pediatric Surgery, Children's Hospital Medical Center, Cincinnati
27. Special Needs of the Pediatric Patient

John A. Windsor, M.D.
Senior Lecturer in Surgery, Faculty of Medicine and Health Science, The University of Auckland School of Medicine; Consultant General Surgeon, Auckland Hospital, Auckland, New Zealand
19. Nutritional Assessment: The Assessment of the Nutritional and Metabolic Status of Surgical Patients

Vernon R. Young, Ph.D., D.Sc.
Professor of Nutritional Biochemistry, Massachusetts Institute of Technology, Cambridge, Massachusetts; Director, Mass Spectrometry Facility, Shriners Burns Institute, Boston
6. Protein and Amino Acid Metabolism

Susan M. Ystueta, M.D.
Resident in Surgery, Massachusetts General Hospital, Boston
4. Energy Metabolism

Yong-Ming Yu, M.D., Ph.D.
Research Fellow, Clinical Research Center, Massachusetts Institute of Technology, Cambridge, Massachusetts; Associate Biochemist, Department of Surgery, Massachusetts General Hospital, Boston
6. Protein and Amino Acid Metabolism

I

General Considerations

Notice. The indications for and dosages of all drugs in this book have been recommended in the medical literature and conform to the practices of the general medical community. The medications described do not necessarily have specific approval by the Food and Drug Administration for use in the diseases and dosages for which they are recommended. The package insert for each drug should be consulted for use and dosage as approved by the FDA. Because standards for usage change, it is advisable to keep abreast of revised recommendations, particularly those concerning new drugs.

1

Body Composition

Danny O. Jacobs
Malcolm K. Robinson

There are four main components to assessing a patient's response to nutritional or metabolic intervention: energy and protein balance, body composition, physiologic function, and the degree of metabolic stress (injury or sepsis) [1]. The interaction of these factors can be conceptualized as a series of circles (Figure 1-1) [2]. Circle A depicts the normal body composition and physiologic function of a healthy subject. Disease induces negative energy and protein balances that are accompanied by changes in body composition

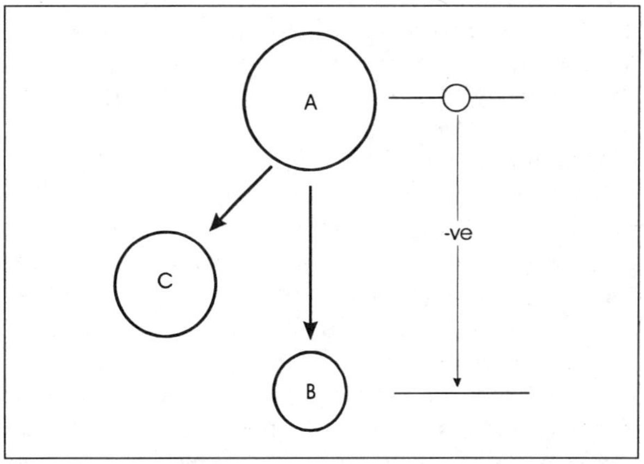

Figure 1-1. A theoretical framework for describing the relationship between energy, protein balance, body composition, and function. The purpose of nutritional assessment is to determine the location, direction, and rate of change of the patient between circles A, B, and C. (From SB Heymsfield, PJ Williams. Nutritional Assessment by Clinical and Biochemical Methods. In ME Shills, UR Young [eds], *Modern Nutrition in Health and Disease* [7th ed]. Philadelphia: Lea & Febiger, 1988.)

and function. Circle B represents the condition where the bodily reserves of fat and protein have been consumed and physiologic function is fatally compromised. Alternatively, major injury or infection may intervene (circle C) and be associated with tissue catabolism and expansion of body water compartments.

This chapter discusses body composition as one component of nutritional and metabolic assessment. A review of various modeling systems is needed to understand the methods used to study the effects of disease. The chapter concludes with a consideration of changes in body composition in the context of the metabolic effects of starvation, stress, and refeeding.

Overview

Nutritional states were originally defined, and still may be most easily understood, in anthropometric terms. Because the traditional goal of nutrition support is to maintain or restore normal body composition, nutritional assessment techniques are currently largely based on tests for changes in body composition. Thus, in the past, changes in composition were indirectly assessed by monitoring changes in body anthropometry.

Anthropometry uses simple measurements of body thicknesses to estimate fat and lean tissue mass. It can estimate both the amount and rate of change of the total energy supply in the body [3]. The major advantages of anthropometry are that it is simple, safe, and inexpensive, and it can be easily performed at the bedside. These relative advantages are outweighed by errors inherent in the method. The person performing the measurements must be well trained, and the measurements should be obtained in a reproducible manner from specific anatomic sites to maximize the accuracy of the technique. Ideally, the same person should perform all the measurements required for a particular patient. In addition, because the measurements are usually compared to those of a reference population, the quality of the reference standards is very important. Even if these factors are accounted for, changes in energy and nitrogen balance during the short term may not be accurately detected by anthropometry, although it may detect large shifts in body composition during a period of months or years. Thus, the variability of the measurements is such that usually only gross changes can be identified as abnormal. Changes in anthropometric indices may not correlate with measurements of changes in total body potassium, believed to be an accurate measure of lean body mass [4,5], or accurately reflect changes in total body nitrogen as measured by neutron activation analysis. In the severely ill, hospitalized patient who is subject to major shifts in body water, anthropometric measurements may be especially hazardous.

Modeling Changes in Body Composition

One- and Two-Compartment Models

The body can be divided into two or more compartments based on anatomic, fluid, or chemical components [6]. Many different models of body composition have been developed and investigated, but cardinal to most models is the measurement of total body water. Water is the single largest component of the body, representing approximately 55% of the total weight of the average, healthy individual [7,8]. Total body water is often divided into intracellular water and extracellular water, which constitute 30% and 25% of body weight, respectively. Extracellular water is further subdivided into plasma volume and interstitial fluid. Blood volume is composed of intracellular (primarily in erythrocytes) and extracellular (i.e., plasma) water (Figure 1-2). Methods for measuring total body water and its subdivisions in vivo are presented in Table 1-1. The most commonly used body composition model is a *two-compartment model* in which the body is divided into fat and lean tissues (Figure 1-3) [9,10].

Various techniques have been developed to measure at least one component of the two-compartment model. In the 1940s, Behnke and col-

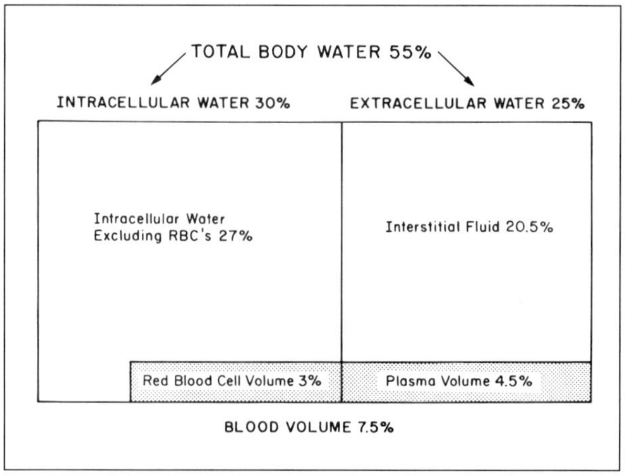

Figure 1-2. Total body water and its divisions. Percentages refer to approximate fraction that each component contributes to total body weight. (Data from FD Moore. *Metabolic Care of the Surgical Patient.* Philadelphia: Saunders, 1959.)

Table 1-1. In Vivo Measurement of Total Body Water and Its Components

Compartment	Technique for Measurement	Explanation
Total body water (TBW)	1. Hydrogen isotopes deuterium oxide tritium oxide	Hydrogen isotopes mix freely with entire water compartment of the body. TBW will approximately equal the amount of isotope given divided by the concentration of the isotope in the plasma after its equilibration in the body.
	2. Bioelectrical impedance analysis (BIA)	Entails passage of a weak electrical current through the body and measurement of the resistance to flow of this current. Whole-body resistance is reciprocally related to the volume of TBW and correlates highly ($r>0.90$) with above isotope dilution techniques.
Extracellular water (ECW)	1. Sodium bromide	Bromide distribution equivalent to chloride distribution in the body, which is primarily limited to the extracellular fluid space. ECW approximately equals amount of bromide given divided by plasma bromide concentration at equilibrium.
	2. Sulfur-35-labeled sulfate	Sulfur is primarily limited to the extracellular space, and this labeled species can be used to calculate ECW using the dilution principle as outlined above for the hydrogen isotopes and sodium bromide.
Intracellular water (ICW)	—	Direct measurement is not done but is calculated from the formula ICW = TBW − ECW.
Plasma volume (PV)	1. I^{131} radiolabeled albumin	Albumin is limited to the plasma space. Dilution of radiolabel in plasma can be measured and used to calculate total plasma volume using same principle as used for nonradioactive isotopes or markers.
	2. Indocyanine green	Also limited to plasma space, but is rapidly cleared by liver. Therefore, one must correct for this factor before calculating plasma volume using isotope/marker dilution principle.
Red cell volume (RCV)	CR^{51}-labeled red blood cells	Labeled cells are distributed among normal red cells in body, allowing calculation of total red cell volume by standard dilution principles.
Blood volume (BV)	—	Determined by adding plasma and red cell volumes, i.e., BV = PV + RCV

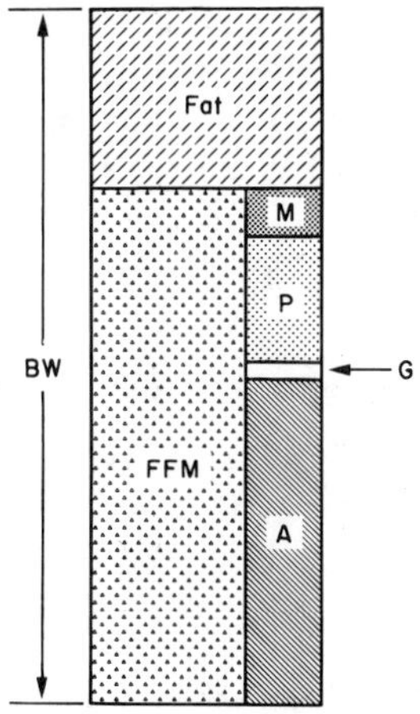

Figure 1-3. Graphic representation of the two-compartment model. According to this approach, fat is either extractable lipid and the remainder of the body weight (BW) is the fat free body mass (FFM). The fat free mass is the sum of four fat-free components: water (A), mineral (M), protein (P), and glycogen (G).

leagues used underwater weighing techniques to estimate *body density* (D_b) [11]. They showed that body density can be expressed as a function of the sum of the densities of its constituent components according to the equation

$$D_b = \left[\sum_{i=0}^{n}\left(\frac{M_i}{M_t} \times \frac{1}{D_i}\right)\right]^{-1}$$

where D_b = body density, M_i = mass of compartment i, M_t = total mass, D_i = density of i.

Therefore, it is possible to estimate the fraction of body weight that is fat if the body's density and the densities of its fat and the "fat-free" masses are known. The fat-free mass is an expression of the composite densities of the body's aqueous, protein, and total mineral components. The density of fat can be estimated from direct measurements performed on tissue specimens. Postmortem studies of animals and humans have been used to derive average values (1.1 g/cc) for the density of the fat-free mass. If one assumes that the densities of fat and the fat-free compartments are known and constant, the fraction of body weight that is fat (fF) can be estimated for an individual using the measured body density (D_b) according to the equation

$$fF = 4.95/D_b - 4.50$$

The fat-free mass (fFFM) is then calculated from the body weight

$$fFFM = \text{body weight} \times (1 - fF)$$

Measurements of residual lung volume are also needed to accurately determine body density.

Because it is impractical to submerge some patients to measure body density, other less cumbersome techniques using water space markers were developed to measure the body's water content. Although there are many compounds that distribute throughout the total body water space and can be used to measure its size, the most common approach is the dilution of labeled water. Three isotopes of water may be used: radioactive tritiated water (^3H_2O) and the stable isotopes deuterium oxide (D_2O) or labeled oxygen ($H_2{}^{18}O$). The labeled water hydrogens and deuterium and tritiated water rapidly exchange with the hydrogens in carboxyl, amide, hydroxyl, and other organic groups that comprise protein, fat, and carbohydrate. As a result of this exchange process, the deuterium and tritiated water dilution volumes are 3% to 5% larger than actual total body water [12]. The stable isotope $H_2{}^{18}O$ differs from the other two isotopes of water because it exchanges with bicarbonate in blood. The labeled bicarbonate ultimately equilibrates with carbon dioxide and is excreted by the respiratory system. Water labeled with ^{18}O also slowly exchanges with minerals and other tissue components such as calcium hydroxyapatite. The $H_2{}^{18}O$ dilution space may be approximately 1% larger than the actual size of the total body water space.

Classically, total body water is measured in vivo by giving a patient a known quantity of one of the hydrogen isotopes deuterium and tritium oxide. Because these compounds freely mix with total body water, after equilibration of the hydrogen isotopes with all body compartments, which takes about 3 hours, total body water will approximately equal the amount of isotope given divided by the concentration of the compound in plasma [13]. Based on research by Pace and Rathbun [14], it is assumed that total body water equals 73.2% of lean body mass. Body fat is then determined by subtracting lean body mass from total body weight. That is,

$$\text{Lean body mass} = \text{total body weight}/0.732$$

and

$$\text{Body fat} = \text{body weight} - \text{lean body mass}$$

Lean body mass is composed of body cell mass and extracellular mass. Body cell mass is defined as "that component of body composition containing the oxygen-exchanging, potassium-rich, glucose-oxidizing, work-performing tissue [15]." Because the "work-performing" tissue resides in this compartment, body cell mass is considered the most important constituent of the body, and its diminution adversely affects the host. Extracellular mass is the difference between body cell mass and lean body mass (i.e., lean body mass minus body cell mass) and consists of extracellular water and extracellular solids such as bone, collagen, and extracellular minerals. Body cell mass represents the total cellular mass and is the living metabolically active component of the body. As such, it performs all the work done by the body and is responsible for all the oxygen consumption and carbon dioxide production. In normal individuals, the body cell mass accounts for 50% of the lean body mass. The extracellular mass is metabolically inactive, and its major functions are transport and support.

By using other isotopes, the dilutional techniques can be extended to derive other components of the body. In one commonly used method, a fixed known amount of tritiated water and ^{22}Na are administered simultaneously. Total body water is determined at equilibrium from the plasma tritium concentration at specific time points after administration [16], and total exchangeable sodium is determined from the specific activity of ^{22}Na. Total exchangeable potassium is then calculated from the measurement of total body water multiplied by a constant R, which is the ratio of the sum of sodium and potassium in a sample of whole blood divided by its water content. The total exchangeable sodium content is then subtracted from this quantity to yield the total exchangeable potassium. Thus,

$$K_e = \text{total body water} \times R\ Na_e$$

The validity of determining exchangeable potassium using this method has been demonstrated in man and animals [17]. Whole body potassium can also be determined from the dilution of its radioactive isotopes. However, a naturally occurring isotope of potassium, ^{40}K, exists in the body at a known abundance of 0.012% compared with total body potassium. This isotope emits a characteristic gamma ray that can be counted by a whole body gamma ray detector, allowing quantification of total body ^{40}K and thus total body potassium [18]. The body's potassium content is more often determined using ^{40}K counting. However, gamma-radiometric equipment for measuring total body potassium is not readily available. The ratio of potassium to the fat-free body mass is derived from studies of both cadaver and in vivo studies [15,19,20]. Dividing this ratio into the subjects, measured total body potassium can be used to estimate the fat-free mass that is calculated as the difference between body weight and the fat-free mass.

Once these quantities are derived, other components of the body can be calculated:

$$\begin{aligned}\text{Body cell mass} &= K_e \times 0.00833\\ \text{Lean body mass} &= \text{total body water}/0.73\\ \text{Extracellular mass} &= \text{lean body mass}\\ &\quad - \text{body cell mass}\\ \text{Body fat} &= \text{body weight} - \text{lean body mass}\end{aligned}$$

To compare the body composition of individuals with different body sizes, the data are usually corrected for body size by expressing the components of body composition relative to the total body water. Table 1-2 lists normal values for various components of body composition.

Although the radioisotope techniques are accurate, multiple blood samples and extensive processing are required. Bioelectrical impedance analysis is increasingly popular as a noninvasive method of determining volumes of body fluids and associated changes in lean body mass [21]. Impedance analysis is noninvasive, safe and painless, and it can easily be performed at the bedside. Little technical training is required to operate the relatively inexpensive equipment needed to perform bioelectrical impedance analysis measurements.

A measurement of impedance consists of the determination of two electrical characteristics of the human body, electrical resistance and reactance. A model of a cylinder containing fluid can be used to explain the rationale of an impedance measurement. When an alternating electrical current is applied to a cylinder, conduction of the current will be opposed by its contents; this ability to oppose current is termed *electrical resistance.* Resistance is defined as the pure opposition to the flow of alternating current and is expressed in ohms. A value of resistance determined across a cylinder is related to its length and inversely related to its diameter [22]. If length and diameter are known, resistance reflects the volume of the cylinder's fluid contents. When a portion of the fluid is replaced by fat, which is a poor conductor, resistance determined across the cylinder will increase. The human body resembles a set of serially connected cylinders (arm, trunk, leg) with a known length and a relatively constant diameter. Thus, resistance measured across the body should reflect its total fluid content. In healthy humans, resistance usually comprises 98% of the impedance signal; these parameters are therefore frequently used interchangeably.

Reactance is the second component of impedance and is thought to reflect capacitive elements

Table 1-2. Normal Adult Body Composition

	Male, 70 kg		Female, 60 kg	
	Absolute	% Body Weight	Absolute	% Body Weight
Body fat[a]	16.0 kg	22.8	19.0 kg	31.7
Lean body mass[b]	54.0 kg	77.1	41.0 kg	68.3
Body cell mass	30.9 kg	44.1	21.7 kg	36.2
Muscle mass	17.4 kg	24.3	9.6 kg	16.0
Extracellular mass	23.1 kg	33.0	19.3 kg	32.1
Total body water	39.4 L	56.3	29.5 L	49.2
Intracellular water	22.1 L	31.6	15.5 L	25.8
Red cell volume	1.93 L	2.8	1.40 L	2.3
Extracellular water	17.3 L	24.7	14.0 L	23.3
Interstitial water	14.3 L	20.4	11.4 L	19.0
Plasma volume	3.15 L	4.5	2.63 L	4.4
Blood volume (plasma + red cell volume)	5.08 L	7.3	4.03 L	6.7

[a]Total body fat = body weight − lean body mass.

[b]Lean body mass = total body water + 0.732.

Source: Data from FD Moore. *Metabolic Care of the Surgical Patient.* Philadelphia: Saunders, 1959; SH Cohn, et al. Compartmental body composition based on total body nitrogen, potassium, and calcium. *Am J Physiol* 239: E524, 1980.

in the body. Also expressed in ohms, reactance contributes very little to whole body impedance (~2%). Cell walls and membranes possess electrical capacity similar to that observed in electrical condensers. Although the clinical value of body reactance is not yet defined, this electrical characteristic may represent cellular health and associated changes in extracellular volume. The following relationship exists between impedance (Z), resistance (R), and reactance (X_c):

$$Z = \sqrt{R^2 + X_c^2}$$

Early investigators appreciated that the outcome of impedance measurements was dependent on the frequency of the alternating current. Studies performed on in vitro models containing blood and plasma suggested that electrical currents of low frequency (~5 kHz) were predominantly conducted by the extracellular compartment (plasma). Using currents of low frequency, erythrocyte membranes acted as a shield and protected the intracellular contents from "penetration" by the electrons. In contrast, cellular membrane capacity during conduction of high frequency currents was thought to be negligible. Thus, impedance obtained at these frequencies reflected both extracellular and intracellular fluid volume. Impedance analysis is usually performed using conduction of alternating current of a high frequency (50 kHz), although some investigators have used measurements obtained at several frequencies. These studies have also suggested that resistance measured after a low frequency (~5 kHz) current may reflect changes in the extracellular water compartment [23,24]. The majority of the body's impedance (60%) is present in a forearm and a lower leg. By bypassing these "high-impedance cylinders" and thus obtaining an impedance value of the "proximal body," impedance measurements may be obtained that more accurately predict total body water and that are more sensitive to acute changes in fluid status [25].

However, limbs resemble a cylinder very closely and may serve as a representative portion of the body. For example, resistance measured just across an arm and a leg accurately predicts the total fluid content of healthy individuals [26,27]. In addition, impedance determined from a limb enables its fat and muscle content to be precisely determined as compared with values derived from CT scanning [28]. An additional advantage of regional measurements is the fact that an (uninjured) limb of a patient is usually easily accessible for serial impedance analysis.

Validation of impedance analysis against a generally accepted method ("gold standard") of body fluid determination such as a dilutional technique did not occur until 1965. At this time, a significant relationship was demonstrated between extracellular water volume measured by bromide dilution and the body's impedance after conduction of a 1 kHz alternating current in a group of normal and edematous patients. Shortly thereafter, body impedance after conduction of high frequency current (100 kHz) was related to total body water volume determined by tritium dilution [29].

Although Hoffer and colleagues [29] were the first to find that the body's resistance and its fluid contents during a steady state were highly related, others have demonstrated a close relationship between acute and chronic changes in body fluids and changes in its electrical conductivity. Orally administered fluids may not be detected, which is probably related to a slow absorption and subsequent redistribution with ongoing production of urine.

The impedance technique has been validated with a number of other body compositional methods, such as dilution of tracers, underwater weighing, anthropometrics, total body electrical conductivity, CT scanning, and total body potassium measurements, in *healthy populations*. Although in most studies a close relationship was demonstrated between the compared techniques, many variables, including electrode placement, body position and geometry, and temperature, may influence the accuracy and reliability of bioelectrical impedance measurements. Daily variation of impedance values in weight-stable individuals is reported to range from 2.0% (expressed as coefficient of variation, defined as standard deviation/mean) to 2.8% [21,30]. The week-to-week variation range is approximately 2.5% [31].

Altered intake of nutrients and release of hormones associated with disease may disrupt the close relationship between body resistance and total body water. A disease itself may also affect conduction of the electrical current. However, the body's drive for homeostasis may result in maintenance of a constant number of conducting particles (electrolytes) per fluid volume. If this were the case, the close relationship between body resistance and fluid contents would be expected to persist during illness. However, one should be cautious when attempting to predict the lean body mass on the basis of the body's impedance during disease. Some investigators have demonstrated an excellent correlation between total body water predicted from body impedance and heavy water dilution in sick patients, whereas others have not [32–34]. In one study, the accuracy of bioelectrical impedance analysis in detecting changes in total body water and potassium was determined in a heterogeneous group of surgical patients [35]. Tritiated water dilution and whole body monitoring were the reference methods for total body water and total body potassium analysis. The authors' results suggested that bioelectrical impedance analysis was of limited value in the estimation of total body water. Furthermore, in another investigation, the impedance technique did not accurately predict fat-free mass in a group of cardiopulmonary and surgical patients [36,37]. However, these studies used regression equations derived from a healthy population that may not be applicable in a specific patient population [38]. The development of disease-specific impedance equations may increase the accuracy of total body water prediction. Although a close relationship between electrical resistance and total body water may be maintained during disease, profound changes in electrical reactance have been reported in patients [39–41]. Bioelectrical impedance appears to provide a noninvasive, safe, rapid, and accurate method for evaluating body composition or large normal populations. It has proved accurate when it is has been compared with dilutional methodology in healthy individuals, but it requires further investigation in patient groups with a normal body compartmentalization.

It should be reemphasized that electrical impedance reflects fluid volumes such as total body water and possibly extracellular water. Various disease processes may alter the relationship between the body's total fluid content and the lean body mass that is more constant during health (total body water = lean body mass $\times$ 0.73). The assumption that the relationship between the total body water and lean body mass is fixed may be invalid. This potential difficulty is inherent to all two-compartment models (e.g., estimation of total body water using dilutional methods, hydrodensitometry, or whole body potassium measurements), where key body components are secondarily derived from the measurement of body water. These methods assume that the chemical components of the fat-free mass occur in the same proportion to each other and in all individuals.

However, the two-compartment model is still useful as a first approximation of the changes that occur during illness. A characteristic response to severe malnutrition and other catabolic stresses is expansion of the extracellular mass relative to the body cell mass that is contracted. The Na_e/K_e ratio, which is a dynamic expression of the extracellular mass expressed as a function of the body cell mass, increases significantly under various conditions, including sepsis, malnutrition, and after major abdominal surgery [42,43]. It is likely a more sensitive index of nutritional or metabolic status than are typical anthropometric and biochemical measurements, and it may accurately predict patients at risk for death after hospitalization [44]. The techniques required to measure the Na_e/K_e ratio accurately are complex and time-consuming, and they require specialized laboratory facilities and specially trained personnel. At this time, they are not suited for routine patient management, but they should be reserved for research purposes.

Although it is clear that patients with a variety of catabolic illnesses have an abnormal Na_e/K_e ratio, it is not as clear whether short-term nutritional repletion (10–14 days) is associated with normalization of this index. Studies of the effect of starvation and stress on the transmembrane potential of myocytes report findings that are similar to studies of the effect of these conditions on Na_e/K_e ratios [45–47]. At the end of 10 days of starvation, the transmembrane potential difference of skeletal muscle falls significantly. A 10-day refeeding period using a standard parenteral nutritional solution with crystalline amino acids and dextrose does not restore a normal potential difference even if nitrogen equilibrium or a positive nitrogen balance is restored.

There are also inherent difficulties in using total body potassium as an index of cellular depletion and repletion. Estimates of body cell mass that use total body potassium measurements generally assume that 3.6% of the cell is nitrogen. The ability to determine body cell mass will vary because the potassium content of the cell changes as a result of changes in intracellular water. These techniques may also be inaccurate if the composition of the cell changes because of alterations in nitrogen content that occur independently of changes in intracellular potassium and water. In other words, a fall in total body potassium is usually interpreted as a change in lean body mass of normal composition, but this is true only if changes in body composition are proportional to changes in body cell mass. In fact, experimental data suggest that changes in intracellular potassium concentrations may occur independently of changes in lean body mass. Changes in intracellular potassium ion activity may be dissociated from changes in intracellular potassium concentration [48]. Thus, the alterations in total body potassium and in intracellular potassium that occur during various dietary manipulations are not necessarily secondary to changes in muscle mass as assessed by measurements of total body nitrogen, but may be the result of changes in cell energy or in membrane characteristics such as permeability and selectivity.

Thus, very different methodologies suggest that there is a persistent defect in cellular membrane function in patients with catabolic illnesses that is not restored by a typical course of intravenous nutritional support. The emphasis in most modern nutritional studies is on whole body and specific tissue changes. However, it is important to consider cellular abnormalities as well. Clearly, *cellular* function is also altered in malnourished and critically ill patients. Cellular responses are increasingly important as clinicians and researchers reconsider the effects of nutritional or metabolic interventions on the metabolism, growth, and function of specific organs, such as skeletal muscle, intestine, liver, lung, and the immune system.

The ability to determine the water and electrolyte content from small samples (~ 30 mg) of muscle tissue is well developed [49–51]. The use of in vitro measurements of skeletal muscle tissue is attractive, because skeletal muscle is quantitatively and metabolically the body's most important protein store. It is also important to consider the contribution of metabolic changes in skeletal muscle to overall changes in whole body composition, because skeletal muscle is a major contributor to the lean body mass. Last, the measurement of changes in intracellular as opposed to extracellular constituents is, at least theoretically, advantageous because these changes may more accurately indicate the body's metabolic state if only because the size of the intracellular compartment is greater.

In vitro analyses of muscle biopsy specimens have confirmed that total water and extracellular water are higher than normal in many hospitalized patients. The intracellular potassium content is typically lower than normal. Changes in distribution of body water and various ions are important to consider when one is evaluating the various stresses imposed on a cell and the efficacy of various therapeutic interventions designed to improve cellular health. There is good evidence that the cellular hydration state is an important factor controlling cellular protein turnover [52]. Decreased activities of various amino acid transporters, Na^+-H^+ antiport or Na^+-K^+-$2Cl^-$ cotransport, dissipation of transmembrane substrate gradients, and opening of K^+ channels under the influence of altered nutrition, hormones, cytokines, oxygen radicals, or other inflammatory mediators may all contribute to cell shrinkage. However, cellular shrinkage may act as the common end path that triggers net protein breakdown.

The energy-dependent membrane system, the Na^+-K^+ pump, is an important marker of energy failure because its activity depends directly on adenosine triphosphate (ATP) concentration [53–55]. Accordingly, because the distribution of sodium and potassium across the cell membrane relies on the availability of ATP to fuel the transmembrane pump, the relationship between changes in the distribution of cations to changes in the cell's energy state is most pertinent. This is especially true, because changes in the distribution of body water parallel changes in the distribution of sodium.

There are also changes in muscle fiber composition and reductions of the key enzymes of glucose oxidation as well as various intracellular substrates [56]. Hypocaloric fasting increases the intracellular calcium content of skeletal muscle and decreases phosphofructokinase and succinate dehydrogenase concentrations. Typically, both type I (high oxidation and low glycolytic capacity) and type II (low oxidation and high glycolytic capacity) fibers are smaller in malnourished patients. Furthermore, the ratio of type II to type I fibers is reduced. The loss of type II fibers may be responsible for the muscle weakness (decreased maximal voluntary grip strength) and fatigue that are commonly seen in malnourished patients [27]. These changes may also be related to the aberrant function of electrically stimulated muscle observed in these individuals. In these studies, a slower maximal relaxation rate and increased muscle fatigability have been demonstrated. These abnormalities in muscle function have been related to changes in intracellular enzymes [57], intracellular substrate [58,59], and cellular chemistry [57]. Shizgal and colleagues did not detect a correlation between body composition (as measured using multiple isotope dilution techniques) and changes in muscle function (as determined by electrical stimulation of the adductor pollicus muscle) [60]. In this study of normal volunteers, changes in muscle function were evident by 24 hours of starvation, but returned to normal within 6 hours of a single normal meal. This observation led the authors to hypothesize that the reaction of skeletal muscle to electrical stimulation does not directly reflect nutritional status, but may be more closely related to energy availability and production.

A primary role of nutrition is the provision of metabolic energy. Figure 1-4 shows one potential relationship between catabolism, changes in body composition and traditional indices of malnutrition, muscle function, and energetics. According to this paradigm, catabolism of skeletal muscle proteins, all of which serve some important structural or functional role, is ultimately responsible for many of the metabolic derangements associated with stress and starvation. This catabolic pro-

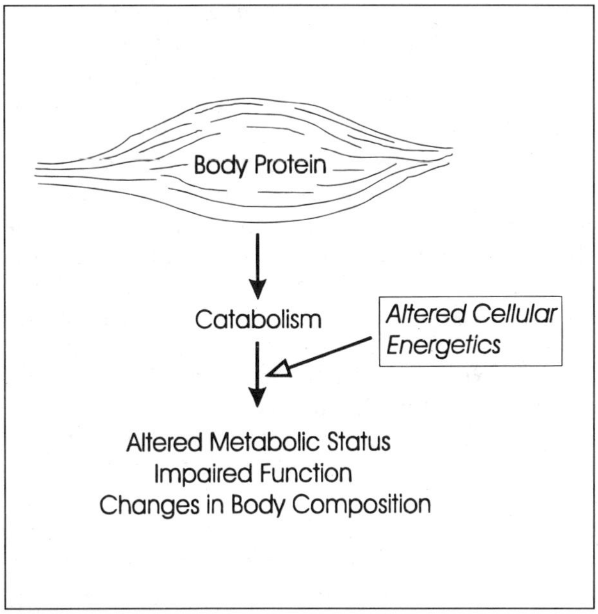

Figure 1-4. A theoretical relationship between protein catabolism and alterations in metabolic status, physiologic functions, and body composition.

cess alters circulating humoral factors, impairs muscle function, and ultimately leads to changes in body composition. Changes in cellular energetics are closely associated with these abnormalities and may antedate changes in body tissue compartments. With respect to skeletal muscle, and perhaps to other organ systems as well, major changes in energy substrates occur with starvation and in other catabolic states [61–63]. Indeed, alterations in muscular energy metabolism may explain many of the abnormalities noted in the electrical stimulation studies, including the decrease in the muscle relaxation rate reported in many studies of the effects of malnutrition. It is likely that the slowing of the muscle relaxation rate observed in malnourished patients is a manifestation of diminished ATP turnover. A decrease in substrate or precursor availability or a decrease in production of high-energy phosphate compounds (or both), in the presence of constant or increased need, could alter muscle energy metabolism and depress muscle energy stores. Changes in energy metabolism and their relationship to alterations in amino acid, water, and ion transport may be critically important in understanding the acute effects of parenteral alimentation, where the appropriate initial therapeutic goal is not to replete existing tissue deficits, but to maximize the cell's ability to respond to the metabolic challenges of disease.

A large body of evidence suggests that muscle energy metabolism and function are altered by malnutrition. The advent of MR spectroscopy has provided a new and powerful tool with which to examine changes in muscle energy metabolism in vivo. Magnetic resonance spectroscopy can be used to detect signals from molecules with an odd number of nuclear particles, such as protons, ^{31}P, ^{15}N, ^{23}Na, and ^{13}C. These elements will align their magnetic poles in the direction of an externally applied magnetic field. They will absorb energy that is applied to the system as specific radio-frequency pulses, which distorts their equilibrium. Once the radio-frequency pulse is discontinued, the molecules will "relax" to their equilibrium state by releasing the absorbed energy. This released energy can be detected and used to detect the amount of the element of interest and its location in specific biologic compounds. Magnetic resonance spectroscopy measurements are well defined in skeletal muscle, where the ^{31}P signal can be used to measure the amount of inorganic phosphate, phosphocreatine, and ATP. The use of phosphonate markers, such as dimethyl methylphosphonate, which distributes in total body water, and phenyphosphonate, which distributes in extracellular water, can be used to study the relationship between changes in cellular energetics, water, and sodium distribution (Figure 1-5).

Multicompartment Models

Body composition can be analyzed at many levels [64]. According to this theoretical framework, there are at least five levels that are relevant to human investigation: atomic, molecular, cellular, tissue-system, and whole-body. Although each can be considered distinct, there are associations within or between levels. For example, total body

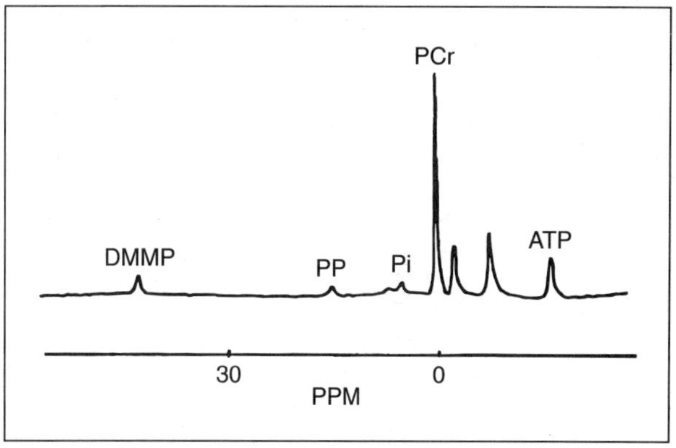

Figure 1-5. A typical high resolution phosphorus magnetic resonance scan of the gastrocnemius muscle of a rat. Peaks that correspond to dimethyl methylphosphonate (DMMP), phenylphosphonate (PP), inorganic phosphate (Pi), phosphocreatine (PCr), and β-ATP are labeled. DMMP is an MRS visible marker that distributes in the total body water whereas PP distributes only in the extracellular compartment.

carbon, lipid content, adipocyte mass, adipose tissue, and skin-fold thickness are all markers of fatness and are related to other tissue components as well as to each other.

Early investigators were unable to quantify the mass of tissues and organs in living subjects. Computed tomography can be used to study human body composition using one of three methods [65]. With the first method, the cross-sectional area of fat, muscle, bone, or a visceral organ can be derived from the reconstructed image using the appropriate software. Representative volumes can then be determined because the slice and distance between each cross-sectional slice is known. Alternatively, when there are no sharp boundaries between structures, but the tissues of interest differ in density, a histogram can be created that separates the picture elements into lean and adipose components. Using these principles, CT has been used to quantify regional and total body muscle and adipose tissue volume [66]. In this regard, MRI techniques can also be used [67]. Examinations with CT are somewhat limited because the procedure exposes the patient to radiation and because of their relatively high cost.

The introduction of *dual-photon absorptiometry* and *neutron activation analysis* have allowed more body compartments to be quantified in vivo. With the introduction of these techniques, multicompartment models that use three to six chemical components have been developed using these new methods in combination with older techniques (Figure 1-6) [68–70]. The main advantage of these more complicated models is that a more complete analysis of the chemical composition of the body is possible [71]. Second, the multicompartment models require fewer assumptions about the relationships among the various body fractions. For example, the major assumption of all body compositional studies is that there is a steady-state relationship between compartments. Although modern multicompartment modeling techniques require some assumptions about the relationship between an element and its parent chemical compound (for example, nitrogen with protein), the two-compartment models assume that the relationships of the main chemical components within the fat-free mass are fixed. As discussed earlier, this assumption may be incorrect, especially in critically ill patients. If the individual components of a multicompartment model are determined independently, errors inherent to methods where body compartments are measured directly are avoided. The original two-compartment models were developed on a theoretical or empirical basis using data derived from animal or a few human necropsy samples. According to the two-compartment approach, the fat component was that which was ether-extractable lipid, whereas the remainder of the body weight represented the fat-free body mass. As was shown earlier, body weight was equal to the sum of the fat and fat-free masses. Multicompartment techniques allow the fat-free compartment to be broken down into as many as five components, e.g., water, bone mineral, cellular mineral, protein, and glycogen. A final advantage of multicompartmental models is that they can (at least) serve as reference methods against which new clinical body compositional techniques such as total body electrical conductivity and bioimpedance analysis are compared. This is particularly important given

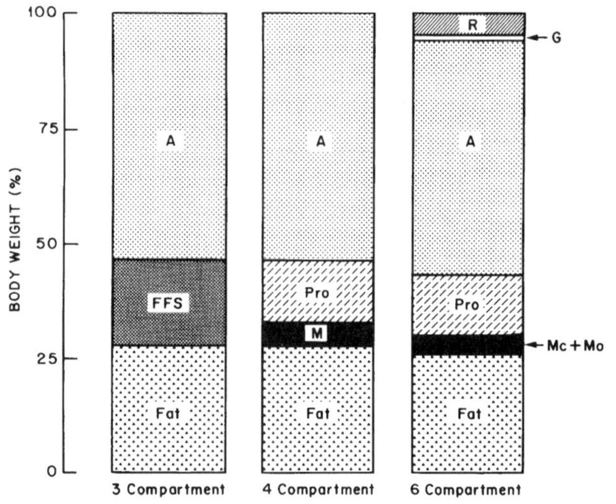

Figure 1-6. Different multicompartment models are shown. A is the aqueous or total body water compartment. FFS = fat free solids; Pro = protein; M = mineral; Mo = osseous mineral; Mc = cellular mineral; G = glycogen; and R = residual "undefined" tissue.

that the later techniques are less expensive and more suitable to repeated measurements in clinical patients.

Dual-Photon Absorptiometry and Dual-Energy X-ray Absorptiometry

Dual photon absorptiometry and dual-energy x-ray absorptiometry (DEXA) systems direct photons of characteristic energy at the person being evaluated. As the beam passes over the patient, some of the photons are absorbed by the body, thus decreasing the original beam strength. The amount of beam attenuation is dependent on the nature of the tissue through which it passes, hence, this technique can be used to quantify the mineral, fat, and fat-free and mineral-free tissue components of the body [72]. Total mineral is calculated directly using data derived from cadavers [73]. Dual-photon absorptiometry systems use a source that generates photons at two energy levels. Newer systems use an x-ray source, so the technique is now usually referred to as DEXA to distinguish it from earlier technologies. Both techniques allow body composition analysis at a level of refinement that was previously unobtainable in the living patient. The use of a dual-energy system increases the ability to discriminate between bone and the soft tissues when areas of variable thicknesses such as the trunk are being analyzed.

Gotfredsen and colleagues [74] used dual-photon absorptiometry to measure lean body mass and total body fat. The accuracy of their method to measure lean body mass was 2.5%. The radiation dose is small (about 5 millirad), which means that dual-photon absorptiometry can be used to follow changes in body composition over time. Current-generation DEXA machines can perform a whole-body scan in about 20 minutes; they also expose patients to very little radiation. Both techniques can be used for serial examinations and are very reliable methods for measuring body compositional changes in vivo.

Studies in healthy, nonobese adults show that there is a very high correlation between the osseous mineral content estimated by dual-photon absorptiometry and the total body calcium content determined by delayed gamma neutron activation. There is also a good agreement between the estimates of total body mineral content determined by dual-photon absorptiometry and neutron activation. The fat content is also accurately estimated using dual-photon absorptiometry as compared with conventional methods such as hydrodensitometry and neutron activation analysis [75]. Thus, the dual-photon absorptiometry or DEXA method is a valuable technique for estimating mineral and fat content in vivo. There are only a few concerns relating to the effects of body thickness on the estimation of mineral and fat contents. One limitation of dual-photon absorptiometry and DEXA is that they have only been calibrated to patients who are less than 35 kg/m^2. For body mass index above this level, changes in variations in tissue thickness may affect photon attenuation.

A major advantage of these methods, which rely on different attenuation coefficients of fat and lean tissue to estimate fat content, is their independence of assumptions regarding biological constancing. The body mass index is not particularly effective for defining fat when it is applied to young humans. It is also subject to variation induced by differences in edema, muscle hypertrophy or atrophy, or disease states. Dual-photon absorptiometry and DEXA, like CT and MRI techniques, slice the body into different pieces and different compartments. They measure body fat within the soft tissue in a manner independent of age or other factors that might affect the chemical composition of the fat-free mass. They appear to be minimally affected by changes caused by age, fluid retention, body density, or muscle potassium content. Unlike underwater weighing and total body water, which have been shown to be excellent measures in healthy homogenous populations, the dual-photon absorptiometry method is convenient. It requires fewer assumptions and may be used in sicker patients.

In Vivo Neutron Activation Analysis

Neutron activation is a process that entails delivery of a beam of neutrons over the subject being studied. Atoms within the body "capture" these neutrons, creating unstable isotopes. When the isotopes return to their original stable state, they emit gamma rays of an energy characteristic of the atom from which it originated. The gamma rays that radiate from the subject are recorded and quantified by a detector [76].

In vivo total body neutron activation analysis is the only technique presently available that allows the multielemental composition of the human body to be measured. The patient receives a moderated beam of fast neutrons when this technique is used. Capture of neutrons by atoms of the target elements creates unstable isotopes such as ^{49}Ca and ^{15}N. The isotopes revert to their stable baseline condition by emission of one or more gamma rays of characteristic energy. The energy emitted identifies the particular element, and the level of activity shows its abundance. From these emissions, the total body content of elements such as calcium, and nitrogen can be measured. Total body bone and cellular mineral, protein, and fat content are then derived from these measurements. Anderson and colleagues [77] originally designed an instrument that provided subjects with a carefully controlled neutron flux of known intensity. The induced activities of three elements (sodium, chloride, and calcium) were then used to quantify their total body mass in vivo. In the late 1960s, Palmer and colleagues [78] described the neutron activation system for estimating total body nitrogen, and thus the protein compartment, by assuming that protein could be estimated by multiplying the total body nitrogen content by 6.25. Currently, when total body protein is quantified, the unstable nitrogen isotope generated has a lifetime of 10 to 15 seconds. For this reason, neutron irradiation and gamma-ray counting must proceed simultaneously. Hence, the technique is usually referred to as *prompt gamma neutron activation analysis*. The method is very precise, with a coefficient of variation of only 2.7% between measurements. A complete study requires about 35 minutes, and the radiation exposure is minimal. The ability to measure protein to quantify whole-body protein content in vivo was a major breakthrough in clinical nutrition research on body composition.

Total body glycogen can be calculated from protein measurements by assuming that the glycogen to protein ratio (as determined from skeletal muscle and liver biopsy specimens) is constant. This estimate may be inaccurate when it is used in patients who have undergone a prolonged fast or who have suffered an acute catabolic injury, because glycogen stores are normally depleted very rapidly under these conditions. Total body mineral content can also be determined using neutron activation analysis, taking advantage of the fact that more than 98% of the body's calcium is in calcium hydroxyapatite of osseous mineral. Irradiation of the patient with the appropriate source generates unstable isotopes of calcium that can be counted and that have half-lives of approximately 9 minutes. This technique, referred to as *delayed gamma neutron activation analysis,* is also very precise and can be expanded to provide separate estimates of osseous mineral and cell mineral. Osseous mineral is calculated from the total body calcium content. Delayed gamma neutron activation and whole-body counting provide estimates of total body sodium and chloride. Total body potassium is estimated by whole-body counting before neutron irradiation. The measurements of these three elements and total body calcium are then used to estimate the amount of cell mineral in the form of six ions (Na^+, K^+, Mg^{++}, $H_2PO_4^-$, HCO_3^-, Cl^-).

The most modern neutron activation systems for measuring total body carbon use a technique known as *inelastic neutron scattering*. This procedure has a precision equivalent to the techniques used to measure nitrogen and calcium and takes approximately 45 minutes. Besides being distributed into the organic skeleton of triglycerides, amino acids, and to a smaller extent glycogen, a small amount of carbon is also present in tissue minerals. The amount of carbon in fat can be calculated by subtracting other carbon sources from the total body calcium. The total quantities of protein, bone mineral, and glycogen are estimated using prompt and delayed gamma neutron activation analysis. The carbon in fat is then determined by subtracting nonlipid sources of carbon from the body's total carbon content. Approximately 77% of human triglyceride is carbon. Thus body fat can be determined by the equation [79]:

$$\text{body fat} = \text{carbon in fat}/0.774$$

Neutron activation models assume that the proportions of carbon, nitrogen, and calcium are known and constant within lipid, protein, and bone mineral, respectively.

Cohn and colleagues at the Brookhaven National Laboratories were among the first to introduce a four-compartment chemical model where body weight was defined as the sum of the aqueous, mineral, protein, and fat compartments [69]. In their model, the water volume was determined by dilution of tritiated water. Total body nitrogen was determined using prompt gamma neutron activation and total body calcium by delayed gamma neutron activation. The body's fat content was equal to the body weight minus the contributions of the other three compartments.

During the last two decades, the method has been refined so that eleven elements (carbon, oxygen, hydrogen, nitrogen, calcium, phosphorus, magnesium, sodium, chloride, iodine, and cadmium) can now be accurately measured in vivo. The multicompartment chemical model is now the benchmark for human body composition research. The chemical model is important because of its central role in studying changes resulting from malnutrition and altered energy metabolism. Six elements (carbon, nitrogen, calcium, potassium, sodium, and chlorine) are used and measured in vivo at the atomic level using neutron activation systems. The classic six-compartment chemical model organizes components into three main chemical groupings: the aqueous compartment or water, mineral, and organic. The minerals are further separated into osseous and extraosseous components.

Heymsfield and colleagues combined neutron activation, total body potassium measurements using a gamma counter, and dilutional methods of body water determinations to develop a multicompartment model of body composition [76]. This model defines greater than 97% of the body's components according to the following formula

$$\text{Body weight} = \text{A} + \text{Mo} + \text{Mc} + \text{Protein} + \text{Fat} + \text{Glycogen} + \text{R}$$

where A = the aqueous or water component, Mo = bone mineral, Mc = cellular mineral, and R = a small residual of "undefined" tissue(s). Figure 1-7 shows the percent contribution to body weight of each of these components. For completeness, glycogen was added to their model, assuming a constant ratio of glycogen to protein. In addition, in their model, fat is estimated from total body carbon as described earlier. Otherwise, the other four compartments are estimated as originally done by Cohn and colleagues [69]. Partitioning the body in this manner has been shown to correlate very highly with estimates of body weight and to account for the overall majority of body weight. Applying these multicompartmental models has yielded useful information regarding some of the assumptions underlying the historical two-compartment modeling techniques. These techniques have shown that there are subtle but significant differences in body composition with age and obesity and in different ethnic groups. For example, healthy black women have significantly higher bone mineral, total body potassium, and density of the fat-free mass as well as the potassium content of the fat-free mass compared with matched white females. Using the conventional constants of the two-compartment modeling technique based on underwater weighing and total body potassium would have significantly underestimated the fat content of black women.

There are two advantages of this new technology. First, the individual components in this model are independently determined, with the exception of glycogen, which is less than 1% of body weight. Second, protein content of the body can be measured. This is a major breakthrough because all protein in the body serves a functional or structural role. Hence, the ability to assess fluctuations in this parameter provides useful information concerning the overall health status of a patient or individual being monitored.

Few facilities are available to measure neutron activation. The technique is quite expensive because it requires a cyclotron and equipment for total body counting. As is true with many techniques that measure body composition, neutron activation may not be very sensitive to short-term fluctuations. Whether it is accurate and important in studying critically ill patients [80] has not been determined, although it is increasingly being shown to be useful in this regard. In the future, these techniques will become the gold standard of in vivo body compositional studies.

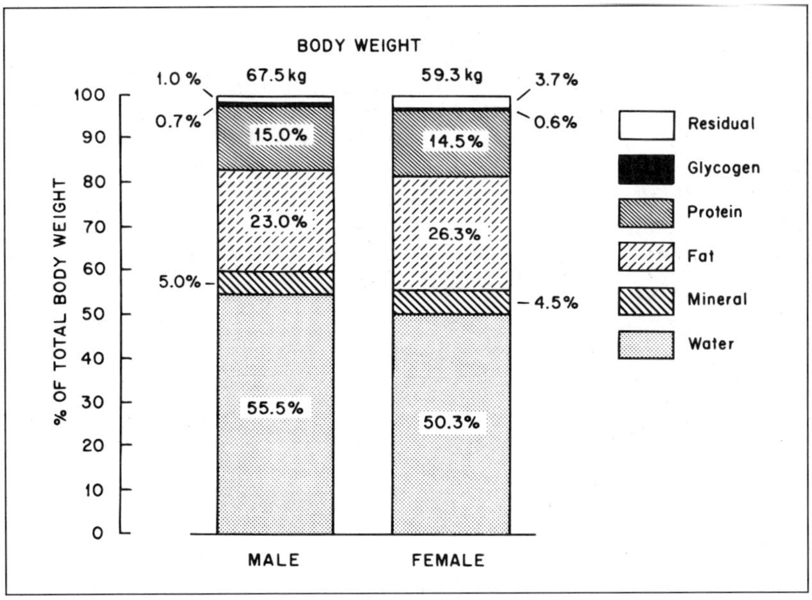

Figure 1-7. Body composition as determined by neutron activation, total potassium measurement and total body water analysis. (Data from SB Heymsfield, et al. Chemical and elemental analysis of humans in vivo using improved body composition models. *Am J Physiol* 261:E190, 1991.)

Body Composition During Illness

Significant changes in body fat, body cell mass, and extracellular mass occur during illness. The body compositions of various catabolic individuals are shown in Figure 1-8 and are compared with the normal body composition. It can be seen that loss of body cell mass and body fat with extracellular fluid accumulation occurs in chronic malnutrition and many illnesses. It should be noted that alterations in total body weight and lean body mass poorly correlate with alterations in body cell mass. This is because *increased interstitial water often masks the severity of body cell mass degradation*. For example, even though body weight and lean body mass are actually greater in septic patients compared with the uncomplicated postoperative patients shown in Figure 1-8, the nutritional status of those with invasive infection is worse because of the diminished body cell mass. This apparent discrepancy is explained by the fact that septic patients have 6.7 L more of extracellular water compared with the surgical patients. Water accumulation commonly occurs during illness, and even if total body weight is decreased, the proportion of body weight that is comprised of water often increases in disease (see Figure 1-8). The reason for water retention and extracellular fluid expansion during these altered states is incompletely understood but likely includes multiple mechanisms. At the cellular level, membrane permeability increases as a result of hypoxia or injury by toxic compounds such as oxygen free radicals [81]. Sepsis and malnutrition have also been associated with alterations in cellular energetics [82,83]. These mechanisms allow efflux of previously nondiffusible solutes from the intracellular space to the interstitium. Endothelial cell function may also be impaired, which allows diffusion of plasma proteins into the interstitial space. Extracellular accumulation of water naturally accompanies these processes because of the increased osmotic pressure exerted by the additional solutes in the interstitium [84], although the physiologic role in albumin and changes in its distribution between plasma and fluid are not fully understood. It is highly likely that hospitalized patients with moderately severe protein energy malnutrition with hypoalbuminemia may suddenly have clinically apparent edema, but the fundamental defect appears to be overhydration of a fat-free body. In patients with protein malnutrition of the kwashiorkor type, overhydration may be more clinically obvious. For example, patients with multiorgan failure and systemic inflammation secondary to infection may have an overexpansion of the total body water space by as much as 10 L [85]. Systemically, the pain and stress as well as the hypovolemia associated with illness can each independently increase release of aldosterone and vasopressin, resulting in increased sodium and water retention. In addition, increased cellular membrane permeability allows movement of sodium and water from the plasma to intracellular space via the interstitium. This shift activates hormonal mechanisms that increase sodium and fluid retention by the kidney to maintain plasma volume [86]. These cellular derangements and hormonal changes in part explain the total body water retention and expansion of the extracellular fluid compartment that occurs during most disease states. In contrast, body cell

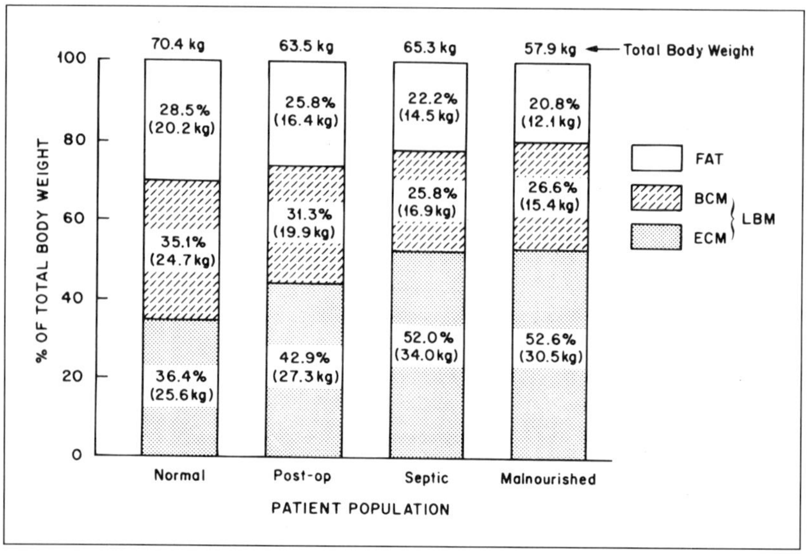

Figure 1-8. Body composition in healthy and catabolic individuals. LBM is lean body mass. BCM is the body cell mass, and ECM is extracellular mass. (Data from HM Shizgal. Nutritional assessment with body composition measurements. *JPEN* 11:42S, 1987; HM Shizgal, MF Martin. Caloric requirement of the critically ill septic patient. *Crit Care Med* 16:312, 1988.)

mass typically decreases during catabolic states. Twenty-five percent of body cell mass is protein; hence, changes in total body protein are indicative of changes in the body cell mass. In healthy, normally nourished individuals, protein synthesis and catabolism are balanced during a 24-hour period. Therefore, body protein mass (and thus body cell mass) is approximately the same from day to day. Any excess protein not needed for structural or functional purposes is broken down when dietary caloric supply exceeds endogenous demands for fuel. The carbon skeletons resulting from protein catabolism in this setting are used for fat synthesis or fuel, whereas the nitrogen is excreted as urea in the urine [87]. Quantifying urinary nitrogen losses is one way of monitoring protein catabolism, and nitrogen balance (total nitrogen intake minus total nitrogen output) has traditionally been used as a marker of overall protein metabolism. Nitrogen balance is usually zero during a 24-hour period in healthy, normally nourished individuals, reflecting the fact that whole-body protein is relatively constant on a daily basis. Negative nitrogen balance is indicative of net protein loss from the body and commonly occurs in all malnourished and moderately to severely injured patients who maintain normal renal function. The magnitude of nitrogen loss varies with the severity of disease, and when this value is multiplied by 6.25, it provides a good estimate of protein losses from the body.

Body fat is decreased during disease and starvation as well. Fat represents a large supply of energy that is needed to fuel recovery from illness or to compensate for the primary lack of adequate caloric intake in the malnourished. Thus, during these states, accelerated lipolysis occurs with diminution of fat stores. Approximately one half of weight loss during catabolic illness is from loss of body fat, whereas the other half is secondary to diminution of the body cell mass [8]. Until recently, in vivo determination of lean body mass and body fat had to be derived from measurement of total body water. However, the assumptions underlying such derivations are less accurate in those with disease when compared with healthy individuals. Neutron activation, dual-photon absorptiometry, and DEXA allow more direct measurement of total body tissue components, as described previously. Although these latter techniques are not practical in the routine clinical setting, they are extremely valuable as a research tool in assessing the severity of many pathologic processes, and more importantly, in assessing the adequacy of various treatment modalities in critically ill patients.

Critical illness results in a variety of complex changes that are the sum of responses to several different perturbations. The metabolic responses characteristic of disease can be grouped as those related to starvation or undernutrition and those related to organ and tissue pathology arising from illness independent of nutrition. As discussed above, loss of body cell mass and body fat with extracellular fluid accumulation occurs in malnutrition and a wide variety of diseases. The metabolic alterations that underlie these changes are described below.

Body Energy Balance and Storage

Body cell mass represents the metabolically active tissue of the body. The protein associated with this mass, in concert with body fat, is also a form of stored energy. In general, long-term gain or loss of body weight indicates positive or negative energy balance, respectively. When one is in positive energy balance, caloric intake exceeds caloric utilization and fat deposition occurs. When one is in negative energy balance, caloric expenditure exceeds caloric intake and body weight decreases as endogenous tissues are broken down to meet fuel needs. During starvation, the body must depend on endogenous sources of energy to meet its fuel requirements. There are three types of tissue that release energy for ATP production when oxidized: fat, protein, and carbohydrate. Fat is the largest depot of energy in the body. Each gram yields 9.3 kcal upon oxidation, and about 80% of potential energy reserves in normal, healthy individuals is in adipose tissue (Table 1-3). Protein is the next-largest energy supply, and each anhydrous gram releases 4.2 kcal when metabolized for fuel. Carbohydrate is stored as glycogen, and although each gram of glucose yields 4.1 kcal upon oxidation, its contribution to energy storage is exceedingly small because there are only 400 g of glycogen in the body. Fat is both calorically dense and lightweight because it is anhydrous. Hence, adipose tissue is ideal for energy storage in humans and other highly mobile animals. Although protein is potentially a large source of energy, *all body protein serves either a structural, enzymatic, or immunologic role* and protein "reserves" do not exist to any appreciable degree. This means that *any protein used for energy needs is lost at the expense of body structure or function*. Because protein utilization beyond certain limits is disadvantageous, one would expect the body to consume fat completely before catabolizing amino acids for energy. However, many organs and cells of the body, including the brain, peripheral nerves, erythrocytes, leukocytes, adrenal medulla, and injured tissue, use glucose, not fat, as a primary fuel. Therefore, a continual supply of glucose is an absolute require-

Table 1-3. Body Composition: Tissue Weight vs. Tissue Caloric Content

	Male		Female	
	Weight (kg)	Kcal (% of total)	Weight (kg)	Kcal (% of total)
Water	37.5	0	29.8	0
Bone mineral	2.9	0	2.3	0
Tissue mineral	0.45	0	0.37	0
Body fat	15.5	144,150 (76.5%)	15.6	145,080 (80.5%)
Body protein	10.1	42,420 (22.5%)	8.6	36,120 (18.6%)
Glycogen	0.44	1804 (1.0%)	0.38	1558 (0.9%)
Residual tissue	0.65	0	2.2	0
TOTAL	67.5	188,374 (100%)	59.3	182,758 (100%)

Source: Adapted from data from SB Heymsfield, et al. Chemical and elemental analysis of humans in vivo using improved body composition models. *Am J Physiol* 261: E190, 1991; GF Cahill. Starvation in man. *N Engl J Med* 282: 668, 1970.

ment for life. The body does not maintain energy in the form of carbohydrate to any appreciable degree, most likely because carbohydrates are heavier and calorically less dense than adipose tissue. In addition, fat cannot be effectively converted to carbohydrate in mammalian tissues. Hence, *in the absence of adequate nutrient intake, endogenous protein must be broken down for conversion to glucose for the host to survive*. This results in simultaneous rather than sequential erosion of body fat and body cell mass in all diseases and conditions where energy expenditure exceeds energy intake.

Metabolic Alterations During Starvation

The basal metabolic rate is defined as the energy expenditure of a person at rest in the postabsorptive state. The metabolic rate can be estimated from oxygen consumption and carbon dioxide production, because energy production is stoichiometrically related to the volume of oxygen consumed and carbon dioxide produced. Determination of oxygen consumption and carbon dioxide production is the basis of indirect calorimetry and is the standard for metabolism studies because it is more practical than and does not differ significantly from direct energy expenditure measurements [88]. The ratio of the volume of carbon dioxide produced to the volume of oxygen consumed is known as the respiratory quotient (RQ). This quotient is used as a general indicator of the type of body fuel being metabolized, and in the steady state it varies between 0.7 and 1.0. Pure fat oxidation (which is approached during prolonged starvation) is associated with an RQ of 0.7, and pure carbohydrate oxidation (which may occur with carbohydrate loading) is associated with an RQ of 1.0. Pure protein oxidation does not occur in vivo, but would have a theoretical RQ of 0.8. When the RQ is greater than 1.0 in the steady state, it represents the conversion of carbohydrate to fat such as occurs when carbohydrate intake exceeds caloric needs. Normally, the RQ is approximately 0.85 in the postabsorptive state under steady-state conditions, which is indicative of mixed substrate utilization. Normograms have been developed for predicting the basal metabolic rate based on age, gender, height, and weight. However, people with illnesses do not meet all the rigid conditions under which the "basal" metabolic rate should be determined. Hence, the metabolic rate in these individuals is often referred to as resting energy expenditure (REE). If the REE is greater than 110% of the predicted basal metabolic rate, the patient is considered hypermetabolic. If the REE is less than 90% of the predicted basal metabolic rate, the patient is considered hypometabolic. Those who are undergoing prolonged starvation usually have a REE less than 90% of the predicted value and therefore are considered hypometabolic. This affords an advantage for the starved individual because it decreases caloric demand and the need to break down endogenous substrates for fuel.

Protein Metabolism

Starvation leads to negative nitrogen balance, reflecting loss of protein from the body. Insulin is central in the control of protein metabolism during health and starvation [89]. During starvation, lack of exogenous nutrients leads to a fall in plasma glucose levels and a decrease in secretion of insulin by pancreatic beta cells. A decrease in plasma insulin has the opposite effect of insulin secretion: protein storage is limited, protein synthesis decreases drastically, and amino acids are released from peripheral tissues, leading to an increase in plasma amino acid concentration. The net effect during starvation is that overall protein synthesis decreases while protein catabolism remains the same, resulting in net degradation of body protein [90]. Skeletal muscle is the major source of this protein loss, and two amino acids, glutamine and alanine, are key in protein metabolism during catabolic states such as starvation [91,92]. These amino acids constitute about 70% of the free amino acid pool in skeletal muscle and greater than 50% of the amino acids released during catabolic states, although they account for only 13% of the amino acids in intact muscle protein. They are synthesized de novo in skeletal muscle from pyruvate and from amino acids obtained from muscle proteolysis. They consequently serve as the major transporters of nitrogen from the periphery to the viscera. Peripherally released glutamine is primarily used for fuel by the gastrointestinal tract and rapidly proliferating cells such as stimulated leukocytes [93,94]. Glutamine is also taken up to a small degree by the liver, where it is used for gluconeogenesis [95]. Alanine released from the periphery is the major amino acid used for hepatic gluconeogenesis. The bowel and kidney also release alanine for hepatic glucose production [96]. Most of these biochemical processes, which are largely initiated by decreased insulin secretion during starvation, obligate nitrogen and thus protein loss from the body. During brief starvation, protein is consumed at the rate of 75 g per day, primarily for the purpose of hepatic gluconeogenesis. If such losses were to proceed unabated, one would only be able to survive for a few weeks before lethal protein depletion occurred. However, previously healthy individuals can survive for months without food because of several metabolic alterations that minimize protein utilization. Decreased nutrient intake in otherwise unstressed individuals leads to a decrease in the metabolic rate and thus lowers caloric requirements. In addition, the majority of body tissues preferentially use fatty acids or ketone bodies for fuel rather than glucose, and this decreases the quantity of amino acids consumed in gluconeogenesis. Tissues that must use carbohydrates often do so by incompletely oxidizing glucose to lactate rather than to water and carbon dioxide. The resulting lactate is transferred to the liver and kidney, where it is converted back into glucose for reuse by glycolytic tissues (the Cori cycle). The energy needed for this resynthesis of glucose is derived from fat oxidation. Hence, in essence, lipid-derived calories are shuttled to glycolytic tissues in the form of glucose, and this decreases irreversible glucose consumption. Finally, and most importantly, the central nervous system adapts to the ketone body utilization for fuel and thus decreases its glucose requirement to 30% to 50% of normal during prolonged starvation [89]. The ability to change from utilization of glucose to ketone bodies for fuel is often referred to as "ketoadaptation." It has a significant protein-sparing effect because decreased glucose consumption by the brain means decreased need for gluconeogenesis from amino acids. Thus, during prolonged starvation, protein utilization may decrease by as much as 75% relative to that found during early starvation. This is associated with a marked improvement in nitrogen balance during prolonged starvation as compared with early starvation, although net nitrogen losses still continue as long as nutrient intake remains inadequate.

Carbohydrate Metabolism

Glucose is stored as glycogen in the liver and skeletal muscle. However, total body glycogen reserves are minimal because any exogenous carbohydrate above that which is needed for energy demands is converted to fat during health. Glycogen stores are rapidly depleted within the first 24 hours of starvation, and thus glucose utilized by tissues thereafter must be synthesized. As discussed previously, certain tissues such as those in the central nervous system require glucose for fuel at all times. Several hormones are involved in maintaining plasma glucose concentration during starvation. The coordinated decrease of insulin and increase in glucagon and cortisol during starvation results in marked enhancement of hepatic glucose production. The glucose produced by this mechanism is consumed by the nervous system (80%) and other glycolytic tissues. As starvation continues, the brain decreases the use of glucose as it ketoadapts for utilization of ketone bodies for fuel. However, the body's need for utilization of glucose as a fuel is never completely eliminated.

Fat Metabolism

The major source for fuel during prolonged starvation is fat. Hence, this condition is characterized by accelerated lipolysis with mobilization of glycerol and free fatty acids from adipose tissue. Although glycerol can be converted to glucose, mammalian cells do not possess the enzymatic machinery necessary for conversion of free fatty acids to carbohydrate. Instead, the fatty acids generated during starvation serve as precursors for acetoacetate, beta-hydroxybutyrate, and acetone, so-called "ketone bodies." Ketone bodies represent a water-soluble by-product of triglycerides that can be easily transported throughout the body for use by various tissues. Fatty acids are converted into ketone bodies in the liver, and these fat metabolites serve as another important signal for tissues to decrease glucose oxidation. The sum of these changes during starvation is that fat becomes the primary energy source, and carbohydrate and protein utilization is minimized.

Summary

There is accelerated skeletal muscle protein degradation with movement of amino acids, predominantly consisting of glutamine and alanine from the periphery to the viscera during starvation. The visceral organs use skeletal muscle protein for fuel production primarily consisting of glucose. Metabolic changes occur in the body to minimize the need for glucose and therefore skeletal muscle protein degradation. Increased lipolysis with mobilization of free fatty acids occurs as well. During starvation, the body adapts for utilization of free fatty acids and ketone bodies that are made from fatty acids, and thus fat is used to meet the majority of fuel requirements.

Metabolic Alterations During Critical Illness

After injury or acute illness, there are changes in the metabolic rate and in protein, carbohydrate, and fat metabolism. Many of these changes are similar to those observed during starvation because some of the hormonal alterations that control cellular events during starvation are also found after injury. However, one of the major differences between injury and simple starvation is the presence of an inflammatory focus. This focus leads to the priming and activation of a variety of cells (e.g., leukocytes) that release a host of compounds that have potent metabolic effects. These compounds are often referred to collectively as "inflammatory mediators" and include the cytokines, prostaglandins, leukotrienes, and platelet-activating factor. In simple starvation the cellular events that are responsible for the complete metabolic response is primarily under hormonal control. In contrast, the cellular changes that result in the metabolic events characteristic of critical illness are orchestrated by inflammatory mediators as well as the classic hormones [97].

Metabolic Rate

Critically ill and injured persons are usually hypermetabolic (i.e., REE greater than 110% of predicted), and the degree of hypermetabolism is related to the severity of the initiating disease process [98]. Metabolism can vary from a 10% to 15% increase in those undergoing elective surgery to more than a 100% increase in those recovering from a major burn. An increase in the metabolic rate is primarily controlled by the counter-regulatory hormones epinephrine, glucagon, and cortisol [99]. Although energy balance is often negative, critically ill patients can acutely gain as well as lose several kilograms of body weight in one day. Weight gain in this setting primarily represents fluid retention rather than accretion of fat or lean tissue. In contrast, decreased weight in this setting indicates loss of fluid as well as loss of body protein and body fat.

Protein Metabolism

As found in starvation, those recovering from mild to moderate injury have a net loss of protein from the body because overall protein synthesis decreases while overall protein catabolism remains unchanged relative to the healthy individual. In contrast, both protein catabolism and protein synthesis are accelerated in severely traumatized and critically ill patients, but the increase in protein catabolism exceeds the increase in protein synthesis, which again results in net protein loss from the body [100,101]. Hence, most patients recovering from illness have a negative nitrogen balance unless attenuated or prevented by an appropriate nutritional support regimen. As with starvation, there is a shift of amino acids from the peripheral tissues, primarily skeletal muscle, to visceral organs, and glutamine and alanine play a key role in this process (Bergström intracellular free amino acid concentration) [102]. Although marked loss of total body protein may occur, visceral organs may lose less protein per gram of tissue than does muscle, and in some instances, such as in the case of the liver and kidney, protein content may significantly increase [103,104]. Degradation of muscle protein has the dual purpose of supplying amino acids for gluconeogenesis (primarily alanine) as well as for synthesis of proteins needed for reparative processes and for defense of the host from microorganisms. Glutamine appears to be the preferred fuel of enterocytes during illness. During starvation, ketoadaptation occurs so that some organs can use ketone bodies instead of glucose for fuel. However, in other catabolic states such as those that occur during recovery from trauma and major illness, ketogenesis is inhibited, and ketoadaptation with its attendant protein-sparing effects is markedly limited. This represents one of the most important differences between the metabolic response to simple starvation and the metabolic response to illness. Hence, the length of survival without adequate nutrition during these conditions is markedly decreased relative to starved individuals. Why this adaptive process does not occur during critical illness is not known. [*Editor's Note*: This, as noted elsewhere in this volume, is the critical question in critical illness. The failure of adaptation to lipid and ketone bodies increases proteolysis and wastage of lean body mass.]

The effects of short-term intravenous nutritional support on body composition are closely related to the interplay of protein metabolism and metabolic expenditure [105]. Patients with moderate to severe body protein depletion and mild to minimal elevations in metabolic expenditure show the greatest tendency to restore body protein stores with intravenous nutrition. Conversely, patients with only mild depletion and elevated metabolic rates tend to have ongoing protein losses despite aggressive intravenous nutritional support. Patients who have normal metabolic expenditures gain more body protein during a 2-week course of total parenteral nutrition as compared with similar patients with elevated metabolic rates.

The physiologic impairments seen in patients with moderate to severe protein-calorie malnutrition are associated with the loss of total body protein. There is a close relationship between the body's protein stores and its physiologic function [106]. When more than 20% of the body's store of protein has been lost, most physiologic functions are significantly impaired, including grip and respiratory muscle strength. These abnormal physiologic functions are also mirrored by changes in circulating protein levels, for example, prealbumin and transferrin. A loss of 20% of body protein is typically mirrored by a 20% decrease in body weight. It is at this degree of weight loss when physiologic impairment is manifest.

Carbohydrate Metabolism

Glycogen stores in the body are very small. Nonetheless, this compound is an important source of energy because it can be rapidly converted to glucose in the liver and muscle and thus be immediately available for fuel requirements during emergency situations. Accordingly, the body avidly maintains these stores under normal circumstances. However, within the first 24 hours of illness, glycogen stores are rapidly depleted, and thus muscle amino acids, glycerol, lactate, and pyruvate released from the periphery are used as precursors for accelerated hepatic gluconeogenesis. The magnitude of increase in glucose production is proportional to the extent of illness. The glucose produced is used by the central nervous system, which specifically requires carbohydrate to meet its energy needs, although its rate of utilization is relatively normal. The kidneys increase their requirement for glucose twofold and therefore consume a large amount of carbohydrate daily. The remainder of the glucose is used for reparative processes in wounds or in other injured tissues. Injured tissue abounds with inflammatory cells, erythrocytes, and fibroblasts. Cells populating such tissue undergo anaerobic metabolism and produce large quantities of lactate. The lactate is then transported back to the liver for resynthesis of glucose that can then be reused by tissues undergoing repair (the Cori cycle).

Fat Metabolism

There is a significant increase in fuel requirements during the metabolic response to injury secondary to hypermetabolism, accelerated gluconeogenesis, mobilization of peripheral substrate, and elevated body temperature. To meet this requirement in part, glycerol and free fatty acids are mobilized from adipose tissue and accelerated lipolysis occurs. These processes are mediated by the sympathetic nervous system, and glucagon, and tumor necrosis factor occurs. Free fatty acids cannot be used by some tissues for energy, which exacerbates the need for protein degradation for gluconeogenic purposes even though lipolysis is increased [107]. Accordingly, both protein and fat stores are rapidly depleted in critically ill patients if they do not receive adequate nutritional support. This is associated with significant increases in morbidity and mortality [108].

Summary

Serious illness and injury initiate the transfer of substrates from the periphery to visceral organs. This enables the body to support the recovery process at the expense of body cell mass and protein. On a short-term basis, the benefits of this homeostatic mechanism far outweigh the negative effects. However, prolonged illness can shift this balance toward adversity, and the body's own response to illness may contribute to further injury and possible death. Strategies have developed to prevent or minimize the effect of infection, inflammation, and malnutrition, all of which slow convalescence and exacerbate catabolic states. More specific treatments are evolving, such as the use of monoclonal antibodies to endotoxin in sepsis syndrome, the addition of glutamine to nutritional regimens to support gut function and vitality, and the provision of growth factors that preserve lean tissue and speed wound healing. It is now clear that the care of the critically ill patient necessarily involves treatment of primary pathologic processes and modulation of the host's metabolic response to injury. This dual approach will likely improve survival, decrease morbidity, and reduce the impact of serious illness.

Effects of Nutritional Repletion

Graham Hill reviewed the effects of parenteral and enteral refeeding in surgical patients [1]. His study and other studies on the effects of nutritional repletion on body composition and function have demonstrated a dissociation between the restoration of lean body mass and the return of normal metabolic functions. For example, 3 to 4 days of parenteral or enteral alimentation of malnourished patients improves many physiologic indices well before a gain in tissue protein can be detected. Muscle grip strength and peak expiratory flow rates are maximally increased in moderate to severely malnourished patients by 4 days of parenteral feeding. No further changes in these indices are observed during an additional 10 days of observation [109]. After this acute period, further improvements in physiologic function observed during several months are accompanied by an increase in body protein.

Although these initial improvements occur rapidly, this does not imply a lack of ongoing improvements in association with restoration of lean body mass and normal body composition. Thus, after an early improvement in physiologic function of approximately 12%, which is significant to be beneficial clinically, additional improvements are related directly to accretion of total body protein. The cellular mechanisms responsible for this early improvement have not been fully worked out. However, it has been suggested that considerable decreases in muscle ATP and adenosine diphosphate that occur in malnourished surgical patients return to normal with nutritional repletion [110].

Whole-body protein synthesis depends on the balance between protein synthesis and catabolism. It is possible to increase whole-body protein synthesis in patients with uncomplicated semistarvation by the enteral or parenteral feeding and induce a positive nitrogen balance. Such is not true in more critically ill patients with sepsis or who have suffered major trauma. However, the protein losses of these individuals can be reduced by up to half if nutrition support is provided [105]. Hill and associates have shown how the response to nutrition support is determined by the relative effects of two opposing processes: protein depletion and metabolic expenditure. For example, patients with moderate to severe protein and calorie malnutrition (defined as 30% or greater depletion of body protein stores) with normal resting metabolic expenditures have the greatest tendency to gain protein with total parenteral nutrition (TPN) [111]. Patients with 10% or less protein depletion and elevated metabolic rates continue to lose protein even in the presence of aggressive nutrition support.

These findings have important implications for the practice of perioperative parenteral and enteral nutrition. The amount of protein accretion and therefore restoration of lean body mass that occurs during a 7- to 14-day period is small and directly influenced by a number of metabolic and nutritional factors. The most severely depleted patients can only be expected to increase their protein stores by 5% with 2 weeks of artificial feeding. However, if the metabolic expenditure is increased in these individuals as a result of sepsis or injury, there may be little or no increase in the body's protein content. These data strongly suggest that the beneficial effects of artificial feeding in these situations are not the result of improvements in body composition per se. A partial explanation may be the salutary effects of physiologic function described earlier. Other important influences may be the effect of TPN on hepatic glycogen, enzyme induction, hormonal responses, amino acid transport, and membrane function.

The effects of nutrition support in critically ill patients can be understood by examining three patient groups: those who undergo major elective operations, those who have suffered major trauma, and those with serious sepsis. Patients who undergo major operations are frequently moderately depleted of body protein preoperatively. In the absence of severe complications, even those who do not receive enteral or parenteral feeding lose only another 5% or 43 g of body protein per day during the first 2 weeks after surgery [112]. Most trauma patients who are not usually depleted can be expected to lose fairly large amounts of body protein (110 g/day) within the first 10 days of injury [1] despite standard nutritional support. Greater losses can be expected to occur in patients with sepsis despite aggressive nutritional support that would normally be expected to result in an increase in total body fat. Overall, TPN appears to significantly increase protein synthesis, but it does not significantly alter protein catabolism [113,114]; the net result of TPN appears to be a decreased rate of protein breakdown. The use of growth factors such as growth hormone or insulin-like growth factor–1 (IGF-1) may significantly modify catabolic responses in critically ill patients. Supplemental growth hormone administration in patients receiving TPN may result in greater protein and lesser fat accretion.

Byrne and colleagues examined the effects of growth hormone in a group of nutritionally compromised surgical patients after operation [115]. Fourteen patients requiring long-term nutritional support received standard nutritional therapy that provided approximately 50 kcal/kg body weight/day and 2 g of protein/kg body weight/day during an initial 7-day equilibrium period. The patients then continued on standard therapy (n = 4) or, in addition, received growth hormone at 0.14 mg/kg/day (n = 10). On day 7 of the equilibrium period and again after 3 weeks of treatment, body fat, mineral content, lean (nonfat- and nonmineral-containing tissue) mass, total body water, extracellular water, and body protein were determined using DEXA and dilutional marker techniques. Daily and cumulative nutrient balance and substrate oxidation studies determined the distribution, efficiency, and utilization of calories for protein, fat, and carbohydrate deposition. The patients treated with growth hormone gained small amounts of body fat and significantly more lean mass and protein than did the patients who received standard TPN. The increase in lean mass was not associated with an inappropriate expansion of extracellular water. In contrast, patients receiving standard therapy retained a greater proportion of body weight as extracellular water and significantly more fat than did the patients who received growth hormone. Growth hormone administration altered substrate oxidation and the use of available energy, which resulted in a 66% increase in the efficiency of protein deposition. Thus, growth hormone may be able to increase protein retention in stable adult patients who receive TPN. The effects of growth hormone in other patient populations are currently under investigation.

Negative mineral balances or abnormal mineral balances during refeeding may also interfere with the body's ability to restore protein mass. Thus, the correction of the total body sodium deficit not only returns the body's hydration status to normal, but also improves its secretion of total body protein. Similar effects are observed in patients with negative potassium or phosphorus balance, or both. The effects of TPN also include partial restoration of type II muscle fibers as well as an increase in activity of the glycolytic enzyme phosphofructokinase.

Conclusions

Modern technologies such as neutron activation and DEXA allow the body's compartments to be measured with great accuracy and precision. Investigators are using these highly advanced techniques and others to improve our understanding of the effects of parenteral and enteral alimentation. Our current understanding suggests that there are two important areas of research and clinical interest: (1) the short-term effects of nutrition support, where the beneficial effects are not related to improvements in body composition, at least in the traditional sense; and (2) the long-term effects of nutrition support, where efforts are being directed toward favorably altering the balance between protein synthesis and breakdown.

References

1. Hill GL. Body composition research: Implications for the practice of clinical nutrition. *JPEN* 16:197, 1992.
2. Heymsfield SB, Williams PJ. Nutritional Assessment by Clinical and Biochemical Methods. In ME Shils, UR Young (eds), *Modern Nutrition in Health and Disease* (7th ed). Philadelphia: Lea & Febiger, 1988. P 823.
3. Heymsfield SB, Casper K. Anthropometric assessment of the adult hospitalized patient. *JPEN* 11:36S, 1987.
4. Forse RA, Shizgal HM. The assessment of malnutrition. *Surgery* 88:17, 1980.
5. Moreiras VO, et al. Nutritional status and food habits assessed by dietary intake and anthropometric parameters in anorexia nervosa. *Int J Vitam Nutr Res* 60:267, 1990.
6. Heymsfield SB, et al. Human body composition: Comparison of two improved four-compartment models that differ in expense, technical complexity, and radiation exposure. *Am J Clin Nutr* 52:52, 1990.
7. Moore FD. *Metabolic Care of the Surgical Patient*. Philadelphia: Saunders, 1959.
8. Moore FD. Energy and the maintenance of the body cell mass. *JPEN* 4:228, 1980.
9. Shizgal HM. Nutritional assessment with body composition measurements. *JPEN* 11:42S,1987.
10. Shizgal HM, Martin MF. Caloric requirement of the critically ill septic patient. *Crit Care Med* 16:312, 1988.
11. Behnke AR, Feen BG, Welham WC. The specific gravity of healthy men. *JAMA* 118:495, 1942.
12. Choller DA, Jones PJH. Measurement of Total Body Water by Isotope Dilution: A Unified Approach to Calculation. In KJ Ellis, S Yasumura, WD Morgan (eds), *In Vivo Body Composition Studies*. London Institute of Physical Sciences in Medicine, 1987. P 131.
13. Schloerb PR, et al. The measurement of total body water in the human subject by deuterium oxide dilution. *J Clin Invest* 29:1296, 1950.

14. Pace H, Rathbun EN. Studies on body composition: III. The body water and chemically combined nitrogen content in relation to fat content. *J Biol Chem* 158:685, 1945.
15. Moore FD, et al. *The Body Cell Mass and Its Supporting Environment: Body Composition in Health and Disease*. Philadelphia: Saunders, 1963.
16. Shizgal HM, Milne CA, Spanier AH. The effect of nitrogen sparing intravenously administered fluids on postoperative body composition. *Surgery* 85:496, 1979.
17. Shizgal HM, et al. Indirect measurement of total exchangeable potassium. *Am J Physiol* 233:F253, 1977.
18. Lukaski HC. Methods for the assessment of human body composition: Traditional and new. *Am J Clin Nutr* 46:537, 1987.
19. Forbes GB. *Human Body Composition*. New York: Springer, 1987. P 5.
20. Pierson RN Jr, Lin DHY, Phillips RA. Total body potassium in healthy men: Effects of age, sex, height and fat. *Am J Physiol* 226:206, 1976.
21. Lukaski HC, et al. Assessment of fat-free mass using bioelectrical impedance measurements of the human body. *Am J Clin Nutr* 41:810, 1985.
22. Nyboer J. *Electrical Impedance Plethysmography*. Springfield: Thomas, 1970. P 349.
23. Sedensky JA, Klein J. Electrical Impedance Derived Measurement of Total Body Water and Extracellular Fluid Volume in Healthy Mongrol Dogs. In *Proceedings of the Seventh Annual Michigan Cardiovascular Research Forum,* 1977. P 45.
24. Thomasset A, et al. Appreciation de la situation electrolytique tissulaire par le rapport dwa impedances globales du corps human en basse et haut frequency. *Rev Med Aeronaut Spaciale* 46:312, 1973.
25. Scheltinga MR, et al. Impedance electrodes positioned on proximal portions of limbs quantify fluid compartments in dogs. *J Appl Physiol* 70:2039, 1991.
26. Fuller NJ, Elia M. Potential use of bioelectrical impedance of the "whole body" and of body segments for the assessment of body composition: Comparison with densitometry and anthropometry. *Eur J Clin Nutr* 43:779, 1989.
27. Baumgarter RN, Chumlea WC, Roche AF. Estimation of body composition from bioelectric impedance of body segments. *Am J Clin Nutr* 50:221, 1989.
28. Brown BH, et al. Determination of upper arm muscle and fat areas using electrical impedance measurements. *Clin Phys Physiol Meas* 9:47, 1988.
29. Hoffer EC, Meador CK, Simpson DC. Correlation of whole body impedance with total body water volume. *J Appl Physiol* 27:531, 1969.
30. Deurenberg P, et al. Factors affecting bioelectrical impedance measurements in humans. *Eur J Clin Nutr* 42:1017, 1988.
31. Schell B, Gross R. The reliability of bioelectrical impedance measurements in the assessment of body composition in healthy adults. *Nutr Rep Intl* 36:449, 1987.
32. Kushner RF, Schoeller DA. Estimation of total body water by bioelectrical impedance analysis. *Am J Clin Nutr* 44:417, 1986.
33. Schols AMWJ, et al. Body composition by bioelectrical impedance analysis compared with deuterium dilution and skinfold anthropometry in patients with chronic obstructive pulmonary disease. *Am J Clin Nutr* 53:421, 1991.
34. Scheltinga MR, et al. Glutamine-enriched intravenous feedings attenuate extracellular fluid expansion following a standard stress. *Ann Surg* 214:385, 1991.
35. Hill GL, et al. Bioelectrical impedance analysis in the measurement of the body composition of surgical patients. *Br J Surg* 78:109, 1991.
36. Schroeder D, Christi PM, Hill GL. Bioelectrical impedance analysis for body composition: Clinical evaluation in general surgical patients. *JPEN* 14:129, 1990.
37. Katch FI, et al. Validity of bioelectrical impedance to estimate body composition in cardiac and pulmonary patients. *Am J Clin Nutr* 43:972, 1986.
38. Scheltinga MR, et al. Altered cellular membrane function can be characterized by measuring body reactance. *Surg Forum* 41:43, 1990.
39. Nyboer J, Sedensky JA. Bioelectrical impedance during renal dialysis. *Proc Dial Trans Forum* 4:214, 1974.
40. Segal KR, et al. Estimation of total body water distribution by bioelectrical impedance. *Fed Proc* 46:1334, 1987.
41. Subramanian R, et al. Total body water in congestive heart failure: A pre- and post-treatment study. *J Assoc Phys Ind* 28:257, 1980.
42. Shizgal HM, Milne CA, Spanier AH. The effect of nitrogen sparing intravenously administered fluids on postoperative body composition. *Surgery* 85:481, 1979.
43. Shizgal HM. Body Composition. In JE Fischer (ed), *Surgical Nutrition*. Boston: Little, Brown, 1983. P 317.
44. Tellado JM, et al. Predicting mortality based on body composition analysis. *Ann Surg* 209:81, 1989.
45. Legaspi A, et al. Effect of starvation and total parenteral nutrition on electrolyte homeostasis in normal man. *JPEN* 12:109, 1988.
46. Legaspi A, et al. The effect of starvation and total parenteral nutrition on skeletal muscle amino acid content and membrane potential difference in normal man. *Surg Gynecol Obstet* 166:233, 1988.
47. Fantini GA, et al. Effect of hormonal and substrate backgrounds on cell membrane function in normal males. *J Appl Physiol* 63:1107, 1987.
48. Pichard C, et al. Intracellular potassium and membrane potential during malnutrition and subsequent refeeding. *Am J Clin Nutr* 54:489, 1991.
49. Bergstrom J, et al. Changes of muscle water and electrolytes with severity of trauma. *Acta Chir Scand* 494:139S, 1979.
50. Bergstrom J, et al. Influence of injury and nutrition on muscle water and electrolytes. *Ann Surg* 193:810, 1981.
51. Bergstrom J, Hultman E. Determination of water and electrolytes in muscle biopsies in the nutritional assessment of clinical disorders. *JPEN* 11:51S, 1987.
52. Häussinger D, et al. Cellular hydration state: An important determinant of protein catabolism in health and disease. *Lancet* 341:1330, 1993.
53. Sayeed MM. The Plasma Membrane in the Pathogenesis of Circulatory Shock. In BM Altura, AM Lefer, W Schumer (eds), *Handbook of Shock and Trauma, Vol 1: Basic Science*. New York: Raven, 1983. P 225.
54. Blum H, et al. Intracellular sodium flux and high-energy phosphorus metabolites in ischemic skeletal muscle. *Am J Physiol* 255:C377, 1988.
55. Glynn IM. The Electrogenic Sodium Pump. In MP Blaustein, M Leiberman (eds), *Electrogenic Transport, Fundamental Principles and Physiological Implications*. New York: Raven, 1984. P 33.
56. Church JM, Choong SY, Hill GL. Abnormalities of muscle

metabolism in histology and malnourished patients awaiting surgery: Effects of a course of intravenous nutrition. *Br J Surg* 71:563, 1984.

57. Russell D, et al. Metabolic and structural changes in skeletal muscle during hypocaloric dieting. *Am J Clin Nutr* 39:503, 1984.
58. Jeejeebhoy KN. Muscle function and nutrition. *Gut* 27:25, 1986.
59. Kobayshi T, Kesselly B, Wilmore D, et al. Starvation Reduces High Energy Phosphate Stores, Work Efficiency, Oxidative Capacity in Skeletal Muscle. *J Parenter Enter Nutr* 15:1S, 1991.
60. Shizgal HM, et al. Nutritional assessment and skeletal muscle function. *Am J Clin Nutr* 44:761, 1986.
61. Symreng T, et al. Nutritional assessment reflects muscle energy metabolism in gastric carcinoma. *Ann Surg* 198:146, 1983.
62. Bergstrom J, Bostrom H. Preliminary studies of energy-rich phosphagens in muscle from severely ill patients. *Crit Care Med* 4:197, 1976.
63. Lennmarken C, Larsson J. Skeletal muscle function and energy metabolites in malnourished surgical patients. *Acta Chir Scand* 152:169, 1986.
64. Wang ZM, Pierson RN Jr, Heymsfield SB. The five level model: A new approach to organizing body composition research. *Am J Clin Nutr* 56:19, 1992.
65. Heymsfield SB, et al. Application of electromagnetic and sound waves in nutritional assessment. *JPEN* 11:64S, 1987.
66. Sjostrom L, et al. Determination of total adipose tissue volume in women by computed tomography: Comparisons with ^{40}K and tritium techniques. *Am J Physiol* 250:E736, 1986.
67. Seidell JC, Bakker CJG, Van derKooy K. Imaging techniques for measuring adipose tissue distribution: A comparison between computed tomography and 1.5 T magnetic resonance. *Am J Clin Nutr* 51:953, 1990.
68. Burkinshaw L, Hill GL, Morgan DN. Assessment of the Distribution of Protein in the Human by In Vivo Neutron Activation Analysis. In *International Symposium on Nuclear Activation Techniques in Life Sciences*. Vienna: IAEA, Publication SM 227/39, 1978. P 787.
69. Cohn SH, et al. Compartmental body composition based on total body nitrogen, potassium and calcium. *Am J Physiol* 239:E524, 1980.
70. Beddoe AH, Hill GL. Clinical measurements of body composition using in vivo neutron activation analysis. *JPEN* 9:504, 1985.
71. Wang Z-M, et al. Body composition in humans: Advances in the development of multicompartment chemical models. *Am J Clin Nutr* 56:19, 1992.
72. Mazes RB, et al. Dual energy x-ray absorptiometry for total body and regional bone mineral and soft tissue composition. *Am J Clin Nutr* 51:1106, 1990.
73. Lichteman S, Heymsfield SB, Kehayias J. Elemental reconstruction of human composition in vivo. *FASEB J* 4:A2261, 1990.
74. Gotfredsen A, et al. Measurement of lean body mass and total body fat using dual photon absorptiometry. *Metabolism* 35:88, 1986.
75. Heymsfield SB, et al. Dual photon absorptiometry: Comparison of bone mineral and soft tissue mass measurements in vivo with established methods. *Am J Clin Nutr* 49:1283, 1989.
76. Heymsfield SB, et al. Chemical and elemental analysis of humans in vivo using improved body composition models. *Am J Physiol* 261:E190, 1991.
77. Anderson J, et al. Neutron activation analysis in men in vivo: A new technique in medical investigation. *Lancet* 2:1201, 1964.
78. Palmer HE, et al. The feasibility of in vivo neutron activation analysis of total body calcium and other elements of body composition. *Phys Med Biol* 13:269, 1968.
79. Heymsfield SB, Waki M. Body composition in humans: Advances in the development of multicompartment chemical models. *Nutr Rev* 49:97, 1991.
80. Pierson RN Jr, et al. Body composition and aging: A study by in vivo neutron activation analysis. *Am J Physiol* 261:E103, 1991.
81. Buckley GB. The role of oxygen free radicals in human disease processes. *Surgery* 94:407, 1983.
82. Jacobs DO, et al. Sepsis alters skeletal muscle energetic and membrane function. *Surgery* 110:318, 1991.
83. Kobayashi T, et al. The effects of growth hormone on muscle energy during short-term starvation. *JPEN* 16:23S, 1992.
84. Fleer CTG, Bhattacharya SS, Singh CM. Solute and water exchanges between cells and extra cellular fluids in health and disturbances after trauma. *JPEN* 4:98, 1980.
85. Street SJ, Beddoe AH, Hill GL. Aggressive nutritional support does not prevent protein loss despite fat gain in septic intensive care patients. *Trauma* 27:262, 1987.
86. Le Quesne LP, Cochrane JPS, Fieldman NR. Fluid and electrolyte disturbances after trauma: The role of adrenocortical and pituitary hormones. *Br Med Bull* 41:212, 1985.
87. Wilmore DW. *The Metabolic Management of the Critically Ill*. New York: Plenum, 1977.
88. de V Weir JB. New methods for calculating metabolic rate with special reference to protein metabolism. *J Physiol* 109:1, 1949.
89. Cahill GF. Starvation in man. *N Engl J Med* 282:668, 1970.
90. Hermann VM, Clarke D, Wilmore DW, et al. Protein metabolism: Effect of disease and altered intake on the stable ^{15}N curve. *Surg Forum* 31:92, 1980.
91. Bergstrom J, Furst P, Vinnars E. Intracellular free amino acid concentration in human muscle tissue. *J Appl Physiol* 36:693, 1974.
92. Ruderman NB, Berger M. The formation of glutamine and alanine in skeletal muscle. *J Biol Chem* 249:5500, 1974.
93. Souba WW, Austgen TR. Interorgan glutamine flow following surgery and infection. *JPEN* 14:90S, 1990.
94. Souba WW, Smith RJ, Wilmore DW. Glutamine metabolism by the intestinal tract. *JPEN* 9:608, 1985.
95. Souba WW, Wilmore DW. Postoperative alteration of arteriovenous exchange of amino acids across the gastrointestinal tract. *Surgery* 94:342, 1983.
96. Bessey PQ. Metabolic Response to Critical Illness. In DW Wilmore, et al (eds), *Care of the Surgical Patient*. New York: Scientific American, 1989.
97. Walters JM, et al. Both inflammatory and endocrine mediators stimulate host response to sepsis. *Arch Surg* 121:179, 1986.
98. Long CL, et al. Metabolic response to injury and illness: Estimation of energy and protein needs from indirect calorimetry and nitrogen balance. *JPEN* 3:452, 1979.

99. Bessey PQ, et al. Combined hormonal infusion simulates the metabolic response to injury. *Ann Surg* 200:264,1984.
100. Birkman RH, et al. Whole-body protein metabolism due to trauma in man as estimated by [^{15}N] alanine. *Am J Physiol* 241:E64, 1981.
101. Aulick LH, Wilmore DW. Increased peripheral amino acid release following burn injury. *Surgery* 85:560, 1979.
102. Ruderman NB, Berger M. The formation of glutamine and alanine in skeletal muscle. *J Biol Chem* 249:5500, 1974.
103. Mealy K, Wilmore DW. Tumor necrosis factor increases hepatic cell mass. *Br J Surg* 78:331, 1991.
104. Goodwin CW, et al. Increased renal perfusion and kidney size in convalescent burn patients. *JAMA* 244:1588, 1980.
105. Hill GL, et al. Protein status and metabolic expenditure determine the response to intravenous nutrition: A new classification of surgical malnutrition. *Br J Surg* 78:109, 1991.
106. Windsor JA, Hill GL. Grip strength: A measure of the proportion of the protein loss in surgical patients. *Br J Surg* 75:880, 1988.
107. Shizgal HM. The effect of malnutrition on body composition. *Surg Gynecol Obstet* 152:22, 1981.
108. Rombeau JL, Rolandelli RH, Wilmore DW. Nutritional Support. In DW Wilmore, et al (eds), *Care of the Surgical Patient*. New York: Scientific American, 1988.
109. Christie PM, Hill GL. Effect of intravenous nutrition and function in acute attacks of inflammatory disease. *Gastroenterology* 99:730, 1990.
110. Kinney JM, Furst P. The Intensive Care Patient: Energy Metabolism. In JM Kinney, et al (eds), *Nutrition and Metabolism in Patient Care*. Philadelphia: Saunders, 1988. P 657.
111. Hill GL, et al. Protein status and metabolic expenditure determine the response to intravenous nutrition: A new classification of surgical malnutrition. *Br J Surg* 78:109, 1991.
112. Streat SJ, Hill GL. Nutrition in the management of critically ill patients in surgical intensive care. *World J Surg* 11:194, 1987.
113. Shaw JHF, Wildbore M, Wolfe RR. Whole body protein kinetics in severely septic patients. *Ann Surg* 205:288, 1987.
114. Shaw JHF, Wolfe RR. An integrated analysis of glucose, fat and protein metabolism in severely traumatized patients. *Ann Surg* 209:63, 1989.
115. Byrne TA, et al. Anabolic therapy with growth hormone accelerates protein gain in surgical patients requiring nutritional rehabilitation. *Ann Surg* 218:400, 1993.

Selected Readings

Heymsfield SB, Waki M, Kehayias J, et al. Chemical and elemental analysis of humans in vivo using improved body composition models. *Am J Physiol* 261:E190, 1991.

Dr. Heymsfield has been at the forefront of modern research in body composition and is a champion of the multicompartment approach.

Hill GL. Body composition research: Implications for the practice of clinical nutrition. *JPEN* 16:197, 1992.

Dr. Hill summarizes most of his seminal work in the field. The synthesis of traditional and modern assessment techniques and their relationship to changes in body composition is well worth reading. More importantly, his investigations highlight one of the most pressing problems facing clinicians and investigators today: the dissociation between large changes in body composition and outcome. This disparity emphasizes the need to examine short-term changes and the mediators of this effect.

Moore FD, et al. *The Body Cell Mass and Its Supporting Environment: Body Composition in Health and Disease*. Philadelphia: Saunders, 1963.

This landmark treatise summarizes Dr. Moore's staggering agglomeration of data describing the effects of disease on the human host. This work set the stage for much of the research in body composition that followed.

Shizgal HM. Body Composition. In JE Fischer (ed), *Surgical Nutrition* 1st ed. Boston: Little, Brown, 1983. P 317.

Dr. Shizgal's chapter shows the type of information that can be obtained using multiple isotope dilution methods.

2

Intestinal Digestion and Absorption of Nutrients

George K. Grimble
Timothy E. Bowling
David B. A. Silk

An early attempt to maintain the nutrition status of a female patient with 15 cm of jejunum anastomosed to the midtransverse colon was described by Althausen and colleagues in 1949 [1]. Despite the limited digestive and absorptive surface, the patient maintained stable body weight on an oral intake of 1610 kcal/d of hospital diet or a synthetic diet containing glucose, cream, hydrolyzed protein, and vitamins and minerals. This form of nutrition support was obviously a clinical tour de force, but it also presaged two factors that have exercised gastroenterologists and clinical nutritionists during subsequent years. The nutrient balance data showed that more than 70% of carbohydrate and 50% of protein was assimilated, and the patient was maintained in slight positive nitrogen balance. In addition, flatulence disappeared during periods when the patient consumed the synthetic diet [2], which clearly suggested that malabsorbed nutrient was no longer reaching the colon. The metabolic significance of colonic fermentation was not fully realized at the time of the study because of the technical problems of measuring colonic gas production, as described in the paper immediately preceding that by Althausen and colleagues in the same issue of *Gastroenterology* [3].

Subsequent efforts to provide diets to patients with severely impaired assimilative function have therefore concentrated on small bowel digestive and absorptive mechanisms. These special "elemental" or "chemically defined diets" are described in more detail elsewhere [4]. It is now clear that the absorptive and digestive mechanisms of the small intestine present a formidable array, with large capacity, to any oral nutrient intake. As a result, the distinction between diets for patients with normal and pathologic intestinal function has become blurred. With our greater understanding of how to define degree of impairment of any aspect of nutrient assimilation, it is possible to use simple dietetic and clinical maneuvers to overcome slight impairment of any of these steps, without reducing the amount of nutrient administered each day.

Despite this, one of the most clinically significant complications of enteral feeding that remains is the onset of diarrhea, the consequence of an insufficient functional absorptive capacity of the intestinal mucosa to deal with the administered nutrient load. This may co-exist with intestinal fluid and electrolyte secretion that is not reversed sufficiently by nutrient absorption. Thus, when discussing present knowledge of the physiology of nutrient, water, and electrolyte assimilation, this chapter will do so based on what is known about the pathogenesis of enteral feeding–related diarrhea.

The Absorptive Capacity of the Intestine

Small Intestine

The reserve capacity or "safety margin" of the small intestine can be defined as the excess over the maximum intake likely to be encountered. In general, the total absorptive area of the small intestine of each animal species suits its *metabolic mass.* Species of similar size, habitat, and diet, but different metabolic mass (e.g., desert wood rat and iguana), have intestines of similar size but with markedly different surface area. This difference can be accounted for by the amplification of surface area by villi and microvilli (1280-fold in the desert rat, much less in the iguana) [5]. Within these morphologic confines lies the possibility of further adaptation, as exemplified by one ingenious study [6]. Mice were rendered hyperphagic by transfer to a 6°C environment and, although the higher nutrient load led to only a modest increase (20%) in digestive and absorptive efficiency, the safety margin was reduced from a range of 220% to 300% to a range of 60% to 90% [6]. This was clearly sufficient to deal with the increased nutrient load and indicates that expression of digestive enzymes [7] and nutrient transporters [8] cannot be infinitely up-regulated; in fact, the process is rather slow [8]. If they were capable of a rapid degree of adaptation, the energy cost of synthesizing enough to meet different individual dietary loads with the same safety margin would probably outweigh the nutritional benefit.

In humans, the safety margin is probably in the range of 4500 to 7000 kcal/d. Indeed, in one ileal intubation study performed in normal human subjects in our laboratory, the constant nasoduodenal infusion of polymeric diet equivalent to 6000 kcal/d was efficiently assimilated [9].

These comments should be borne in mind when considering studies that appear to show impairment of absorptive function (e.g., reduced exocrine pancreatic secretion, reduced brush-border membrane hydrolase specific activities, or altered kinetics of substrate uptake) in different disease states. Few of these studies have addressed the question of whether such changes give rise to *clinically* significant impairment of nutrient uptake. Because of the overlap between the luminal and brush-border membrane phases of digestion, the degree of impairment has to be profound before clinically significant malabsorption will occur. Thus, malabsorption of some nutrients may occur only if 90% impairment of organ function has occurred, for example, in exocrine pancreatic disease [10–12]. In other situations, malabsorption may occur as a vitamin deficiency state or as diarrhea resulting from malabsorption of macronutrients and their fermentation by the colonic luminal microflora [2]. It is also important to consider whether impaired digestive or absorptive function in a patient who is receiving enteral nutrition support will affect the global clinical or nutritional outcome. Thus, in a prospective, randomized, controlled trial of enteral feeding with a polymeric or predigested chemically defined formula diet, we could find no differences in any nutritional parameter in patients with moderately impaired gasrointestinal function [13]. This suggests that polymeric diets will be efficiently assimilated in many patients with moderately impaired gastrointestinal function who are receiving 24-hour nasoenteral infusions of diet.

Despite this, malabsorption may occur if digestive and absorptive systems are overwhelmed by too high a luminal nutrient concentration for a sustained period. This "load" can be defined as the product of the rate of administration of a nutrient and the resulting luminal concentration, *in relation to mouth-to-cecum transit time.* An oral intake of food will slow transit, measured by lactulose-H_2 breath test, quite considerably [14]. Thus, nasogastric infusion of a significant proportion of daily nutrient requirements over a short time (e.g., 30 minutes) may result in transient malabsorption of part of the diet.

Lactose and its hydrogenated derivative, lactitol, provide a good example of this concept. Lactitol is not absorbed to any appreciable extent in the human small intestine and will traverse the small intestine intact (accompanied by water) to be rapidly fermented by luminal microflora [15], and at a high dose, lactitol will elicit a laxative effect [16]. Lactose can be hydrolyzed by β-galactosidase to galactose and glucose that are absorbed, but in lactase-deficient patients a bolus of lactose will cause diarrhea [17], whereas continuous nasogastric infusion of lactose-containing enteral diets will not [18]. The difference can be explained by the fact that in alactasic patients, brush-border β-galactosidase is never entirely absent but is insufficient to hydrolyze a lactose bolus (high "load") within the orocecal transit time. During continuous infusion, the load is low and residual β-galactosidase activity is not saturated by the rate of delivery.

This concept can be applied to the patient on supplemental feeding who has gastrointestinal symptoms that are not antibiotic related. A slower nasoenteral nutrient infusion rate over an extended period of the day may resolve the problem without recourse to "half-strength" regimes, which limit nutrient intake.

Large Intestine

As will be discussed, the colon has the important function of salvaging water and electrolytes, and this process is often considered in relation to mucosal mechanisms that also exist in the small intestine. In reality, the large bowel is two organs: the first is the colon itself with several functional compartments, and the second is the colonic microflora that have been termed an "organ within an organ." Although the large bowel is sterile at birth, development of the microflora is accompanied by the establishment of six characteristics (Table 2-1). This has been nicely demonstrated by Midtvedt and colleagues [19] in relation to short-chain fatty acid production, whose rate of development depends on the colonic substrate load that is increased during formula-feeding compared with breast-feeding.

Table 2-1. Development of Colonic Microflora-Associated Activities During Early Life

Mucin breakdown
Regulation of fecal trypsin activity
Conversion of bilirubin to urobilinogen
Cholesterol catabolism
Fermentation of malabsorbed carbohydrate and protein to organic acids, including short-chain fatty acids
Recycling of urea back into host amino acid metabolism

Although the normal colonic microflora play no *direct* role in water and electrolyte salvage, they do so *indirectly* by fermenting malabsorbed nutrient to a form whose colonic mucosal absorption is accompanied by water and electrolyte uptake. Therefore, any consideration of colonic reserve capacity must take these two aspects of colonic physiology into account. Thus, rapid intracolonic infusion of more than 500 ml of isotonic saline has been shown to provoke diarrhea in normal subjects [20] and suggests an upper limit of fluid-absorbing capacity. In addition, the healthy colon has the capacity to assimilate up to 70 to 80 g/d of nonabsorbed lactitol, sorbitol, or lactulose [16,21] before diarrhea ensues. Impairment of colonic microflora function by antibiotics (e.g., ampicillin) has been shown to reduce fermentation of oral doses of lactulose (which did not increase stool volume) to the point where inefficient fermentation and salvage led to osmotic diarrhea [22].

These two factors are therefore essential to any consideration of enteral feeding–related diarrhea and will be discussed in a later section.

Small Intestinal Nutrient Assimilation

Protein Absorption

Assimilation of dietary protein proceeds by two complementary phases. Luminal digestion produces small peptides and free L-amino acids that are then subject to further hydrolysis or absorption at the enterocyte brush border.

Gastric Luminal Protein Digestion

Gastric acid denaturation of the diet renders previously stable protein structures susceptible to proteolysis. It is often assumed that the gastric pepsins have a low pH optimum (~pH 2), but in fact it is somewhat higher for soluble oligopeptide substrates (~pH 4–5). The combined effects of gastric-acid denaturation and dicarboxylic acid side-chain protonation will expose more internal peptide bonds to pepsin hydrolysis, which more than offsets the reduction in activity caused by the lower pH. This highly cooperative mechanism is an efficient means by which pepsin converts dietary protein to large soluble oligopeptides [23] and accounts for the fact that the functional pH optimum of pepsin is approximately pH 2. This soluble oligopeptide mixture is a susceptible substrate for luminal digestion by pancreatic endopeptidases and exopeptidases, whose pH optimum is much higher. The peptide-bond specificities of the three endopeptidases and two exopeptidases are cooperative and will release large amounts of free amino acid and small peptides [24,25].

Some dietary proteins are poorly solubilized in the stomach, casein in particular. Retrograde reflux of gastric contents along the feeding tube can lead to casein precipitation, tube blockage [26], or even esophageal obstruction [27]. In one study [28], casein-based diets led to a higher incidence of gastric residuals and side effects than did a highly soluble soy-protein hydrolysate. Whole protein is more slowly cleared from the gastric lumen than are protein hydrolysates [29], although this has not been observed in all studies [30].

Intestinal Nitrogen Assimilation

Dietary and Endogenous Protein

The rapid appearance of amino acids in blood after a protein meal suggests that the proximal jejunum is the major site of dietary protein assimilation [31–33]. In addition, there is an increasing gradient of specific activity of all major brush-border peptidases from jejunum to ileum, which has considerable digestive capacity [34–36]. Taken together with functional differences in the ability of the jejunum and ileum to assimilate amino acids and dipeptides [37], this suggests a difference in the source of amino acids absorbed at these two sites. It would not be unreasonable to suggest that assimilation of endogenous proteins (i.e., from intestinal secretions, secreted plasma proteins, and desquamated cells) occurs at more distal sites, although the distinction is not clear-cut. Adibi and colleagues have shown that some electrophoretically identifiable protein will survive passage to the ileum 4 hours after a meal containing bovine serum albumin [38]. The colon is also a major site of assimilation of endogenously derived protein, in view of evidence of stomal protein losses in ileostomy patients [39]. Indeed, as discussed below, the luminal microflora of the colon have considerable capacity for digesting endogenous and dietary proteins in vitro and in vivo [40–42]. There is a cooperative interaction between protein fermentation (producing short-chain fatty acids, isomeric short-chain fatty acids, and copious amounts of NH_4^+) and carbohydrate fermentation that consumes NH_4^+ [41]. It should be noted that this synergism has been exploited in the treatment of chronic hepatic encephalopathy with nonabsorbable disaccharides such as lactulose or lactitol [43].

Other Modes of Nitrogen Uptake

One other source of nitrogen assimilation in the large intestine has often been overlooked. The human large intestine has a significant capacity to utilize urea as a source of nitrogen for resynthesis of the α-NH_2 of amino acids (see Table 2-1). Urea hydrolysis by colonic microflora will liberate NH_4^+ that can be absorbed and incorporated into amino acids via the glutamate dehydrogenase reaction. Stable-isotope studies with $^{15}N^{15}N$-urea have shown that this occurs in significant amounts in man, approximately 2.6 g nitrogen/d (of which 1.4 g/d is recycled into amino acids) in comparison to a daily urea production rate of 8.5 g nitrogen from 14 g nitrogen protein intake [44–46]. This source of NH_4^+ is in addition to that derived from metabolic consumption of glutamine by the gastrointestinal tract [47,48].

Free Amino Acid Transport

There are four major Na^+-dependent, group-specific, active transport systems in the brush-border membrane of the mammalian enterocyte: (1) monoamino, monocarboxylic (neutral amino acids); (2) glycine, proline, hydroxyproline; (3) dibasic amino acids and cystine; and (4) dicarboxylic (acidic) amino acids [8,49]. In addition, there are other transporters present in the basolateral membrane that are also present in the plasma membrane of other tissues (Table 2-2).

A good example of this complexity is shown by the dibasic amino acids, which include arginine, a possible nutritional immune modulator [50]. Where uptake is impaired by a genetically inherited lesion in the transport protein (e.g., in cystinuria), patients will exhibit a characteristically high urinary excretion of all dibasic amino acids and cystine. Uptake of dibasic amino acids is never entirely abolished because a component of uptake is passive and nonsaturable [51]. Amino acids that do not share the same transporter (e.g., leucine) or metabolically related compounds (e.g., polyamines, α-ketoglutarate) can also stimulate dibasic amino acid uptake via a countertransport mechanism [52–54].

All dibasic amino acids stimulate net water secretion in the perfused jejunum, but the most potent amino acid, arginine, has a local effect [55]. It may be that arginine, absorbed from the intestinal lumen, is stoichiometrically converted to ornithine and citrulline (and urea) during passage through the enterocyte [56]. It would be tempting to speculate that this unique metabolic adaptation represents an adaptive response to excessive stim-

Table 2-2. Macronutrient Transporters in the Small Intestine

	Membrane Location		Coupling			
Transporter	Brush Border	Basolateral	Na^+	H^+	Typical Substrates	Comments
Monosaccharides						
SGLT1	Yes	No	Yes	No	Glucose/galactose	Main glucose/galactose transporter. Unrelated to GLUT family. Inducible by luminal glucose.
System 2	Yes	No	Yes	No	Glucose	
GLUT2	No	Yes	No	No	Glucose/fructose	Liver type, low affinity, high capacity. Modulated by glycemia/diabetes.
GLUT3	?	?	No	No	Glucose/galactose	Brain type, moderate affinity/capacity. Predominantly expressed in tissues with high glucose demand.
GLUT5	Yes	No	No	No	Fructose	Intestine type, high abundance. High affinity for fructose, little for glucose.
Amino Acids						
NBB	Yes	No	Yes	No	Neutral amino acids	Also known as system B [49].
IMINO	Yes	No	Yes	No	Imino acids	
PHE	Yes	No	Yes	No	Phe, Met	
β	Yes	No	Yes	No	β-ala	May be two types (ileum and jejunum).
X^-G,A	Yes	(Yes)	Yes	No	Glu, Asp	High affinity, more than one Na^+ per amino acid transported.
Y^+	Yes	No	Yes	No	Lys, Cys, Arg, Orn	Electrogenic.
y^+	Yes	Yes	No	No	Lys, Cys, Arg, Orn	Electrogenic.
L	Yes	Yes	No	No	Neutral, Cys	Not usually inducible. Sodium independent transport.
A	No	Yes	Yes	No	Short-chain polar	Inducible by starvation, hormones, growth factors.
ASC	No	Yes	Yes	No	Ala, Cys, Ser, Thr	Not usually inducible.
asc	No	Yes	No	No	Ala, Cys, Ser, Thr	
N	No	Yes	Yes	No	Glx, His, Asx	
Peptides						
Dipeptide	Yes	Yes	No	Yes	Dipeptides and tripeptides	Unclear whether this is a single transporter or a family (cf. GLUT transporter) or whether the brush-border and basolateral transporters are the same [66, 68].

GLUT = glucose transporters; SGLUT = sodium-glucose linked transporters.

Note: Bracketed numbers correspond with references.

Source: Data adapted from BH Hirst. Dietary regulation of intestinal nutrient carriers. *Proc Nutr Soc* 52:315, 1993; JD McGivan, M Pastor-Anglada. Regulatory and molecular aspects of mammalian amino acid transport. *Biochem J* 299:321, 1994; Y-J Fei et al. Expression cloning of a mammalian proton-coupled oligopeptide transporter. *Nature* 368:563, 1994; J Dyer et al. Glycyl-L-proline transport in rabbit enterocyte basolateral-membrane vesicles. *Biochem J* 269:565, 1990; and GW Gould, GD Holman. The glucose transporter family: Structure, function and tissue-specific expression. *Biochem J* 295:329, 1993.

ulation of local motility effects by the arginine metabolite, nitric oxide [57].

Peptide Transport

Brush-border membrane hydrolysis of peptides and their uptake are closely related phenomena that are consistent with a dual mode of peptide-bound amino acid transport. A dipeptide or tripeptide can be absorbed intact by a system, distinct from any amino acid transporter, and will be hydrolyzed intracellularly (Figure 2-1). Alternatively, constituent amino acids (or smaller peptide fragments) may be absorbed after brush-border membrane hydrolysis of the peptide. As indicated in Figure 2-1, there is also the possibility that dipeptides and tripeptides that are resistant to brush-border and intracellular peptidases may translocate intact into the portal circulation to be hydrolyzed by blood or tissue peptidases [58].

This transport system has unique characteristics (see Table 2-2): it is H^+-dependent [59] and is stimulated by the low pH in the submucosal layer adjacent to the brush-border membrane [60]. This transport mechanism has fairly wide tissue distribution, being present in the brush-border membrane of the small intestine and renal tubule [61] as well as the placental membrane [62]. In addition, cephalosporin antibiotics containing a peptide bond share the same transport system [63], elegantly investigated by Kramer and colleagues, who covalently tagged and isolated a brush-border membrane protein of 127,000 Da [64,65]. When reconstituted into synthetic liposomes, it proved to have all the characteristics of dipeptide transport and is likely to be either the peptide transporter system itself or a part of it. A cDNA probe to this transporter (PepT1) that has now been sequenced [66] showed that it is expressed in rabbit duodenum, jejunum, kidney, and, to a lesser extent, liver [66]. The possibility that the liver may be able to absorb dipeptides and tripeptides intact from portal blood is intriguing, because most evidence suggests that membrane hydrolysis and amino acid uptake is the major route of liver assimilation [67]. This may raise the possibility of liver targeting of oral or intravenous peptides. It is likely that the enterocyte basolateral membrane peptide

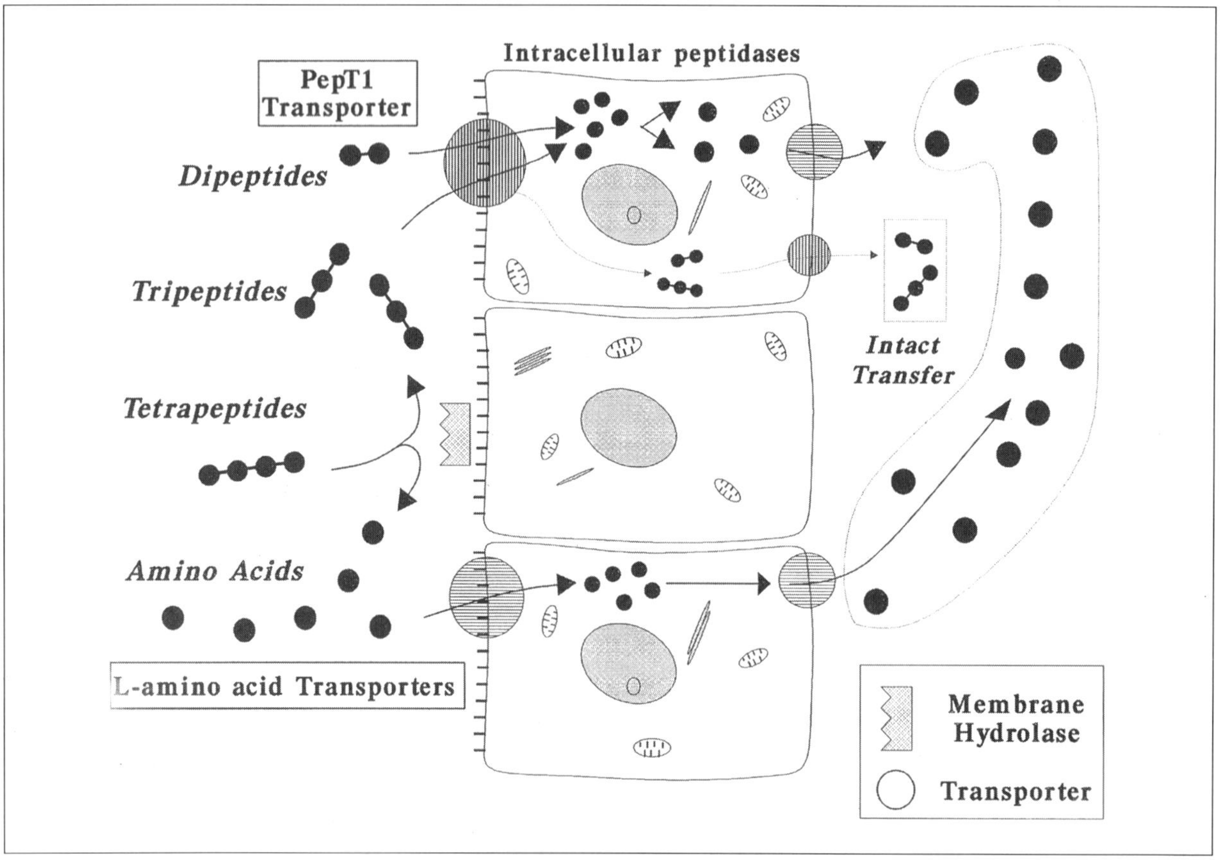

Figure 2-1. Mechanisms of amino acid and peptide uptake in the small intestine. An idealized view of the intestinal wall is shown. The two major mechanisms of amino acid transfer (L-amino acid transport, dipeptide and tripeptide uptake) is shown, together with the minor pathway of intact translocation of peptidase-resistant di- and tripeptides.

transporter described by Dyer and colleagues is the same transport protein [68]. This would explain why basolateral membrane efflux of dipeptides and tripeptides that have escaped intracellular hydrolysis can occur. Daniel and colleagues [69] showed that in terms of its kinetic characteristics, peptide uptake by renal brush-border membrane vesicles has the following structural requirements:

1. A free terminal α-NH_2 and COOH group.
2. α-Configuration for both termini.
3. A *trans*- rather than *cis*-peptide bond.
4. L-amino acid isomers at both termini, although hydrophobic D-amino acids are acceptable at the N-terminus.
5. Chain-length of two or three amino acids only.

As shown in Figure 2-1, amino acids absorbed by either route will efflux from the basolateral membrane via transporters whose kinetic characteristics are sensitive to circulating amino acid concentrations [52].

These differences between L-amino acid and peptide transport are highly significant. Free L-amino acid transport often works "uphill" against a transmembrane concentration gradient, whereas dipeptide and tripeptide uptake is "downhill" because the high activity of intracellular peptidases rapidly removes peptides from the intracellular compartment. Indeed, it has proved remarkably difficult to identify any intracellular pool of small peptides in tissues [70]. In contrast, the ratio of luminal/mucosal intracellular amino acids after a protein meal is less than 1 for several amino acids, for whom transport would have to be concentrative or "uphill" [38]. A second consideration is that stimulation of Na^+ and water uptake by dipeptides is less strong than that by amino acids [71], because transport of the latter is generally Na^+-dependent (see Table 2-2). We have observed that hydrolysates containing more than 70% dipeptides and tripeptides had a rather weak effect on Na^+ (and water) uptake, in contrast to tetrapeptide and pentapeptide preparation or free L-amino acids [72]. Thus, the clinical use of hydrolysates designed to promote maximum nitrogen absorption (dipeptides and tripeptides) may not give optimal water and Na^+ uptake.

Quantitative Aspects of Dietary Protein Assimilation

Absorptive Characteristics of Dietary Peptides and Amino Acids

Dipeptide transport predominates over free L-amino transport during early growth [73,74]. It is less sensitive to the effects of starvation [75], which up-regulates brush-border peptidase activity [36,75]. Sepsis down-regulates amino acid transport [76], but at present there are no data on comparative effects on peptide transport. Curiously, dipeptide transport is up-regulated by dietary nitrogen intake, regardless of whether it is in the form of free L-amino acids, peptides, or whole protein [77]. The same phenomenon has been observed for free L-amino acid transport, except that L-amino acid diets reduced brush-border peptidase levels [78]. At present, the nature of the proximate regulatory signal is not clear because the substrates for one transport system will stimulate the other.

This could imply that peptide assimilation in the small intestine is strongly conserved when dietary amino acid supply may be rate-limiting to growth. It would also suggest that in the absence of protein intake, efficient assimilation of endogenous secretions is necessary. In addition, human and animal intestinal-perfusion studies have shown that in most [79–83], but not all, cases [84] the rate of absorption of individual amino acid residues was faster and more even from partially hydrolysed protein than from its equivalent free amino acid mixture. These findings suggest that there may be an absorptive advantage in using protein hydrolysates rather than free amino acids in enteral diets.

Several factors affect uptake. The starter protein, the method of enzymic hydrolysis, and the chain length of constituent peptides have all been shown to have profound effects on uptake of amino acid residues [82,83,85]. A small increase in the chain length of ovalbumin, casein, and whey hydrolysates from dipeptides and tripeptides to tetrapeptides and pentapeptides (Figure 2-2) markedly reduced nitrogen uptake from these preparations at both high and low perfused concentrations [72,86,87]. As in previous animal studies [88], in the absence of luminal pancreatic enzymes, brush-border hydrolysis of tetrapeptides and pentapeptides is rate-limiting to the uptake of constituent nitrogen.

It would clearly be profitable to investigate the effect of other hydrolysis variables in similar detail, as we have proposed before [89]. For example, the sequence and hydrophobicity of the constituent peptides of a protein hydrolysate will profoundly influence uptake [69]. Thus, two hydrolysates of the same protein and of identical chain-length profile produced by two groups of peptidases with different bond specificity may have different absorption characteristics. Some evidence for this hypothesis has been gained from animal feeding studies in which casein that was partially hydrolysed by pepsin and pancreatic pro-

Figure 2-2. Effect of peptide chain-length on nitrogen assimilation in the perfused human jejunum. The effect of enrichment with dipeptides and tripeptides, of partial hydrolysates of ovalbumin, casein, or whey protein on nitrogen uptake from the perfused human jejunum is shown. (Data for ovalbumin, casein, and whey protein from GK Grimble, et al. The effect of peptide chain-length on absorption of egg-protein hydrolysates in the normal human jejunum. *Gastroenterology* 92:136, 1987; AH Raimundo, et al. The influence of fat and carbohydrate on absorption of partial enzymic hydrolysates of casein in the normal human jejunum. *Gastroenterology* 94:A988, 1988; GK Grimble, et al. The influence of whey hydrolysate peptide chain length on nitrogen and carbohydrate absorption in the perfused human jejunum. *Clin Nutr* 14 [Suppl]:46, 1994, respectively.)

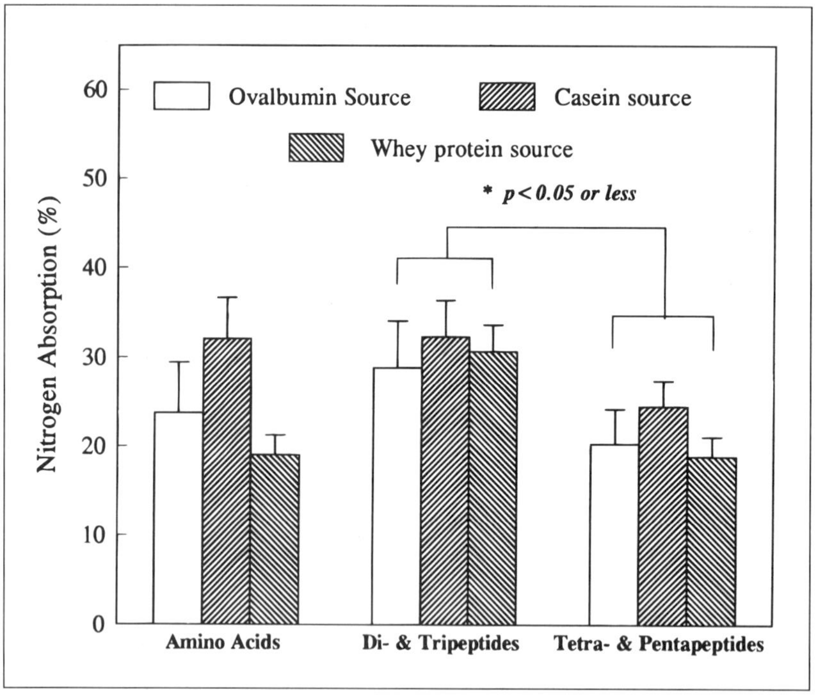

teases yielded better nitrogen retention than did bovine albumin hydrolysed to small peptides by bacterial proteases [90]. Although this study did not compare like with like, it indicates that there may be scope for "tailoring" protein hydrolysates. A second reason is that we were surprised to observe that one short-chain hydrolysate reduced glucose uptake from a co-perfused maltodextrin [91] by a direct inhibitory effect on one of the brush-border α-glucosidases [92]. One cannot, therefore, assume that the "perfect" protein hydrolysate for enteral feeding exists at present.

Nutritional Characteristics of Whole Protein, Peptides, and Amino Acids

There are many published "formula trials" comparing clinical benefit from enteral diets based on protein hydrolysates, free L-amino acids, or whole proteins [28,30,93–95] in which the diets were not balanced in terms of energy or nitrogen intake. Indeed, in only two have the amino acid composition of the hydrolysate and protein been matched [29,96]. There are few *clinical* data on strict comparisons of the relative nutritional efficacy of different forms of enteral nitrogen.

Diets based on casein or the identical amino acid mixture produce equal growth rates in young, healthy rats [97]. Similar long-term comparisons in healthy volunteers showed that regardless of the degree of hydrolysis of lactalbumin, nitrogen balance remained the same [98]. Similarly, in postsurgical patients [99] or short-bowel patients [100] receiving nasoenteral diets based on a protein hydrolysate or its equivalent free L-amino acids, there was no difference in whole-body protein turnover or nitrogen balance.

A degree of skepticism should be exercised over enthusiastic use of any particular form of enteral nitrogen (e.g., peptides) because of claimed specific benefits. This is not because specific advantages do not exist—they may—but the appropriate controlled studies have not, in many cases, been performed.

In one study demonstrating better nitrogen retention in burned guinea pigs with a whole-protein–based diet versus a diet based on the equivalent free amino acids [101], the difference was in the content of specific amino acids. As we have found, it is very difficult to balance the exact amino acid content of the diets, in particular that of glutamine and asparagine. There are technical reasons for this [89], but if not accounted for, this imbalance may lead to a 20% difference in the nitrogen content of the diets. Even where this correction has been made, no nutritional differences have been observed in the ability of casein, its partial hydrolysate, or L-amino acid mixture to support rat growth [97]. Where this correction has not been made, nutritional efficacy appears to be unaltered, but a diet containing a whey-protein (glutamine-containing) hydrolysate caused marked cecal hypertrophy compared with the "equivalent" free L-amino acid–based diet [102] of the same magnitude as in pectin-supplemented rats [103]. A degree of caution should be exercised in considering clinical trials that claim metabolic advantages for enteral diets based on whole protein, hydrolysates, or free amino acids in stressed patients if this simple correction has not been made. [*Editor's Note:* This point, which might be stressed, should be made for intravenous nutritional studies as well.]

In only one study has a metabolic advantage been claimed for oral peptides vs. free amino acids when rats received their diet as short intragastric infusions of 10 to 15 minutes, twice daily [104]. The marked increases in growth and protein deposition are probably related to the more rapid aminoacidemia that follows oral bolus of hydrolysates [32], because insulinemia was markedly increased during peptide feeding [105]. During continuous 24-hour nasoenteral infusion, absorptive differences between peptides and amino acids are likely to be minimal because the "load" is modest. However, with increased use of cyclical nasoenteral nutrition, these absorptive differences may be accentuated, as suggested by a recent trial in postsurgical patients [29].

Effect of Gastrointestinal Function on Protein Assimilation

The large reserve capacity of the small intestine is highlighted by the lack of nutritional difference between diets based on lactalbumin, a partial hydrolysate of lactalbumin, or an equivalent free amino acid mixture fed to healthy volunteers [98]. Even in nasoenterally fed patients with moderately impaired gastrointestinal function, polymeric and predigested diets were of similar nutritional efficacy [13]. Similar results have been obtained in patients with markedly reduced absorptive area (60–150 cm of remaining jejunum) [106]. In patients with inadequate short-bowel syndrome (50–80 cm jejunum), we have observed no differences in nitrogen balance, nitrogen absorption, or ^{13}C-leucine kinetics during 5-day feeding periods with a whey-protein, hydrolysate-based, or equivalent amino acid–based enteral diet [107]. These data point to the capacity of the digestive and transport mechanisms of the remaining small bowel to adapt to adequate nutrient loads [108,109].

Severe impairment of pancreatic function can affect nitrogen assimilation, but in one study of patients with total pancreatectomy, 91% of nitrogen from a lactalbumin hydrolysate–based diet was absorbed, compared with only 61% from a similar diet based on intact lactalbumin [96]. The remarkable feature of this study was that more than half the protein was assimilated in the absence of measurable luminal pancreatic enzymes, and the remainder was partly reutilized by large-bowel fermentation. This study confirms the high capacity and versatility of the brush-border peptidases toward oligopeptides liberated during the gastric phase of digestion [110,111].

Carbohydrate Absorption

Carbohydrate assimilation proceeds in two phases: starch undergoes luminal hydrolysis by pancreatic amylase, and the end products are hydrolyzed (together with other dietary disaccharides) by brush-border glycosidases to monosaccharides that can be absorbed. The carbohydrate source of enteral diets usually comprises partially hydrolysed cornstarch or "maltodextrins" that are produced by the action of bacterial and fungal α-amylase, glucoamylase, and pullulanase [112].

Digestion and Absorption of Dietary Carbohydrate

Dietary carbohydrate is predominantly absorbed in the proximal small intestine, approximately 75% of absorption occurring in the first 70 cm [113]. The luminal hydrolysis of starch is catalyzed by two α-amylases (salivary and pancreatic) whose pH optimum of 7 corresponds to the luminal pH of the duodenum and upper jejunum [114]. Both α-amylases are endoglycosidases, with an absolute specificity for α-1,4 glucose linkages with two adjacent α-1,4 linkages, and will not hydrolyze lactose or sucrose (Figure 2-3). Thus, the end products of starch digestion are maltose, maltotriose, and the α-limit dextrins, with no free glucose release. The α-limit dextrins are branched structures containing both α-1,4 and α-1,6 linkages; the smallest that can be produced by α-amylase attack is a pentasaccharide comprising maltotriose linked by an α-1,6 bond to maltose at the central glucose moiety [115]. Further hydrolysis of this compound can only occur through the action of brush-border glucoamylase. The chain length of the linear, α-1,4 linked dextrins in the lumen after a starch meal depends on the extent to which α-amylase digestion has gone to completion, but it is probably in the range of 5 to 10 glucose units, similar to the chain-length profile of maltodextrins used in enteral diets.

Membrane Digestion and the Brush-Border Oligosaccharidases

The final stages of the digestion of dietary disaccharides and the products of luminal amylase di-

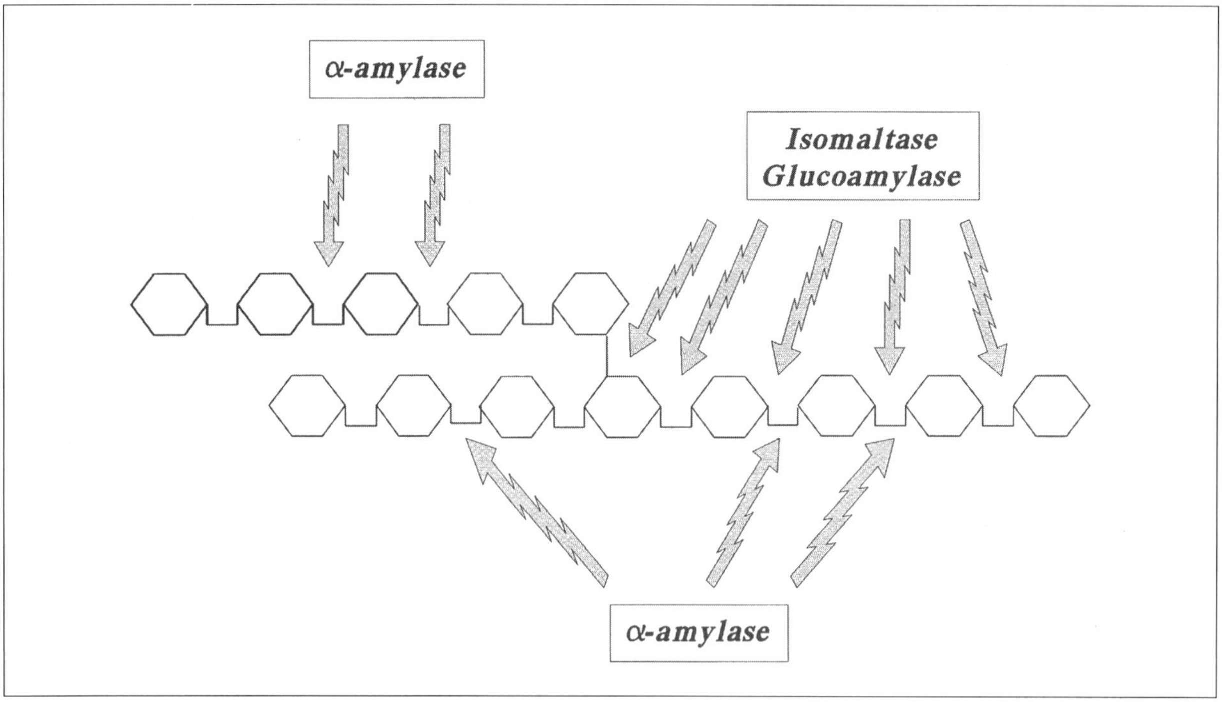

Figure 2-3. Sites of starch hydrolysis by luminal and brush-border α-glucosidases. The branch point of starch is shown and the different glucosyl-bond specificities of intestinal α-glucosidases are indicated.

gestion of starch involve brush-border hydrolysis (by several saccharidases) to produce monosaccharides (Figure 2-4). These enzymes are all inserted as multisubunit structures into the brush-border membrane via a hydrophobic domain, whereas the hydrophilic domains contain the active site of the enzyme [116–119].

A classification of the brush-border α-glucosidases is shown in Table 2-3. Various names have been given to them, but all are capable of hydrolyzing external α-1,4 glycosidic linkages at the nonreducing end of maltose, maltotriose, amylose, or amylopectin [120,121]. Maltases Ib, II, and perhaps III also have activity toward α-1,6 linkages, that is, the branch points of the α-limit dextrins and in amylopectin [111]. Sucrase-isomaltase is a hybrid enzyme with two activities. The isomaltase moiety has the ability to split α-1,6 linked glucose oligomers, albeit at a slower rate than α-1,4 linkages. In contrast, the sucrase moiety has activity toward α-1,4 linkages (e.g., maltose) in addition to that of sucrose [111]. Lactase or β-galactosidase exists as two forms in a dimeric structure, both of which can cleave lactose to glucose and galactose [111].

Thus, hydrolysis of starch to glucose at the brush border uses all the "maltases," of which sucrase-isomaltase is the most important (approximately 80% of total activity). The isomaltase moiety alone accounts for 50% of total activity, and maltase II (glucoamylase) has considerable activity toward oligosaccharides [122]. These considerations help explain why starch assimilation can proceed after total pancreatectomy.

Rate-Limiting Steps in Carbohydrate Assimilation

The glycemic response to 50 g of glucose, maltose, a maltodextrin, or starch has been shown to vary little [123]. When an α-amylase inhibitor was used to completely inhibit luminal amylase, most but not all starch was assimilated [124]. These data suggest that glucose polymer chain length has a slight effect on assimilation in the presence of normal pancreatic secretions and that brush-border saccharidase activity is high. Even where the linkage of the glucose polymer was varied from its usual form (α-1,4) to α-1,6 (dextran 40,000 Da molecular weight), we were able to show that it was almost completely assimilated by healthy volunteers [125]. Because dextran is completely resistant to luminal α-amylase hydrolysis, this finding implies that the brush-border glucosidases of the small intestine have extremely high efficiency and activity and are unlikely to be rate-limiting toward

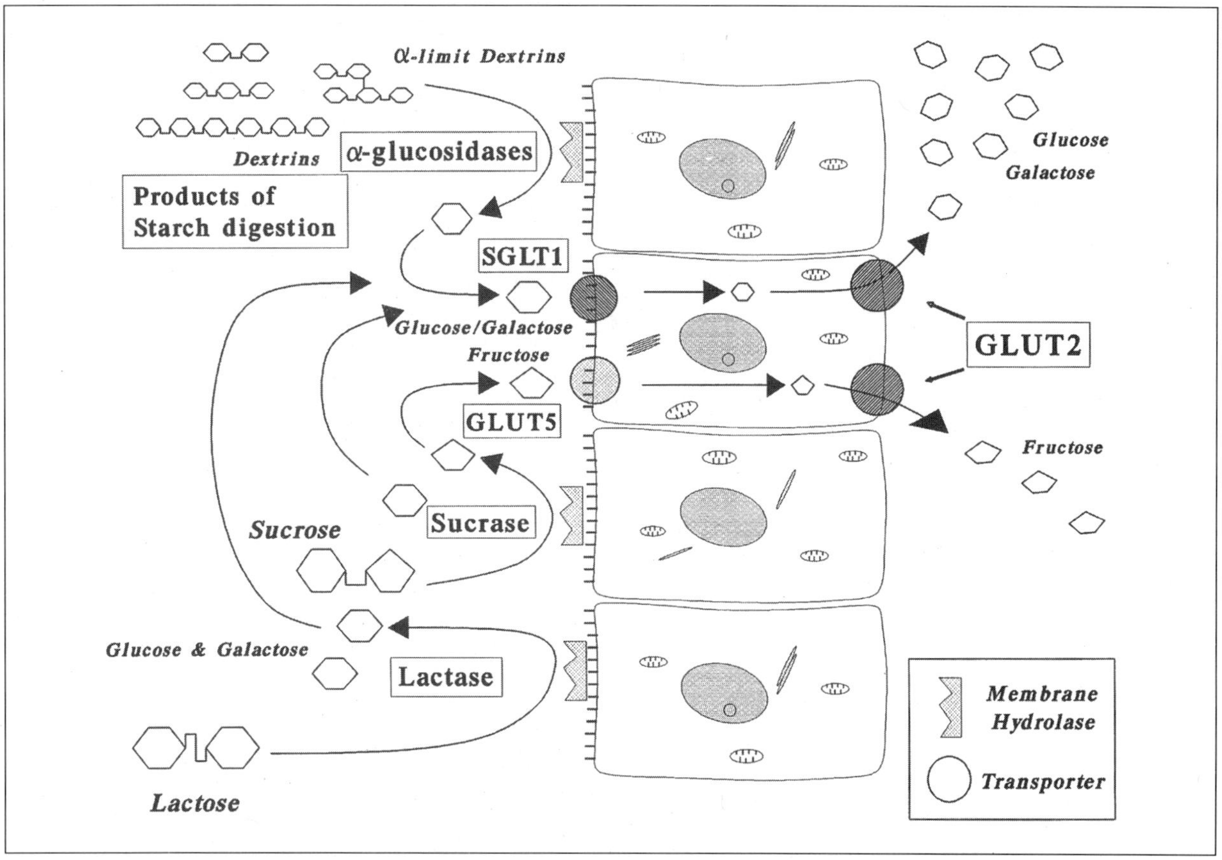

Figure 2-4. Mechanisms of carbohydrate uptake in the small intestine. An idealized view of the intestinal wall is shown. The major mechanisms of brush-border membrane hydrolysis of common dietary disaccharides and starch digestion products are shown together with major monosaccharide transport mechanisms. GLUT = glucose transporters; SGLUT = sodium-glucose linked transporters.

soluble maltodextrins unless the absorptive area is markedly reduced.

The Route of Mucosal Monosaccharide Uptake

Despite persistent claims that a large part of glucose uptake is by a mechanism of "solvent drag" via the tight-junctional pathways [126] and that this may modulate peptide uptake [127], most recent evidence suggests that this is not so. The evidence for this is twofold. Pappenheimer was puzzled that luminal glucose concentrations were much higher than the K_m of the sodium-glucose linked transporter (SGLT1; see Table 2-2). It appeared that another pathway of glucose uptake was necessary to explain this discrepancy [126]. In reality, postprandial luminal glucose concentrations rarely exceed 50 mmol/L [128]. During perfusion of the human small intestine with high glucose concentrations, Fordtran, Fine, and colleagues could detect no stimulation of net uptake of urea and passively absorbed sugar probes [129], which should have occurred if Fisher's original proposal for solvent drag was correct [130]. We have confirmed this in steady-state human jejunal perfusion studies in which enteral diets with different peptide profiles were used [87]. As can be seen in Figure 2-5, little free glucose was liberated by brush-border hydrolysis, implying that rates of mucosal glucose liberation and uptake are well matched in man.

It can therefore be accepted that in humans the most significant mode of transmucosal passage of dietary carbohydrate is by specific monosaccharide transporters. This is not to say that disaccharides and oligosaccharides cannot permeate the brush-border membrane (transcellular route) or pass through the tight junction (paracellular route), but the amount is small [15]. This phenomenon has been exploited as a useful noninvasive marker for increased intestinal permeabil-

Table 2-3. Membrane Digestion of Dietary Starch

Enzyme Trivial Name	Alternative Name	Enzyme Number	Substrate	Product	Comments
Sucrase	Maltase Ia	3.2.1.48	Sucrose	Glucose, fructose	Multienzyme complex, each subunit has high degree of sequence homology with acid α-glucosidase (EC 3.2.1.3) in liver and other tissues [118, 119].
Isomaltase	Maltase Ib	3.2.1.10	Maltose, α-1,4/α-1,6 linked oligomers	Glucose	
Glucoamylase	Maltase II	3.2.1.20	Starch, α-1,4 >> α-1,6	Glucose	Multienzyme complex, may be similar enzymes but slightly different activities [117, 120, 121].
Maltase	Maltase III	3.2.1.20	Maltose, α-1,4 linked oligomers	Glucose	
Other Membrane Saccharidases					
Lactase	β-D-galactosidase	3.2.1.23 3.2.1.62	Lactose	Glucose, galactose	Expression of this enzyme is genetically determined [17]. Can be induced by high intake of disaccharides [148], not monosaccharides [238].

Note: Bracketed numbers correspond with references.

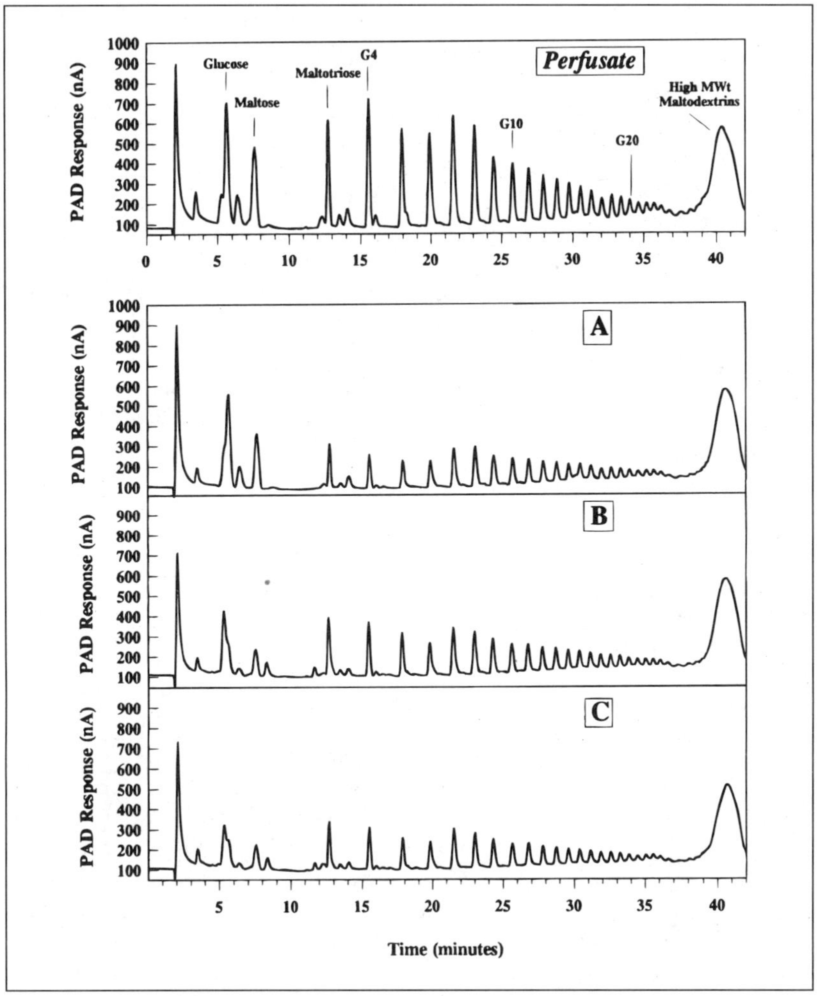

Figure 2-5. High-performance anion-exchange liquid chromatography (Carbopak PA-100, Pulsed Amperometric Detection [PAD]) of maltodextrins in human jejunal perfusate and aspirates, when co-perfused with a short **(B)** or medium-chain whey hydrolysate **(C)**, or its equivalent free L-amino acid mixture **(A)**. (Data taken from GK Grimble, et al. The influence of whey hydrolysate peptide chain length on nitrogen and carbohydrate absorption in the perfused human jejunum. *Clin Nutr* 14[Suppl]:46, 1994.)

ity to sugar probes (e.g., lactulose, lactitol) in inflammatory illness, such as Crohn's disease [131–133].

Monosaccharide Transport

Glucose transport occurs via the Na^+-linked transporter SGLT1, which is unrelated to the GLUT family of glucose transporters, as reviewed elsewhere [134]. It is very closely related to the glucose transporter in the renal tubular brush-border membrane [135]; the kinetic and biochemical properties of this tetramer with 73,000 Da subunits are reviewed elsewhere [136]. Expression of this transporter can be up-regulated by luminal glucose concentrations, that is, the nutrient "load" [137].

In contrast, uptake of fructose occurs by a distinct transporter, GLUT5 (see Table 2-2). This carrier-mediated system is not inhibited by phlorhizin or metabolic inhibitors [138]. A second component is electrogenic and can be inhibited by phlorhizin, a specific inhibitor of the Na^+-glucose cotransporter [139].

The process of glucose uptake by membranes of different tissues has been described in much greater detail and several closely related GLUT transporters have been identified [134]. The liver-type transporter GLUT2 (see Table 2-2) is responsible for facilitated diffusion exit of glucose from the basolateral membrane of mucosal cells of the intestine and renal tubule as well as uptake into liver cells [140]. This transporter (indeed the whole GLUT family) is responsive to hormonal and substrate regulation. Thus, the density of GLUT2 on the basolateral membrane of intestinal cells is modulated by circulating glucose concentration being up-regulated in patients with diabetes [52]. This may be a key control point for intracellular compartmentation of glucose and its uptake by the enterocyte, because only a small fraction of the glucose is metabolized during passage through the absorptive cell [141].

Absorption of Carbohydrates From Enteral Diets

We have expended considerable effort in defining the composition of the maltodextrins used in elemental diets by developing chromatographic methods of increasing power [142]. Although maltodextrins can be defined by a single value for their dextrose equivalent (DE), this masks the fact that they are a very heterogenous mixture of glucose polymers. This is shown for the base material used in one of our jejunal perfusion studies (see Figure 2-5). As a result, it is impossible to describe the material simply as "maltodextrin" without referring to its absorptive characteristics.

In vitro, glucose uptake from a short-chain maltodextrin (4–9 glucose units) by a rabbit jejunal preparation in an Ussing chamber was significantly slower than from free glucose solutions [143]. Although this suggests that brush-border hydrolysis is rate-limiting to uptake (see discussion on peptide transport above), we have not observed the same in the perfused human jejunum. These studies were performed with fractionated maltodextrins having an average size ranging from less than 10 glucose units or more than 10 glucose units. In the absence of luminal α-amylase, the lower molecular weight glucose polymers were assimilated more rapidly than higher molecular weight glucose polymers and seemed to be conferring a kinetic advantage on glucose uptake. An α-amylase hydrolysate of the low molecular weight glucose polymer fraction (<10 glucose molecules) conferred the expected kinetic advantage on glucose transport, and the high molecular weight fraction (osmolality one fifth of the starting material) was surprisingly well absorbed even in the absence of α-amylase. In addition, the low molecular weight polymer was as rapidly assimilated as maltose and maltotriose and more efficiently than equivalent concentrations of free glucose [144–146]. Thus, the energy content of enteral diets can be *increased* and diet osmolality *reduced* by substituting the (commonly used) heterogenous starch hydrolysates with purified high molecular weight fractions. In one diet (Tolerex, Sandoz), this concept has been used, with a subsequent lowering of osmolality from 830 to 630 mOsmol/kg. Where digestive and absorptive functions are both severely impaired, a low molecular weight maltodextrin could be used.

Sucrose and Enteral Nutrition

In patients with a very short small intestine that has not adapted, the remaining digestive and absorptive capacity of the mucosal surface may limit uptake of glucose from glucose polymer mixtures. Jejunal perfusion studies have shown that if glucose transport from glucose polymers is saturated, sugar absorption can be enhanced if the disaccharide sucrose is added [147]. This is because although sucrose and maltodextrin hydrolysis is by the same hybrid brush-border hydrolase, sucrase-isomaltase (see Table 2-3), the absorption of fructose is by GLUT5 and not SGLT1 (glucose/galactose carrier). Furthermore, both GLUT5 and sucrase activity can be induced by dietary sucrose [138,148]. The linkage between brush-border hydrolysis of sucrose and absorption of the monosaccharides fructose and glucose appears to confer a kinetic advantage on fructose uptake, because in one study 8 of 10 subjects malabsorbed 50 g of fructose, and none malabsorbed 100 g of sucrose [149]. Thus, adding sucrose to enteral diets can further enhance carbohydrate uptake, in addition to its beneficial taste properties.

Fat Absorption

The major dietary fats are triglycerides, cholesterol, and the fat-soluble vitamins. Triglycerides are fatty acid triesters of glycerol, which may contain long-chain fatty acids (C16–C18: long-chain triglycerides) or medium-chain fatty acids (C6–C12: medium-chain triglycerides), and inclusion of either in the fat source of enteral diets is related to the physiology of fat digestion and absorption.

Triglycerides are insoluble in water, and if absorption were solely on the basis of direct uptake of triglycerides at the brush-border membrane, it would be severely limited by the droplet-size of the triglyceride emulsion and by the limited permeability of fat droplets across the mucosal barrier and unstirred water layer. The efficiency of lipid assimilation is ensured by exogenous (e.g., bile acids) or endogenous (e.g., fatty acids, monoglycerides released in situ) chemical emulsificants that produce an emulsion with high surface area/volume for efficient enzyme hydrolysis. The actions of lingual lipase and gastric mechanical activity combine to provide some emulsification, with enzymic release of free fatty acid and diglyceride [150]. Transfer of fat-rich gastric contents to the duodenum has two consequences:

1. H^+-stimulated secretin stimulates pancreatic water and HCO_3 secretion into the duodenum, raising the pH to 6 to 7.
2. Luminal free fatty acids in the duodenum stimulate cholecystokinin-pancreozymin (CCK-PZ) release by duodenal epithelial cells. This signals contraction of the gallbladder and release of bile acids into the intestinal lumen.

The higher pH of the duodenal contents aids in further emulsification and facilitates the action of pancreatic lipase. At pH 6 to 7, bile salts are soluble in water, but above a certain concentration (critical micellar concentration), they will form pure bile salt micelles. Fatty acids, monoglycerides, and phospholipids interdigitate with this structure, forming mixed micelles with a hydrophobic core and hydrophilic outer surface. This has been reviewed in detail elsewhere [151–154]. Pancreatic colipase binds tightly to the surface of mixed micelles and acts as electrostatic anchor for lipase, which has considerable specificity for the 1,3 positions of triglycerides.

In addition to lingual and pancreatic lipase, a third and distinct mucosal acid-active intestinal lipase has been partially characterized and found in the villus tips in the proximal intestine [155], that is, the most mature population of enterocytes engaged in the absorption and transport of dietary lipid. Its binding to the brush border involves heparin [156], which allows fatty acids and monoglycerides to be generated in close proximity to the intestinal membrane before absorption.

Osmotic and other pressures generated within the micelle by extensive triglyceride hydrolysis cause budding of smaller micelles from the surface of these structures. The resulting smaller micelles are then available for uptake of monoglycerides and fatty acids at the microvilli surface. Lipolysis products are absorbed in the proximal intestine, whereas bile salts are absorbed at the distal ileum, so mixed micelles must dissociate.

The acidic microenvironment adjacent to the brush-border membrane is important in promoting lipid absorption because protonation of fatty acids allows their diffusion through the membrane [157]. Within the enterocyte, the higher intracellular pH results in their ionization, thus reducing the likelihood of back-diffusion. However, mucosal uptake of long-chain fatty acids is now known to occur as a result of binding to a specific intestinal membrane binding protein that is a member of a family of cytoplasmic hydrophobic ligand-binding proteins [158,159]. This intestinal fatty acid binding protein is thought to participate in the uptake, intracellular targeting, and metabolic processing of fatty acids within the intestinal epithelial cell.

Within the enterocyte, fatty acids are transferred by their specific cytoplasmic carrier proteins to the smooth endoplasmic reticulum for re-esterification to triglycerides [152]. These triglycerides are transferred, along with cholesterol, phospholipids, and fat soluble vitamins, to the Golgi apparatus where they combine with apolipoproteins to form chylomicrons and very low density lipoproteins. The Golgi apparatus is transferred to the enterocyte lateral membrane and fuses with it. Subsequent rupture of the fused vesicle by exocytosis results in the release of lipid into the lymphatic system.

Table 2-4. Mechanisms Involved in Transfer of Dietary Lipid Into the Circulation

Emulsification
Lipolysis
Micellar formation
Membrane transport
Intracellular triglyceride resynthesis
Chylomicron formation
Transfer into lymphatic system

Although probably not of any clinical significance, not all the neutral lipid absorbed from the lumen of the intestine is destined for packaging and transport via the lymphatics in chylomicrons [160,161]. Experimental animal studies indicate that nearly half of neutral lipids may be transported out of the enterocytes via nonlymphatic pathways (presumably via the portal vein). These are postulated to require prior hydrolysis by a specific, nonpancreatic, alkaline-active lipase.

Medium-chain triglycerides appear to "short circuit" some of these processes because they are more water soluble than long-chain triglycerides and may either be absorbed intact or undergo considerably more rapid lipase hydrolysis than do long-chain triglycerides, with subsequent direct uptake of monoglycerides and fatty acids. There is no absolute requirement for mixed micelle formation with bile acids and, within the enterocyte, short- and medium-chain fatty acids are generally not re-esterified to triglycerides and incorporated into chylomicrons, but may be released directly into the portal circulation where they bind to albumin [152]. These mechanisms are summarized in Table 2-4.

Absorption of Water and Electrolytes

The approximate amounts of water and electrolytes handled by the normal human intestine during a 24-hour period are summarized in Table 2-5. As can be seen, these are considerable because combined small-intestinal luminal intake of fluid from the diet and secretions from the salivary glands, stomach, pancreas, biliary tree, and intestinal mucosa amounts to about 9 L. Of this, about 1 to 5 L pass the ileocecal valve, with less than 200 ml escaping into the stool [162]. There are no specific active transport processes for the absorption of water. The intestinal mucosa acts as a semi-

Table 2-5. Approximate Quantities of Water and Electrolytes Handled by the Intestine Each Day in Healthy Subjects

	Water (ml)	Sodium (mmoles)	Chloride (mmoles)	Potassium (mmoles)
Input				
Diet	1500	150	150	80
Gut Secretions	7500	1000	750	40
Total	9000	1150	900	120
Absorption				
Small intestine	7500	950	800	110
Colon	1350	195	97	−3
Output	150	5	3	13

permeable membrane through which water flows in either direction in response to differences in osmotic pressure. Thus, luminal nutrient digestion renders the bulk phase hypertonic, and water moves from the intestinal fluid into the gut lumen [163]; nutrient absorption, however, renders it more hypotonic such that water is absorbed along with these solutes. In this way, the luminal contents are adjusted to near isotonicity throughout the small bowel.

Mucosal permeability varies along the length of the intestine; permeability is highest in jejunum, intermediate in the ileum, and lowest in the colon [163]. Therefore, the jejunum affects the rapid equilibration of osmotic pressure gradients created by the digestion and absorption of nutrients. The lower permeability of the colonic mucosa prevents water from leaking back into the lumen when the mainly ionic solutes are actively absorbed, although this mechanism has specific properties [164]. Water has difficulty passing across the lipid membrane of the epithelial cells, and it is now clear that most of it passes between cells rather than through them [165]. Therefore, the differences in permeability throughout the intestine depend on the different permeabilities of the "tight" junctions between cells. It has been calculated that the pores through which water passes in the jejunum are about twice the diameter of those in the ileum [163]. Thus, water absorption in the upper intestine is determined largely by absorption of nutrients; however, in the ileum, and particularly in the colon, the absorption of salt is the main driving force for water absorption and resulting dehydration of colonic contents.

Electrolytes

The gut has extremely efficient mechanisms for conserving Na^+ intake, as shown in Table 2-5. In the duodenum and upper jejunum, simple diffusion of sodium and chloride occurs down concentration gradients producing luminal concentrations similar to those in plasma. When a sodium chloride solution that is isotonic with plasma is perfused in the normal human jejunum, no net uptake of sodium or chloride ions occurs [166]. Sodium uptake is, however, stimulated in the presence of glucose [167], amino acids, dipeptides and tripeptides [166] as well as bicarbonate ions (168) through the action of Na^+-nutrient cotransporters [136]. Bicarbonate is removed as carbon dioxide by reaction with actively secreted hydrogen ions. Hydrogen ion is secreted by exchange with absorbed sodium on a specific cation-exchange carrier. In addition to nutrient- and bicarbonate-stimulated absorption in the jejunum, sodium and chloride ions are also thought to move in response to solvent drag (see above). A lower luminal nutrient concentration in the ileum results in the greater significance of active absorption processes, such as ion exchange of H^+ and Cl^- for HCO_3^- [165,169]. The ileal mucosa is less permeable to ions than in the jejunum, so once absorbed only limited back-diffusion occurs into the lumen.

In the colon, 1.5 to 2.6 L of water are absorbed daily, compared with a reserve capacity of 3 to 4 times this amount. It is only when this absorptive capacity is overwhelmed acutely that diarrhea results [20,162]. The absorption of water is dermined largely by absorption of sodium and chloride ions and short-chain fatty acids [170,171]. Between species, there are marked differences in colonic water absorption that affect the water content of normal stool. As Bleakman and Naftalin suggested, pure mechanical contractile forces are not capable of dehydrating the fecal stream, because the force necessary to reduce water content from 85% to less than 65% is equivalent to 5 to 10 atm. Clearly, some other osmotic mechanism operates to ensure efficient water salvage. Their proposal is that water and Na^+ passage is differentiated between the crypt cells and adjacent colonocytes. Active uptake of Na^+ and its passage via cells to the base of the crypt will produce a region of hyperosmolarity (>1000 mOsm/kg) around the crypt (Figure 2-6), which is sufficient to provide the motive force for water passage from the colonic lumen and through the crypt lumen and crypt cells [164,172]. Na^+ and Cl^-, but not water, may then leak back into the colonic lumen via a passive route. Collapse of the crypt in the face of these considerable forces is prevented by its mucus plug. Na^+ uptake by adjacent colonocytes may therefore be stimulated by uptake of solutes such as the short-chain fatty acids that are generated within the lumen by bacterial fermentation (see below).

This system of necessity requires expenditure of metabolic energy to maintain the active transport of Na^+ against a concentration gradient, and any factor that inhibits this or stimulates passive permeation of Na^+ or Cl^- back into the colonic lumen will result in impaired water uptake and diarrhea [165].

Colonic Fermentative Activities that Stimulate Water and Electrolyte Salvage

Development of Colonic Fermentation Capacity in Humans

The colonic luminal bacteria have been described as an "organ-within-an-organ" that slowly develops during the first 2 years of life in human infants [19] before establishment of the adult microflora, which remain remarkably stable [173]. These luminal functions of the colon are bacterial and comprise mucin breakdown, regulation of fecal tryptic activity, conversion of bilirubin to urobilinogen, cholesterol catabolism, and finally the generation of short-chain fatty acids and other organic acids (see Table 2-1). The rate of adaptation is driven by the pattern of fermentable substrates that enter the cecum and, although carbohydrate fermentation is rapidly established, indicators of pro-

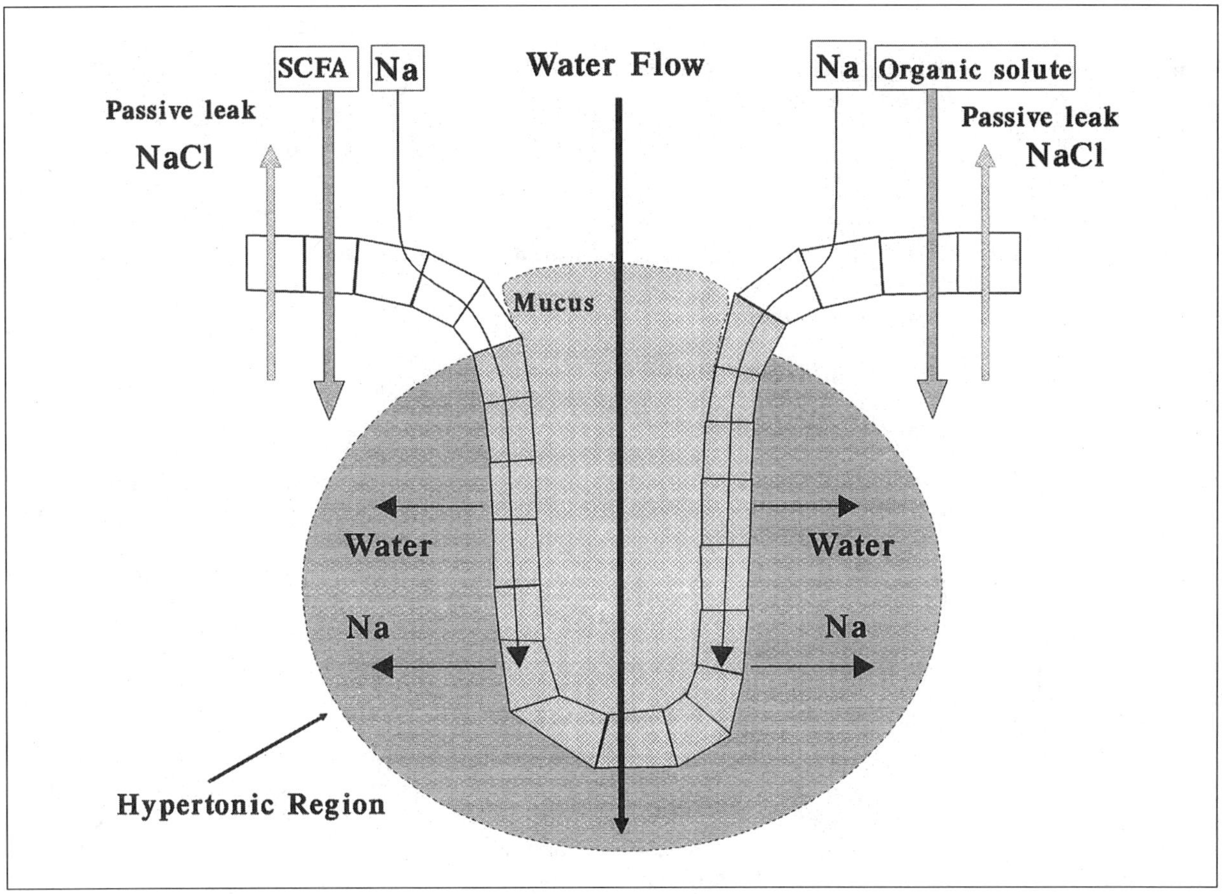

Figure 2-6. Hypothetical mechanism for water and electrolyte uptake in the colon. A cross-section of one colonic crypt is shown. Substrate-stimulated Na^+ uptake is transferred by inter-colonocyte movement to the submucosal region. This stimulates net water uptake against the countervailing force of the dehydrated fecal stream. SCFA = short-chain fatty acids.

tein fermentation (*iso*- and *n*-valeric acids) are not complete until 16 months of life [19]. Acetate-producing bacteria are rapidly established, and the resulting luminal "acetate-buffer" is strongly bacteriostatic for some gram-negative bacteria. The adult pattern of colonic luminal metabolism requires development of a population of butyrate-producing bacteria at the expense of acetate production. This is essentially a reductive metabolic pathway that uses H_2 as substrate [174], as do nitrate- and sulphate-reducing bacteria that are substrate inducible [175,176]. In addition, carbon dioxide reduction to CH_4 consumes H_2, and the significance of the methanogenic bacteria varies among individuals [177].

Metabolic Activities of Colonic Microflora

The relationship between bacteria and the colon is therefore truly symbiotic. The host makes a significant contribution to the growth of luminal bacteria by providing both fermentable carbohydrate (dietary sources, mucins) and nitrogen (urea, endogenous proteins, malabsorbed dietary protein) that act synergistically [178,179]. Establishment of this symbiosis may be retarded by antibiotic treatment in early life that allows the establishment of *Clostridium difficile* colonies, which may be detected by the presence of *iso*-caproic acid in fecal samples. Malabsorption of components of formula diet by infants, because of their strong buffering capacity, will tend to oppose establishment of an acetate buffer and thus allow establishment of coliform and streptococcal colonies. It is estimated that in adult humans, approximately 70 g/d fermentable carbohydrate would be required to produce the bacterial mass of daily stool [180].

Metabolic Activities of the Colonocyte

Of the short-chain fatty acids, butyrate has the most pronounced effects on the epithelial cells of the cecum and colon. It provides the function of a precursor for ketone production, which is not shared with acetate and propionate [181,182], and of the possible metabolic fuels (e.g., glucose and glutamine) it appears to be preferentially used by colonocytes [183]. Butyrate promotes proliferation and differentiation of colonic epithelial crypt cells toward the mature, highly polarized form that expresses apical membrane hydrolases at the top of the crypt [184–187]. In vivo studies in rats have confirmed that it is the fermentation products of dietary fiber (i.e., short-chain fatty acids) and not its effects in lowering luminal pH [188] or the presence of bulk in the intestinal lumen that increase crypt-cell proliferation rates in the rat colon [189,190]. Butyrate also appears to modulate the cell cycle at the level of gene transcription, because it can down-regulate N-*ras* oncogene expression and the proliferative potential of cultured human colon tumor cell lines [185,191,192]. In addition, addition of butyrate to the medium induces greater differentiation in terms of expression of surface hydrolases and glycosylated cell-surface components [193] and reduces expression of surface tumor-specific antigens [185].

A further unique feature of butyrate production by the colonic luminal microflora is that it provides for the unique polarity of butyrate uptake by the colonocyte. Rolandelli and colleagues and Kripke and colleagues showed that healing of the colon in a rat model of surgical resection and reanastomosis was accelerated by luminal butyrate [194,195] but not by intravenous administration, according to Koruda and colleagues [196].

In contrast, acetate, the major short-chain fatty acid produced by fermentation, has the most marked stimulatory effects on colonic blood flow [197–199]. In general, absorption of luminal nutients is accompanied by increased regional blood flow to the intestine in health [200–202] and after injury [203,204]. However, it is difficult to disentangle the contribution of direct metabolic trophism of the short-chain fatty acids and the consequences of regional stimulation of the intestine through increased blood flow.

Short-Chain Fatty Acids and Colonic Water and Electrolyte Uptake

Colonic (and jejunal) mucosal transport of short-chain fatty acids is accompanied by water and Na^+ uptake that appears to be mediated by two mechanisms. First, active uptake of unprotonated short-chain fatty acids and Na^+ occurs in exchange for Cl^- and H^+, respectively. The second mode of uptake is probably by passive diffusion of protonated short-chain fatty acids down a concentration gradient [171,205,206]. The latter may explain why inflammatory bowel disease reduces colonic uptake of other actively transported organic anions, but has a lesser impact on short-chain fatty acid uptake [207]. The capacity of the colonic luminal bacteria to ferment nonabsorbed disaccharides such as lactulose [21] and lactitol [16] and for the colon to absorb short-chain fatty acids is limited (approximately 80 g/d), and above this level of intake, osmotic diarrhea will ensue. Thus, at lower levels of intake of fermentable carbohydrate, short-chain fatty acids generated by luminal bacteria aid the process of dehydrating the fecal stream and salvage 90% of the water and electrolytes that enter the colon from the small intestine (approximately 1350 ml/d).

Enteral Feeding–Related Diarrhea: A Failure of Colonic Water and Substrate Salvage?

These considerations should therefore be borne in mind when considering the characteristics of diarrhea associated with tube feeding in patients, which has now been quite carefully defined. We would propose that enteral feeding–related diarrhea is multifactorial, but has the common mechanism of failure of the colon to efficiently salvage a normal or increased water and electrolyte load. Apart from infectious diarrhea, several other factors have been noted (Table 2-6). There is a close association of diarrhea with concurrent antibiotic therapy [18] and not with the lactose content of enteral feeds or the rate of infusion [208] or the digestibility of the protein source [30,209]. In addition, diarrhea may be a consequence of enteral diet malabsorption, aberrant small and large bowel motility, and aberrant large bowel secretory response to the mode of nasoenteral feeding used.

Antibiotics

Antibiotic administration has been shown to elicit symptoms of diarrhea in healthy volunteers consuming a 20-g dose of lactulose that had not previously altered stool output [22]. Antibiotics will inhibit many of the functions of the colonic luminal microflora and thus impair its function as "an organ within an organ." Evidence for this is that some antibiotics (most notably ampicillin, erythromycin, clindamycin, and metronidazole) will suppress indices of colonic bacterial fermentation, such as breath H_2 output [22], acidification of the cecum [210], urinary excretion of D-amino acids derived from colonic bacteria [211], and in vitro production of short-chain fatty acids by fecal inoculates [212]. In addition, metronidazole therapy has been shown to be of significant clinical benefit in reducing the colonic production of short-chain fatty acids in children with inborn errors of methylmalonate and propionate metabolism [213]. It is likely that the effects of impaired microbial function are twofold. First, reduced fermentation will reduce salvage of osmotically active colonic luminal nutrients and thus impair water uptake. Second, impaired generation of short-chain fatty acids will lead to reduced water and electrolyte uptake.

Malabsorption

A series of reports have demonstrated the link between carbohydrate malabsorption and impaired salvage in enterally fed postsurgical patients, because a rise in breath H_2 concentrations preceded the onset of diarrhea by several hours [214]. This mechanism may be complex. Although antibiotics *reduce* colonic fermentation and breath H_2 production in the clinical setting [212] and would be expected to *impair* salvage of an increased colonic substrate load, some antibiotics (e.g., erythromycin) can significantly shorten

Table 2-6. Causes of Noninfectious Diarrhea in Enterally Fed Patients

Causative Agents	Mechanism	Suggested Solution
Inappropriate feeding techniques		
Too-rapid diet infusion (e.g., bolus-feeding)	Will result in high "load" that overwhelms the digestive or absorptive capacity of the small intestine.	Use lower infusion rate
Too-slow diet infusion	Fails to elicit postprandial motility response (i.e., slowing of transit).	Use higher infusion rate (e.g., cyclical feeding)
Impaired digestive or absorptive function	Malabsorption of macronutrients. Osmotic diarrhea.	Use predigested diets or enzyme supplements
Low sodium content in enteral diet	Poor water and Na^+ uptake in small intestine.	Increase Na^+ to >90 mmol/L [147]
Failure of colonic salvage		
Antibiotics	Inhibition of short-chain fatty acid production by luminal microflora. Removal of stimulus for water/Na^+ uptake.	
Altered small-bowel motility patterns	Failure to convert fasting to fed motility pattern with nasogastric feeding?	The relationship of this to enteral-feeding diarrhea is unclear at present [226]
Colonic secretion	A consequence of nasogastric feeding?	

Note: Bracketed numbers correspond with references.

mouth-to-cecum transit time [215] and may directly contribute to malabsorption resulting from increased motility.

Altered Small Bowel and Large Bowel Motility

As described above, nutrient assimilation in humans takes place predominantly in the upper small intestine. It follows that if gastric emptying is impaired, the intragastric route of nutrient administration cannot be considered. Severe impairment of gastric emptying or gastric atony is not uncommonly encountered in patients requiring enteral feeding, and when present it will lead to nausea, vomiting and regurgitation, and aspiration of diet. Gastric atony related to enteral nutrition occurs in association with a number of disorders (Table 2-7).

Efficient absorption of nutrients from chyme in the upper small intestine requires a repetitive mixing action in which the mucosa dips into the chyme, minimizing the diffusion barrier to absorption. This movement is accompanied by villous contractions whose propelling action aids blood and lymphatic flow to carry away the products of digestion and absorption. Interposed with these repetitive segmenting movements are erratic propulsive movements that rapidly propel chyme 10 to 30 cm distally, and the segmenting process recommences [216]. Our understanding of how such complex patterns of motor activity are organized has advanced considerably in recent years, mainly as a consequence of improved monitoring techniques that allow the small intestinal and colonic motility patterns in the fasting and fed state to be measured in ambulatory subjects.

In the fasting state, small intestinal motility is characterized by a period of inactivity (phase I) followed by phase II, a period of irregular spike activity lasting (like phase I) for 30 to 40 minutes [217]. Pressure activity increases steadily during the later half of phase II, ushering in phase III, during which there are intense, repetitive high-amplitude contractions. Phase III lasts for about 4 to 6 minutes of irregular activity (phase IV) and then gives way to a new phase I. The whole cycle of activity migrates down the upper small intestine at 4 to 6 cm/min, slowing distally to 1 to 2 cm/min in the terminal ileum. This migrating motor complex (MMC) is thought to have the function of sweeping debris down the small intestine and does not occur until 4 to 6 hours after a meal. The fasting pattern of motility is disrupted by feeding, and irregular activity is seen throughout the small intestine. It resembles that seen during phase II of the MMC and hence is called "type II activity." Contraction frequency and speed is reduced by nutrients, thereby prolonging transit time [218]. The intestine appears able to discriminate between different nutrients because there are qualitative differences in motor response as a result of particularly intense nonpropagating clustered contractions, which are generated by luminal fat, whose function is presumably to aid emulsification and hence absorption. In essence, therefore, the fasting function of the motility response is to propagate debris distally, and the fed response is basically nonpropagative in type to aid digestion and absorption of nutrients [219].

Studies of the small intestinal response to enteral feeding are in their infancy. We have recently shown that constant infusion of a polymeric diet intragastrically at 1.38 kcal/min (equivalent to the constant infusion of 2 L of diet or 1.0 kcal/ml over 24 hours) does *not* elicit the normal fed response, in that propagating MMCs are seen throughout diet infusion [9]. A similar effect has been noted by others in dogs when the infusion rate is less than 1.5 kcal/min [220]. In humans, intraduodenal infusion of the same and higher loads of nutrients elicited the change from the normal fasting to fed response with an abolition of MMCs throughout feeding [9]. Most recently, we have shown that intragastric and intraduodenal infusion of standard loads of 1.38 kcal/min resulted in a persistence of the normal fasting motility response in the distal colon [221]. This response was significantly diminished during intragastric and intraduodenal infusion of higher loads of nutrients [222].

The clinical significance of these findings is yet uncertain. Clearly, intragastric infusion of enteral diets elicits an "abnormal" small intestinal and colonic motility response [9,222]. Bearing in mind that one of the functions of the normal fed motor pattern is to aid luminal and membrane digestion, there may be grounds for prescribing predigested chemically defined elemental diets to patients who are perceived to have disordered small intestinal motility. The problem is that neither the small

Table 2-7. Patient Groups and Diseases Associated With Gastric Atony

Diabetes with neuropathy
Hypothyroidism
Head injuries and neurosurgical patients
Multiple trauma
Post–abdominal surgery patients
Intraabdominal sepsis
Intensive care patients on ventilators
Some patients with neuromotor deglutition disorders
Some patients after a cerebrovascular accident

intestinal nor colonic motility responses in response to enteral feeding have been monitored in sick patients as yet. This is therefore a fruitful area for future research.

Altered Colonic Secretory Responses

As described above, nasogastric feeding failed to elicit the normal switch from fasted to fed patterns of motility [9]. It is possible that prepyloric diet infusion is insufficient in terms of nutrient load and osmolarity to stimulate the small intestinal receptors that are responsible for motility changes [223,224]. An interesting observation of our studies was that subjects being fed prepylorically invariably developed diarrhea, whereas those fed postpylorically did not [9]. Furthermore, in a series of in vivo colonic perfusion studies in normal human subjects, we observed a marked secretion of water (160 ml/hr), Na^+, and Cl^- in the ascending colon during prepyloric infusion of enteral diet [225]. This did not occur during postpyloric diet infusion. The site of diet infusion did not alter distal colonic motor activity from the fasting pattern, implying that it was not primarily involved in the pathogenesis of diarrhea. In the clinical setting, if this rate of secretion were to persist for 24 hours, total secretion of 3.8 L would ensue. Although this is within the capacity of the colon to absorb water [20], under normal circumstances the ascending colon would handle the load. Our observation that net secretion occurred in the ascending, not the distal colon, would suggest that colonic water absorptive capacity is overwhelmed. It is likely that this response originates from the proximal gastrointestinal tract and is probably neurohormonal in nature. Further studies are awaited to confirm this.

An additional study has demonstrated that this colonic secretion is reversed by cecal infusion of short-chain fatty acids [226]. Given the stimulatory effect of short-chain fatty acids on colonic water and electrolyte uptake (see above), this result is not surprising. It has been noted in animal models that inclusion of fermentable fibers in the diet will lead to increased cecal short-chain fatty acid production as well as net increases in uptake of short-chain fatty acids, electrolytes, and ammonia derived from urea hydrolysis [197,227]. This effect appears also to move the site of colonic salvage more distally.

Within the context of enteral nutrition, these results are intriguing because they provide a basis for the use of fermentable fiber in liquid formulas as a means of moderating symptoms of diarrhea, as is reviewed in detail elsewhere [228,229]. It will be necessary to perform controlled clinical trials to see if postpyloric feeding has a beneficial effect on enteral feeding–related diarrhea.

Perspectives

Protein Assimilation

A significant proportion of dietary nitrogen is absorbed in the form of dipeptides and tripeptides, for which the transport protein has been identified. This is an exciting possibility because it will allow thorough investigation of factors that affect the expression of the PepT1 transporter at the molecular level to be correlated with more traditional quantitative methods of intestinal perfusion. Duplication of amino acid uptake through this system and that of the brush-border membrane L-amino acid transporters is clearly an efficient means of ensuring maximum absorption of the products of luminal protein digestion. In the intestine, there may be several good reasons for this duplication of amino acid transport. Luminal protein digestion never proceeds to completion (i.e., free amino acids) within the time frame of orocecal transit time. In addition, pancreatic and other secretions produce luminal protein *distal* to the major site of luminal hydrolysis, the duodenum and jejunum. These secretions are by nature resistant to pancreatic proteolytic attack, and the coupling of peptide uptake to brush-border peptidases with different specificity may provide an efficient means for their salvage. This is especially true if one considers that dietary protein assimilation is a jejunal event, whereas endogenous protein secretions are assimilated more distally as reflected by the increasing gradient of brush-border endopeptidases and exopeptidases toward the ileocecal valve [34]. Thus, adaptation that will occur in the remaining intestine after resection has more limited scope for maintenance of protein assimilation [230,231].

A second reason for duplication is that peptide transport serves to relieve competition for transport between free amino acids that share the same carrier. This may be especially true in cases where poor protein quality and malabsorption coexist with a high requirement for essential amino acid residues (e.g., rapid growth in infants).

Carbohydrate Assimilation

We now have a clearer understanding of the molecular biology of the brush-border membrane protein responsible for hydrolysis of dietary carbohydrate to monosaccharides and their translocation from apical to basolateral membranes of the enterocyte. In addition, the reserve capacity of the small intestine for carbohydrate assimilation has been defined by different experimental strategies. Current knowledge suggests that it is 2 to 3 times the maximum nutrient intake that is likely to be used in enteral feeding and would comfortably exceed the necessary intake of a hypermetabolic, severely burned patient. Where absorptive function has been severely reduced by distal small bowel resection, remaining reserve capacity is often sufficient to allow complete assimilation of carbohydrate [1,106] as opposed to protein [39]. The reason for this difference is that carbohydrate assimilation is primarily duodenal and jejunal, as shown by the negative longitudinal distribution gradient for the brush-border disaccharidases and the Na^+-glucose co-transporter [34,232].

Fat Assimilation

Normal lipid digestion and absorption is dependent on a host of mechanisms, the most important of which appear to be adequate luminal levels of pancreatic lipase and bile salts as well as sufficient absorptive area. In some patients, some or all of these factors may be limiting, and diets containing excessive amounts of long-chain triglycerides should be avoided to prevent essential fatty acid and vitamin deficiency caused by competition for uptake by other long-chain fatty acids [233]. Such patients include those with severe exocrine pancreatic insufficiency (chronic pancreatitis and cystic fibrosis), severe abnormalities of intestinal mucosa (untreated celiac disease), or extensive small bowel resection [152]. Although medium-chain triglycerides have been proposed as an efficiently absorbed fat source in these cases [234,235], they do not contain linoleic acid, and exclusive use of medium-chain triglycerides may provoke essential fatty acid deficiency [236]. Thus, for this group, and especially in infants, it is preferable to use a combination therapy of diets containing mixtures of medium-chain and long-chain triglycerides as well as oral, enteric-coated pancreatic enzyme supplements that enhance utilization of long-chain and medium-chain triglycerides and reduce steatorrhea [12,237].

Colonic Water and Electrolyte Conservation

Colonic water and electrolyte conservation is now better understood from the point of view of mucosal physiology and gastrointestinal motility. In addition, several lines of evidence have converged to indicate the importance of the luminal microflora, their substrates (including fiber) and products (short-chain fatty acids) and how impairment of their function by antibiotics will affect colon function. There is exciting new evidence that nasogastric diet infusion may provoke abnormal colonic water and electrolyte secretion. Together with metabolic and physiologic data (see Table 2-6), such studies give promise of providing a rational basis not only for enteral diet formulation, but also to its optimum form of administration in the patient with impaired bowel function.

References

1. Althausen TL, Uyeyama K, Simpson RG. Digestion and absorption after massive resection of the small intestine: I. Utilization of food from a "natural" versus a "synthetic" diet and a comparison of intestinal absorption tests with nutritional balance studies in a patient with only 45 cm of small intestine. *Gastroenterology* 12:795, 1949.
2. Hammer HF, et al. Carbohydrate malabsorption: Its measurement and its contribution to diarrhea. *J Clin Invest* 86:1936, 1990.
3. Kirk E. The quantity and composition of human colonic flatus. *Gastroenterology* 12:782, 1949.
4. Randall HT. Enteral nutrition: Tube feeding in acute and chronic illness. *JPEN* 8:113, 1984.
5. Ferraris RP, Lee PP, Diamond JM. Origin of regional and species differences in intestinal glucose uptake. *Am J Physiol* 257:G689, 1989.
6. Toloza EM, Lam M, Diamond J. Nutrient extraction by cold-exposed mice: A test of digestive safety margins. *Am J Physiol* 261:G608, 1991.
7. Le Heuron-Luron I, et al. Molecular aspects of enzyme synthesis in the exocrine pancreas with emphasis on development and nutritional regulation. *Proc Nutr Soc* 52:301, 1993.
8. Hirst BH. Dietary regulation of intestinal nutrient carriers. *Proc Nutr Soc* 52:315, 1993.
9. Raimundo AH, et al. Colonic in-flow and small bowel motility during intraduodenal enteral nutrition. *Gut* 29:A1469, 1988.
10. Crane CW. Studies on the Absorption of ^{15}N Labelled Yeast in Normal Subjects and Patients with Malabsorption. In HN Munro (ed), *The Role of the Gastrointestinal Tract in Protein Metabolism.* Philadelphia: Davis, 1964. P 333.
11. DiMagno EP, Go VLW, Summerskill WHJ. Relations between pancreatic enzyme outputs and malabsorption in severe pancreatic insufficiency. *N Engl J Med* 288:813, 1973.
12. Bronstein MN, et al. Pancreatic insufficiency, growth, and nutrition in infants identified by newborn screening as having cystic fibrosis. *J Pediatr* 120:533, 1992.
13. Rees RGP, et al. Do patients with moderately impaired gastrointestinal function requiring enteral nutrition need a predigested nitrogen source? A prospective crossover controlled clinical trial. *Gut* 33:877, 1992.
14. Ladas SD, et al. Reproducible lactulose hydrogen breath test as a measure of mouth-to-cecum transit time. *Dig Dis Sci* 34:919, 1989.
15. Grimble GK, Patil DH, Silk DBA. Assimilation of lactitol, an "unabsorbed" disaccharide in the normal human colon. *Gut* 29:1666, 1988.
16. Patil DH, Grimble GK, Silk DBA. Lactitol, a new hydrogenated lactose derivative: Intestinal absorption and laxative threshold in normal human subjects. *Br J Nutr* 57:195, 1987.

17. O'Keefe SJD, et al. Nutritional support of malnourished lactose-intolerant African patients. *Gut* 25:942, 1984.

18. Keohane PP, et al. The roles of lactose and Clostridium difficile in the pathogenesis of enteral feeding-associated diarrhea. *Clin Nutr* 1:259, 1983.

19. Midtvedt A-C, Midtvedt T. Production of short-chain fatty acids by the intestinal microflora during the first two years of human life. *J Pediatr Gastroenterol Nutr* 15:395, 1992.

20. Debongnie JC, Phillips SF. Capacity of the human colon to absorb fluid. *Gastroenterology* 74:698, 1978.

21. Hammer HF, et al. Studies of osmotic diarrhea induced in normal subjects by ingestion of polyethylene glycol and lactulose. *J Clin Invest* 84:1056, 1989.

22. Rao SS, et al. Impaired colonic fermentation of carbohydrate after ampicillin. *Gastroenterology* 94:928, 1988.

23. Foltmann B. Pepsin, Chymosin and Their Zymogens. In P Desnuelle, H Sjostrom, O Noren (eds), *Molecular and Cellular Basis of Digestion.* Amsterdam: Elsevier, 1986. P 491.

24. Desnuelle P. Chemistry and Enzymology of Pancreatic Endopeptidases. In P Desnuelle, H Sjostrom, O Noren (eds), *Molecular and Cellular Basis of Digestion.* Amsterdam: Elsevier, 1986. P 195.

25. Puigserver A, Chapus C, Kerfelec B. Pancreatic Exopeptidases. In P Desnuelle, H Sjostrom, O Noren (eds), *Molecular and Cellular Basis of Digestion.* Amsterdam: Elsevier, 1986. P 235.

26. Marcuard SP, Perkins AM. Clogging of feeding tubes. *JPEN* 12:403, 1988.

27. Turner JS, et al. Esophageal obstruction during nasogastric feeding. *Intensive Care Med* 17:302, 1991.

28. Viall C, et al. A double-blind clinical trial comparing the gastrointestinal side effects of two enteral feeding formulas. *JPEN* 14:265, 1990.

29. Ziegler F, et al. Efficiency of enteral nitrogen support in surgical patients: Small peptides vs. non-degraded proteins. *Gut* 31:1277, 1990.

30. Mowatt-Larssen CA, et al. Comparison of tolerance and nutritional outcome between a peptide and a standard enteral formula in critically ill, hypoalbuminemic patients. *JPEN* 16:20, 1992.

31. Craft IL, et al. Absorption and malabsorption of glycine and glycine peptides in man. *Gut* 9:425, 1968.

32. Silk DBA, et al. Comparison of oral feeding of peptide and amino acid meals to normal human subjects. *Gut* 20:291, 1979.

33. Chung YC, et al. Protein digestion and absorption in human small intestine. *Gastroenterology* 76:1415, 1979.

34. Skovbjerg H. Immunoelectrophoretic studies on human small intestinal brush border proteins: The longitudinal distribution of peptidases and disaccharidases. *Clin Chim Acta* 112:205, 1981.

35. Triadou N, Bataille J, Schmitz J. Longitudinal study of the human intestinal brush border membrane proteins: Distribution of the main disaccharidases and peptidases. *Gastroenterology* 85:1326, 1983.

36. Tarvid I. Effect of early postnatal long-term fasting on the development of peptide hydrolysis in chicks. *Comp Biochem Physiol A* 101:161, 1992.

37. Silk DBA, et al. Functional differentiation of human jejunum and ileum: A comparison of the handling of glucose, peptides and amino acids. *Gut* 15:444, 1974.

38. Adibi SA, Mercer DW. Protein digestion in human intestine as reflected in human mucosal and plasma amino acid concentrations after meals. *J Clin Invest* 52:1586, 1973.

39. Chacko A, Cummings JH. Nitrogen losses from the human small bowel: Obligatory losses and the effect of physical form of food. *Gut* 29:809, 1988.

40. Mortensen PB, Rasmussen HS, Holtug K. Lactulose detoxifies in vitro short-chain fatty acid production in colonic contents induced by blood: Implications for hepatic coma. *Gastroenterology* 94:750, 1988.

41. Mortensen PB, et al. The degradation of amino acids, proteins, and blood to short-chain fatty acids in colon is prevented by lactulose. *Gastroenterology* 98:353, 1990.

42. MacFarlane GT, Cummings JH, Allison C. Protein degradation by human intestinal bacteria. *J Gen Microbiol* 132:1647, 1986.

43. Morgan MY. The treatment of chronic hepatic encephalopathy. *Hepatogastroenterology* 38:377, 1991.

44. Moran BJ, Jackson AA. Metabolism of ^{15}N-labeled urea in the functioning and defunctioned human colon. *Clin Sci* 79:253, 1990.

45. Moran BJ, Jackson AA. ^{15}N-urea metabolism in the functioning human colon: Luminal hydrolysis and mucosal permeability. *Gut* 31:454, 1990.

46. Hibbert JM, Forrester T, Jackson AA. Urea kinetics: Comparison of oral and intravenous dose regimens. *Eur J Clin Nutr* 46:405, 1992.

47. Windmueller HG. Glutamine utilization by the small intestine. *Adv Enzymol* 53:201, 1982.

48. Souba WW. Intestinal glutamine metabolism and nutrition. *J Nutr Biochem* 4:2, 1993.

49. McGivan JD, Pastor-Anglada M. Regulatory and molecular aspects of mammalian amino acid transport. *Biochem J* 299:321, 1994.

50. Kirk SJ, Barbul A. Role of arginine in trauma, sepsis and immunity. *JPEN* 14:226S, 1990.

51. Milliner DS. Cystinuria. *Endocrinol Metab Clin North Am* 19:889, 1990.

52. Cheeseman C. Role of intestinal basolateral membrane in absorption of nutrients. *Am J Physiol* 263:R482, 1992.

53. Medina MA, et al. Diamines interfere with the transport of L-ornithine in Ehrlich-cell plasma-membrane vesicles. *Biochem J* 280:825, 1991.

54. Payne-James J, et al. Jejunal absorption of ornithine-oxoglutarate (OKGA) in man. *JPEN* 13:22S, 1989.

55. Hegarty JE, et al. Jejunal water and electrolyte secretion induced by L-arginine in man. *Gut* 22:108, 1981.

56. Rérat A, et al. Amino acid absorption and production of pancreatic hormones in non-anaesthetised pigs after duodenal infusions of a milk enzymic hydrolysate or of free amino acids. *Br J Nutr* 60:121, 1988.

57. Calignano A, et al. Involvement of endogenous nitric oxide in the regulation of rat intestinal motility in vivo. *Eur J Pharmacol* 229:273, 1992.

58. Gardner ML, et al. Intestinal absorption of the intact peptide carnosine in man, and comparison with intestinal permeability to lactulose. *J Physiol* 439:411, 1991.

59. Ganapathy V, Leibach FK. Is intestinal transport energised by a proton gradient? *Am J Physiol* 249:G153, 1985.

60. Lucas ML, et al. Direct measurement by pH-microelectrode of the pH microclimate in rat proximal jejunum. *Proc R Soc Lond* 192:39, 1975.

61. Ganapathy V, Mendicino JF, Leibach FH. Transport of glycyl-L-proline into intestinal and renal brush border vesicles from rabbit. *J Biol Chem* 256:118, 1981.

62. Ganapathy ME, et al. Dipeptide transport in brush-border membrane vesicles isolated from normal term human placenta. *Am J Obstet Gynecol* 153:83, 1985.
63. Okano T, et al. H^+ gradient-dependent transport of aminocephalosporins in rat intestinal brush-border membrane vesicles. *Biochem Pharmacol* 35:1781, 1986.
64. Kramer W. Identification of identical binding polypeptides for cephalosporins and dipeptides in intestinal brush-border membrane vesicles by photoaffinity labeling. *Biochim Biophys Acta* 905:65, 1987.
65. Kramer W, et al. Direct photoaffinity labelling of binding proteins for β-lactam antibiotics in rabbit intestinal brush border membranes with [^{3}H]benzylpenicillin. *Biochem Pharmacol* 37:2427, 1988.
66. Fei Y-J, et al. Expression cloning of a mammalian proton-coupled oligopeptide transporter. *Nature* 368:563, 1994.
67. Grimble GK. The Significance of Peptides in Clinical Nutrition. In RE Olson, DM Bier, DB McCormick (eds), *Annual Review of Nutrition,* Vol 14. Palo Alto: Annual Reviews, 1994. P 419.
68. Dyer J, et al. Glycyl-L-proline transport in rabbit enterocyte basolateral-membrane vesicles. *Biochem J* 269:565, 1990.
69. Daniel H, Morse EL, Adibi SA. Determinants of substrate affinity for the oligopeptide/H^+ symporter in the renal brush border membrane. *J Biol Chem* 267:9565, 1992.
70. Botbol V, Scornik OA. Measurement of instant rates of protein degradation in the livers of intact mice by the accumulation of bestatin-induced peptides. *J Biol Chem* 266:2151, 1991.
71. Cook GC. Comparison of intestinal absorption rates of glycine and glycylglycine in man and the effect of glucose in the perfusing fluid. *Clin Sci* 43:443, 1972.
72. Rees RG, et al. Peptide based nitrogen source of enteral diets: Studies with casein hydrolysates in man. *JPEN* 12:21S, 1988.
73. Guandalini S, Rubino A. Development of dipeptide transport in the intestinal mucosa of rabbits. *Pediatr Res* 16:99, 1982.
74. Miller PM, et al. Kinetics of uptake of L-leucine and glycylsarcosine into normal and protein malnourished young rat jejunum. *Pediatr Res* 18:504, 1984.
75. Vasquez JA, Morse EL, Adibi SA. Effect of starvation on amino acid and peptide transport and peptide hydrolysis in humans. *Am J Physiol* 249:G563, 1985.
76. Gardiner K, Barbul A. Intestinal amino acid absorption during sepsis. *JPEN* 17:277, 1993.
77. Ferraris RP, Diamond J, Kwan WW. Dietary regulation of intestinal transport of the dipeptide carnosine. *Am J Physiol* 255:G143, 1988.
78. Ferraris RP, Kwan WW, Diamond J. Regulatory signals for intestinal amino acid transporters and peptidases. *Am J Physiol* 255:G151, 1988.
79. Silk DBA, et al. Absorption of amino acids from an amino acid mixture simulating casein and a tryptic hydrolysate of casein in man. *Clin Sci Mol Med* 45:715, 1973.
80. Fairclough PD, et al. Comparison of the absorption of two protein hydrolysates and their effects on water and electrolyte movements in the human jejunum. *Gut* 21:829, 1980.
81. Silk DBA, et al. Use of a peptide rather than free amino acid nitrogen source in chemically defined "elemental" diets. *JPEN* 4:548, 1980.
82. Grimble GK, et al. Effect of peptide chain-length on amino acid and nitrogen absorption from two lactalbumin hydrolysates in the normal human jejunum. *Clin Sci* 71:65, 1986.
83. Keohane PP, et al. Influence of protein composition and hydrolysis method on intestinal absorption of protein in man. *Gut* 26:907, 1985.
84. Hegarty JE, et al. Effects of concentration on in vivo absorption of a peptide containing protein hydrolysate. *Gut* 23:304, 1982.
85. Friedrich M, et al. Absorption of enzymatic protein hydrolysates and equimolar amino acid mixtures in the perfused small intestine of the rat [in German]. *Biomed Biochim Acta* 43:117, 1984.
86. Grimble GK, et al. The effect of peptide chain-length on absorption of egg-protein hydrolysates in the normal human jejunum. *Gastroenterology* 92:136, 1987.
87. Grimble GK, et al. The influence of whey hydrolysate peptide chain length on nitrogen and carbohydrate absorption in the perfused human jejunum. *Clin Nutr* 14(Suppl):46, 1994.
88. Adibi SA, Morse EL. The number of glycine residues which limits intact absorption of glycine oligopeptides in human jejunum. *J Clin Invest* 60:1008, 1977.
89. Grimble GK, Silk DBA. Peptides in human nutrition. *Nutr Res Rev* 2:87, 1989.
90. Cezard JP, et al. Effects of two protein hydrolysates on growth, nitrogen balance and small intestine adaptation in growing rats. *Biol Neonate* 65:60, 1994.
91. Raimundo AH, et al. The influence of fat and carbohydrate on absorption of partial enzymic hydrolysates of casein in the normal human jejunum. *Gastroenterology* 94:A988, 1988.
92. Grimble GK, et al. Use of high performance liquid chromatography with pulsed amperometric detection (PAD-HPLC) to investigate an interaction between peptide and maltodextrin assimilation in the perfused human jejunum. *Clin Nutr* 14(Suppl):32, 1994.
93. Zaloga GP, Ward KA, Prielipp RC. Effect of enteral diets on whole body and gut growth in unstressed rats. *JPEN* 15:42, 1991.
94. Balogh D, et al. Differentiated enteral feeding in the post-aggression phase in polytrauma patients: Comparison of a high calorie nutritionally defined diet (whole protein high calorie diet) with a peptide diet [in German]. *Infusionsther Klin Ernahr* 16:52, 1989.
95. Chlebowski RT, et al. Long-term effects of early nutritional support with a new enterotrophic peptide-based formula vs. standard enteral formula in HIV-infected patients: Randomized prospective trial. *Nutrition* 9:507, 1993.
96. Steinhardt HJ, et al. Nitrogen absorption in pancreatectomised patients: Protein versus protein hydrolysate as substrate. *J Lab Clin Med* 113:162, 1989.
97. Itoh H, Kishi T, Chibata I. Comparative effects of casein and amino acid mixture simulating casein on growth and food intake in rats. *J Nutr* 103:1709, 1973.
98. Moriarty KJ, et al. Relative nutritional value of whole protein, hydrolysed protein and free amino acids in man. *Gut* 26:694, 1985.
99. Velasco N, et al. Whole-body protein kinetics in elective surgical patients receiving peptide or amino acid solutions. *Nutrition* 7:28, 1991.
100. Grimble GK, et al. Are enterally fed peptides better utilised than free amino acids in the short-bowel syndrome? *Clin Nutr* 5(Suppl):50, 1986.
101. Trocki O, et al. Intact protein versus free amino acids

in the nutritional support of thermally injured animals. *JPEN* 10:139, 1986.

102. Grimble GK, et al. Trophic effects of dietary peptides on the rat intestinal tract. *JPEN* 13:6S, 1989.

103. Koruda MJ, et al. The effect of a pectin-supplemented elemental diet on intestinal adaptation to massive small bowel resection. *JPEN* 10:343, 1986.

104. Monchi M, et al. Net protein utilisation after duodenal infusion of small peptides of free amino acids in growing rats. *Clin Nutr* 10(Suppl):31, 1991.

105. Monchi M, Rérat AA. Comparison of net protein utilization of milk protein mild enzymatic hydrolysates and free amino acid mixtures with a close pattern in the rat. *JPEN* 17:355, 1993.

106. McIntyre PB, Fitchew M, Lennard-Jones JE. Patients with a high ileostomy do not need a special diet. *Gastroenterology* 91:25, 1986.

107. Rees RG, et al. Influence of orally administered amino acids and peptides on protein turnover kinetics in the short bowel syndrome. *Gut* 28:A1397, 1988.

108. Schmitz J, et al. Perfusion Study of Disaccharide Absorption After Extensive Intestinal Resection. In JWL Robinson, RH Dowling, EO Riecken (eds), *Mechanisms of Intestinal Adaptation.* Lancaster, England: MTP, 1982. P 413.

109. Dowling RH. Small bowel adaptation and its regulation. *Scand J Gastroenterol* 17(Suppl 74):53, 1982.

110. Tobey N, et al. Human intestinal brush-border peptidases. *Gastroenterology* 88:913, 1985.

111. Noren O, et al. The Enzymes of the Enterocyte Plasma Membrane. In P Desnuelle, H Sjostrom, O Noren (eds), *Molecular and Cellular Basis of Digestion.* Amsterdam: Elsevier, 1986. P 335.

112. Pedersen S, Norman BE. Enzymatic Modification of Food Carbohydrates. In AT Andrews (ed), *Chemical Aspects of Food Enzymes.* London: Royal Society of Chemistry, 1987. P 156.

113. Johansson C. Studies of gastrointestinal interactions: VII. Characteristics of the absorption pattern of sugar, fat and protein from composite meals in man: A quantitative study. *Scand J Gastroenterol* 10:33, 1975.

114. Meldrum SJ, et al. pH profile of gut as measured by a radiotelemetry capsule. *Br Med J* 2:104, 1972.

115. Gray GM. Carbohydrate digestion and absorption. *Gastroenterology* 58:96, 1970.

116. Kenny AJ, Maroux S. Topology of microvillar membrane hydrolases of kidney and intestine. *Physiol Rev* 62:91, 1982.

117. Semenza G. Anchoring and biosynthesis of stalked brush border membrane proteins: Glycosidases and peptidases of enterocytes and renal tubuli. *Annu Rev Cell Biol* 2:255, 1986.

118. Hoefsloot LH, et al. Primary structure and processing of lysosomal alpha-glucosidase; homology with the intestinal sucrase-isomaltase complex. *EMBO J* 7:1697, 1988.

119. Hoefsloot LH, et al. Characterization of the human lysosomal α-glucosidase gene. *Biochem J* 272:493, 1990.

120. Sivakami S, Radhakrishnan AN. Kinetic studies on glucoamylase of rabbit small intestine. *Biochem J* 153:321, 1976.

121. Pereira B, Sivakami S. A comparison of the active site of maltase-glucoamylase from the brush-border of rabbit small intestine and kidney by chemical modification studies. *Biochem J* 274:349, 1991.

122. Gray GM. Carbohydrate digestion and absorption: Role of the small intestine. *N Engl J Med* 292:1225, 1975.

123. Wahlqvist ML, et al. The effect of chain length on glucose absorption and the related metabolic response. *Am J Clin Nutr* 31:1998, 1978.

124. Layer P, Sinmeister AR, DiMagno EP. Effect of decreasing intraluminal amylase activity on starch digestion and post-prandial gastrointestinal functions in humans. *Gastroenterology* 91:41, 1986.

125. Grimble GK, Collins S, Silk DBA. In vivo and in vitro assimilation of orally administered dextran 40KDa in man. *Proc Nutr Soc* 51:120A, 1992.

126. Pappenheimer JR. Paracellular intestinal absorption of glucose, creatinine, and mannitol in normal animals: Relation to body size. *Am J Physiol* 259:G290, 1990.

127. Atisook K, Madara JL. An oligopeptide permeates intestinal tight junctions at glucose-elicited dilatations: Implications for oligopeptide absorption. *Gastroenterology* 100:719, 1991.

128. Ferraris RP, et al. Luminal glucose concentrations in the gut under normal conditions. *Am J Physiol* 259:G822, 1990.

129. Fine KD, et al. Effect of D-glucose on intestinal permeability and its passive absorption in human small intestine in vivo. *Gastroenterology* 105:1117, 1993.

130. Fisher RB, Parsons DS. Glucose absorption from surviving rat small intestine. *J Physiol* 110:281, 1949.

131. Maxton DG, et al. Lactulose, ^{51}Cr-labelled ethylenediaminetetra-acetate, L-rhamnose and polyethyleneglycol 400 [corrected] as probe markers for assessment in vivo of human intestinal permeability. *Clin Sci* 71:71, 1986. [Published erratum appears in *Clin Sci* 1986 Dec;71(6): following xxi].

132. Maxton DG, Catt SD, Menzies IS. Combined assessment of intestinal disaccharidases in congenital asucrasia by differential urinary disaccharide excretion. *J Clin Path* 43:406, 1990.

133. Katz KD, et al. Intestinal permeability in patients with Crohn's disease and their healthy relatives. *Gastroenterology* 97:927, 1989.

134. Gould GW, Holman GD. The glucose transporter family: Structure, function and tissue-specific expression. *Biochem J* 295:329, 1993.

135. Pajor AM, Hirayama BA, Wright EM. Molecular biology approaches to comparative study of Na(+)-glucose cotransport. *Am J Physiol* 263:R489, 1992.

136. Stevens BR. Vertebrate intestine apical membrane mechanisms of organic nutrient transport. *Am J Physiol* 263:R458, 1992.

137. Minami H, et al. Inhibition of glucose absorption by phlorizin affects intestinal function in rats. *Gastroenterology* 105:692, 1993.

138. Crouzoulon G, Korieh A. Fructose transport by rat intestinal brush border membrane vesicles: Effect of high fructose diet followed by return to standard diet. *Comp Biochem Physiol A* 100:175, 1991.

139. Milla PJ, et al. Fructose absorption and the effects of other monosaccharides on its absorption in the rat jejunum in vivo. *Gut* 18:A425, 1977.

140. Thorens B, et al. Liver glucose transporter: A basolateral protein in hepatocytes and intestine and kidney cells. *Am J Physiol* 259:C279, 1990.

141. Fernandez Lopez JA, et al. Intestinal handling of a glucose gavage by the rat. *Mol Cell Biochem* 113:43, 1992.

142. Grimble GK. Ion chromatography in clinical research: A neglected technique? *Analyt Proc* 29:468, 1992.

143. Heitlinger LA, et al. Transport of glucose polymer-derived glucose by rabbit jejunum. *Gastroenterology* 102:443, 1992.

144. Jones BJM, et al. Energy dense enteral feeds: The use of high molecular weight glucose polymers. *JPEN* 5:567, 1981.

145. Jones BJM, et al. Glucose absorption from starch hydrolysates in the human jejunum. *Gut* 24:1152, 1984.

146. Jones BJM, Higgins BE, Silk DBA. Glucose absorption from maltotriose and glucose oligomers in the human jejunum. *Clin Sci* 72:409, 1987.

147. Spiller RC, Jones BJM, Silk DBA. Jejunal water and electrolyte absorption from two proprietary enteral feeds in man: Importance of sodium content. *Gut* 28:681, 1986.

148. Samulitis-dos Santos BK, Goda T, Koldovsky O. Dietary-induced increases of disaccharidase activities in rat jejunum. *Br J Nutr* 67:267, 1992.

149. Rumessen JJ, Gudmand Hoyer E. Absorption capacity of fructose in healthy adults: Comparison with sucrose and its constituent monosaccharides. *Gut* 27:1161, 1986.

150. Hamosh M, et al. Pharyngeal lipase and digestion of dietary triglyceride in man. *J Clin Invest* 55:908, 1975.

151. Gluckman RM. Fat absorption and malabsorption. *Clin Gastroenterol* 12(2):323, 1983.

152. Stremmel W. Intestinal Absorption of Fat and Fat-Soluble Vitamins. In G Dietze, A Grunert, G Wolfram (eds), *Clinical Nutrition and Metabolic Research.* Basel: Karger, 1986. P 118.

153. Hauton JC. A Quantitative Dynamic Concept of the Role of Bile in Fat Digestion. In P Desnuelle, H Sjostrom, O Noren (eds), *Molecular and Cellular Basis of Digestion.* Amsterdam: Elsevier, 1986. P 147.

154. Caspary WF. Physiology and pathophysiology of intestinal absorption. *Am J Clin Nutr* 55:299S, 1992.

155. Rao RH, Mansbach CM. Acid lipase in rat intestinal mucosa: Physiological parameters. *Biochim Biophys Acta* 1043:273, 1990.

156. Bonner MS, et al. Heparin-modulated binding and pancreatic lipase and uptake of hydrolysed triglycerides in the intestine. *J Biol Chem* 264:20261, 1989.

157. Shiau Y. Mechanism of intestinal fatty acid uptake in the rat: The role of an acidic environment. *J Physiol* 421:463, 1990.

158. Sacchettini JC, Gordon JI, Banaszak LJ. Refined apoprotein of rat intestinal fatty acid binding protein produced in Escherichia coli. *Proc Natl Acad Sci USA* 86:7736, 1989.

159. Iseki S, Kondo H. Light microscopic localization of HFABP proteins mRNA in jejunal epithelia in rats using in situ hybridization, immunohistochemical, and autoradiographic techniques. *J Histochem Cytochem* 38:111, 1990.

160. Mansbach CM, Arnold A, Cox MA. Factors influencing triacylglycerol delivery into mesenteric lymph. *Am J Physiol* 249:G642, 1985.

161. Tipton AD, Frase S, Mansbach CM. Isolation and characterisation of a mucosal triacylglycerol pool undergoing hydrolysis. *Am J Physiol* 257:G871, 1989.

162. Phillips SF, Giller J. The contribution of the colon to electrolyte and water conservation in man. *J Lab Clin Med* 81:733, 1973.

163. Fordtran JS, et al. Permeability characteristics of the human small intestine. *J Clin Invest* 44:1935, 1965.

164. McKie AT, Goecke IA, Naftalin RJ. Comparison of fluid absorption by bovine and ovine descending colon in vitro. *Am J Physiol* 261:G433, 1991.

165. Turnberg L. Cellular basis of diarrhoea: The Croonian lecture 1989. *J R Coll Physicians* 25:53, 1991.

166. Silk DBA, et al. A study of relations between the absorption of amino acids, dipeptides, water and electrolytes in the normal human jejunum. *Clin Sci Mol Med* 49:401, 1975.

167. Sladen GE, Dawson AM. Inter-relationship between the absorption of glucose, sodium and water by the normal human jejunum. *Clin Sci* 36:119, 1969.

168. Sladen GE, Dawson AM. Effect of bicarbonate on sodium absorption by the human jejunum. *Nature* 218:267, 1968.

169. Turnberg LA, et al. Inter-relationships of chloride bicarbonate sodium and hydrogen transport in the human ileum. *J Clin Invest* 49:557, 1970.

170. Devroede GJ, Phillips SF. Conservation of sodium, chloride and water by the human colon. *Gastroenterology* 56:101, 1969.

171. Ruppin H, et al. Absorption of short chain fatty acids by the colon. *Gastroenterology* 78:1500, 1980.

172. Bleakman D, Naftalin RJ. Hypertonic fluid absorption from rabbit descending colon in vitro. *Am J Physiol* 258:G377, 1990.

173. Weaver GA, et al. Constancy of glucose and starch fermentations by two different human faecal microbial communities. *Gut* 30:19, 1989.

174. Grimble GK. Fibre, fermentation, flora and flatus. *Gut* 30:6, 1989.

175. Gibson GR, Cummings JH, MacFarlane GT. Use of a three-stage continuous culture system to study the effect of mucin on dissimilatory sulphate reduction and methanogenesis by mixed populations of human gut bacteria. *Appl Environ Microbiol* 54:2750, 1988.

176. Gibson GR, MacFarlane GT, Cummings JH. Occurrence of sulphate-reducing bacteria in human faeces and the relationship of dissimilatory sulphate reduction to methanogenesis in the large gut. *J Appl Bacteriol* 65:103, 1988.

177. Flourié B, et al. Site and substrates for methane production in human colon. *Am J Physiol* 260:G752, 1991.

178. Mortensen PB, et al. Colonic fermentation of Ispaghula, wheat bran, glucose and albumin to short-chain fatty acids and ammonia evaluated in vitro in 50 subjects. *JPEN* 16:433, 1992.

179. Mueller KJ, et al. Estimation of fecal nitrogen in patients with liver disease. *JPEN* 7:266, 1983.

180. Smith CJ, Bryant MP. Introduction to metabolic activities of intestinal bacteria. *Am J Clin Nutr* 32:149, 1979.

181. Windmueller HG, Spaeth AE. Identification of ketone bodies and glutamine as the major respiratory fuels in vivo for postabsorptive rat small intestine. *J Biol Chem* 253:69, 1978.

182. Henning SJ, Hird FJR. Concentrations and metabolism of volatile fatty acids in the fermentative organs of two species of kangaroo and the guinea-pig. *Br J Nutr* 24:145, 1970.

183. Roediger WEW. Role of anaerobic bacteria in the metabolic welfare of the colonic mucosa in man. *Gut* 21:793, 1980.

184. Young GP, Gibson P. Contrasting Effects of Butyrate on Proliferation and Differentiation of Normal and Neoplastic Cells. In AF Roche (ed), *Short Chain Fatty Acids: Metabolism and Clinical Importance. Report of 10th Ross Conference on Medical Research.* Columbus, Ohio, 1991, Ross Laboratories. P 50.

185. Niles RM, et al. The effect of sodium butyrate and retinoic acid on growth and CEA production in a series of human colorectal tumor cell lines representing different states of differentiation. *Cancer Invest* 6:39, 1988.

186. Scheppach W, et al. Effect of short-chain fatty acids on the human colonic mucosa in vitro. *JPEN* 16:43, 1992.

187. Sakata T. Stimulatory effect of short-chain fatty acids on epithelial cell proliferation in the rat intestine: A possible explanation for trophic effects of fermentable fibre, gut microbes and luminal trophic factors. *Br J Nutr* 58:95, 1987.

188. Lupton JR, Coder DM, Jacobs LR. Influence of luminal pH on rat large bowel epithelial cell cycle. *Am J Physiol* 249:G382, 1985.

189. Goodlad RA, et al. Effects of an elemental diet, inert bulk and different types of dietary fibre on the response of the intestinal epithelium to refeeding in the rat and relationship to plasma gastrin, enteroglucagon and PYY concentrations. *Gut* 28:171, 1987.

190. Goodlad RA, et al. Does dietary fibre stimulate intestinal epithelial cell proliferation in germ free rats? *Gut* 30:820, 1989.

191. Kruh J, Defer N, Tichonicky L. Molecular and Cellular Effects of Sodium Butyrate. In AF Roche (ed), *Short Chain Fatty Acids: Metabolism and Clinical Importance. Report of the 10th Ross Conference on Medical Research.* Columbus, Ohio, 1991, Ross Laboratories. P 45.

192. Tanaka Y, et al. Enhancement of butyrate-induced differentiation of HT-29 human colon carcinoma cells by 1,25-dihydroxyvitamin D_3. *Biochem Pharmacol* 38:3859, 1989.

193. Siddiqui B, Kim YS. Effects of sodium butyrate, dimethyl sulfoxide, and retinoic acid on glycolipids of human rectal adenocarcinoma cells. *Cancer Res* 44:1648, 1984.

194. Rolandelli RH, et al. Effects of intraluminal infusion of short-chain fatty acids on the healing of colonic anastomoses in the rat. *Surgery* 100:198, 1986.

195. Kripke SA, et al. Stimulation of intestinal mucosal growth with intracolonic infusion of short-chain fatty acids. *JPEN* 13:109, 1989.

196. Koruda MJ, et al. Effect of parenteral nutrition supplemented with short-chain fatty acids on adaptation to massive small bowel resection. *Gastroenterology* 95:715, 1988.

197. Remesy C, Demigne C. Specific effects of fermentable carbohydrates on blood urea flux and ammonia absorption in the rat cecum. *J Nutr* 119:560, 1989.

198. Mortensen FV, et al. Short chain fatty acids dilate isolated human colonic resistance arteries. *Gut* 31:1391, 1990.

199. Kvietys PR, Granger DN. Effect of volatile fatty acids on blood flow and oxygen uptake by the dog colon. *Gastroenterology* 80:962, 1981.

200. Crissinger KD, Burney DL. Influence of luminal nutrient composition on hemodynamics and oxygenation in developing intestine. *Am J Physiol* 263:G254, 1992.

201. Buckley NM, Frasier ID. Regional circulatory responses to intestinal work in developing swine. *Am J Physiol* 258:H1119, 1990.

202. Qamar MI, Read AE, Mountford R. Increased superior mesenteric artery blood flow after glucose but not lactulose ingestion. *Q J Med* 60:893, 1986.

203. Flynn WJJ, Gosche JR, Garrison RN. Intestinal blood flow is restored with glutamine or glucose suffusion after hemorrhage. *J Surg Res* 52:499, 1992.

204. Lang CH, et al. Increased glucose uptake by intestinal mucosa and muscularis in hypermetabolic sepsis. *Am J Physiol* 261:G287, 1991.

205. Binder HJ, Mehta P. Short-chain fatty acids stimulate active sodium chloride absorption in vitro in the rat distal colon. *Gastroenterology* 96:989, 1989.

206. Watson AJM, et al. Acetate absorption in the normal and secreting rat jejunum. *Gut* 31:170, 1990.

207. Vernia P, et al. Organic anions and the diarrhea of inflammatory bowel disease. *Dig Dis Sci* 33:1353, 1988.

208. Rees RGP, et al. Tolerance of elemental diet administered without starter regimen. *Br Med J* 290:1869, 1985.

209. Kemen M, et al. Is intact protein superior for post-operative enteral nutrition than hydrolysed protein? *Clin Nutr* 10(Suppl):37, 1991.

210. Patil DH, et al. Comparative modes of action of lactitol and lactulose in the treatment of hepatic encephalopathy. *Gut* 28:255, 1987.

211. Konno R, Niwa A, Yasumura Y. Intestinal bacterial origin of D-alanine in urine of mutant mice lacking D-amino-acid oxidase. *Biochem J* 268:263, 1990.

212. Clausen MR, et al. Colonic fermentation to short-chain fatty acids is decreased in antibiotic-associated diarrhea. *Gastroenterology* 101:1497, 1991.

213. Thompson GN, et al. The use of metronidazole in management of methylmalonic and propionic acidaemias. *Eur J Pediatr* 149:792, 1990.

214. Homann H-H, et al. The role of carbohydrate malabsorption in the pathogenesis of diarrhea during postoperative enteral nutrition. *J Clin Nutr Gastroenterol* 7:54, 1992.

215. Lehtola J, et al. Effect of erythromycin on the oro-caecal transit time in man. *Eur J Clin Pharmacol* 39:555, 1990.

216. Cannon WB. The movements of the intestines studied by means of the roentgen rays. *Am J Physiol* 6:251, 1902.

217. Szurszewiski JJ. A migrating electrical complex of canine small intestine. *Am J Physiol* 217:1757, 1969.

218. Schemann M, Ehrlein HJ. Post prandial patterns of canine jejunal motility and transit of luminal contents. *Gastroenterology* 90:991, 1986.

219. Silk DBA, Spiller RC. The Small Intestine. In J Kyle, LC Carey (eds), *Scientific Foundations of Surgery* (4th ed). Oxford: Heineman, 1989. P 409.

220. Ehrlein HJ, Schmid HR, Feinle C. Recording of intestinal motility is a useful control of enteral nutrition. *Clin Nutr* 11(Suppl):62, 1992.

221. Raimundo AH, et al. The effect of enteral nutrition on distal colonic motility. *Gastroenterology* 102:A573, 1992.

222. Bowling TE, et al. The effect of enteral feeding on colonic motility in man. *Gut* 34:S64, 1993.

223. Snape WJ, Matarazzo SA, Cohen S. Effect of eating and gastrointestinal hormones on human colonic myoelectrical and motor activity. *Gastroenterology* 75:373, 1978.

224. Wiley J, et al. Participation of gastric mechanoreceptors and intestinal chemoreceptors in the gastrocolonic response. *Gastroenterology* 94:1144, 1988.

225. Bowling TE, Raimundo AH, Silk DBA. Effect of enteral feeding on colonic water absorption in man. *Gastroenterology* 104:A610, 1993.

226. Bowling TE, et al. Reversal by short-chain fatty acids of colonic fluid secretion induced by enteral feeding. *Lancet* 342:1266, 1993.

227. Demigne C, Levrat MA, Remesy C. Effects of feeding fermentable carbohydrates on the cecal concentrations of minerals and their fluxes between the cecum and blood plasma in the rat. *J Nutr* 119:1625, 1989.

228. Silk DBA. Progress report: Fibre and enteral nutrition. *Gut* 30:246, 1989.

229. Silk DBA. Fibre and enteral nutrition. *Clin Nutr* 12:S106, 1993.

230. Curtis KJ, Sleisenger MH, Kim YS. Protein digestion and absorption after massive small bowel resection. *Dig Dis Sci* 29:834, 1984.

231. Bristol JB, Williamson RCN. Nutrition, operations, and intestinal adaptation. *JPEN* 12:299, 1988.

232. Haase W, et al. Characterization and histochemical localization of the rat intestinal Na^+-D-glucose co-transporter by monoclonal antibodies. *Eur J Cell Biol* 52:297, 1990.

233. Dodge JA, Yassa JG. Essential fatty acid deficiency after prolonged treatment with elemental diet. *Lancet* 2:1256, 1980.

234. Dodge JA. Nutrition in cystic fibrosis: A historical overview. *Proc Nutr Soc* 51:225, 1992.

235. Durie PR, Pencharz PB. Cystic fibrosis: Nutrition. *Br Med Bull* 48:823, 1992.

236. Pettei MJ, Daftary S, Levine JJ. Essential fatty acid deficiency associated with the use of a medium-chain-triglyceride infant formula in pediatric hepatobiliary disease. *Am J Clin Nutr* 53:1217, 1991.

237. Hamosh M, et al. Fat absorption in premature infants: Medium-chain triglycerides and long-chain triglycerides are absorbed from formula at similar rates. *J Pediatr Gastroenterol Nutr* 13:143, 1991.

238. Collins AJ, James PS, Smith MW. Sugar-dependent selective induction of mouse jejunal disaccharidase activities. *J Physiol* 419:157, 1989.

Selected Readings

Bowling TE, et al. Reversal by short-chain fatty acids of colonic fluid secretion induced by enteral feeding. *Lancet* 342:1266, 1993.

The high incidence of diarrhea in enterally fed patients is associated with concurrent antibiotic therapy, but it may also arise as a consequence of altered large-bowel motility from other causes. This study attempted to explain the high incidence of diarrhea in nasogastrically fed volunteers, which was not observed when diet was infused into the jejunum. A long perfusion tube was used to intubate the small and large intestine, and regional water and electrolyte flows were measured by use of ^{3}H- and 14C-polyethylene glycol. Nasogastric feeding stimulated ileocolonic inflow, but not in amounts sufficient to explain the diarrhea. Nasogastric feeding, however, initiated a net *efflux* of water and electrolyte into the lumen of the ascending colon at approximately 60 ml/hr. The addition of short-chain fatty acids to the solution perfusing the colonic lumen reversed this to an uptake of 96 ml/hr. These highly significant data suggest the presence of a systemic effect of nasogastric feeding that elicits an inappropriate colonic secretory response. It is possible that continuous nasogastric feeding, which was developed to overcome the many technical problems of feeding patients who could otherwise not eat, may be less appropriate than more physiologic methods such as cyclical enteral nutrition, which more nearly approaches the normal pattern of "three square meals each day."

Fei Y-J, et al. Expression cloning of a mammalian proton-coupled oligopeptide transporter. *Nature* 368:563, 1994.

The quantitative significance of dipeptide and tripeptide uptake by the human small intestine has been established by numerous in vivo studies and in vitro transport studies on isolated brush-border membrane vesicles. This paper describes the isolation and characterization of the peptide transporter itself, or at least a significant part of it. The DNA coding for a transport protein containing 707 amino acids was isolated and expressed in *Xenopus laevis* oocytes. Incorporation of this protein (which has the provisional title of PepT1) into the cell membrane increased uptake of glycylsarcosine 64-fold and also transported the antibiotic, cephalexin. Modeling of the amino acid sequence showed the possibility of 12 membrane-spanning domains (with helical structure). In addition, rabbit tissues probed with ^{32}P-cDNA showed strongest expression in the intestine (jejunum > duodenum), followed by the liver plasma membrane, the kidney, and a small amount in the brain. This is highly significant because the presence of a transporter in liver suggests the presence of substrate for transport, that is, dipeptides and tripeptides in blood. If this were so, then current ideas about the interorgan transport of amino acids as *free* L-amino acid may require revision. Furthermore, as antibiotics containing a peptide bond use this transporter, further detailed studies of the structure and function of this transport protein may allow more rational design of oral antibiotics that can be targeted to specific organs.

Midtvedt A-C, Midtvedt T. Production of short-chain fatty acids by the intestinal microflora during the first 2 years of human life. *J Pediatr Gastroenterol Nutr* 15:395, 1992.

Human babies are germ-free at birth and slowly acquire colonic bacteria that provide the five major characteristics of adult-pattern colonic metabolism. None of these (e.g., mucin degradation or cholesterol catabolism) are fully established by 6 months. This study investigated short-chain fatty acid concentrations in fresh feces from 30 children during their first two years of life who received breast milk only, breast milk and formula-feed, or formula only. Total short-chain fatty acid concentration had reached adult concentrations by 6 months for all groups combined. Formula-feeding hastened this process (1 month), whereas breast-feeding delayed it (9 months). Organic acids, whose presence indicated luminal protein fermentation (*iso*- and *n*-valeric acids) did not reach adult concentrations for at least 16 months. Antibiotic treatment delayed establishment of adult-pattern short-chain fatty acid production and selectively increased butyrate at the expense of acetate. These data are consistent with better absorption of breast milk, which provides less substrate for colonic luminal fermentation. The dominance of acetate among the short-chain fatty acids provides a buffer that is strongly bacteriostatic for some gram-negative species. Formula diets tend to prevent this process through the buffering capacity of malabsorbed dietary components. This may in turn lead to establishment of *Escherichia coli* and streptococci colonies, which allows subsequent colonization by other aerobes and anerobes. The interest of this paper lies in the power of such longitudinal studies to allow inferences to be made. Clearly, colonic microflora and their fermentation products constitute an ecosystem of great complexity and flexibility. Overall bacterial growth can be increased by substrate supply, but this is hardly surprising. What is of particular interest is that reduced substrate availability as well as antibiotic treatment will antagonize this process and may allow selective growth of potentially harmful pathogens. The challenge for the future is to modulate this process by dietary means, to the clinical benefit of the patient.

Moran BJ, Jackson AA. Metabolism of ^{15}N-labeled urea in the functioning and defunctioned human colon. *Clin Sci* 79:253, 1990.

Colonic luminal fermentation of protein has long been suspected as a source of ammonia production, which is unwelcome in patients with alcoholic liver disease and encephalopathy. Curiously, the likelihood that part of this may come from urea hydrolysis has been overlooked. Certainly, early studies showed that infants fed marginally inadequate diets could be put into nitrogen balance if urea was included in the diet. In this study, double-labeled urea (^{15}N^{15}N urea) was placed in the colonic lumen through a colostomy. It was found that some of the label was recovered in urine or stool as $^{14}N^{15}N$ urea, indicating that hydrolysis had occurred and that released ammonia had been transferred to the liver and reincorporated into urea together with unlabeled (^{14}N) ammonia. It also confirms that the colon is permeable to the intact urea molecule, which on hydrolysis will liberate ammonia that can be absorbed and reincorporated into the amino acid α-NH_2 pool. In quantitative terms, this form of urea recycling is highly significant, and further studies from Jackson and colleagues suggest that it may be as much as 80% of total urea production in infants and 40% in adults. These data may explain why the nitrogen requirements of enterally fed patients are higher than can be explained by their degree of catabolism. Concurrent antibiotic therapy may inhibit this useful means of conserving dietary nitrogen intake.

Toloza EM, Lam M, Diamond J. Nutrient extraction by cold-exposed mice: A test of digestive safety margins. *Am J Physiol* 261:G608, 1991.

The "safety margin" of the small intestine is defined as the excess absorption and digestion of the intestine over prevailing daily intake. This safety margin has been assumed to be very large, in which case its maintenance would cause an energy burden. This ingenious study increased nutrient intake in mice, not by force-feeding, but by transferring the animals from an environment at 22°C to one at 6°C. The resulting hyperphagia of the animals in response to increased shivering and nonshivering energy expenditure showed as a 68% increase in intake by 12 hours and by a 150% increase at 2 days. Resulting changes in food intake, apparent digestive efficiency, intestinal morphometrics, and intestinal brush-border uptake capacities for D-glucose and L-proline were measured during a 28-day period. Apparent digestive efficiency remained unchanged, even within the first 12 hours, and intestinal transit times also remained unchanged, implying the existence of at least some safety margin. The mass of the small and large intestine, liver, kidney and spleen nevertheless increased within 4 days by 16% to 20%. Glucose and proline uptake (μmoles/mg intestine) increased by approximately 5%, and thus the intestine's summed uptake capacity for these solutes increased by 24% to 26%. A comparison of calculated summed uptake capacities with measured dietary intake suggests that at 22°C, the safety margin was approximately 220% to 300% and was reduced to 27% to 50% on initial transfer to 6°C. Subsequent adaptation restored this to 60% to 88%.

3

Mediators, Hormones, and Control of Metabolism: Regulation of Protein, Carbohydrate, and Lipid Metabolism in Critical Illness

Per-Olof Hasselgren

The control of metabolism is complex and can occur at the organ/tissue level, cellular/subcellular level, and molecular level. For example, changes in blood flow to an organ or tissue in response to sepsis or any other noxious insult can influence metabolism, although under normal conditions, it is usually the metabolic needs of the tissue that determine blood flow. However, under certain circumstances, total body circulatory requirements compete with regional blood flow; severe injury, burn, sepsis, and cardiac failure may result in hypoperfusion of such organs as liver and intestine, with significant metabolic and functional consequences.

Regulation of metabolism can also occur at a cellular/subcellular level. Cellular control may be at least in part at the membrane level. For example, transport of amino acids and glucose across the cell membrane can influence intracellular protein and carbohydrate metabolism. Metabolic control may also take place at the membrane of intracellular organelles, e.g., the mitochondrion and the Golgi apparatus; changes of the mitochon-

Supported in part by NIH grants DK37908, DK44201, and DK40644, and grants 15851, 15859, and 15861 from the Shriners of North America.

drial membrane may have pronounced effects on cellular energy metabolism, whereas changes of the Golgi membranes may influence the metabolism/processing of intracellular proteins [1]. Cellular metabolism is also influenced by enzyme concentrations and the regulation of the activity or amount of receptors (e.g., hormone receptors) and membrane transporters (e.g., amino acid transporters), or both.

Two additional important mechanisms for metabolic control are substrate availability and end product inhibition. For example, increased availability of lactate and the gluconeogenic amino acids stimulates hepatic gluconeogenesis. In contrast, acetoacetate and β-hydroxybutyrate formed during starvation serve as a negative feedback signal to different tissues to decrease glucose utilization and proteolysis, thus being an example of end product inhibition.

The recent, almost explosive development in the field of recombinant DNA technology has opened up the possibility to study the molecular regulation of metabolism, and there are numerous examples in the literature of metabolic processes in which regulation at the molecular level have already been elucidated. There is reason to believe that the field of molecular biology will continue to increase its impact on the understanding of metabolic regulation in various pathophysiologic conditions. This aspect of metabolic control will be exemplified in greater detail in subsequent sections of this chapter.

Hormones and various mediators, including cytokines, nitric oxide (NO), oxygen radicals, and prostaglandins, play an important role in the regulation of metabolism in various organs and tissues. These substances can exert their control of metabolism at the different levels discussed above. Both groups of substances (hormones and mediators) are important for the regulation of metabolism in patients with severe injury, inflammation, or sepsis. In this chapter, the role of mediators (in particular cytokines) and hormones in the control of metabolism during these conditions is discussed. First, however, the response of hormones and cytokines to injury and sepsis is described to give a better understanding of their influence on different metabolic processes. Although pronounced changes in intermediary metabolism occur in other conditions as well, such as starvation, cancer, and various endocrine disorders, the role of cytokines and their interaction with hormones have been most extensively studied after injury, infection, and inflammation. Therefore, this chapter primarily describes metabolic control related to these conditions.

Dividing regulatory substances into hormones and mediators may seem artificial. However, the term *hormones* is used in this chapter to describe the classical hormones such as glucocorticoids, glucagon, insulin, etc., although they of course are also mediators of metabolic changes. The other substances, *mediators,* refer to signal substances released by tissues other than the endocrine organs; some of these substances may actually be regarded as hormones as well. For example, cytokines can be looked upon as hormones of the immune system. For the most part, however, the classical hormones are endocrine, i.e., they circulate in the bloodstream and achieve their actions as delivered by the circulation. In contrast, cytokines are mainly thought of as autocrine or paracrine, i.e., they act on adjacent cells or the same cell in which they are produced. When cytokines circulate in the bloodstream, it is probably mainly an overflow phenomenon, although there is some evidence they can act in an endocrine fashion as well.

Responses to Injury and Sepsis

In this section, the influence of injury and sepsis on the release of hormones and cytokines is described. The metabolic consequences of these conditions are also reviewed.

Neuroendocrine Response

It is well established that injury and sepsis promote a neuroendocrine response with an initial pronounced sympathoadrenal discharge, stimulating the release of the counter-regulatory hormones glucagon, epinephrine, norepinephrine, growth hormone (GH), and cortisol [2]. This group of hormones are called counter-regulatory because they respond to hypoglycemia and play a role in *glucose counter-regulation* [3]. Some of these hormones have a catabolic effect in different organs and tissues and are therefore called *catabolic hormones.* Usually, these hormones are elevated early after injury, during the *ebb-phase,* but they may remain increased into the *flow phase* during sustained injury, such as burn injury [4].

Different stimuli that can activate the neuroendocrine response in critical illness include (1) hemodynamic changes (caused by hemorrhage, dehydration, third-space losses, etc.); (2) changes in pH, P_{O_2}, and P_{CO_2} in tissues and blood; (3) pain; (4) anxiety; (5) changes in substrate availability (e.g., changes in plasma glucose or amino acid concentrations); (6) changes in ambient or body temperature; and (7) infection [5]. In the presence of severe injury or sepsis, several stimuli act simultaneously to induce the neuroendocrine response. The regulation of this response is summarized in Figure 3-1.

From a metabolic standpoint, cortisol is probably the most important of the counter-regulatory hormones with widespread effects on the metabolism of glucose, amino acids, and fatty acids. Glucocorticoids do not only induce metabolic changes by themselves, but they also act as a permissive agent to other mediators. Stress results in hypothalamic stimulation with release of corticotropin releasing factor (CRF), which stimulates pituitary release of corticotropin (ACTH). The ACTH, in turn, regulates the synthesis and release of cortisol from the adrenal cortex. The importance of the central nervous system for the glucocorticoid response to injury was demonstrated in a number of early studies [6,7].

Among the other counter-regulatory hormones, glucagon is increased in patients after trauma, burn injury, infection, and sepsis [8–11]. Several studies have shown that catecholamines are released after injury [12,13] and in patients with severe infection [14]. Secretion of GH is stimulated after a number of stressful situations, including hypoglycemia, exercise, hemorrhage, surgery, burn, infection, and starvation [15,16], although conflicting results have been reported [17,18]. Synthesis and release of GH in the pituitary gland is stimulated by the growth hormone releasing hormone (GHRH) and is inhibited by insulin-like growth factor-1 (IGF-1). Growth hormone exerts most, if not all, of its metabolic effects through IGF-1. The fact that IGF-1 levels are reduced in critically ill patients, despite increased GH levels [15,19], suggests that the liver (where IGF-1 is produced under the influence of GH) becomes resistant to GH during critical illness or that IGF-1 is degraded more rapidly. Plasma levels of IGF-1 may also be affected by changes in IGF-binding proteins or production of the hormone in tissues other than the liver.

In addition to changes in the counter-regulatory hormones, sepsis and trauma influence the plasma concentrations of other hormones as well, most notably insulin and thyroid hormone. Although plasma insulin levels are normally reduced during the early ebb phase after injury, they subsequently rise and usually peak during the maximal catabolic *flow phase* [2]. At this time, the insulin levels are inappropriately high for the plasma glucose levels [4,20], supporting the concept of "insulin resistance" in peripheral tissues, well described during sepsis and after trauma [2,21]. The mechanism of the elevated insulin release is not known but may reflect a potentiation of glucose-stimulated insulin secretion by amino acids; at this stage after injury and during sepsis, several plasma amino acid levels are elevated [22], including arginine, which is a potent stimulator of insulin secretion [23].

Reduced serum levels of triiodothyronine (T_3) are frequently present in injured and septic patients [24]. The mechanism of this *low T_3 syndrome* is not completely understood, but a defect in the peripheral conversion of thyroxine (T_4) to T_3 has been suggested [25]. An alternative explanation may be that the cellular uptake of T_3 in various organs and tissues is increased. In a recent study, muscle levels of T_3 were unchanged or increased in septic rats, despite reduced serum levels of the hormone [26]. Increased tissue levels of T_3 may be one of the mechanisms of the catabolic response to injury and sepsis, because many of the metabolic changes seen in these conditions resemble those observed during hyperthyroidism.

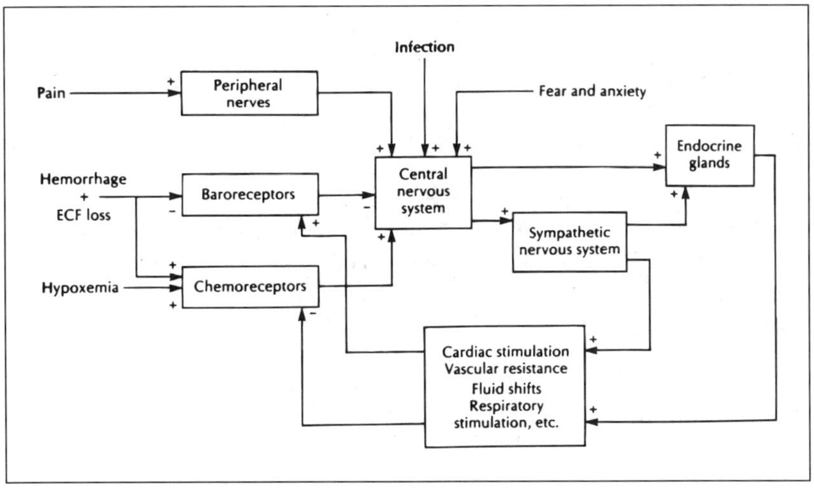

Figure 3-1. Overview of the neuroendocrine reflexes induced by shock and trauma. There are at least seven stimuli to the neuroendocrine response to trauma and shock. These include changes in the circulating body fluids; changes in the concentrations of hydrogen ions, oxygen, and carbon dioxide in tissues; pain; emotional arousal; changes in substrate availability; changes in ambient temperature or core temperature; and infection. Of these stimuli, a reduction in the effective circulating volume is of prime importance because it is almost always present. (From DS Gann et al. Neuroendocrine Response to Stress, Injury, and Sepsis. In JH Davis et al. *Surgery—A Problem Solving Approach*. St. Louis: Mosby, 1995.)

A recent study in injured pigs suggests that catecholamines may stimulate the cellular uptake of thyroid hormone [27].

Although several of the metabolic changes seen in critical illness may reflect increased levels of counter-regulatory hormones, part of the response may also be caused by a diminished influence of anabolic hormones, as exemplified by insulin resistance [21] or reduced levels of IGF-1 [15,19].

Release of Cytokines in Critical Illness

In addition to the counter-regulatory hormones, the cytokines are another group of substances that are released after injury and severe infection and participate in the control of metabolism. Cytokines are regulatory proteins of low molecular weight (the majority less than 20 kDa) that can be released from a variety of cells, although after trauma and sepsis, macrophages are probably the predominant source. Cytokines primarily act locally in an autocrine or paracrine fashion, although increased plasma levels of the substances in injured and septic patients and experimental animals [28–31] suggest that the cytokines may have a hormone-like function as well. Indeed, the cytokines may be looked upon as the hormones of the immune system. A possible biologic role of circulating cytokines was supported in experiments in which interleukin-6 (IL-6) injected into rats was found to accumulate in the liver because of binding to specific IL-6 receptors on hepatocytes [32]. The major role of IL-6 in the regulation of hepatocyte acute-phase protein synthesis is well documented [33].

In addition to their control of various metabolic processes, the cytokines influence survival after injury and sepsis, possibly because of their hemodynamic effects [30,34–36]. There is evidence that the neuroendocrine system and cytokines interact at different levels during the response to injury, inflammation, and sepsis. The production and release of the two groups of substances are interrelated; in addition, hormones and cytokines interact in the control of metabolism. The interaction between the neuroendocrine and cytokine systems is discussed further in subsequent sections of this chapter.

During sepsis and endotoxemia and after injury, cytokines are released in a sequential fashion with an early release of tumor necrosis factor (TNF), followed by subsequent production of IL-1 and IL-6 [31,37,38]. This cascade-like cytokine response is partly due to the fact that TNF can stimulate the release of IL-1 and that both IL-1 and TNF can stimulate the release of IL-6 [39–41]. The pattern of an early TNF release followed by increased production of IL-1 and IL-6 has been observed in a number of different clinical and experimental conditions, including burn injury [28], sepsis [42], and experimental endotoxemia, both in nonhuman primates and in humans [43]. The proximal position of TNF in the cytokine cascade was illustrated in a study in which antibodies to TNF reduced IL-1β and IL-6 appearance during lethal bacteremia [44]. It should be noted that although increased plasma levels of the cytokines were observed in the various conditions described above, the role of circulating cytokines is somewhat unclear. Because cytokines are thought to act primarily in an autocrine or paracrine fashion, it is possible that cytokines released into the circulation represent an overflow phenomenon caused by high local production rates in certain tissues. Evidence for local production of cytokines has been found in various tissues. For example, increased production of IL-1α was noted in mucosa of the small intestine after administration of endotoxin in mice [45]. In other studies, intestinal epithelial cell IL-1β gene expression was increased during inflammation [46]. Evidence of splanchnic production of TNF after administration of endotoxin in humans has been reported [47]. Because in those studies the splanchnic output was assessed from differences between arterial and hepatic venous TNF concentrations, it was not known from which organ or tissue the TNF originated. A cell-associated form of TNF in liver tissue of burned and infected rats has been identified [48].

A correlation between plasma levels of cytokines, in particular those of TNF and IL-6, and mortality rates in sepsis was noted in several recent studies [28,29,35], and from such observations it has been implied that these cytokines may account for the high mortality in these conditions. A recent study suggests that it may be the persistence of TNF and IL-6 in the serum, rather than the peak levels of the cytokines, that predicts a poor outcome in patients with septic shock [30].

Another factor that may influence the outcome in sepsis is the balance between the cytokines and their naturally occurring inhibitors. Soluble cytokine receptors or receptor fragments have been demonstrated in serum and urine, most likely representing shedding of receptors from the cell surface. Receptor shedding may reduce cytokine action by removing binding sites from target cells and by providing soluble inhibitors that bind to circulating cytokines. Soluble forms of receptors for TNF, IL-1, IL-6, and IFN-γ have been identified [49–52]. Two structurally distinct soluble TNF receptors have been found, and in vitro studies have shown that these binding proteins protect cells from TNF-mediated toxicity [49,50]. The complementary DNAs (cDNAs) for the two soluble TNF receptors were recently cloned and expressed as recombinant soluble TNF-binding proteins [53]. In a recent study of patients with severe meningococcemia, the ratio between serum levels of TNF-α and the soluble TNF receptors was higher in patients with fatal outcome than in survivors, supporting the concept that naturally occurring TNF inhibitors may play an important role in modulating the biologic activity of TNF in critical illness [54]. It should be noted, however, that preliminary clinical studies using recombinant soluble TNF receptors in septic patients have not been successful.

Because a correlation has been found between high cytokine levels and mortality in patients with sepsis and meningitis, attempts have been made to improve outcome by using cytokine antibodies or receptor antagonists. A protective effect of anti-TNF antibodies was demonstrated in rabbits [55] and mice [56] given otherwise lethal doses of endotoxin and in baboons with sepsis [57]. Improved survival after treatment of endotoxemic mice with anti-IL-6 antibodies was reported by Starnes and associates [58]. Although an initial study using IL-1 receptor antagonist (IL-1ra) was encouraging in showing improved survival in septic patients [59], a subsequent controlled, multicenter, prospective double-blind study did not confirm the beneficial effects of IL-1ra in septic patients [60]. A detailed analysis of the results in that study, however, indicate that a subgroup of patients with more severe sepsis may benefit from treatment with IL-1ra. That hypothesis is presently being tested in a new controlled study.

Although the discussion in this section has focused on TNF, IL-1, and IL-6 (mainly because most information regarding the regulation of metabolism has been gathered for these cytokines), it is likely that other cytokines are involved in the pathophysiology of inflammation and sepsis, including IL-4, IL-7, IL-8, IL-10, and IFN-γ [61-63].

Mechanisms of Sepsis/Endotoxin-Induced Production of Cytokines

The regulation of cytokine production/release during sepsis and after injury is not fully understood. In a recent study, the increases in serum TNF and IL-6 activities were proportional to tissue injury induced by surgical trauma and shock in rats, suggesting that the cytokine production is regulated by factors released from necrotic or injured tissue [64]. Other results suggest that the release of TNF during severe infection is modulated by the complement component C5 [65]. As discussed above, however, one must bear in mind that there is a question as to whether increased circulating levels of cytokines represent a physiologic action or merely a pathologic overflow phenomenon.

The cellular stimulation by endotoxin (lipopolysaccharide [LPS]) of macrophages and other cell types to produce cytokines requires three important steps: (1) LPS-cell interaction; (2) intracellular signaling; and (3) molecular regulation of cytokine synthesis. All these aspects have been the subject of recent research and have been reviewed more extensively elsewhere [66,67].

There is evidence that endotoxin binds to macrophages on specific LPS receptors [67,68]. At least three different groups of LPS receptors have been identified: the CD11/CD18 group, the CD14 receptor, and the acetyl–low-density lipoprotein or *scavenger* receptor. The binding of endotoxin to CD14 receptor is the most important mechanism for induction of cytokines. Recent studies demonstrated that endotoxin first must form a complex with the LPS binding protein (LBP) before it binds to CD14 [69]. Binding of the LBP + LPS complex to the CD14 receptor triggers the synthesis and release of cytokines.

The activation of cellular processes by external stimuli after binding to the receptor is accomplished by second messenger pathways. Two major intracellular signal pathways have been identified. One uses cyclic adenosine monophosphate (cAMP) and protein kinase A, and the other uses inositol triphosphate and diacylglycerol, which activate calmodulin-dependent (CaM) kinase and protein kinase C (PKc), respectively (Figure 3-2). By using specific inhibitors of the different pathways, it has been possible to establish that the synthesis of IL-1 is regulated both by the PKc and CaM kinase pathway, whereas TNF is regulated only by PKc (Figure 3-3) [70].

The synthesis of cytokines after stimulation with endotoxin is regulated both at the transcriptional and translational level. The addition of LPS to macrophages triggers an increase in gene transcription as well as translation of "stored" and newly synthesized messenger RNA (mRNA). In the absence of stimulation, macrophages usually do not express detectable levels of cytokine mRNA. However, cytokine genes are rapidly induced after treatment with endotoxin; IL-1β mRNA expression was induced as early as 1 hour after endotoxin stimulation, reached a peak at 6 hours, and remained elevated for at least 16 hours [71]. In other studies, TNF-α mRNA levels peaked at 90 minutes after endotoxin treatment of macrophages [72]. When blockers of either the PKc or CaM kinase

Figure 3-2. Signal transduction pathway through cyclic AMP (cAMP) and protein kinase A *(left)* and through CaM kinase and protein kinase C *(right)*. External signals arrive through interaction with cell surface receptors, which initiates membrane associated and intracellular pathways, activating the different kinases. (Reprinted with permission from EJ Kovacs. Control of IL-1 and TNFα Production at the Level of Second Messenger Pathways. In ES Kimball [ed], *Cytokines and Inflammation.* Boca Raton: CRC, 1991. Copyright CRC Press, Boca Raton, Florida.)

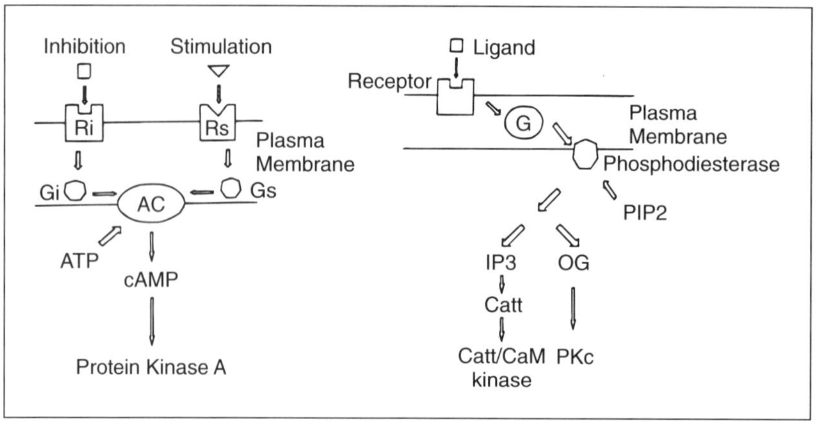

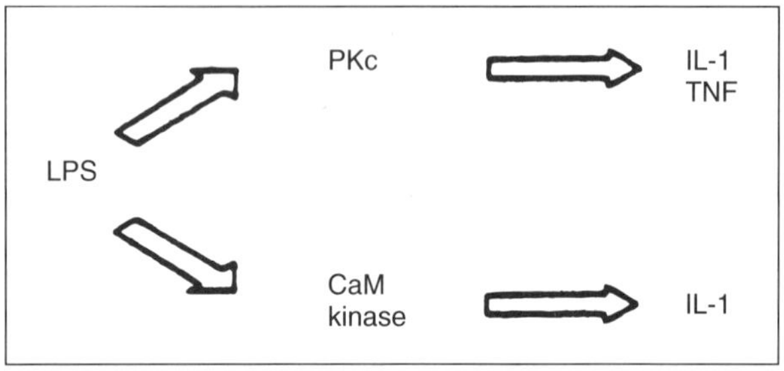

Figure 3-3. Second messenger pathways involved in the control of IL-1 and TNF mRNA expression in monocytes following treatment with LPS. (Reprinted with permission from EJ Kovacs. Control of IL-1 and TNFα Production at the Level of Second Messenger Pathways. In ES Kimball (ed), *Cytokines and Inflammation.* Boca Raton: CRC, 1991. Copyright CRC Press, Boca Raton, Florida.)

were used, the induction of IL-1 gene expression induced by endotoxin was inhibited. In contrast, only the PKc dependent pathway was required for LPS induction of TNF-α mRNA expression, supporting the concept that CaM-dependent kinase is not involved in the LPS-stimulated production of TNF (see Figure 3-3).

In a recent report, the molecular regulation of IL-1 production after injection of endotoxin was studied in mice both by Northern analysis of total RNA and by in situ hybridization using murine cDNA probes [46]. During endotoxemia, a dramatic induction of IL-1 mRNA was noted in the small bowel. In situ hybridization showed increased signals after endotoxin in the lamina propria and in the bottom of the crypts, suggesting that endotoxin up-regulates IL-1 gene expression in macrophages in the lamina propria and in intestinal crypt cells. Using similar techniques, Radema and colleagues [73] found that experimental colitis in rats was associated with an early up-regulation of IL-1β mRNA levels and that this occurred predominantly in undifferentiated cells in the basal parts of the mucosal crypts. In a more recent study, administration of endotoxin in rats resulted in elevated serum IL-6 levels and increased mRNA levels for IL-6 in the spleen, pituitary gland, and adrenals, suggesting that this cytokine is also regulated at the transcriptional level [74]. Interestingly, in the same study, treatment of rats with corticosterone blocked the increase of IL-6 in serum and tissue levels of IL-6 mRNA, suggesting that the endotoxin-induced IL-6 gene expression is subject to glucocorticoid suppression [74].

Interaction Between Hormones and Cytokines: The Immune-Neuroendocrine Network

Several lines of evidence suggest that the neuroendocrine and immune (cytokines) systems interact at different levels. The proinflammatory cytokines TNF, IL-1, and IL-6 stimulate the hypothalamic-pituitary-adrenal axis, resulting in the release of ACTH and glucocorticoids [75–77]. Administration of TNF to normal human subjects results in a pronounced stress hormone response with elevated plasma levels of ACTH, cortisol, catecholamines, GH, and glucagon. In addition to stimulating the hypothalamic-pituitary-adrenal axis, there is evidence that at least IL-1 has a direct effect on the adrenals. In a recent study, the capacities of IL-1, IL-6, and TNF to stimulate the release of ACTH and corticosterone were compared in rats; all three cytokines stimulated the pituitary-adrenal axis, but IL-1 was most potent [37].

In addition to a stimulatory effect of cytokines on the pituitary-adrenal axis, glucocorticoids inhibit the release of cytokines from macrophages and other cells, consistent with a negative feedback mechanism between the two systems [78]. This may be a mechanism by which the body is protected from dangerously high levels of cytokines during trauma and sepsis. In recent studies, glucocorticoids reduced cytokine mRNA transcription rates in various cell types [79]. A similar regulatory mechanism was demonstrated in vivo; treatment of rats with corticosterone completely blocked the endotoxin-induced increase in IL-6 mRNA levels in spleen, adrenals, and hypophysis [74], suggesting that the IL-6 gene contains sequences that respond to glucocorticoids and bind the glucocorticoid-receptor complex. In studies using cultured HeLa cells, evidence was found that glucocorticoid repression of IL-6 gene expression involves direct binding of the glucocorticoid receptor to functional DNA elements in the IL-6 promoter [80].

In contrast to inhibited production of cytokines by glucocorticoids, there is evidence that the binding of cytokines to cell surface receptors is stimulated by steroids. For example, the binding of IL-1 to human neutrophils was increased in the presence of dexamethasone, and this response was the result of an increase in IL-1 receptor numbers rather than a change in binding affinity [81].

An additional example of the interaction between the endocrine and immune systems is the reduced serum T_3 levels after administration of TNF [82] or IL-1 [83]. These results suggest that cytokines, in addition to or perhaps in combination with catecholamines [27], are important for the development of the "low T_3 syndrome" in sepsis and after trauma [24].

Metabolic Responses to Injury and Sepsis

Regulation of protein, carbohydrate, and lipid metabolism under normal conditions is discussed in detail in other chapters of this book (Chapters 6 to 8). A brief description of the metabolic responses to injury, sepsis, and inflammation is given here to provide a background to the role of hormones and mediators in the control of metabolism.

Ebb and Flow

The metabolic response to injury and sepsis is usually divided into an ebb and flow phase followed by a convalescence phase (Figure 3-4). This metabolic pattern is better defined after injury than during sepsis, because there is a well-defined time sequence starting at the time of injury, whereas the septic insult can be more prolonged and can fluctuate in intensity during its course. This was illustrated in a recent study in which hormone levels and energy production rates were measured on a daily basis during the first week after admission to the hospital in 12 consecutive patients with severe sepsis [18]. The specific pattern of the endocrine and metabolic responses commonly seen after injury did not occur in the septic patients.

The ebb phase is characterized by glycogenolysis and lipolysis [2], providing the organism with readily available energy for "fight or flight." The ebb phase is followed by the *catabolic phase* or

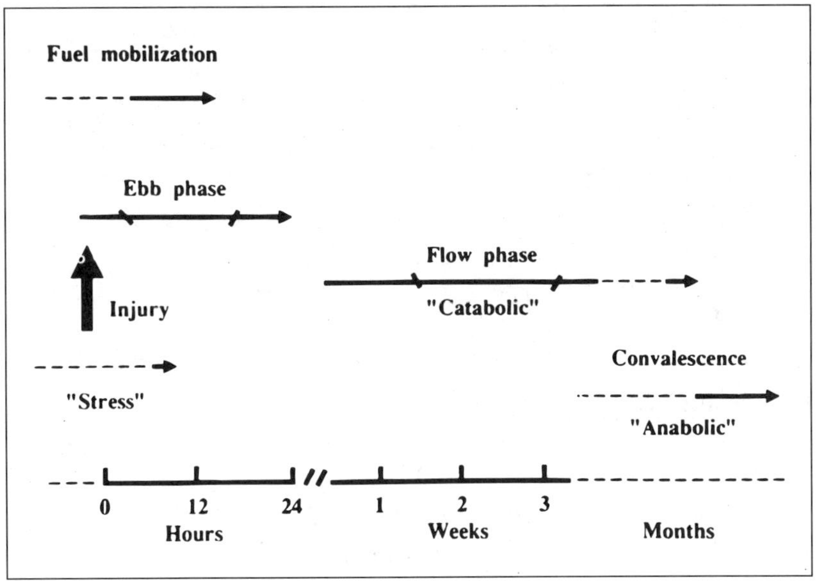

Figure 3-4. Phases of the response to injury. The duration of each phase is variable and representative figures only are given. The course of the metabolic response to sepsis is seldom as well defined as outlined in this figure (see text). (Redrawn from KN Frayn. Hormonal Control of Metabolism in Trauma and Sepsis. *Clin Endocrinol* 24:577, 1986.)

flow phase, characterized by increased metabolic rate, elevated body temperature and pulse rate, increased urinary nitrogen excretion and muscle catabolism. The subsequent anabolic convalescence phase can last from weeks to months.

During sepsis, the typical features of the ebb and flow phases are usually more reflective of severity of the condition, rather than of the time course. Patients with severe sepsis or septic shock usually exhibit many of the characteristics of the ebb phase, whereas patients with more chronic and less severe sepsis display the hypermetabolism and catabolism of the flow phase *(hypermetabolic sepsis).*

Carbohydrate Metabolism

The early metabolic response to endotoxemia and sepsis is characterized by an elevated rate of glucose appearance, mainly reflecting increased hepatic glucose production and stimulated glucose utilization by multiple tissues [84]. In the fed state, hepatic glucose production results from an early stimulation of glycogenolysis followed by increased gluconeogenesis. The rate of glucose appearance usually exceeds the rate of glucose disposal, resulting in increased plasma glucose levels during this phase of endotoxemia and sepsis. An additional mechanism of hyperglycemia is the insulin resistance in muscle and fat that results in a relative inhibition of glucose uptake in those tissues [21].

The increased glucose disposal during sepsis and endotoxemia primarily reflects increased uptake of glucose by macrophage-rich tissues and certain muscles. When hypermetabolic sepsis or endotoxemia was induced in rats, whole-body glucose disposal increased, mainly reflecting enhanced rate of glucose removal by some (but not all) muscles, liver, spleen, small intestine, and skin (Figure 3-5) [85,86]. In the same study, glucose uptake was increased in the diaphragm, whereas other muscles (gastrocnemius, heart) did not increase their glucose uptake. Studies by Spitzer and colleagues [87] demonstrated that the increased uptake of glucose by the liver during endotoxemia reflects increased glucose utilization by nonparenchymal cells (Kupffer cells and endothelial cells). In addition, endotoxemia was associated with a substantial inflow of neutrophils into the liver, and these cells also contributed to the increase in glucose uptake. In contrast, glucose uptake by the hepatocytes was not increased during endotoxemia. Thus, during endotoxemia, the different cell populations in the liver respond in an opposite way with respect to glucose kinetics; glucose production is increased in the hepatocyte, at least during early endotoxemia and sepsis, reflecting glycogenolysis and gluconeogenesis, whereas glucose uptake is increased in nonparenchymal cells. The net effect of these changes, however, is increased release of glucose from the liver as a whole during early endotoxemia and hypermetabolic sepsis.

During protracted and more severe endotoxemia and septic shock, hypoglycemia usually devel-

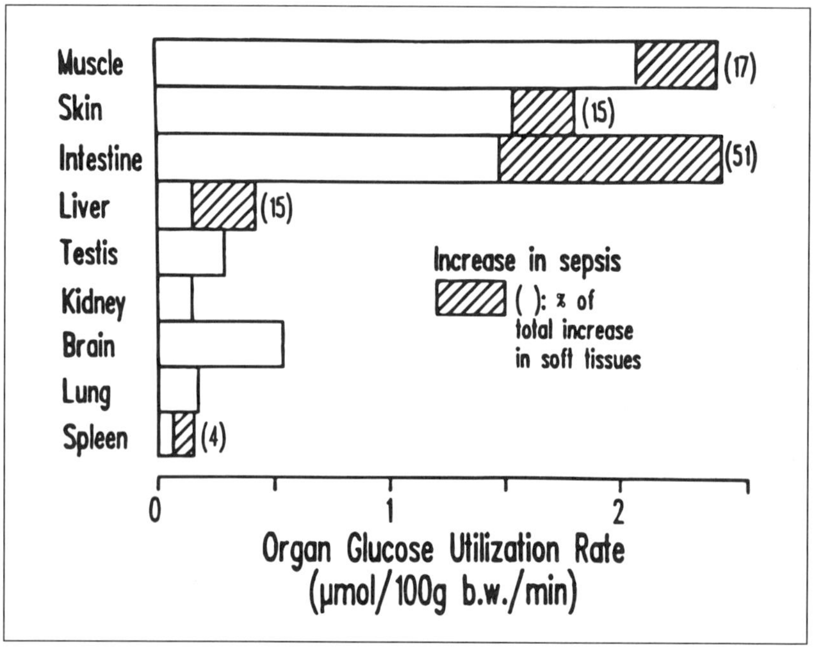

Figure 3-5. In vivo glucose utilization by individual organs in septic and nonseptic rats. Hypermetabolic sepsis was induced by subcutaneous injections of live *E. coli* bacteria. Glucose utilization rate of tissue was determined by the 2-deoxyglucose tracer method. Open bars show glucose utilization by whole organs and organ systems in nonseptic rats. Hatched bars represent the increase induced by sepsis. (From JJ Spitzer et al. Alterations in lipid and carbohydrate metabolism in sepsis. *JPEN* 12:535, 1988.)

ops [88]. This is primarily the result of reduced hepatic production of glucose. During a prolonged septic course, the glycogen stores in the liver are depleted; the glucose production has to rely on gluconeogenesis and this may also fail. Evidence of inhibited gluconeogenesis during endotoxemia has been found both in perfused liver and isolated hepatocytes [89]. The inhibited gluconeogenesis is caused by a combination of reduced levels of gluconeogenic substrates and altered enzyme activities. Although some studies suggest that impaired gluconeogenesis reflects reduced activity of the enzyme phosphoenolpyruvate carboxykinase, other reports indicate that stimulated phosphofructokinase-1 activity is more important for impairment of hepatic gluconeogenesis during sepsis and endotoxemia [89].

Studies in septic rats demonstrated that the increased uptake of glucose by several macrophage-rich tissues (liver, spleen, lung, ileum, and skin) persists even when plasma glucose levels are low [90]. This, of course, worsens the hypoglycemia that may ultimately contribute to mortality in septic shock.

The relationship between the severity of endotoxemia and the changes in glucose kinetics was illustrated in a study by Lang and associates [91]. When rats were injected with endotoxin at doses that induced hypotension and reduced cardiac output (endotoxin ranging from 10 to 1,000 μg/100 g body weight), early increases in plasma glucose levels and glucose appearance rate were followed subsequently by reduced glucose appearance and hypoglycemia. In contrast, smaller doses of endotoxin (ranging from 0.01 to 1 μg/100 g body weight), which did not induce hemodynamic alterations (but did induce a febrile response), gave rise to a delayed and sustained increase in glucose appearance and hyperglycemia.

A recent study compared the changes in carbohydrate metabolism induced by sepsis or endotoxemia in rats [92]. Sepsis, induced by cecal ligation and puncture (CLP), gave rise to a similar metabolic pattern as seen after the intravenous injection of endotoxin (16.7 mg/kg), i.e., an early increase in plasma glucose levels followed later by hypoglycemia, although (as expected) the metabolic changes after CLP developed more slowly. The results are important because they support the concept that the metabolic changes seen during sepsis are mediated by endotoxin.

The changes in glucose metabolism during early and late sepsis/endotoxemia are summarized in Figure 3-6.

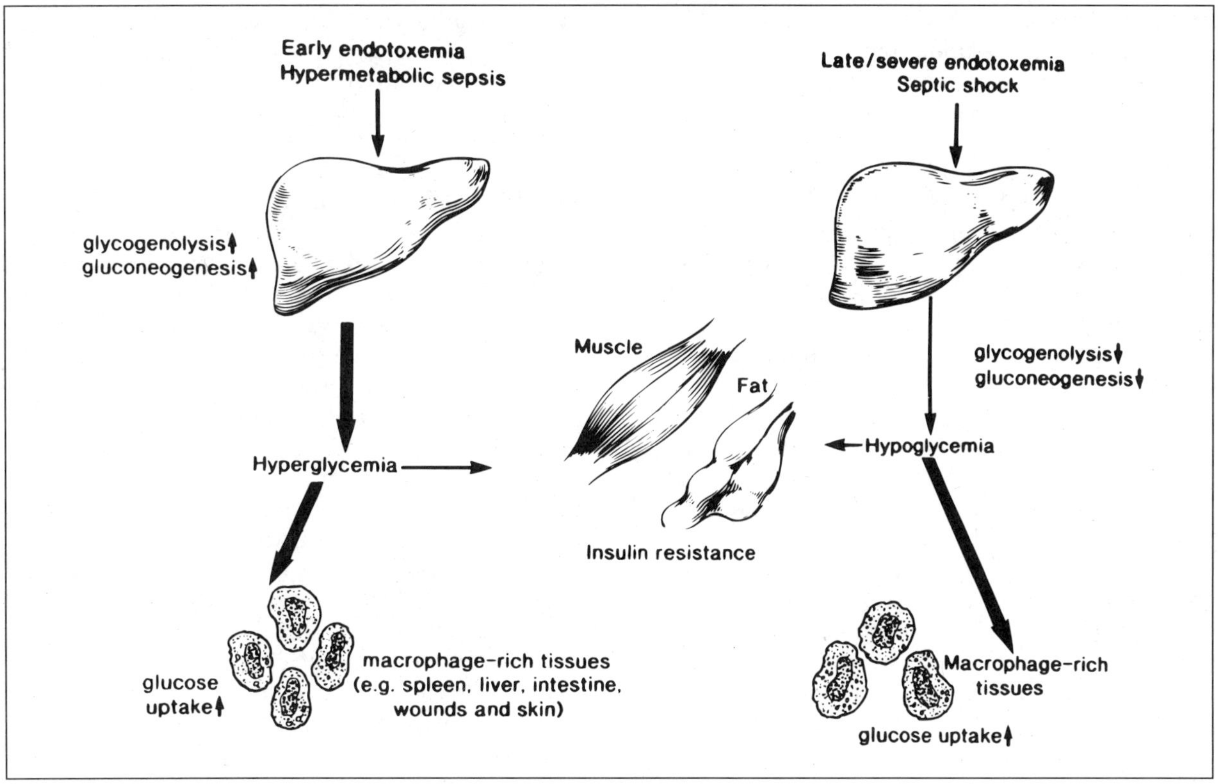

Figure 3-6. Summary of carbohydrate metabolism during early endotoxemia/hypermetabolic sepsis *(left)* and late endotoxemia/septic shock *(right)*.

Lipid Metabolism

Injury and sepsis are associated with increased fat metabolism manifested by increased circulating levels of free fatty acids, triglycerides, and cholesterol [2,93–95]. The changes in lipid metabolism seen in patients with metabolic stress are caused by a combination of several factors. Reduced activity of the enzyme lipoprotein lipase in muscle and adipose tissue decreases the clearance of triglyceride-rich lipoproteins [96]. Increased lipolysis in adipose tissue contributes to the hyperlipidemia. Stimulated synthesis in the liver of apolipoproteins and triglycerides, however, are probably the major mechanisms of hypertriglyceridemia after injury and infection. Two mechanisms support the increased synthesis of triglycerides in the liver during sepsis: (1) increased flux of fatty acids to the liver resulting from stimulated lipolysis in adipose tissue and (2) increased de novo synthesis of fatty acids in the liver. Although increased synthesis of triglycerides in the liver during sepsis is well agreed upon, the influence of sepsis and endotoxemia on the secretion of triglycerides is controversial, with both unchanged and decreased secretion being reported.

Impaired perfusion of adipose tissue during severe sepsis or endotoxic shock may result in reduced lipolysis and can explain why plasma levels of free fatty acids are not always increased under those circumstances. Another reason why plasma levels of fatty acids and triglycerides are not always increased after injury and sepsis is that the rate of fatty acid clearance (peripheral oxidation) can be higher than the rate of appearance (lipolysis) or production (hepatic lipogenesis).

From a teleologic standpoint, inhibition of lipid deposition in adipose tissue and mobilization of lipid stores, in combination with increased hepatic synthesis of fatty acids and triglycerides, provide lipid substrates for oxidation in other tissues, including muscle and the immune system, thereby sparing glucose for the nervous system. Another important aspect of the sepsis- and endotoxin-induced changes in lipid metabolism is the observation that lipoproteins, including very low-density lipoproteins, can bind endotoxin [97]. Studies have shown that this binding of endotoxin by lipoproteins can protect animals from the toxic and lethal effects of endotoxin [98]. One result of the binding of endotoxin to lipoproteins is inhibited ability of endotoxin to stimulate secretion of cytokines by macrophages [99]; this may be one of the mechanisms by which lipoproteins can prevent mortality after endotoxin. In addition to binding endotoxin, lipoproteins bind a number of different viruses and can reduce the toxic effects of these viruses [100].

Protein Metabolism

The metabolic changes that have probably been most widely described after injury and severe infection are those that affect protein metabolism. Although critical illness can influence protein turnover in virtually all organs and tissues, the metabolic changes that occur in skeletal muscle, liver, intestine, and lungs have attracted the greatest interest. Closely related to changes in protein metabolism are changes in amino acid transport and metabolism; alterations in uptake and intracellular metabolism of amino acids can result in changes in cellular amino acid concentrations that in turn may influence protein synthesis and breakdown rates. Changes in the intracellular concentrations of certain amino acids, such as alanine, leucine, and glutamine, may have particularly great impact on protein turnover rates. Any discussion of regulation of protein metabolism, therefore, must also include considerations of amino acid transport and metabolism. Changes in protein and amino acid metabolism during sepsis were reviewed recently [101] and will only be briefly summarized here.

In studies by Sir David Cuthbertson, published more than 60 years ago, increased urinary excretion of nitrogen, phosphate, and sulphate was noticed in injured patients [102]. A number of subsequent studies provided evidence that skeletal muscle is the major source of these substances, and negative nitrogen balance and muscle catabolism are now well recognized metabolic responses to sepsis and injury.

The catabolic condition in muscle that develops during critical illness is multifactorial and is caused by a combination of reduced protein synthesis, increased protein breakdown, and inhibited amino acid uptake [101]. From a quantitative standpoint, the increase in protein breakdown seems to be the most important component of muscle catabolism during critical illness. Of particular interest is the pronounced increase in myofibrillar protein breakdown as evidenced by urinary excretion of 3-methylhistidine (3-MH; an amino acid present only in the myofibrillar proteins actin and myosin) in injured and septic patients [103] and by increased release of 3-MH by incubated muscles from septic rats [104]. The breakdown of myofibrillar proteins may partly explain the muscle weakness of catabolic patients and may severely impair the recovery in these patients.

The intracellular and molecular mechanisms of muscle proteolysis during catabolic conditions have been explored only recently. Muscle cells contain multiple proteolytic pathways that are regulated by specific enzymes and serve different physiologic functions [105,106]. Principally, pro-

Table 3-1. Different Intracellular Proteolytic Pathways in Skeletal Muscle

Pathway	Enzymes
Lysosomal	Cathepsin B, H, L
Nonlysosomal	
Energy dependent	
Ubiquitin dependent	26S protease
Ubiquitin independent	600-kDa protease
Energy independent	
Ca dependent	Calpain I, II

Source: PO Hasselgren. *Protein Metabolism in Sepsis.* Austin: Landes, 1993.

teins are degraded by lysosomal or nonlysosomal mechanisms (Table 3-1). The nonlysosomal proteolytic pathways include energy-dependent and energy-independent pathways. Among the different proteolytic pathways, the lysosomal and the energy–ubiquitin-dependent pathways are probably the most important mechanisms for regulation of protein degradation during various physiologic and pathophysiologic conditions. The different proteolytic pathways are responsible for the breakdown of different classes of proteins (Figure 3-7).

The ubiquitin-dependent system for protein degradation is a relatively newly described mechanism of protein breakdown [107]. Ubiquitin is a 76-amino acid residue polypeptide present in all eukaryotic cells that is required for the activity of an adenosine triphosphate (ATP)–dependent, nonlysosomal proteolytic pathway. In addition to a role in nonlysosomal protein breakdown, the ubiquitin system is involved in a number of other cellular processes such as cell cycle control, DNA repair, ribosome biosynthesis, and the stress response.

Proteins that are degraded in the ubiquitin system are first conjugated to ubiquitin, whereafter they are degraded by a high molecular weight 26S protease complex [108,109]. After proteolysis, free and reusable ubiquitin is released from the polyubiquitin chain and can be reused in the proteolytic pathway. The different steps in the ubiquitin-dependent proteolytic pathway are summarized in Figure 3-8. Of note is the fact that ATP is required for at least three steps in the ubiquitin system. Different aspects of the ubiquitin system have been reviewed extensively in several reports, including molecular genetics [110], various biologic roles, biochemistry and enzymology [108], and involvement in pathologic conditions [111]. More than 40 gene products are involved in trafficking ubiquitin, and several of the genes encoding ubiquitin and the various ubiquitin-activating enzymes have been sequenced.

Recent studies from our group suggest that muscle proteolysis during sepsis is at least partly caused by activation of the ubiquitin system and that this activation occurs at the transcriptional level [112]. By using specific blockers of the different proteolytic pathways, we found evidence that sepsis stimulates a nonlysosomal, energy-dependent mechanism, and Northern analysis of muscle RNA extracts revealed increased levels of ubiquitin mRNA in muscle from septic rats (Figure 3-9). Evidence for ubiquitin-dependent muscle proteolysis has been reported in other catabolic conditions as well, including denervation [113] and starvation [114].

One of the consequences of stimulated protein breakdown and inhibited protein synthesis is increased release of amino acids from muscle. Inhibited cellular uptake of amino acids further contributes to the peripheral release of amino acids [115,116]. Of particular interest is the release of

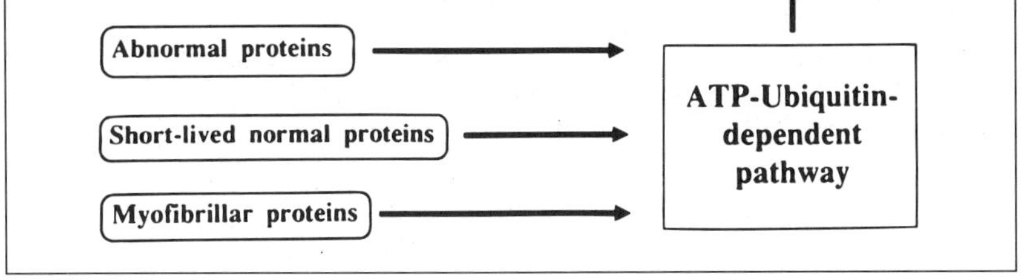

Figure 3-7. Different types of intracellular proteins are predominantly degraded by the lysosomal or the nonlysosomal, energy and ubiquitin-dependent pathway. (From PO Hasselgren. *Protein Metabolism in Sepsis.* Austin: Landes, 1993.)

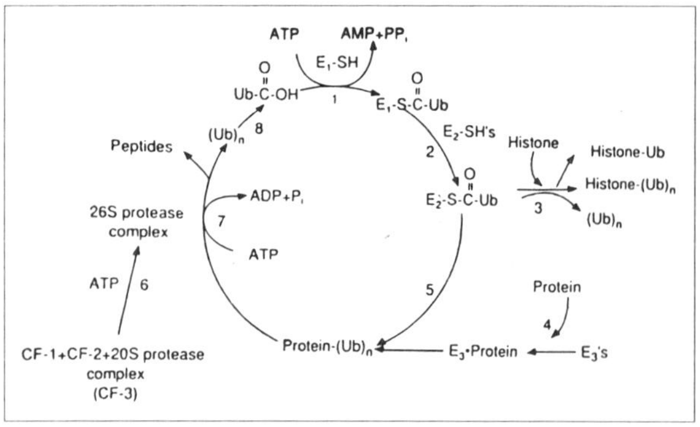

Figure 3-8. Simplified scheme of events in the ubiquitin (Ub) proteolytic pathway. (Reproduced, with permission, from the *Annual Review of Biochemistry,* Volume 61, © 1992, by *Annual Reviews Inc.*)

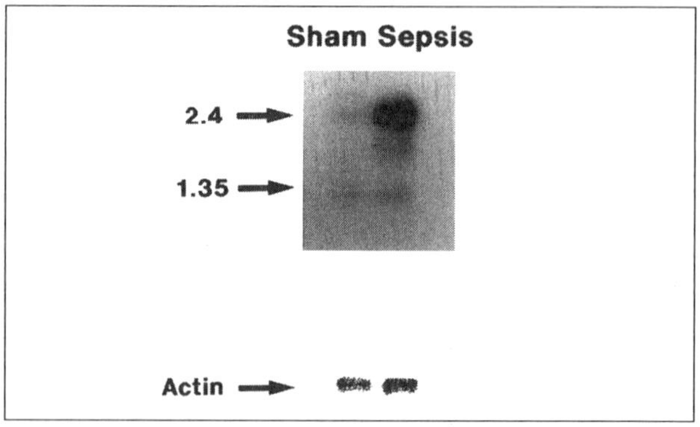

Figure 3-9. Northern blot analysis of ubiquitin (Ub) mRNA and smooth muscle actin mRNA in 5 pooled muscles from sham-operated and septic rats (16 hours after CLP).

glutamine from skeletal muscle, resulting in reduced intracellular concentrations of this amino acid. The reduced glutamine levels may be one of the mechanisms of increased muscle proteolysis and inhibited protein synthesis after injury and sepsis and during starvation [117,118]. Another important biologic consequence of the release of glutamine is that the amino acid is made available to cells that rely on this amino acid for optimal function and energy production, such as intestinal epithelial cells [119] and cells in the immune system [120].

There is also evidence that a large proportion of amino acids released from muscle during sepsis and other critical illness is taken up by the liver [121]. These amino acids support hepatic gluconeogenesis and, perhaps more importantly, the synthesis of acute-phase proteins. Increased hepatic protein synthesis has been reported after trauma and during sepsis in a number of previous studies in patients and experimental animals [122–127].

The acute-phase proteins are a heterogenous group of plasma proteins with various biologic functions. They serve a number of different roles in inflammation and in restoring homeostasis after injury and sepsis. The biologic functions of different acute-phase proteins were reviewed recently [128]. Considering the wide variety of important biologic functions ascribed to these proteins, it is not surprising that they are important for the outcome in sepsis and inflammation. Clowes and colleagues [129] reported that survival in septic patients was dependent on a well-maintained acute-phase response in the liver, i.e., an effective extraction of amino acids and protein synthesis. Other studies also found that the risk for fatal outcome in surgical patients with sepsis was increased when the synthesis of acute-phase proteins was impaired [130].

Studies on the cellular mechanisms of acute-phase protein synthesis suggest that sepsis and inflammation do not affect all hepatocytes in a homogenous fashion. Thus, at least during the early phase of the acute-phase response, protein synthesis is stimulated mainly in the periportal hepatocytes [131]. A recent study suggests that the inhibition of synthesis of albumin (a "negative" acute-phase reactant) also affects hepatocytes in a heterogenous fashion, with the most pronounced changes noted in the periportal hepatocytes [132]. This distribution of hepatocytes ("zonation") with altered protein synthesis rates may be caused by gradients in oxygen, nutrients, and perhaps more importantly, inflammatory mediators, as described in subsequent sections of this chapter.

Other studies have provided evidence that although not all hepatocytes are recruited for the acute-phase response, at least not initially, each individual hepatocyte that participates in the acute-phase response is capable of exhibiting a full response, i.e., simultaneously increasing the synthesis of multiple acute-phase proteins and reducing the production of albumin [133]. In this context, it is worth pointing out that the reduction in albumin synthesis during the acute-phase response may be relatively short-lived; studies in a chronic model of sepsis indicate that albumin synthesis is quickly restored, perhaps as early as 24 to 48 hours after onset of sepsis [126].

The genes for several acute-phase proteins have been cloned, making it possible to study the molecular regulation of the acute-phase response. In humans, C-reactive protein (CRP) is a major acute-phase reactant. The CRP gene has been cloned by several groups [134,135]. A schematic representation of the CRP gene is given in Figure 3-10. The CRP gene is present on human chromosome 1 and is 2263 bases long. The gene has a 278 base pair (bp) unique intron. The length of the spliced mature CRP mRNA is approximately

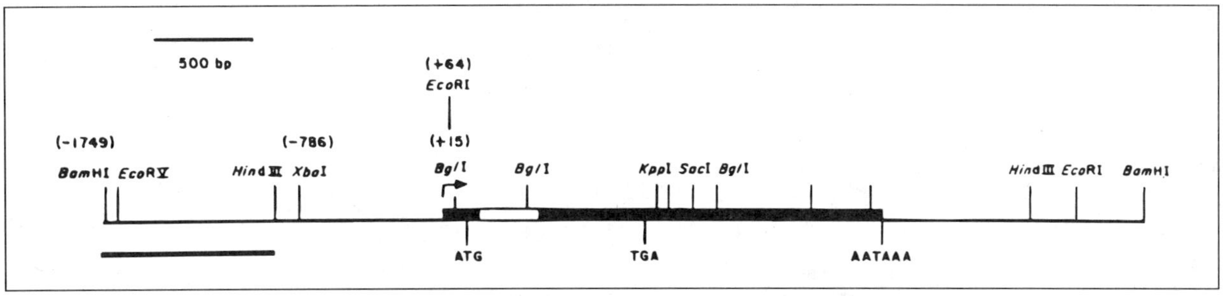

Figure 3-10. Structure of the human CRP gene. Restriction map of a 5.6 kb *Bam*HI-*Bam*HI genomic fragment carrying the CRP gene. Filled boxes represent exons. Open box represents the unique intron. The bar at the bottom indicates the *Bam*HI-*Hind*III fragment used as a probe in the mapping of DNase I-hypersensitive sites. (From C. Toniatti et al. Regulation of the human C-reactive protein gene, a major marker of inflammation and cancer. *Mol Biol Med* 7:199, 1990.)

2000 bases and is detectable in liver tissue of individuals during inflammation but not in liver samples of normal subjects [136].

Increased concentrations in liver tissue of mRNA for positive acute-phase proteins and reduced levels of mRNA for albumin (a negative acute-phase reactant) during inflammation are consistent with regulation of acute-phase protein synthesis at the transcriptional level [137], although changes in mRNA stability can give rise to similar results. Although transcriptional regulation seems to be important for acute-phase protein synthesis, there is evidence that regulation occurs at the posttranscriptional level as well. For example, in the rat, plasma levels of α_2-macroglobulin increase nearly 100-fold during the acute-phase response. This increase is preceded by an approximately 70-fold increase in cytoplasmic mRNA. Nuclear run-on experiments showed that the α_2-macroglobulin gene transcription is increased only 4- to 5-fold during inflammation [138], suggesting that in addition to an increase in transcription rate, posttranscriptional mechanisms are probably involved in the increased levels of α_2-macroglobulin mRNA.

Although the intestine has one of the highest protein turnover rates in the body, accounting for 10% to 15% of total body protein production under normal conditions, it is not until recently that the influence of injury and sepsis on protein turnover in the gastrointestinal tract has been examined. Results from those studies suggest that sepsis stimulates protein synthesis in mucosa of the small intestine [139]. Measurement of protein turnover rates in isolated jejunal enterocytes demonstrated that both sepsis (induced by CLP in rats) and endotoxemia stimulate protein synthesis in enterocytes from different levels of the villi, although the increase in protein synthesis was most pronounced in cells from the lower parts of the villi and the crypts [140]. In addition to enterocytes, intestinal mucosa contains a number of other cell types such as lymphocytes, macrophages, and endothelial cells. The response to sepsis and inflammation of protein turnover in these cells has not been reported.

The mechanisms of increased mucosal protein synthesis during sepsis is not fully understood at present. The response may partly reflect increased cellular turnover, secondary to cell loss from the tips of the villi [141]. Other mechanisms are probably involved as well, and it is possible that the response in part reflects increased synthesis of specific proteins. In recent studies, the production of certain gut peptides, i.e., vasoactive intestinal peptide and peptide YY, was increased in enterocytes isolated from septic rats [142]. Thus, the increased circulating levels of these and other gastrointestinal hormones observed during sepsis and endotoxemia [143] may be caused by increased synthesis of these substances in mucosa of the small intestine.

The changes in protein metabolism in various organs and tissues may be an integrated response to sepsis supporting the body's defense against invading bacteria and tissue injury. For example, increased protein breakdown in muscle and lung results in increased release of glutamine and other amino acids, supporting protein synthesis and other functions in the liver, intestine, and immune system. This concept of an integrated response was discussed in more detail elsewhere [101] and is summarized in Figure 3-11. The fact that several of the metabolic changes depicted in Figure 3-11 are subject to the same control mechanisms (discussed below) further supports the notion that changes in protein metabolism and amino acid fluxes are part of an integrated response and serve an important purpose in critical illness. During prolonged and severe illness, several of the meta-

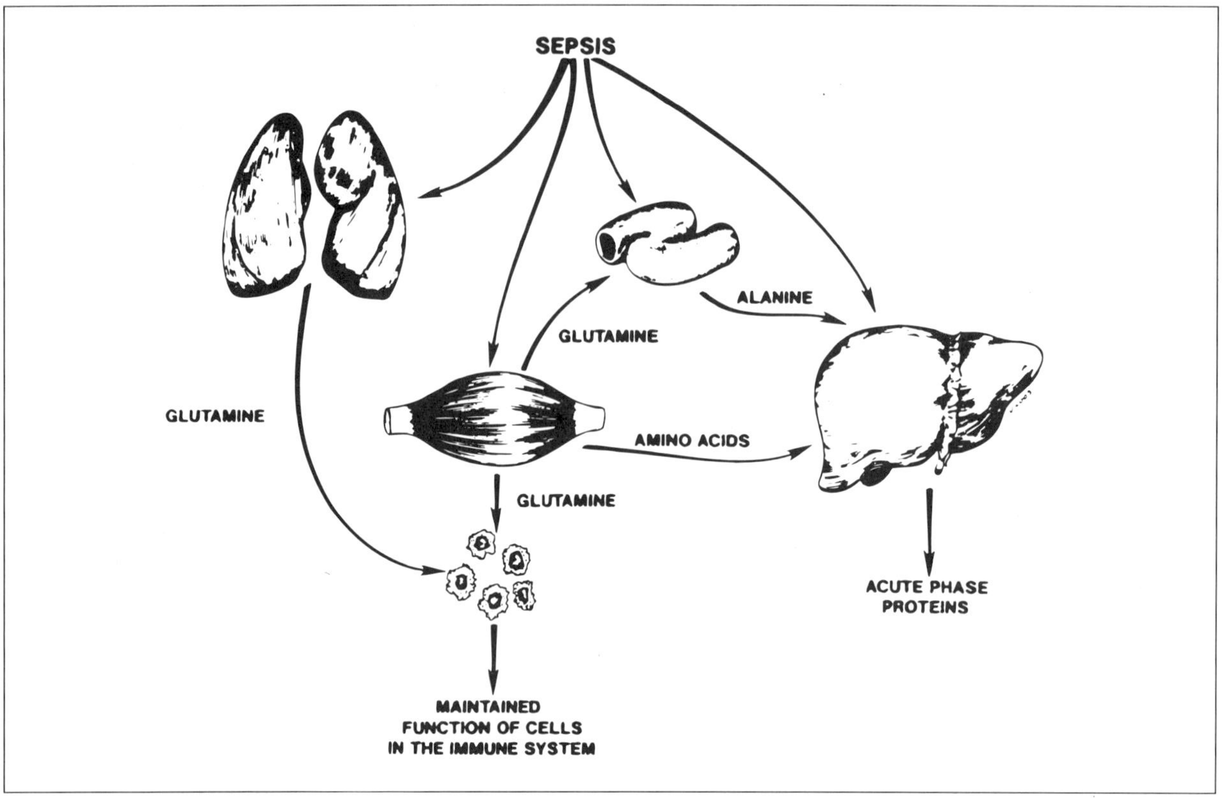

Figure 3-11. Integrated concept of sepsis-induced changes in protein metabolism. The function of cells in the immune system and synthesis of acute-phase proteins are supported by changes in protein turnover in skeletal muscle, liver, intestine, and lungs. (From PO Hasselgren. *Protein Metabolism in Sepsis.* Austin: Landes, 1993.)

bolic changes may "get out of control" and multiple organ failure may be the result. One of the features of the integrated response is that at least in the liver, acute-phase reactants may be synthesized at the expense, as it were, of structural and repair proteins. It is possible that a prolonged failure to synthesize structural proteins may at least in part contribute to the hepatic failure of sepsis.

Control of Metabolism

The focus of this section is to describe the role of hormones and cytokines in the regulation of intermediary metabolism. The interaction between the endocrine and immune systems in the control of metabolism will also be reviewed. In addition, the metabolic effects of nitric oxide, prostaglandins, and oxygen radicals will be discussed.

Hormones

Mechanisms of Action

Humans possess several hundred different hormones that interact with an even larger number of different cell types throughout the body. Hormones can act on cells remote from the production site (endocrine effect), on adjacent cells (paracrine effect), or on the secretory cell itself (autocrine effect).

The genetic control of hormone formation and the molecular pathways of hormone action have been extensively studied in recent years. Some of the results from those studies will be briefly described here. More extensive reviews can be found elsewhere [144–146].

Polypeptide hormones are a group of hormones consisting of approximately 100 small proteins and peptides ranging in size from as few as three amino acids (thyrotropin releasing hormone [TRH]) to 192 amino acids (GH). Most of the genes encoding these hormones have been cloned. The production of nonpeptide hormones such as catecholamines, thyroid hormones, and steroid hormones is regulated by multiple enzymes and is therefore controlled by the expression of multiple genes.

The steps involved in the cellular synthesis of peptide hormones are depicted in Figure 3-12 and are, of course, common for the synthesis of any peptide or protein. The formation of polypeptide

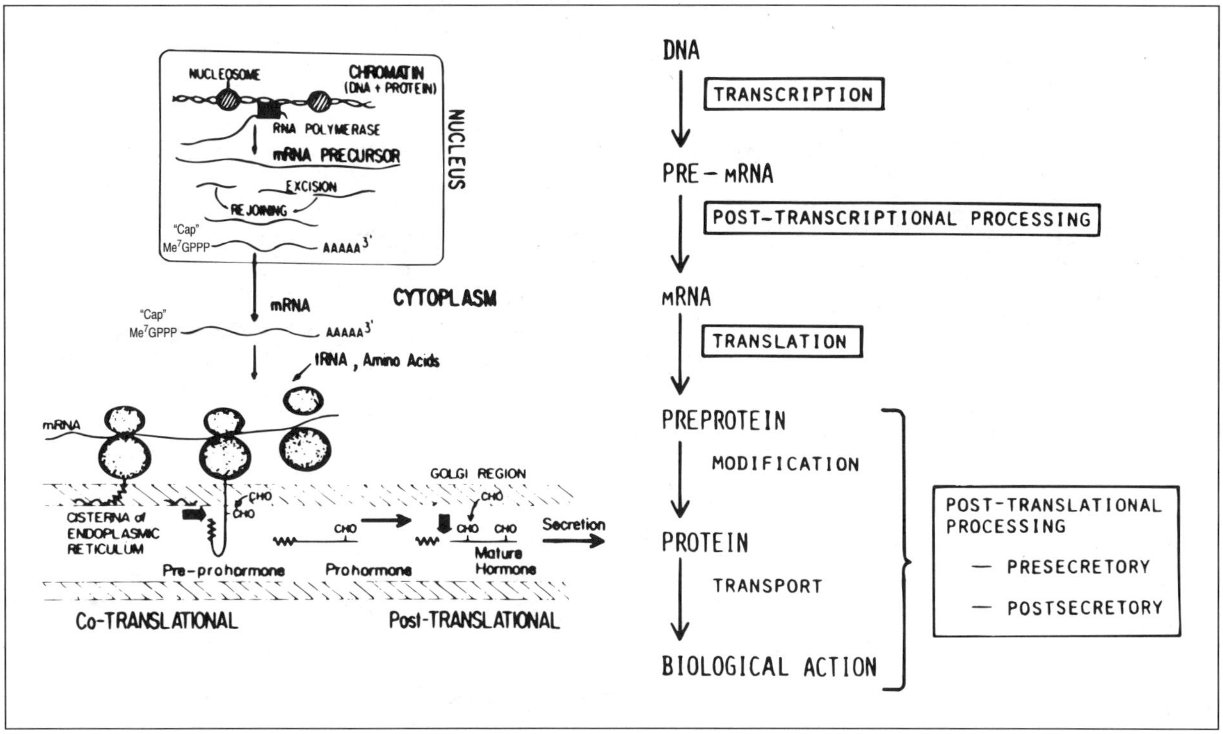

Figure 3-12. Steps in the cellular synthesis of polypeptide hormones. Steps that take place within the nucleus include transcription of genetic information into an mRNA precursor (pre-mRNA) followed by posttranscriptional processing, which includes RNA cleavage, excision of introns, and rejoining of exons, resulting in formation of mRNA. The cytoplasmic mRNA is assembled with ribosomes. Amino acids, carried by aminoacylated transfer RNAs (tRNAs), are then polymerized into a polypeptide chain. The final step in the synthesis of polypeptide hormones is that of posttranslational processing. (From JF Habener. Genetic Control of Hormone Formation. In JD Wilson, DW Foster [eds], *Williams Textbook of Endocrinology.* Philadelphia: W.B. Saunders Company, 1992.)

hormones can be regulated at one or more levels in the pathway of hormone biosynthesis [144]. For example, the regulation of the synthesis of parathyroid hormone by calcium takes place at the levels of DNA synthesis and cell division. Prolactin synthesis is regulated by TRH at the transcriptional level. Cortisol stimulates the synthesis of growth hormone by increasing the rate of gene transcription and by stabilizing GH mRNA. The synthesis of insulin is enhanced by glucose by increased efficiency of initiation of translation of proinsulin mRNA. Posttranslational modification is important for the synthesis of most peptide hormones by cleavages of hormone precursors in the Golgi apparatus of the secretory cells.

Hormones induce metabolic changes in the target cells after binding to specific receptors. Peptide hormones and catecholamines bind to membrane-associated receptors. This reaction results in the activation of an intracellular second messenger system, two examples of which are the diacylglycerol-protein kinase C pathway and the cAMP-protein kinase A pathway (see Figure 3-2). A cascade of intracellular reactions follows, leading to the formation of a phosphoprotein. This phosphoprotein, acting as a transcription factor, interacts with regulating sites (hormone response elements) on a gene, activating transcription and gene expression, which in turn results in the synthesis of a peptide or protein that can influence cellular metabolism or function. The molecular mechanisms by which a membrane-active hormone can activate gene expression in a target cell are summarized in Figure 3-13.

Other hormones bind to intracellular receptors that are found in cytoplasm and the nucleus. Steroid hormones enter most cells by diffusion, whereas thyroid hormones are actively transported across the cellular and nuclear membranes before binding to the receptor. Binding of the hormone to the receptor results in conformational changes of the receptor, and the activated hormone-receptor complex then activates gene expression through a series of reactions that are summarized in Figure 3-14. The hormone-receptor complex acts as a transcription factor, binding

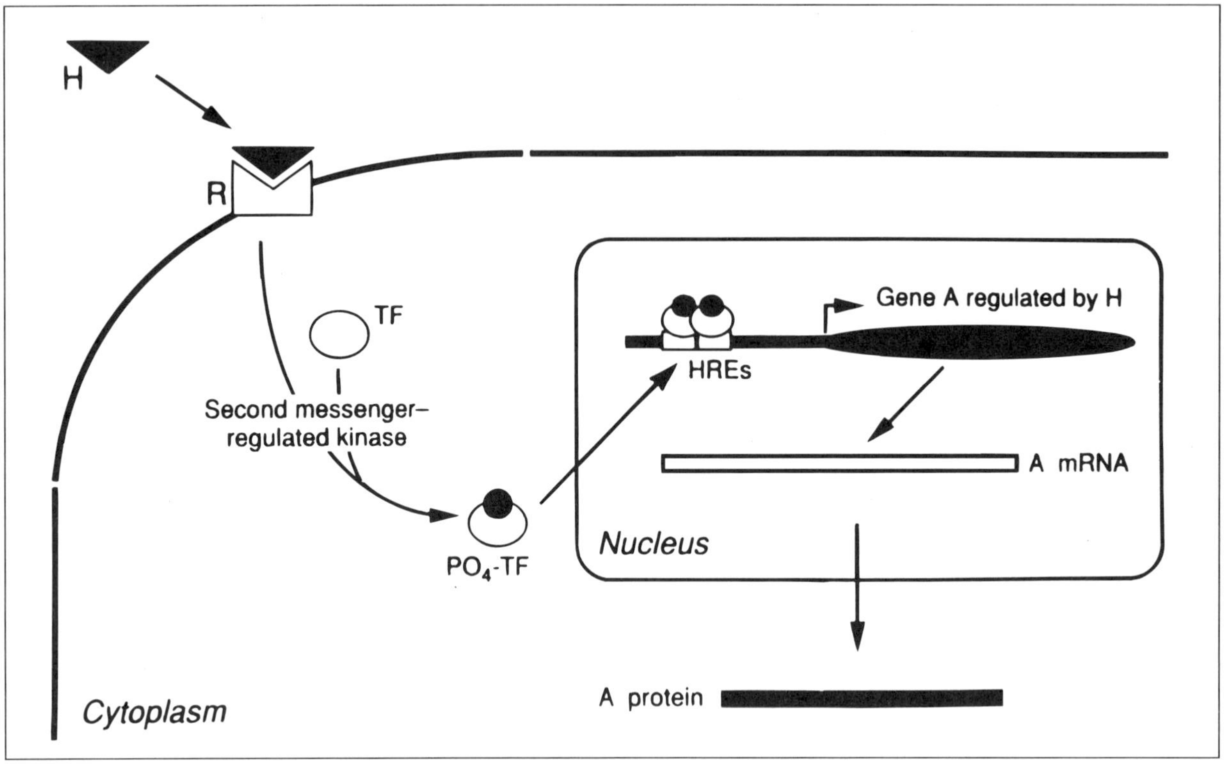

Figure 3-13. General scheme of peptide hormone regulation of gene expression. Interaction of hormone (H) with its target cell surface receptor (R) results ultimately in the production of second messengers. These molecules may activate cytoplasmic kinases that, in turn, can phosphorylate transcription factors (TFs). Such modified TFs (PO_4-TFs) can then act in the nucleus to modulate gene expression by binding to hormone response elements (HREs) in gene-regulatory regions, often as dimers (as shown). Altered rates of gene transcription may lead to changes in steady-state levels of corresponding mRNA and protein. (From CR Kahn et al. Mechanism of Action of Hormones That Act at the Cell Surface. In JD Wilson, DW Foster [eds], *Williams Textbook of Endocrinology.* Philadelphia: W.B. Saunders Company, 1992.)

to a specific hormone receptor binding site of the gene. These hormone response elements are enhancer elements with profound effect on transcriptional activity when stimulated by the hormone-receptor complex. Hormone response elements have been described for each of the known ligand-activated cytoplasmic and nuclear receptors and have been identified as glucocorticoid response element, thyroid hormone response element, etc.

Not all effects of hormones are mediated through gene activation. For example, hormones such as insulin can influence amino acid and glucose transport by acting on transporters that are already present in the cell. This hormone action, then, does not require gene transcription and synthesis of new proteins. Considering the diverse and complex actions of hormones, it is not surprising that the time course of different events in hormone action varies from seconds to several hours (Figure 3-15).

Carbohydrate Metabolism

During critical illness, carbohydrate metabolism is regulated both by the counter-regulatory hormones and by insulin. The counter-regulatory hormones (glucagon, epinephrine, norepinephrine, GH, and cortisol) are released at increased rates during conditions of reduced plasma glucose levels, e.g., severe sepsis and endotoxemia, starvation, or after the administration of insulin [2,3]. Each of the counter-regulatory hormones has metabolic actions that may reverse hypoglycemia. In humans, the major counter-regulatory hormones are glucagon and catecholamines [147]. The role of the counter-regulatory hormones in the regulation of metabolism during critical illness was supported in experiments in which the infusion of a combination of some of these hormones (glucagon, epinephrine, cortisol) resulted in alterations in whole-body carbohydrate metabolism similar to those seen in sepsis and other critical illness

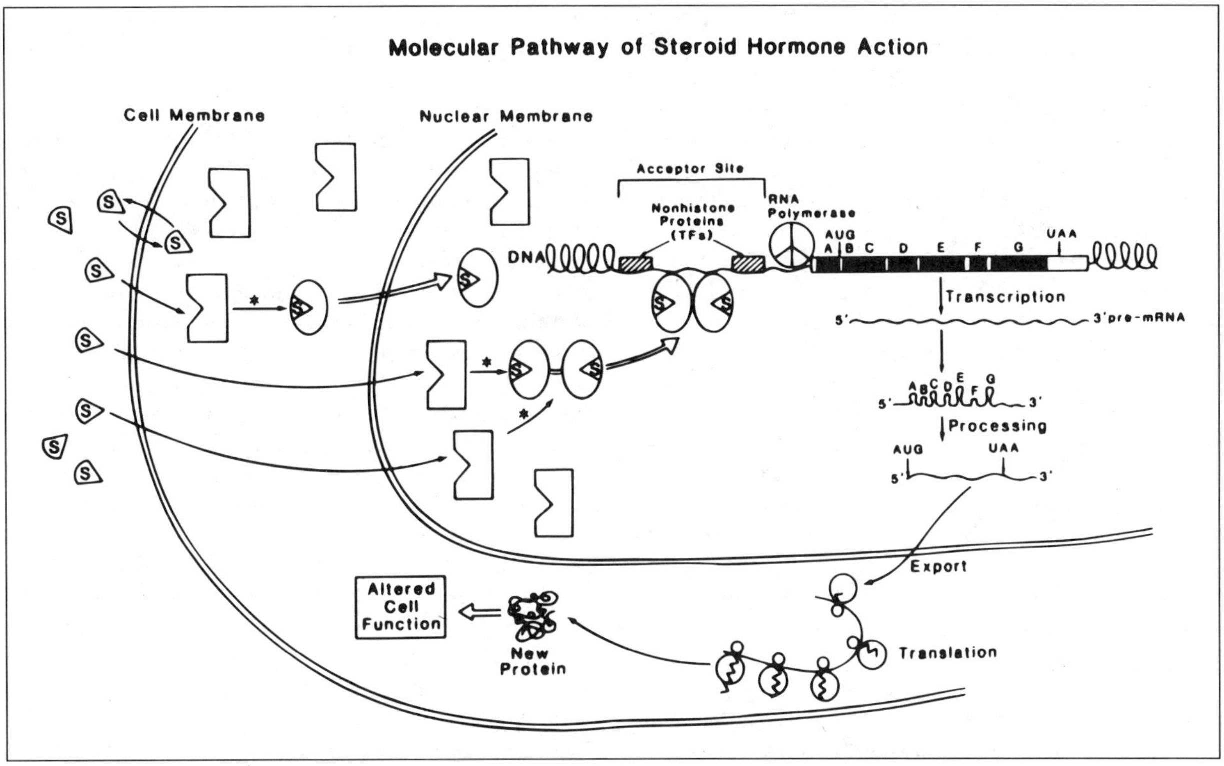

Figure 3-14. Scheme of the molecular pathway of steroid hormone action. Steroids bind to receptors in the cytoplasm or in the nucleus. (From JH Clark et al. Mechanisms of Action of Steroid Hormones. In JD Wilson, DW Foster [eds], *Williams Textbook of Endocrinology.* Philadelphia: W.B. Saunders Company, 1992.)

SECONDS
- Binding to receptor
- Conformation change in receptor
- Receptor aggregation
- Activation of receptor kinase
- Change in ion flux

MINUTES
- Receptor internalization
- Generation of possible "mediator" substances
- Stimulation of glucose transport
- Stimulation of phospholipid turnovers
- Activation of intracellular enzymes

HOURS
- Activation of amino acid transport
- Stimulation of protein and lipid synthesis
- Stimulation of RNA synthesis
- Stimulation of DNA synthesis

Figure 3-15. Time course of events in the cellular action of insulin. (Reproduced, with permission, from the *Annual Review of Medicine,* Volume 36, © 1985, by Annual Reviews Inc.)

[148,149]. In a recent study, the catabolic effects of "triple hormone infusion" were amplified when insulin levels were suppressed [150].

It is an old observation that catecholamines are important for the control of carbohydrate metabolism [151]. Infusion of epinephrine stimulates hepatic glucose production and inhibits the metabolic clearance rate of glucose. The increased rate of glucose production after epinephrine infusion is caused by an early increase in hepatic glycogenolysis followed by stimulated gluconeogenesis [152]. In addition to these direct effects of the hormone, epinephrine can also influence carbohydrate metabolism by modulating the release of other hormones that can influence glucose kinetics. Epinephrine stimulates the release of glucagon and inhibits insulin secretion [153]. Evidence for a role of catecholamines in the increased hepatic glucose production during endotoxemia was reported by Hargrove and colleagues [154]. They found that combined α- and β-adrenergic blockade prevented the hyperglycemia and increased glucose turnover in endotoxin-treated rats. Treatment of burned patients with phentolamine and propranolol reduced whole-body metabolic rate [155], further illustrating the role of catecholamines in the regulation of metabolism after injury.

Interestingly, the sympathetic nervous system seems to be less important in sepsis. Adrenergic blockade did not abolish the elevated rates of gluconeogenesis or glucose turnover in septic rats [156]. In contrast, there is evidence that glucagon plays an important role in the control of carbohydrate metabolism during sepsis, at least in the regulation of hepatic glucose production. The role of glucagon for the regulation of glucose metabolism is illustrated by pronounced and sustained increase in plasma glucagon levels during sepsis [11]. When the hyperglucagonemia induced by sepsis in rats was blocked by infusion of somatostatin, the elevated rate of glucose production was reduced to control values [157]. In contrast, the increased disposal rate of glucose was not influenced by treatment with somatostatin, suggesting that the two aspects of carbohydrate metabolism (hepatic glucose production and glucose clearance) are controlled by different mechanisms during sepsis.

Although the evidence discussed above suggests that hyperglucagonemia is important for increased hepatic glucose production during hypermetabolic sepsis, infusion of glucagon alone has only transient effects on glucose production [158]. Thus, additional hormones or other mediators are probably required to potentiate the glucagon-induced increase in glucose production. In previous studies, glucocorticoids interacted synergistically with glucagon to increase glucose production [148,158]. Wolfe and Shaw [159] found that adrenergic antagonists potentiated the inhibitory effect of somatostatin on glucose production in septic animals, suggesting that catecholamines as well interact with glucagon to increase hepatic gluconeogenesis.

The mechanisms of the differential role of catecholamines in the regulation of carbohydrate metabolism in sepsis versus other catabolic conditions was studied by Hargrove and colleagues [160]. Results in that study suggest that the influence of catecholamines on hepatic glucose production is blunted during sepsis because of increased plasma insulin levels, in turn caused by reduced epinephrine-induced inhibition of insulin secretion.

In addition to the counter-regulatory hormones, insulin plays an important role in the regulation of carbohydrate metabolism in injury and sepsis. During early sepsis, plasma levels of insulin are reduced in relationship to the degree of hyperglycemia [2,5]. One of the mechanisms of inappropriate insulin secretion, despite high plasma glucose levels, is a reduction of pancreatic β-cell sensitivity to glucose secondary to the combined effects of catecholamines, somatostatin, glucocorticoids, and reduced pancreatic blood flow. During the flow phase after injury or hypermetabolic sepsis, β-cells regain their sensitivity and insulin concentrations rise. Despite increased insulin concentrations, however, hyperglycemia may persist, consistent with insulin resistance. The presence of insulin resistance was also evident from reduced hormone response when exogenous insulin was administered to septic or injured patients [21].

Insulin Resistance

Because of its importance for the metabolic regulation in critical illness, the phenomenon of insulin resistance is discussed in some detail here. Insulin resistance can be defined as any situation in which a certain concentration of the hormone induces a less-than-normal biologic response [161]. Although insulin resistance has been best characterized regarding its effect on carbohydrate metabolism, particularly peripheral (muscular) glucose uptake, other metabolic processes can also become resistant to the hormone under certain circumstances [162].

From a theoretical standpoint, insulin resistance can be caused by alterations that block the hormone from reaching the receptor (prereceptor), from changes in the binding of insulin or signal transduction by the receptor, or from impairment of any of the postreceptor steps in insulin action [161].

Because most metabolic responses occur with only a small fraction of total receptors occupied, there are "spare receptors" available for insulin action. Therefore, insulin resistance at the receptor level usually results in a rightward shift of the dose-response curve, i.e., decreased hormone sensitivity (Figure 3-16). In contrast, if the insulin resistance is caused by a postreceptor defect, the maximal response is decreased even when insulin is present at high concentrations (decreased responsiveness) (see Figure 3-16).

Injury and sepsis are associated with peripheral insulin resistance, and there is evidence that the hormone resistance is at the postreceptor level (reduced responsiveness) in these conditions [21,162]. The mechanism of insulin resistance in critical illness is probably multifactorial and may be mediated both by β-adrenoreceptor activity [163,164] and TNF [165]. Another possible mechanism of hormone resistance is prolonged hormonal stimulation of target tissue. When adipocytes were cultured in the presence of glucose plus insulin, the insulin responsiveness of glucose transport was decreased because of an impairment of translocation of glucose transporters to the cell surface rather than by reducing the total number of cellular glucose transporters [166].

Injury and sepsis induce insulin resistance not only in peripheral tissue, but in the liver as well. The increased gluconeogenesis seen in hypermetabolic sepsis (flow phase), despite near-normal insulin levels, is consistent with a state of insulin resistance in the liver. Infusion of insulin in septic rats failed to suppress hepatic glucose output, supporting the concept of insulin resistance in the liver during sepsis [167].

Lipid Metabolism

Hormonal control of lipid metabolism occurs in both adipose and other tissues. Frequently, the regulation by the same hormone is different in various tissues. In general, hormone-induced changes in lipid metabolism, with the exception of those induced by catecholamines, are not similar to those that occur during sepsis and other critical illness. The role of hormonal control of lipid metabolism in these conditions, therefore, is probably less prominent than is the hormonal

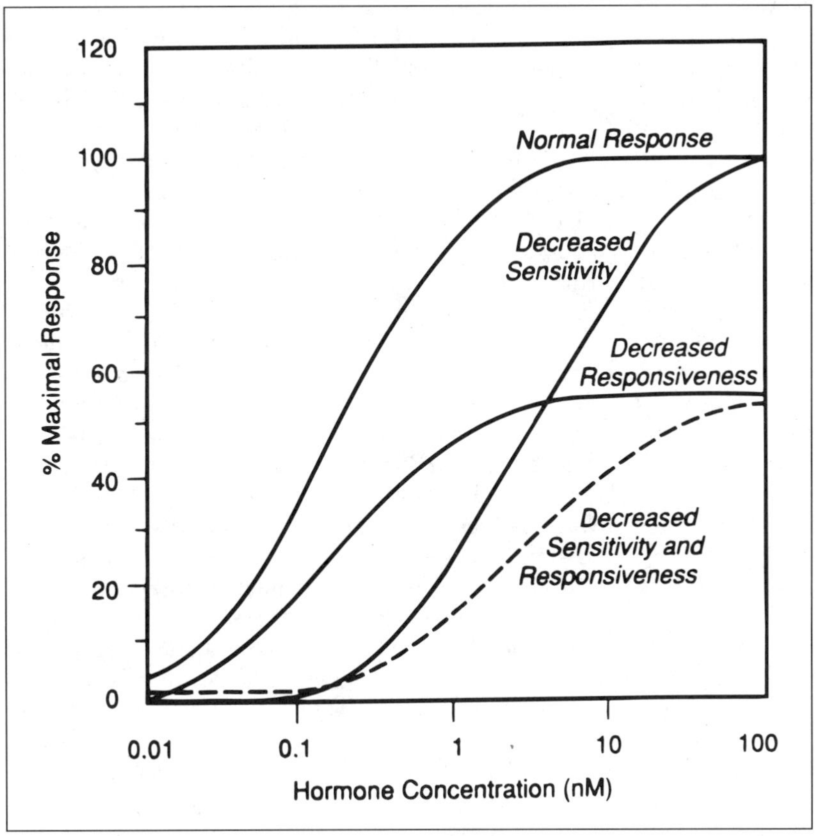

Figure 3-16. Types of resistance to hormone action. In hormone-resistant states there may be a rightward shift of the dose-response curve (decreased sensitivity), a decrease in maximal response (decreased responsiveness), or a combination of the two. Decreased sensitivity indicates a defect at a non-rate-limiting step (often the receptor), whereas decreased responsiveness indicates a defect at a rate-limiting step (usually postreceptor). (From CR Kahn et al. Mechanism of Action of Hormones That Act at the Cell Surface. In JD Wilson, DW Foster [eds], *Williams Textbook of Endocrinology.* Philadelphia: W.B. Saunders Company, 1992.)

control of protein and carbohydrate metabolism; other mediators, such as cytokines, may be more important for the regulation of lipid metabolism in injury, inflammation, and severe infection.

Among the counter-regulatory hormones, glucagon and glucocorticoids have been found to influence lipid metabolism. Administration in vivo of hydrocortisone in rats resulted in reduced activities of the enzymes fatty acid synthetase and acetyl-CoA carboxylase in adipose tissue [168]. Both these substances are key enzymes in the biosynthesis of fatty acids. The inhibition of fatty acid synthetase activity was caused by reduced synthesis and amount of the enzyme rather than a change in catalytic activity. In the same study, fatty acid synthetase and acetyl-CoA carboxylase activities in the liver were unchanged after treatment with glucocorticoids. Thus, glucocorticoids did not induce the metabolic pattern of sepsis and other critical illness with increased lipid metabolism and hepatic lipogenesis.

When glucagon was administered in vivo to rats, fatty acid synthetase and acetyl-CoA carboxylase activities decreased in liver and were unchanged in adipose tissue [169], again unlike the situation in sepsis. Treatment of isolated hepatocytes with glucagon in vitro inhibited fatty acid synthesis, and cAMP was required as a second messenger for this response [170]. More recent studies suggest that the effects of glucagon on the synthesis and secretion of lipids by hepatocytes may be biphasic; no change or reduced lipogenesis was noted during the first 12 hours of incubation of hepatocytes with glucagon followed by increased synthesis of various lipids during more extended (12 to 24 hours) incubation [171]. Although these results could be consistent with a role of glucagon in stress-induced changes in fat metabolism, at least in the liver, a study in septic dogs found evidence that glucagon was not responsible for increased fatty acid synthesis [159]. In the same study, evidence was found that catecholamines may be involved in the control of lipid metabolism during sepsis; when a combined α- and β-adrenergic blockade was induced with propranolol and phentolamine, the sepsis-induced increase in palmitate appearance was blocked. This is consistent with other reports that catecholamines stimulate lipolysis in adipose tissue [172].

Several studies have shown that insulin stimulates fatty acid synthesis in the hepatocyte [173]. The effect of insulin alone may be less important than the balance between insulin and glucagon. Insulin reduces the glucagon-induced increase in cAMP levels and inhibits some of the reduction of fatty acid synthesis caused by glucagon. This balance between insulin and glucagon may be important for the development of hepatic steatosis during total parenteral nutrition. Administration of glucagon to rats receiving total parenteral nutrition prevented the accumulation of lipid in the liver [174].

Protein Metabolism

A number of hormones participate in the regulation of whole-body protein metabolism, both under normal and various pathophysiologic conditions such as starvation, diabetes, hyperthyroidism, and cancer. During metabolic stress induced by injury, inflammation, and sepsis, the counter-regulatory hormones play a particularly important role in the control of protein and amino acid metabolism.

Muscle

Among the counter-regulatory hormones, there is evidence that glucocorticoids are most important for the induction of muscle protein breakdown. Administration of glucocorticoids in humans [175] or rats [176,177] results in increased muscle protein degradation. Of note is the observation that myofibrillar proteins are particularly sensitive to the influence of glucocorticoids [177]. Thus, in this respect, the effect of glucocorticoids resembles the effects of sepsis [104] and burn injury [178].

In a recent study, the role of glucocorticoids in the regulation of sepsis-induced muscle proteolysis was tested by treating septic rats with the glucocorticoid receptor blocker RU38486 [179]. RU38486 is the first known antiglucocorticoid that can fully block the hormonal effects in vivo and in vitro in different tissues without agonist activity even at high concentrations [180]. When septic rats were pretreated with this drug (5 mg/kg administered by gavage 2 hours before induction of sepsis by CLP), total protein breakdown, measured as release of tyrosine by incubated extensor digitorum longus muscles, was reduced by 28%, and myofibrillar protein breakdown, measured as release of 3-MH, was inhibited by 44% (Figure 3-17) [179]. The finding that muscle proteolytic rates were reduced but not normalized after treatment of septic rats with RU38486 suggests that sepsis-induced muscle proteolysis is not controlled by glucocorticoids alone. Muscle protein synthesis was not influenced by RU38486, neither in control nor septic rats, suggesting that muscle protein synthesis and degradation are regulated by different mechanisms during sepsis.

The mechanism by which glucocorticoids stimulate muscle proteolysis is not fully known. Recent studies suggest, however, that glucocorticoids may exert their control of muscle proteolysis at the

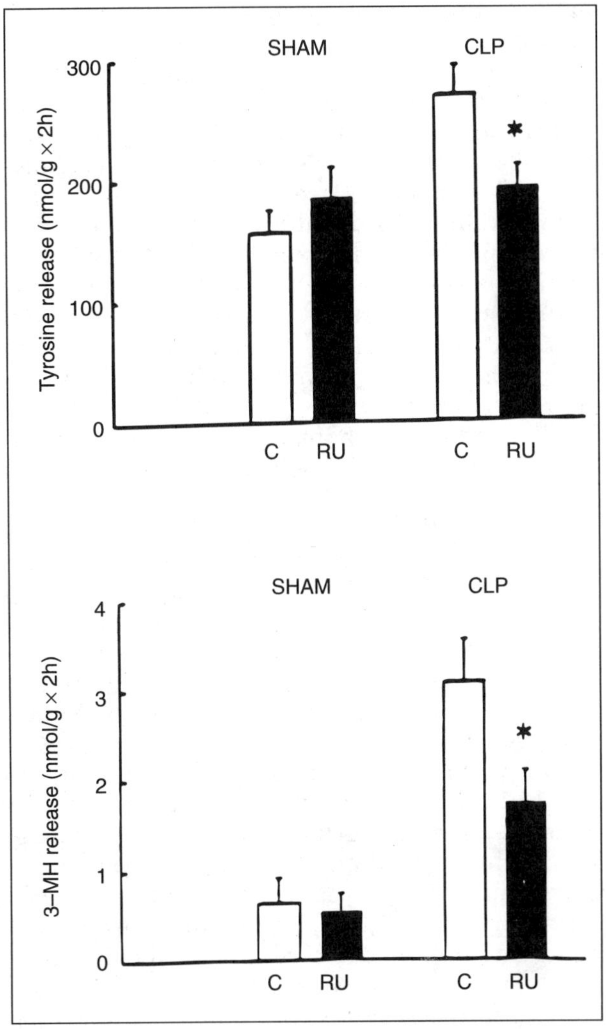

Figure 3-17. Total (upper panel) and myofibrillar (lower panel) protein breakdown rates in incubated EDL muscles from sham-operated and septic (CLP) rats treated with 5 mg/kg RU 38486 (RU) or control gavage (C) 2 hours before sham-operation or CLP. *$p < 0.05$ vs. control gavage. (From M Hall-Angerås et al. Effect of the glucocorticoid receptor antagonist RU 38486 on muscle protein breakdown in sepsis. *Surgery* 109:468, 1991.)

transcriptional level. During starvation in rats, the ubiquitin-dependent proteolytic pathway was stimulated, as evidenced by increased levels in muscle of ubiquitin-conjugated proteins and ubiquitin mRNA [114]. This response to starvation was blocked in adrenalectomized rats, but was restituted by the administration of dexamethasone. Thus, it is possible that the activated glucocorticoid-receptor complex acts as a transcription factor on the ubiquitin gene in skeletal muscle. It remains to be determined whether sepsis-induced increase in ubiquitin gene transcription is regulated by glucocorticoids.

In addition to influencing protein degradation, there is evidence that glucocorticoids affect glutamine transport and metabolism in skeletal muscle. After treatment of rats with dexamethasone, Hundal and associates [181] noted a 45% reduction in muscle glutamine concentration, mainly caused by increased net efflux of the amino acid. The uptake of glutamine in muscle by system N^m was substantially reduced in glucocorticoid-treated rats, reflecting a decrease in both V_{max} and K_m for the glutamine transporter and further contributing to the reduction in muscle glutamine levels. In the same report, almost identical changes could be induced by adding dexamethasone to the medium of perfused rat hindquarters, suggesting that glucocorticoids may have a direct effect on muscle glutamine transport.

Other studies also support a role of glucocorticoids in the control of glutamine transport in muscle. Increased net release of glutamine from extremities of human subjects and experimental animals was observed after treatment with glucocorticoids [175-177]. Parry-Billings [182] reported increased release of glutamine and reduced concentrations of the amino acid in muscle of dexamethasone-treated rats.

Not only transport of glutamine but metabolism of the amino acid as well is regulated by glucocorticoids. Thus, increased glutamine synthetase activity in skeletal muscle was reported after treatment of rats with dexamethasone [183]. This effect was probably induced at the transcriptional level, because glutamine synthetase mRNA levels were increased after treatment with dexamethasone.

In contrast to the role of glucocorticoids for the regulation of muscle glutamine transport (by system N^m), there is evidence that amino acid transport by system A is not controlled by glucocorticoids, at least not during sepsis [184]. The biologic importance of this is not clear, because recent reports suggest that system A plays only a minor role in overall muscle amino acid transport [185].

Additional hormones that are important for the regulation of muscle protein and amino acid metabolism during sepsis and other catabolic conditions include thyroid hormones, GH, IGF-1, and insulin. Previous studies, both in vivo and in vitro, provided evidence that thyroid hormones regulate muscle protein turnover [186]. Whereas physiologic concentrations of thyroid hormone are necessary for normal growth of muscle and other tissues, high hormone concentrations result in muscle catabolism. Elevated thyroid hormone levels induce muscle catabolism mainly by stimulating protein degradation, whereas the influence on muscle protein synthesis is controversial. Previous studies suggest that both lysosomal and nonlysosomal, energy-dependent proteolytic pathways are influenced by thyroid hormone [186].

Although reduced serum levels of T_3 during sepsis and other critical illnesses (low T_3 syndrome) would suggest that T_3 (the metabolically active thyroid hormone) is not involved in the control of muscle catabolism during these conditions, thyroid hormones may indeed participate in the regulation of muscle protein metabolism during sepsis. The inhibition of muscle protein synthesis observed in septic rats was completely abolished in thyroidectomized rats and the increase in muscle protein breakdown was significantly blunted [26]. A role of T_3 in sepsis-induced muscle proteolysis, despite reduced serum levels of the hormone, may partly reflect increased uptake of T_3 by muscle during sepsis [26]. From a metabolic standpoint, tissue levels of the hormone are more important than serum levels. Thus, it is possible that uptake of T_3 by skeletal muscle is increased during critical illness and that this phenomenon may contribute to the low T_3 syndrome and reduced synthesis and stimulated breakdown of muscle protein. Further studies are needed, however, to test that hypothesis.

The anabolic effects of GH in skeletal muscle have been documented in several reports. There is evidence that the hormone promotes protein synthesis but does not block protein degradation in muscle [187]. Improved nitrogen balance after the administration of GH has been demonstrated in patients with a variety of catabolic conditions such as surgical injury [188], burn [189], critical illness [190], in patients receiving parenteral nutrition [191], and in healthy volunteers treated with glucocorticoids [192].

Recent studies have made it clear that the anabolic effects of GH are mediated by IGF-1, which is primarily produced in the liver. Muscle tissues possess abundant receptors for IGF-1, and the anabolic effects of IGF-1 have been documented in incubated rat muscles [186] and cultured myoblasts [193]. Improved protein balance was noted after the in vivo administration of IGF-1 in lambs with TNF-induced catabolism [194].

The regulatory role of IGF-1 on muscle protein turnover is supported by reduced plasma levels of the hormone in critically ill patients [15]. Interestingly, in the same study, plasma levels of GH were increased, suggesting that the biosynthesis of IGF-1 in the liver becomes resistant to GH during catabolic conditions. In recent studies, administration of IGF-1 prevented weight loss after burn injury [195], inhibited protein breakdown during starvation [196], and blocked protein loss induced by TNF [194]. Thus, it is possible that administration of IGF-1 could have a role in the treatment of patients with severe infection and other catabolic conditions.

Although the regulatory effects of insulin on muscle protein turnover and amino acid transport have been known for many years, the mechanisms by which insulin improves muscle protein balance are still evolving. In recent studies in healthy human volunteers, insulin was found to promote muscle protein anabolism mainly by inhibiting protein breakdown, rather than by stimulating protein synthesis [197]. Other studies have shown that the anabolic effects of insulin may at least in part be mediated by changes in amino acid concentrations [198].

The cellular mechanisms by which insulin regulates muscle protein metabolism were reviewed previously [161,199]. Protein synthesis is stimulated by insulin mainly at the translational level by enhanced peptide-chain initiation, although increased capacity for protein synthesis, secondary to increased amounts of ribosomes, may also play a role. The inhibitory effect of insulin on muscle protein breakdown reflects inhibition of lysosomal proteolysis as well as reduced formation of autophagosomes.

Previous studies suggest that the mechanisms by which insulin controls muscle protein metabolism are impaired during various catabolic conditions. Thus, regulation of muscle protein synthesis or degradation becomes resistant to the hormone after burn injury [200], blunt trauma [201], and denervation [202]. We recently found evidence of insulin resistance in muscle from septic rats with respect to the regulation of protein degradation [203]. Dose-response curves for insulin concentration in incubation medium and the inhibition of protein degradation in incubated muscles suggested that the insulin resistance of protein breakdown in septic muscle reflected a reduced responsiveness, i.e., was caused by a postreceptor defect. This was further supported by the finding that the stimulatory effects of the hormone on protein synthesis and amino acid uptake were not impaired in septic muscle [203].

Administration of insulin to injured patients [204] or animals [205] inhibited whole-body or forearm protein catabolism, and the use of insulin to reduce the catabolic response to trauma was proposed. The improvement of nitrogen balance after treatment of injured patients with insulin, however, was short-lasting [204], perhaps because of insulin resistance of protein metabolism.

Liver and Other Tissues

Counter-regulatory hormones control both protein turnover and amino acid transport and metabolism in the liver. Evidence for a role of catecholamines in the synthesis of acute-phase proteins, in particular α-macrofetoprotein, was reported in rats [206]. Other studies suggest that catecholamines stimulate hepatocyte amino acid transport and that this effect is mediated by α-receptors [207].

A role of glucagon in the control of hepatic protein synthesis was observed in experiments in which the hormone stimulated synthesis of the acute-phase protein α_1-glycoprotein in isolated rat hepatocytes [208]. A stimulatory effect of glucagon on amino acid uptake by system A was reported in freshly isolated and cultured hepatocytes. There is evidence that this effect requires the synthesis of new transporters and is regulated at the transcriptional level [209]. In addition to system A, there is evidence that the glutamine transporting system N as well is stimulated by glucagon [210].

The role of glucocorticoids in the control of amino acid transport has been examined by treating isolated rat hepatocytes in vitro with dexamethasone. Results from those experiments demonstrated that system A amino acid transport was stimulated by the glucocorticoid [211,212]. The stimulation of system A transport by glucocorticoids required RNA and protein synthesis, suggesting that the hormonal effect was caused by synthesis of new transporter proteins, perhaps regulated at the transcriptional level. In other experiments, evidence was found that system N as well is stimulated by steroids [210].

Glucocorticoids are important for the control of acute-phase protein synthesis. In most studies, however, glucocorticoids alone did not influence expression of plasma proteins, but acted as an important co-factor to various cytokines. The interaction between glucocorticoids and cytokines in the regulation of acute-phase protein synthesis is discussed in a subsequent section of this chapter. Glucocorticoids can also exert a permissive effect on other hormones, in particular glucagon, in hepatocytes.

Growth hormone affects amino acid transport by systems A and N in the liver [213]. The effect of GH is biphasic, with an acute (within hours) increase in hepatic amino acid transport and a delayed (after treatment for days) inhibition of amino acid transport.

In addition to muscle and liver, intestine and lungs have been studied with respect to hormonal control of metabolism after injury, inflammation, and infection. Among the counter-regulatory hormones, glucocorticoids have been most extensively studied for the regulation of intestinal amino acid (in particular glutamine) transport and metabolism. Results, however, have been contradictory, and the exact role of glucocorticoids in the regulation of amino acid metabolism in the gut remains unclear. Both increased [214], inhibited [215], and unchanged [216] intestinal glutamine uptake have been reported after administration of dexamethasone in different species. In experiments in our laboratory [unpublished results], treatment of rats with RU38486 did not influence the sepsis-induced increase in mucosal protein synthesis, and injection of dexamethasone in normal rats did not affect protein synthesis in the small intestine, suggesting that glucocorticoids may not play an important role in the regulation of intestinal protein metabolism during critical illness.

Results from experiments in which the direct effect of glucocorticoids on amino acid transport was tested have also been contradictory. Dexamethasone inhibited glutamine transport when added to cultured Caco-2 cells (a human intestinal epithelial cell line) [217], but it did not influence glutamine transport when added to perfused small intestine [216].

In other studies, the Na^+-dependent transport of alanine in the small intestine was stimulated after treatment of neonatal piglets with dexamethasone, whereas the Na^+-independent alanine uptake and lysine transport (probably by system L and y^+) were unaffected [218]. These results suggest that glucocorticoids may regulate the activity of different amino acid transporters individually.

Certain enzymes involved in the metabolism of amino acids in the gut are controlled by glucocorticoids. Intestinal glutaminase activity was stimulated after treatment of rats with dexamethasone [219,220], and this effect may be regulated at the transcriptional level because glutaminase mRNA levels in intestinal mucosa were increased as early as 4 hours after the injection of dexamethasone.

The activity of glutamine synthetase may be regulated by glucocorticoids. Treatment of rats with RU38486 prevented the endotoxin-induced increase in mucosal glutamine synthetase activity [221]. In the same report, addition of dexamethasone to cultured Caco-2 cells increased both glutamine synthetase mRNA levels and the activity of the enzyme.

The metabolic response to sepsis and endotoxemia in the lung is that of catabolism as evidenced by increased efflux of amino acids, in particular glutamine and alanine. This response has been observed in patients with sepsis [222] and in experimental animals with sepsis and endotoxemia [223]. Although increased release of amino acids may reflect reduced protein synthesis or increased protein breakdown, increased release of glutamine may also be caused by stimulated de novo synthesis of the amino acids. This is supported by increased activity of the enzyme glutamine synthetase in lung tissue during sepsis and endotoxemia [224].

Glucocorticoids may be involved in the regulation of the catabolic response in the lung. Thus, increased release of glutamine and alanine from the lungs was noted in rats after treatment with dexamethasone [225,226]. In the same studies, treatment of rats with dexamethasone stimulated glutamine synthetase activity by 20% to 30%. In subsequent experiments, the increase in enzyme activity was preceded by increased levels of glutamine synthetase mRNA, suggesting that dexamethasone stimulates enzyme gene transcription [227].

Cytokines

Although cytokines may be involved in the regulation of metabolism in a variety of pathophysiologic conditions, such as cancer cachexia and inflammatory bowel disease, it is primarily in the fields of trauma, sepsis, and endotoxemia that new information regarding cytokines and metabolic control has appeared in recent years. Despite the fact that knowledge about the role of cytokines for the regulation of intermediary metabolism is relatively recent, a great amount of information is available, and this field is rapidly expanding. Cytokines have been implicated in the control of both carbohydrate, lipid, and protein metabolism.

Carbohydrate Metabolism

Among the cytokines, TNF has been most extensively studied for its role in the regulation of carbohydrate metabolism. In several reports in humans and experimental animals, administration in vivo of TNF enhanced glucose metabolism in a manner similar to that seen after endotoxin challenge and during hypermetabolic sepsis, with evidence for increased hepatic production of glucose, hyperglycemia, and stimulated glucose utilization by macrophage-rich tissues and diaphragm [228–231]. The effect of TNF on glucose kinetics is dose dependent, with hyperglycemia developing after relatively modest doses and hypoglycemia after larger doses. Thus, also in this respect, TNF can induce changes that resemble the situation in patients with hypermetabolic sepsis or septic shock. The hypoglycemia seen after high doses of TNF can at least in part be explained by increased peripheral glucose utilization, although impaired hepatic gluconeogenesis may also contribute.

When TNF was administered in healthy postabsorptive men, glucose turnover increased and hyperglycemia developed [229]. From those and

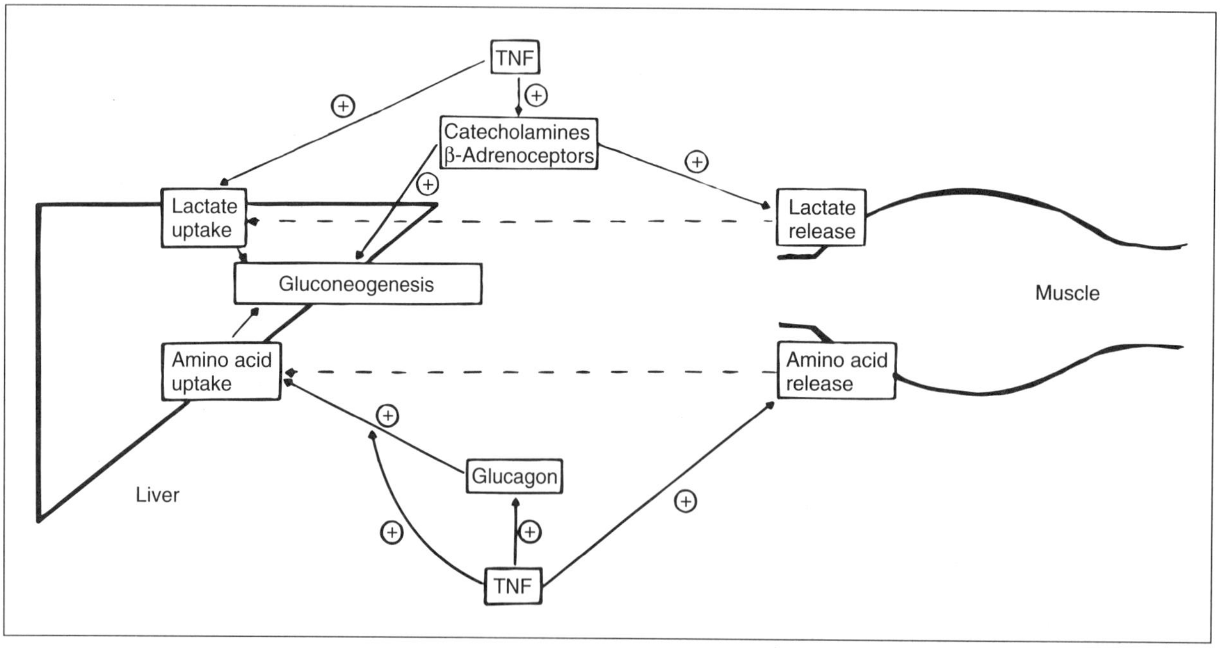

Figure 3-18. TNF enhances gluconeogenesis in vivo by β-adrenergic stimulation. The supply of the gluconeogenic precursors alanine and lactate is increased by the stimulation of their release from muscle by TNF. TNF increases the uptake of amino acids and lactate by the liver. Hepatic amino acid uptake is stimulated by TNF through increasing glucagon levels and potentiating the effect of glucagon on the liver. (From T van der Poll, HP Sauerwein. Tumour necrosis factor-α: Its role in the metabolic response to sepsis. *Clin Sci* 84:247, 1993.)

other in vivo studies, it is not known if the changes in carbohydrate metabolism reflect a direct or indirect effect of TNF. Because administration of TNF induced a stress response, it is possible that the increase in glucose metabolism is secondary to increased secretion of catecholamines, glucagon, and cortisol. It is also possible that TNF influences gluconeogenesis by modulating the effect of these hormones, for example, by stimulating glucagon-mediated hepatic amino acid uptake. Studies by Rofe and colleagues [232] suggest that TNF does not influence hepatic glucose production by a direct effect. Similarly, Bagby and associates [233] reported evidence that the TNF-induced increase in hepatic glucose production is mediated by catecholamines; infusion of phentolamine and propranolol prevented the increase in glucose appearance noted in rats treated with TNF. An additional explanation for the effect of propranolol may be that the TNF-induced increase in hepatic glucose production is flow mediated, because propranolol decreases portal blood flow. An integrated picture of the role of TNF in gluconeogenesis was provided recently by van der Poll and Sauerwein (Figure 3-18) [234].

In contrast to the effect in the liver, TNF can have a direct effect on cellular glucose kinetics in peripheral tissues. Evidence for increased glucose uptake after stimulation in vitro with TNF was found in cultured L6 myotubes [235] and 3T3-L1 preadipocytes [236]. The molecular regulation by TNF of glucose transport was examined recently by Cornelius and colleagues [236]. In those studies, exposure of cultured murine 3T3-L1 preadipocytes to TNF resulted in a dose- and time-dependent increase in glucose transport, measured as uptake of 2-deoxyglucose (Figure 3-19). The effect of TNF on the amount of glucose transporter protein in plasma and intracellular membranes was determined by Western blot analysis. After 30 minutes of exposure of the cells to TNF, the amount of glucose transporter was increased at the plasma membrane but was decreased within the intracellular membrane, suggesting that TNF stimulates glucose transport on an acute basis by promoting translocation of the glucose transporter from intracellular membranes to the plasma membrane. After prolonged (16 hr) exposure to TNF, the amount of glucose transporter was increased at the plasma and intracellular membranes (Figure 3-20 and Table 3-2). Northern blot analysis in the same cell system showed that the amount of mRNA for the glucose transporter was increased early (after 30 min exposure) and late (after 8 to 16 hr) after exposure of the cells to TNF (Figure 3-21). Increased mRNA levels may reflect the increased transcription rate of the gene

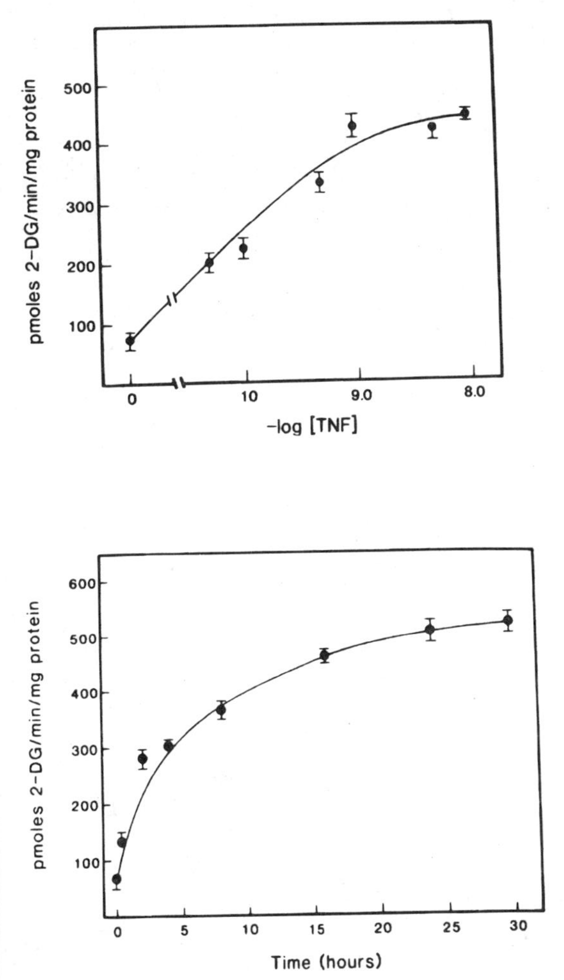

Figure 3-19. Stimulation by TNF of 2-deoxyglucose uptake in 3T3-L1 cells is dose *(top)* and time *(bottom)* dependent. (From P Cornelius et al. The growth factor-like effects of tumor necrosis factor-α: Stimulation of glucose transport activity and induction of glucose transporter and immediate early gene expression in 3T3-L1 preadipocytes. *J Biol Chem* 265:20506, 1990.)

or the increased stability of the mRNA (or combinations thereof). To dissect these possibilities, the authors measured the transcription rate of the glucose transporter gene, using run-on assay on isolated nuclei. Results from those experiments showed that transcription of the glucose transporter gene was activated early, within 15 minutes of exposure to TNF, but thereafter returned to basal rates. Thus, the early increase in mRNA levels (see Figure 3-21) probably reflected the increased transcription rate, whereas the late peak in mRNA levels must have been caused by an alternative mechanism, for example, increased stability of mRNA. To test that possibility, the decline in glucose transporter mRNA levels were measured during 2 hours of incubation of 3T3-L1

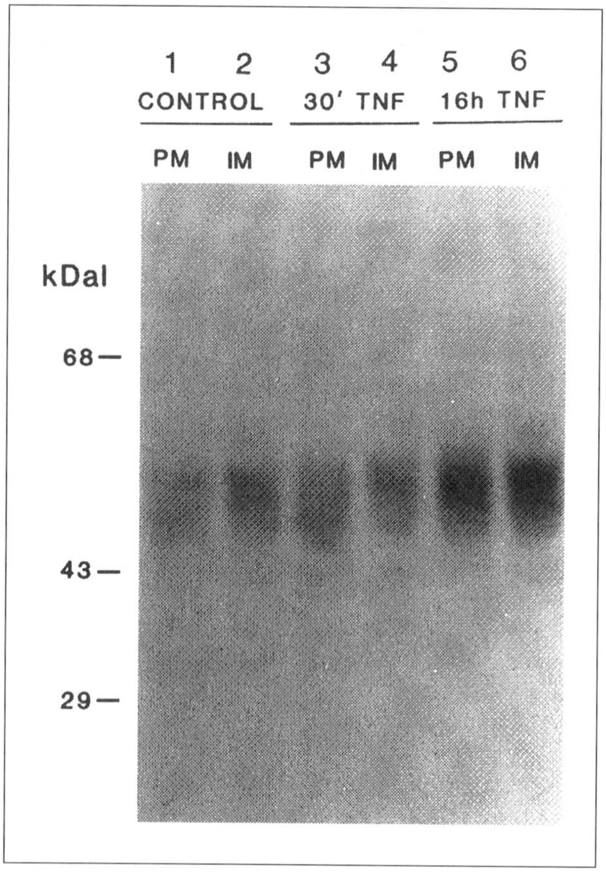

Figure 3-20. Effect of TNF on the amount of glucose transporter protein in plasma and intracellular membranes. Plasma membranes (PM) or intracellular membranes (IM) were isolated from quiescent 3T3-L1 cells (CONTROL), or those exposed to 5.0 nM TNF for the indicated times and subjected to Western blot analysis. The figure shows a representative experiment independently performed three times with similar results. (From P Cornelius et al. The growth factor-like effects of tumor necrosis factor-α: Stimulation of glucose transport activity and induction of glucose transporter and immediate early gene expression in 3T3-L1 preadipocytes. *J Biol Chem* 265:20506, 1990.)

Table 3-2. Quantitation of Glucose Transporters in Plasma Membrane and Intracellular Membrane Fractions Isolated From Quiescent 3T3-L1 Fibroblasts in the Presence and Absence of TNF*

Membrane Fraction	Time (hr)	Cytochalasin B Bound (pmol/mg Membrane Protein)
Plasma membrane	0	16.6 ± 2.9
	0.5	31.7 ± 5.8
	16.0	30.4 ± 4.3
Intracellular membrane	0	27.0 ± 2.3
	0.5	19.0 ± 2.1
	16.0	24.0 ± 3.2

*Quiescent 3T3-L1 cells were incubated for the indicated periods of time in the presence of 2.5 nM TNF. For the two incubations, cells from 25- to 100-mm culture plates were harvested, and the plasma membrane and intracellular membrane fractions were prepared. D-glucose-displaceable binding of cytochalasin B was determined in triplicate. Results are expressed as picomoles of D-glucose-displaceable cytochalasin B bound per mg membrane protein ± S.E. with n (number of independent experiments) = 4.

Source: P Cornelius et al. The growth factor-like effects of tumor necrosis factor-α: Stimulation of glucose transport activity and induction of glucose transporter and immediate early gene expression in 3T3-L1 preadipocytes. *J Biol Chem* 265:20506, 1990.

cells that had been exposed to 2.5 nM TNF for 8 hours or cultured under control conditions. During the 2-hour incubation period, actinomycin D was added to the cells to block transcription. The decline in mRNA levels under those conditions therefore reflected breakdown of mRNA. Results from those experiments showed that glucose transporter mRNA from TNF-treated cells was more

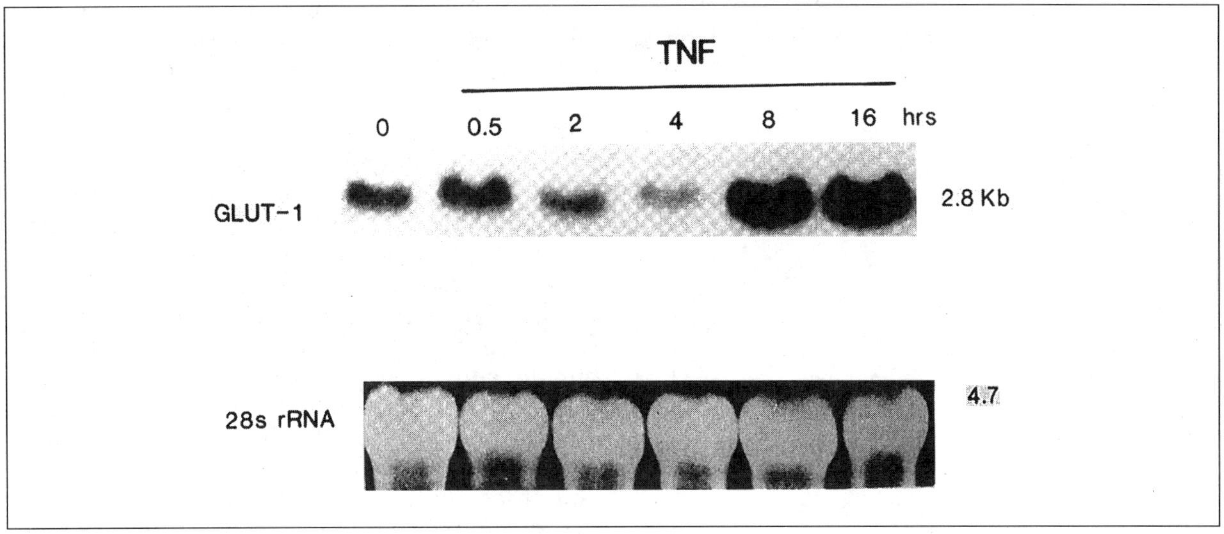

Figure 3-21. Regulation of glucose transporter (GLUT-1) mRNA by TNF. Following treatment of quiescent 3T3-L1 cells with 2.5 nM TNF, total RNA was isolated at the indicated times. 20 μg of RNA was subjected to Northern blot analysis. The panels were generated from the same blot, which was sequentially hybridized, stripped, and rehybridized with a probe for 28s rRNA to control for equal loading. (From P Cornelius et al. The growth factor-like effects of tumor necrosis factor-α: Stimulation of glucose transport activity and induction of glucose transporter and immediate early gene expression in 3T3-L1 preadipocytes. *J Biol Chem* 265:20506, 1990.)

stable than mRNA from control cells (Figure 3-22). Thus, TNF stimulates glucose transport in cultured 3T3-L1 cells by different mechanisms, i.e., by an initial translocation of the glucose transporter to the cell surface, followed by stimulated transcription of the transporter gene and finally by stabilization of glucose transporter mRNA. These elegant experiments have been described in detail here to illustrate how different techniques can be used to study the influence of cytokines on metabolic events at the molecular level.

Although a number of studies suggest that sepsis-like changes in carbohydrate metabolism can be induced by TNF, the exact role of the cytokine in the development of metabolic changes during sepsis and endotoxemia remains unclear. In a recent study, pretreatment of septic or endotoxemic rats with anti-TNF antibodies did not modify the changes in whole-body carbohydrate metabolism assessed from measurements of plasma glucose and lactate levels and rates of glucose appearance and clearance [237]. The results were interpreted as indicating that endogenous production of TNF is not a requirement for the increase in hepatic glucose production and whole-body glucose disposal seen in endotoxemia and hypermetabolic sepsis.

In addition to TNF, IL-1 can influence carbohydrate metabolism. Administration of IL-1 in rats reduces plasma glucose levels, and this effect of IL-1 is even more pronounced than that of TNF [37]. In the same study, intracerebroventricular injection of IL-1 in mice resulted in hypoglycemia despite the fact that the same amount of the cytokine (0.5 ng per mouse) did not induce changes in plasma glucose levels when administered intraperitoneally. These results suggest that the hypoglycemic effect of IL-1 is at least in part integrated at the central nervous system.

The exact mechanisms by which IL-1 induces hypoglycemia are not known, but it is possible that the response reflects both reduced hepatic glucose production and increased peripheral glucose transport and utilization. IL-1 partially inhibits the in vitro glucocorticoid induction of phosphoenol pyruvate carboxykinase, the rate-limiting enzyme in gluconeogenesis [238]. In other studies, evidence was found that supernatants from activated macrophages containing IL-1 (in addition to other cytokines) stimulate glucose oxidation in fat tissue [239]. Furthermore, IL-1 may stimulate glucose transport in adipocytes [240] and increase the whole-body glucose clearance rate [241].

Lipid Metabolism

A large number of in vivo and in vitro studies support a role of cytokines in the control of lipid metabolism. Perhaps the most extensively studied

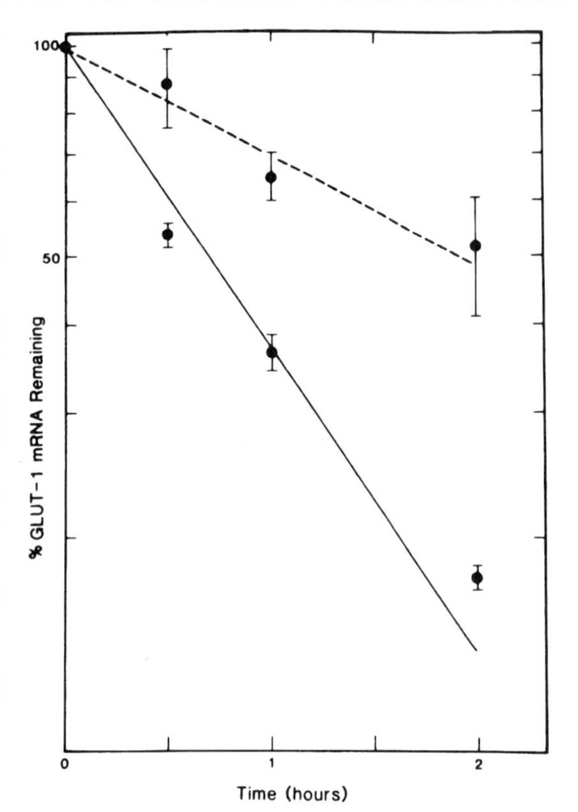

Figure 3-22. Effect of TNF on the stability of GLUT-1 mRNA. Total RNA was isolated from control (quiescent) and TNF-treated (8 h, 2.5 nM) 3T3-L1 cells at the indicated times following the addition of actinomycin D to a final concentration of 5 μg/ml. 20 μg of total RNA were subjected to Northern blot analysis using the GLUT-1 cDNA probe. The results were quantified by laser densitometry of the x-ray film and are presented as the percent of GLUT-1 mRNA remaining after actinomycin-D treatment, for either control cells (solid line) or those exposed to TNF for 8 h (dashed line). The half-life of GLUT-1 mRNA was calculated by linear estimation from the best fit of each line on the logarithmic plot. (From P Cornelius et al. The growth factor-like effects of tumor necrosis factor-α: Stimulation of glucose transport activity and induction of glucose transporter and immediate early gene expression in 3T3-L1 preadipocytes. *J Biol Chem* 265:20506, 1990.)

cytokine in this respect is TNF. Indeed, early studies demonstrated that the same factor was responsible both for the cachexia and hyperlipidemia that frequently accompany infection and tumors, and this factor was called cachectin; subsequent studies showed cachectin and TNF to be the same substance [242].

TNF and Lipid Metabolism

A number of studies have shown that TNF can induce several of the changes in lipid metabolism commonly seen in sepsis or injury. Tumor necrosis factor injected in rats resulted in hypertriglyceridemia within 2 hours after administration of the cytokine [243]. A similar response was seen after administration of the cytokine to patients with cancer [244]. When TNF was injected intravenously in normal subjects, plasma levels of free fatty acids and glycerol were increased, consistent with stimulated lipolysis, and the free fatty acid turnover was increased up to fourfold [229].

As mentioned earlier, one of the mechanisms of hypertriglyceridemia is down-regulation of lipoprotein lipase activity. An inhibitory effect of TNF on adipocyte lipoprotein lipase was noted in 3T3-L1 preadipocytes [245] and was also observed in human adipose organ cultures, in which TNF down-regulated lipoprotein lipase gene expression [246]. Administration of TNF in vivo reduced lipoprotein lipase activity in adipose tissue of rats and other species [247]. Although TNF inhibits lipoprotein lipase, there is evidence that reduced activity of this enzyme is not the principal factor in the development of hypertriglyceridemia after TNF administration. Thus, in one study, serum levels of triglycerides were increased long before a decreased lipoprotein lipase activity could be detected in adipose tissue after administration of TNF to rats [248].

As in sepsis, the most important mechanism of hypertriglyceridemia after TNF administration is probably increased hepatic synthesis of triglycerides. Administration of TNF to rats resulted in both increased synthesis and secretion of triglycerides in the liver [249]. One of the mechanisms of stimulated synthesis of triglycerides is increased availability of free fatty acids. In fact, unchanged activities of the enzymes involved in the esterification of fatty acids to glycerol after administration of TNF suggest that the increase in triglyceride production in the liver is the result primarily of availability of the rate-limiting substrate, fatty acids. This can be achieved by release of fatty acids from adipose tissue caused by lipolysis and by synthesis of fatty acids in the liver. There is evidence that TNF can regulate both these processes. In vivo and in vitro studies suggest that TNF stimulates lipolysis [242]. Other reports demonstrated that TNF induces a rapid increase in fatty acid synthesis in the liver [243].

Interestingly, the effect of TNF on fatty acid synthesis is site-specific. Whereas TNF increased fatty acid synthesis in the liver, it did not influence this process in muscle, fat tissue, or small intestine [243]. One reason why TNF has a differential effect on fatty acid synthesis in various tissues may be differences in enzyme activities. In liver, TNF mediates the increase in fatty acid synthesis by increasing the activities of the enzymes acetyl-CoA carboxylase (secondary to increased citrate levels) and fatty acid synthetase [250], but similar effects of the cytokines have not been reported in other tissues.

The cellular mechanisms by which TNF influences lipid metabolism are not fully understood. Evidence for a direct effect of TNF on cellular lipid metabolism was found in Hep-G2 cells [251] and in cultured preadipocytes [245]. It is possible that the counter-regulatory hormones are also involved in the TNF-induced regulation of lipid turnover; for example, evidence for an interaction between catecholamines and the cytokine was found in a study in which preincubation of isolated rat hepatocytes with TNF increased the epinephrine-stimulated lipolysis [232]. In addition, nutritional status is important for the mechanism by which TNF induces hypertriglyceridemia [252]. In chow-fed rats, TNF increased the availability of fatty acids by increasing lipolysis in adipose tissue, whereas in sucrose-fed rats, TNF markedly stimulated hepatic de novo synthesis of fatty acids. Both conditions resulted in increased triglyceride production by the liver. The observation that TNF can stimulate hepatic triglyceride synthesis and increase plasma triglyceride levels through multiple mechanisms supports the concept that changes in lipid metabolism play an important role in the overall response to infection and inflammation.

Other Cytokines and Lipid Metabolism

In addition to TNF, other cytokines can influence the various aspects of lipid metabolism. Interleukin-1, IFN-α, IFN-β, and IFN-γ have been shown to stimulate lipolysis and reduce lipoprotein lipase activity in cultured adipocytes [253,254]. The inhibitory effect of IL-1 on lipoprotein lipase activity in cultured 3T3-L1 adipocytes was caused by reduced synthesis of the enzyme [254]. Administration in vivo of TNF-α, TNF-β, IL-1, IL-6, or IFN-α resulted in increased synthesis in the liver of fatty acids [255]. When the effects of TNF, IL-1, and IFN-α were compared, the stimulation of hepatic fatty acid synthesis peaked approximately 2 hours after administration of each cytokine, and the most pronounced stimulation was found after IFN-α (Figure 3-23) [255].

Different classes of cytokines increase hepatic fatty acid synthesis through different mechanisms [256]. Tumor necrosis factor, IL-1, and IL-6 increase hepatic levels of citrate, which is an activator of acetyl-CoA carboxylase, the rate-limiting enzyme in fatty acid synthesis. In contrast, IFN-α does not alter hepatic citrate levels, and the mechanism of IFN-α-stimulated hepatic fatty acid synthesis has not yet been clarified [256].

The fact that different cytokines influence hepatic fatty acid synthesis through different mechanisms can explain some of the interactions between the cytokines. For example, an additive effect of IFN-α was observed when the cytokine was administered together with either TNF or IL-1. In contrast, maximal doses of TNF and IL-1 given together (presumably working through the same mechanism) did not further increase fatty acid synthesis (Figure 3-24).

Interestingly, recent studies suggest that not only do different classes of cytokines stimulate

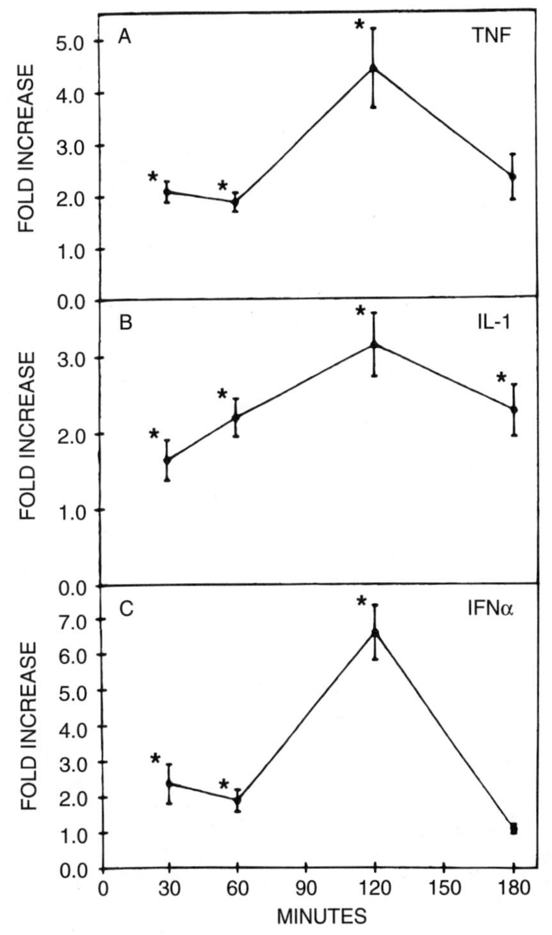

Figure 3-23. Time course of cytokine stimulation of hepatic fatty acid synthesis. Zero, 30, 60, and 120 minutes after the im. administration of a cytokine or vehicle alone, animals were injected ip. with 20 mCi tritiated water. Thirty minutes (0 and 30 minute groups) or 60 minutes (60 and 120 minute groups) later the animals were killed, and the incorporation of tritiated water into fatty acids was determined. The difference between the cytokine and control groups was statistically significant. **(A)** TNFα (5 μg/mouse); **(B)** IL-1 (200 ng/mouse); **(C)** IFNα (50 μg/mouse). * = $p < 0.05$ vs. control. (From KR Feingold et al. Multiple cytokines stimulate hepatic lipid synthesis in vivo. *Endocrinology* 125:267, 1989. Copyright The Endocrine Society.)

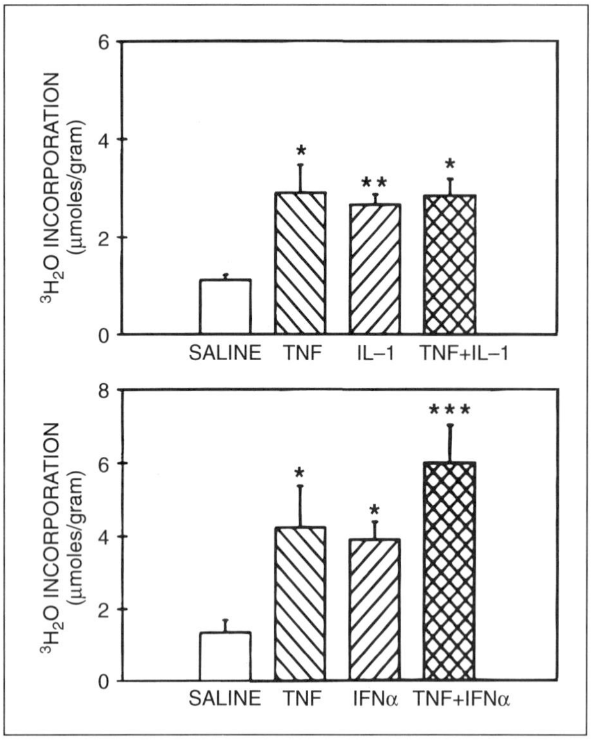

Figure 3-24. The effect of cytokines alone and in combination on hepatic fatty acid synthesis in mice. *Upper:* * = $p < 0.02$ vs. saline; ** = $p < 0.05$ vs. saline. *Lower:* * = $p < 0.02$ vs. saline; *** = < 0.0001 vs. saline. (From C Grunfeld et al. Evidence for two classes of cytokines that stimulate hepatic lipogenesis: Relationships among tumor necrosis factor, interleukin-1 and interferon-alpha. *Endocrinology* 127:46, 1990. Copyright The Endocrine Society.)

hepatic lipogenesis through different mechanisms, but certain cytokines may have an inhibitory effect. Interleukin-4 was found to inhibit the stimulation of hepatic fatty acid synthesis induced by TNF, IL-1, or IL-6 [257]. Interleukin-4 did not have an effect by itself and did not influence the IFN-α-stimulated hepatic fatty acid synthesis. These results also support the concept that different cytokines induce hepatic lipogenesis through distinct mechanisms, as described above.

Protein Metabolism

Cytokines may affect protein and amino acid metabolism in all tissues of the body. The most compelling evidence for a role of cytokines in the control of protein metabolism, at least during sepsis and other critical illness, has been generated for skeletal muscle and liver.

Skeletal Muscle

The two scientific reports that have probably been most important in terms of generating an interest in the field of cytokines, protein metabolism, and sepsis are the reports by Clowes and colleagues [258] and Baracos and colleagues [259] published back to back in the same issue of *New England Journal of Medicine* in 1983. Both papers proposed a role of IL-1 as a mediator of muscle proteolysis during sepsis.

Clowes and colleagues [258] demonstrated that addition of plasma from injured and septic patients to incubated muscles from normal rats or to muscle fibers from nonseptic patients resulted in an increase in protein degradation, similar to that induced by sepsis itself (Figure 3-25). The authors found evidence of an active factor in plasma, which they called proteolysis inducing factor (PIF). The factor had a molecular weight of 4200 Da and was proposed to be an active cleavage product of IL-1.

In the study by Baracos and colleagues [259], addition of IL-1, purified from supernatant from endotoxin-stimulated monocytes, to incubated rat muscles increased total protein breakdown. In the same report, addition of indomethacin to the incubation medium blocked the cytokine-induced muscle proteolysis, and it was suggested that prostaglandin E_2 mediates the effect of IL-1 on muscle protein breakdown. It should be noted that in this report [259], purified IL-1 was used, and it is possible that the preparation contained a number of other biologically active substances released from the monocytes. In subsequent studies from the same laboratory, the direct effect of IL-1 on protein breakdown in incubated muscles could not be duplicated when a recombinant form of the cytokine was used [260].

Studies from our group confirmed the presence of a proteolysis-inducing factor in plasma from septic rats or patients [261]. However, the septic plasma did not induce the typical sepsis-like response of a predominant increase in myofibrillar protein breakdown, and the response to the septic plasma was seen only in muscles from starved rats and under very specific in vitro conditions. Thus, the role of PIF in the sepsis-induced muscle proteolysis remains unclear.

The possible direct effect of IL-1, TNF, and other cytokines on muscle protein degradation has been tested in a number of reports in which varying concentrations of recombinant cytokines were added to incubated muscles from rats or mice [260–263]. Although results in most of those studies were negative, i.e., no evidence of increased protein breakdown was found, not even at very high cytokine concentrations, they do not rule out the possibility of a direct effect of cytokines in muscle tissue. It is possible, for example, that the cytokines require a specific milieu, present in the septic organism but difficult to reproduce in vitro, to be able to induce muscle proteolysis. Indeed,

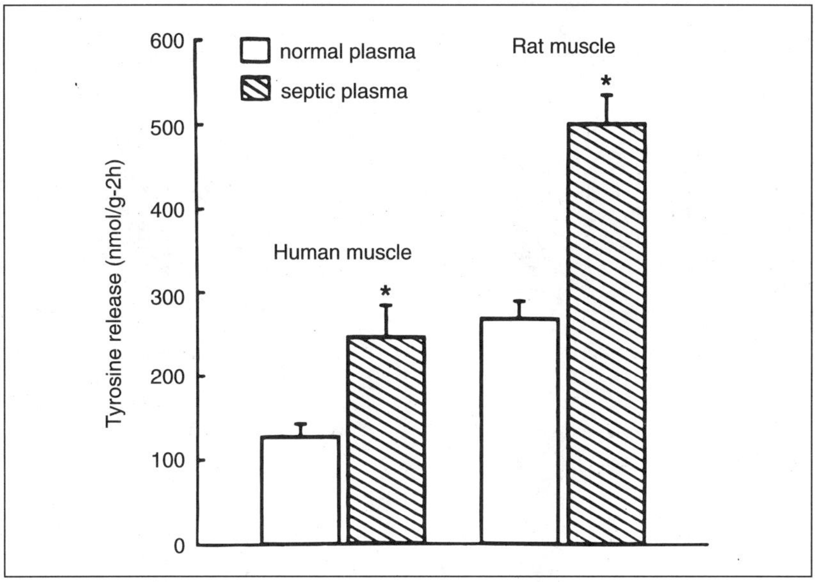

Figure 3-25. Protein breakdown rates in human muscle biopsies and in rat soleus muscles incubated in the presence of normal plasma or plasma from septic patients. *$p < 0.05$. (Reprinted, by permission of *The New England Journal of Medicine,* from GHA Clowes et al. Muscle proteolysis induced by a circulating peptide in patients with sepsis or trauma. *N Engl J Med* 308:545, 1983. Copyright Massachusetts Medical Society.)

there is evidence that the regulation of muscle proteolysis during sepsis is complex and that cytokines exert their effect in muscle only in the presence of essential co-factor(s).

The in vivo role of cytokines in the regulation of muscle protein turnover has been tested with two different experimental approaches, i.e., either by administering cytokines to normal animals or to nonseptic humans, or by treating septic animals or patients with cytokine antibodies or receptor blockers.

Previous studies, in which cytokines were administered to normal rats or mice, gave rise to conflicting results. Whereas some authors found evidence of muscle catabolism after administration of IL-1 or TNF [264–266], others failed to demonstrate increased muscle proteolysis after administration of various cytokines [263,267]. In experiments in our laboratory, treatment of rats with rTNF-α (total dose of 300 μg/kg divided into three equal intraperitoneal injections over 16 hours) or identical doses of rIL-1α resulted in increased protein breakdown in incubated extensor digitorum longus muscles (Figure 3-26) [268–271]. Of interest was the finding that the increase in myofibrillar protein breakdown (3-MH release) was more prominent than the increase in total protein breakdown (tyrosine release). Thus, in this respect the cytokines gave rise to a sepsis-like metabolic pattern in skeletal muscle. In the same studies, the cytokines did not influence muscle protein synthesis rates, measured as incorporation of ^{14}C-phenylalanine into protein, suggesting that muscle protein synthesis and breakdown are subject to different control mechanisms.

Further evidence for a role of TNF in the control of muscle protein breakdown was found in experiments in which pretreatment of septic rats with anti-TNF antibodies significantly blunted the sepsis-induced increase in muscle protein breakdown (Figure 3-27) [268]. In the same study, treatment with anti-TNF antibodies did not influence the reduced protein synthesis noted in septic rats, further supporting the concept that protein synthesis and breakdown in muscle are regulated by different mechanisms during sepsis.

In other experiments, endotoxemic or septic rats were treated with a recombinant form of the naturally occurring IL-1ra [272]. This treatment blunted the increase in muscle proteolysis (Figure 3-28), supporting the role of IL-1 as a mediator of muscle proteolysis during sepsis and endotoxemia.

Thus, both TNF and IL-1 may participate in the regulation of muscle protein breakdown during sepsis or endotoxemia. Because TNF can induce release of IL-1 [39], the effects caused by TNF injection in normal rats or by administration of anti-TNF antibodies in septic rats may have reflected a regulatory role of IL-1. Both TNF and IL-1 may also exert their effects through another mediator or mediators, for example, cytokines such as IL-6. The complex interaction between the various cytokines is further illustrated by the cytokine cascade described above and by the release during sepsis and endotoxemia of endogenous inhibitors of the cytokines [49–52].

An additional mechanism by which cytokines may exert their catabolic effect could be inhibition of an anabolic factor or factors. One such factor

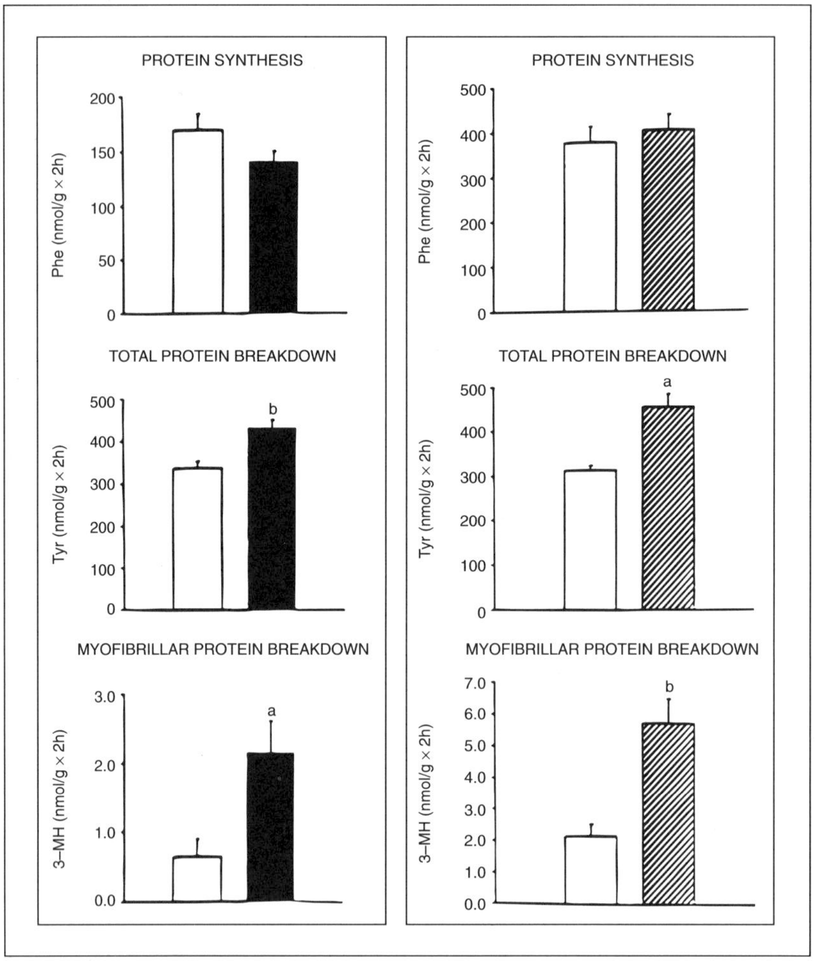

Figure 3-26. *Left:* Protein synthesis, total protein breakdown, and myofibrillar protein breakdown in incubated extensor digitorum longus (EDL) muscles from control rats (open bars) and from rats treated with rTNFα, three ip. injections of 100 μg/kg each over 16 hours (solid bars).
[a]$p < 0.05$.
[b]$p < 0.01$.
(From O Zamir et al. Evidence that tumor necrosis factor participates in the regulation of muscle proteolysis during sepsis. *Arch Surg* 127:171, 1992. Copyright 1992, American Medical Association.)
Right: Effect of rIL-1α injected ip. in rats at a dose of 100 μg/kg three times over 16 hours on protein synthesis, total protein breakdown, and myofibrillar protein breakdown in incubated EDL muscles from control rats (open bars) and from rIL-1α treated rats (hatched bars).
[a]$p < 0.05$.
[b]$p < 0.01$.
(From O Zamir et al. In vivo administration of interleukin-1α induces muscle proteolysis in normal and adrenalectomized rats. *Metabolism* 42:204, 1993.)

may be IGF-1. Previous studies have shown that IGF-1 inhibits muscle protein breakdown and stimulates protein synthesis [186,193,194]. In other reports, the anabolic effects of IGF-1 in chondrocytes were blocked by cytokines, most effectively by TNF [273]. Further studies will be important to define the interaction between IGF-1 and cytokines in the regulation of muscle proteolysis.

Liver

Among the cytokines, IL-6 is the most important regulator of the acute-phase response in the liver. The role of IL-6 in the acute-phase response was reviewed more extensively elsewhere [33]. Interleukin-6 is the same substance that was previously called hepatocyte stimulating factor or INF-β_2.

Evidence for the important role of IL-6 in the acute-phase response has been generated both in vivo and in vitro. Administration in vivo of IL-6 to rats increased hepatic mRNA levels for α_2-macroglobulin, β-fibrinogen, cystein protease inhibitor, and α_1-acid glycoprotein, and decreased albumin mRNA concentrations, indicating that an almost complete acute-phase response can be induced by this cytokine [274]. Added in vitro to cultured human hepatocytes, IL-6 stimulated acute-phase protein synthesis, consistent with a direct effect of IL-6 on the hepatocyte [275].

The effects induced by IL-6 (and other cytokines) may be receptor mediated. Baumann and associates [276] reported the presence of IL-6 receptors on liver cells. A large increase in acute-phase protein synthesis, despite a relatively low number of IL-6 receptors, is consistent with an efficient amplification system. The most important source of IL-6 during sepsis and inflammation is probably the Kupffer cell, although other cell types, including the hepatocyte itself, have been found to secrete IL-6. Recent studies in our laboratory have shown that the enterocyte is another potential source of IL-6 [unpublished observations]. This may be of biologic significance because IL-6 produced in the intestine reaches the liver directly through the portal vein, and there

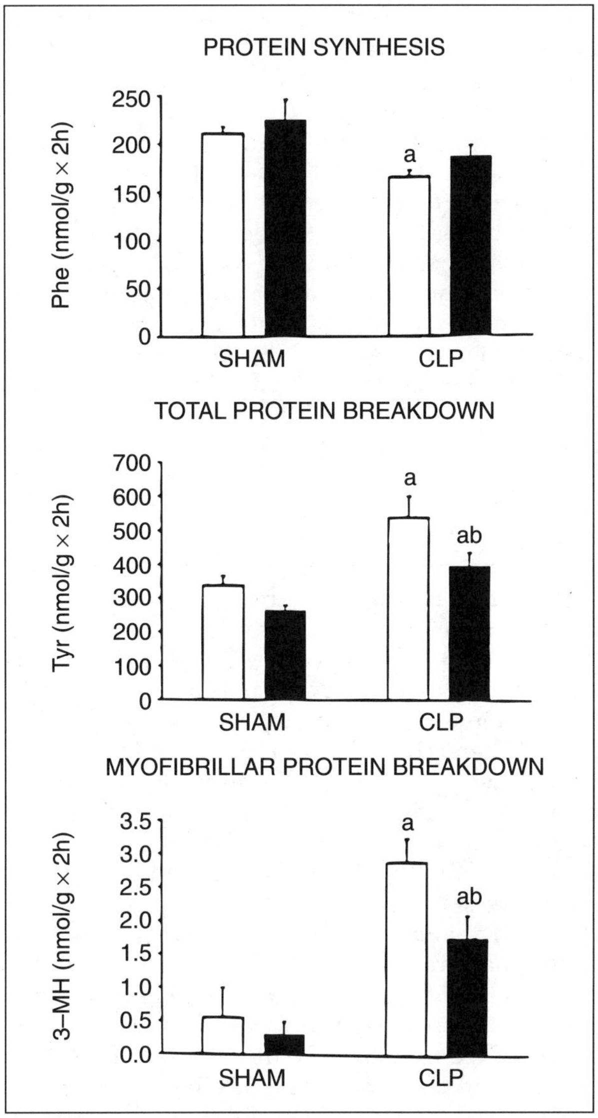

Figure 3-27. Protein synthesis, total protein breakdown, and myofibrillar protein breakdown in incubated extensor digitorum longus (EDL) muscles from sham-operated and septic (CLP) rats. Rats were treated with control serum (open bars) or anti-TNF antiserum (solid bars) 2 hours before sham-operation or CLP.
[a]$p < 0.05$ vs. corresponding sham-operated group.
[b]$p < 0.05$ vs. control injected CLP.
(From O Zamir et al. Evidence that tumor necrosis factor participates in the regulation of muscle proteolysis during sepsis. *Arch Surg* 127:171, 1992. Copyright 1992, American Medical Association.)

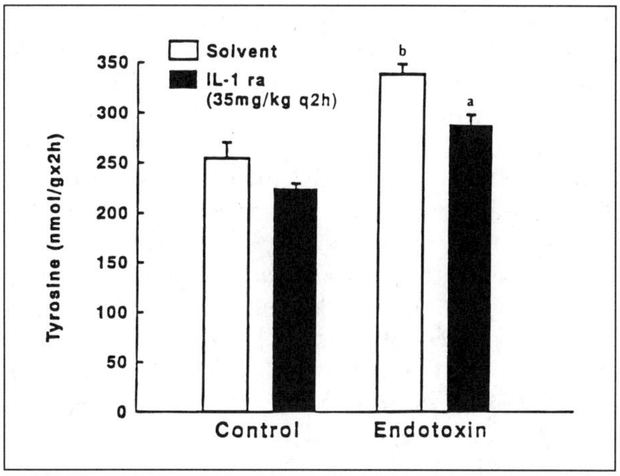

Figure 3-28. Total protein breakdown rates in incubated extensor digitorum longus (EDL) muscles from control and endotoxin (1 mg/kg) injected rats. Muscles were incubated 4 hours after control or endotoxin injection. Groups of rats were treated with rIL-1ra (35 mg/kg every 2 hours) or corresponding volumes of solvent.
[a]$p < 0.05$ vs. endotoxin/solvent.
[b]$p < 0.05$ vs. all other groups.
(From O Zamir et al. Muscle protein breakdown during endotoxemia in rats and after treatment with interleukin-1 receptor antagonist (IL-1ra). *Ann Surg* 216:381, 1992.)

is abundant evidence of the importance of gut (and pancreas) flow on hepatic function, particularly biosynthetic activity.

The important role of IL-6 in the acute-phase response has been documented in several clinical studies. High circulating levels of IL-6 were observed in patients with severe sepsis [277,278]. The correlation between IL-6 levels and CRP concentrations observed in septic patients further supports a role of IL-6 as a mediator of acute-phase protein synthesis [278].

The molecular regulation of acute-phase protein synthesis by IL-6 has been extensively studied in recent years and is briefly summarized here. In principle, similar mechanisms are involved in the regulation of acute-phase protein synthesis by IL-1, TNF, and glucocorticoids.

After binding of IL-6 to its receptor on the hepatocyte, nuclear proteins (transcription factors) bind to an IL-6 responsive region of the acute-phase gene. This region, the IL-6 response element (IL-6RE), is present on the promoter of the acute-phase gene and has been described for the genes encoding human and rat haptoglobin, human hemopexin, human CRP, and rat α_2-macroglobulin [279–283]. Other studies suggest that the cytokine response elements of acute-phase protein genes are complexes of several interacting regulatory sequences [284].

Several different transcription factors induced by IL-6 have been described, including the so-called IL-6RE binding protein [285–287]. The sequence of events that occur between binding of the cytokine to its receptor and activation of the transcription factor(s) are not completely understood, but intracellular second messenger systems, including activation of protein kinases (see previous sections of this chapter), are probably involved. Interleukin-6 induction of acute-phase protein gene expression is not inhibited by cycloheximide, suggesting that the induction does not require de novo synthesis of transcription factors, but may involve posttranslational modification of preexisting nuclear proteins [28]. After binding of the transcription factor to the response element, transcription of mRNA is initiated. There is evidence that transcriptional induction of acute-phase protein expression is a very fast process. C-reactive protein mRNA was detectable as early as 2 hours after injection of endotoxin in transgenic mice [288] and 2 hours after exposure of cells to IL-6 in vitro [135]. The induction of acute-phase protein genes by IL-6 is summarized in Figure 3–29 in a highly simplified scheme.

Two major classes of acute-phase protein genes have been identified. Class 1 genes are regulated by IL-1, combinations of IL-1 and IL-6, and by combinations of these two cytokines with glucocorticoids [289,290]; this class includes the rat haptoglobin, C3, α_1-acid glycoprotein, and human CRP. Class 2 genes are primarily controlled by IL-6 and leukemia inhibitory factor and by combinations of these cytokines and glucocorticoids; fibrinogen, α_1-antitrypsin, α_1-antichymotrypsin, and α_2-macroglobulin genes belong to class 2 [280]. A recent study by Hocke and colleagues [291] found further evidence that IL-6 activates two different classes of acute-phase genes. This activation was mediated by at least two different nuclear DNA-binding proteins (transcription factors) that in turn bind to two different types (types 1 and 2) of response elements.

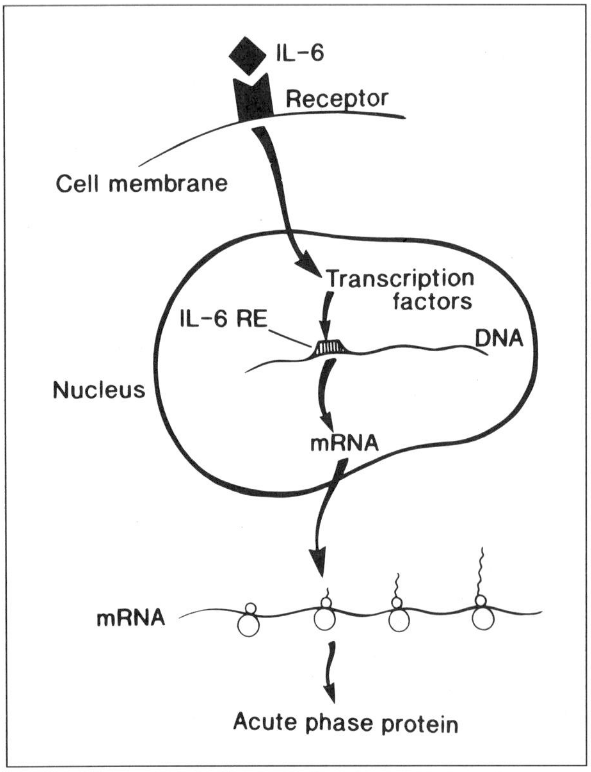

Figure 3-29. Simplified scheme of the molecular regulation of IL-6-induced acute-phase protein synthesis.

Although IL-6 is the most important cytokine in the regulation of acute-phase protein synthesis [33], other cytokines may also control hepatic protein synthesis. In early studies, infusion of leukocytic endogenous mediator (LEM) resulted in increased amino acid uptake and protein synthesis in the liver and elevated plasma concentrations of acute-phase proteins [292]. Although it was assumed that most of the activity of LEM was caused by IL-1, the LEM preparations probably contained a number of other biologically active substances in addition to IL-1.

In subsequent studies using recombinant forms of IL-1, results supported a role of this cytokine in the control of acute-phase protein synthesis, although it is not the major regulator. A partial acute-phase response after infusion of rIL-1 in rats was reported by Flores and colleagues [265]. Increased mRNA levels in liver for serum amyloid A was noted after treatment of mice with rIL-1 [293]. When rIL-1α was administered to rats during 3 days, the synthesis of total secreted proteins, complement component C3, and α_1-acid glycoprotein was increased in perfused liver, whereas the synthesis of albumin was unchanged and not reduced as expected [294]. These results suggest that IL-1 regulates part of, but not the complete, acute-phase response.

Treatment of cultured rat hepatoma cells with TNF in vitro resulted in stimulated synthesis of α_1-acid glycoprotein and reduced production of albumin, and these changes may have been regulated at the transcriptional level because mRNA levels for α_1-acid glycoprotein and albumin were increased and reduced, respectively [295]. In the same report, TNF had no effect on fibrinogen mRNA, suggesting that TNF does not regulate the complete acute-phase response. In recent experiments in our laboratory, pretreatment of endotoxemic rats with anti-TNF antibodies almost completely abolished the increase in hepatic protein synthesis (Figure 3-30). This result is consistent with TNF being a "proximal" mediator in the cytokine cascade. A recent study by Bankey and associates [296] provided evidence that the role of TNF in vivo in the regulation of acute-phase protein synthesis is indirect.

In addition to IL-6, IL-1, and TNF, other cytokines may be involved in the regulation of acute-phase protein synthesis. Those cytokines include IFN-γ, transforming growth factor β, leukemia inhibiting factor, IL-11, and oncostatin M [297–299]. The large number of substances that modulate the

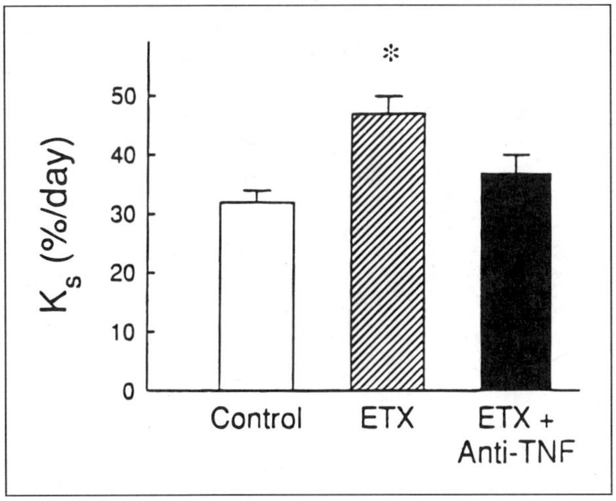

Figure 3-30. Hepatic protein synthesis rate in vivo, determined by flooding dose technique, in control and endotoxemic rats and in endotoxemic rats treated with anti-TNF antiserum. * = $p < 0.05$ vs. other groups by ANOVA. (From unpublished studies in our laboratory.)

acute-phase response illustrates the complexity of this system.

Other Tissues

Although less well established than for muscle and liver, cytokines may be involved in the regulation of protein turnover in other tissues as well. Administration of TNF or IL-1 to rats resulted in increased protein synthesis in the mucosa of small intestine, similar to the response seen during sepsis and endotoxemia [139]. A number of observations suggest that IL-1 may be the most important cytokine for regulation of intestinal metabolism. Administration to rats of IL-1, but not TNF, induced a sepsis-like increase in the biosynthesis of intestinal polyamines [300]. In vitro treatment of cultured IEC-6 cells with IL-1, but not TNF, stimulated the expression and activity of ornithine decarboxylase (ODC), the rate-limiting enzyme in the polyamine biosynthesis [301].

Further evidence for a differential effect of TNF and IL-1 was reported by Austgen and associates [302]. They found that administration of rIL-1α to normal rats resulted in inhibited glutamine uptake by the intestine. This effect of the cytokine was caused by reduced extraction of glutamine because intestinal blood flow was not affected by IL-1. In addition, treatment with rIL-1α reduced mucosal glutaminase activity. In contrast to the effects of IL-1, administration of rTNF-α to normal rats did not increase intestinal glutamine uptake or mucosal glutaminase activity [302].

Argiles and colleagues [303] measured brush-border transport by system A by determining the absorption of carbon 14 alpha amino isobutyric acid (^{14}C-AIB) administered orally to rats. Intestinal absorption of AIB was inhibited after treatment of rats with IL-1, whereas TNF did not significantly affect intestinal absorption of the amino acid.

The role of cytokines in the regulation of protein metabolism in the lungs is not known. However, cytokines may influence amino acid transport and metabolism in different cell types present in the lungs [304].

Interaction Between Cytokines and Hormones in the Control of Metabolism

As discussed earlier, the release of hormones and cytokines during sepsis and other critical illness is interrelated. In addition, certain cytokines can stimulate the synthesis and release of other cytokines. In this section, evidence will be discussed that hormones and cytokines interact in the control of metabolism in various organs and tissues.

The interaction between glucocorticoids and cytokines in the control of acute-phase protein synthesis has been well documented. In several previous studies, glucocorticoids acted as an important or essential co-factor to IL-6 or other cytokines in the control of hepatocyte protein synthesis. In a report by Koj and associates [305], cytokines from endotoxin-stimulated human monocytes increased the production of α_2-macroglobulin and fibrinogen and inhibited albumin synthesis in isolated rat hepatocytes only when dexamethasone was present in the medium. In other in vitro studies, Baumann and colleagues [306] found that dexamethasone alone did not affect the production of acute-phase proteins in human hepatoma cells, but potentiated the effect of IL-1 or IL-6 several-fold. Administration in vivo of IL-6 to rats stimulated the acute-phase protein expression in liver, but glucocorticoids were necessary to get a maximal response to IL-6 [307]. These results are consistent with a permissive role of glucocorticoids in the acute-phase response in liver. In a previous report from our laboratory, the stimulated acute-phase protein synthesis seen after treatment with rIL-1α was blunted in adrenalectomized rats [294], further supporting the concept that glucocorticoids are necessary for a complete acute-phase response.

The complexity involved in the metabolic control of the acute-phase response is further illustrated by the fact that certain acute-phase proteins are regulated individually by specific substances, whereas some acute-phase proteins require the interaction between two or more mediators. Thus, whereas fibrinogen mRNA levels increased several-fold in a rat hepatoma cell line after the addition of IL-6, other cytokines (IL-1β and TNF-α) had no effect on fibrinogen gene transcription, but instead led to a substantial increase in α_1-acid glycoprotein mRNA [295]. All three cytokines reduced albumin mRNA concentrations. In the same study, dexamethasone potentiated the induction of fibrinogen mRNA and was required for the increase in α_1-acid glycoprotein mRNA.

Although the molecular mechanisms of the interaction between glucocorticoids and cytokines in the acute-phase response are not fully understood at present, the synergism may reflect activation by glucocorticoids of a gene that regulates the synthesis of cytokine response element-binding proteins [291].

In skeletal muscle, an interaction between hormones, in particular glucocorticoids, and cytokines may be important for the control of protein metabolism. Support for this concept was found in a study in which treatment of rats with rTNF-α (200 μg/kg) stimulated total and myofibrillar protein breakdown only when the cytokine was administered together with corticosterone and when the treatment resulted in increased plasma levels of corticosterone [308]. When adrenalectomized rats were identically treated, plasma corticosterone levels did not increase and muscle protein degradation rates were unaffected by the cytokine, further supporting the concept that TNF-induced muscle proteolysis is mediated by glucocorticoids or by an interaction between TNF and glucocorticoids at the cellular level.

The role of glucocorticoids in cytokine-induced muscle proteolysis was further tested in a recent study by treating rats with the glucocorticoid receptor antagonist RU38486 [270]. In that study, the TNF-induced increase in muscle proteolysis was almost completely abolished by RU38486, suggesting that TNF-induced muscle proteolysis is mediated by glucocorticoids or that TNF requires the presence of glucocorticoids as a co-factor for its catabolic effect in muscle. In contrast, stimulated muscle proteolysis induced by IL-1 was not blocked by RU38486, suggesting that IL-1 induces muscle protein breakdown through a glucocorticoid-independent pathway. The finding that IL-1 increases muscle proteolysis in adrenalectomized rats [271] is also consistent with a glucocorticoid-independent pathway through which IL-1 can induce muscle proteolysis. Our current understanding of the interaction between TNF, IL-1, and glucocorticoids in the regulation of muscle protein breakdown is summarized in Figure 3-31.

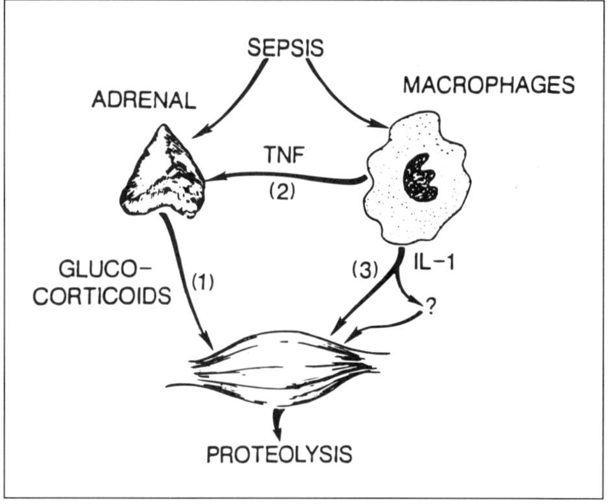

Figure 3-31. Proposed interaction between (1) glucocorticoids, (2) TNF, and (3) IL-1 in the regulation of sepsis-induced muscle proteolysis. The effect of TNF on muscle proteolysis is primarily mediated by glucocorticoids, whereas IL-1 regulates muscle proteolysis by glucocorticoid-independent pathway(s). (From PO Hasselgren. *Protein Metabolism in Sepsis.* Austin: Landes, 1993.)

Studies in other laboratories have provided evidence that glucocorticoids are necessary for the TNF-induced muscle catabolism. Mealy and colleagues [309] reported that administration of TNF to normal rats resulted in reduced carcass nitrogen content and impaired nitrogen balance; when TNF was infused in adrenalectomized rats, the urinary nitrogen loss was blunted. Although protein turnover rates were not measured in that study, the results were interpreted as indicating that TNF stimulates muscle proteolysis and that this effect of the cytokine is glucocorticoid-dependent.

The observation that IL-1 increases muscle proteolysis independently of glucocorticoids does not necessarily mean that IL-1 has a direct effect on muscle tissue. In fact, a number of previous studies failed to demonstrate a direct effect of IL-1 when the cytokine was added to incubated muscles at different concentrations [260–263]. Interleukin-1 may stimulate muscle proteolysis through some other substance than a glucocorticoid, perhaps another cytokine. In this respect, IL-6 may be one possible candidate as a "second messenger" of IL-1, considering the important role of this cytokine for the control of protein metabolism in other tissues. There is evidence that IL-1 can stimulate the release of IL-6 and that metabolic effects and mortality induced by IL-1 may be mediated by IL-6 [40,58]. The effect of IL-6 on muscle protein turnover remains to be determined.

An additional mechanism by which IL-1 may

induce muscle catabolism could be inhibited release or counteraction of IGF-1. The anabolic effect of IGF-1 in muscle tissue is well established (discussed above). In a recent study, treatment of mice with IL-1α, but not TNFα, resulted in reduced circulating levels of free and total IGF-1 [310]. Other studies, discussed earlier in this chapter, provided evidence that cytokines, including TNF, IL-1, and IL-6, may counteract the anabolic effects of IGF-1 at the cellular level [273].

Other Mediators

In addition to hormones and cytokines, other substances that may be involved in the regulation of metabolism during critical illness include prostaglandins, free oxygen radicals, and nitric oxide (NO). Some of these substances may interact with each other and may also interact with hormones and cytokines in the control of metabolism. In this section, the roles of prostaglandins, oxygen radicals, and NO are briefly discussed.

Prostaglandins

The possible role of prostaglandins in the regulation of metabolism has been studied in liver and, more extensively, in muscle. A direct effect of prostaglandin E_1 (PGE_1) on the synthesis of the acute-phase protein α_2-macroglobulin has been suggested [311]. In that study, induction of inflammation in rats by subplantar injection of a carrageenin suspension resulted in increased serum levels of α_2-macroglobulin. A similar response was seen after the injection of PGE_1, and the increase in serum α_2-macroglobulin after PGE_1 injection was dose- and time-dependent. When PGE_1 was added to incubated liver slices, incorporation of ^{14}C-leucine into α_2-macroglobulin increased, and the results were interpreted as indicating a direct effect of PGE_1 on hepatocyte acute-phase protein synthesis. Some of the results in that study, however, were contradictory and make it less likely that prostaglandins directly control acute-phase protein synthesis in the hepatocyte. In contrast to the effect of PGE_1 in normal rats, administration of PGE_1 to rats with inflammation reduced serum α_2-macroglobulin levels. A similar inhibitory effect of PGE_1 was noted when the substance was added in vitro to incubated liver slices from rats with inflammation. In vivo and in liver slices, the possible role of the Kupffer cells needs to be taken into account. Several studies have shown that cytokine production by Kupffer cells, and other macrophages as well, is regulated by prostaglandins [312]. It is possible that the seemingly contradictory results observed after administration of PGE_1 to normal or inflamed rats may reflect differences in cytokine production by Kupffer cells that were present either in a nonstimulated or stimulated state. Prostaglandins may participate in the regulation of acute-phase protein synthesis, but this is probably not the result of a direct effect on the hepatocyte.

A role of prostaglandins in the control of muscle protein metabolism was proposed by Goldberg and co-authors [259,313]. Addition in vitro of PGE_2 or arachidonic acid to incubated rat muscles was reported to stimulate protein degradation. In other experiments in the same laboratory, treatment of incubated rat muscles in vitro with purified IL-1 increased PGE_2 production and protein breakdown, and both effects were blocked with the prostaglandin synthesis inhibitor, indomethacin [259]. From these observations, the authors proposed that PGE_2 is a mediator of muscle proteolysis, distal to IL-1, and that prostaglandin synthesis inhibitors may be useful in the treatment of muscle catabolism during fever and infection.

Experiments in other laboratories, however, have not confirmed a role of prostaglandins in the regulation of muscle protein turnover, neither under normal nor catabolic conditions. Addition of PGE_2 or arachidonic acid to incubated rat or mouse muscles did not stimulate protein breakdown in a report by Barnett and Ellis [314]. In another study, indomethacin blocked PGE_2 production in muscles from burned rats, but did not affect muscle protein breakdown rates [315].

In our laboratory as well, we have been unable to find evidence of a role of PGE_2 in the control of muscle protein degradation [316–318]. In those studies, both total and myofibrillar protein breakdown rates were unaffected by the addition of PGE_2 or arachidonic acid to incubated rat muscles. Indomethacin blocked the production of PGE_2 without affecting proteolysis in incubated muscles from control or septic rats. Also, when PGE_2 production was inhibited by indomethacin in vivo, total and myofibrillar protein breakdown rates remained increased in rats with sepsis.

One possible explanation why stimulated protein breakdown after the addition of PGE_2 or arachidonic acid to incubated muscles observed in earlier studies [259,313] have not been reproduced could be the presence of contaminants that are no longer present in the highly purified reagents that are currently available. This could also explain why the effect of PGE_2 could not be reproduced in subsequent studies in Goldberg's own laboratory [319].

Oxygen Radicals

One mechanism by which proteins are degraded at an increased rate is substrate modification. Proteins can be altered by a number of different mechanisms, including mutations, errors in biosynthesis, nonenzymatic glycosylation, and spontaneous deamidation. It is well known that such "abnormal proteins" are rapidly degraded within cells, mainly via the ATP-ubiquitin-dependent proteolytic pathway.

An additional mechanism by which proteins can be altered is by reactions with oxygen free radicals [320]. The generation of oxygen free radicals during reperfusion of ischemic tissue and the important role of the free radicals in the development of postischemic tissue/organ injury is well established. Improvement of protein synthesis in the postischemic liver after treatment with allopurinol [321] suggests that oxygen radicals may induce changes in protein metabolism. Previous studies suggest that oxygen free radicals may also be responsible for pathophysiologic changes observed during sepsis and endotoxemia [322] and, in fact, it is possible that tissue ischemia and reperfusion occur in these conditions as well. Other studies suggest that cytokines may amplify the generation of free radicals [323].

Although most previous evidence for a role of oxygen radicals in the pathogenesis of endotoxemia and septic shock was indirect after treatment with various oxygen radical scavengers, a recent study provided direct evidence of oxygen radical production during septic shock in nonhuman primates by using electron spin resonance spectroscopy and spin-trapping techniques [324]. In the same study, evidence was found that TNF is involved in the generation of oxygen radicals during sepsis.

Previous studies provided evidence that oxidant-damaged proteins are degraded by intracellular proteolytic systems at increased rates [325]. In a report by Davies [320], exposure of proteins to oxygen radicals, in particular the hydroxyl radical, resulted in aggregation or fragmentation of proteins, altered net electrical charge, and modifications of amino acids in the proteins. Simple denaturation, i.e., unfolding of proteins with increased accessibility of peptide bonds to proteases, also occurred after exposure to oxygen radicals. Most of the oxidatively damaged proteins were degraded in cell-free extracts of erythrocytes and reticulocytes up to 50 times faster than untreated proteins, and the degradation was conducted by nonlysosomal energy-independent proteolytic enzymes.

Recent studies performed in our laboratory in collaboration with Dr. Julie Fagan suggest that sepsis increases the amount of oxidatively damaged proteins in skeletal muscles assessed as the amount of sulfhydryl-containing proteins. The role of these changes in the increased total and myofibrillar protein breakdown rates during sepsis and other critical illness remains to be determined. It is interesting to note, however, that most previous studies of muscle proteolysis in various catabolic conditions have focused on the activity of different proteolytic pathways. It is possible that alterations of the substrates (proteins) may be equally important for the increase in muscle protein breakdown during critical illness.

Nitric Oxide (NO)

The role of NO as a mediator of hemodynamic and metabolic consequences of sepsis, endotoxemia, and inflammation has become increasingly prominent over the last few years; NO can probably be regarded as the "molecule of the decade" as far as the regulation of the inflammatory response is concerned.

L-Arginine is the substrate for NO production and nitrite/nitrate (NO_2/NO_3) are the stable end products together with citrulline (Figure 3-32). Because of the short half-life of NO, NO_2/NO_3 are usually measured to assess the production of NO. Nitric oxide is released from a number of different cell types, including endothelial cells, Kupffer cells and other macrophages, cerebellar neurons, and neutrophils [p. 326 provides a review]. The produc-

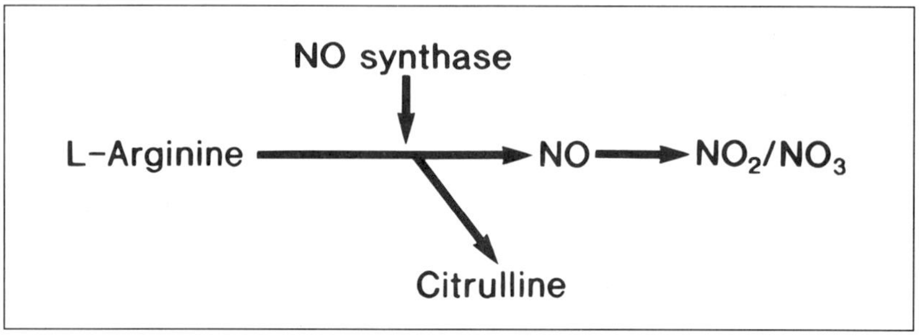

Figure 3-32. Arginine-dependent pathway for the production of nitric oxide (NO). The reaction is catalyzed by the enzyme NO synthase.

tion of NO from arginine is regulated by the enzyme NO synthase. Two forms of this enzyme have been described, i.e., the constitutive, calcium-dependent and the inducible, calcium-independent enzymes. The human inducible NO synthase gene was cloned recently [327,328]. Relaxation of vascular smooth muscle, inhibition of platelet aggregation and adherence, and inactivation of complex I and II of the electron transport chain are some of the biologic functions that have been ascribed to NO. Most of the cellular effects of NO are exerted through activation of soluble guanylate cyclase, resulting in increased cellular levels of cyclic guanosine monophosphate (cGMP).

Extensive studies regarding the involvement of NO in the control of metabolism have been performed with respect to hepatocyte protein synthesis. There is evidence that the direct effect of NO in vitro on hepatocyte protein synthesis is different than the influence of NO in vivo, possibly reflecting hemodynamic and other effects of the substance in vivo.

The regulation by NO in vitro of hepatocyte protein synthesis has been examined in a number of studies by Simmons, Billiar, and co-workers. When endotoxin was added to a co-culture of hepatocytes and Kupffer cells, the production of NO_2/NO_3 and citrulline increased, whereas hepatocyte protein synthesis decreased [329]. The inhibition of protein synthesis was dependent on the concentration of L-arginine and was prevented by the NO synthase inhibitor N^G-monomethyl-L-arginine (NMA). The results in that study were consistent with the concept that NO, released from endotoxin-stimulated Kupffer cells, inhibited protein synthesis in the hepatocyte.

In subsequent experiments in the same laboratory, evidence was found that not only Kupffer cells, but the hepatocyte as well can produce NO under certain circumstances [330]. Addition to cultured hepatocytes of supernatant from Kupffer cells that had been stimulated by endotoxin and IFN-γ stimulated release of NO from the hepatocytes and, at the same time, inhibited protein synthesis in the hepatocytes. These results suggest that hepatocyte protein synthesis may be regulated by NO in an autocrine fashion in addition to the paracrine effect of NO released from Kupffer cells. Also, after in vivo stimulation, evidence has been found that both Kupffer cells and hepatocytes can produce NO [331].

In the experiments described above, the evidence for an inhibitory effect of NO on hepatocyte protein synthesis was indirect, i.e., it was based on a correlation between NO_2/NO_3 levels and protein synthesis and on the effects of the NO synthase inhibitor NMA. More direct evidence for the concept that NO inhibits hepatocyte protein synthesis, at least in vitro, was found in experiments in which exposure of cultured rat hepatocytes to authentic NO or the NO-generating compound S-nitroso-N-acetylpenicillamine (SNAP) inhibited total protein synthesis in a dose-dependent fashion [332]. In the same study, albumin synthesis was reduced after exposure of the hepatocytes to NO, but albumin mRNA levels were unchanged, indicating that the inhibition of protein synthesis by NO is posttranscriptional. Exposure of the hepatocytes to NO resulted in high concentrations of cGMP (as expected), but because addition of the cGMP analogue 8-bromo-cGMP to the hepatocytes did not reduce protein synthesis, it was concluded that the inhibitory effect of NO on protein synthesis is not mediated by cGMP.

Although the experiments described above were performed in rat hepatocytes, other studies suggest that similar regulatory mechanisms may be present in humans as well. Increased plasma levels of NO_2/NO_3 have been reported in patients with sepsis [333], and NO production was induced in human hepatocytes by a mixture of TNF, IL-1, IFN-γ, and endotoxin [334].

Although in vitro experiments with cultured hepatocytes and Kupffer cells have been important in determining the direct effect of NO on hepatocyte protein synthesis, the results do not necessarily reflect the role of NO in vivo for the regulation of hepatic protein synthesis. Whereas NO in vitro impairs hepatocyte protein synthesis, other studies suggest that NO has a protective effect on the liver in vivo during sepsis and inflammation [335]. We recently found evidence that NO may participate in the up-regulation of hepatic protein synthesis during sepsis and endotoxemia [336]. In those experiments, circulating levels of NO_2/NO_3 and hepatic protein synthesis rates were increased after injection of endotoxin in rats. When NO production was blocked with the NO synthase inhibitor N^G-nitro-L-arginine (NNA), plasma levels of NO_2/NO_3 in endotoxemic rats were almost normalized, and hepatic protein synthesis decreased. These results are consistent with the concept that NO may actually stimulate hepatic protein synthesis in vivo. The mechanism of this effect of NO is not known, but it may reflect improved liver blood flow at the microcirculatory level, secondary to the vasodilatory effect of the substance, or to prevention of platelet aggregation and adhesion.

Further support for a protective role of NO during sepsis and endotoxemia has been found in recent studies in which blockade of NO synthase was deleterious and resulted in increased mortality rates [337]. A recent study from our laboratory suggests that increased mortality in endotoxemic rats after blockade of NO synthase may be caused by a dramatic increase in cytokine production, in particular that of IL-6 [338]. These results could be consistent with a negative feedback between NO and cytokine production by Kupffer cells and other macrophages so that when NO levels are reduced, cytokine production increases. Recent in vitro experiments support such a mechanism [338,339]. These results also serve to illustrate the complexity of the response to sepsis, endotoxemia, and inflammation with respect to the release of various mediators and the interaction between different types of mediators. They also emphasize that interference with the acute-phase response by biologic agents is a double-edged sword and may be deleterious.

One possible explanation why previous studies on the role of NO in vitro and in vivo seem to be contradictory may be that they reflect different severity levels of sepsis. Increased hepatic protein synthesis in the in vivo studies [336] most likely reflected an acute-phase response. In contrast, inhibited protein synthesis after exposure of hepatocytes to NO in vitro [329,332] may reflect a more severe state of sepsis with multiple organ failure, including failure of liver functions. In fact, some of the results observed in vitro may support that hypothesis. For example, exposure of cultured hepatocytes to NO resulted in inhibited synthesis of both albumin and fibrinogen [332], which contrasts to the acute-phase response of reduced albumin synthesis and increased synthesis of other proteins, including fibrinogen. Furthermore, addition of high concentrations of the cGMP analogue 8-bromo-cGMP to cultured hepatocytes increased protein synthesis [332], supporting the concept that NO may up-regulate hepatocyte protein synthesis, at least under certain circumstances. If the improved hepatic protein synthesis that was associated with high NO_2/NO_3 levels in vivo [336] reflected improved liver perfusion, this effect of NO, of course, could not be detected in vitro.

References

1. Fries E, Gustafson L, Peterson PA. Four secretory proteins synthesized by hepatocytes are transported from endoplasmic reticulum to Golgi complex at different rates. *EMBO J* 3:147, 1984.
2. Frayn KN. Hormonal control of metabolism in trauma and sepsis. *Clin Endocrinol* 24:577, 1986.
3. Cryer PE. Glucose counterregulation in man. *Diabetes* 30:261, 1981.
4. Batstone GF, et al. Metabolic studies in subjects following thermal injury. *Burns* 2:207, 1976.
5. Gann DS, Amaral JF, Caldwell MD. Neuroendocrine Response to Stress, Injury, and Sepsis. In JH Davis (ed), *Clinical Surgery.* St Louis: Mosby, 1987.
6. Gann DS, Dallman MF, Engeland WC. Reflex Control and Modulation of ACTH and Corticosteroids. In SM McCann (ed), *Endocrine Physiology III: International Review of Physiology.* Baltimore: University Park, 1981.
7. Frohman LA. CNS peptides and glucoregulation. *Annu Rev Physiol* 45:95, 1983.
8. Lindsey A, et al. Pancreatic alpha-cell function in trauma. *JAMA* 227:757, 1974.
9. Wilmore DW, et al. Hyperglucagonaemia after burns. *Lancet* 1:73, 1974.
10. Goschke H, et al. Glucagon, insulin, cortisol, and growth hormone levels following major surgery: Their relationship to glucose and free fatty acid elevations. *Horm Metab Res* 10:465, 1978.
11. Siegel JH, et al. Physiological and metabolic correlations in human sepsis. *Surgery* 86:163, 1979.
12. Goodall MC, Stone C, Haynes BW. Urinary output of adrenaline and noradrenaline in severe thermal burns. *Ann Surg* 145:479, 1957.
13. Wilmore DW, et al. Catecholamines: Mediator of the hypermetabolic response to thermal injury. *Ann Surg* 180:653, 1974.
14. Groves AC, et al. Plasma catecholamines in patients with serious postoperative infection. *Ann Surg* 178:102, 1973.
15. Ross R, et al. Critically ill patients have high basal growth hormone levels with attenuated oscillatory activity associated with low levels of insulin like growth factor-I. *Clin Endocrinol* 35:47, 1991.
16. Newsome HH, Rose JC. The response of human adrenocorticotrophic hormone and growth hormone to surgical stress. *J Clin Endocrinol Metab* 33:481, 1971.
17. Voerman HJ, Strack van Schijndel RJM, Thijs LG. Endocrine Disturbances in the Critically Ill: The Role of Growth Hormone and Cortisol. In JL Vincent (ed), *Update in Intensive Care and Emergency Medicine.* Berlin: Springer, 1990.
18. Voerman HJ, et al. Time course and variability of the endocrine and metabolic response to severe sepsis. *Surgery* 114:951, 1993.
19. Dahn MS, Lange MP, Jacobs LA. Insulin-like growth factor I production is inhibited in human sepsis. *Arch Surg* 123:1409, 1988.
20. Frayn KN, et al. Metabolic control in non-septic patients with musculo-skeletal injuries. *Injury* 16:73, 1984.
21. Black PR, et al. Mechanisms of insulin resistance following injury. *Ann Surg* 196:420, 1982.
22. Askanazi J, et al. Muscle and plasma amino acids following injury. Influence of intercurrent infection. *Ann Surg* 192:78, 1980.
23. Fajans SS, et al. Effect of amino acids and proteins on insulin secretion in man. *Recent Prog Horm Res* 23:617, 1967.
24. Wartofsky L, Burman KD. Alterations in thyroid function in patients with systemic illness: The "euthyroid sick syndrome." *Endocrine Rev* 3:164, 1982.
25. Aun F, et al. The effect of major trauma on the pathways of thyroid hormone metabolism. *J Trauma* 23:1048, 1983.
26. Hasselgren PO, et al. Studies on the possible role of thyroid hormone in altered muscle protein turnover during sepsis. *Ann Surg* 206:18, 1987.
27. Madsen M, Smeds S, Lemnquist S. Relationships between thyroid hormone and catecholamines in experimental trauma. *Acta Chir Scand* 152:413, 1986.
28. Drost AC, et al. Plasma cytokines after thermal injury and their relationship to infection. *Ann Surg* 218:74, 1993.

29. Marano MA, et al. Serum cachectin/tumor necrosis factor in critically ill patients with burns correlates with infections and mortality. *Surg Gynecol Obstet* 170:32, 1990.

30. Pinsky MR, et al. Serum cytokine levels in human septic shock: Relation to multiple-system organ failure and mortality. *Chest* 103:565, 1993.

31. Ertel W, et al. The complex pattern of cytokines in sepsis: Association between prostaglandins, cachectin, and interleukins. *Ann Surg* 214:141, 1991.

32. Soune O, et al. Cellular targets and receptors for interleukin-6: I. In vivo and in vitro uptake of IL-6 in liver and hepatocytes. *Eur J Clin Invest* 20:366, 1990.

33. Heinrich PC, Castell JV, Andus T. Interleukin-6 and the acute phase response. *Biochem J* 265:621, 1990.

34. Waage A, Halstensen A, Espevik T. Association between tumor necrosis factor in serum and fatal outcome in patients with meningococcal disease. *Lancet* 1:355, 1987.

35. Sullivan JS, et al. Correlation of plasma cytokine elevations with mortality rate in children with sepsis. *J Pediatr* 120:510, 1992.

36. Mozes T, et al. Serum levels of tumor necrosis factor determine the fatal or non-fatal course of endotoxic shock. *Immunol Lett* 27:157, 1991.

37. Del Rey A, Besedovsky HO. Metabolic and neuroendocrine effects of pro-inflammatory cytokines. *Eur J Clin Invest* 22(Suppl 1):10, 1992.

38. Molloy RG, Mannick JA, Rodrick ML. Cytokines, sepsis and immunomodulation. *Br J Surg* 80:289, 1993.

39. Dinarello CA, et al. Tumor necrosis factor (cachectin) is an endogenous pyrogen and induces production of interleukin-1. *J Exp Med* 163:1433, 1986.

40. McIntosh JK, et al. In vivo induction of IL-6 by administration of exogenous cytokines and detection of de novo serum levels of IL-6 in tumor-bearing mice. *J Immunol* 143:162, 1989.

41. Tracey KJ. Tumor necrosis factor (cachectin) in the biology of septic shock syndrome. *Circ Shock* 35:123, 1991.

42. Waage A, et al. The complex pattern of cytokines in serum from patients with meningococcal septic shock. *J Exp Med* 169:333, 1989.

43. Hesse DG, et al. Cytokine appearance in human endotoxemia and primate bacteremia. *Surg Gynecol Obstet* 166:147, 1988.

44. Fong Y, et al. Antibody to cachectin/tumor necrosis factor attenuates interleukin-1 beta and interleukin-6 appearance during overwhelming bacteremia. *J Exp Med* 170:1627, 1989.

45. Mester M, et al. Intestinal production of interleukin-1α during endotoxemia in the mouse. *J Surg Res* 54:584, 1993.

46. Mester M, et al. Lipopolysaccharide inducible IL-1 gene expression in the crypts of Lieberkühn. *Gastroenterology* 100:A600, 1991.

47. Fong Y, et al. The acute splanchnic and peripheral tissue metabolic response to endotoxin in humans. *J Clin Invest* 85:1896, 1990.

48. Keogh C, et al. Identification of a novel tumor necrosis factor α/ cachectin from the livers of burned and infected rats. *Arch Surg* 125:79, 1990.

49. Engelmann H, et al. A tumor necrosis factor-binding protein purified to homogeneity from human urine protects cells from tumor necrosis factor toxicity. *J Biol Chem* 264:11974, 1989.

50. Engelmann H, Novick D, Wallach D. Two tumor necrosis factor-binding proteins purified from human urine. *J Biol Chem* 265:1531, 1990.

51. Giri JG, Newton RC, Horuk R. Identification of soluble interleukin-1 binding protein in cell-free supernatants. *J Biol Chem* 265:17416, 1990.

52. Novick D, et al. Soluble cytokine receptors are present in normal human urine. *J Exp Med* 170:1409, 1989.

53. Gray PW, et al. Cloning of human tumor necrosis factor (TNF) receptor cDNA and expression of recombinant soluble TNF-binding protein. *Proc Natl Acad Sci USA* 87:7380, 1990.

54. Girardin E, et al. Imbalance between tumour necrosis factor α and soluble TNF receptor concentrations in severe meningococcaemia. *Immunology* 76:20, 1992.

55. Mathison JC, Wolfson E, Ulevitch RJ. Participation of tumor necrosis factor in the mediation of gram-negative bacterial lipopolysaccharide-induced injury in rabbits. *J Clin Invest* 81:1925, 1988.

56. Buetler B, Milsark IW, Cerami AC. Passive immunization against cachectin/tumor necrosis factor protects mice from lethal effect of endotoxin. *Science* 229:869, 1985.

57. Hinshaw L, Olson P, Kuo G. Efficacy of post-treatment with anti-TNF monoclonal antibody in preventing the pathophysiology and lethality of sepsis in the baboon. *Circ Shock* 27:362, 1989.

58. Starnes HF, et al. Anti-IL-6 monoclonal antibodies protect against lethal *Escherichia coli* infection and lethal tumor necrosis factor challenge in mice. *J Immunol* 145:4185, 1990.

59. Fisher CJ, et al. Initial evaluation of human recombinant interleukin-1 receptor antagonist in the treatment of sepsis syndrome: A randomized, open-label, placebo-controlled trial. *Crit Carc Med* 22:12, 1994.

60. Fisher CJ, et al. Recombinant human interleukin-1 receptor antagonist in the treatment of patients with sepsis syndrome: Results from a randomized, double-blind, placebo-controlled trial. *JAMA* 271:1836, 1994.

61. Redmond HP, et al. Inhibition of macrophage-activating cytokines is beneficial in the acute septic response. *Ann Surg* 214:502, 1991.

62. Howard M, et al. Interleukin 10 protects mice from lethal endotoxemia. *J Exp Med* 177:1205, 1993.

63. Van Zee K, et al. IL-8 in septic shock, endotoxemia and after IL-1 administration. *J Immunol* 146:3478, 1991.

64. Bitterman H, et al. Acute release of cytokines is proportional to tissue injury induced by surgical trauma and shock in rats. *J Clin Immunol* 11:184, 1991.

65. Barton PA, Warren JS. Complement component C5 modulates the systemic tumor necrosis factor response in murine endotoxin shock. *Infect Immun* 61:1474, 1993.

66. Kovacs EJ. Control of IL-1 and TNFα Production at the Level of Second Messenger Pathways. In ES Kimball (ed), *Cytokines and Inflammation.* Boca Raton: CRC, 1991.

67. Burd RS, Cody CS, Dunn DL. *Immunotherapy of Gram-Negative Bacterial Sepsis.* Austin: Landes, 1992.

68. Wright S. Multiple receptors for endotoxin. *Curr Opin Immunol* 3:83, 1991.

69. Tobias P, Soldau K, Ulevitch R. Isolation of a lipopolysaccharide-binding acute phase reactant from rabbit serum. *J Exp Med* 164:777, 1986.

70. Kovacs EJ, et al. Differential biochemical pathways involved in the expression of interleukin-1 (IL-1) and tumor necrosis factor (TNF) mRNAs in mouse peritoneal macrophages. *J Immunol* 141:3031, 1988.

71. Matsushima K, et al. Intracellular localization of human monocyte associated interleukin 1 (IL-1) activity and release of biologically active IL-1 by trypsin and plasmin. *J Immunol* 136:2883, 1986.

72. Kunkel SL, et al. Production and regulation of tumor necrosis factor-α: A cellular and molecular analysis. *Methods Achiev Exp Pathol* 13:240, 1988.
73. Radema SA, van Derenter SJH, Cerami A. Interleukin-1β is expressed predominantly by enterocytes in experimental colitis. *Gastroenterology* 100:1180, 1991.
74. Schöbitz B, et al. Regulation of interleukin 6 gene expression in rat. *Endocrinology* 132:1569, 1993.
75. Besedovsky H, del Rey A. Neuroendocrine and metabolic responses induced by interleukin-1. *J Neurosci Res* 18:172, 1987.
76. Naitoh Y, et al. Interleukin-6 stimulates the secretion of adrenocorticotropic hormone in conscious, freely-moving rats. *Biochem Biophys Res Commun* 155:1459, 1988.
77. Sharp BM, et al. Tumor necrosis factor-α is a potent ACTH secretagogue: Comparison to interleukin-1β. *Endocrinology* 124:131, 1989.
78. Besedovsky HO, et al. Immunoregulatory feedback between interleukin-1 and glucocorticoid hormones. *Science* 233:652, 1986.
79. Waage A, Slupphaug G, Shalaby R. Glucocorticoids inhibit the production of IL-6 from monocytes, endothelial cells and fibroblasts. *Eur J Immunol* 20:2439, 1990.
80. Ray A, La Forage KS, Sehgal PB. On the mechanism for efficient repression of the interleukin-6 promoter by glucocorticoids: Enhancer, TATA box, and RNA start site (infr motif) occlusion. *Mol Cell Biol* 10:5736, 1990.
81. Shieh JH, Peterson RHF, Moore MAS. Cytokines and dexamethasone modulation of IL-1 receptors on human neutrophils in vitro. *J Immunol* 150:3515, 1993.
82. Ozawa M, et al. Effects of tumor necrosis factor-α/cachectin on thyroid hormone metabolism in mice. *Endocrinology* 123:1461, 1988.
83. Dubuis JM, et al. Human recombinant interleukin-1β decreases plasma thyroid hormone and thyroid stimulating hormone levels in rats. *Endocrinology* 123:2175, 1988.
84. Spitzer JJ, et al. Altered control of carbohydrate metabolism in endotoxemia. *Prog Clin Biol Res* 286:145, 1989.
85. Spitzer JJ, et al. Alterations in lipid and carbohydrate metabolism in sepsis. *JPEN* 12:53S, 1988.
86. Mészáros K, et al. In vivo glucose utilization by individual tissues during nonlethal hypermetabolic sepsis. *FASEB J* 2:3083, 1988.
87. Spitzer JJ, et al. Increased Glucose Uptake and Superoxide Anion Production After Priming or Activation of Hepatic Phagocytes: A Potential Source of Liver Damage. In G Schlag et al (eds), *Shock, Sepsis, and Organ Failure.* Berlin: Springer, 1991.
88. Filkins JP. Phases of glucose dyshomeastasis in endotoxicosis. *Circ Shock* 5:347, 1978.
89. Knowles RG, et al. The characteristics and site of inhibition of gluconeogenesis in rat liver cells by bacterial endotoxin. *Biochem J* 242:721, 1987.
90. Lang CH, Dobrescu C. Sepsis-induced increases in glucose uptake by macrophage-rich tissues persist during hypoglycemia. *Metabolism* 40:585, 1991.
91. Lang CH, Bagby GJ, Spitzer JJ. Glucose kinetics and body temperature after lethal and non-lethal doses of endotoxin. *Am J Physiol* 248:R471, 1985.
92. Yelich MR. Glucoregulatory, hormonal, and metabolic responses to endotoxicosis or cecal ligation and puncture sepsis in the rat: A direct comparison. *Circ Shock* 31:351, 1990.
93. Douglas RG, Shaw JHF. Metabolic response to sepsis and trauma. *Br J Surg* 76:115, 1989.
94. Gallin JE, Kay D, O'Leary WM. Serum lipids in infection. *N Engl J Med* 281:1081, 1969.
95. Kaufmann RL, Matson CF, Beisel WR. Hypertriglyceridemia produced by endotoxin: Role of impaired triglyceride disposal mechanisms. *J Infect Dis* 133:548, 1976.
96. Robin AP, et al. Lipoprotein lipase activity in surgical patients: Influence of trauma and infection. *Surgery* 90:401, 1981.
97. Van Lenten BJ, et al. The role of lipoproteins and receptor-mediated endocytosis in the transport of bacterial lipopolysaccharide. *Proc Natl Acad Sci USA* 83:2704, 1986.
98. Harris HW, et al. Human VLDL and chylomicrons can protect against endotoxin-induced death in mice. *J Clin Invest* 86:696, 1990.
99. Cavaillon JM, et al. Cytokine response by monocytes and macrophages to free and lipoprotein-bound lipopolysaccharide. *Infect Immunol* 58:2375, 1990.
100. Huemer HP, et al. Herpes simplex virus binds to human serum lipoproteins. *Intervirology* 29:68, 1988.
101. Hasselgren PO. *Protein Metabolism in Sepsis.* Austin: Landes, 1993.
102. Cuthbertson DP. Observations on the disturbance of metabolism produced by injury to the limbs. *Q J Med* 1:233, 1932.
103. Long CL, et al. Urinary excretion of 3-methylhistidine: An assessment of muscle protein catabolism in adult normal subjects and during malnutrition, sepsis, and skeletal trauma. *Metabolism* 30:765, 1981.
104. Hasselgren PO, et al. Total and myofibrillar protein breakdown in different types of rat skeletal muscle: Effects of sepsis and regulation by insulin. *Metabolism* 38:634, 1989.
105. Khairallah EA, Bond JS, Bird JWC. *Intracellular Protein Catabolism.* New York: Liss, 1985.
106. Mayer R, Doherty F. Intracellular protein catabolism: State of the art. *FEBS Lett* 198:181, 1986.
107. Hershko A, Ciechanover A. The ubiquitin system for protein degradation. *Annu Rev Biochem* 61:761, 1992.
108. Waxman L, Fagan J, Goldberg AL. Demonstration of two distinct high molecular weight proteases in rabbit reticulocytes, one of which degrades ubiquitin conjugates. *J Biol Chem* 262:2451, 1987.
109. Fagan JM, Waxman L, Goldberg AL. Skeletal muscle and liver contain a soluble ATP and ubiquitin-dependent proteolytic system. *Biochem J* 243:335, 1987.
110. Jentsch S, Seufert W, Hauser HP. Genetic analysis of the ubiquitin system. *Biochim Biophys Acta* 1089:127, 1991.
111. Mayer RJ, et al. Ubiquitin in health and disease. *Biochim Biophys Acta* 1089:141, 1991.
112. Tiao G, et al. Sepsis stimulates non-lysosomal, energy-dependent proteolysis and increases ubiquitin mRNA levels in rat skeletal muscle. *J Clin Invest* 94:2255, 1994.
113. Furuno K, Goodman MN, Goldberg AL. Role of different proteolytic systems in the degradation of muscle proteins during denervation atrophy. *J Biol Chem* 265:8550, 1990.
114. Wing SS, Goldberg AL. Glucocorticoids activate the ATP-ubiquitin-dependent proteolytic system in skeletal muscle during fasting. *Am J Physiol* 264:E668, 1993.
115. Hasselgren PO, James JH, Fischer JE. Inhibited muscle amino acid uptake in sepsis. *Ann Surg* 203:360, 1986.
116. Hasselgren PO, et al. Reduced muscle amino acid uptake in sepsis and the effects in vitro of septic plasma and interleukin-1. *Surgery* 100:222, 1986.
117. Jepson MM, et al. Relationship between glutamine con-

centration and protein synthesis in rat skeletal muscle. *Am J Physiol* 255:E166, 1988.

118. MacLennan PA, et al. Inhibition of protein breakdown by glutamine in perfused rat skeletal muscle. *FEBS Lett* 237:133, 1988.

119. Windmueller HG, Spaeth AE. Respiratory fuels and nitrogen metabolism in vivo in small intestine of fed rats. *J Biol Chem* 255:107, 1980.

120. Newsholme EA, Parry-Billings M. Properties of glutamine release from muscle and its importance for the immune system. *JPEN* 14:63S, 1990.

121. Rosenblatt S, et al. Exchange of amino acids by muscle and liver in sepsis. *Arch Surg* 118:167, 1983.

122. Hasselgren PO, et al. Changes of protein metabolism in liver and skeletal muscle following trauma complicated by sepsis. *J Trauma* 24:224, 1984.

123. Pedersen P, Seeman T, Hasselgren PO. Protein synthesis and degradation in liver tissue following induction of septic peritonitis in rats. *Acta Chir Scand* 152:29, 1986.

124. Pedersen P, Säljö A, Hasselgren PO. Protein and energy metabolism in liver tissue following intravenous infusion of live *E. Coli* bacteria in rats. *Circ Shock* 21:59, 1987.

125. Sax HC, et al. Increased synthesis of secreted hepatic proteins during abdominal sepsis. *J Surg Res* 44:109, 1988.

126. von Allmen D, Hasselgren PO, Fischer JE. Hepatic protein synthesis in a modified septic rat model. *J Surg Res* 48:476, 1990.

127. Aronsen KF, et al. Sequential changes of plasma proteins after surgical trauma. *Scand J Clin Lab Invest* 29:127, 1972.

128. Kushner I. The acute phase response: An overview. *Methods Enzymol* 163:373, 1988.

129. Clowes GHA, et al. Survival from sepsis: The significance of altered protein metabolism regulated by proteolysis inducing factor, the circulating cleavage product of interleukin-1. *Ann Surg* 202:446, 1985.

130. Dominioni L, et al. Sepsis score and acute phase protein response as predictors of outcome in septic surgical patients. *Arch Surg* 122:142, 1987.

131. Macintyre SS, Schultz D, Kushner I. Biosynthesis of C-reactive protein. *Ann NY Acad Sci* 389:76, 1982.

132. Ballmer PE, et al. Acute suppression of albumin synthesis in systemic inflammatory disease: An individually graded response of rat hepatocytes. *J Histochem Cytochem* 40:201, 1992.

133. Courtoy PJ, et al. Synchronous increase in four acute phase proteins synthesized by the same hepatocytes during the inflammatory reaction. *Lab Invest* 44:105, 1981.

134. Woo P, Korenberg JR, Whitehead AS. Characterization of genomic and complementary DNA sequence of human C-reactive protein, and comparison with the complementary DNA sequence of serum amyloid P component. *J Biol Chem* 260:13384, 1985.

135. Toniatti C, et al. Regulation of the human C-reactive protein gene, a major marker of inflammation and cancer. *Mol Biol Med* 7:199, 1990.

136. Whitehead AS, et al. Isolation of human C-reactive protein complementary DNA and localization of the gene to chromosome 1. *Science* 221:69, 1983.

137. Primen JMG, et al. Direct evidence of transcriptional control of fibrinogen and albumin synthesis in rat liver during the acute phase response. *Biochem Biophys Res Commun* 102:717, 1981.

138. Northemann W, et al. Molecular cloning of cDNA sequences for rat α_2-macroglobulin and measurement of its transcription during experimental inflammation. *J Biol Chem* 260:6200, 1985.

139. von Allmen D, et al. Increased intestinal protein synthesis during sepsis and following the administration of tumor necrosis factor α or interleukin-1α. *Biochem J* 286:585, 1992.

140. Higashiguchi T, et al. Protein synthesis in isolated enterocytes from septic or endotoxemic rats: Regulation by glutamine. *Clin Sci,* in press.

141. Rafferty JA, et al. Sepsis in rats stimulates cellular proliferation in mucosa of the small intestine. *Gastroenterology* 107:121, 1994.

142. Higashiguchi T, et al. Sepsis increases production of total secreted proteins, vasoactive intestinal peptide, and peptide YY in isolated rat enterocytes. *Am J Surg* 168:251, 1994.

143. Zamir O, et al. Effect of sepsis or cytokine administration on release of gut peptides. *Am J Surg* 163:181, 1992.

144. Habener JF. Genetic Control of Hormone Formation. In JD Wilson, DW Foster (eds), *Williams Textbook of Endocrinology.* Philadelphia: Saunders, 1992.

145. Clark JH, Schrader WT, O'Malley BW. Mechanisms of Action of Steroid Hormones. In JD Wilson, DW Foster (eds), *Williams Textbook of Endocrinology.* Philadelphia: Saunders, 1992.

146. Kahn CR, Smith RJ, Chin WW. Mechanism of Action of Hormones That Act at the Cell Surface. In JD Wilson, DW Foster (eds), *Williams Textbook of Endocrinology.* Philadelphia: Saunders, 1992.

147. Gerich J, Cryer P, Rizza R. Hormonal mechanisms in acute glucose counterregulation: The relative roles of glucagon, epinephrine, norepinephrine, growth hormone, and cortisol. *Metabolism* 29:1164, 1980.

148. Bessey PQ, et al. Combined hormonal infusion simulates the metabolic response to injury. *Ann Surg* 200:264, 1984.

149. Gelfand RA, et al. Role of counterregulatory hormones in the catabolic response to stress. *J Clin Invest* 74:2238, 1984.

150. Bessey PQ, Lowe KA. Early hormonal changes affect the catabolic response to trauma. *Ann Surg* 218:476, 1993.

151. Rizza R, Cryer P, Gerich J. Role of glucagon, catecholamines, and growth hormone in human glucose counterregulation: Effects of somatostatin and combined α and β adrenergic blockade on plasma glucose recovery and glucose flux rates following insulin-induced hypoglycemia. *J Clin Invest* 64:62, 1979.

152. Sacca L, et al. Role of gluconeogenesis in epinephrine-stimulated hepatic glucose production in humans. *Am J Physiol* 245:E294, 1983.

153. Porte D, Smith PH, Eusinck JW. Neurohumoral regulation of the pancreatic islet A and B cells. *Metabolism* 25:1453, 1976.

154. Hargrove DM, et al. Adrenergic blockade prevents endotoxin-induced increases in glucose metabolism. *Am J Physiol* 255:E629, 1988.

155. Wilmore DW, et al. Catecholamines: Mediator of the hypermetabolic response to thermal injury. *Ann Surg* 180:653, 1974.

156. Hargrove DM, et al. Adrenergic blockade does not abolish elevated glucose turnover during bacterial infection. *Am J Physiol* 254:E16, 1988.

157. Lang CH, et al. Importance of hyperglucagonemia in eliciting the sepsis-induced increase in glucose production. *Circ Shock* 29:181, 1989.

158. Eigler N, Sacca L, Sherwin RS. Synergistic interactions of physiologic increments of glucagon, epinephrine and cortisol in the dog. *J Clin Invest* 63:114, 1979.

159. Wolfe RR, Shaw JHF. Glucose and FFA kinetics in sepsis: Role of glucagon and sympathetic nervous system activity. *Am J Physiol* 248:E236, 1985.

160. Hargrove DM, et al. Role of insulin in the blunted glucose metabolic response of septic rats to epinephrine. *Metabolism* 39:1180, 1990.

161. Kahn CR. The molecular mechanism of insulin action. *Annu Rev Med* 36:429, 1985.

162. Raymond RM, et al. Skeletal muscle insulin unresponsiveness during chronic hyperdynamic sepsis in the dog. *J Trauma* 25:845, 1985.

163. Hasselgren PO, Fischer JE. Regulation by insulin of muscle protein metabolism during sepsis and other catabolic conditions. *Nutrition* 8:434, 1992.

164. Bessey PQ, Wilmore DW. β-Adrenergic regulation of glucose disposal: A reciprocal relationship with insulin release. *J Surg Res* 34:404, 1983.

165. Lang CH, Dobreson C, Bagby GJ. Tumor necrosis factor impairs insulin action on peripheral glucose disposal and hepatic glucose output. *Endocrinology* 130:43, 1992.

166. Garvey WT, et al. Glucose and insulin co-regulate the glucose transport system in primary cultured adipocytes: A new mechanism of insulin resistance. *J Biol Chem* 262:189, 1987.

167. Iochida LC, et al. Insulin resistance in septic rats: A study by the euglycemic clamp technique. *Life Sci* 45:1567, 1989.

168. Volpe JJ, Marasa JC. Hormonal regulation of fatty acid synthetase, acetyl-CoA carboxylase and fatty acid synthesis in mammalian adipose tissue and liver. *Biochim Biophys Acta* 380:454, 1975.

169. Klain GJ. In vivo effects of glucagon on fatty acid synthesis in fasted and refed rats. *J Nutr* 107:942, 1977.

170. Geelen MJH, et al. Short-term effects of insulin and glucagon on lipid synthesis in isolated rat hepatocytes. *FEBS Lett* 95:326, 1978.

171. Hermier D, Hales P, Brindley DN. Biphasic effects of glucagon and cyclic AMP on the synthesis and secretion of lipids by rat hepatocytes. *Biochem J* 279:705, 1991.

172. Himms-Hagen J. Adrenergic receptors for metabolic responses in adipose tissue. *Fed Proc* 29:1388, 1970.

173. Geelen MJH, Gibson DM. Lipogenesis in maintenance cultures of rat hepatocytes. *FEBS Lett* 58:334, 1975.

174. Li S, et al. Increasing dextrose concentrations in total parenteral nutrition (TPN) causes alterations in hepatic morphology and plasma levels of insulin and glucagon in rats. *J Surg Res* 44:639, 1988.

175. Darmann D, Mathews DE, Bier DM. Physiological hypercortisolemia increases proteolysis, glutamine, and alanine production. *Am J Physiol* 255:E366, 1988.

176. Tomas FM, Munro HN, Young VR. Effect of glucocorticoid administration on the rate of muscle protein breakdown in vivo in rats, as measured by urinary excretion of N^{τ}-methylhistidine. *Biochem J* 178:139, 1979.

177. Kayali AG, Young VR, Goodman MN. Sensitivity of myofibrillar proteins to glucocorticoid-induced muscle proteolysis. *Am J Physiol* 252:E621, 1987.

178. Downey RS, et al. Protein dynamics in skeletal muscle after trauma: Local and systemic effects. *Surgery* 99:265, 1986.

179. Hall-Angerås M, et al. Effect of the glucocorticoid receptor antagonist RU 38486 on muscle protein breakdown in sepsis. *Surgery* 109:468, 1991.

180. Philibert D. RU 38486: An Original Multifaceted Antihormone In Vivo. In MK Agarwal (ed), *Adrenal Steroid Antagonism.* Hawthorne: de Gruyter, 1984.

181. Hundal HS, et al. Effects of corticosteroid on the transport and metabolism of glutamine in rat skeletal muscle. *Biochim Biophys Acta* 1092:376, 1991.

182. Parry-Billings M. *Studies of Glutamine Release From Skeletal Muscle* (Thesis). Oxford, England, 1989.

183. Max SR, et al. Dexamethasone regulates glutamine synthetase expression in rat skeletal muscles. *Am J Physiol* 255:E397, 1988.

184. Zamir O, et al. Evidence that inhibition of muscle amino acid uptake during endotoxemia is not mediated by glucocorticoids. *Metabolism* 42:1190, 1993.

185. MacKenzie B, Ahmed A, Rennie M. Muscle Amino Acid Metabolism and Transport. In MS Kilberg, D Häussinger (eds), *Mammalian Amino Acid Transport, Mechanism and Control.* New York: Plenum, 1992.

186. Kettelhut IC, Wing SS, Goldberg AL. Endocrine regulation of protein breakdown in skeletal muscle. *Diabetes Metab Rev* 4:751, 1988.

187. Manson JM, Smith RJ, Wilmore DW. Growth hormone stimulates protein synthesis during hypocaloric parenteral nutrition. *Ann Surg* 208:136, 1988.

188. Jiang ZM, et al. Low-dose growth hormone and hypocaloric nutrition attenuate the protein-catabolic response after major operation. *Ann Surg* 210:513, 1989.

189. Herndon DN, et al. Effects of recombinant human growth hormone on donor-site healing in severely burnt children. *Ann Surg* 212:424, 1990.

190. Douglas RG, et al. Metabolic effects of recombinant human growth hormone: Isotopic studies in the postabsorptive state and during total parenteral nutrition. *Br J Surg* 77:785, 1990.

191. Ponting GA, et al. Protein and energy metabolism with biosynthetic human growth hormone in patients on full intravenous nutritional support. *JPEN* 14:437, 1990.

192. Harber FF, Haymond MW. Human growth hormone prevents the protein catabolic side-effects of prednisolone in humans. *J Clin Invest* 86:265, 1990.

193. Ballard JF, et al. Binding properties and biological potencies of insulin-like growth factor in L6 myoblasts. *Biochem J* 233:223, 1986.

194. Douglas RG, et al. Effects of recombinant IGF-1 on protein and glucose metabolism in rTNF-infused lambs. *Am J Physiol* 261:E606, 1991.

195. Strock LL, et al. The effect of insulin-like growth factor I on postburn hypermetabolism. *Surgery* 108:161, 1990.

196. O'Sullivan U, et al. Insulin-like growth factor I (IGF-I) in mice reduced weight loss during starvation. *Endocrinology* 125:2793, 1989.

197. Gelfand RA, Barrett EJ. Effect of physiologic hyperinsulinemia on skeletal muscle protein synthesis and breakdown in man. *J Clin Invest* 80:1, 1987.

198. Tessari P, et al. Differential effects of hyperinsulinemia and hyperaminoacidemia on leucine-carbon metabolism in vivo: Evidence for distinct mechanisms in regulation of new amino acid deposition. *J Clin Invest* 79:1062, 1987.

199. Kimball SR, Jefferson LS. Cellular mechanisms involved in the action of insulin on protein synthesis. *Diabetes Metab Rev* 4:773, 1988.

200. Newman JJ, et al. Altered protein metabolism in diaphragms from thermally injured rats. *J Surg Res* 36:177, 1984.

201. Tischler ME, Fagan JM. Response to trauma of protein,

amino acid, and carbohydrate metabolism in injured and uninjured rat skeletal muscles. *Metabolism* 32:853, 1983.

202. David TA, Karl IE. Resistance of protein and glucose metabolism to insulin in denervated rat muscle. *Biochem J* 254:667, 1988.

203. Hasselgren PO, et al. Effect of insulin on amino acid uptake and protein turnover in skeletal muscle from septic rats: Evidence for insulin resistance of protein breakdown. *Arch Surg* 122:228, 1987.

204. Woolfson AMJ, Heatley RV, Allison SP. Insulin to inhibit protein catabolism after injury. *N Engl J Med* 300:14, 1979.

205. Tannuri U, Amaral LA, Maksoud JG. Effect of insulin on protein catabolism after injury in young animals. *J Pediatr Surg* 17:296, 1982.

206. Van Gool J, et al. Glucocorticoid and catecholamines as mediators of acute-phase proteins, especially rat α-macrofetoprotein. *Biochem J* 220:125, 1984.

207. Canivet B, Fehlmann M, Freychet P. Glucocorticoid and catecholamine stimulation of amino acid transport in rat hepatocytes. *Mol Cell Endocrinol* 19:253, 1980.

208. Jeejeebhoy KN, et al. Effects of hormones on the synthesis of α_1 (acute phase) glycoprotein in isolated rat hepatocytes. *Biochem J* 168:347, 1977.

209. Kilberg MS, Häussinger D. Amino Acid Transport in Liver. In MS Kilberg, D Häussinger (eds), *Mammalian Amino Acid Transport, Mechanisms and Control.* New York: Plenum, 1992.

210. Gebhardt R, Kleeman E. Hormonal regulation of amino acid transport system N in primary cultures of rat hepatocytes. *Eur J Biochem* 166:339, 1987.

211. Le Cam A, Freychet P. Effect of glucocorticoids on amino acid transport in isolated rat hepatocytes. *Mol Cell Endocrinol* 9:205, 1977.

212. Kletzien RF, et al. A "permissive" effect of dexamethasone on the glucagon induction of amino acid transport in cultured hepatocytes. *Nature* 256:46, 1975.

213. Pacitti AJ, et al. Growth hormone regulates amino acid transport in human and rat liver. *Ann Surg* 216:353, 1992.

214. Souba WW, Smith RJ, Wilmore DW. Effects of glucocorticoids on glutamine metabolism in visceral organs. *Metabolism* 34:450, 1985.

215. Heitmann RN, Bergmann AE. Glutamine metabolism, interorgan transport, and glucogenicity in the sheep. *Am J Physiol* 234:E197, 1978.

216. Plauth M, et al. Effects of dexamethasone on glutamine metabolism in the isolated vascularly perfused rat small intestine. *Res Exp Med* 191:349, 1991.

217. Souba WW, Copeland EM. Cytokine modulation of Na^+-dependent glutamine transport across the brush border membrane of monolayers of human intestinal Caco-2 cells. *Ann Surg* 215:536, 1992.

218. James PS, et al. Dexamethasone selectively increases sodium-dependent alanine transport across neonatal piglet intestine. *J Physiol* 393:569, 1987.

219. Ardawi MSM, Majzoub M, Newsholme EA. Effect of glucocorticoid treatment on glucose and glutamine metabolism by the small intestine of the rat. *Clin Sci* 75:93, 1988.

220. Sarantos P, Abouhanze A, Souba WW. Glucocorticoids regulate intestinal glutaminase expression. *Surgery* 112:278, 1992.

221. Sarantos P, Souba WW. Glucocorticoids regulate intestinal glutamine synthetase gene expression in endotoxemia. *Arch Surg* 129:59, 1994.

222. Plumley DA, et al. Accelerated lung amino acid release in hyperdynamic septic surgical patients. *Arch Surg* 125:57, 1990.

223. Ardawi MSM. Glutamine and alanine metabolism in lungs of septic rats. *Clin Sci* 81:603, 1991.

224. Ardawi MSM. Glutamine-synthesizing activity in lungs of fed, starved, acidotic, diabetic, injured and septic rats. *Biochem J* 270:829, 1990.

225. Souba WW, et al. Effects of glucocorticoids on lung glutamine and alanine metabolism. *Surgery* 108:213, 1990.

226. Ardawi MSM. Glutamine metabolism in the lungs of glucocorticoid-treated rats. *Clin Sci* 81:37, 1991.

227. Sarantos P, Howard D, Souba WW. Dexamethasone regulates glutamine synthetase expression in rat lung. *Metabolism* 42:795, 1993.

228. Mészáros K, et al. Tumor necrosis factor increases in vivo glucose utilization of macrophage-rich tissues. *Biochem Biophys Res Commun* 149:1, 1987.

229. Van der Poll T, et al. Tumor necrosis factor mimics the metabolic response to acute infection in healthy humans. *Am J Physiol* 261:E457, 1991.

230. Evans DA, Jacobs DO, Wilmore WW. Tumor necrosis factor enhances glucose uptake by peripheral tissues. *Am J Physiol* 257:R1182, 1989.

231. Bagby GJ, et al. Glucose kinetics in rats infused with endotoxin-induced monokines or tumor necrosis factor. *Circ Shock* 24:111, 1988.

232. Rofe AM, et al. The effects of recombinant tumor necrosis factor (cachectin) on metabolism in isolated rat adipocyte, hepatocyte, and muscle preparations. *Biochem J* 247:789, 1987.

233. Bagby GJ, et al. Attenuation of glucose metabolic changes resulting from TNF-α administration by adrenergic blockade. *Am J Physiol* 262:R628, 1992.

234. Van der Poll T, Sauerwein HP. Tumour necrosis factor-α: Its role in the metabolic response to sepsis. *Clin Sci* 84:247, 1993.

235. Lee MD, et al. Effect of endotoxin-induced monokines on glucose metabolism in the muscle cell line L6. *Proc Natl Acad Sci USA* 84:2590, 1987.

236. Cornelius P, et al. The growth factor-like effects of tumor necrosis factor-α: Stimulation of glucose transport activity and induction of glucose transporter and immediate early gene expression in 3T3-L1 preadipocytes. *J Biol Chem* 265:20506, 1990.

237. Bagby GJ, et al. Regulation of glucose metabolism after endotoxin and during infection is largely independent of endogenous tumor necrosis factor. *Circ Shock* 39:211, 1993.

238. Hill MR, Stith RD, McCallum RE. Human recombinant IL-1 alters glucocorticoid receptor function in Reuber hepatoma cells. *J Immunol* 141:1522, 1988.

239. Filkins JP. Endotoxin-enhanced secretion of macrophage insulin-like activity. *J Reticuloendothelial Soc* 27:507, 1980.

240. Garcia-Welsh A, Schneiderman JS, Baly DL. Interleukin-1 stimulates glucose transport in the rat adipose cells: Evidence for receptor discrimination between IL-1 beta and alpha. *FEBS Lett* 269:421, 1990.

241. Flores EA, et al. Effect of interleukin-1 and tumor necrosis factor/cachectin on glucose turnover in the rat. *Metabolism* 39:783, 1990.

242. Beutler BA, Cerami A. Cachectin and tumor necrosis factor as two sides of the same biological coin. *Nature* 320:584, 1986.

243. Feingold KR, Grunfeld C. Tumor necrosis factor-alpha stimulates hepatic lipogenesis in the rat in vivo. *J Clin Invest* 80:184, 1987.
244. Feinberg B, et al. A phase I trial of intravenously-administered recombinant tumor necrosis factor-alpha in cancer patients. *J Clin Oncol* 6:1328, 1988.
245. Kawakami M, et al. Human recombinant TNF suppresses lipoprotein lipase activity and stimulates lipolysis in 3T3-L1 cells. *J Biochem* 101:331, 1987.
246. Fried SK, Zechner R. Cachectin/tumor necrosis factor decreases human adipose tissue lipoprotein mRNA levels, synthesis, and activity. *J Lipid Res* 30:1917, 1989.
247. Semb H, et al. Multiple effects of tumor necrosis factor on lipoprotein lipase in vivo. *J Biol Chem* 262:8390, 1987.
248. Grunfeld C, et al. Effect of tumor necrosis factor administration in vivo on lipoprotein lipase activity in various tissues of the rat. *J Lipid Res* 30:579, 1989.
249. Feingold KR, et al. Tumor necrosis factor stimulates hepatic lipid synthesis and secretion. *Endocrinology* 124:2336, 1989.
250. Grunfeld C, et al. Mechanisms by which tumor necrosis factor stimulates hepatic fatty acid synthesis. *J Lipid Res* 29:1327, 1988.
251. Grunfeld C, Dinarello CA, Feingold KR. Tumor necrosis factor-α, interleukin-1, and interferon-α stimulate triglyceride synthesis in Hep G2 cells. *Metab Clin Exp* 40:894, 1991.
252. Feingold KR, et al. Diet affects the mechanisms by which TNF stimulates hepatic triglyceride production. *Am J Physiol* 259:E177, 1990.
253. Patton JS, et al. Interferons and tumor necrosis factors have similar catabolic effects on 3T3-LI cells. *Proc Natl Acad Sci USA* 83:8313, 1986.
254. Price SR, Mizel SB, Pekala PH. Regulation of lipoprotein lipase synthesis and 3T3-LI adipocyte metabolism by recombinant interleukin-1. *Biochim Biophys Acta* 889:374, 1986.
255. Feingold KR, et al. Multiple cytokines stimulate hepatic lipid synthesis in vivo. *Endocrinology* 125:267, 1989.
256. Grunfeld C, et al. Evidence for two classes of cytokines that stimulate hepatic lipogenesis: Relationships among tumor necrosis factor, interleukin-1 and interferon-alpha. *Endocrinology* 127:46, 1990.
257. Grunfeld C, et al. Interleukin-4 inhibits stimulation of hepatic lipogenesis by tumor necrosis factor, interleukin-1 and interleukin-6 but not by interferon-α_1. *Cancer Res* 51:2803, 1991.
258. Clowes GHA, et al. Muscle proteolysis induced by a circulating peptide in patients with sepsis or trauma. *N Engl J Med* 308:545, 1983.
259. Baracos V, et al. Stimulation of muscle protein degradation and prostaglandin E_2 release by leukocyte pyrogen (interleukin-1). *N Engl J Med* 308:553, 1983.
260. Goldberg AL, et al. Activation of protein breakdown and prostaglandin E_2 production in rat skeletal muscle in fever is signaled by a macrophage product distinct from interleukin-1 or other known monokines. *J Clin Invest* 81:1378, 1988.
261. Hasselgren PO, et al. Is there a circulating proteolysis-inducing factor during sepsis? *Arch Surg* 125:510, 1990.
262. Hummel RP, et al. In vitro effects of TNF, IL-1α, and other monokines on skeletal muscle amino acid uptake and protein degradation. *Surg Forum* 38:13, 1987.
263. Moldawer LL, et al. Interleukin-1 and tumor necrosis factor do not regulate protein balance in skeletal muscle. *Am J Physiol* 253:C766, 1987.
264. Fong Y, et al. Cachectin/TNF or IL-1α induces cachexia with redistribution of body proteins. *Am J Physiol* 256:R659, 1989.
265. Flores EA, et al. Infusion of tumor necrosis factor/cachectin produces muscle catabolism in the rat: A synergistic effect with interleukin-1. *J Clin Invest* 83:1614, 1989.
266. Goodman MN. Tumor necrosis factor induces skeletal muscle protein breakdown in rats: *Am J Physiol* 260:E727, 1991.
267. Kettelhut IC, Goldberg AL. Tumor necrosis factor can induce fever in rats without activating protein breakdown in muscle or lipolysis in adipose tissue. *J Clin Invest* 81:1384, 1988.
268. Zamir O, et al. Evidence that tumor necrosis factor participates in the regulation of muscle proteolysis during sepsis. *Arch Surg* 127:170, 1992.
269. Zamir O, et al. The effect of interleukin-1α and the glucocorticoid receptor blocker RU 38486 on total and myofibrillar protein breakdown in skeletal muscle. *J Surg Res* 50:579, 1991.
270. Zamir O, et al. Tumor necrosis factor (TNF) and interleukin-1 (IL-1) induce muscle proteolysis through different mechanisms. *Mediat Inflam* 1:247, 1992.
271. Zamir O, et al. In vivo administration of interleukin-1α induces muscle proteolysis in normal and adrenalectomized rats. *Metabolism* 42:204, 1993.
272. Zamir O, et al. Muscle protein breakdown during endotoxemia in rats and after treatment with interleukin-1 receptor antagonist (IL-1ra). *Ann Surg* 216:381, 1992.
273. Lazarus DD, Moldawer LL, Lowry SF. Insulin-like growth factor-1 activity is inhibited by interleukin-1α, tumor necrosis factor-α and interleukin-6. *Lymphokine Cytokine Res* 12:219, 1993.
274. Geiger T, et al. Induction of rat acute phase proteins by interleukin-6 in vivo. *Eur J Immunol* 18:717, 1988.
275. Castell JV, et al. Interleukin-6 is the major regulator of acute-phase protein synthesis in adult human hepatocytes. *FEBS Lett* 242:232, 1989.
276. Baumann H, et al. Phorbol ester modulates interleukin-6 and interleukin-1 regulated expression of acute phase plasma proteins in hepatoma cells. *J Biol Chem* 263:17390, 1988.
277. Calandra T, et al. High circulating levels of interleukin-6 in patients with septic shock: Evolution during sepsis, prognostic value, and interplay with other cytokines. *Am J Med* 91:23, 1991.
278. Damas P, et al. Cytokine serum levels during severe sepsis in human: IL-6 as a marker of severity. *Ann Surg* 215:356, 1992.
279. Prowse KR, Baumann H. Hepatocyte-stimulating factor, β_2 interferon and interleukin-1 enhance expression of the rat α_1-acid glycoprotein gene via a distal upstream regulatory region. *Mol Cell Biol* 8:42, 1988.
280. Northemann W, et al. Structure and acute-phase regulation of the rat α_2-macroglobulin gene. *Biochemistry* 27:9194, 1988.
281. Kunz D, et al. Identification of the promoter sequences involved in the interleukin-6 dependent expression of the rat α_2-macroglobulin gene. *Nucleic Acids Res* 17:1121, 1989.
282. Marinkovic S, Baumann H. Structure, hormonal regulation, and identification of the interleukin-6 and dexamethasone-responsive element of the rat haptoglobin gene. *Mol Cell Biol* 10:1573, 1990.
283. Baumann H, et al. Transcriptional regulation through

cytokine and glucocorticoid response elements of rat acute phase plasma protein genes by C/EBP and Jun B. *J Biol Chem* 266:20390, 1991.

284. Won KA, Baumann H. The cytokine response element of the rat α_1-acid glycoprotein gene is a complex of several interacting regulatory sequences. *Mol Cell Biol* 10:3965, 1990.

285. Ito T, et al. Nuclear factors interacting with an interleukin-6 responsive element of rat α_2-macroglobulin gene. *Nucleic Acids Res* 17:9425, 1989.

286. Poli V, Cortese R. Interleukin-6 induces a liver-specific nuclear protein that binds to the promoter of acute-phase genes. *Proc Natl Acad Sci USA* 86:8202, 1989.

287. Hattori M, et al. Acute-phase reaction induces a specific complex between hepatic nuclear proteins and the interleukin-6 response element of the rat α_2-macroglobulin gene. *Proc Natl Acad Sci USA* 87:2364, 1990.

288. Ciliberto G, et al. Inducible and tissue-specific expression of human c-reactive protein in transgenic mice. *EMBO J* 6:4017, 1987.

289. Baumann H. Hepatic acute phase reaction in vivo and in vitro. *In Vitro Cell Dev Biol* 25:115, 1989.

290. Baumann H, Gauldie J. Regulation of hepatic acute phase plasma protein genes by hepatocyte stimulating factors and other mediators of inflammation. *Mol Biol Med* 7:147, 1990.

291. Hocke GM, Barry D, Fey GH. Synergistic action of interleukin-6 and glucocorticoids is mediated by the interleukin-6 response element of the rat α_2 macroglobulin gene. *Mol Cell Biol* 12:2282, 1992.

292. Kampschmidt RF, et al. Multiple biological activities of a partially purified leukocytic endogenous mediator. *Am J Physiol* 224:530, 1973.

293. Weinstein JA, Taylor JM. Interleukin-1 and the acute phase response: Induction of mouse liver serum amyloid A mRNA by murine recombinant interleukin-1. *J Trauma* 27:1227, 1987.

294. Pedersen P, et al. Synthesis of acute phase proteins in perfused liver following administration of recombinant interleukin-1α to normal or adrenalectomized rats. *J Surg Res* 45:333, 1988.

295. Andus T, et al. Regulation of synthesis and secretion of major rat acute phase proteins by recombinant human interleukin-6 (BSF-2/IL-6) in hepatocyte primary cultures. *Eur J Biochem* 173:287, 1988.

296. Bankey PE, et al. Hepatic acute phase protein synthesis is indirectly regulated by tumor necrosis factor. *J Trauma* 30:1181, 1990.

297. Mackiewicz A, et al. Transforming growth factor β_1 regulates production of acute-phase proteins. *Proc Natl Acad Sci USA* 87:1491, 1990.

298. Baumann H, Wong GG. Hepatocyte-stimulating factor III shares structural and functional identity with leukemia-inhibitory factor. *J Immunol* 143:1163, 1989.

299. Baumann H, Schendel P. Interleukin-11 regulates the hepatic expression of the same plasma protein genes as interleukin-6. *J Biol Chem* 266:20424, 1991.

300. Noguchi Y, et al. Influence of sepsis and endotoxemia on polyamine metabolism in mucosa of small intestine in rats. *Metabolism,* in press.

301. Chung DH, et al. Cytokine regulation of gut ornithine decarboxylase gene expression and enzyme activity. *Surgery* 112:364, 1992.

302. Austgen TR, et al. Cytokine regulation of intestinal glutamine utilization. *Am J Surg* 163:174, 1992.

303. Argiles JM, et al. Comparative effects of tumour necrosis factor-α (cachectin), interleukin-1-β and tumour growth on amino acid metabolism in the rat in vivo. *Biochem J* 261:357, 1989.

304. Souba WW, et al. Cytokine modulation of glutamine transport by pulmonary artery endothelial cells. *Surgery* 110:295, 1991.

305. Koj A, et al. The acute phase response of cultured rat hepatocytes. *Biochem J* 224:505, 1984.

306. Baumann H, Richards C, Gauldie J. Interaction among hepatocyte-stimulating factors, interleukin-1, and glucocorticoids for regulation of acute phase plasma proteins in human hepatoma (Hep G2) cells. *J Immunol* 139:4122, 1987.

307. Marinkovic S, et al. IL-6 modulates the synthesis of a specific set of acute phase plasma proteins in vivo. *J Immunol* 142:808, 1989.

308. Hall-Angerås M, et al. Interaction between corticosterone and tumor necrosis factor stimulated protein breakdown in rat skeletal muscles, similar to sepsis. *Surgery* 108:460, 1990.

309. Mealy K, et al. Are the catabolic effects of tumor necrosis factor mediated by glucocorticoids? *Arch Surg* 125:42, 1990.

310. Lazarus DD, Lowry SF, Moldawer LL. Cytokines acutely decrease circulating insulin-like growth factor-1 (IGF-1) and IGF binding protein-3 (IGFBP-3). *Surg Forum* 43:92, 1992.

311. Anbalagan K, Sadique J. Role of prostaglandins in acute phase proteins in inflammation. *Biochem Med* 31:236, 1984.

312. Kunkel SL, et al. Prostaglandin E_2 regulates macrophage-derived tumor necrosis factor gene expression. *J Biol Chem* 263:5380, 1988.

313. Rodemann HP, Goldberg AL. Arachidonic acid, prostaglandin E_2 and $F_{2\alpha}$ influence rates of protein turnover in skeletal and cardiac muscle. *J Biol Chem* 257:1632, 1982.

314. Barnett JG, Ellis S. Prostaglandin E_2 and the regulation of protein degradation in skeletal muscle. *Muscle Nerve* 10:556, 1987.

315. McKinley CJ, Turinsky J. Prostaglandin E_2 and muscle proteolysis: Effect of burn injury and cycloheximide. *Am J Physiol* 250:R207, 1986.

316. Hasselgren PO, et al. Effect of indomethacin on proteolysis in septic muscle. *Ann Surg* 202:557, 1985.

317. Hasselgren PO, et al. Further evidence that accelerated muscle protein breakdown during sepsis is not mediated by prostaglandin E_2. *Ann Surg* 207:399, 1988.

318. Hasselgren PO, et al. Prostaglandin E_2 does not regulate total or myofibrillar protein breakdown in incubated skeletal muscle from normal or septic rats. *Biochem J* 270:45, 1990.

319. Fagan JM, Goldberg AL. Progress in Leukocyte Biology. In MJ Kluger, JJ Oppenheim, MC Powanda (eds), *The Physiologic, Metabolic and Immunological Actions of Interleukin-1.* New York: Liss, 1985.

320. Davies KJA. Intracellular proteolytic systems may function as secondary antioxidant defenses: An hypothesis. *J Free Rad Biol Med* 2:155, 1986.

321. Nordström G, Seeman T, Hasselgren PO. Beneficial effect of allopurinol in liver ischemia. *Surgery* 97:679, 1985.

322. Manson NH, Hess ML. Interaction of oxygen free radicals and cardiac sarcoplasmic reticulum: Proposed role in the pathogenesis of endotoxin shock. *Circ Shock* 10:205, 1983.

323. Klebanoff SJ, et al. Stimulation of neutrophils by tumor necrosis factor. *J Immunol* 136:4220, 1986.

324. Lloyd SS, et al. Free radicals and septic shock in primates: The role of tumor necrosis factor. *J Free Rad Biol Med* 14:233, 1993.

325. Fagan JM, Waxman L. Purification of a protease in red blood cells that degrades oxidatively-damaged hemoglobin. *Biochem J* 277:779, 1991.

326. Moncada S. The L-arginine:nitric oxide pathway. *Acta Physiol Scand* 145:201, 1992.

327. Geller DA, et al. Molecular cloning and expression of inducible nitric oxide synthase from human hepatocytes. *Proc Natl Acad Sci USA* 90:3491, 1993.

328. Geller DA, Billiar TR. Should surgeons clone genes? The strategy behind the cloning of the human inducible nitric oxide synthase gene. *Arch Surg* 128:1212, 1993.

329. Billiar TR, et al. An L-arginine-dependent mechanism mediates Kupffer cell inhibition of hepatocyte protein synthesis in vitro. *J Exp Med* 169:1467, 1989.

330. Curran RD, et al. Hepatocytes produce nitrogen oxides from L-arginine in response to inflammatory products of Kupffer cells. *J Exp Med* 170:1769, 1989.

331. Billiar TR, et al. Inducible cytosolic enzyme activity for the production of nitrogen oxides from L-arginine in hepatocytes. *Biochem Biophys Res Commun* 168:1034, 1990.

332. Curran RD, et al. Nitric oxide and nitric oxide generating compounds inhibit hepatocyte protein synthesis. *FASEB J* 5:2085, 1991.

333. Ochoa JB, et al. Nitrogen oxide levels in patients after trauma and during sepsis. *Ann Surg* 214:621, 1991.

334. Nussler AK, et al. Stimulation of the nitric oxide synthase pathway in human hepatocytes by cytokines and endotoxin. *J Exp Med* 176:261, 1992.

335. Billiar TR, et al. Modulation of nitrogen oxide synthesis in vivo: N^G-monomethyl-L-arginine inhibits endotoxin-induced nitrite/nitrate biosynthesis while producing hepatic damage. *J Leukoc Biol* 48:565, 1990.

336. Frederick JA, et al. Nitric oxide may upregulate in vivo hepatic protein synthesis during endotoxemia. *Arch Surg* 128:152, 1993.

337. Minnard EA, et al. Inhibition of nitric oxide (N:O) synthesis is detrimental during endotoxemia. *Arch Surg* 129:142, 1994.

338. Tiao G, et al. Detrimental effect of nitric oxide synthase inhibition during endotoxemia may be caused by high levels of TNF and IL-6. *Surgery* 116:332, 1994.

339. Stadler J, et al. Endogenous nitric oxide inhibits the synthesis of cyclooxygenase products and interleukin-6 by rat Kupffer cells. *J Leukoc Biol* 53:165, 1993.

Selected Readings

Besedovsky H, et al. Immunoregulatory feedback between interleukin-1 and glucocorticoid hormones. *Science* 233:652, 1986.

Evidence was found that there is a close relationship between the immune system and the neuroendocrine system that is of great importance for the metabolic response to injury and sepsis. Administration of IL-1 to mice or rats increased blood levels of ACTH and glucocorticoids. Combined with results in other papers in which glucocorticoids inhibited the release of cytokines, the data strongly supported the existence of an immunoregulatory feedback circuit in which cytokines act as an afferent and glucocorticoids as an efferent hormonal signal.

Bessey PQ, et al. Combined hormonal infusion simulates the metabolic response to injury. *Ann Surg* 200:264, 1984.

This is another classic paper in the field of mediators of metabolic changes after injury. This paper reports that a combined infusion of the "stress hormones" cortisol, glucagon, and epinephrine gives rise to several metabolic changes similar to those seen after injury, that is, hypermetabolism, negative nitrogen and potassium balance, glucose intolerance, hyperinsulinemia, insulin resistance, sodium retention, and peripheral leukocytosis. Additional studies with single hormone infusions indicated that these responses resulted from both additive and synergistic interactions among the hormones. This experimental approach—*triple hormone infusion*—has been used by several other research groups as well with similar conclusions.

Clowes GHA, et al. Muscle proteolysis induced by a circulating peptide in patients with sepsis or trauma. *N Engl J Med* 308:545, 1983.

This classic paper discusses regulators of metabolism after injury and during sepsis. The paper describes the presence of a factor in plasma from septic and injured patients that induces muscle proteolysis. This proteolysis inducing factor was suggested to be a cleavage product of IL-1. Although several other laboratories have not been able to reproduce some of the results, the paper is important because it generated a great amount of interest in the field of mediators of sepsis- and trauma-induced metabolic changes.

Hesse DG, et al. Cytokine appearance in human endotoxemia and primate bacteremia. *Surg Gynecol Obstet* 166:147, 1988.

This paper is important because it demonstrates the presence of a cascade-like response of cytokines after induction of endotoxemia. The authors documented an early (within the first few hours after endotoxin injection) peak in circulating TNF levels, followed by subsequent release of other cytokines such as IL-1 and IFN-γ. This concept of a cascade-like response of cytokines with an early release of TNF followed by subsequent release of other cytokines is now well accepted as an important part of the response to injury, inflammation, and severe infection.

4

Energy Metabolism

Naji N. Abumrad
Susan M. Ystueta
Patricia Molina
Simon Bursztein

Metabolism may be defined as the sum of complex and integrated chemical reactions by which the cells of the body are capable of deriving energy from the environment and synthesizing the organic compounds necessary for the establishment and maintenance of biologic processes [1]. The sole source of energy for the human body is food derived from the external environment, ingestion of which may be expressed in terms of caloric intake. Upon ingestion of food in the form of carbohydrates, proteins, or fats, these nutrients are either oxidized to produce immediate chemical free energy via adenosine triphosphate (ATP) production or are otherwise transformed to long-term storage forms of free energy, such as glycogen or fat [2–7]. The *first law of thermodynamics* states that the total energy of a system and its surroundings is constant [8]. Based on this fundamental principle that "energy may neither be created nor destroyed," the human body is in a constant state of energy equilibrium, actively combusting food from its own reserves or from dietary intake and transforming this energy to produce mechanical work and heat. According to various conditions such as nutritional status, presence of illness, age, sex, level of physical activity, time of the day, environmental factors, and psychological status, the human body will modify its energy metabolism to satisfy its metabolic needs and energy balance. Surgical intervention (whether elective or emergent), trauma, malnutrition, and infection all disrupt the

This work was supported by NIH grants DK30515 and GM29327.

normal physiologic and metabolic pathways of the human body [4–7,9]. Essential to the comprehension of the modifications in energy metabolism that occur as a result of these afflictions is a firm basis of knowledge in physiologic energy metabolism. Once this is accomplished, the surgeon may then apply his knowledge to the assessment and management of nutritional status in the surgical patient.

Sources of Energy: Hydrolysis of ATP

The human body requires the continuous input of free energy that is derived from the external environment via the ingestion of food for the establishment and maintenance of biologic processes. The principal source of immediate chemical free energy in the body is ATP. Adenosine triphosphate is a nucleotide consisting of one molecule of adenine, one of ribose, and three molecules of phosphate linked by pyrophosphate bonds (Figure 4-1). Adenosine triphospate is continuously produced and consumed at a very high turnover rate (Table 4-1). The rate of ATP consumption varies (see Table 4-1) [8]. The high turnover rate of ATP is essential to life, because the energy derived from the hydrolysis of ATP is necessary for processes such as biosynthesis, motion, active transport, and signal transduction.

Because of the two high-energy phosphoanhydride bonds found in the triphosphate unit [10], ATP is referred to as a "high-energy" phosphate compound. The bonds are referred to as *high energy* because upon hydrolysis, a relatively large amount of free energy (denoted as G) is generated.

Table 4-1. Estimated ATP Turnover Rates

Condition	Amount
Rest	~40 kg ATP per 24 hr
Strenuous exercise	~700 kg ATP per 24 hr

The hydrolysis of any phosphorylated compound may yield free energy, the extent to which depends on the substrate in question (Table 4-2). In general, two categories of phosphorylated compounds have been recognized. The high-energy bond compounds consist of substrates such as ATP, pyrophosphate, creatine phosphate (CrP), and phosphoenolpyruvate (PEP). In contrast, the low-energy bond compounds include adenosine monophosphate (AMP), which yields 3 kcal/mol, and glycerophosphate, which yields 2.5 kcal/mol [8].

Note that not all of the energy released upon hydrolysis of these phosphorylated compounds is available to do work. This "unavailable" energy is that which is spent to maintain randomness or disorder of the system, which is referred to as entropy, denoted by S. The entropy of a closed system and its surroundings will always increase for a spontaneous reaction [8,11]. The energy nec-

Table 4-2. Energy Yield of Phosphorylated Compounds

High Energy Compounds	Energy Yield (kcal/mol)
ATP	7.3
Pyrophosphate	8.0
Creatine P	10.3
Phosphoenolpyruvate	14.8

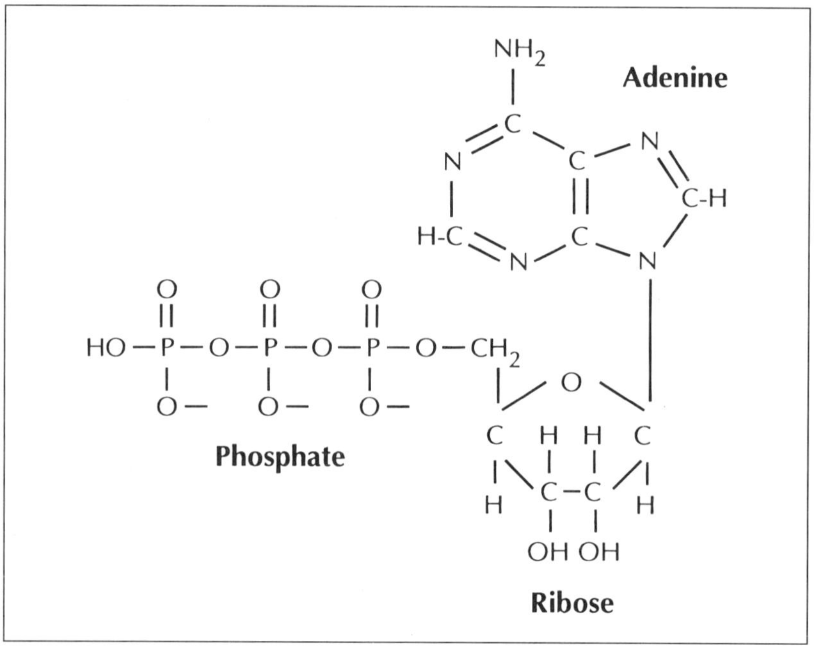

Figure 4-1. Schematic structure of ATP.

essary to maintain this randomness may be expressed as TS (where T represents the temperature measured in degrees Kelvin). Enthalpy, denoted by H, defines the heat content or internal energy of a physical object or body. Using the quantitative values of entropy (S) and enthalpy (H), the maximum amount of energy that is available to do work, or Gibb energy (G), may be calculated. This is expressed as:

$$G = H - TS$$

The driving force of a reaction is more accurately described as the change in free energy represented as ΔG:

$$\Delta G = H - T\Delta S$$

Thus, the change in free energy (ΔG) of a reaction depends on the change in the internal energy or heat content of the system and the change in the energy necessary to maintain disorder in the system.

Calculation of ΔG is necessary in determining whether a reaction is capable of proceeding spontaneously or not. Quite simply, a reaction may only proceed spontaneously if ΔG is negative (−). If ΔG is positive (+), then an input of free energy is required to drive that reaction. If ΔG is zero, then the system is at equilibrium [11]. For the reaction below:

$$A + B \rightarrow C + D$$

calculation of ΔG may be expressed as:

$$\Delta G = \Delta G^\circ + RT \log \{[C] \times [D]\} \{[A] \times [B]\}$$

where ΔG° of the reaction is the change in free energy under standard conditions in which the reactants are each present at 1.0 M concentrations. R is the gas constant (1.98×10^{-3} kcal·mol^{-1} ·deg^{-1}), and T is the absolute temperature (298° K) [8]. At equilibrium, where ΔG = 0, the above equation becomes:

$$\Delta G^\circ = -RT \log \{[C] \times [D]\} \{[A] \times [B]\}$$

or

$$\Delta G = \Delta G^\circ + RT \log \{[C] \times [D]\} \{[A] \times [B]\}$$

The equilibrium constant under standard conditions, denoted by Keq, is expressed as:

$$Keq = \{[C] \times [D]\} \{[A] \times [B]\}$$

Thus, the equation for ΔG° may be simply expressed as:

$$\Delta G^\circ = -2.303\ RT\log_{10} Keq$$

Note that ΔG is dependent on the nature and concentrations of the reactants; however, it is independent of the molecular mechanism of the transformation [8]. Although it is true that a thermodynamically unfavorable reaction, in which ΔG is positive (+), will not proceed spontaneously on its own, it may be driven by a thermodynamically favorable reaction, in which ΔG is negative (−). The total free energy change for a chemically coupled series of reactions may be determined by the sum of the individual free energy changes. If the free energy change for a coupled reaction is negative, then the net reaction may proceed spontaneously. As an example:

$A + B \rightleftarrows C + D$	$\Delta G^\circ = +6.3$ kcal/mol
$C \rightleftarrows E$	$\Delta G^\circ = -9.4$ kcal/mol
$A + B \rightleftarrows D + E$	$\Delta G^\circ = -3.1$ kcal/mol

This exemplifies the concept of energy coupling, which is central to understanding the role of ATP in metabolism. The free energy (ΔG), liberated by the hydrolysis of ATP, is used to drive otherwise thermodynamically unfavorable reactions. It is in this capacity that ATP serves as the principal source of free energy for the human body.

Regeneration of the high-energy phosphate bonds of ATP is essential for the maintenance of these biochemical reactions and processes, and ultimately for the maintenance of life. The regeneration of ATP from adenosine diphosphate (ADP) and Pi (inorganic phosphate) occurs by means of harnessing the energy liberated by the oxidation of ingested carbohydrates, fats, and proteins. In addition, ATP is regenerated from the hydrolysis of creatine phosphate to creatine, which occurs in skeletal muscle (Figure 4-2). This coupling of the oxidation with the phosphorylation of ADP to yield ATP is called oxidative phosphorylation.

Overview of Metabolism

Energy production and utilization are two features that are absolutely essential for survival. Most of that energy is derived from ingested foodstuffs. Hans A. Kreb described three states essential to the extraction of this energy (Figure 4-3) [8].

The first stage consists of the breakdown of foodstuffs to its smaller constituents. Carbohydrates are broken down into simple sugars, fats are hydrolyzed to glycerol and fatty acids, and proteins are degraded to amino acids. *Essentially no energy production occurs during this stage. On the contrary, most of these processes require energy.*

The second stage of metabolism consists of further degradation of fuel molecules to a few key substrates that play a central role in energy metabolism. Pyruvate, with its subsequent conversion to acetyl-CoA, is one such key player that is common to carbohydrate, fat, and protein metabo-

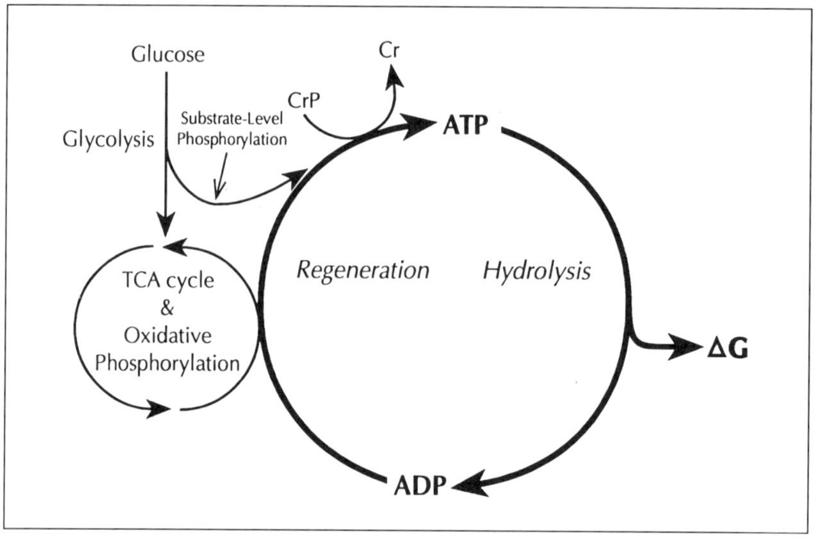

Figure 4-2. Schematic representation of possible pathways of regeneration and hydrolysis of ATP. Regeneration occurs primarily via two pathways. The first one is related to the process of glycolysis, and the second, and quantitatively more important, is associated with the tricarboxylic acid cycle (TCA). A minor pathway, which is usually operational during periods of exhaustive exercise, is that related to the dephosphorylation of creatine phosphate to creatine, which occurs primarily in skeletal muscle.

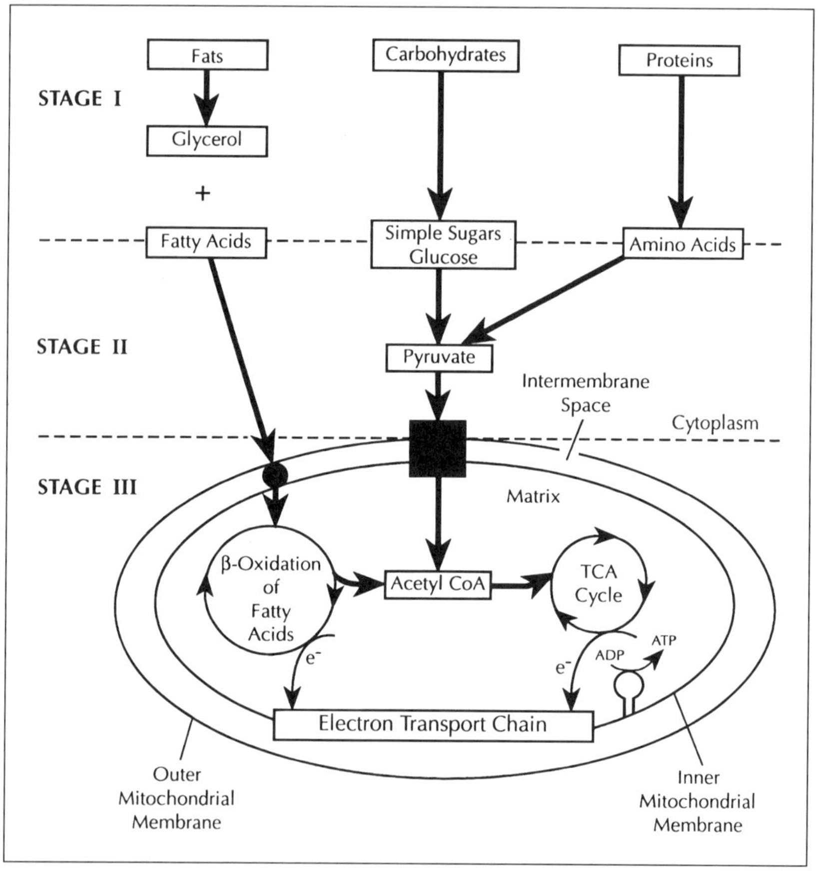

Figure 4-3. The three stages of energy metabolism as first defined by H. Krebs. Stage I involves the breakdown of fats into glycerol and fatty acids, carbohydrates into simple sugars, and proteins into amino acids. In Stage I, energy is required. In Stage II, the simple sugars are broken down into pyruvate. Energy is generated during this stage, but the amount of ATP produced is small in comparison to that produced from the complete oxidation of foodstuffs during Stage III, in the TCA cycle, and via the process of oxidative phosphorylation. The metabolic activities associated with Stage III occur within the mitochondria.

lism. Some energy in the form of ATP is generated during this second stage of metabolism; however, the amount produced is small in comparison to that produced from the complete oxidation of foodstuffs via oxidative phosphorylation.

During the third stage of metabolism, the acetyl-CoA molecules derived from the previous stages undergo oxidation in the tricarboxylic acid cycle (TCA). The oxidation of acetyl-CoA and other substrates generates high-energy electron carriers that then enter the electron transport chain, so named because electrons are transferred from high-energy electron carriers to a series of protein complexes, with the ultimate transfer of the electrons to oxygen (Figure 4-4) [12]. The energy liberated during this electron transfer is the energy used to generate the high-energy phosphate bond of ATP. Because many of the processes of metabolism take place in the mitochondria of the cell, further knowledge of the structure of the mitochondrion is essential to the understanding of energy metabolism.

Mitochondrion: Structure-Function Relationships

The mitochondrion is often referred to as the "powerhouse of the cell," because within this highly specialized organelle the majority of ATP is produced. The intracellular location of the mitochondria and their number vary with the species and tissues under consideration. Typically, these oval-shaped organelles are found in the cytoplasm and measure approximately 2μm in length and 0.5–1 μm in diameter [13–16]. Structurally, mitochondria consist of an outer membrane and an extensively folded inner membrane (Figure 4-5). The internal folds are called cristae. The presence of these membranes compartmentalizes the mitochondrion into the intermembrane space located between the outer and inner membranes and the matrix that comprises the space internal to the inner membrane. The TCA cycle and fatty acid oxidations take place in the matrix, and oxidative phosphorylation occurs in the inner mitochondrial membrane.

Mitochondria contain many proteins, most of which are bound to the mitochondrial membranes, and all of which assume major roles in the transport of substrates and ions required for mitochondrial oxidation to occur. Approximately 95% of the mitochondrial proteins are encoded by nuclear DNA. Once produced, the proteins are directed to the mitochondrial membranes by a specific presequence leader segment that addresses the protein to its specific membrane receptor site. Those proteins designed to reside in the outer membrane are anchored in place, and all other mitochondrial-destined proteins are transported across the outer membrane. Some of these proteins are further di-

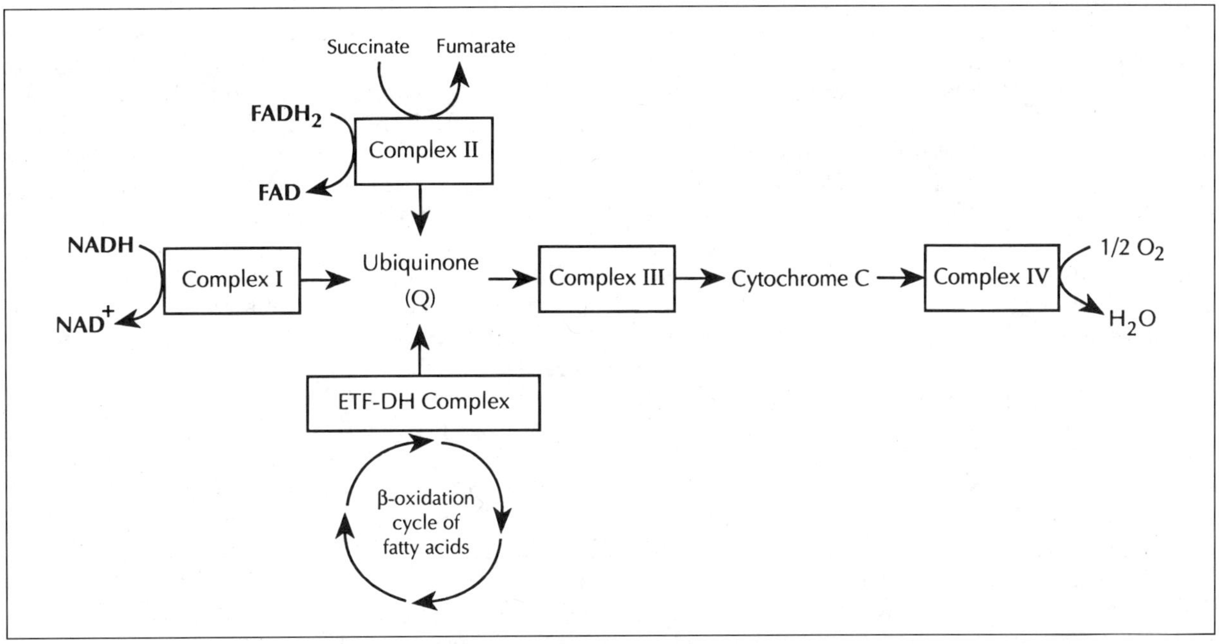

Figure 4-4. Schematics of the mitochondrial respiratory chain. Electrons from NADH are transferred to Complex I (known as NADH-ubiquinone, CoQ oxireductase). Electrons from flavoproteins are transferred to Ubiquinone (Q) either via Complex II (known as succinate-ubiquinone, CoQ, oxireductase), or via ETF (known as Electron Transfer Flavoprotein). ETF assumes a more important role in the transfer of electrons from the oxidation of fats, via beta-oxidation cycle through ETF dehydrogenase (DH). Complex III is known as cytochrome C reductase and oxidizes ubiquinol. The electrons are transferred via cytochrome C to Complex IV, known as cytochrome C oxidase. In the process of electron transfer from Complex III to Complex IV, four electrons (4 e^-) are donated to oxygen (O_2), and four protons (4 H^+) are derived from the matrix to form water. Complex V is known as ATP Synthase. The overall reactions catalyzed by this chain is: 2[NADH + H^+] + $O_2 \rightarrow NAD^+ + 2H_2O$ and $2FPH_2 + O_2 \rightarrow 2FP + 2H_2O$. (From HSA Sherratt. Mitochondria: Structure and function. *Rev Neurol* 147:417, 1991.)

Figure 4-5. Schematic diagram of a mitochondrion.

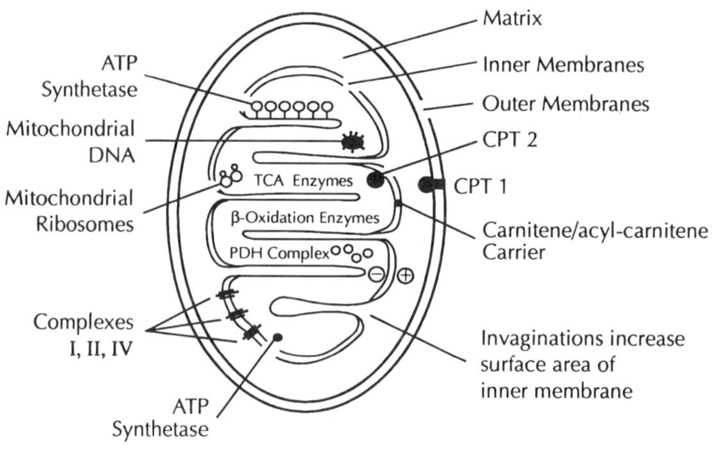

rected to the inner membrane, where they are then anchored in place, and yet other proteins will reside unbound in the mitochondrial matrix [17].

The mitochondrial proteins undergo processing that specifies their functional activity, particularly as it relates to redox potential and oxidative phosphorylation. This may entail covalent or noncovalent modifications with the insertion of specific prosthetic groups such as flavin mononucleotide (FMN), flavin adenine dinucleotide (FAD), or heme A, B, or C that are essential to oxidative phosphorylation. Final processing of the proteins occurs with the incorporation of the mitochondrial-derived proteins, encoded by mitochondrial DNA (mtDNA), which constitutes the remaining 5% of the mitochondrial proteins. This mtDNA is essential to the proper functioning of oxidative phosphorylation in the electron transport chain.

It is well established that mtDNA encodes for seven peptides of complex I, one peptide of complex III, three peptides of complex IV, and two peptides of complex V of the respiratory electron chain. Mitochondrial DNA possesses a rapid replication rate, and as such, is subject to a high tendency toward mutation. The expression of mitochondrial-derived protein mutations requires surpassing a threshold level within the cell. Once exceeded, phenotypic expression of mutated mitochondrial oxidative phosphorylation occurs. *These mutations of mtDNA may potentially result in metabolic acidosis, lactic acidosis, encephalopathy, myopathy, optic neuropathy, ataxia, cardiomyopathy, and other abnormal physiologic and pathologic states.* Several syndromes based on these oxidative phosphorylation genetic mutations have been described [18–20]. Thus, it is conceivable that a mutation in either one of these proteins, or a deformation in their anchoring mechanisms, may be responsible for some of the disease conditions associated with energy metabolism during periods of stress, injury, and infection.

The major high-energy electron carriers essential in the oxidation of fuel substrates are nicotinamide adenine nucleotide (NAD^+) and FAD. NAD^+ acts as an electron carrier because of the presence of its nicotinamide group that is capable of accepting two electrons and a hydrogen ion, forming NADH, the reduced form of NAD^+ [8]. The other high-energy electron carrier, FAD, acts as an electron carrier because of the presence of its isoalloxazine ring that is capable of accepting two electrons along with two hydrogen ions, forming $FADH_2$, the reduced form of FAD. The reduced forms of these electron carriers, NADH and $FADH_2$, are responsible for providing the energy necessary for ATP production. The determination of the amount of ATP produced per molecule of substrate is defined by the P/O ratio, which is the ratio of Pi (inorganic phosphate) consumed in ATP production for each oxygen (O) consumed [21,22]. It has been determined that for every molecule of NADH that enters the electron transport chain, three molecules of ATP are produced. For every molecule of $FADH_2$, two molecules of ATP are produced. Hence, the P/O ratios for NADH and $FADH_2$ are 3 and 2, respectively. Knowledge of these P/O ratios is important in determining total energy production derived from the combustion of foodstuffs.

Fat Metabolism

Fats are a class of structurally diverse compounds consisting almost exclusively of carbon and hydrogen. The three main forms of fat found in the human diet and in the body are the glycerides, phospholipids, and sterols. Fats serve as the greatest source of fuel in the body for energy-requiring processes, generating 9.3 kcal/g upon complete oxidation, compared with the oxidation of carbohydrates and proteins, which only generate approximately 4 kcal/g [23,24]. An average 70-kg man has approximately 16 kg of fat stored in adipose tissue, which can yield nearly 150,000 kcal upon combustion. The enormity of this potential energy may be more appropriately appreciated when one considers that this energy is sufficient to allow an individual to survive for two months at an average expenditure of approximately 2500 kcal per day.

The major form of fat is triglycerides (TG), accounting for approximately 95% to 98% of both dietary fat and storage fat in the human body [1]. Triglycerides are composed of three fatty acid molecules and a glycerol molecule. The main stores of TG are found in adipose tissue. Adipose cells are highly specialized for the synthesis and storage of TG. The hormone-sensitive lipase of adipose cells is responsible for the hydrolysis of TG, termed *lipolysis,* which liberates fatty acids from their main storage depots in TG. Fatty acids are a class of compounds containing a long hydrocarbon chain and a terminal carboxylate group. Those tissues capable of using fatty acids as an energy source include the liver, kidney, heart, and skeletal muscle. The oxidation of fatty acids by these tissues yields acetyl-CoA that may then enter the citric acid cycle (TCA) to complete oxidation and energy formation. If the rate of acetyl-CoA formed exceeds that of acetyl-CoA use as may occur in starvation and other pathologic states, then the liver may produce ketone bodies. Ketone bodies may subsequently be used by extrahepatic tissues as fuel for biologic processes.

The discussion that follows will focus on those aspects of fat metabolism most relevant to energy metabolism in the human body: fatty acid oxidation and ketone body metabolism.

Triglyceride Hydrolysis and Fatty Acid Oxidation

As stated above, the first step in the utilization of stored fat as an energy source is the hydrolysis of TG by hormone-sensitive lipases found in the adipose cells (Figure 4-6). The most potent lipase-activating hormone is epinephrine. Other lipolytic hormones include norepinephrine, growth hormone, glucagon, thyroid hormone, and corticotropin (ACTH). These hormones act by stimulating adenylate cyclase in adipose tissues to convert ATP to cyclic AMP (cAMP). The increase in cAMP in turn stimulates a protein kinase that phosphorylates the adipose cell lipase, thereby activating it. In contrast, the inhibition of lipolysis occurs by the action of mediators that dephosphorylate the hormone-sensitive lipase in adipose tissues, thereby inactivating it. These mediators include insulin and somatomedins. Further control of lipid metabolism is exerted through the association between increased lipolysis and decreased lipid synthesis. The activated protein kinase of lipolysis serves to phosphorylate the enzyme used in fatty acid biosynthesis, acetyl-CoA carboxylase, resulting in its inactivation and hence a decrease in lipid formation.

Lipolysis results in the liberation of three molecules of fatty acids and one molecule of glycerol for each TG compound. The glycerol released from the adipose cells travels to the liver, and to a lesser degree to the kidney, where it is phosphorylated to form glycerol-3-phosphate. For every two moles of glycerol-3-phosphate, one mole of glucose can be synthesized in gluconeogenesis. Alternatively, the glycerol-3-phosphate may enter the glycolytic pathway with its subsequent conversion into py-

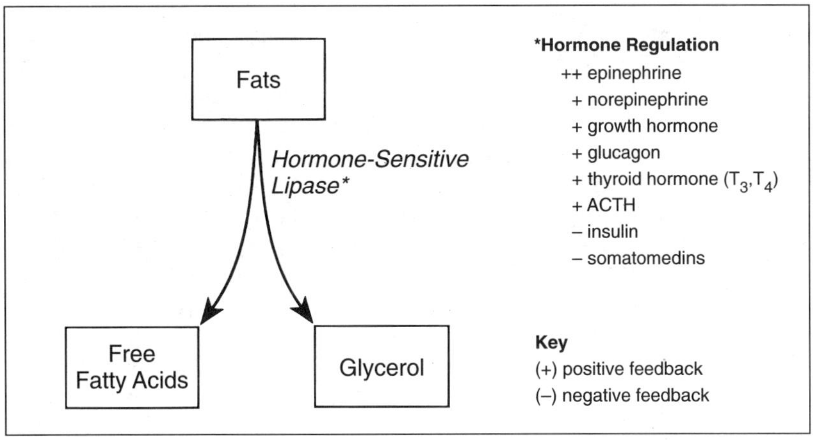

Figure 4-6. Hormonal regulation of lipolysis.

ruvate. In addition, glycerol-3-phosphate serves as a precursor to TG synthesis.

The fatty acids liberated from the adipose cells act as fuel molecules for specific tissues by the oxidation of their β-carbon atom, hence the term *β-oxidation of fatty acids.* This principal route for the catabolism of fatty acids occurs in the mitochondria. β-Oxidation requires the activation of fatty acids and their transport across the mitochondrial membranes into the matrix (see Figure 4-6). This occurs by the enzymatic activity of acyl-CoA synthetase, which is located on the outer mitochondrial membrane. This enzyme links fatty acids to the sulfhydryl group of CoA, creating fatty-acyl-CoA at the expense of two molecules of ATP.

Long-chain fatty-acyl-CoA molecules formed on the outer mitochondrial membrane cannot readily traverse the inner mitochondrial membrane. The activated long-chain fatty acids therefore must bind to carnitine, a transport protein, to produce fatty-acyl-carnitine, a reaction catalyzed by carnitine palmitoyl transferase I (CPT I) as shown in Figure 4-7. This complex converts carnitine to acyl-carnitine. The acyl-carnitine is then translocated to the inner border of inner mitochondrial membrane using a translocase. Once inside, CPT II catalyzes the reverse reaction, thereby liberating fatty-acyl CoA within the mitochondria [25].

Once inside the mitochondrial matrix, the fatty acids undergo β-oxidation, a process that essentially consists of a sequence of four reactions (Figure 4-8). Each pass through the β-oxidation cycle results in the removal of two carbon atoms from the fatty acid in the form of acetyl-CoA. The remaining fatty acid (less two carbon atoms) subsequently re-enters β-oxidation, and the cycle continues until oxidation to acetyl-CoA molecules is complete. Most biologic fatty acids contain an even number of carbon atoms, therefore resulting simply in a factor of acetyl-CoA molecules. However, in the case of odd-numbered fatty acid chains, β-oxidation continues until a three-carbon fatty-acyl-CoA, named *propionyl-CoA,* is produced [26]. This molecule may subsequently be converted to succinyl-CoA and enter the TCA cycle.

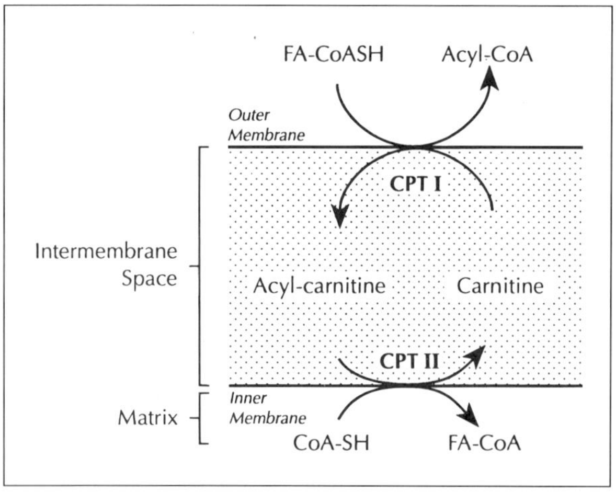

Figure 4-7. Schematic diagram of fatty acid transport across the mitochondrial membranes. CPT depicts carnitine palmitoyl transferase enzymes.

In addition to the generation of acetyl-CoA, each pass through the cycle generates one molecule of $FADH_2$ and one molecule of NADH. The $FADH_2$ and NADH will subsequently undergo oxidative phosphorylation in the electron transport chain. The acetyl-CoA produced from the β-oxidation of fatty acids may have three fates: it may enter the TCA cycle for completion of oxidation and the generation of energy; it may serve as substrate for the production of ketone bodies in the liver; or it may serve as a substrate in the synthesis of fatty acids and TG. Of special note is the fact that humans and other mammals do not possess the enzymes necessary for the conversion of acetyl-CoA or fatty acids into glucose. The particular fate of the acetyl-CoA will be dependent on the nutritional state of the body and its energy needs.

Ketone Body Metabolism

Ketone bodies are produced by the liver from acetyl-CoA whenever the rate of acetyl-CoA formation exceeds its utilization by the TCA cycle. The entry of acetyl-CoA into the TCA cycle depends on the activity of carbohydrate degradation for the generation of TCA cycle intermediates, specifically oxaloacetate, to which acetyl-CoA combines to form citrate. Citrate then proceeds to be oxidized in the TCA cycle. If fat breakdown predominates over carbohydrate degradation, as occurs during prolonged starvation, then the unavailability of oxaloacetate precludes the entrance of acetyl-CoA into the cycle. In addition, the enzyme acetyl-CoA, which catalyzes the rate-controlling step in the synthesis of fatty acids, is inhibited by the absence of citrate. Therefore, yet another potential route of acetyl-CoA utilization is inhibited and acetyl-CoA accumulates in the liver. The accumulated acetyl-CoA is then utilized to produce the ketone bodies acetoacetate and β-hydroxybutyric acid. Negative feedback regulates excess acetyl-CoA production. Elevated levels of ketone bodies in the blood signify an abundance of acetyl units that stimulate negative feedback mechanisms, resulting in a decrease in the rate of lipolysis in adipose tissue. Hence, there is a decrease in fatty acid generation and subsequent acetyl-CoA production.

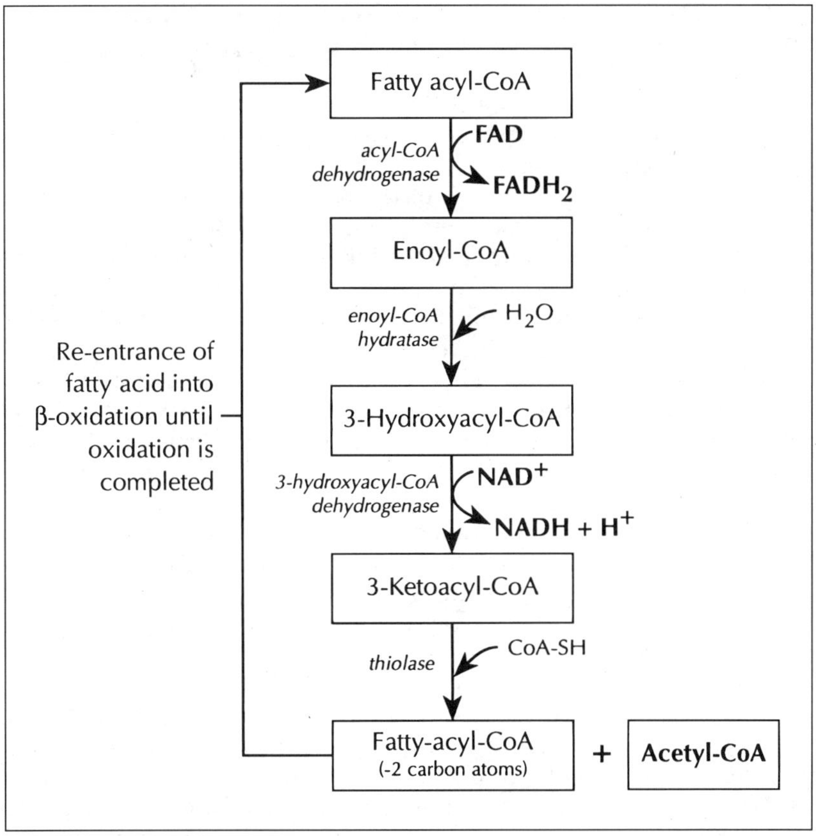

Figure 4-8. Pathways of mitochondrial beta-oxidation of fatty acids.

Once formed, the ketone bodies diffuse from the liver into the bloodstream and are transported to extrahepatic tissues for use as fuel. Ketone bodies are converted into two molecules of acetyl-CoA, which then enter the TCA cycle. Those tissues capable of utilizing acetoacetate and β-hydroxybutyrate include skeletal muscle, cardiac muscle, renal cortex, and brain. Normally, the brain uses glucose as its major source of fuel. However, the brain has the enormous capacity to adapt to the utilization of acetoacetate during prolonged starvation, during which such use accounts for nearly 75% of its energy needs.

Despite regulatory mechanisms that attempt to control the rate of acetyl-CoA and ketone body production, ketonemia and ketosis may occur. Ketosis occurs whenever the rate of hepatic ketone body production exceeds the rate of extrahepatic utilization. This may occur during severe carbohydrate deficiency, the main underlying mechanism for diabetic ketoacidosis, alcoholic ketoacidosis, and starvation ketosis. The presence of severe ketonemia overwhelms the buffering capacity of the serum proteins, resulting in metabolic acidosis, characterized by increased anion gap with the unmeasured anions represented by β-hydroxybutyric acid and acetoacetate. To prevent ketosis it is recommended that the adult diet contain a minimum of 100 g or 400 kcal of carbohydrate daily, which will generate enough oxaloacetate to maintain the TCA cycle.

Protein Metabolism

Proteins are a class of molecules that serve a multitude of key roles in nearly all biologic processes. The basic structural unit of proteins, the amino acids, consists of an amino group, carboxyl group, hydrogen atoms, and a side chain that denotes the physical and chemical activity of the amino acid. Amino acids are linked together by an amide bond, or peptide bond, to form a polypeptide chain, or protein. In comparison to fats and carbohydrates, proteins play a small role in energy metabolism in the well-nourished individual, providing only approximately 12% of the daily energy need [23]. Furthermore, in contrast to fats and carbohydrates, amino acids in excess of those needed for protein synthesis cannot be stored. The 11 kg of protein present in an average 70-kg man, 40% of which may be present in muscle solely, represents functional or structural proteins [23]. The protein present in the human body may serve as a source of carbon for glucose production via gluconeogenesis during periods of fasting, and indeed during starvation protein serves as the major source of carbon for glucose production. However, it is inaccurate to refer to this protein as storage protein because such use of structural and functional protein present in human tissue always occurs with the resultant loss of bodily structure or function.

Amino acids from dietary intake, although not capable of serving directly as a storage form of metabolic fuel, do serve as substrates for the generation of metabolic fuel. Excess amino acids are degraded and subsequently converted to fatty acids, ketone bodies, and glucose.

Amino acid catabolism is quite complex and highly integrated with multiple metabolic pathways (Figure 4-9) [27]. The discussion that follows will simply provide a general overview of protein catabolism as it relates to energy metabolism rather than to attempt to describe the intricate catabolic pathways of each individual amino acid.

Complete amino acid catabolism occurs primarily in the liver and secondarily in the kidney [3,27,28]. Most other tissues are capable of only partial amino acid catabolism. The initial step in amino acid catabolism is the removal of the α-amino acid group from the carbon skeleton of the amino acid, resulting in an α-keto acid and the generation of ammonia. The most common mechanism for the removal of the α-amino group is transamination, which is catalyzed by a transaminase or aminotransferase. The most essential of these enzymes include aspartate aminotransferase and alanine aminotransferase. Most of the ammonia formed as a result of the deamination is converted by the liver to urea, which is then secreted into the urine.

The fate of the carbon skeleton of the α-keto acid that remains after deamination is the conversion to one of a limited member of key metabolic intermediates. Based on the particular amino acid in question, the carbon skeleton may be converted to a TCA cycle intermediate such as α-ketoglutarate, succinyl-CoA, fumarate, and oxaloacetate. Alternatively, the carbon skeleton may be converted to acetyl-CoA or to a precursor of acetyl-CoA such as pyruvate and acetoacetyl-CoA, a ketone body. Based on their individual capacities to be degraded to these metabolic intermediates, the amino acids are classified as glucogenic, ketogenic, or glucogenic/ketogenic. Amino acids capable of conversion to oxaloacetate, pyruvate, α-ketoglutarate, succinyl-CoA, and fumarate are termed *glucogenic,* because these metabolites can be converted to glucose via gluconeogenesis. Those amino acids capable of conversion to acetyl-CoA and acetoacetyl-CoA are termed *ketogenic,* because these metabolites can be converted to ketone bodies but not to glucose. Amino acids capable of conversion to both types of intermediates are termed ketogenic/glucogenic. Ultimately, all the

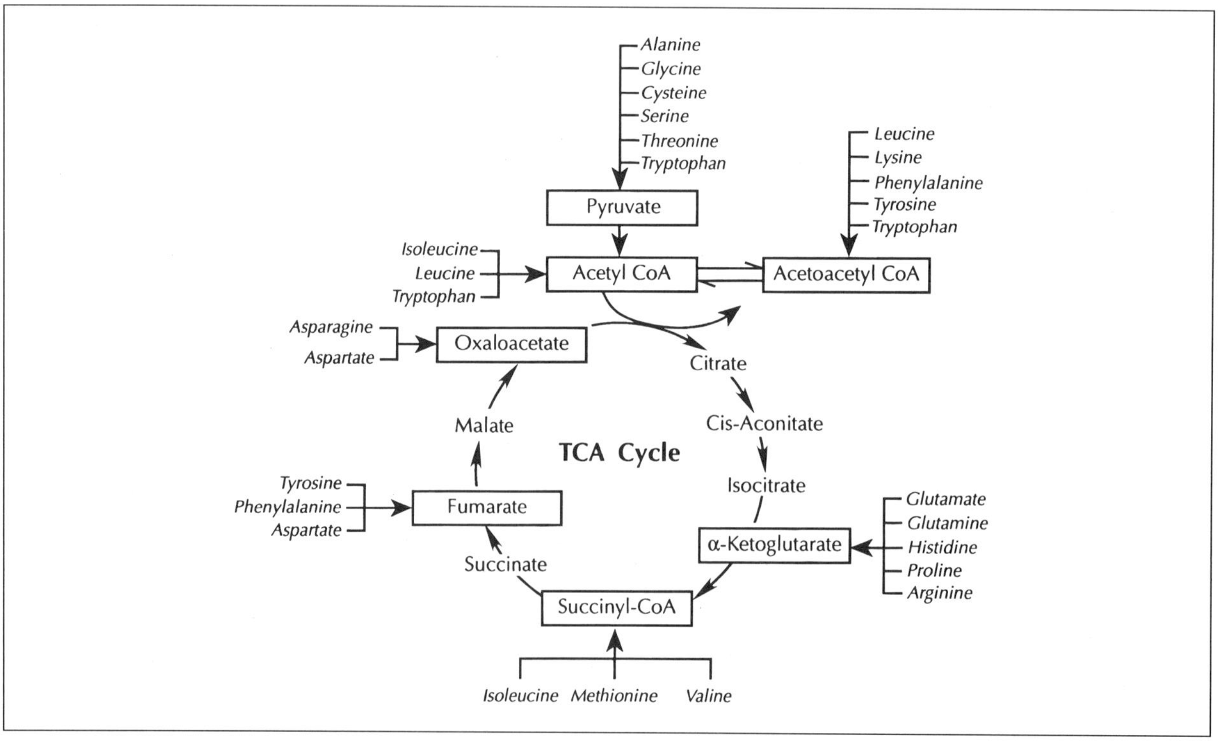

Figure 4-9. Pathways of amino acid catabolism.

carbon skeletons of the amino acids can be oxidized in the TCA cycle for the generation of metabolic fuel.

Amino acid metabolism is regulated by hormonal control. Insulin inhibits gluconeogenesis from amino acids and stimulates protein synthesis [28,29]. Somatomedins, growth hormone, thyroid hormones, and androgens also promote protein synthesis. Glucocorticoids, on the contrary, enhance gluconeogenesis from amino acids. During fasting, the gluconeogenic action of glucocorticoids predominates, depleting the body's functional and structural proteins for the production of glucose for use by the brain and other tissues. If left unchecked, this protein depletion would eventually become life-threatening. Therefore, the body possesses another mechanism by which it adapts to starvation and reduces its need for protein-dependent gluconeogenesis. This is accomplished via the stimulation of ketone body formation, which serves as an alternative fuel to glucose for most tissues, including the brain. To avoid protein catabolic gluconeogenesis, it is recommended that the adult diet consist of at least 100 g of carbohydrate daily. This is the same daily dietary amount that is recommended to prevent excess ketone body formation.

Carbohydrate Metabolism

Carbohydrates are polyhydroxylated compounds containing at least three carbon atoms and an aldehyde or ketone group, denoting the carbohydrates as aldoses or ketoses, respectively. The storage form of glucose is glycogen, consisting of branched polymers of glucose residues. The main stores of glycogen are found in the liver skeletal muscle, where glycogen is present in the cytosol in the form of granules. Although the average 70-kg man has only approximately 40 kcal of energy derived from the glucose in body fluids, the total body glycogen energy content is approximately 1000 to 3000 kcal [30]. The glucose derived from the breakdown of glycogen via the process of *glycogenolysis* is available for immediate use between meals and during exercise. However, the storage form of glucose is of little long-term value. The liver stores of glycogen are only sufficient enough to supply the body with glucose for up to 24 hours during fasting. Therefore, during prolonged fasting, glucose must be derived from noncarbohydrates such as lactate, pyruvate, amino acids, and glycerol, via the process of *gluconeogenesis*.

Dietary carbohydrates consist mainly of polysaccharides, which are carbohydrate polymers consisting of at least ten monosaccharide units, and the disaccharides such as sucrose and lactose. Only a small amount of dietary carbohydrate consists of the monosaccharides, glucose and fructose; however, the principal monosaccharide derived from the hydrolysis of dietary carbohydrates is glucose. Glucose serves as the principal fuel for the generation of energy in metabolism. Consequently, we have chosen to elaborate in greater detail on the various carbohydrate-related pathways involved in ATP generation.

Glycolysis

The process by which glucose is broken down to pyruvate with the concomitant production of energy is called *glycolysis* (Figure 4-10) [31,32]. Glycolysis takes place within the cytoplasm of the cell. Note that all the intermediates of glycolysis contain at least one phosphate group. The energy derived from the hydrolysis or dephosphorylation of these intermediates is that energy used to phosphorylate ADP to produce ATP.

The first energy-consuming step in glycolysis is the irreversible phosphorylation of glucose by *hexokinase* to produce glucose-6-phosphate. This reaction consumes one mole of ATP and requires Mg^{++} as an essential co-factor, which is common to all phosphorylation reactions. This step represents one of the rate-limiting steps in glycolysis. Abundance of glucose-6-phosphate will inhibit hexokinase and therefore inhibit further glucose-6-phosphate production in the cytoplasm. The abundance of glucose-6-phosphate in the cytoplasm will stimulate the activity of *glucokinase,* an enzyme present in the liver that acts in a similar fashion by phosphorylating glucose to produce glucose-6-phosphate. Hexokinase in the liver is only effective when glucose is abundant in the cell, and the glucose-6-phosphate produced in this way will be used for the synthesis of glycogen, the storage form of glucose.

After the conversion of glucose-6-phosphate to fructose-6-phosphate via *phosphoglucose isomerase,* a second mole of ATP is consumed in the irreversible phosphorylation of fructose-6-phosphate by *phosphofructokinase* (PFK) to produce fructose-1-6-bisphosphate. This reaction essentially commits glucose to glycolysis, because it is the first irreversible reaction unique to the glycolytic pathway [33,34]. Up until this step, glucose-6-phosphate may be used as a substrate for glycogen production or as a substrate for the production of NADPH, a reducing agent in reductive biosynthesis.

This reaction further serves as the key rate-limiting step in glycolysis. Phosphofructokinase is an allosteric enzyme, and its level of activity is regulated by several substrates. The enzyme is inhibited by high levels of ATP by decreasing its

Figure 4-10. Glycolytic pathways for carbohydrate metabolism.

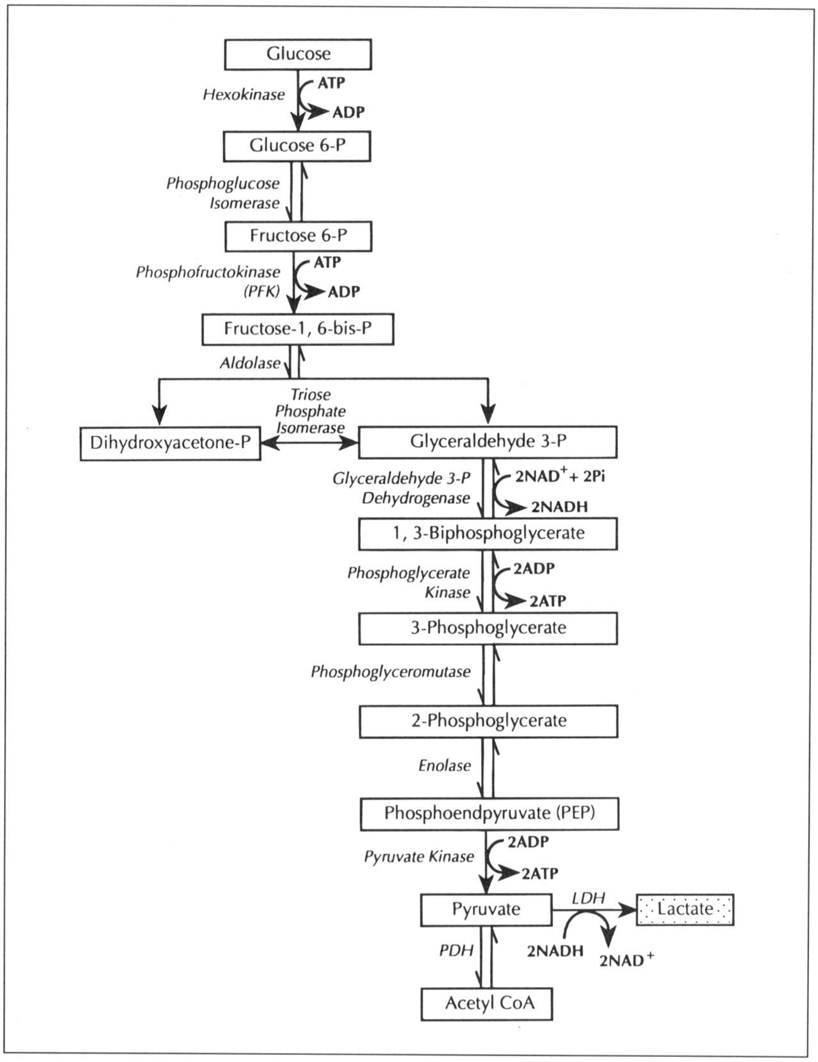

affinity for fructose-6-phosphate. Conversely, AMP diminishes the inhibitory effect of ATP. Therefore, the level of activity of PFK is increased when the ratio of ATP to AMP fall [33,34], thus stimulating more energy production via glycolysis. Phosphofructokinase is also inhibited by the presence of H^+, which halts excess formation of lactate that would aggravate the acidosis. The inhibition of PFK by citrate is related to another function of glycolysis, the provision of carbon skeletons for biosynthesis of other substrates. If the carbon skeletons are in abundance, the consequent abundance of citrate will inhibit PFK by enhancing the inhibitory effect of ATP, thus blunting any further unnecessary glucose breakdown [33,34].

Phosphofructokinase is further regulated by yet another substrate, fructose-2,6-bisphosphate. Fructose-2,6-bisphosphate is formed via the phosphorylation of fructose-6-phosphate by *phosphofructokinase 2* (PFK-2). Note that this enzyme is distinguished from PFK-1. In the presence of abundant fructose-6-phosphate, the activity of PFK-2 is stimulated, which leads to enhanced production of fructose-2,6-bisphosphate. The increased abundance of fructose-2,6-bisphosphate in turn stimulates PFK-1, therefore stimulating further glycolysis.

The next step in glycolysis converts the hexose, fructose-1,6-bisphosphate, to two triose phosphates, dihydroacetone-phosphate (DHAP) and glyceraldehyde-3-phosphate. The DHAP is then isomerized to form another molecule of glyceraldehyde-3-phosphate. Thus, for every molecule of fructose-1,6-bisphosphate, two molecules of glyceraldehyde-3-phosphate are formed.

Next, each molecule of glyceraldehyde-3-phosphate is converted into a molecule of 1,3-bisphosphoglycerate. During this step, the energy thus far contained in the phosphorylated substrates of glycolysis is used to generate a total of two molecules of the high-energy electron carrier, NADH. The phosphate group used to phosphorylate glyceraldehyde-3-phosphate is inorganic phosphate (Pi), and therefore no ATP is consumed during this phosphorylation reaction.

The next reaction generates the first ATP molecule in glycolysis. The removal of a high-energy phosphate group from each molecule of 1,3-bisphosphoglycerate by phosphoglycerate kinase yields one molecule of 3-phosphoglycerate plus one molecule of ATP, for a total of two ATP molecules produced at this step for every molecule of glucose. The ATP production occurring in the cytoplasm is referred to as substrate-level phosphorylation. This is distinguished from ATP production via the process of oxidative phosphorylation that occurs in the mitochondria.

During the next series of reactions, each molecule of 3-phosphoglycerate is converted into 2-phosphoglycerate and then subsequently to phosphoenolpyruvate (PEP). The next energy-producing step is that of the conversion of PEP to pyruvate, catalyzed by *pyruvate kinase,* which generates one mole of ATP from each mole of PEP. As shown in the previous discussion on free energy, PEP is a very high-energy phosphate compound with a $\Delta G°$ of -14.8 kcal/mol. Its hydrolysis, therefore, easily drives ATP production, which has a ΔG of $+7.3$ kcal/mol. This step represents the third irreversible and rate-limiting step in glycolysis.

There are three forms, or isoenzymes, of pyruvate kinase, which differ in their regulatory mechanisms. In the liver, one of the isoenzymes is inhibited by an abundance of ATP, therefore inhibiting further glycolysis and ATP production. Glycolysis is further inhibited at this step during hypoglycemia. This regulatory mechanism prevents further breakdown of glucose by the liver so that the small amount of serum glucose present may be preferentially used by the brain. Conversely, pyruvate kinase is stimulated by fructose-1,6-bisphosphate, a preceding glycolytic intermediate. It thus serves to signal pyruvate kinase to maintain a high level of enzymatic activity for the oncoming glycolytic intermediates.

The process of glycolysis, with the conversion of glucose to pyruvate, therefore has a net production of two ATP and two NADH molecules. The ATP molecules generated are available immediately to do work as free energy. The NADH molecules will subsequently be utilized to produce ATP via oxidative phosphorylation.

The fate of pyruvate formed by the process of glycolysis in the cytoplasm is dependent on the presence or absence of oxygen in the cell. In tissues with an adequate oxygen supply, pyruvate is transported from the cytosol to the mitochondrial matrix via an electroneutral antiporter found on the inner mitochondrial membrane. This pyruvate carrier exchanges one molecule of pyruvate for a hydroxyl group (OH^-). The pyruvate/OH^- antiporter acts as a "gateway" through which the entry of pyruvate into the mitochondrial matrix is regulated. This regulation occurs during periods of excessive production of pyruvate, such as glycogenolysis and glycolysis. The excessive production of pyruvate essentially saturates the antiporter. As a result, a significant portion of the pyruvate is then reduced to lactic acid, catalyzed by the *lactate dehydrogenase* (LDH) complex. The lactate is then transported to the liver to be used as a substrate for gluconeogenesis. This regulatory mechanism works well, for it results in the generation of more glucose in the face of increased glucose demand. However, under conditions of severe exercise, injury, or hypoxia, the rate of lactate formation exceeds the capacity of gluconeogenesis. As a result, lactic acid accumulates in the bloodstream, and if left unchecked, may result in lactic acidosis.

Under aerobic conditions, once transported into the mitochondrial complex matrix, pyruvate is decarboxylated, oxidized, and then combined with a coenzyme A to form acetyl-CoA. This series of reactions is catalyzed by the pyruvate dehydrogenase (PDH) complex. As should be expected, the activity of this enzyme complex is strictly regulated. Its activity is inhibited by acetyl-CoA, NADH, and guanosine triphosphate (GTP). Conversely, its activity is stimulated by CoA, NAD^+, and AMP. Once formed, acetyl-CoA then enters the TCA cycle and subsequently undergoes oxidative phosphorylation.

Under anaerobic conditions, such as in exercising muscle or inadequately perfused tissues, the pyruvate formed from glycolysis does not enter the TCA cycle nor undergo oxidative phosphorylation. Rather, pyruvate is reduced to lactate by the LDH complex using the NADH generated by glycolysis as the reducing agent. Under anaerobic conditions, therefore, there is no net production of NADH. The lactate generated diffuses into the bloodstream to the liver. The liver oxidizes lactate back to pyruvate, where the pyruvate may then be metabolized aerobically. If lactate is produced excessively by anaerobic tissues such that it exceeds the liver's capacity to oxidize it, then this, too, may result in lactic acidosis.

The Common Final Pathway in Substrate Metabolism: The TCA Cycle

The TCA cycle, also known as the Krebs cycle after Hans A. Krebs, has been referred to as the "central hub" in metabolism, because it often serves as the common final pathway for glycolysis, fatty acid oxidation, and amino metabolism (Figure 4-11). It is named the tricarboxylic acid cycle because many of the intermediates of the cycle have three carboxyl groups. In essence, the TCA cycle oxidizes acetyl-CoA completely to form two moles of CO_2, three molecules of NADH, one molecule of $FADH_2$, and one molecule of GTP. The NADH and $FADH_2$ produced then feed into the electron transport chain to complete the process of oxidative-phosphorylation of foodstuffs for the generation of ATP. In addition to the cycle's primary function in energy generation, it also serves as a source of intermediates for substrate synthesis. The following discussion of the TCA cycle will focus on those aspects most relevant to energy metabolism.

The first step of the TCA cycle combines oxaloacetate with acetyl-CoA, generating citrate. This step controls the rate of the cycle, because the enzyme citrate synthase is allosterically inhibited by ATP. Citrate is subsequently isomerized to *cis*-aconitate and then to isocitrate. Isocitrate subsequently undergoes oxidation and decarboxylation to α-ketoglutarate, leading to the production of NADH, CO_2, and H^+. This is a rate-controlling step in the cycle, because isocitrate dehydrogenase is activated by high levels of ADP and inhibited by high levels of NADH and ATP.

The next step in the cycle results in the decarboxylation and dehydrogenation of α-ketoglutarate to produce succinyl-CoA, with the concomitant production of NADH, CO_2, and H^+. This enzyme complex, α-ketoglutarate dehydrogenase, functions similarly to the PDH complex. It is allosterically inhibited by high levels of succinyl-CoA, NADH, and ATP.

The only substrate level phosphorylation to occur in the TCA cycle is represented by the next reaction. The hydrolysis of the high-energy bond of succinyl-CoA, with a $\Delta G°$ of approximately 8 kcal/mol, drives the phosphorylation of guanosine diphosphate (GDP) to generate GTP. This reaction is catalyzed by succinyl-CoA synthetase and produces succinate. The subsequent series of reactions consists of the oxidation, hydration, and repeated oxidation of succinate to ultimately lead to the production of oxaloacetate and one mole each of $FADH_2$, NADH, and H^+.

Overall, the TCA cycle generates three moles of NADH + H^+, one mole of $FADH_2$, and one mole

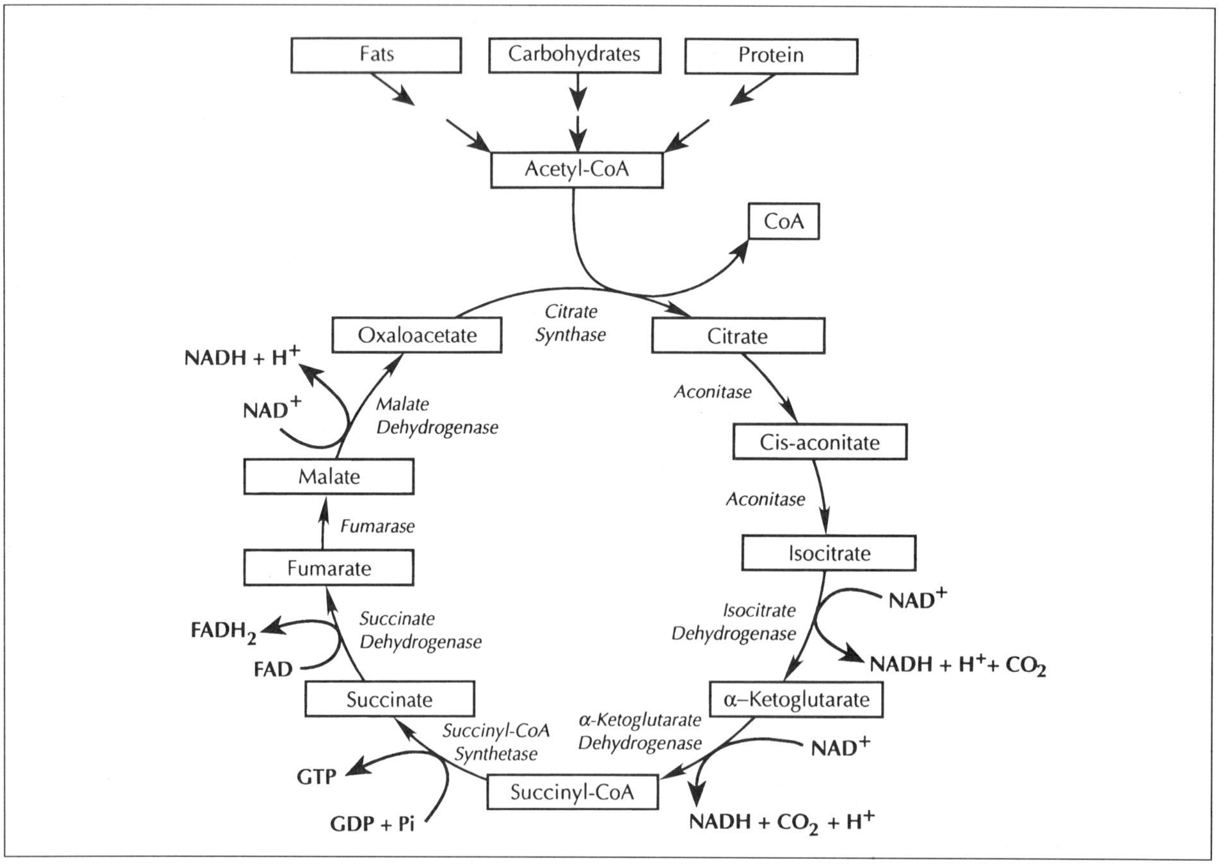

Figure 4-11. The pathways involved in the tricarboxylic acid cycle (TCA).

of GTP for every mole of acetyl-CoA it oxidizes [8]. The net reaction may be written as:

$$\text{Acetyl-CoA} + 3\,NAD^+ + FAD + GAP + Pi + 2H_2O \rightarrow 2CO_2 + 3\,NADH + FADH_2 + GTP + 2H^+ + CoA$$

The GTP generated is immediately available to do work as free energy. The NADH and $FADH_2$ will enter the electron transport chain.

Note that the TCA cycle may only function in the presence of oxygen, unlike glycolysis, which may proceed either aerobically or anaerobically. Aerobic conditions are obligatory for the TCA cycle because only in the presence of oxygen may NAD^+ and FAD be regenerated to maintain the cycle. The regeneration of NAD^+ and FAD is discussed below.

Mitochondrial Respiration and the Generation of ATP: Oxidative Phosphorylation

Oxidative phosphorylation is the process by which the majority of ATP is generated from the combustion of foodstuffs. It occurs by the transfer of electrons from the high-energy electron carriers NADH and $FADH_2$ produced by glycolysis, the TCA cycle, and fatty acid oxidation, to molecular oxygen (O_2) via a series of alternating oxidative and reductive reactions as shown in Figures 4-12 and 4-13. This respiratory electron transport chain (also shown in Figure 4-4) is composed of a series of electron carriers and enzyme complexes

Table 4-3. Respiratory Enzyme Complexes

I	NADH-ubiquinone (CoQ) oxidoreductase
II	Succinate-ubiquinone (CoQ) oxidoreductase
III	Cytochrome c reductase
IV	Cytochrome c oxidase
V	ATP synthase

(complexes I–V) located in the matrix and inner membrane of the mitochondria. The five respiratory complexes (Table 4-3) are multiple polypeptide enzyme complexes consisting of protein subunits provided by both nuclear DNA and mtDNA. The complexes are located in the mitochondrial inner membrane.

Mitochondrial Respiration

The transfer of electrons through these carriers leads to the pumping of protons out of the mitochondrial matrix, generating a *proton motive force* (PMF) [35,36]. The PMF provides the drive by which protons flow back to the mitochondrial matrix through the enzyme complex, ATP synthetase (complex V), with the concurrent phosphorylation of ADP to produce ATP shown in Figure 4-13. The oxidation of the electron carriers is coupled to the phosphorylation of ADP, hence the term oxidative phosphorylation.

Most of the NADH and $FADH_2$ that will provide electrons for the electron respiratory chain are generated via the TCA cycle and fatty acid oxidation. These processes occur in the mitochon-

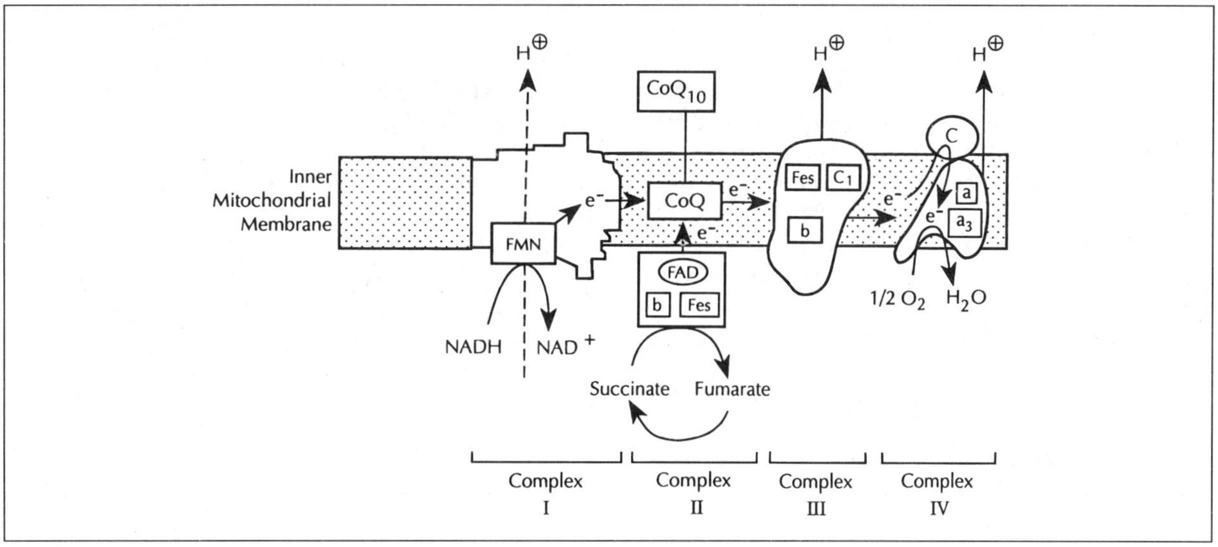

Figure 4-12. Schematic representation of the respiratory chain. The complexes are anchored in the inner mitochondrial membrane. FMN denotes flavin mononucleotide; CoQ_{10} denotes coenzyme Q_{10}. FES denotes iron-sulfur group. Cytochromes are designated as b, C_1, C, a, and a_3.

Figure 4-13. Schematic representation of Complex V or ATP synthase and ATP synthesis and exchange across the inner mitochondrial membrane. The enzyme complex is made of a base piece (F_0) that is connected to a spherical headpiece (F_1) by a stalk.

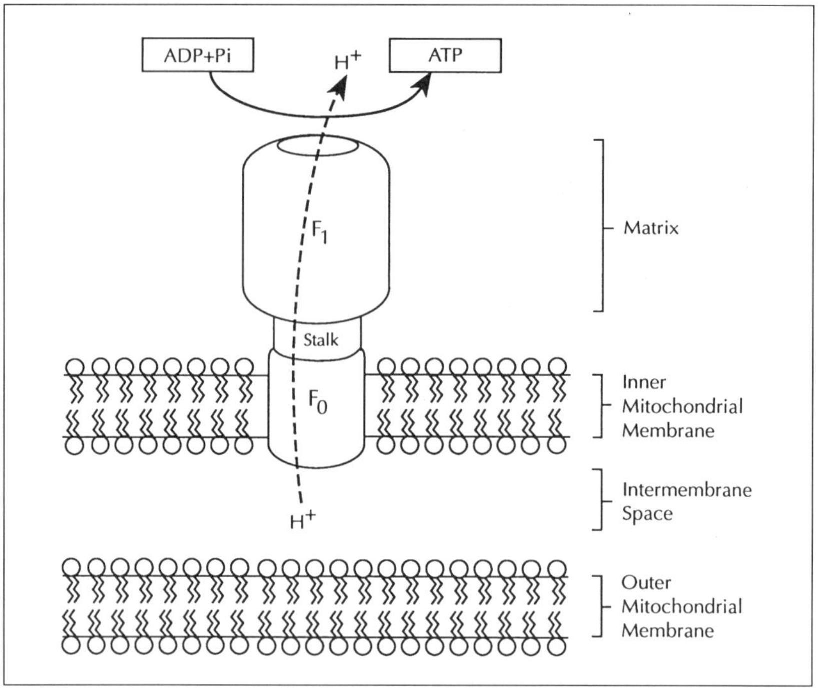

drial matrix, and as such these high-energy electron carriers are appropriately positioned and readily available to undergo oxidative phosphorylation. In contrast, the NADH molecules produced as a result of glycolysis are situated in the cytoplasm of the cell, and NADH is not capable of crossing the mitochondrial membrane. Therefore, a transport mechanism must be used.

Two transport mechanisms exist for NADH: the malate-aspartate shuttle and the glycerol phosphate shuttle. These shuttles transport the electrons from NADH, rather than transporting NADH itself, across the mitochondrial membrane [8]. The malate-aspartate shuttle, used by the liver and heart, transfers electrons from cytoplasmic NADH to mitochondrial NAD^+, generating NADH and thus conserving the P/O ratio. In contrast, the glycerol phosphate shuttle transfers electrons from cytoplasmic NADH to mitochondrial FAD, with the resulting generation of $FADH_2$. As shown earlier, $FADH_2$ possesses a P/O ratio of only 2. Therefore, two moles of ATP are generated per NADH molecule produced by glycolysis when the glycerol phosphate shuttle is used.

The electrons of NADH and $FADH_2$ enter the respiratory chain at different sites. The electrons of NADH enter the chain at NADH-ubiquinone (Q) reductase (complex I). Two electrons are transferred from NADH to the FMN prosthetic group of this enzyme complex, yielding the reduced form $FMNH_2$. Subsequently, $FMNH_2$ transfers the electrons to the iron-sulfur clusters (Fe-S) of the complex, reducing Fe^{+++} to Fe^{++}. Electrons from the Fe-S group are then transferred to ubiquinone (complex II), also known as coenzyme Q, yielding ubiquinol (QH_2). The NADH-Q reductase complex furthermore serves as one of three proton pumps in the electron chain, generating energy for the PMF.

The electrons of $FADH_2$ are not capable of entry at complex I. Rather, these electrons enter at succinate-Q reductase (complex II). The enzyme that catalyzes the reaction in the TCA cycle that generates the $FADH_2$ is actually part of the succinate-Q reductase complex of the respiratory chain. The electrons of $FADH_2$ are transferred to the Fe-S prosthetic group and then to coenzyme Q of complex II, forming QH_2. In contrast to NADH-Q reductase, succinate-Q reductase does not serve as a proton pump. Therefore, less energy is generated for the PMF with entry at complex II in comparison to entry at complex I. For this reason, less ATP is produced from the oxidation of $FADH_2$ compared with NADH.

The next step in the transfer of electrons in the respiratory chain is the cytochrome c reductase complex (complex III). A cytochrome is a hemeprotein capable of carrying electrons. The cytochrome c reductase complex transfers the electrons from QH_2 to the Fe-S group of the complex, reducing Fe^{+++} to Fe^{++}. Next, the electrons are transferred to cytochrome cl, and subsequently to cytochrome c. Cytochrome b of the enzyme complex also participates in the transfer of electrons. The cytochrome c reductase complex serves as the second of the three proton pumps in the respiratory chain.

Cytochrome c of complex III is a mobile electron carrier capable of shuttling electrons from cytochrome c reductase to cytochrome c oxidase (complex IV), the last complex of the electron transport chain. This complex is responsible for donating its electrons to O_2, the final electron acceptor in the respiratory chain. The electrons from cytochrome c are transferred to the heme a-copper (Cu) A prosthetic group of the complex. The heme a-CuA then transfers its electron to the heme a3-CuB complex, resulting in the reduction of Fe^{+++} and Cu^{++} to Fe^{++} and Cu^{+}, respectively. The Fe^{++} and Cu^{+} groups each donate an electron to O_2. Complete reduction of oxygen yields H_2O, with the utilization of $4H^{+}$ from the matrix, according to the reaction:

$$4e^{-} + O_2 + 4H^{+} \rightarrow 2H_2O$$

The cytochrome c oxidase complex serves as the third of the three complexes capable of pumping protons across the mitochondria membrane into the mitochondrial matrix, further generating the PMF necessary for the subsequent formation of ATP.

The mechanism by which electrons are transferred across the various complexes remains unclear. It is speculated, however, that the specific transfer is highly dependent on the number of peptide subunits of each complex, and most importantly, on the number and type of prosthetic groups present within each complex.

Oxidative Phosphorylation

As already stated, oxidative phosphorylation is dependent on the proton gradient generated across the inner mitochondrial membrane as a result of three enzyme complexes of the electron transport chain. The energy of this proton gradient (PMF) is used to produce ATP from ADP and Pi.

This mechanism was first proposed by Peter Mitchell in 1961 as the chemosmotic hypothesis. He postulated that electron transport along the respiratory chain results in free energy changes in the matrix and conformational changes in the membrane enzyme complexes that result in the pumping of protons out of the mitochondrial matrix into the intermembrane space. As a result, the inner aspect of the inner membrane becomes negative in relation to the outer aspect of the membrane, establishing an electrical gradient. Furthermore, the movement of protons across the membrane results in a pH gradient, wherein the matrix is alkaline relative to the intermembrane space. The gradient that is established is therefore both an electrical gradient and a chemical gradient. This PMF acts to drive protons back across the mitochondrial membrane through a special enzyme complex known as ATP synthase (complex V), located in the inner mitochondrial membrane. This movement of protons drives the synthesis of ATP from AMP and Pi within the enzyme complex.

The ATP synthase enzyme responsible for the generation of ATP projects from the inner mitochondrial membrane (see Figure 4-13). It is a tripartite complex consisting of: F_0, a hydrophobic segment that spans the inner mitochondrial membrane and functions as the proton channel of the complex; F_1, the head piece, which catalyzes the synthesis of ATP; and a stalk, which connects the F_0 and F_1 subunits and functions to regulate proton flow and ATP synthesis.

Studies have shown that the PMF itself does not generate the synthesis of ATP. Rather, the role of the PMF is to release the ATP already formed and bound to the ATP synthase enzyme complex. The release of ATP from the enzyme complex is dependent on the conformational form of ATP synthase, which in turn is dependent on the interactions between the three catalytic sites of F_1. These three catalytic sites all exist in different conformation forms at any one time and are directly regulated by the F_0 subunit according to the state of the mitochondrion.

There are five mitochondrial states. *State 1* is characterized by a slow respiratory rate limited by the availability of ADP. *State 2* represents starved mitochondria, with total consumption of substrates and hence a slow respiratory rate. *State 3* occurs when all substrates are abundant, thus displaying a rapid respiratory rate. The availability of ADP in this state stimulates electron transport by utilizing the PMF for ATP generation. *State 4* is best described as a state of respiratory control, because the mitochondria have abundant substrate, oxygen, and Pi, but low quantities of ADP, resulting in a slow rate of electron transport. In this state there is complete reduction of NADH, whereas flavoproteins (FAD) and cytochrome b and c will show only partial reduction. *State 5* is the result of anoxia, wherein all available oxygen has been consumed.

The ratio of state 3 oxygen uptake to state 4 oxygen uptake has been termed the *respiratory control index* and serves as a measure of the integrity of mitochondrial suspension in vitro. From this measurement it has been inferred that the availability of ADP is extremely important in regulating the rate of oxidative phosphorylation. Essentially, electrons do not flow through the electron-transport chain to O_2 unless ADP is available to generate ATP. Furthermore, electrons will not flow through the electron transport chain from fuel molecules unless the cell signals the need for ATP. In vivo, the mitochondria are usually found between states 3 and 4.

The ATP synthesized within the mitochondria is used primarily in the cytoplasm. However, ATP cannot freely traverse the mitochondrial membrane. Therefore, a specific transport protein located in the mitochondrial membrane is utilized, called the ATP-ADP translocase, which couples the entry of ADP to the exit of ATP. Transport is driven by the membrane potential generated by the electron transport chain. This ATP-ADP transport is very energetically expensive, consuming approximately one fourth of the energy yield of electron transport to regenerate the membrane potential that is used by this exchange process.

Overall, the thermodynamic efficiency of electron transport is approximately 40%. This is determined by calculating the free energy released by the oxidation of a particular substrate as determined by calorimetry and comparing it to the amount of free energy stored in the specific number of ATP molecules generated by its oxidation. For example, the complete oxidation of glucose yields 36 to 38 moles of ATP per molecule of glucose, depending on which shuttle is used to transfer the electrons from cytoplasmic NADH into the mitochondria. Given a $\Delta G^{\circ\prime}$ of -7.3 kcal/mol of ATP, the total free energy stored in 36 ATP is 263 kcal. $\Delta G^{\circ\prime}$ for the oxidation of glucose is -686 kcal. Therefore, the overall efficiency of ATP formation from the complete oxidation of glucose under standard conditions is 263/686 (38%). In comparison, under anaerobic conditions, only two moles of ATP are produced in anaerobic glycolysis. Tissues that derive their free energy under anaerobic conditions must metabolize glucose at a much greater rate compared with aerobic tissues to attempt to compensate for this small energy yield.

The energy yield derived from the oxidation of fatty acids under standard conditions approximates the efficiency of glycolysis, the TCA cycle, and oxidative phosphorylation.

Certainly, the specific energy production will depend on the number of carbon atoms present in the particular fatty acid, which in turn determines the number of β-oxidation passes required for complete oxidation. For example, the 16-carbon palmitoyl-CoA requires seven passes through β-oxidation. The net yield from the complete oxidation of palmitate is 129 ATP, which has a total free energy storage of -940 kcal. The $\Delta G^{\circ\prime}$ of the oxidation of palmitoyl-CoA is -2340 kcal. Hence, the efficiency of ATP formation from fatty acid oxidation under standard conditions is about 40%.

Energy Expenditure in Humans

Measurements of energy in human beings has been of interest to many physiologists and nutritionists. Such measurements have been performed since the turn of the century. Although energy expenditure can be evaluated accurately by *direct calorimetry,* measuring heat loss [37], the method of choice for acutely ill patients often connected to respirators, infusion pumps, and other devices, is indirect calorimetry, measuring heat production obtained from measurements of V_{O_2}, V_{CO_2}, and nitrogen excretion. These measurements allow the measurements of energy balance and composition of stored energy in both healthy and critically ill patients. Hence, energy balance in humans (and mammals) is equal to energy stored + energy expended = energy intake, or:

$$\text{Stored energy} = \text{Energy taken in} - \text{energy expenditure}$$

Indirect calorimetry is thus based on two principles: The first is the *law of conservation of energy,* and the second is that the *energy produced in the body by the oxidation of foodstuffs is equivalent to the energy produced by the combustion of these foodstuffs in the bomb calorimeter.* For fat and for carbohydrates, the end products in the bomb calorimeter and in the body are the same (H_2O and CO_2), producing respectively 9.5 kcal and 4.1 kcal (3.74 for glucose), whereas in the bomb calorimeter proteins are totally oxidized to CO_2, H_2O, SO_4, and nitrogen, with a production of about 5.7 kcal. From these measurements, stoichiometric equations can be derived for carbohydrates (ΔCH), proteins (ΔP), and fat (ΔF) using the well-established constants represented in Table 4-1 [38]:

Carbohydrate:

$$1\text{ g }\Delta CH + 0.829L\ O_2 \rightarrow 0.829L\ CO_2 + 0.67\text{ g }H_2O + 4.17\text{ kcal}$$

Protein:

$$1\text{ g }\Delta P + 0.966L\ O_2 \rightarrow 0.782L\ CO_2 + 0.41\text{ g }H_2O + 4.4\text{ kcal}$$

Fat:

$$1\text{ g }\Delta F + 2.019L\ O_2 \rightarrow 1.427L\ CO_2 + 1.07\text{ g }H_2O + 9.3\text{ kcal}$$

The three equations shown above represent fuel oxidation in the body, and the three nutrients are probably metabolized simultaneously in different proportions according to patient's condition and to many other factors, most of which are not well known.

The oxygen consumed in a certain period of time is the amount of oxygen that was used for the oxidation of given quantities of carbohydrate, protein, and fat, each of these nutrients using 0.829 L, 0.966 L, and 2.019 L of oxygen, respectively, per gram of metabolized substance. During the same period of time, carbon dioxide is produced in the amounts of 0.829 L, 0.782 L, and 1.427 L per gram of carbohydrate, protein, and fat, respectively. When the three nutrients are being metabolized, there is also a heat production of 4.1 kcal for each gram of carbohydrate, 4.1 kcal for each gram of protein, and 9.3 kcal for each gram of fat metabolized.

The above-mentioned facts can be expressed by the following equations, representing events happening in the same period of time, and can thus be considered as a system of three equations with 4 unknowns. For solving these equations for ΔCH, ΔP, ΔF, and EE (energy expenditure), the classical method is to derive the value of ΔP from the amount of urea excreted in the 24-hour urinary output. Because 30 grams of muscle is considered to contain 6.25 grams of proteins and because 1 gram of metabolized nitrogen (NM) is considered to have been produced by 6.25 grams of protein, the system of 3 equations with 4 unknowns becomes a system of 4 equations with 4 unknowns that can be solved:

$$V_{O_2}\ (L) = 0.829\ \Delta CH + 0.966\ \Delta P + 2.019\ \Delta F$$

$$V_{CO_2}\ (L) = 0.829\ \Delta CH + 0.782\ \Delta P + 1.427\ \Delta F$$

$$EE\ (kcal) = 4.17\ \Delta CH + 4.4\ \Delta P + 3\ \Delta F$$

$$\Delta P\ (g) = 6.25\ NM$$

Because the amount of metabolized proteins (ΔP) is already known from the measured urea or nitrogen in the urine, the resolution of this system of equations allows the calculation of EE, ΔCH, and ΔF as a function of V_{O_2}, V_{CO_2}, and NM as shown below:

$$EE\ (kcal) = 3.586\ V_{O_2} + 1.433\ V_{CO_2} - 1.180\ NM$$

$$\Delta CH\ (g) = 4.113\ V_{CO_2} - 2.907\ V_{O_2} - 2.544\ NM$$

$$\Delta F\ (g) = 1.689\ (V_{CO_2} - V_{O_2}) - 1.943\ NM$$

When ΔCH, ΔP, and ΔF are known, the water of oxidation (H_2OM) produced by the metabolism of ΔCH, ΔP, and ΔF can be calculated with the constants shown in Table 4-1:

$$H_2OM\ (g) = 0.67\ \Delta CH + 0.41\ \Delta P + 1.07\ \Delta F$$

By solving the equation, H_2OM can also be calculated as a function of V_{O_2}, V_{CO_2}, and NM:

$$H_2OM\ (g) = 0.949\ V_{CO_2} - 0.141\ V_{O_2} - 1.220\ NM$$

The indirect calorimetry method for monitoring metabolic data is based on the measurements of V_{O_2}, V_{CO_2}, and NM. Although V_{O_2} and V_{CO_2} could be measured by the Fick method, metabolic measurements are performed by totally noninvasive methods, consisting of volumes and concentration measurements of respiratory gases and by solving the following equations:

$$V_{O_2} = (V_I \times FiO_2) - (V_E \times FeO_2)$$

$$V_{CO_2} = (V_E \times FeCO_2) - (V_I \times Fi_{CO_2})$$

where V_I and V_E are the inspired and the expired respiratory volumes, respectively, over a determined period of time, and FiO_2 and FeO_2 are the inspired and expired concentrations of oxygen. It is important to note that $FiCO_2$ is usually neglected because it is close to zero. The NM can be derived from measurements of urea in the 24-hour urinary excretion as was explained previously. Finally, information that can also be recorded in metabolic monitoring includes the respiratory quotient (RQ) or the ratio between V_{CO_2} and V_{O_2}. Information can also be obtained as a function of the concentrations of O_2 in inspired and expired air (FiO_2 and FeO_2) and from the concentration of CO_2 in expired air ($FeCO_2$) [39]:

$$RQ = (V_{CO_2}/V_{O_2})$$

$$\text{or } RQ = [FeCO_2\ (1 - FiO_2)] \div [FiO_2(1 - FeCO_2) - FeO_2]$$

In critically ill patients, the measurement of V_{O_2} is not easy, particularly if the patient requires high concentrations of O_2 in inspired air [40]. The V_{CO_2} is easier to measure, but it is much more sensitive than is V_{O_2} to any modification in the patient's respiratory pattern. Energy expenditure can only be evaluated if the amount of CO_2 exhaled over a given period of time corresponds to the amount of CO_2 produced by the metabolism over the same period of time. These difficulties can be solved if the given period of time lasts 20 to 30 minutes. Because the techniques were developed for measuring "respiratory exchange" by Tissot in 1904 and by Douglas in 1911, several improvements have been performed in the measurements of V_{O_2} and V_{CO_2}, and about 10 different tools are today available on the market, with different problems and different levels of accuracy. Some of them are easy to calibrate and handle [41].

Although V_{O_2} and V_{CO_2} correspond directly to the O_2 consumed and to the CO_2 produced by the oxidation of nutrients during the measurement, the nitrogen measured in the urine does not correspond to the protein breakdown during the same period of time. There are indeed great variations of hourly urea excretions in a single day, and therefore the determination of protein breakdown from nitrogen excretion has to be performed over a 24-hour period.

It has to be emphasized that for EE, measurement of the factor NM may be neglected if we look at the following equation:

$$EE\ (\text{kcal}) = 3.586\ V_{O_2} = 1.443\ V_{CO_2} - 1.180\ NM$$

Assuming a V_{O_2} of 0.250 L/min, a V_{CO_2} of 0.225 L/min, and a NM of 0.01 g/min, which are in normal range for these values, this would give us an EE of 1775.52 kcal/day. A 10% error in V_{O_2} would cause a 7% error in EE, a 10% error in V_{CO_2} would cause an error of 3% in EE, and a 100% error in NM would only be responsible for a 1% error in EE. For acutely ill patients in a hypercatabolic state with large and variable protein breakdown, EE can be calculated from V_{O_2} and V_{CO_2} only, with a maximum error of no more than 2%, in using the following equation [42]:

$$EE\ (\text{kcal/d}) = 3.586\ V_{O_2}\ (\text{L/d}) + 1.443\ V_{CO_2}\ (\text{L/d}) - 2.15$$

Although it is obvious that EE can be accurately measured without measuring nitrogen excretion, this information is most important for evaluating the magnitude of protein breakdown and for estimating nitrogen daily requirements.

Energy Expenditure Estimation From Standard Formulas

In trying to adapt nutritional supply to needs, most dieticians and nutritionists will estimate EE from standard formulas like those of Harris and Benedict, which are derived from sex, weight (W), height (H), and age (A) as follows:

$$\text{Men: } EE = 66.4730 + 13.7513\ W + 5.0033\ H + 6.7750\ A$$

$$\text{Women: } EE = 655.0955 + 9.5634\ W + 1.8496\ H + 4.6756\ A$$

The values for EE obtained by these formulas are considered to be the basal metabolic rate or the basal energy expenditure for normal individuals and were established from measurements performed in 1919 on 136 normal men, 103 normal women, and 94 infants. The values obtained with this method for normal individuals are accurate within approximately 10% when compared to measured values. When corrected for the degree of stress or for the type of disease, the estimated EE is not adapted at all for critically ill patients and even less for patients with multiple organ failure, because they may easily present a variability of their EE of 50% or more from one patient to the other or in the same patient from one day to another. On the other hand, estimated values will not vary from one day to another: in applying Harris and Benedict formulas, the only factor that may change is weight. Because in multiple organ failure weight is influenced by several factors such as water and natrium balance, inducing overhydration or underhydration will artificially change body weight, and it will usually change much less than does eventually the EE. A better estimation could be obtained taking into account lean body mass, but this is not common practice for clinical purposes. Estimated EE, even corrected according to patient condition, can by no means be considered as a way of monitoring metabolic response in critically ill patients, neither for evaluating the degree of hypermetabolism nor for nutritional purposes.

Nutritional problems arise in critically ill patients when they are unable to be adequately nourished orally. The major problems in determining the optimal amounts of essential nutrient administration concern the macronutrients, carbohydrates, fat, and protein. It is important to emphasize that maintenance and regulation of body cell mass (BCM) requires adequate intake of all other essential nutrients provided for the most part on a daily basis. For instance, omission from an otherwise adequate diet of either potassium, phosphate, or nitrogen will convert markedly positive nitrogen and potassium balances to negative balances within one day. Little is known about whether stress or malnutrition changes requirements of vitamins or trace elements, although problems of malabsorption or increased intestinal losses may require increased intravenous intake. Fat requirements are limited to the dietary essential fatty acid, linoleic acid, and these are estimated to be about 10 g/d. This is usually met by administration of 200 ml of a 10% fat emulsion, which is approximately equal to 10% of total energy requirements. As for the other essential fatty acid, linolenic acid, the daily requirements are not presently known. It is noteworthy to emphasize the fact that normal adults have reserves equivalent to about a one-year supply of these two fatty acids, which in normal postabsorptive periods are released daily. There is no absolute requirement for carbohydrate in the diet, because it can be synthesized from protein or to a limited extent from fat. However, there is a requirement for glucose by the brain and nervous tissues, which comprise 20% of the resting energy expenditure (REE). In the absence of carbohydrate, this need for glucose can be met by providing 200 g of protein/d, roughly 450 mg of nitrogen per kilogram per day, which is not easily administered and is much better met by providing 100 to 150 g of carbohydrate. Injured or septic patients are glucose- and insulin-resistant and may require lesser amounts of carbohydrates, or alternatively higher amounts of insulin, administered with the carbohydrate load, to be able to utilize these substrates quite effectively. Therefore, at least 25% of the REE should be provided as carbohydrate. However, both carbohydrates and proteins have marked effects on respiration. Administration of hypercaloric glucose-based TPN can cause doubling of CO_2 production and a corresponding increase in minute ventilation (VE). Protein or amino acid infusion causes an increase in respiratory response or sensitivity to CO_2, so that administration of too much protein adds to the respiratory effects of carbohydrate. For patients with inadequate pulmonary reserve, this may induce respiratory distress and prevent weaning from ventilators [43,44]. [*Editor's Note:* These studies were carried out in very depleted septic patients who were suddenly given relatively large amounts of glucose, a setting which is not often duplicated. The problem posed probably occurs far less than it is mentioned. Nonetheless, although I personally do not limit carbohydrate to 25% to 50% of calories, in patients with marginal pulmonary function, excessive carbohydrate may make weaning more difficult by increasing CO_2 production.] In patients with respiratory problems and mainly in patients with chronic obstructive pulmonary disease, carbohydrate intake should be kept between 25% and 50% of caloric supply. When nitrogen is administered, the increased sensitivity to CO_2 it causes should be taken into account.

Recommendations for the Septic or Injured Patient

1. If EE is measured, provide energy (carbohydrate, fat, and proteins) at 1.33 times REE, with the nonprotein calories given as 50% carbohydrates and 50% as fat. The calorie-to-nitrogen ratio should be 150 kcal per gram of nitrogen. This ratio, however, can be lower (75 kcal per gram of nitrogen) if insulin is infused with the TPN solution.
2. If EE is not measured, provide 2800 kcal/d or 40 $kcal/kg \cdot d^{-1}$ with a calorie-to-nitrogen ratio of 150 kcal per gram of nitrogen.

Recommendations for Malnourished Patients

1. If EE is measured, provide energy at 1.25 times REE for bedridden patients and at 1.5 times REE for ambulatory patients. The calorie-to-nitrogen ratio should be 100 kcal per gram nitrogen.
2. If energy expenditure is not measured, provide 2000 kcal/d or 32 $kcal/kg \cdot d^{-1}$ to bedridden patients and 2400 kcal/d or 39 $kcal/kg/d^{-1}$ to ambulatory patients. The calorie-to-nitrogen ratio should also be 100 kcal per gram of nitrogen given.

Patients who are septic or injured and malnourished have a better response to nutrients than have the patients who are septic or injured who are well nourished. Those malnourished and at the same time stressed patients are usually hypercatabolic and should be given energy at the same rates as those recommended for the injured and septic patients, but with a calorie-to-nitrogen ratio of 100 as used with the malnourished patients. (*Editor's Note:* Authorities will differ slightly in situations in which patients undergo severe stress or sepsis, and this should not be surprising. My view differs somewhat. I believe that 20% or 30% of lipid is optimal for hepatic protein synthesis, which is most important. Calories should be maintained at 32 to 35 kcal/kg/d. In severe sepsis, caloric requirements are apt to be shifted by what the patient can tolerate. I agree that in sepsis, a ratio of 100:1 is probably more appropriate. One will find, however, that for the most part it really is very heavily dependent on what the patient can tolerate.)

These recommendations should be used only as guidelines. Indeed, with contraindications such as renal failure or respiratory failure, the amounts of calories or nitrogen, or both, should be reduced. In patients with respiratory failure the proportion of carbohydrate should be reduced, and during the weaning procedure nutrition should be maintained at a minimum level. Although these recommendations seem reasonable to us, they are arbitrary, and other recommendations may seem equally reasonable to others. Much larger amounts of nutrients have been given many years ago, with great success and without major complications. [*Editor's Note:* Looking back on the late 1960s and early 1970s, I'm not certain we didn't have major complications, or perhaps we didn't recognize them.]

Summary

Until we have serious clinical studies of the effects of various amounts of nutrients on morbidity and mortality, uncertainty about the optimal amounts of nutrients to be administered will persist. However, what seems to be evident is that adequate nutrition should always be prescribed on a daily basis except when resumption to oral feeding is expected within 2 to 4 days. Both enteral and parenteral feeding techniques have risks that can be minimized if administered by specialized teams that are well experienced with all modes of nutritional support.

References

1. Cahill G Jr. Starvation in man. *N Engl J Med* 282:669, 1970.
2. Cahill GF Jr, et al. Hormone-fuel interrelationships during fasting. *J Clin Invest* 45:1751, 1966.
3. Owen OE, et al. Liver and kidney metabolism during prolonged starvation. *J Clin Invest* 48:574, 1969.
4. Owen OE, et al. Brain metabolism during fasting. *J Clin Invest* 46:1589, 1967.
5. Felig P, et al. Amino acid metabolism in prolonged starvation. *J Clin Invest* 48:584, 1969.
6. Elwyn DH, et al. Influence of increasing carbohydrate intake on glucose kinetics in injured patients. *Ann Surg* 190:117, 1979.
7. Kinney JM, Elwyn DH. Protein metabolism and injury. *Annu Rev Nutr* 3:433, 1983.
8. Stryer L. Generation and Storage of Metabolic Energy. In *Biochemistry* (3rd ed). New York: Freeman, 1988. P 313.
9. Wilmore DW, Aulick LH. Metabolic changes in burned patients. *Surg Clin North Am* 58:1173, 1976.
10. Jobsis FF. Basic Processes in Cellular Respiration. In WO Fenn, H Rahn (eds), *Handbook of Physiology, Vol 1: Respiration.* Baltimore: Waverly, 1964 P 63.
11. Friedman PJ. *Biochemistry: A Review With Questions and Explanations* (4th ed). Boston: Little, Brown, 1992. P 45.
12. Sherratt HSA. Mitochondria: Structure and function. *Rev Neurol* 147:417, 1991.
13. Sherratt HSA, et al. Methods used for the study of normal and abnormal skeletal muscle mitochondria. *Methods Biochem Anal* 33:243, 1988.
14. Sherrat HSA, Turnbull DM. Mitochondrial Oxidation and ATP Synthesis in Muscle. In JB Harris, DM Turnbull (eds), *Muscle Metabolism.* London: Balliere Tindall, 1993.
15. Harold FM. *The Vital Force: A Study of Bioenergetics.* New York: Freeman, 1986.
16. Nicholls DG. *Bioenergetics: An Introduction to the Chemiosmotic Theory.* New York: Academic, 1982.
17. Beasley EM, Clemens W, Schatz G. Putting energy into mitochondrial protein import. *Curr Opin Cell Biol* 4:646, 1992.
18. Zevianni M, et al. Mitochondrial diseases. *Neurol Clin* 7:123, 1989.
19. Breningstall GN. Approach to diagnosis of oxidative metabolism disorders. *Pediatr Neurol* 9:81, 1992.
20. Shoffner JM, Wallace DC. Oxidative Phosphorylation. In H Harris et al (eds), *Advances in Human Genetics.* New York: Plenum, 1990.
21. Chance B, William GR. Respiration enzymes in oxidative phosphorylation. *J Biol Chem* 217:383, 1955.
22. Lardy HA, Ferguson SM. Oxidative phosphorylation in mitochondria. *Annu Rev Biochem* 38:991, 1969.
23. Linder MC. Nutrition and Metabolism of Carbohydrates, Fat and Proteins. In *Nutritional Biochemistry and Metabolism With Clinical Applications.* New York: Elsevier, 1985. P 15.
24. Amaral JF, Caldwell MD. Metabolic Response to Starvation, Stress and Sepsis. In TA Miller (ed), *Physiologic Basis of Modern Surgical Care.* St Louis: Mosby, 1988. P 1.
25. Zeviani M, et al. Mitochondrial Diseases. In WG Johnson (ed), *Neurologic Clinics: Neurogenic Diseases.* Philadelphia: Saunders, 1989.
26. Wallace DC. Mitochondrial genes and diseases. *Hosp Pract* 21:77, 1986.
27. Williams PE, et al. Surgical Models to Measure Organ Amino Acid Metabolism. In S Nissen (ed), *Modern Methods in Protein Nutrition and Metabolism.* San Diego: Academic, 1992. P 167.
28. Abumrad NN, et al. Role of insulin in the regulation of leucine kinetics in the conscious dog. *J Clin Invest* 70:1031, 1982.
29. Stevenson RW, et al. Insulin Action in Vivo. In KGMM Alberti, LP Krall (eds), *Annual Review of Diabetes.* Amsterdam: Elsevier, 1985. P 418.
30. Nilsson L, Hultman E. Liver glycogen in man: The effect of total starvation or a carbohydrate-poor diet followed by carbohydrate refeeding. *Scand J Clin Lab Invest* 32:325, 1973.
31. Krebs H, et al. The fate of isotopic carbon in kidney cortex synthesizing glucose from lactate. *Biochem J* 101:242, 1966.
32. Strisower E, Kohler G, Chaikoff I. Incorporation of acetate carbons into glucose by liver slices of normal and alloxan diabetic rats. *J Biol Chem* 198:115, 1952.
33. Pilkis SJ, Granner DK. Molecular physiology of the regulation of hepatic gluconeogenesis and glycolysis. *Annu Rev Physiol* 54:885, 1992.
34. Pilkis SJ, Claus TH. Hepatic gluconeogenesis/glycolysis: Regulation and structure/function relationships of substrate cycle enzymes. *Annu Rev Nutr* 11:465, 1991.
35. Mitchell P. Coupling of phosphorylation to electron and hydrogen transfer by a chemiosmotic type of mechanism. *Nature* 191:144, 1961.
36. Mitchell P, Moyle J. Respiratory-driven proton translocation in rat liver mitochondria. *Biochem J* 105:1147, 1967.
37. Acheson KJ, et al. Nutritional influences on lipogenesis and thermogenesis after a carbohydrate meal. *Am J Physiol* 246:E62, 1984.
38. Livesey G, Elia M. Food energy value of artificial feeds for man. *Clin Nutr* 4:99, 1985.
39. Bursztein S, et al. The Theoretical Framework of Indirect Calorimetry and Energy Balance. In *Energy Metabolism: Indirect Calorimetry and Nutrition.* Baltimore: Williams & Wilkins, 1989. P 47.
40. Ultman JS, Bursztein S. Analysis of error in the determination of respiratory gas exchange at varying FIO_2. *J Appl Physiol* 50:210, 1981.
41. Bursztein S, et al. Evaluation of Metabolic Measurement Equipment. In TH Grayson, C Eckhart (eds), *Energy Metabolism: Indirect Calorimetry and Nutrition.* Baltimore: Williams & Wilkins, 1989. P 211.
42. Bursztein S, et al. Determination of energy metabolism from respiratory function alone. *J Appl Physiol* 42:117, 1977.
43. Askanazi J, et al. Nutrition for the patients with respiratory failure, glucose versus fat. *Anesthesiology* 54:373, 1980.
44. Askanazi J, et al. Effects of increasing protein intake on ventilatory drive. *Anesthesiology* 60:106, 1984.

Selected Readings

Cahill G Jr. Starvation in man. *N Engl J Med* 282:669, 1970.

This classic article reviews the changes in interorgan fluxes of various substrates and the dependence of organs on specific substrates during the progression of humans into starvation.

Felig P, et al. Amino acid metabolism in prolonged starvation. *J Clin Invest* 48:584, 1969.

This is a continuation of the work that was already in progress in the laboratory of Dr. George Cahill that examined the substrate metabolism and utilization by various organs during prolonged starvation. This article addresses the interorgan relationships during starvation.

Kinney JM, Elwyn DH. Protein metabolism and injury. *Annu Rev Nutr* 3:433, 1983.

This article is a review of the changes that occur in protein and amino acid metabolism by various organs during periods of injury. The review examines in more detail the extensive work done by the principal investigator, Dr. John Kinney, in the metabolic unit at Columbia University Medical Center.

Mitchell P. Coupling of phosphorylation to electron and hydrogen transfer by a chemiosmotic type of mechanism. *Nature* 191:144, 1961.

This classic study examined the mechanism by which coupling of electron and hydrogen transfer occur across the mitochondrial membranes that enable the body to couple the various metabolic aspects of oxidative phosphorylation.

Owen OE, et al. Liver and kidney metabolism during prolonged starvation. *J Clin Invest* 48:574, 1969.

This article examines the switch in the metabolism of the liver and kidneys during fasting in humans.

Owen OE, et al. Brain metabolism during fasting. *J Clin Invest* 46:1589, 1967.

This article is unique and examines the switch of the brain from a predominantly glucose-based substrate during feeding and early fasting to a primary dependence on ketone bodies during periods of prolonged starvation.

Sherratt HSA. Mitochondria: Structure and function. *Rev Neurol* 147:417, 1991.

This review article examines the up-to-date information regarding the structure-function interrelationships of the role of mitochondria in the handling of various aspects of substrate and energy metabolism. This review is all-encompassing of the recent developments in this field. In particular, it sets the stage for the understanding of the electron motive force (EMF) concept of coupling of energy and electron transfer as previously proposed by Mitchell.

5

Growth Factors

R. Daniel Beauchamp
E. Aubrey Thompson

History and General Concepts

The Beginning

The systematic study of peptide growth factors began in the 1950s with the work of Levi-Montalcini, Hamburger, and Cohen on what became known as nerve growth factor (NGF). The subsequent discovery of epidermal growth factor (EGF) by Cohen followed shortly thereafter. These investigators were awarded the Nobel Prize for their pioneering work that opened the door to the discovery of many more peptide growth factors. In the 1960s, shortly after the seminal discoveries of EGF and NGF, Judah Folkman postulated the existence of an angiogenic growth factor that was produced by tumors. This eventually led to the discovery of the fibroblast growth factor (FGF) family of peptides. Transforming growth factors (TGFs) were reported in 1978 by DeLarco and Todaro [1]. These are but a few of the many peptide growth factors that have been characterized during the nearly 40 years since the initial discovery of NGF.

This field has stimulated great interest because of the multiple clinically relevant problems that potentially involve peptide growth factors. Peptide growth factors have central roles in such seemingly diverse areas as embryologic and postnatal development, commitment to differentiation, normal epithelial cell turnover, chemotaxis, hematopoiesis, wound healing, inflammatory responses, and cancer. Much has been learned of the mechanisms by which these factors elicit their

Supported by grants from the National Institutes of Health (R01 CA64750, R37 CA24347, P01 AG10514).

actions on a variety of cells, but there remain vast gaps in our understanding.

Limited Nomenclature and Diverse Actions

Growth factors include a group of peptide hormones that regulate cell proliferation. Many, probably all, of these principles also regulate cellular metabolic activity. Consequently, any distinction between growth factors and other types of hormones is purely operational, and any attempt to systematically define growth factors, as a separate class of hormones, is likely to be more confusing than helpful. Insulin, for example, is a potent regulator of cell proliferation, yet insulin is seldom discussed within the context of growth factors. Many lymphokines have both metabolic and mitotic regulatory properties, yet these are not called growth factors. Steroid hormones regulate proliferation but are never classified as growth factors. In this review, we will focus upon the properties of a subset of the growth factors, including EGF/TGF-α, TGF-β, and the FGF family.

Historically, growth factors have been named on the basis of the biologic activity that resulted in their discovery. Consequently, the name of the factor does not reflect the variety of potential roles and often does not reflect the most important role that the molecule may have in vivo. For example, EGF was discovered and named because it stimulated epithelial cell growth in the newborn mouse eyelid. Further investigation revealed that EGF is also a potent mitogen for fibroblast cells. Transforming growth factor-β (TGF-β) was so named for the ability to cause cultured fibroblasts to grow in soft agar and acquire monolayer morphology that was suggestive of transformation. The effects of TGF-β on fibroblasts are completely reversible and do not reflect true transformation. The name *transforming growth factor* also does not reflect that the predominant biologic effect of TGF-β on most cell types in culture is growth inhibition.

Growth factors often have multiple biologic actions that are seemingly independent of growth. For example, EGF and the related TGF-α are potent inhibitors of gastric acid secretion. Transforming growth factor-β has multiple effects on cells that are not directly related to growth: regulation of extracellular matrix, modulation of the acute-phase response, and modulation of macrophage and lymphocyte activity. The predominant action of a growth factor may be growth stimulation in a particular cell type and a completely different action in other cell types or in the same cell type under different circumstances. Tumor necrosis factor (TNF) is a potent inducer of apoptosis in some cell types, can act as growth factors on specific cell types, and has potent and clinically important biologic effects on other cell types during the systemic inflammatory response. Similar functional diversity can be ascribed to the interleukins and other cytokines, monokines, lymphokines, and colony-stimulating factors. The properties of these important growth-regulatory peptides are considered in chapters 3 and 21 and will not be discussed in depth in this chapter. For further information regarding many of the cytokine peptides, the reader is referred to an excellent recent review by Fong and Lowry [2].

Improved understanding of the mechanisms that underlie the actions of these growth factors is vital to fully exploit their potential in clinical practice. Some of these growth factors are already being used in clinical practice, and many others are under development. For example, erythropoietin is an endocrine growth factor produced in the kidney that stimulates bone marrow production of erythrocytes. Recombinant human erythropoietin is now used to stimulate erythrocyte production in patients (e.g., renal failure patients) in which the endogenous erythropoietin is deficient. Numerous growth factors (e.g., PDGF, bFGF, TGF-β) are under investigation, and several show promise as agents to promote the healing of wounds in compromised patients. Many other potential clinical applications for growth factors will be forthcoming as scientific investigation reveals regulatory pathways that can be subjected to pharmacologic regulation and as specific receptor binding agonists and antagonists are developed from the knowledge gained about ligand and receptor structure and biochemistry.

In this chapter, several of the major classes of peptide growth factors will be briefly described, and their potential biologic roles will be discussed (Table 5-1). Common properties and mechanisms of action for the group of growth factors that primarily stimulate mitogenesis through activation of the tyrosine kinase receptors will be described. In addition to these primarily growth-stimulatory growth factors, the TGF-β family of peptides, which act through serine–threonine kinase receptors and have widely divergent actions, will be presented in considerably more detail to illustrate major concepts and complexity of molecular regulation of cell functions by the peptide growth factors.

Cell Cycle Regulation: The Key to Growth Responses

Their very names indicate that the peptide growth factors act on cells to stimulate a proliferative response. Implied in growth factor actions is that

Table 5-1. In Vivo Effects of Growth Factors

Epidermal growth factor
- Eyelid opening
- Incisor eruption
- Mandibular development
- Lung maturation
- Skin development
- Cutaneous wound healing
- Inhibition of gastric acid secretion
- Healing of gastric mucosal injury
- Tumor promoter

Transforming growth factor-α
- Same as epidermal growth factor, and autocrine stimulation of some cancers
- Induction of breast cancer and hepatomas in transgenic mice

Amphiregulin, *cripto,* poxvirus growth factors
- Unknown

Insulin-like growth factor-1
- Reversal of growth hormone deficient state
- Decreases catabolic effects of trauma and sepsis
- Prevents gut atrophy and bacterial translocation

Platelet-derived growth factor
- Blood vessel growth and repair
- Vasoconstriction
- Trophic for brain tissue
- Tumor initiation and promotion

Fibroblast growth factors
- Capillary growth (angiogenesis)
- Wound healing (skin, gut, bone)
- Mesodermal induction during embryogenesis
- Tumor initiation and promotion

Transforming growth factor-β
- Promotion of wound healing
- Induction of granulation tissue
- Pathologic fibrosis (pulmonary fibrosis, hepatic cirrhosis, tumor-associated fibrosis, etc.)
- Renal glomerulosclerosis
- Leukocyte and fibroblast chemoattractant
- Modulates (primarily down-regulation) the systemic inflammation response
- Immunosuppression
- Enhancement of tumor invasiveness and metastasis

they are capable of regulating machinery in the cell that controls DNA synthesis and subsequent mitosis (or meiosis). An understanding of the actions of growth factors requires some background information about what is known of the cell cycle (Figure 5-1). Cell replication is a highly regulated process, otherwise cell renewal could not occur when needed (e.g., wound healing, gut and skin epithelial turnover, hematopoiesis). Conversely, unrestricted cell proliferation would lead to chaotic disruption of normal function (e.g., hyperplasia, cancer).

Our current understanding of the cell cycle suggests that regulation of cell proliferation consists in three more or less separate events, all of which appear to be initiated and maintained by growth factors. The first of these, in a kinetic sense, is the acquisition of proliferative capacity. Cell proliferation is also regulated at the level of the commitment to DNA synthesis, and the mech-

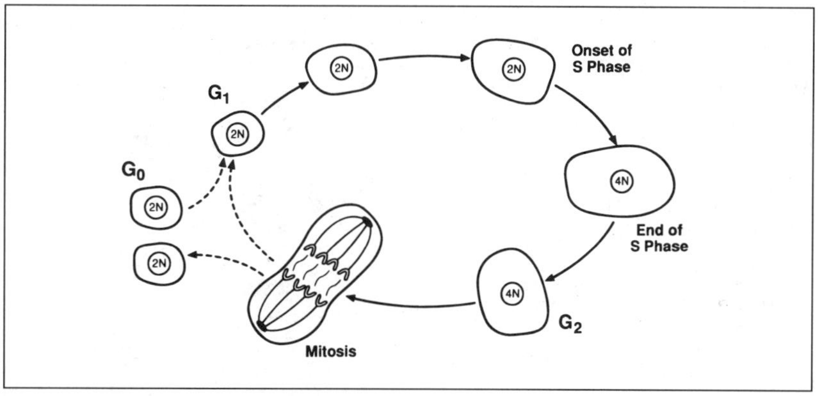

Figure 5-1. Traverse through the cell cycle. G_0 is a nonproliferating state. In G_1 the cell is preparing to undergo DNA synthesis (S phase). During G_0 and G_1 the cell nucleus contains the normal diploid (2N) content of chromosomal DNA. G_2 is a usually brief interval after the S phase, in which the cell has two copies (4N) of each of its DNA molecules. Actual nuclear and cell division occur during the mitosis (M) period. The S, G_2 and M periods are fairly constant in length: about 7 hours, 3 hours, and 1 hour, respectively. G_1 is variable and can last from a few hours to several days. Some cells can be recruited into G_1 from the G_0 stage, while others may be constantly dividing. (From RD Beauchamp, HL Moses. *Regul Pept Lett* 2:1, 1990. Reproduced with permission from M.E.D. Communications, Woodbridge, NJ.)

anism(s) that govern this aspect of cell proliferation appear to be distinct from those that prepare the cell for proliferation. Finally, there appears to be a set of distinct regulatory mechanisms that facilitate withdrawal from the cell cycle. All three of these processes are almost certainly regulated by growth factors.

Growth factors clearly convey the ability to proliferate, and the most obvious manifestation of this is the rapid induction of a subset of genes upon addition of growth factors to cells that have withdrawn from the cell cycle. By analogy with viral gene expression programs, these rapidly induced genes are called *immediate early* genes. Activation of these does not require protein synthesis, and the mechanistic implications of this observation will be discussed below. Most of these immediate early genes are proto-oncogenes (e.g., c-*fos*, c-*jun*, c-*myc*).

The products of the immediate early genes convey proliferative capacity, but the commitment to DNA synthesis and to cell division involves a different set of regulatory principles whose original function in lower eukaryotes may have been to ensure orderly progression through the cell cycle. Maintenance of ploidy demands that the cell cycle proceed strictly in order. A cell must not divide until it has replicated its DNA and completed the S phase, lest the genomic complement be reduced. Likewise, a cell must not replicate its genome until it has completed cell division during the M phase, lest the genomic complement be increased. This orderly progression from G1 to S to G2 to M in proliferating cells is governed by programmed expression of a family of serine/threonine protein kinases that consist of a catalytic subunit (the cyclin-dependent kinases [CDKs]) and a regulatory subunit (the cyclins) [3]. Cyclins and CDKs also appear to regulate whether a cell that is quiescent (in G0) will enter the G1 phase of the cell cycle so that replication may occur.

There are at least 20 CDKs, of which the products of the *cdc2* (also known as *cdk1*), *cdk2*, and *cdk4* genes are the best characterized and will be discussed in more detail here [3–6]. The *cdc2* kinase (also designated as $p34^{cdc2}$) is critical for M-phase progression, whereas the products of the *cdk2* and *cdk4* loci ($p33^{cdk2}$ and $p34^{cdk4}$, respectively) appear to govern entry into the S phase. The substrates of these kinases are largely unknown, although there is evidence that both $p33^{cdk2}$ and $p34^{cdk4}$ can phosphorylate $p105^{Rb}$, the product of the retinoblastoma susceptibility gene *Rb-1* [7]. Hyperphosphorylation of $p105^{Rb}$ occurs during late G1 and appears to be required for entry into the S phase, whereas accumulation of underphosphorylated $p105^{Rb}$ prevents DNA synthesis [8,9]. It has been proposed that phosphorylation of $p105^{Rb}$ causes dissociation of complexes containing essential transcription factors such as E2F [10]. The transcription factor E2F has been shown to stimulate expression of several proliferation-associated genes (Figure 5-2) [11], whereas the E2F-$p105^{Rb}$ complex appears to inhibit transcription [12,13]. These observations indicate that regulation of CDK activity and substrate specificity are central to cell-cycle progression. The activity and perhaps the specificity of CDKs are controlled by

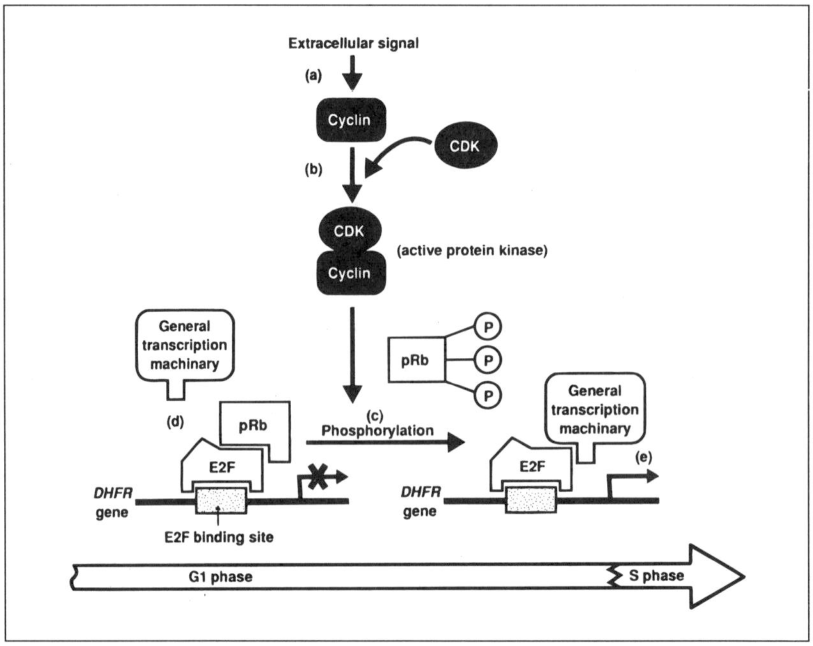

Figure 5-2. Model for the regulation of gene expression by the cyclin-CDKs through Rb. Rb regulates the activity of several transcription factors. **(a)** In response to environmental stimuli, G1 cyclins are synthesized or activated, and **(b)** combine with CDKs to yield active protein kinases. **(c)** Phosphorylation of Rb by these kinases renders it unable to regulate the transcription factors. **(d)** Factors that had been repressed by Rb, such as E2F, **(e)** can then promote transcription of cell division stimulators; factors that had been activated by Rb, such as ATF-2, are then incapable of promoting transcription of cell division inhibitors (not shown). Rb functions other than those involved in the regulation of transcription factors may also be controlled by cyclin-CDK catalyzed phosphorylation. (Note that although this figure indicates that the Rb-E2F complex still binds DNA, this point is not yet clear.) (From RE Hollingsworth et al. *Curr Opin Cell Biol* 5:194, 1993. Reproduced with permission from Current Science, London.)

Table 5-2. ***cdc2*****-Related cDNAs and Associated Cyclins**

Name	Identity to *cdc2* Kinase Domain (%)	Cyclin Bound
cdc1 (CDK1)	100	B-types
CDK2	65	A-,D-, and E-types
CDK3	66	Unknown
CDK5 (PSSALRE)	57	D-types
PICTAIRE (1–3)	51–55	Unknown
CDK4 (PSKJ3)	44	D-types
PLSTIRE (CDK6)	47	D-types
PITAIRE	42	Unknown
$p58^{GTA}$	42	Unknown
$p40^{Mo15}$	40	Unknown

Source: From J Pines. Cyclins and cyclin-dependent kinases: Take your partners. *Trends Biochem Sci* 18:195, 1993. With permission from Elsevier Trends Journals, Cambridge, UK.

a family of regulatory subunits: the cyclins (Table 5-2).

Cyclins were first identified in marine invertebrate embryos as labile proteins that are synthesized in each cell cycle and destroyed at mitosis [8,9]. This cyclic pattern of synthesis and degradation accounts for the name given these regulatory subunits. At least 12 mammalian cyclins have been identified [6,14]. These cyclins are classified according to their presumed function at specific points in the cell cycle. The G1 cyclins (cyclins C, D, and E) are believed to control initiation of the S phase, and the M phase cyclins (cyclins A and B) control mitosis (Figure 5-3).

The best-characterized cyclin is cyclin B, a 48-kDa protein encoded by the *CcnB* gene. Cyclin B is synthesized late in the S phase or early in the M phase and associates with its catalytic subunit, $p34^{cdc2}$ [3,4,14,15]. Association between cyclin B and $p34^{cdc2}$ triggers a series of phosphorylation–dephosphorylation reactions that result in activation of the cyclin B/$p34^{cdc2}$ kinase during the M phase. Although the physiologically relevant substrates of the cyclin B/$p34^{cdc2}$ complex are unknown, it is clear that this entity is the principal promoter of M-phase progression. Cyclin B is degraded late in the M phase, and $p34^{cdc2}$ is inactivated as a result. Degradation of the M cyclins at the end of the M phase prevents the cell from dividing again in the absence of DNA replication. Similar mechanisms probably exist for G1 cyclins, some of which regulate S-phase progression.

Two types of G1 cyclins, cyclin C and cyclin E, exhibit classic cyclic patterns of synthesis and degradation, as observed with cyclins A and B [5,6]. Both cyclins C and E are synthesized in G1 and degraded in S. The catalytic partner of cyclin C is unknown. Cyclin E binds $p33^{cdk2}$ during late G1, activating the kinase. Activation of $p33^{cdk2}$ precedes phosphorylation of $p105^{Rb}$ and entry into the S phase. Overexpression of cyclin E shortens the G1 interval [16]. It is not known whether expression of cyclin C or E is essential for entry into the S phase, but one may infer that G1 cyclins, such as cyclins C and E, contribute to the formation of an "S-phase progression factor," which is analogous to the classic M-phase progression factor (MPF) formed by association of cyclin B and $p34^{cdc2}$. Although much remains to be learned about cell-cycle progression factors, it is clear that in a general sense the programmed synthesis and degradation of cyclins accounts for ordered progression through the cell cycle.

The D-type cyclins are central to the ability of cells to respond to a wide variety of growth factors. The prototype for cyclins of this class is

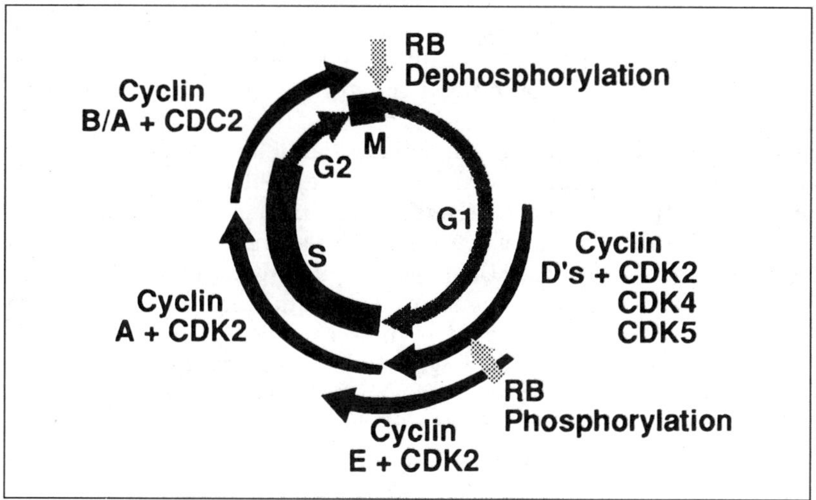

Figure 5-3. Combinatorial interactions of cyclins and CDKs during the cell cycle [CJ Sherr. Mammalian G_1 cyclins. *Cell* 73: 1059, 1993. Reproduced with permission from *Cell,* Cambridge, MA]. The G1 cyclins (D cyclins and cyclin E) and their cognate CDKs are induced and/or activated during G1. This leads to phosphorylation of RB and RB-related proteins, a necessary step for progression to the S phase. Interactions of cyclin A and CDK2 are necessary for DNA synthesis, and their levels and activities are increased, beginning near the G1/S transition through the S phase. The G2/M cyclins are increased during late S phase and through their interactions with CDC2 regulate M-phase progression. RB dephosphorylation occurs near the end of the M phase.

cyclin D1, a 35-kDa protein encoded by the *CcnD1* locus [6]. Sherr and co-workers cloned this gene from colony-stimulating factor-1 (CSF-1)–stimulated macrophages. Cyclin D1 is not expressed in quiescent, G0 macrophages, but it is rapidly induced upon mitotic stimulation. Withdrawal of CSF-1 causes cyclin D1 to disappear and macrophages re-enter the quiescent G0 state. Cyclin D1 is also induced upon serum-stimulation of quiescent fibroblasts, and microinjection of antisense oligonucleotides into serum-stimulated fibroblasts blocks the mitogenic response [17].

There are at least three different D-type cyclins, which are encoded by *CcnD1, CcnD2,* and *CcnD3* loci [6]. Some cells express all three of the D-type cyclin genes, whereas others express a more limited repertoire. In general, one observes that quiescent cells express low, often undetectable levels of D cyclin messenger RNA (mRNA) and protein [18]. Cyclin D expression is induced rapidly upon addition of growth factors, and dividing cells contain abundant cyclin D mRNA and protein, irrespective of the phase of the cell cycle. This noncyclic pattern of expression suggests that regulation of D cyclins, and perhaps the function of D cyclins, may be different from that of the M cyclins or the true G1 cyclins (such as cyclins C and E). Cyclin E (and perhaps C) is likely to be a component of an S-phase progression factor that regulates initiation of DNA synthesis. D cyclins function at an earlier stage in G1 progression and appear to be required for cells to remain in a proliferative state. Inhibition of D cyclin expression causes withdrawal from the cell cycle and accumulation in G1 [18], whereas overexpression of cyclin D1 shortens the G1 phase of the cell cycle [19]. The relationship between D-type cyclin expression and growth factor stimulation as well as the probable role of D cyclins in preventing G0 arrest suggests that D cyclins may play important roles in development, differentiation, and malignant transformation.

Cyclins D1 and D2 have been identified as proto-oncogenes [6,20]. Cyclin D1 is identical to the oncogene *PRAD/bcl1* that has been mapped to chromosome 11q13. Chromosomal rearrangement of the 11q13 locus results in overexpression of cyclin D1 in some forms of B-cell lymphomas and in parathyroid adenomas. Approximately 20% of primary breast cancers and even more squamous cell carcinomas of the head and neck exhibit amplification of *CcnD1* and overexpression of cyclin D1. Overexpression of cyclin D1 has been correlated with progression of experimentally induced skin tumors. Cyclin D2 has been identified as the proto-oncogene *vin1* [6].

The mechanisms by which the D-type cyclins act to enable a cell to respond to growth factors and progress through G1 into the S phase are not well understood. It is clear that the D-type cyclins can interact with several of the CDKs such as *cdk2, cdk4, cdk5,* and *cdk6.* Several proteins that associate with and inhibit the activities of the cycline kinase complexes have been identified and cloned. These cyclin kinase inhibitors add yet another level of regulation to this complex process. One potential mechanism by which the D-type cyclins appear to regulate G1 progression is suggested by the observations that D cyclins and their catalytic partner *cdk4* can associate with and phosphorylate the tumor suppressor $p105^{Rb}$, an event that is necessary for progression to the S phase [21–24]. The mechanisms by which the growth factors induce and activate the D cyclins and their catalytic subunits have not yet been determined. Nevertheless, it is tempting to speculate that D-type cyclins play an important role in maintaining cells in a proliferative state. According to this hypothesis, inhibition of D-cyclin expression, either by growth factor withdrawal or by direct action of an antagonist, causes withdrawal from the cell cycle.

The role of the cyclins in growth factor regulation of cell proliferation is just beginning to emerge. There are data that indicate that the effects of TGF-β are mediated by changes in cyclin or cyclin-dependent kinase activity (discussed below). Although there is presently confusion concerning the precise mechanisms, it is very likely that the effects of all of the growth factors will ultimately come to be understood in terms of their effects on those serine/threonine protein kinases that regulate cell-cycle progression.

Growth Factor Receptors

Peptide growth factors act on target cells by binding to specific cell surface protein receptors that, in turn, transduce their signals to the cell nucleus. The binding of the growth factor ligand to its receptor triggers a series of intracellular events that result in immediate and delayed biologic actions, some of which control the cell cycle. The receptors for peptide ligands are transmembrane proteins. Most receptors have an extracellular domain that binds to the peptide ligand (i.e., the growth factor), a transmembrane domain, and an intracellular domain that is linked to the signal transduction system. A few peptide receptors have been identified as proteoglycan molecules that have no capacity for signal transduction. These nontransducing receptors are often characterized by high binding capacity and relatively lower binding affinity, and they may function to bind ligands to the cell surface so that they are accessible to the transducing receptors under appropriate conditions.

Cell surface receptors are generally classified according to the ligands to which they bind (e.g., EGF receptor, TGF-β receptor). Receptors may also be classified by virtue of their intracellular signaling apparatus. Protein activities are modulated through conformational changes that result from the enzyme-catalyzed transfer of the γ phosphoryl group of ATP to serine, threonine, or tyrosine residues within the protein substrate [25]. Growth factor receptors that catalyze this transfer of phosphoryl groups are protein kinases. There are two distinct types of protein kinases; those that phosphorylate serine or threonine residues are different from those that phosphorylate tyrosine residues. (A few protein kinase receptors can phosphorylate both serine–threonine and tyrosine residues.) Most receptors for mitogenic growth factors possess intrinsic tyrosine kinase activity evidenced by ligand-dependent autophosphorylation of tyrosine residues located within the intracellular domain of the receptor. Such receptors can also catalyze ligand-dependent tyrosine phosphorylation of intracellular proteins. Many of the growth factor receptors are also phosphorylated on serine and threonine residues, probably as a result of feedback loops involving activation of signal transducing serine–threonine kinases. Dephosphorylation of both serine–threonine and tyrosine residues on the receptors also plays an important role in signal transduction, but less is known about these reactions. These phosphorylation–dephosphorylation reactions normally serve to regulate receptor availability and activity. Mutations that modify or abrogate these regulatory constraints or that allow overexpression of the receptors or their ligands have been shown to result in unrestrained proliferation and malignant transformation. Mutational impairment of receptor function often results in defects in development [25].

Most of the tyrosine kinase receptors fall into one of two major categories based on structural similarity; these categories may be subdivided into groups with even greater similarity (Figure 5-4A). The first category defines a group of receptors with cysteine-rich regions in the extracellular domain and an intracellular kinase domain that is discontinuous. The EGF receptor, c-*erb*B2/*neu*, and HER3/*erbB3* receptors are representative of one group of the first category. The second major category contains receptors that have regularly spaced cysteines and regions that appear analogous to immunoglobulin variable and constant regions in their extracellular domains. The receptors that constitute this category vary with respect to the numbers of immunoglobulin-like domains. The insulin receptor, the insulin-like growth factor-1 (IGF-1) receptor, the hepatocyte growth factor (HGF) receptor (also known as c-*met*), as well as the receptors for PDGF, CSF-1, c-*kit*, and FGF belong to this category. The *trk* gene product, recently identified as the NGF receptor, and related proteins such as *trkB* belong to a third category of tyrosine kinase receptors that contain neither cysteine-rich regions nor immunoglobulin-like regions. A fourth category of tyrosine kinase receptors that are activated by cytokines (e.g., the IL-2 receptor) have no catalytic component in the cytoplasmic domain, but they form complexes with cytoplasmic *src* family tyrosine kinases that activate the transduction cascade [26].

Tyrosine kinase receptors are activated upon binding to their specific growth factor ligands. Ligand binding results in rapid formation of receptor dimers and rapid activation of tyrosine kinase activity, which is manifest by autophosphorylation and by the phosphorylation of specific substrates. These initial tyrosine phosphorylation reactions initiate a cascade of phosphorylation reactions in which at least three protein kinases activate each other in series. Our current understanding is that autophosphorylation facilitates the association of a macromolecular complex involving the receptor and several other proteins. One group of proteins appears to interact with receptor tyrosine kinase receptors through protein-protein interactions that involve conserved *src*-homology-2 (SH2) domains [27,28]. The SH2 domain is a conserved sequence of approximately 100 amino acids that is found in several intracellular signaling proteins, including phospholipase C-γ1, phosphatidylinositol 3-kinase (PI-3-kinase), $p21^{ras}$GTPase activating protein (GAP, a molecule that modulates the GTPase activity of Ras protein), and $p60^{c\text{-}src}$ (see Figure 5-4B). The SH2 domains bind to tyrosine-phosphorylated peptide sequences with high affinity. This appears to be the rate-limiting step in formation of a complex in which the *Raf1* gene product is activated by association with the product of the *Ras* gene [29]. *Raf1* is believed to phosphorylate Mek (also known as mitogen-activated protein [MAP] kinase), which, in turn, phosphorylates, MAP kinases (also known as ERKs) [31]. The MAP kinase phosphorylates ribosomal protein kinases ($p90^{rsk}$ and $p70^{S6K}$), leading to their activation; both MAP kinase and ribosomal protein kinases phosphorylate the transcription factor AP-1 [31]. Phosphorylation of AP-1 and other

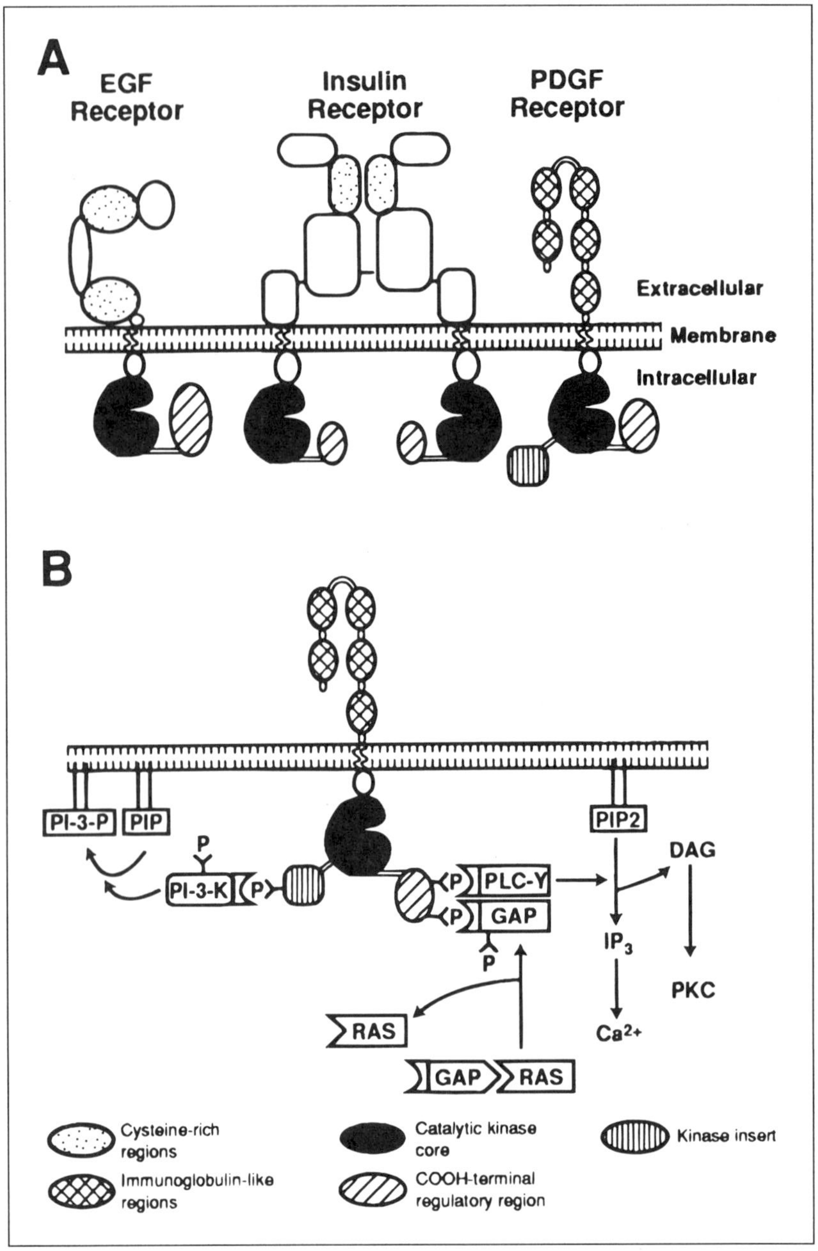

Figure 5-4. **(A)** Structural models of three protein tyrosine kinase receptors. **(B)** Protein-protein interactions between autophosphorylated protein tyrosine kinase receptors and proteins that contain SH2 domains. The PDGF receptor binds PI-3-kinase (PI-3-K) via the kinase insert region; PLC-γ and RAS-GAP are bound via the COOH-terminus. All three are tyrosine phosphorylated. (From DL Cadena, GN Hill. *FASEB J* 6:2332, 1992. Reproduced with permission.)

transcription factors may precipitate the immediate early response.

Autophosphorylation of tyrosine kinase receptors results in activation of phospholipase C-γ1 [25,27]. Although the mechanism is not clear, activation of phospholipase C-γ1 results in rapid hydrolysis of phosphatidylinositol 4,5-bisphosphate (PIP_2) with the generation of inositol trisphosphate (IP_3) and diacylglycerol (DAG) as second messengers. The increase in intracellular IP_3 results in release of intracellular free Ca^{++} stores and the activation of multiple calcium-dependent proteins. Diacylglycerol is an endogenous activator of protein kinase C (PKC). Although this pathway is clearly important for both cell growth and metabolic regulation by growth factors, the mechanistic linkage remains to be discovered. It is known that PKC can phosphorylate and activate *Raf1* [32,33], but it is almost certain that many of the effects of activation of PKC and the Ca^{++}/IP_3 pathway are not mediated by MAP kinase. We do not yet know how these pathways contribute to the commitment to initiate DNA synthesis or to maintain the proliferative state. These define the critical questions that must be answered if we are to understand the molecular details of growth factor regulation of cell proliferation.

Epidermal Growth Factor and Related Peptides

The EGF Family of Transmembrane Growth Factors

Epidermal growth factor is the prototypical member of a family of peptides that bind to and activate the EGF receptor (Figure 5-5). The family includes EGF, TGF-α, heparin-binding EGF (HB-EGF), amphiregulin (AR), *cripto,* poxvirus growth factors (PVGF), and betacellulin [34–36]. Heregulin,

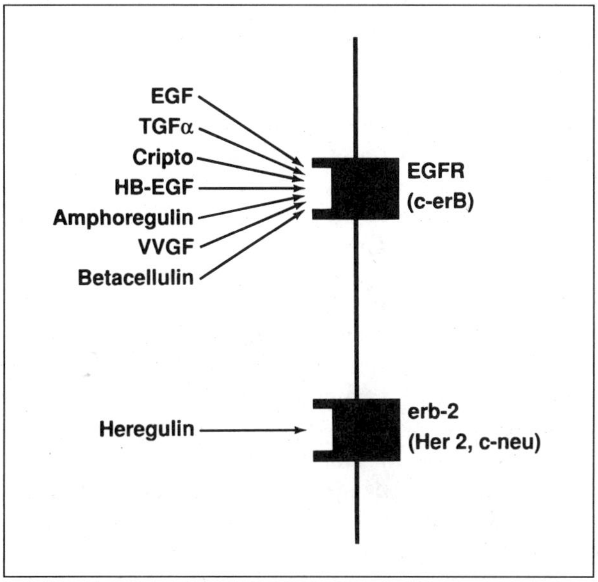

Figure 5-5. TGF-α/EGF family of ligands and receptors. (From RJ Coffey et al. *J Cell Biochem* [suppl.] 16G:111, 1992. Reproduced with permission from Wiley-Liss, a division of John Wiley and Sons, Inc., New York, copyright © 1992.)

a ligand for the EGF receptor–related tyrosine kinase p185[erbB2] (also known as *Her-2* and c-*neu*) is also a member of the EGF family [37]. The EGF-like peptides are defined by similarities in their primary structures. The mature EGF-related peptides consist of 50 to 60 amino acid residues and exhibit strict conservation of six cysteines that contribute to tertiary structure by the formation of disulfide bridges. The spacing of these cysteines and intervening amino acids follows the characteristic scheme: $X_nCX_7CX_{2-3}GXCX_{10-13}CXCX_3$-$YXGXRCX_4LX_n$ according to the single letter coding for amino acids (X can represent any amino acid) [35].

All of these EGF-related peptides are synthesized as precursor molecules that are anchored to the cell membrane, and the mature peptides (located in the extracellular domains) are released via proteolytic cleavage at the NH2- and COOH-terminal peptides of the mature peptides (Figure 5-6). For example, cleavage sites in proTGF-α that generate the NH2-terminus and COOH-terminus of mature TGF-α are both located between alanine and valine and are targets for an elastase-like enzyme [38]. Enzymatic cleavage of the membrane-anchored proTGF-α can be activated in response to serum factors or tumor-promoting phorbol esters, thereby releasing soluble TGF-α [39]. Heregulin differs from other members of the EGF family in that its release requires only a single cleavage COOH-terminal to the conserved cysteine cluster, to produce the mature peptide [37]. Interestingly, the membrane-bound precursors of EGF and TGF-α have been shown to be capable of activating EGF receptors on adjacent cells [40–42]. The term *juxtacrine activity* has been

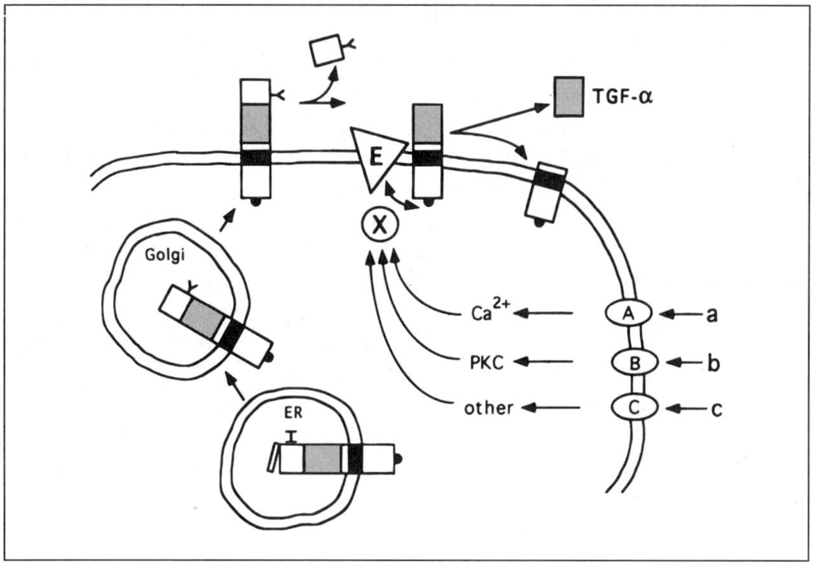

Figure 5-6. Biosynthesis and regulated cleavage of proTGF-α. The primary translation product undergoes signal sequence cleavage and cotranslational N-glycosylation (I) in the endoplasmic reticulum (ER) followed by maturation of sugar chains (Y) in the Golgi compartment and transport to the plasma membrane. Soon after reaching the cell surface, proTGF-α loses the N-terminal glycosylated region. Cleavage at the C-terminus of the mature TGF-α sequence with release of soluble factor occurs at or near the cell surface and involves a proteolytic system (E) that is activated in response to various agonists (a, b, c) that act through independent signaling mechanisms and converge into a common effector (X). The signal that targets proTGF-α for recognition by this cleavage system is its C-terminal valine (dot). (From J Massague, A Pandiella. Membrane-anchored growth factors. *Annu Rev Biochem* 62:515, 1993. Reproduced with permission from Annual Reviews Inc., Palo Alto, CA.)

coined to describe this mechanism of ligand-receptor interaction [38].

Epidermal Growth Factor

Epidermal growth factor was originally detected in extracts from mouse submaxillary glands and was characterized by its ability to induce precocious eyelid opening and incisor eruption [43]. It is abundantly expressed in salivary glands, lacrimal glands, Brunner's glands of the duodenum, megakaryocytes, mature luminal ductal cells of the breast, and kidney, with smaller amounts expressed in the exocrine pancreas [35,44]. Epidermal growth factor immunoreactivity is abundant in the saliva, colostrum, milk, and urine, and high concentrations are found in the α granules of platelets, where it is found along with several other growth factors (including platelet-derived growth factor [PDGF], TGF-α, and TGF-β) that appear to be important in wound repair. It is not normally produced in the intestine (except in Brunner's glands). However, after injury to the gastrointestinal tract, EGF (along with several other growth factors) is expressed in regenerating crypts adjacent to the area of ulceration and is likely important in gut epithelial repair [45].

The EGF receptors are ubiquitous, and EGF is mitogenic for many different cell types in cell culture models. Biologically important roles for EGF are suggested by the locations in which it is expressed and are supported by demonstrations of the biologic activity through exogenous administration of EGF. In addition to the effects on eyelid opening and incisor eruption, EGF has multiple biologic actions in various animal models [35,46,47]. Epidermal growth factor promotes lung maturation in fetal rats, rabbits, and lambs. It stimulates the proliferation of gastric mucosal cells in suckling rats and the growth of intestinal epithelium in adult rats maintained on total parenteral nutrition. The normal development of the mouse mandible requires the local expression of EGF. Epidermal growth factor infusion increases hepatic DNA synthesis in normal rats. It also accelerates the development of skin in fetal lambs, and treatment with EGF can enhance the healing of wounds of the skin corneal epithelium, mesentery, and tympanic membrane in animal models [48]. Clinical trials in humans suggest that EGF may be useful in promoting healing of skin graft harvest sites, chronic wounds, and corneal injuries [48].

Many cancers exhibit overexpression of the EGF receptor, but relatively few have been found to express EGF. Expression of EGF has been demonstrated in pleomorphic adenomas of the salivary glands (86%) and prostate carcinomas (68%) as well as in small numbers of pancreatic cancers and gastric carcinomas [49]. It is not yet clear what role, if any, EGF has in carcinogenesis.

TGF-α and EGF Have Similar Actions, but Different Distribution

Transforming growth factors were originally identified in a partially purified form from cell culture medium conditioned by Rous sarcoma virus–transformed fibroblasts [1]. Activity of TGF was originally defined by the biologic effects on fibroblast cells in culture. The activity caused the fibroblast cells to undergo a reversible change in their morphology to a pattern that appeared similar to transformed cells. Activity of TGF also caused the normally anchorage-dependent fibroblasts to acquire anchorage independence and to form colonies in soft agar, another characteristic of transformed cells. Upon further purification of the TGF activity in the conditioned media, it was found that two different peptides (TGF-α and TGF-B) were responsible for the observed effects on fibroblast cells. The peptide TGF-α is an EGF-related 50–amino acid peptide cleaved from a 160–amino acid transmembrane precursor. Initially, TGF-α was thought to be an embryonic growth factor that was inappropriately expressed in neoplasia. Subsequent studies have demonstrated expression of TGF-α in numerous normal adult tissues. Expression has been detected in skin keratinocytes, activated macrophages, mammary epithelium, brain, bronchus, pituitary, ovary, testis, kidneys, and most gastrointestinal tissues [44,49,50]. In most of these locations there is no detectable expression of EGF under normal conditions.

The biologic activities of EGF and TGF-α that result from the activation of the EGF receptor are qualitatively similar, although several quantitative differences have been observed [51,52]. Both EGF and TGF-α stimulate the migration of epithelial cells and both induce proliferation in a variety of cell types [34,35,53].

Both EGF and TGF-α appear to have important roles in the gastrointestinal tract. Both peptides are acid stable [54,55], and both suppress gastric acid production and induce mucus production [56–61]. Administration of either EGF [62–64] or TGF-α [65] is protective against experimentally induced gastric ulceration. Although EGF is not detectable in the stomach, TGF-α mRNA and immunoreactive peptide are detected in the normal gastric mucosa, especially in parietal cell–enriched fractions [44,66]. After gastric injury, there is rapid release of TGF-α immunoreactivity into the gastric lumen, followed by a subsequent increase in TGF-α mRNA levels and DNA synthesis [66]. Transforming growth factor-α is also found in the intestinal epithelium where, under normal conditions, it is localized primarily in the epithelium near the villus tips. When there is intestinal ulceration, TGF-α becomes more widely distributed throughout the entire gland and villus [45]. A similar situation prevails in the stomach after acute mucosal injury [R.J. Coffey, personal communication].

There is substantial experimental evidence to suggest that TGF-α has an important role in carcinogenesis and in the growth of established tumors [34,36]. Overexpression of TGF-α by transfection leads to transformation in cells that also express relatively high numbers of EGF receptors. Transfection of *Rat-1* fibroblasts with TGF-α expression vectors resulted in a transformed phenotype that could be reversed by addition of antibodies to TGF-α. Expression of EGF receptor and concomitant TGF-α expression are found in several types of naturally existing human cancers, including those from the breast, pancreas, stomach, and lung [34,49,67]. The significance of the TGF-α/EGF receptor autocrine stimulatory loop is suggested by recent observations that TGF-α antisense RNA blocked estrogen-induced production of TGF-α and inhibited proliferation in estrogen-responsive human breast cancer cells [68]. Expression of TGF-α in transgenic mice has been shown to cause breast carcinomas in postlactational female mice; hepatomas occurred with an even higher frequency than did breast cancers in some transgenic strains [34].

Both EGF and TGF-α have been shown to function as tumor promoters in experimental models of carcinogenesis. Tumor promoters, by definition, have little or no carcinogenic activity when tested alone, but they can enhance tumor formation when applied after a low dose of carcinogen (initiator). A classic example of a tumor promoter is 12-0-tetradecanoyl-phorbol-13-acetate (TPA). Treatment with TPA and EGF receptor activation both result in intracellular PKC activation [34]. Pittelkow and associates [69] found that TPA administration to keratinocytes resulted in a 20-fold induction of TGF-α mRNA and protein expression. Thus, some of the tumor-promoting effects of TPA may be the result of induction of TGF-α. Spontaneous mammary carcinomas occur with high frequency in some strains of C3H female mice, and this incidence can be reduced by fivefold by removal of salivary glands (sialadenectomy) in virgin females. This removes the greatest source of endogenous EGF, and administration of exogenous EGF to the sialadenectomized mice significantly increased the incidence of mammary carcinoma [34,49]. Treatment with EGF also resulted in a threefold increase in the incidence of squamous cancer of the anus in mice that received an initiating dose of dimethylhydrazine. Further support for a tumor-promoting role for TGF-α comes from observations that virgin MMTV-TGF-α transgenic mice given a single initiating dose of the carcinogen 7,12-dimethyl-benzanthracene at 8 weeks of age have a high incidence (>50%) of mammary carcinomas as compared with their nontransgenic littermates (none) by age 220 days [34]. In contrast, spontaneous mammary tumors did not occur before age 320 days in the same line of transgenic mice.

Other EGF Family Members

Amphiregulin has been detected in many normal human tissues, including placenta, ovary, breast, testis, lung, colon, skin keratinocytes, and kidney, as well as in carcinoma cells from breast, ovary, pancreas, colon, rectum, and stomach [70–74]. In addition, there is an increase in amphiregulin mRNA in the hyperplastic epidermal lesions of psoriasis in humans [75]. Amphiregulin appears to be a bifunctional growth regulator. It inhibits growth of several human carcinoma cell types in culture, and it stimulates the proliferation of other tumor cell lines as well as nontransformed human fibroblasts, keratinocytes, and mammary epithelial cell lines [71,73,74]. Amphiregulin mRNA and protein were found to be overexpressed in 60% to 70% of human primary and metastatic colorectal carcinomas [70], and immunohistochemical analysis revealed that most adenomas and well-differentiated carcinomas of the colon and rectum were positive for amphiregulin expression [76].

The *cripto* gene was identified and cloned from a human teratocarcinoma cell line [77]. The expression of *cripto* is more restricted than TGF-α and amphiregulin. *Cripto* mRNA expression has been detected in undifferentiated mouse and human embryonal carcinoma cells, midgestation mouse embryos, adult mouse brain and lung, and human hepatomas, but not in other normal adult mouse or human tissues [77]. Like amphiregulin, *cripto* is expressed in the majority of human colon cancer cell lines and in primary colorectal tumors and hepatic metastases from colorectal carcinomas. Unlike amphiregulin, *cripto* was not found in normal colon specimens [70,76]. Expression of *cripto* has also been reported in gastric carcinomas [49]. Further evidence for a role of *cripto* comes from experiments in which transfection of the *cripto* cDNA expression vector into mouse NIH-

3T3 fibroblasts or into normal mouse mammary epithelial cells results in malignant transformation of the cells [70,77].

Several members of the poxviruses have been found to express peptides with homology to EGF, and most of these growth factors have been named according to their viral origin. Vaccinia virus growth factor (VVGF) was the first to be identified and characterized. It is expressed by infected cells in the early phase of the virus replicative cycle; it binds to the EGF receptor and stimulates EGF receptor autophosphorylation, and it is mitogenic for keratinocytes and fibroblasts [38,78]. Other related peptides are expressed by myxoma virus, Shope fibroma virus, and the molluscum contagiosum virus; all are members of the poxvirus family [34,49].

Insulin-Like Growth Factors

The insulin-like growth factors (IGF-1 and IGF-2) are growth-regulatory polypeptides that share structural homology with proinsulin [79–81]. The insulin and IGF receptors to which these ligands bind also share structural and functional similarity. Insulin and IGFs exert their growth stimulatory actions by virtue of their capacity to bind to and activate the IGF-1 receptor, although insulin and IGFs bind with significantly different affinities. Both IGF-1 and IGF-2 bind to the type 2 IGF/mannose-6-phosphate receptor, the insulin receptor, and high-affinity IGF binding proteins (IGFBPs).

IGFs are thought to be important in the regulation of growth and differentiation in various tissues. Insulin-like growth factor-1 acts as a progression factor for the cell cycle in selected cell types. It acts in concert with competence factors such as PDGF, EGF, and FGF. The mitogenic effects of IGF-1 in late G1 appear to require the participation of *Ras* proteins, whereas G0–G1 transition events, induced by the competence factors PDGF or EGF, do not require *Ras* [82]. IGF-1 induces c-Ha-*ras* mRNA expression early during the G0–G1 phase transition [83]. Anti-*Ras* antibody microinjected into NIH 3T3 cells blocked IGF-1–stimulated cell-cycle progression to the S phase from mid to late G1. The anti-*Ras* IgG did not block c-*fos* induction (a G0–G1 transition event) by PDGF or EGF. In contrast, an antibody to the α subunit of the G protein inhibited c-*fos* induction by PDGF or EGF [82].

The IGFs are produced in most tissues (although in varying concentrations) and are found in abundance in the circulation. The liver is the major source for circulating IGFs. The amount of IGF-1 in adults exceeds that of IGF-2. The rate of production of IGF-1 is approximately 10 mg/d [84]. In the process of purification of IGF-1 and IGF-2, investigators found that the IGFs were usually bound to higher molecular weight proteins known as the IGFBPs. Six forms of IGFBPs have been identified and characterized, and they are designated IGFBP-1 through IGFBP-6. The IGFBPs are expressed in numerous tissues to varying degrees, and there is some variation in the binding affinities for the IGFs among the family. The most abundant IGFBP in the circulating plasma is IGFBP-3, and it has high affinities for both IGF-1 and IGF-2. More than 95% of IGF in the circulation is bound to IGFBP-3. The IGFBPs prevent catabolism of IGFs and prolong their half-lives, and they may be important in transporting IGFs to specific tissues. At the cellular level, IGFBPs may either inhibit or potentiate the biologic effects of the IGFs. Although the inhibition of IGF action may be the result of binding with IGFBPs that prevent receptor interactions, the ability of IGFBPs to potentiate proliferative actions of the IGFs in selected cell systems appears to be more complex. Some cell types appear capable of post-translational processing of the IGFBPs (e.g., phosphorylation) that can alter their affinities for the IGFs [85,86].

Growth hormone (GH) regulates the synthesis and circulating concentrations of IGF-1. Most (but not all) of the growth defects that result from growth hormone deficiency are effectively treated by infusion of IGF-1. For example, infusion of IGF-1 in GH-deficient rats stimulates body weight gain and bone growth, but with less potency than GH treatment [80]. Considerable insight has been gained from transgenic experiments. Transgenic mice that overexpress the IGF-1 gene have increased body weight compared with controls, but less than those of littermates that overexpress the GH gene. When IGF-1 transgenic mice are crossbred with a line of GH-deficient mice, the offspring that express IGF-1 grow at a rate similar to littermates that are not GH deficient. Analysis of organ growth revealed some differences between the effects of GH and IGF-1. Growth hormone results in normal liver growth, and IGF-1 stimulates brain growth [87].

There is also evidence that IGF-1 has a role in renal growth and function [79–81]. Both IGF-1 and IGFBP-1 are colocalized in the kidney, and the levels are regulated by GH. Expression of IGF-1, IGF-1 receptor, and IGF-2 receptor are increased in the remnant kidney after unilateral nephrectomy in immature rats. In adult rats, there is an increase in the levels of IGF-1 in the remnant kidney after unilateral nephrectomy. Infusion of exogenous IGF-1 increases kidney size in rats, and it also increases glomerular filtration and renal plasma flow rates in humans.

Evidence is accumulating for multiple other biologic or potential therapeutic roles for IGF [48,79–81]. Both plasma and platelets have substantial levels of IGF-1, where it is ideally located to participate in wound repair. Insulin-like growth factor-1 is a potent chemotactic agent for vascular endothelial cells, and it synergizes with other PDGFs in the stimulation of fibroblast, osteocyte, and chondrocyte proliferation during wound healing. Exogenous infusion of pharmacologic doses of IGF-1 may have beneficial effects in reversing the catabolic effects of major trauma, burns, or sepsis, based on recent studies in animal models [88,89]. Further, the proliferative effects on intestinal epithelial cells appear to prevent atrophic changes in the gut and to decrease bacterial translocation in burned rats [90]. On the other hand, there is an accumulating body of evidence to suggest that production of IGFs, IGF receptors, and IGFBPs may have important roles in the growth of many different types of human tumors [91–93]. The therapeutic value of IGF agonist or antagonist therapy in humans awaits further studies.

Platelet-Derived Growth Factor

The PDGF was initially discovered by Ross and colleagues, who found that serum was more mitogenic for cultured fibroblasts than plasma [94–96]. The PDGF found in serum is released from α-granules of platelets. Subsequent studies revealed that PDGF is synthesized and released by many different normal and transformed cell types. Platelet-derived growth factor is a disulfide-bonded dimer (30 kDa) consisting of A and B PDGF polypeptide chains. The A and B subunits are products of separate genes, and there is about 60% identity of the amino acid sequence of the A and B polypeptides. The active growth factor is a dimer of A–A, B–B, or A–B polypeptide chains. Alternative splicing of the primary transcript may result in addition of basic residues at the COOH terminus, and this structural difference may be important for regulation of peptide secretion or interaction with extracellular matrix.

Vascular endothelial growth factor (VEGF) is another member of the PDGF family that has been recently isolated, purified, and characterized. A 45-kDa heparin-binding protein, VEGF exists as a disulfide-linked homodimer, the subunits of which have 24% amino acid sequence identity to the PDGF B chain. It is mitogenic for endothelial cells, but not other PDGF-responsive cells in cell culture. It is angiogenic in vivo [48].

There are two PDGF receptors (α and β) that share structural similarity; each has two extracellular immunoglobulin-like domains and a split intracellular tyrosine kinase domain. The α receptor binds all three types of PDGF dimers, and the β receptor binds only PDGF dimers containing B chains (B–B and A–B) [97]. There is rapid turnover of PDGF receptors at the cell surface under basal conditions, with a marked increase in turnover in the presence of high concentrations of PDGF. Saturating concentrations of PDGF cause almost complete internalization and down-regulation of PDGF receptors. PDGF receptors are found in a variety of cell types, including fibroblasts, vascular smooth muscle, mesangial cells, glial cells, and microvascular endothelial cells [48]. Although PDGF has been considered to be primarily a mitogen for mesenchymal cells, cutaneous injury results in expression of PDGF receptors in keratinocytes. Most cells expressing PDGF receptors express both types of receptor (α and β), but their expression appears to be regulated independently. For example, TGF-β down-regulates α-receptors in cultured cells, but it does not affect β-receptor expression. A very few cells express exclusively α or β receptors. The oligodendrocyte 0-2A progenitor cells, mesothelial cells, and liver capillary cells express only α receptors; whereas capillary endothelial cells of the brain, neurons, meningeal cells, and Schwann cells express only β-receptors [97,98].

Platelet-derived growth factor is primarily a mitogen for cells of mesenchymal origin [48]. The mitogenic effects of PDGF for smooth muscle cells and fibroblasts are potentiated by IGF-1 [97]. Exposure of smooth muscle cells to PDGF results in a decrease in the synthesis of the contractile protein, α-actin, and transition from a contractile to a synthetic phenotype that is less differentiated [97]. It is chemotactic for both vascular smooth muscle cells and fibroblasts [48,97].

Smooth muscle cells express predominantly the PDGF A chain, and A chain mRNA in these cells is induced by angiotensin II and TGF-β. Platelet-derived growth factor probably directly mediates the mitogenic effects of these peptides on smooth muscle cells [95–98]. There is an increasing body of evidence that PDGF has important roles in blood vessel growth and repair. There is an increase in the release of PDGF from smooth muscle cells derived from the proliferating neointima of injured rat arteries compared with cells from normal arteries.

Platelet-derived growth factor has been implicated in atherogenesis and hypertension [95,97]. Increased expression of PDGF and PDGF receptors has been observed in atherosclerotic segments of human artery, injured blocked vessels, healing vascular grafts, atherosclerotic plaque, and vascular smooth muscle cells cultured from hypertensive rats. It is also a potent vasoconstricting agent for rat aortic rings.

Platelet-derived growth factor is released by several cell types that are important for wound healing, including placental cells, fibroblasts, vascular smooth muscle cells, and vascular endothelial cells [48]. High concentrations of PDGF are released into wounds by platelets, where it likely aids in hemostasis because of its vasoconstrictor effects. It also attracts and activates leukocytes, which are required for microbicidal action [99]. It induces transient increases in fibroblast expression of immediate-early proliferation-associated genes such as JE, KC, c-*fos,* and c-*myc.* Interleukin-6 expression and prostaglandin E_2 synthesis are also increased by PDGF [99].

There appear to be important roles for PDGF in the nervous system. Most of the cells that comprise the central and peripheral nervous systems have PDGF receptors. Furthermore, expression of PDGF has been demonstrated in several cell types within the nervous system. Neurons and Schwann cells produce PDGF-B, and type 1 astrocytes produce PDGF-A. It has recently been shown to be trophic for brain tissue *in vivo* [98].

There is considerable evidence that PDGF has important roles in cancer. The PDGF-B-chain is virtually identical to the transforming protein $p28^{sis}$ (or v-*sis*) of the simian sarcoma retrovirus [96]; PDGF-B is therefore the c-*sis* proto-oncogene. The transforming potential of c-*sis*/PDGF-B has been found to be identical to that of v-*sis*, and transformation by c-/v-*sis* occurs only in cells that express PDGF receptors [96,98]. Numerous cancer cell lines arising from neural or mesenchymal cells express both PDGF receptors and the PDGF ligand, and therefore have potential autocrine growth stimulation [96]. Paracrine effects of PDGF expressed by some types of cancers may be important in stimulating tumor stroma and desmoplasia. For example, human scirrhous gastric carcinoma [100], breast cancer cells [101], pancreatic ductal carcinoma cells [102], and human carcinoid tumor cells [103] all express PDGF, and stromal cells express PDGF receptors [104].

The Fibroblast Growth Factor Family

The FGF family contains at least seven members: acidic FGF (aFGF); basic FGF (bFGF); the *int*-2 gene product, Kaposi sarcoma FGF (K-FGF); the product of the *hst*-1 oncogene; FGF-5; and FGF-6; and keratinocyte growth factor (KGF) [48,105,106]. Members of the FGF family are 35% to 55% identical in amino acid sequence, and the genes have similar structures and organization [105]. The first members of the FGF family to be purified and characterized were aFGF and bFGF, and three of the FGF genes (int-2, K-FGF/*hst*-1, and FGF-5) were first isolated as oncogenes [105,106]. Basic and acidic FGFs were initially purified from bovine pituitary and brain on the basis of mitogenic effects on fibroblasts [105]. The FGFs have been found to be mitogenic for epithelial, fibroblast, and endothelial cells, with the exception of KGF (FGF-7). Keratinocyte growth factor is expressed by connective tissue cells adjacent to epithelia, but stimulates only epithelial cells in a paracrine interaction. Both aFGF and bFGF lack a secretory signal sequence, and the mechanism of secretion is not well understood. The remainder of the FGFs have functional signal sequences. Interestingly, aFGF and bFGF share 25% to 27% amino acid homology with interleukin (IL)-1α and IL-1β; the IL-1 proteins also lack signal peptide sequences.

Acidic and basic FGFs have been purified from many different tissues, including brain, pituitary and adrenal glands, bone, cartilage, corpus luteum, hypothalamus, placenta, prostate, retina, testis, and thymus. Both basic and acidic FGFs are mitogenic for a wide variety of cell types of mesenchymal and neurectodermal origin. Both FGFs have a high affinity for heparin, and this property led to the development of standardized affinity purification protocols using heparin affinity chromatography [105]. Of particular importance is the ability of both acidic and basic FGFs to act as mitogens and chemoattractants for endothelial cells in culture. The biologic relevance of this effect on endothelial cells is supported by the angiogenic effect that has been observed in vivo [107].

The FGFs have been implicated in both normal and aberrant angiogenesis in vivo. For example, there are probable roles in healing of cutaneous, gastrointestinal, and skeletal wounds [48]. There is evidence to suggest roles for FGFs in pathologic angiogenesis in tumors and in vascular diseases such as diabetic retinopathy. In combination with TGF-β, bFGF can induce formation of tube-like endothelial cell cords reminiscent of capillary sprouts in vitro. Transgenic mouse studies reveal the potential importance of FGF production in multistep tumorigenesis [108]. Transgenic mice carrying the bovine papilloma virus type 1 transgene develop a progressive dermal disease that is initially seen as mild fibromatosis and progresses to aggressive fibromatosis and finally fibrosarcoma. Basic FGF was detected in normal dermal fibroblasts and in those from mice bearing all three cutaneous lesions, but there was a change in the localization of bFGF. The growth factor is normally bound to the surface of cells, but it was released from the cells derived from lesions of aggressive fibromatosis and fibrosarcoma. This tendency to secrete bFGF, rather than retain it bound to the cell, was correlated with a high degree of neovascularity in the aggressive lesions.

Roles for bFGF in the gastrointestinal tract have been proposed. Folkman and colleagues [109] found that bFGF is produced in gastric and duodenal mucosa, but it is very sensitive to degradation by gastric acid (Figure 5-7). A recombinant derivative of bFGF (called bFGF-mutein) that is resistant to acid degradation can speed healing of experimental peptic ulcers in rats. Aluminum sucrose octasulfate (Sucralfate) has a molecular structure similar to heparin and, like heparin, binds bFGF with high affinity. Oral Sucralfate apparently binds to intragastric bFGF and protects it from acid degradation. This is thought to elevate the local concentration of bFGF in the peptic ulcer bed. In this manner, Sucralfate increases local angiogenesis and promotes ulcer healing. Similarly, neutralization of gastric acid (pH 6.4–7.2) by cimetidine results in increased levels of biologically active bFGF in experimentally induced ulcers.

The FGF family has important roles in embryonic development [105,106]. The FGFs play a critical role in embryonic mesodermal induction in *Xenopus,* and disruption of FGF signaling by mutation of the FGF receptor results in defective formation of mesodermal tissues. The expression of *int*-2 appears to be necessary for the development of the otic vesicle of the inner ear. The FGF-4 appears to be critical in early limb bud development [110]. It is likely that all of the FGFs have important roles during development.

Four FGF receptors have been identified and named FGFR-1 through FGFR-4 [48,105,106]. Each is encoded by a separate gene, although the receptors are highly related, with 60% to 70% amino acid sequence identity. The FGF receptors share structural similarity; all have three extracellular, FGF-binding immunoglobulin-like loops, a transmembrane domain, and a cytoplasmic tyrosine kinase domain. The FGF receptors range in mass from approximately 95 kDa to 150 kDa. Binding of FGFs to their receptors results in autophosphorylation. Both FGFR-1 and FGFR-2 bind both aFGF and bFGF with equal affinity. The K-FGF binds to FGFR-1 with a 20-fold lower affinity than bFGF, whereas both ligands bind to FGFR-2 with similar affinity. Both aFGF and bFGF can activate FGFR-3. The FGFR-4 binds aFGF with approximately 100-fold higher affinity than bFGF [106,111]. Differential temporal and spatial regulation of FGFs and their receptors, along with considerable redundancy of both ligands and receptors, appears to be an important determinant for biologic actions during development and in adult tissues.

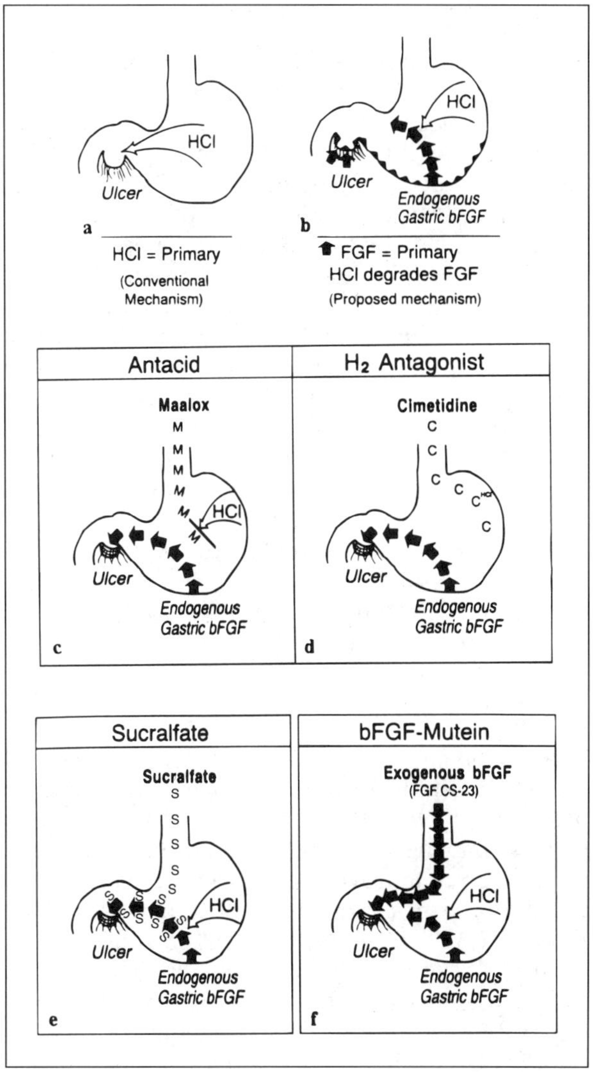

Figure 5-7. Models of ulcer formation and anti-ulcer therapy. **(a)** A conventional model in which HCl is believed to directly cause duodenal ulcers. **(b)** A proposed mechanism in which endogenous bFGF in the stomach and duodenum may act to prevent ulceration unless this peptide is excessively degraded by HCl. **(c)** A hypothetical model of anti-ulcer therapy in which neutralization of HCl permits increased availability of endogenous bFGF in the ulcer bed. **(d)** A hypothetical model of anti-ulcer therapy in which an H_2 antagonist decreases secretion of HCl, thus interfering with degradation of bFGF in the gastric mucosa in the ulcer bed. **(e)** A hypothetical model of anti-ulcer therapy in which Sucralfate binds and protects available endogenous bFGF without affecting levels of HCl. **(f)** A hypothetical model of anti-ulcer therapy by oral delivery of an angiogenic peptide that has been made acid resistant (bFGF CS-23). In this model, exogenous bFGF can be considered as replacement therapy for endogenous bFGF undergoing degradation by HCl. (From J Folkman et al. Duodenal ulcer: Discovery of a new mechanism and development of angiogenic therapy that accelerates healing. *Ann Surg* 214:414, 1991. Reproduced with permission from J.B. Lippincott Co., Philadelphia, PA.)

Transforming Growth Factor-β

The TGF-βs are 25-kDa homodimeric polypeptides belonging to a superfamily of growth-regulatory molecules that includes mullerian-inhibiting substance, activins, inhibins, and bone morphogenetic proteins, among others [112–115]. Three isoforms of TGF-β (TGF-β1, TGF-β2, and TGF-β3) have been identified in mammals. These isoforms share 70% to 75% amino acid sequence identity, bind to and activate the same receptors, and have identical biologic activities, with few exceptions. In this chapter, the term TGF-β refers to any or all three of the isoforms. The TGF-βs regulate a diversity of biologic processes that include cellular proliferation, cell migration, differentiation, and extracellular matrix deposition. The growth-regulatory effects of TGF-β appear to be cell-type specific; TGF-β promotes proliferation of many types of mesenchymal cells, and TGF-β is a potent inhibitor of proliferation for most epithelial, endothelial, and hematopoietic cell types.

TGF-β Activation

The TGF-βs are released from most cultured cell types in a latent form [116,117]. The biochemical basis by which TGF-β is maintained in a latent form is that the active mature C-terminal peptide remains in a noncovalent association with the N-terminal precursor form (called latency-associated protein [LAP]), thereby masking the ability to recognize TGF-β receptors (Figure 5-8). The 75 kDa LAP is often covalently linked to a 135-kDa binding protein. The latent TGF-β complex can be activated by sialidase and glycosidases, which probably disrupt interaction of the active dimer from the glycosylated large LAP-binding protein complex. The TGF-β is also activated by exposure to an acidic environment. Proteases such as plasmin and cathepsin can also activate latent TGF-β, and it appears that TGF-β binding to mannose-6-phosphate/IGF-2 receptors is an important component in this protease activation process at the cell surface (Figure 5-9). Sato and Rifkin [118] have demonstrated that co-culture of endothelial cells and their adjacent pericytes results in activation of latent TGF-β1. Studies of transfected fibrosarcoma cells and transfected mouse fibroblasts revealed that overexpression of latent TGF-β1 yields responses consistent with the actions of mature, active TGF-β; in vivo activation of latent TGF-β may result in biologically important autocrine and paracrine effects [119,120].

TGF-β Receptors

There are three types of TGF-β receptors (type 1, type 2, and type 3) that were originally classified according to size on affinity crosslinking experiments [112,121,122]. The complementary DNAs corresponding to all three receptors have been cloned. The type 1 (a 53-kDa protein) and the type 2 (73-kDa) receptors both appear to be necessary for signal transduction. Both receptors have cytoplasmic serine–threonine kinase domains [123,124]. These two receptors form a heterodimeric complex in the presence of TGF-β, and it appears that the ratios of type 1 to type 2 receptors may determine the range of biologic responses to TGF-β. There is evidence of interdependence among these two types of receptors. In mutant cell

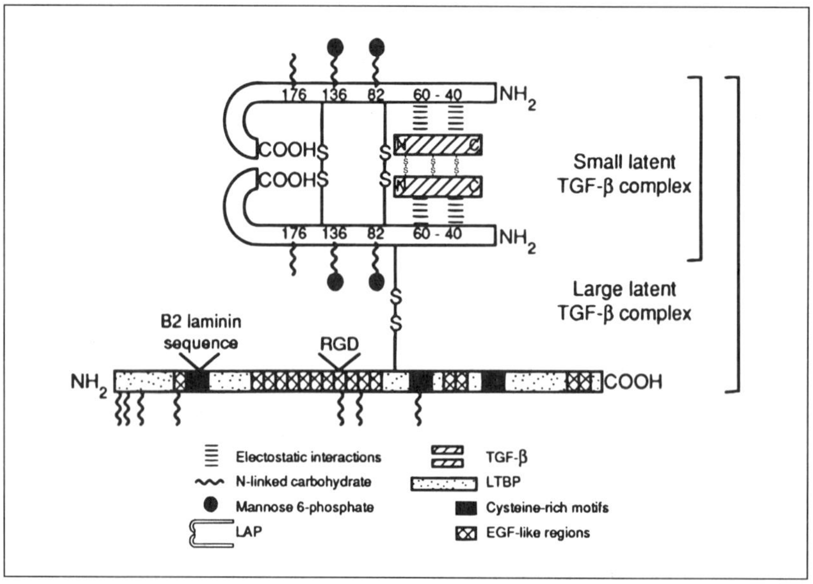

Figure 5-8. Structures of the small and large latent TGF-β complexes. The electrostatic interactions and the exact number and precise location of intra- and intermolecular disulfide bonds are not known. The glycosylated residues of LTBP are predicted by the cDNA sequence (not shown). (From JG Harpel et al. Control of transforming growth factor-β activity: Latency vs. activation. *Prog Growth Factor Res* 4:321, 1992. Reproduced with kind permission from Pergamon Press Ltd, Headington Hill Hall, Oxford 0X3 0BW, UK, copyright© 1992.)

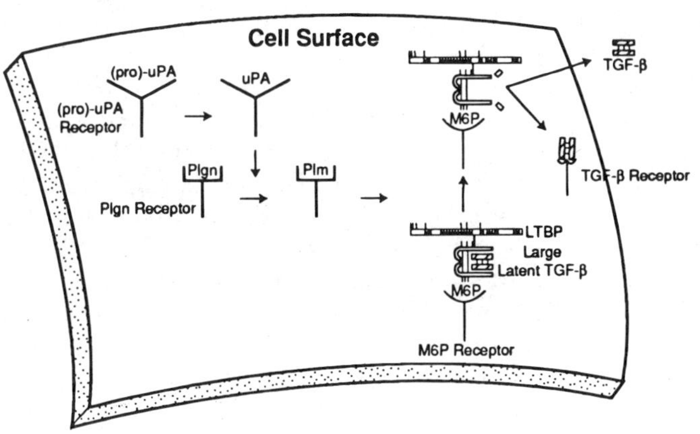

Figure 5-9. A model for the surface activation of latent TGF-β by the PA/plasmin system. Receptor-bound uPA activates receptor-bound plasminogen (plgn) to plasmin (plm). Plasmin proteolytically liberates mature TGF-β from the latent complex bound to the cell surface via the M6P receptor. The role of LTBP during activation is unknown. It is possible that unidentified cell surface or ECM binding sites exist for LTBP. (From JG Harpel et al. Control of transforming growth factor-β activity: Latency vs. activation. *Prog Growth Factor Res* 4:321, 1992. Reproduced with kind permission from Pergamon Press Ltd, Headington Hill Hall, Oxford 0X3 0BW, UK, copyright© 1992.)

lines of mink lung epithelial cells, loss of the type 2 receptors is always accompanied by loss of the type 1 receptors (according to affinity crosslinking studies). Transfection of type 2 receptors back into the receptor-deficient mutants resulted in the appearance of both types of receptors [125]. This led to the conclusion that the type 1 receptor requires the type 2 receptor for transport to the cell surface, TGF-β binding, or both [123,125]. It is also possible that the type 2 receptor is required to stabilize the type 1 receptor.

There is evidence that the type 2 receptor subtype is required for the growth inhibitory responses to TGF-β. Several studies have shown an association between loss of the type 2 TGF-β receptor and loss of growth inhibition in response to TGF-β [126–128]. Growth inhibition by TGF-β was restored in TGF-β-resistant hepatoma cells (that lack the type 2 receptor) after transfection of the TGF-β type 2 receptor cDNA [128]. Functional inactivation of the type 2 receptors in mink lung epithelial cells by overexpression of a mutant type 2 receptor (truncated in the cytoplasmic domain) resulted in loss of growth inhibitory response to TGF-β, although TGF-β-dependent induction of *jun*-B, fibronectin, and plasminogen activator inhibitor-type 1 (PAI-1) (presumably through activation of the type 1 receptor) were retained [126].

The type 3 receptor in most cells is a proteoglycan with a 100-kDa protein core (β-glycan) and a short cytoplasmic domain [112,122]. Another type 3 receptor proteoglycan (endoglin) has been found on endothelial cells and contains a disulfide-linked homodimer of 95-kDa subunit polypeptides [129]. β-glycan binds to all three types of TGF-β, whereas endoglin binds to TGF-β1 and TGF-β3 but not to TGF-β2. These proteoglycan type 3 receptors are thought to be incapable of signal transduction, but they may be important for presenting TGF-β to the signaling type 1 and 2 receptors [112,122,130].

TGF-β and Mechanisms of Cell Growth Regulation

Transforming growth factor-β can regulate the growth of many cell types in culture [112–114]. Several recent studies have begun to provide insight into the mechanisms of growth regulation by TGF-β. It appears to be an indirect mitogen for AKR-2B mouse fibroblasts and for aortic smooth muscle cells. In the aortic smooth muscle cells, TGF-β induced the synthesis of PDGF-A [131], and TGF-β stimulation of DNA synthesis could be blocked with neutralizing antibodies to PDGF-AA. In AKR-2B cells, the transcription of c-*sis* (PDGF-B) increased rapidly after TGF-β treatment. A series of studies by Howe and Leof [132–134] suggest that c-*sis* induction and growth stimulation may occur through coupling of the TGF-β receptor to guanine nucleotide-binding regulatory proteins (G proteins), whereas other actions of TGF-β, such as induction of fibronectin expression, are not mediated by G proteins.

Although mitogenic for selected mesenchyme-derived cells in culture, TGF-β is a growth inhibitor for most other cell types, including mesenchymal, epithelial, endothelial, hematopoietic, myogenic, and neural tissues [112–114,121]. Most data indicate that TGF-β blocks cell-cycle progression in middle to late G1, before the initiation of DNA synthesis. It does not interfere with the binding of mitogenic growth factors or the activation of mitogenic growth factor receptors.

The induction of immediate early genes that mark G0 to G1 transition after mitogenic stimulation of quiescent cells is also not prevented by TGF-β [135]. As discussed above, the phosphorylation of the retinoblastoma gene product ($p105^{Rb}$) appears to be necessary for cells to enter the S phase (DNA synthesis) [8,9]. The TGF-β prevents phosphorylation of $p105^{Rb}$ [136,137], and appears to regulate the activity of the cyclins and cyclin-dependent kinases (including $p34^{cdk4}$ and $p33^{cdk2}$) that phosphorylate $p105^{Rb}$ and related proteins [136,138]. In some cell types (e.g., mouse keratinocytes), the ability of TGF-β to inhibit cell growth also appears to be linked with its ability to down-regulate expression of the c-*myc* gene [138,139].

TGF-β and Intestinal Epithelial Cells

The intestinal epithelium is one of the most rapidly proliferating tissues in the body; it is able to replicate every 3 to 8 days. There is normally a dynamic equilibrium between cell proliferation at the base of the crypt and cell extrusion at the tip of the villus. Cells in the crypt are rapidly proliferating and less differentiated, whereas cells nearer the villus tip are terminally differentiated and do not divide. This continual process of mucosal renewal is tightly regulated and is altered during malignant transformation. In experimental models of colon carcinogenesis, there is an increase in the proliferative compartment that is thought to be, in part, the result of loss of normal inhibitory controls. This aberrant regulation leads to intestinal hyperplasia and subsequent formation of adenoma, carcinoma in situ, and finally invasive carcinoma [140,141].

Intestinal crypt cell proliferation is thought to be regulated by autocrine and paracrine peptide growth factors [35–37, 39–43] that stimulate or inhibit proliferation. Among these factors, the TGF-β family of peptides appears to have a major role in differentiation and growth inhibition of the intestinal epithelium. Because TGF-β is a potent inhibitor of cultured rat intestinal crypt cell proliferation, it has been postulated that TGF-β may be an important physiologic regulator of normal intestinal cell proliferation and a suppressor of uncontrolled gut growth [127,135,142–144]. It is also a potent stimulant of intestinal cell migration and possibly has a role in repair of epithelial wounds [145].

The TGF-β1 mRNA is expressed and TGF-β bioactivity is secreted by a normal rat intestinal crypt cell line, IEC-6 [135,142,144]. The TGF-β1 inhibits proliferation of IEC-6 cells and induces their differentiation, as evidenced by stimulation of sucrase activity [144], immunoglobulin A secretory component production, and major histocompatibility complex class I antigen expression [146].

Although TGF-β1 appears to be an important negative regulator of intestinal cell replication, the mechanisms are not fully understood. It inhibits intestinal crypt (IEC-6) cell proliferation by blocking cell-cycle progression at a point in the middle of the G1 phase of the cell cycle (Figure 5-10). It does not block early G1 events, such as induction of c-*myc* or other immediate early genes [135]. However, TGF-β blocks induction of *cdc2,* during the G1/S transition. The specific G1 event that is directly regulated by TGF-β to cause growth inhibition is not known.

Transforming growth factor-β is found in the gut epithelium, and has inhibitory growth effects on intestinal cell cultures. There is increased ex-

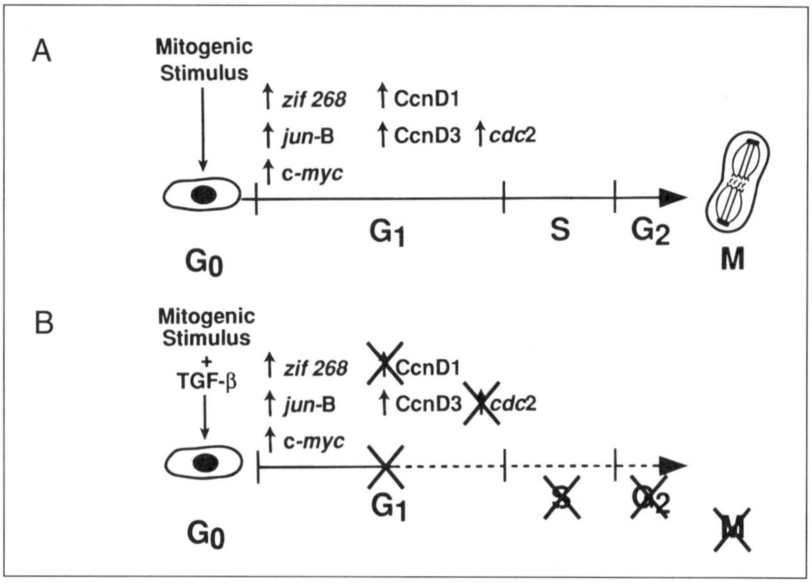

Figure 5-10. TGF-β blocks progression through the cell cycle in IEC-6 cells. **(A)** Addition of a mitogenic stimulus (e.g., serum) to quiescent (G_0). IEC-6 cells result in rapid induction of immediate early genes (e.g., zif 268, *jun*-B, c-*myc*) followed by an increase in *cdc2* and DNA synthesis (S phase) by 12 hours, then cell division (M phase). **(B)** TGF-β treatment, added simultaneously with serum, interrupts the cell cycle in mid-G_1 and prevents the increase in *cdc2* and subsequent DNA synthesis. In addition, we have recently found that the G_1 cyclins D1 (*CcnD1*) and D3 (*CcnD3*) are increased during G_1. TGF-β treatment blocks the induction of *CcnD1* in mid-G_1, but does not alter *CcnD3* levels (unpublished data).

pression of TGF-β1 mRNA in rat intestinal cells, as they migrate from crypt to the villus tip [147], establishing a reciprocal relationship between TGF-β expression and proliferation. This crypt-to-villus distribution was recently confirmed by immunohistochemical analysis in which Barnard and colleagues [148] demonstrated that TGF-β1, 2, and 3 were all expressed in the epithelium of the small and large bowel (Figures 5-11 and 5-12). The TGF-βs were found predominantly in the villus tip cells that had stopped dividing and had undergone terminal differentiation and were not detected in the proliferating crypt compartment [148]. These findings support the current view that TGF-β is the major autocrine or paracrine regulator of intestinal cell proliferation and differentiation and accounts for the phenotypic changes that occur as intestinal epithelial cells migrate from the crypt toward the villus.

TGF-β and Liver

The TGF-β may regulate liver cell proliferation as well as expression of liver-specific genes. When parenterally administered, TGF-β1 or TGF-β2 can delay the first wave of DNA synthesis in the regenerating rat liver; however, regeneration of liver mass (measured after 8 days) is not delayed [149]. The TGF-β1 also inhibits the growth of nontransformed hepatocytes in primary culture [150,151]. Expression of TGF-β1 is low in quiescent adult liver and increases early (4 hours after partial hepatectomy) during hepatic regeneration [152]. These observations indicate that although TGF-β is expressed early during hepatic regeneration, it is not clear that its primary role is the inhibition of liver cell proliferation. Processes other than cell proliferation that are important for the establishment of reconstituted tissue may be equally im-

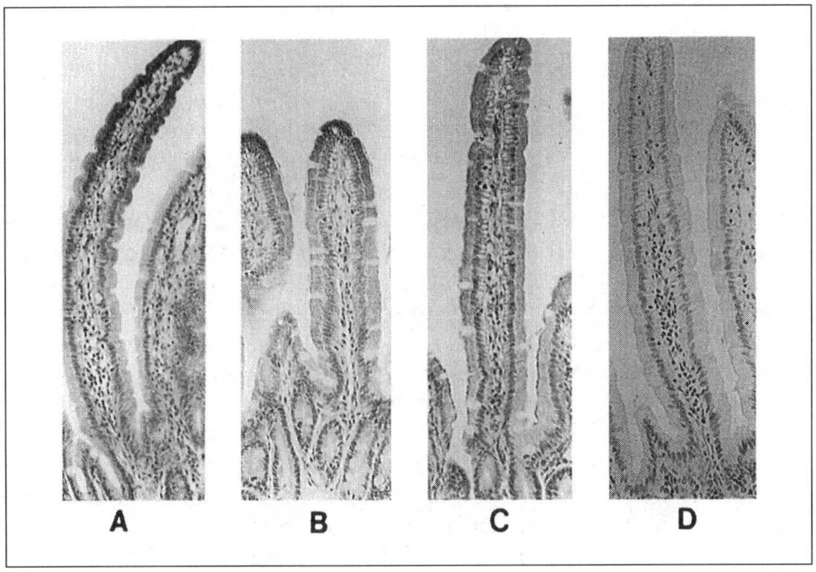

Figure 5-11. Immunohistochemistry showing the expression of TGF-β1, TGF-β2, and TGF-β3 proteins along the normal adult mouse jejunal crypt-villus axis. Secretions were incubated with affinity-purified polyclonal antibodies to TGF-β1 **(A)**, TGF-β2 **(B)**, TGF-β3 **(C)**, and isotypic IgG **(D)**, and color was developed using the avidin-peroxidase system. In **(A)–(C)** expression is primarily epithelial and most prominent at the villus tip. No staining is seen in **(D).** (From JA Barnard et al. Localization of transforming growth factor β isoforms in the normal murine small intestine and colon. *Gastroenterology* 105:67, 1993. Reproduced with permission from W.B. Saunders Co., Orlando, FL.)

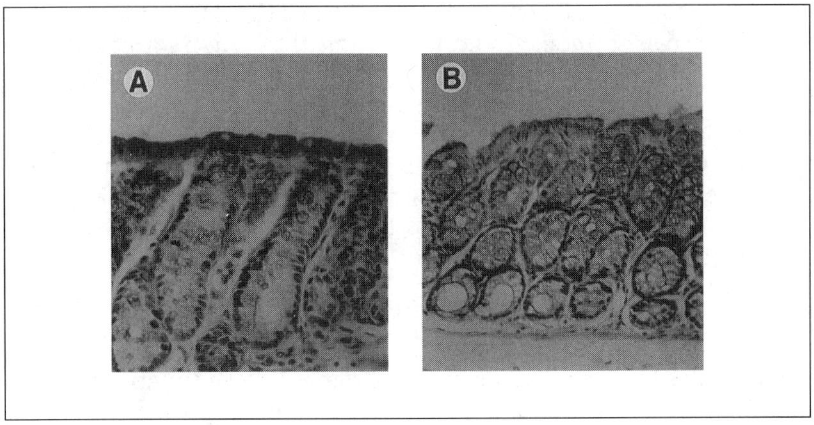

Figure 5-12. Immunohistochemistry showing the expression of TGF-β2 in the mouse colon (midcolon) **(A)**. No staining was seen in sections incubated with isotypic IgG **(B)**. Expression is most prominent in surface colonocytes. Immunopositive cells are also seen in cells near the neck of mucus glands, but cells at the base of the glands are immunonegative. Goblet cells and mucosal lymphocytes are negative. (From JA Barnard et al. Localization of transforming growth factor β isoforms in the normal murine small intestine and colon. *Gastroenterology* 105:67, 1993. Reproduced with permission from W.B. Saunders Co., Orlando, FL.)

portant targets of TGF-β action. For example, TGF-β regulates extracellular matrix and can regulate differentiated cell function in other systems [121,153]. Increased expression of TGF-β has also been implicated in hepatic fibrosis in rodents [154] and in humans [155]. Furthermore, active TGF-β in the circulation is rapidly cleared ($T_{1/2}$ 2 to 3 min) and metabolized by the liver [156,157], whereas the latent TGF-β complex has a greatly extended plasma half-life (> 100 min) and remains largely confined to the circulating plasma pools [157].

Regulation of Inflammation, Tissue Repair and Development

There appear to be numerous other biologically important effects of TGF-β, in both normal physiology and pathophysiology. Despite the well-described growth inhibitory actions of TGF-β in cell culture, expression of TGF-β in vivo is often greatest in tissues that are actively growing [112–115,121,158,159]. Perhaps this represents a constant brake on growth. It may also be that other actions of TGF-β are important for tissue regeneration and repair. The most concentrated source of TGF-β in the body is in the α granules of platelets, and TGF-β is released at sites of tissue injury. Transforming growth factor-β is also released by other cells such as activated macrophages, lymphocytes and fibroblasts that are abundant in tissue that is injured and undergoing repair. Release of TGF-β is increased from circulating monocytes of severely injured patients in association with the immunosuppressed state [160]. One target of the cytokines (including TGF-β) released after injury is the liver.

The TGF-β may act as a regulator of the hepatic acute-phase response [161–163]. Secretion of some of the positive acute-phase reactants (α_1-protease inhibitor and α_1-antichymotrypsin) from human hepatoma cells is increased by TGF-β1 treatment [162]. There are also negative acute-phase reactants, including albumin, whose concentrations decrease after injury [164]. The TGF-β1 decreases albumin mRNA abundance and inhibits albumin secretion in human hepatoma cells [161–163] and in primary cultures of normal adult human hepatocytes [161]. The decrease in albumin and α-fetoprotein mRNA occurs primarily at the post-transcriptional level [165].

Expression of TGF-β in the developing embryo and fetus is greatest in sites undergoing intense developmental morphogenesis and remodeling [114,158,159]. The TGF-β has important roles in tissue repair in adult organisms [48,112,114, 115,166], because it is stored in platelet α granules and expressed in activated macrophages, where it can be delivered to sites of injury and inflammation. The combined actions of TGF-β, including the induction of extracellular matrix, chemoattraction of fibroblasts and monocytes, promotion of epithelial cell migration, and regulation of chondrocyte and bone cell proliferation and function, all contribute to the wound-healing actions of TGF-β. In experimental animal models, TGF-β has been shown to be effective in promoting the healing of cutaneous wounds, bone fractures, and retinal detachment. On the other hand, excessive production of TGF-β appears to contribute to pathologic fibrosis in numerous organs and tissues including the eye, lungs, kidneys, and liver.

The regulation of the inflammatory response appears to be among the more important actions of TGF-β [112,114,115]. The effects on the inflammatory response are pleiotropic. The TGF-β is a potent chemoattractant for leukocyte infiltration into wounds, and it appears to be involved in the early activation of monocytes and T lymphocytes. Conversely, the predominant overall effects of TGF-β seem to be both anti-inflammatory and immunosuppressive through the inhibition of lymphocyte proliferation, suppression of the functions of activated macrophages, and inhibition of cytokine expression and actions. A striking example of the importance of TGF-β in modulating the inflammatory response was recently demonstrated through the creation of mice with a nonfunctional TGF-β1 gene [167,168]. These mice did not express functional TGF-β1 protein, but were born without any obvious gross developmental defect. Within two to three weeks of age, they began to die from a diffuse inflammatory syndrome that was characterized by massive mononuclear cell infiltration of multiple organ systems. Although it was surprising that these mice did not have gross developmental defects, it is likely that the redundancy of expression of other TGF-β isoforms adequately replaced the TGF-β1 during development. It is interesting that this redundancy did not extend to regulation of the inflammatory response in TGF-β-deficient mice. This is one of the few examples of physiologically relevant functional differences among the TGF-β isoforms. Transgenic ablation studies have not been reported for the other TGF-β isoforms.

TGF-β Regulation of Gene Expression

Transforming growth factor-β regulates the expression of several genes whose functions do not appear to be directly related to growth inhibition

[112,114,115,158,159]. It suppresses transcription of the transin–stromelysin gene and the myogenic regulatory gene Myo D1. In contrast, TGF-β increases the transcription of several other genes, including α2(I) collagen [169], plasminogen activator inhibitor type-1 [170], *jun*-B [171], fibronectin [172], and TGF-β1 itself [173,174]. In some cases, TGF-β-responsive *cis*-acting elements have been identified [169,173], and the *trans*-acting proteins that interact with those elements are under examination. For example, a nuclear factor-1 binding site mediates the transcriptional activator of the α2(I) collagen promoter [169].

A group of transcriptional regulatory proteins called the *activating protein complex* (AP-1) appears to be involved in mediating some of the transcriptional effects of TGF-β [173,175]. The AP-1 complex is a family of dimeric nuclear proteins that were originally discovered to mediate transcriptional regulation by phorbol esters (TPA or PMA) [176–179]. Genes that are induced by PMA have a consensus DNA sequence (TGA[C/G]TCA) in the regulatory region that can bind to the AP-1 protein complex, and this interaction regulates transcription. The AP-1 complex can comprise either homodimers of JUN protein or heterodimers of JUN and FOS proteins. The c-*jun* proto-oncogene is the cellular homologue of the transforming v-*jun* gene, first isolated from a retrovirus that causes tumors in chickens. Three separate but homologous members of the *jun* proto-oncogene family have been identified and are called c-*jun*, *jun*-B, and *jun*-D. In differentiated myocytes, the rapid transcriptional induction of *jun*-B by TGF-β is independent of protein synthesis and is among the earliest responses to TGF-β [171].

The other component of the AP-1 complex is the FOS protein. The *fos* family includes c-*fos* [176–179] and more recently identified genes encoding homologous proteins: *fos*-B, *fra*-1, and *fra*-2. FOS:JUN protein heterodimers form more stable complexes with the AP-1 site than JUN:-JUN homodimers. Any JUN protein can interact with any FOS protein. Although induction of *jun* expression is among the earliest responses to TGF-β in most cell types [171,180], TGF-β also induces *fos*-B expression in mouse hepatocytes [181]. Many of the actions of TGF-β probably result from the activation of AP-1.

TGF-β and Cancer

Loss of responsiveness to the inhibitory effects of TGF-β appears to be an important event in the loss of normal growth control that attends malignant transformation. For example, TGF-β regulation of intestinal cell proliferation is altered during malignant transformation. TGF-β is a potent growth suppressor of nontumorigenic human colonic adenoma cells [182]. However, conversion of adenoma to a tumorigenic adenocarcinoma is associated with a decreased response to the inhibitory actions of TGF-β [182]. Transformation of a normal rat intestinal epithelial cell line (IEC-18) to a tumorigenic phenotype by overexpression of H-*ras* gene results in a loss of TGF-β-mediated growth regulation [127]. Studies in human colon carcinoma cell lines have demonstrated strong correlation between the degree of differentiation of the tumor and sensitivity to the antiproliferative and differentiation-promoting effects of TGF-β [183]. Although TGF-β inhibits the growth of most epithelial and lymphoid cells, malignant transformation results in escape from normal growth control that often involves loss of TGF-β responsiveness [184].

Manning and colleagues [182] found that loss of responsiveness to growth inhibitory actions of TGF-β may contribute to tumor progression in colonic neoplasia. In a reported histopathologic analysis of human colon mucosal and adenocarcinoma specimens, the TGF-β1 distribution was limited to the surface of normal colonic epithelium [185]. This distribution was identical to that found in normal mouse colon by Barnard and colleagues [148]. In epithelium immediately adjacent to carcinomas, the TGF-β was diffusely distributed throughout the colonic gland, 46 of 48 cancers, and 9 of 10 adenomas. Tumors grow despite this high level of exposure to a potent growth inhibitor. Progression from a colon adenoma cell line to carcinoma in tissue culture coincides with the development of resistance to the growth-inhibitory actions of TGF-β [182]. Goyette and colleagues [186] have shown that the loss of the candidate tumor suppressor gene DCC (deleted in colon cancer) may be involved in the loss of TGF-β responsiveness in colorectal carcinomas. The DCC gene shares homology with the neural cell adhesion molecule (N-CAM). Other potential mechanisms of TGF-β resistance have been identified in cultured cells. Functional knockout of the type 2 TGF-β receptors by overexpression of a truncated mutant type 2 receptor results in loss of the growth-inhibitory responsiveness to TGF-β in mink lung epithelial cells [126]. Intestinal epithelial cells transformed with the Ha-*ras* oncogene develop resistance to the growth-inhibitory actions of TGF-β and exhibit loss of type 2 receptors [127].

Other mechanisms by which cells may acquire resistance to the growth-inhibitory actions of

TGF-β may involve abrogation of part of the signal transduction pathway. Pietenpol and associates [187] observed that human foreskin keratinocytes that were transformed with DNA tumor virus (either HPV-16, HPV-18, or SV-40) were resistant to the growth-inhibitory actions of TGF-β. This loss of TGF-β responsiveness appears to result from the failure of TGF-β to down-regulate c-*myc* expression in the transformed cells. The loss of c-*myc* regulation could be induced by transient expression of transforming proteins and appears to indicate disruption of the normal signal transduction process [139,188].

Suardet and associates [189], in a study of colon cancer cell lines, proposed that TGF-β responsiveness may correlate inversely with TGF-β production, so that TGF-β resistant cells may be selected in the environment of tumors that produce high amounts of TGF-β. One may speculate that TGF-β resistance may arise spontaneously with a finite frequency because of the genomic instability that is characteristic of neoplastic cells. An apparent paradoxical relationship may exist in which TGF-β production in tumor cells that have lost the growth-inhibitory responsiveness to TGF-β may actually be a critical determinant in the ability of the tumor to grow. Torre-Amione and associates [120] demonstrated that expression of TGF-β by tumor cells suppresses the immune responses directed against those tumors in vivo. Sieweke and co-workers [190] implicated TGF-β expression in the mediation of wound-related Rous sarcoma virus tumorigenesis, in which wounding leads to nearly 100% tumor incidence in Rous sarcoma virus–infected chickens. Wounding results in the local expression of TGF-β, and subcutaneous administration of TGF-β1 can substitute for wounding in the induction of the sarcomas. Production of TGF-β promotes growth and metastatic potential of fibrosarcomas and mammary adenocarcinomas in vivo [191–193]. Steiner and Barrack [194] demonstrated that rat prostate cancer cells that were transfected and overexpressed the latent TGF-β1 protein demonstrated enhanced tumor growth in vivo. Thus, it seems reasonable to conclude that, before malignant transformation, TGF-β acts to inhibit epithelial cell growth but, after transformation, TGF-β appears to promote tumor growth and invasiveness through several mechanisms. It seems likely that if we can understand the mechanistic basis of these paradoxical effects of TGF-β, we will have come a long way toward understanding the physiologic and pathologic bases of TGF-β action. This is an area of active research at this time, and exciting new developments are to be expected over the next few years.

Summary

The term *growth factors* is loosely applied to a diverse group of polypeptide hormones that have the ability to influence mitotic activity. In most cases, the proliferative effects of these substances have been defined in tissue culture. In very few cases is it clear that regulation of cell proliferation is the only, or even the most important, effect of these factors in vivo. Many, perhaps all, growth factors have the ability to regulate the metabolic activity of cells, and it is certain that cellular metabolism has a direct influence on cellular renewal processes. The relationship between cellular energy charge, nucleotide biosynthetic processes, and initiation of DNA synthesis is a classic example that serves to make the point that growth promotion need not necessarily emanate from a change in the expression of some critical regulatory principle, such as a proto-oncogene or some other cell-cycle progression factor. Although such changes in gene expression are characteristic of the response to growth factors, this does not mean that the primary effect of the growth factor is to stimulate the expression of such genes. Indeed, there are many cases in which the expression of cell-cycle progression factors changes as a result of stimulation of cell proliferation, rather than as a cause. It is well to bear in mind that the growth-promoting properties of some growth factors may come to be understood in terms of metabolic, rather than transcriptional, regulation.

It is also the case that some growth factors exert their effects by directly regulating the expression of genes that encode key cell-cycle progression factors. Transforming growth factor-β is one of the most likely candidates for such a factor, and a number of laboratories are actively involved in studying the molecular mechanisms of TGF-β action in several different types of cells. The results are a bit confusing at this time. If the reports in the literature are taken at face value, then different cell types must respond in significantly different ways. One is inclined to believe that we have not yet identified the primary effect of TGF-β, from which a more diverse set of responses may emanate. This remains to be seen.

We are beginning to gain insight into the molecular mechanisms of action of growth factors. The purpose of this review is to highlight a number of very interesting questions that can be raised with respect to this class of substances. It is certain that growth factors are essential modulators of metabolism, differentiation, and proliferation of cells both in culture and in vivo. Growth factors impinge on normal physiologic processes and are certain to be important mediators of some metabolic disorders. Loss of growth factor responsiveness is one of the hallmarks of malignant transformation. One might suppose that we would know a lot more about the etiology of cancer if we understood how growth factors worked. One is entitled to expect that the study of growth factors will provide exciting new insights into cellular physiology, gene regulation, and a number of very important disease processes.

References

1. Delarco J, Todaro GJ. Growth factors from murine sarcoma virus-transformed cells. *Proc Natl Acad Sci USA* 75:4001, 1978.
2. Fong Y, Lowry SF. Cytokines and the Cellular Response to Injury and Infection. In DW Wilmore et al (eds), *American College of Surgeons Care of the Surgical Patient,* Vol 1. New York: Scientific American, 1988. Pp 1–22.
3. Meyerson M, et al. The cyclin-dependent kinase family. *Cold Spring Harb Symp Quant Biol* 56:177, 1991.
4. Pines J. Cyclins and cyclin-dependent kinases: Take your partners. *Trends Biochem Sci* 18:195, 1993.
5. Reed SI. The role of p34 kinases in the G1 to S-phase transition. *Annu Rev Cell Biol* 8:529, 1992.
6. Sherr CJ. Mammalian G_1 cyclins. *Cell* 73:1059, 1993.
7. Kato JY, et al. Direct binding of cyclin D to the retinoblastoma gene product (pRb) and pRb phosphorylation by the cyclin D-dependent kinase CDK4. *Genes Dev* 7:331, 1993.
8. Nevins JR, et al. E2F transcription factor is a target for the RB protein and the cyclin A protein. *Cold Spring Harb Symp Quant Biol* 56:157, 1991.
9. Nigg EA. Targets of cyclin-dependent protein kinases. *Curr Opin Cell Biol* 5:187, 1993.
10. Chellappan SP, et al. The E2F transcription factor is a cellular target for the RB protein. *Cell* 65:1053, 1991.
11. Nevins JR. E2F: A link between the Rb tumor suppressor protein and viral oncoproteins. *Science* 258:424, 1992.
12. Hamel PA, et al. Transcriptional repression of the E2-containing promoters EIIaE, c-*myc,* and RB1 by the product of the RB1 gene. *Mol Cell Biol* 12:3431, 1992.
13. Hiebert SW, et al. The interaction of RB with E2F coincides with an inhibition of the transcriptional activity of E2F. *Genes Dev* 6:177, 1992.
14. Pines J. Cyclins: Wheels within wheels. *Cell Growth Differ* 2:305, 1991.
15. Draetta G. Cell cycle control in eukaryotes: Molecular mechanisms of *cdc*2 activation. *Trends Biochem Sci* 15:378, 1990.
16. Ohtsubo M, Roberts JM. Cyclin-dependent regulation of G_1 in mammalian fibroblasts. *Science* 259:1908, 1993.
17. Baldin V, et al. Cyclin D1 is a nuclear protein required for cell cycle progression in G1. *Genes Dev* 7:812, 1993.
18. Matsushime H, et al. Identification and properties of an atypical catalytic subunit ($p34^{PSK-J3}$/cdk4) for mammalian D type G1 cyclins. *Cell* 71:323, 1992.
19. Quelle DE, et al. Overexpression of mouse D-type cyclins accelerates G1 phase in rodent fibroblasts. *Genes Dev* 7:1559, 1993.
20. Motokura T, Arnold A. Cyclins and oncogenesis. *Biochim Biophys Acta* 1155:63, 1993.
21. Dowdy SF, et al. Physical interaction of the retinoblastoma protein with human D cyclins. *Cell* 73:499, 1993.
22. Ewen ME, et al. Functional interactions of the retinoblastoma protein with mammalian D-type cyclins. *Cell* 73:487, 1993.
23. Hall FL, et al. Two potentially oncogenic cyclins, cyclin A and cyclin D1, share common properties of subunit configuration, tyrosine phosphorylation and physical association with the Rb protein. *Oncogene* 8:1377, 1993.
24. Xiong Y, Zhang H, Beach D. D type cyclins associate with multiple protein kinases and the DNA replication and repair factor PCNA. *Cell* 71:505, 1992.
25. Cadena DL, Gill GN. Receptor tyrosine kinases. *FASEB J* 6:2332, 1992.
26. Hatakeyama M, et al. Interaction of the IL-2 receptor with the src-family kinase p561ck: Identification of novel intermolecular association. *Science* 252:1523, 1991.
27. Carpenter G. Receptor tyrosine kinase substrates: *src* homology domains and signal transduction. *FASEB J* 6:3283, 1992.
28. Siddle K. The insulin receptor and type I IGF receptor: Comparison of structure and function. *Prog Growth Factor Res* 4:301, 1992.
29. Crews CM, Erikson RL. Extracellular signals and reversible protein phosphorylation: What to Mek of it al. *Cell* 74:215, 1993.
30. Crews CM, Alessandrini A, Erikson RL. Erks: Their fifteen minutes has arrived. *Cell Growth Differ* 3:135, 1992.
31. Pelech SL, Sanghera JS. Mitogen-activated protein kinases: Versatile transducers for cell signaling. *Trends Biochem Sci* 17:233, 1992.
32. Kolch W, et al. Protein kinase C alpha activates RAF-1 by direct phosphorylation. *Nature* 364:249, 1993.
33. Sozeri O, et al. Activation of the c-Raf protein kinase by protein kinase C phosphorylation. *Oncogene* 7:2259, 1992.
34. Coffey RJ, et al. Transforming growth factors and related peptides in gastrointestinal neoplasia. *J Cell Biochem Suppl* 16G:111, 1992.
35. Podolsky DK. Peptide growth factors in the gastrointestinal tract: An overview. *Regul Pept Lett* 5:10, 1993.
36. Shing Y, et al. Betacellulin: A mitogen from pancreatic β cell tumors. *Science* 259:1604, 1993.
37. Holmes WE, et al. Identification of heregulin, a specific activator of $p185^{erbB2}$. *Science* 256:1205, 1992.
38. Massague J, Pandiella A. Membrane-anchored growth factors. *Annu Rev Biochem* 62:515, 1993.
39. Pandiella A, Massague J. Cleavage of the membrane precursor for transforming growth factor alpha is a regulated process. *Proc Natl Acad Sci USA* 88:1726, 1991.
40. Brachmann R, et al. Transmembrane TGF-α precursors activate EGF/TGF-α receptors. *Cell* 56:691, 1989.
41. Dobashi Y, Stern DF. Membrane-anchored forms of EGF stimulate focus formation and intercellular communication. *Oncogene* 6:1151, 1991.
42. Wong ST, et al. The TGF-α precursor expressed on the cell surface binds to the EGF receptor on adjacent cells, leading to signal transduction. *Cell* 56:495, 1989.
43. Cohen S. Isolation of a mouse submaxillary gland protein accelerating incisor eruption and eyelid opening in the new born animal. *J Biol Chem* 237:1555, 1962.
44. Beauchamp RD, et al. Localization of TGFα and its receptor in gastric mucosal cells: Implications for a regulatory role in acid secretion and mucosal renewal. *J Clin Invest* 84:1017, 1989.
45. Ahnen DJ, Wright NA. Growth factors, the ulcer associated cell lineage, and the repair of gastrointestinal mucosal injury. *Regul Pept Lett* 5:18, 1993.

46. Burgess AW. Epidermal growth factor and transforming growth factor α. *Bri Med Bull* 45:401, 1989.
47. Fisher DA, Lakshmanan J. Metabolism and effects of epidermal growth factor and related growth factors in mammals. *Endocrine Rev* 11:418, 1990.
48. Bennett NT, Schultz GS. Growth factors and wound healing: Biochemical properties of growth factors and their receptors. *Am J Surg* 165:728, 1993.
49. Prigent SA, Lemoine NR. The type 1 (EGFR-related) family of growth factor receptors and their ligands. *Prog Growth Factor Res* 4:1, 1992.
50. Malden LT, Novak U, Burgess AW. Expression of transforming growth factor alpha messenger RNA in the normal and neoplastic gastrointestinal tract. *Int J Cancer* 43:380, 1989.
51. Derynck R. Transforming growth factor-α: Structure and biological activities. *J Cell Biol* 32:293, 1986.
52. Schreiber AB, Winkler ME, Derynck R. Transforming growth factor-α: A more potent angiogenic mediator than epidermal growth factor. *Science* 232:1250, 1986.
53. Derynck R. Transforming growth factor alpha. *Cell* 54:593, 1988.
54. Cohen S, Carpenter G. Human epidermal growth factor: Isolation and chemical and biological properties. *Proc Natl Acad Sci USA* 72:1317, 1975.
55. Roberts AB, et al. Transforming growth factors: Isolation of polypeptides from virally and chemically transformed cells by acid/ethanol extraction. *Proc Natl Acad Sci USA* 77:3494, 1980.
56. Dempsey PJ, et al. Possible role of transforming growth factor α in the pathogenesis of Menetrier's disease: Supportive evidence from humans and transgenic mice. *Gastroenterology* 103:1950, 1992.
57. Finke U, et al. Effects of epidermal growth factor on acid secretion from guinea pig gastric mucosa: In vitro analysis. *Gastroenterology* 88:1175, 1985.
58. Gonzalez A, Garrido I, Vial ID. Epidermal growth factor inhibits cytoskeleton-related changes in the surface of parietal cells. *J Cell Biol* 88:108, 1981.
59. Gregory H, et al. The contribution of the C-terminal undecapeptide sequence of urogastrone-epidermal growth factor to its biological action. *Regul Pept Lett* 22:217, 1988.
60. Konturek SJ, et al. Effects of epidermal growth factor on gastrointestinal secretions. *Am J Physiol* 246:G580, 1984.
61. Rhodes JA, et al. Transforming growth factor-α inhibits secretion of gastric acid. *Proc Natl Acad Sci USA* 83:3844, 1986.
62. Konturek SJ, et al. Role of epidermal growth factor in healing of chronic gastroduodenal ulcers in rats. *Gastroenterology* 94:1300, 1988.
63. Konturek SJ, et al. Gastric cytoprotection by epidermal growth factor. *Gastroenterology* 81:438, 1981.
64. Skinner KA, Soper BD, Tepperman BL. Effect of sialoadenectomy and salivary gland extracts on gastrointestinal mucosal growth and gastrin levels in the rat. *J Physiol* 351:1, 1984.
65. Romano M, et al. Transforming growth factor alpha protection against drug-induced injury to the rat gastric mucosa in vivo. *J Clin Invest* 90:2409, 1992.
66. Polk WH Jr, et al. Increased production of transforming growth factor alpha following acute gastric injury. *Gastroenterology* 102:1467, 1992.
67. Derynck R, et al. Synthesis of messenger RNAs for transforming growth factors α and β and the epidermal growth factor receptor by human tumors. *Cancer Res* 47:707, 1987.
68. Kenney NJ, et al. Expression of transforming growth factor α antisense mRNA inhibits the estrogen-induced proliferation of estrogen-responsive human breast cancer cells. *J Cell Physiol* 156:497, 1993.
69. Pittelkow MR, et al. Induction of transforming growth factor-α expression in human keratinocytes by phorbol esters. *J Biol Chem* 264:5164, 1989.
70. Ciardiello F, et al. Differential expression of epidermal growth factor–related proteins in human colorectal tumors. *Proc Natl Acad Sci USA* 88:7792, 1991.
71. Cook PW, et al. A heparin sulfate-regulated human keratinocyte autocrine factor is similar or identical to amphiregulin. *Mol Cell Biol* 11:2547, 1991.
72. Plowman GD, et al. The amphiregulin gene encodes a novel epidermal growth factor-related protein with tumor-inhibitory activity. *Mol Cell Biol* 10:1969, 1990.
73. Shoyab M, et al. Amphiregulin: A bifunctional growth-modulating glycoprotein produced by the phorbol 12-myristate 13-acetate-treated human breast adenocarcinoma cell line MCF-7. *Proc Natl Acad Sci USA* 85:6528, 1988.
74. Shoyab M, et al. Structure and function of human amphiregulin: A member of the epidermal growth factor family. *Science* 243:1074, 1989.
75. Cook PW, et al. Amphiregulin messenger RNA is elevated in psoriatic epidermis and gastrointestinal carcinomas. *Cancer Res* 52:3224, 1992.
76. Saeki T, et al. Differential immunohistochemical detection of amphiregulin and cripto in human normal colon and colorectal tumors. *Cancer Res* 52:3467, 1992.
77. Ciccodicola A, et al. Molecular characterization of a gene of the "EGF family" expressed in undifferentiated human NTERA2 teratocarcinoma cells. *EMBO J* 8:1987, 1989.
78. Stroobant P, et al. Purification and characterization of vaccinia virus growth factor. *Cell* 42:383, 1985.
79. Clemmons DR, Underwood LE. Nutritional regulation of IGF-I and IGF binding proteins. *Annu Rev Nutr* 11:393, 1991.
80. Cohick WS, Clemmons DR. The insulin-like growth factors. *Annu Rev Physiol* 55:131, 1993.
81. LeRoith D (ed). *Insulin-like Growth Factors: Molecular and Cellular Aspects.* Boca Raton: CRC, 1991.
82. Lu K, Campisi J. Ras proteins are essential and selective for the action of insulin-like growth factor 1 late in the G_1 phase of the cell cycle in BALB/c murine fibroblasts. *Proc Natl Acad Sci USA* 89:3889, 1992.
83. Lu KH, Levine RA, Campisi J. c-ras-Ha gene expression is regulated by insulin or insulin-like growth factor and by epidermal growth factor in murine fibroblasts. *Mol Cell Biol* 9:3411, 1989.
84. Guler HP, et al. Insulin-like growth factors I and II in healthy man: Estimations of half-lives and production rates. *Acta Endocrinol* 121:753, 1989.
85. Frost RA, Tseng L. Insulin-like growth factor-binding protein-1 is phosphorylated by cultured human endometrial stromal cells and multiple protein kinases in vitro. *J Biol Chem* 266:18082, 1991.
86. Jones JI, et al. Phosphorylation of insulin-like growth factor (IGF)-binding protein 1 in cell culture and in vivo: Effects on affinity for IGF-I. *Proc Natl Acad Sci USA* 88:7481, 1991.
87. Behringer RR, et al. Expression of insulin-like growth factor I stimulates normal somatic growth in growth hormone-deficient transgenic mice. *Endocrinology* 127:1033, 1990.
88. Dong Y-L, et al. Impact of exogenous insulinlike growth

factor 1 on hepatic energy metabolism in burn injury. *Arch Surg* 128:703, 1993.

89. Strock LL, et al. The effect of insulin-like growth factor I on postburn hypermetabolism. *Surgery* 108:161, 1990.
90. Huang KF, Chung DH, Herndon DN. Insulin-like growth factor 1 (IGF-1) reduces gut atrophy and bacterial translocation after severe burn injury. *Arch Surg* 128:47, 1993.
91. Cullen KJ, et al. Insulin-like growth factor-II overexpression in MCF-7 cells induces phenotypic changes associated with malignant progression. *Mol Endocrinol* 6:91, 1992.
92. Guo Y-S, et al. Insulin-like growth factor-binding protein modulates the growth response to insulin-like growth factor 1 by human gastric cancer cells. *Gastroenterology* 104:1595, 1993.
93. Macaulay VM. Insulin-like growth factors and cancer: *Br J Cancer* 65:311, 1992.
94. Casscells W. Smooth muscle cell growth factors. *Prog Growth Factor Res* 3:177, 1991.
95. Heldin C-H, Westermark B. Possible in vivo effect and clinical utility of platelet-derived growth factor and PDGF antagonists. *Transplant Proc* 25:2074, 1993.
96. Khachigian LM, Chesterman CN. Platelet-derived growth factor and alternative splicing: A review. *Pathology* 24:280, 1992.
97. Westermark B, Claesson-Welsh L, Heldin C-H. Structural and functional aspects of the receptors for platelet-derived growth factor. *Prog Growth Factor Res* 1:253, 1989.
98. Westermark B, Heldin C-H. Platelet-derived growth factor: Structure, function and implications in normal and malignant cell growth. *Acta Oncologica* 32:101, 1993.
99. Rappolee DA, Werb Z. Macrophage-derived growth factors. *Curr Top Microbiol Immunol* 181:87, 1992.
100. Tahara E. Growth factors and oncogenes in human gastrointestinal carcinomas. *J Cancer Res Clin Oncol* 116:121, 1990.
101. Gullick WJ. Growth factors and oncogenes in breast cancer. *Prog Growth Factor Res* 2:1, 1990.
102. Beauchamp RD, et al. Expression of and response to growth regulatory peptides by two human pancreatic carcinoma cell lines. *Pancreas* 5:369, 1990.
103. Beauchamp RD, et al. Human carcinoid cell production of paracrine growth factors that can stimulate fibroblast and endothelial cell growth. *Cancer Res* 51:5253, 1991.
104. Funa K, et al. Expression of platelet-derived growth factor beta-receptors on stromal tissue cells in human carcinoid tumors. *Cancer Res* 50:748, 1990.
105. Johnson DE, Williams LT. Structural and functional diversity in the FGF receptor multigene family. *Adv Cancer Res* 60:1, 1993.
106. Partanen J, et al. Diverse receptors for fibroblast growth factors. *Prog Growth Factor Res* 4:69, 1992.
107. Folkman J, Klagsburn M. Angiogenic factors. *Science* 235:442, 1987.
108. Kandel J, et al. Neovascularization is associated with a switch to the export of bFGF in the multistep development of fibrosarcoma. *Cell* 66:1095, 1991.
109. Folkman J, et al. Duodenal ulcer: Discovery of a new mechanism and development of angiogenic therapy that accelerates healing. *Ann Surg* 214:414, 1991.
110. Niswander L, Martin GR. FGF-4 and BMP-2 have opposite effects on limb growth. *Nature* 361:68, 1993.
111. Jaye M, Schlessinger J, Dionne CA. Fibroblast growth factor receptor tyrosine kinases: Molecular analysis and signal transduction. *Biochim Biophys Acta* 1135:185, 1992.
112. Massague J, et al. Transforming growth factor-β. *Cancer Surv* 12:81, 1992.
113. Moses HL, et al. Regulation of Fibroblastic and Epithelial Cell Function by Transforming Growth Factors. In C Etievant, J Cros, YM Rustum (eds), *New Concepts in Cancer: Metastasis, Oncogenes, and Growth Factors.* London: MacMillan, 1990. Pp 218–230.
114. Sporn MB, Roberts AB. Transforming growth factor-β: Recent progress and new challenges. *J Cell Biol* 119:1017, 1992.
115. Wahl SM. Transforming growth factor beta (TGF-β) in inflammation: A cause and a cure. *J Clin Immunol* 12:61, 1992.
116. Harpel JG, et al. Control of transforming growth factor-β activity: Latency vs. activation. *Prog Growth Factor Res* 4:321, 1992.
117. Lyons RM, Moses HL. Transforming growth factors and the regulation of cell proliferation: A review. *Eur J Biochem* 187:467, 1990.
118. Sato Y, Rifkin DB. Inhibition of endothelial cell movement by pericytes and smooth muscle cells: Activation of a latent TGFβ1-like molecule by plasmin during coculture. *J Cell Biol* 109:309, 1989.
119. Beauchamp RD, et al. Phenotypic alterations in fibroblasts and fibrosarcoma cells that overexpress latent transforming growth factor-β1. *Endocrinology* 130:2476, 1992.
120. Torre-Amione G, et al. A highly immunogenic tumor transfected with a murine TGF-β1 cDNA escapes immune surveillance. *Proc Natl Acad Sci USA* 87:1486, 1990.
121. Massague J. The transforming growth factor-β family. *Annu Rev Cell Biol* 6:597, 1990.
122. Massague J. Receptors for the TGF-β family. *Cell* 69:1067, 1992.
123. Ebner R, et al. Cloning of a type I TGF-β receptor and its effect on TGF-β binding to the type II receptor. *Science* 260:1344, 1993.
124. Lin HY, et al. Expression cloning of the TGF-β type II receptor, a functional transmembrane serine/threonine kinase. *Cell* 68:775, 1992.
125. Wrana JL, et al. TGF beta signals through a heteromeric protein kinase receptor complex. *Cell* 71:1003, 1992.
126. Chen R-H, Ebner R, Derynck R. Inactivation of the type II receptor reveals two receptor pathways for the diverse TGF-β activities. *Science* 260:1335, 1993.
127. Filmus J, Zhao J, Buick RN. Overexpression of H-*ras* oncogene induces resistance to the growth-inhibitory action of transforming growth factor beta-1 (TGF-β1) and alters the number and type of TGF-β1 receptors in rat intestinal epithelial cell clones. *Oncogene* 7:521, 1992.
128. Inagaki M, et al. Growth inhibition by transforming growth factor β (TGF-β) type I is restored in TGF-β-resistant hepatoma cells after expression of TGF-β receptor type II cDNA. *Proc Natl Acad Sci USA* 90:5359, 1993.
129. Cheifitz S, et al. Endoglin is a component of the transforming growth factor-β receptor system in human endothelial cells. *J Biol Chem* 267:19027, 1992.
130. Lopez-Casillas F, Wrana JL, Massague J. Betaglycan presents ligand to the TGF beta signaling receptor. *Cell* 73:1435, 1993.
131. Battegay EJ, et al. TGF-β induces bimodal proliferation of connective tissue cells via complex control of an autocrine PDGF loop. *Cell* 63:515, 1990.

132. Howe PH, et al. Regulation of transforming growth factor beta 1 action by multiple transducing pathways: Evidence for both G protein-dependent and -independent signaling. *Cancer Res* 49:6024, 1989.
133. Howe PH, Cunningham MR, Leof EB. Distinct pathways regulate transforming growth factor beta 1-stimulated proto-oncogene and extracellular matrix gene expression. *J Cell Physiol* 142:39, 1990.
134. Howe PH, Cunningham MR, Leof EB. Inhibition of mink lung epithelial cell proliferation by transforming growth factor-beta is coupled through a pertussis-toxin-sensitive substrate. *Biochem J* 266:537, 1990.
135. Ko TC, et al. Transforming growth factor β inhibits rat intestinal cell growth by regulating cell cycle specific gene expression. *Am J Surg,* in press.
136. Koff A, et al. Negative regulation of G1 in mammalian cells: Inhibition of cyclin E-dependent kinase by TGF-β. *Science* 260:536, 1993.
137. Laiho M, et al. Growth inhibition by TGF-beta linked to suppression of retinoblastoma protein phosphorylation. *Cell* 62:175, 1990.
138. Ewen ME, et al. TGFβ inhibition of cdk4 synthesis is linked to cell cycle arrest. *Cell* 74:1009, 1993.
139. Pietenpol JA, et al. Transforming growth factor beta 1 suppression of c-*myc* gene transcription: Role in inhibition of keratinocyte proliferation. *Proc Natl Acad Sci USA* 87:3758, 1990.
140. Fearon ER. Genetic alterations underlying colorectal tumorigenesis. *Cancer Surv* 12:119, 1992.
141. Sporn MB, Roberts AB. Autocrine growth factors and cancer. *Nature* 313:745, 1985.
142. Barnard JA, et al. Regulation of intestinal epithelial cell growth by transforming growth factor type β. *Proc Natl Acad Sci USA* 86:1578, 1989.
143. Ko TC, et al. Mechanism of action of transforming growth factor-β on rat jejunal cells. *Surg Forum* 43:135, 1992.
144. Kurokowa M, Lynch K, Podolsky DK. Effects of growth factors on an intestinal epithelial cell line: Transforming growth factor β inhibits proliferation and stimulates differentiation. *Biochem Biophys Res Commun* 142:775, 1987.
145. Ciacci C, Lind SE, Podolsky DK. Transforming growth factor β regulation of migration in wounded rat intestinal epithelial monolayers. *Gastroenterology* 105:93, 1993.
146. Howe PH, Draetta G, Leof EB. Transforming growth factor beta 1 inhibition of p34cdc2 phosphorylation and histone H1 kinase activity is associated with G1/S-phase growth arrest. *Mol Cell Biol* 11:1185, 1991.
147. Babyatsky MW, Podolsky DK. Growth and Development in the Gastrointestinal Tract. In T Yamada et al (eds), *Textbook of Gastroenterology.* Philadelphia: Lippincott, 1991. Pp 475–501.
148. Barnard JA, Warwick GJ, Gold LI. Localization of transforming growth factor β isoforms in the normal murine small intestine and colon. *Gastroenterology* 105:67, 1993.
149. Russell WE, et al. Type β transforming growth factor reversibly inhibits the early proliferative response to partial hepatectomy in the rat. *Proc Natl Acad Sci USA* 85:5126, 1988.
150. Carr BI, et al. Inhibition of DNA synthesis in rat hepatocytes by platelet-derived type β transforming growth factor. *Cancer Res* 46:2330, 1986.
151. Nakamura T, et al. Inhibitory effect of transforming growth factor-β on DNA synthesis of adult rat hepatocytes in primary culture. *Biochim Biophys Res Commun* 133:1042, 1985.
152. Braun L, et al. Transforming growth factor β mRNA increases during liver regeneration: A possible paracrine mechanism of growth regulation. *Proc Natl Acad Sci USA* 85:1539, 1988.
153. Sporn MB, Roberts AB. Transforming growth factor-β: Multiple actions and potential clinical applications. *JAMA* 262:938, 1989.
154. Czaja MJ, et al. In vitro and in vivo association of transforming growth factor-β1 with hepatic fibrosis. *J Cell Biol* 108:2477, 1989.
155. Castilla A, Prieto J, Fausto N. Transforming growth factors β1 and α in chronic liver disease: Effects of interferon alpha therapy. *N Engl J Med* 324:933, 1991.
156. Coffey RJ Jr, et al. Hepatic processing of transforming growth factor β in the rat: Uptake, metabolism, and biliary excretion. *J Clin Invest* 80:750, 1987.
157. Wakefield LM, et al. Recombinant latent transforming growth factor β1 has a longer plasma half-life in rats than active transforming growth factor β1, and a different tissue distribution. *J Clin Invest* 86:1976, 1990.
158. Barnard JA, Lyons RM, Moses HL. The cell biology of transforming growth factor beta. *Biochim Biophys Acta* 1032:79, 1990.
159. Roberts AB, Sporn MB. Transforming Growth Factor-Betas. In MB Sporn, AB Roberts (eds), *Peptide Growth Factors and Their Receptors.* Heidelberg: Springer, 1990. Pp 419–472.
160. Miller-Graziano CL, et al. Role of elevated monocyte transforming growth factor beta (TGF β) production in post-trauma immunosuppression. *J Clin Immunol* 11:95, 1991.
161. Busso N, et al. Transforming growth-factor-β (TGF-β) inhibits albumin synthesis in normal human hepatocytes and in hepatoma HepG2 cells. *Biochem Biophys Res Commun* 171:647, 1990.
162. Mackiewicz A, et al. Transforming growth factor β1 regulates production of acute-phase proteins. *Proc Natl Acad Sci USA* 87:1491, 1990.
163. Morrone G, Cortese R, Sorrentino V. Posttranscriptional control of negative acute phase genes by transforming growth factor beta. *EMBO J* 8:3767, 1989.
164. Kushner I, Ganapathi M, Schultz D. The acute phase response is mediated by heterogeneous mechanisms. *Ann NY Acad Sci* 557:19, 1989.
165. Beauchamp RD, et al. Posttranscriptional regulation of albumin and α-fetoprotein messenger RNA by transforming growth factor-β1 requires *de novo* RNA and protein synthesis. *Mol Endocrinol* 6:1789, 1992.
166. Bennett NT, Schultz GS. Growth factors and wound healing: Part II. Role in normal and chronic wound healing. *Am J Surg* 166:74, 1993.
167. Kulkarni AB, et al. Transforming growth factor beta 1 null mutation in mice causes excessive inflammatory response and early death. *Proc Natl Acad Sci USA* 90:770, 1993.
168. Shull MM, et al. Targeted disruption of the mouse transforming growth factor-β1 gene results in multifocal inflammatory disease. *Nature* 359:693, 1992.
169. Rossi P, et al. A nuclear factor 1 binding site mediates the transcriptional activation of a type I collagen promoter by transforming growth factor-β. *Cell* 52:405, 1988.
170. Riccio A, et al. The regulatory region of the human plasminogen activator inhibitor type-1 (PAI-1) gene. *Nucleic Acids Res* 16:2805, 1988.
171. Li L, Hu J-S, Olson EN. Different members of the jun proto-oncogene family exhibit distinct patterns of expression in response to Type β transforming growth factor. *J Biol Chem* 265:1556, 1990.

172. Blatti SP, et al. Induction of fibronectin gene transcription and mRNA is a primary response to growth-factor stimulation of AKR-2B cells. *Proc Natl Acad Sci USA* 85:1119, 1988.

173. Kim S-J, et al. Autoinduction of transforming growth factor beta 1 is mediated by the AP-1 complex. *Mol Cell Biol* 10:1492, 1990.

174. Kim S-J, et al. Promoter sequences of the human transforming growth factor-β1 gene responsive to transforming growth factor-β1 autoinduction. *J Biol Chem* 264:7041, 1989.

175. Westerhausen DR Jr, Hopkins WE, Billadello JJ. Multiple transforming growth factor-β-inducible elements regulate expression of the plasminogen activator inhibitor type-1 gene in HepG2 cells. *J Biol Chem* 266:1092, 1991.

176. Curran T, Franza BR Jr. Fos and jun: The AP-1 connection. *Cell* 55:395, 1988.

177. Kraft AS. So what's new with jun? *Am J Med Sci* 302:176, 1991.

178. Ransone LJ, Verma IM. Nuclear proto-oncogenes fos and jun. *Annu Rev Cell Biol* 6:539, 1990.

179. Schule R, Evans RM. Cross-coupling of signal transduction pathways: Zinc finger meets leucine zipper. *Trends Genet* 7:377, 1991.

180. Zentella A, et al. Early gene responses to transforming growth factor-β in cells lacking growth-suppressive RB function. *Mol Cell Biol* 11:4952, 1991.

181. Beauchamp RD, et al. Transforming growth factor (TGF)-β stimulates hepatic *jun*-B and *fos*-B proto-oncogenes and decreases albumin mRNA. *Ann Surg* 216:300, 1992.

182. Manning AM, et al. Differential sensitivity of human colonic adenoma and carcinoma cells to transforming growth factor β (TGF-β): Conversion of an adenoma cell line to a tumorigenic phenotype is accompanied by a reduced response to the inhibitory effects of TGF-β. *Oncogene* 6:1471, 1991.

183. Hoosein NM, et al. Differential sensitivity of subclasses of human colon carcinoma cell lines to the growth inhibitory effects of transforming growth factor-β1. *Exp Cell Res* 181:442, 1989.

184. Roberts AB, Sporn MB. Physiological actions and clinical applications of transforming growth factor-β (TGF-β). *Growth Factors* 8:1, 1993.

185. Avery A, et al. TGF-β expression in the human colon: Differential immunostaining along crypt epithelium. *Br J Cancer* 68:137, 1993.

186. Goyette MC, et al. Progression of colorectal cancer is associated with multiple tumor suppressor gene defects but inhibition of tumorigenicity is accomplished by correction of any single defect via chromosome transfer. *Mol Cell Biol* 12:1387, 1992.

187. Pietenpol JA, et al. TGF-beta 1 inhibition of c-*myc* transcription and growth in keratinocytes is abrogated by viral transforming proteins with pRB binding domains. *Cell* 61:777, 1990.

188. Pietenpol JA, et al. Factor-binding element in the human c-*myc* promoter involved in transcriptional regulation by transforming growth factor β1 and by the retinoblastoma gene product. *Proc Natl Acad Sci USA* 88:10227, 1991.

189. Suardet L, et al. Responsiveness of three newly established human colorectal cancer cell lines to transforming growth factors β1 and β2. *Cancer Res* 52:3705, 1992.

190. Sieweke MH, et al. Mediation of wound-related Rous sarcoma virus tumorigenesis by TGF-β. *Science* 248:1656, 1990.

191. Chang H-L, et al. Increased transforming growth factor β expression inhibits cell proliferation *in vitro*, yet increases tumorigenicity and tumor growth of Meth A sarcoma cells. *Cancer Res* 53:4391, 1993.

192. Schwarz LC, et al. Aberrant TGF-β production and regulation in metastatic malignancy. *Growth Factors* 3:115, 1990.

193. Welch DR, Fabra A, Nakajima M. Transforming growth factor β stimulates mammary adenocarcinoma cell invasion and metastatic potential. *Proc Natl Acad Sci USA* 87:7678, 1990.

194. Steiner MS, Barrack ER. Transforming growth factor-β1 overproduction in prostate cancer: Effects on growth in vivo and in vitro. *Mol Endocrinol* 6:15, 1992.

Selected Readings

Cadena DL, Gill GN. Receptor tyrosine kinases. *FASEB J* 6:2332, 1992.

This is a review of receptor tyrosine kinases. The authors very nicely condense a tremendous amount of information that has been published regarding receptor tyrosine kinases. They describe similarities and differences in tyrosine kinase receptor structure; what is known of the mechanisms of ligand recognition and binding; receptor activation; and signal transduction. Roles of receptor tyrosine kinase (and mutations thereof) in development and cancer are discussed to emphasize the biologic relevance.

Delarco J, Todaro GJ. Growth factors from murine sarcoma virus-transformed cells. *Proc Natl Acad Sci USA* 75:4001, 1978.

This landmark article reported the discovery of TGFs that were found in medium conditioned by fibrosarcoma cells in culture. The TGFs were operationally defined as peptides that reversibly induce nonneoplastic fibroblasts to express the transformed phenotype, determined by loss of density-dependent inhibition of growth and acquisition of anchorage-independent growth. As it turned out, the TGF activity contained two very different families of peptide growth factors, the TGF-α and TGF-β families.

Pledger WJ, et al. An ordered sequence of events is required before BALB/c-3T3 cells become committed to DNA synthesis. *Proc Natl Acad Sci USA* 75:2839, 1978.

These authors found that a serum factor (PDGF) was capable of inducing mouse fibroblasts to become competent to enter the cell cycle and proliferate. However, the cells would not progress through G1 and enter S phase in the absence of a progression factor. A factor in platelet-poor plasma (later determined to be IGF-1) induced these competent cells to progress through G1 and enter the S phase. Once cells progress past a late growth arrest point in late G1, they are committed to DNA synthesis.

Sherr CJ. Mammalian G_1 cyclins. *Cell* 73:1059, 1993.

This is a concise but thorough review of one of the most exciting and rapidly advancing areas of cell biology: the regulation of cell proliferation by G1 cyclins. Sherr is one of the leading investigators in this field and provides an overview and framework for understanding the complexities of cell cycle regulation.

Tucker RF, et al. Growth inhibitor from BSC-1 cells closely related to platelet type β transforming growth factor. *Science* 226:705, 1984.

The purified growth inhibition from African green monkey (BSC-1) cells and TGF-β purified from human platelets were found to be nearly identical and competed for binding to the same cell membrane receptor. This was the first report that TGF-β could either stimulate or inhibit cell proliferation, depending on the cell type and experimental conditions.

II

Intermediary Metabolism

6

Protein and Amino Acid Metabolism

Vernon R. Young
Yong-Ming Yu

During the course of biologic evolution, animal cells lost their enzymatic capacity to synthesize certain organic molecules that were required for their growth and for the maintenance of tissue function [1]. These molecules are the essential dietary nutrients, which include dietary proteins or, more specifically, certain amino acids and the nitrogen that is used for the synthesis of other physiologically important nitrogen-containing compounds [2]. In this chapter, we will focus attention on the metabolism of proteins (nitrogen) and amino acids with a more practical goal in mind: the nutritional needs for these nutrients and their metabolic basis under varying pathophysiologic states. The emphasis will be on the biochemistry and physiology of human protein and amino acid metabolism and on the flows of amino acids and their derivatives through metabolic pathways and the impact of nutritional and other factors that affect them. However, it is also appropriate that we briefly consider the cellular and subcellular pathways responsible for the formation of proteins and amino acids, their movement to particular sites, and interconversion and degradation, together with details of the molecular mechanisms by which these processes take place. Some of these specific biochemical topics are dealt with more extensively in Chapters 3 and 4, and the nutritional needs and characteristics of the surgical patient are specific topics in Chapters 13, 19, 29, and 30. This chapter will also discuss protein and amino acid metabolism without extensive reference to pathologic states (these are considered in Chapters 3, 22, and 25).

Amino acids serve as the currency of the nitrogen and protein economy of the host, and so we will consider a number of them in some detail. Although there are hundreds of amino acids in nature [3], only 20 of these appear in proteins via charging by its cognate transfer RNA (tRNA), with subsequent recognition of a codon on the messenger RNA (mRNA) (or 21 in the case of selenocysteine-containing proteins, in which case it is restricted via a UGA codon) [4]. Other amino acids, such as hydroxyproline, hydroxylysine, N^{τ}-methylhistidine, and two rare amino acids, 3-hydroxyaspartic acid and 3-hydroxyasparagine, are also present in proteins because of posttranslational modification of specific amino acids residues, and this aspect of protein metabolism will be discussed below. However, the common 20 amino acids, together with a few others that are not present in the body in peptide-bound form (such as ornithine, citrulline, and taurine), are of major quantitative importance in the maintenance of nitrogen economy and nutritional status of the human subject. Further, whereas all plants can synthesize the 18 amino acids and two amides commonly found in proteins, the animal kingdom, from protozoa up to mammals, is dependent on at least eight of the amino acids being supplied from exogenous sources. These are the essential or indispensable amino acids [2]. For these eight, we will revisit briefly the concept of "essentiality" in the nutritional segment of this chapter. We will consider the interrelations between the various sources of amino acid nitrogen, and we will attempt to provide a contemporary metabolic framework on which the nutritional and metabolic significance of the dietary amino acids might be best understood.

Cystine was the first amino acid to be discovered, apparently by Woolaston in 1810 [3], and it was later given its name by the Swedish chemist, Jac Berzelius, in about 1833. This impressive scientist is also credited with proposing the name "protein" in a letter of July 10, 1838, sent to the Dutch chemist G. Mulder, in Rotterdam. In turn, Mulder formally accepted the term in his communication in the *Bulletin des Sciences physiques et naturelles en Néerlande,* July 30, 1838 [5].

Amino Acid and Protein Functions

The nutritionally relevant amino acids serve multiple and diverse physiologic functions. Some of these are listed in Table 6-1, together with those functions that are met by the proteins, which are elaborated from the precursor amino acid pools.

Table 6-1. Some Functions of Amino Acids and of Their Products, Including Proteins

Function	Example
Amino Acids	
Substrates for protein synthesis	Those for which there is a codon
Regulators of protein turnover	Leucine; arginine?
Regulators of enzyme activity (allosteric)	Arginine and NAG synthetase; Phe and PAH activation
Precursor of signal transducer	Arginine and nitric oxide
Methylation reactions	Methionine
Neurotransmitter	Tryptophan (serotonin); glutamate
Ion fluxes	Taurine; glutamate
Precursor of "physiologic" molecules	Arg (creatinine); glut (NH_2)-purines
Transport of nitrogen	Alanine; glut (NH_2)
Proteins	
Enzymatic catalysis	Branched-chain ketoacid dehydrogenase
Transport	B_{12} binding proteins; ceruloplasmin; apolipoproteins; albumin
Messengers/signals	Insulin; growth hormone
Movement	Kinesin; actin
Structure	Collagens; elastin
Storage/sequestration	Ferritin; metallothionein
Immunity	Antibodies; TNF; interleukins
Growth; differentiation; gene expression	Peptide growth factors; transcription factors

NAG = N-acetyl glutamate; PAH = phenylalanine hydroxylase; glut (NH_2) = glutamine; TNF = tumor necrosis factor; Phe = phenylalanine

While carrying out their physiologic and functional roles, the proteins and amino acids turn over, and part of their nitrogen and carbon is irretrievably lost via the excretory pathways, including carbon dioxide in expired air and urea and ammonia in urine. To maintain an adequate body protein and amino acid status, these losses must be balanced by an appropriate exogenous or dietary supply of (1) a usable source of nitrogen to support cell and organ function and (2) the indispensable amino acids and, under specific states, the "conditionally indispensable" amino acids. These are used to replace those that are lost during their daily metabolic transactions or deposited in new tissues during growth, repair, and body protein repletion. We will consider first the nature of the metabolic systems that are responsible for determining these dietary needs, and we will subsequently explore some of the changes in these systems when various physiologic or pathologic factors intervene. Because our emphasis is on human protein and amino acid metabolism, we will include a brief description and analysis of methods that are, or might be, applied in the in vivo human and clinical setting for investigating protein/amino acid metabolism.

The Major Systems

The principal metabolic systems responsible for the maintenance of body protein and amino acid homeostasis are protein synthesis, protein breakdown or degradation, amino acid oxidation with elimination of carbon dioxide, and urea production and amino acid synthesis, in the case of the nutritionally dispensable or conditionally indispensable amino acids (Figure 6-1). At the organ level, amino acid transport is also important, as discussed briefly below. Dietary factors and various other nutritional characteristics also determine the status of protein and amino acid metabolism. These include considerations of intake levels relative to protein and amino acid requirements, the form and route of delivery (i.e, parenteral and enteral nutritional support), and timing of intake, particularly in relation to that of the major energy-yielding substrates. Some of these issues will be discussed below. Changes in the rates of these systems lead to an adjustment in whole-body nitrogen (protein) balance and retention, with the overall direction and extent depending on the strength of the prevailing factor(s), some of which are listed in Table 6-2.

The synthesis of proteins may be controlled at the level of gene transcription or mRNA translation, and the amount of cell proteins is determined by the balance between their rates of synthesis and breakdown. This latter phase is also an important control point in protein metabolism, and so we begin now with a short overview of the processes of gene transcription, translation, and protein breakdown. Later, we will attempt to apply this information within physiologic and nutritional contexts.

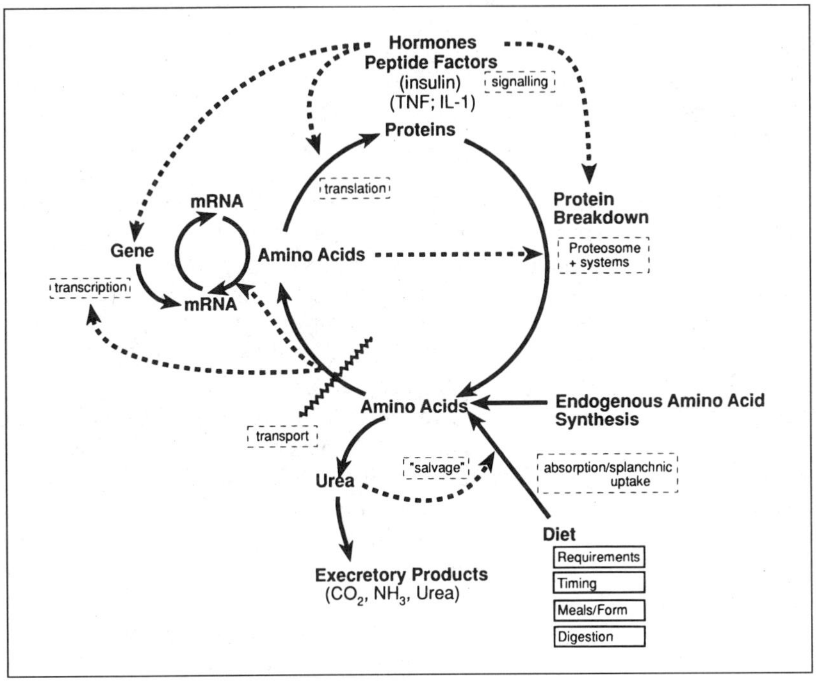

Figure 6-1. The major systems involved in and responsible for the maintenance of body protein and amino acid homeostasis.

Table 6-2. Some Factors Influencing the Status of Whole-Body Protein, Organ Protein, and Amino-Acid Metabolism

Agent (Diet)	Host
Nitrogen intake and form	Genetic and inherited disease
Amino acid intake and balance	Physiologic
Energy supply and sources	Metabolic state; developmental state; age
Other nutrients	
Route of delivery (enteral; parenteral)	Hormonal factors
	Pathologic
	Infection; trauma cancer; diabetes

Transcription

Three classes of eukaryotic genes exist, differing in their organization, the proteins that regulate their transcription, and the RNA polymerase that transcribes the gene [6]. Class 1 genes encode 18S and 28S ribosomal RNA molecules; class 2 genes encode a wide variety of mRNA molecules that are translated into the cellular proteins; and class 3 genes encode the small tRNA molecules involved in translational phase of protein synthesis as well as the 5S RNA of the ribosome. Each class expresses different *cis*-acting DNA sequences within its promoter (various regulatory elements, generally with fixed orientations that are close to the start of transcription) and enhancer (groups of regulatory elements that are distant from the initiation site of transcription). The transcription factors interact with these different *cis*-acting DNA sequences, creating a transcription complex [6]. Other transcription factors that are not sequence-specific DNA-binding proteins interact with the DNA-binding proteins present at the promoter and enhancer to create a multiprotein DNA complex. Figure 6-2 illustrates the assembly of a transcription complex on the promoter of a eukaryotic gene and the processing of the transcript [7]. Recurrent structural motifs in DNA-binding domains provide the basis for the classification of the various transcription factors [6,8]. More than 80% of these factors contain one of four motifs: helix-turn-helix (HTH), zinc finger, leucine zipper, or helix-loop-helix (HLH) (Figure 6-3). Although positively acting transcription factors have received a great deal of attention, negative regulation of transcription is claimed to be an equally vital process in the modulation of gene expression; transcription factors may be positive or negative depending on the cellular and sequence context [9].

After transcription of a protein-encoding gene into an RNA copy in the nucleus, a number of steps remain in the eventual readout of the genetic information (see Figure 6-2). First, both ends of the single-stranded RNA are modified. At the 5′ end, the cell adds a special nucleotide structure, called a cap [7], which increases the efficiency of mRNA translation by enhancing ribosomal binding to the transcript. At the 3′ end, a nuclease recognizes a sequence rich in adenine and uridine in the noncoding portion of the transcript. The enzyme trims about 20 bases from the downstream end of the RNA. Next, another enzyme modifies the newly cleaved 3′ end of the transcript by adding a stretch of adenine bases. This so-called *polyA tail* probably stabilizes the RNA molecule and affects translational efficiency [10]. The modified RNA transcript then undergoes a highly regulated process called splicing. In higher organisms, most protein-coding gene sequences are interrupted by stretches of noncoding sequences, called *introns,* and these must be removed to form a continuous chain of exons or coding sequences. The translation of a protein then follows.

Translation

Initiation

The translation of the genetic message is usually referred to as the process of polypeptide chain or protein synthesis, and it is divided into three phases: initiation, elongation, and termination. The reactions in each phase are promoted by soluble protein factors (Table 6-3) [11] that interact transiently with the ribosome, mRNA, and aminoacyl-tRNAs [12, 13]. Translation involves a series of noncovalent binding interactions among the protein and RNA components and the hydrolysis of pyrophosphate bonds in adenosine triphosphate (ATP) and guanosine triphosphate (GTP). Although more detail is needed concerning the structures of the intermediates involved and the underlying basis for the particular protein and nucleic acid interactions, the major steps in the pathway leading to the formation of the initiation

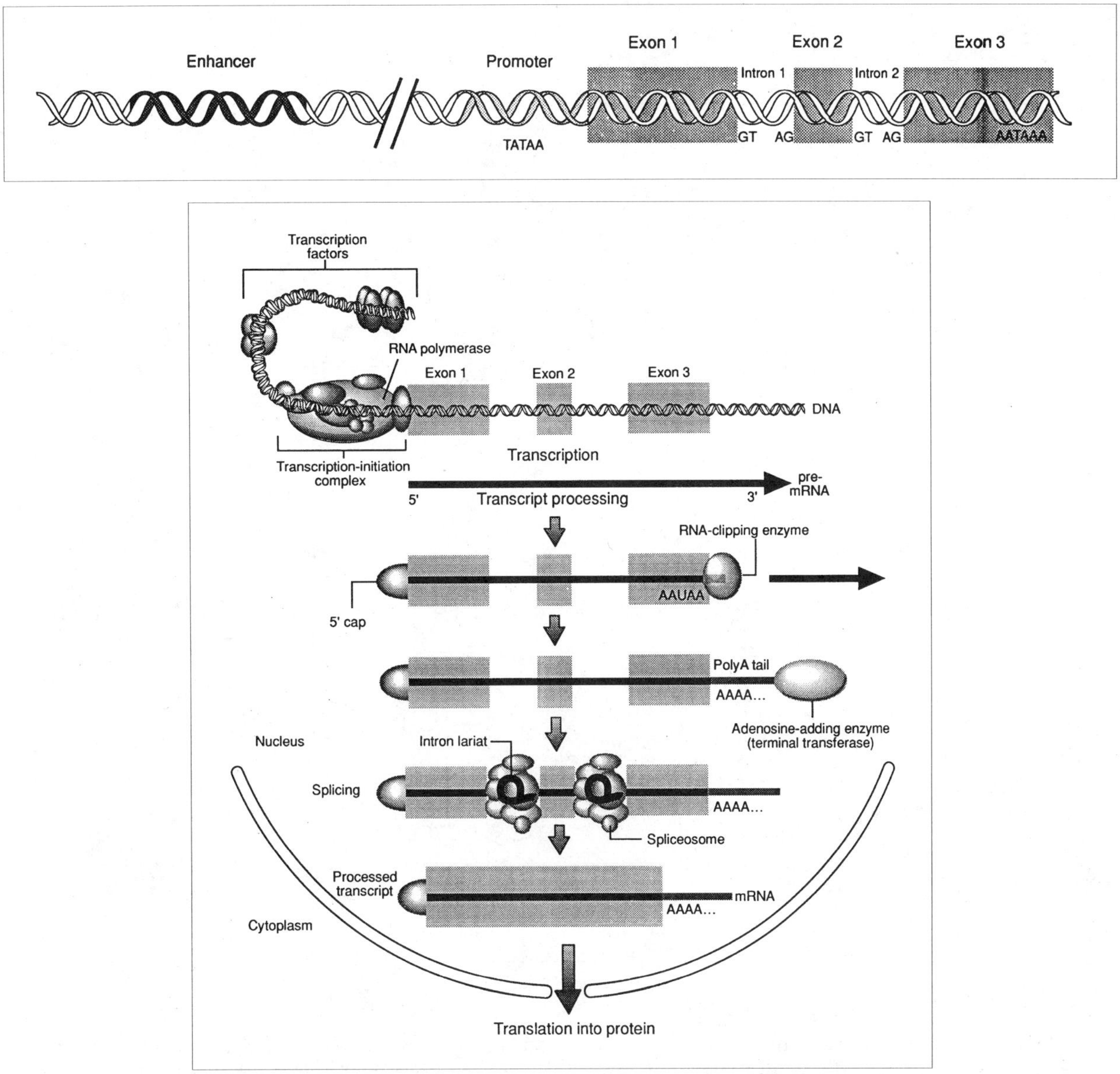

Figure 6-2. Gene structure (top) and expression (bottom) in higher organisms: The sequences of DNA transcribed include introns and exons, with expression beginning with binding of multiple protein factors to enhancer and promotor sequences. The RNA transcript is subjected to posttranscriptional processes prior to the entry of a mature, spliced mRNA molecule which leaves the nucleus for translation within the cytoplasm. (From N Rosenthal. Regulation of gene expression. *N Engl J Med* 331:931, 1994.)

complex are schematically outlined in Figure 6-4 [14].

The rate-limiting step of translation is usually, but not always, located within the initiation phase. As summarized by Hershey [12], the intrinsic activity or strength of most mRNAs is determined first by (1) the accessibility of the capped 5′-terminus to initiation factors; (2) the ability of the 40S ribosomal subunit to bind and scan the mRNA distally, and (3) the frequency of recognition of the initiator codon and surrounding context. Additionally, an important regulator of the expression of specific mRNAs is the mobilization of mRNAs from repressed messenger ribonucleoprotein particles (mRNPs) into active polysomes. This appears to be controlled separately from ribosome initiation on polysomes.

The dominant mechanism of control of global protein synthesis is phosphorylation/dephosphorylation of translational components, primarily of initiation and elongation factors [12,13,15]. Apparently the stimulation of protein synthesis is particularly related to eIF-4F (the mRNA cap-binding protein complex), which is a major phos-

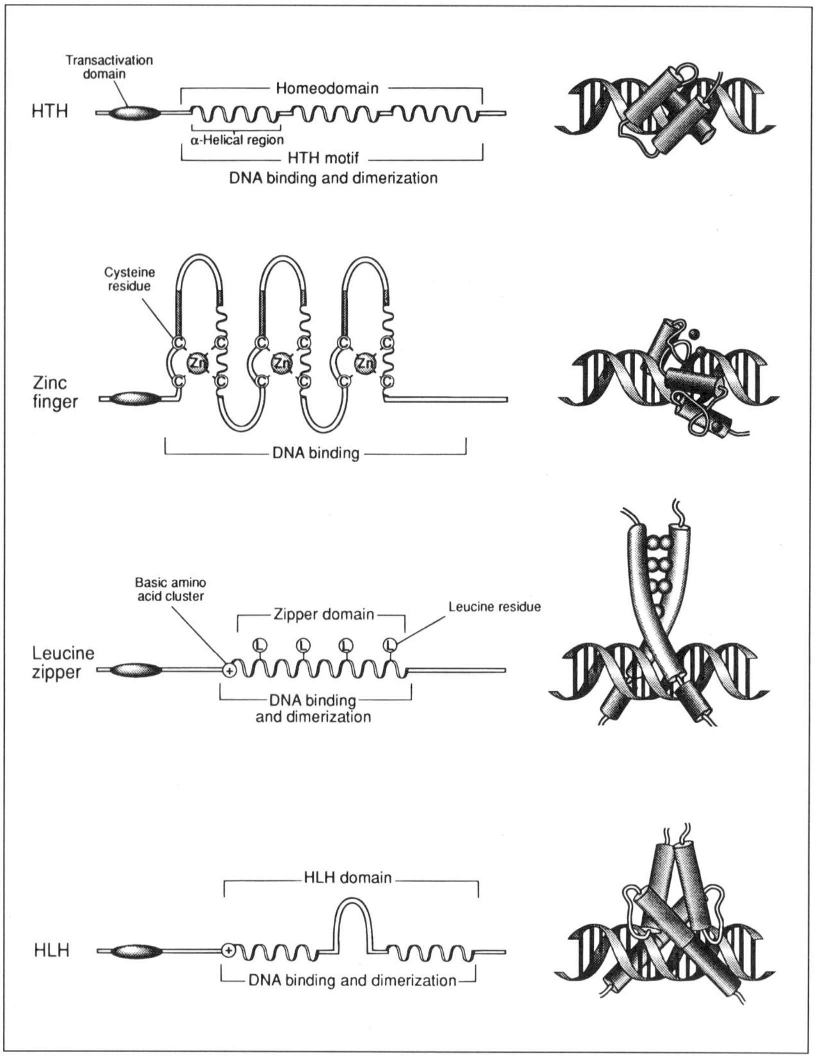

Figure 6-3. Transcription factors and their interactions with DNA, indicating the four major classes of these factors. (From AG Papavassiliou. Transcription factors. *N Engl J Med* 332:45, 1995.)

phorylation target, although phosphorylation of other proteins such as eIF-3, eIF-4B, and ribosomal protein S6 can be important also [12,13]. Phosphorylation also causes repression of protein synthesis, normally by modifying the α-subunit of initiation factor eIF-2 or the elongation factor eEF-2 [15]. Indeed, phosphorylation of eIF-2α appears to be a general mechanism for inhibiting initiation of translation, whereas EF-2 phosphorylation affects elongation rates and may be used less frequently. In general, a complex set of interactions, some redundant or overlapping, serve to link the rate of translation to the overall metabolic state of the cell. For example, insulin has been shown to alter the phosphorylation state of four initiation factors, eIF-2, eIF-2B, eIF-3, and eIF-4 [15].

In the context of the nutritional supply of amino acids, a deficient intake level or availability of one or more of these nutrients can affect the transcriptional phase of protein synthesis. For example, the levels of mRNA for albumin, transferrin, transthyretin, the β-chain of fibrinogen, and apolipoprotein E are reduced in livers obtained from rats after 3 days of protein depletion [16]; rat refeeding experiments have also revealed that changes in mRNA levels may occur more slowly than do changes in actual rates of protein synthesis [16]. As already implied, alterations in mRNA levels may be the result of changes in transcription rates, mRNA splicing and its delivery to the cytoplasmic compartment, or mRNA stability; however, much remains to be learned about the quantitative impact of different nutritional and pathophysiologic factors, such as cytokines, on these various sites and processes and their quantitative significance. Of course, it is highly unlikely that the concentration and profile of different amino acids function as the sole protein/amino acid nutritional regulator of translation and transcription. There is now considerable evidence that

Table 6-3. Protein Factors Required for mRNA Translation in Eukaryotes

Factor	Function(s)
Initiation	
eIF-1	Stimulates formation of and stabilizes 43S and 48S initiation complexes
eIF-1A	Stimulates formation of and stabilizes 43S and 48S preinitiation complexes
eIF-2	GTP-dependent binding of initiator Met-tRNA to 43S
eIF-2B	See GEF
eIF-3	Formation of native 43S ribosome
GEF	GT:GDP exchange on eIF-2
Elongation	
eEF-1α	GTP-dependent binding of aminoacyl-tRNA
eEF-1$\beta\gamma$	GTP:GDP exchange of eEF-1α
eEF-2	Translocation
Termination	
eRF	Chain termination and polypeptide release
Initiation	
eIF-3A	Formation of native 60S ribosomal subunit
eIF-4A	ATP-dependent RNA helicase
eIF-4B	Stimulates RNA binding to 43S preinitiation complexes
eIF-4C	See eIF-1A
eIF-4D	See eIF-5A
eIF-4E	Cap recognition; stimulates mRNA binding to 43S preinitiation complex
eIF-4F	Recognition of 5-cap structure; binding of mRNA to 43S preinitiation complex; ATP-dependent RNA helicase
eIF-5	GTP-dependent release of bound factors upon joining 60S subunit to the 43S complex
eIF-5A	Stimulates ribosomal subunit joining and enhances 80S-bound Met-tRNA, reactivity with puromycin
eIF-6	See eIF-3A

GTP = guanosine triphosphate; GDP = guanosine diphosphate; Met = methionine

Source: Abstracted from CG Proud. Protein phosphorylation in translational control. *Curr Top Cell Regul* 32:243, 1992.

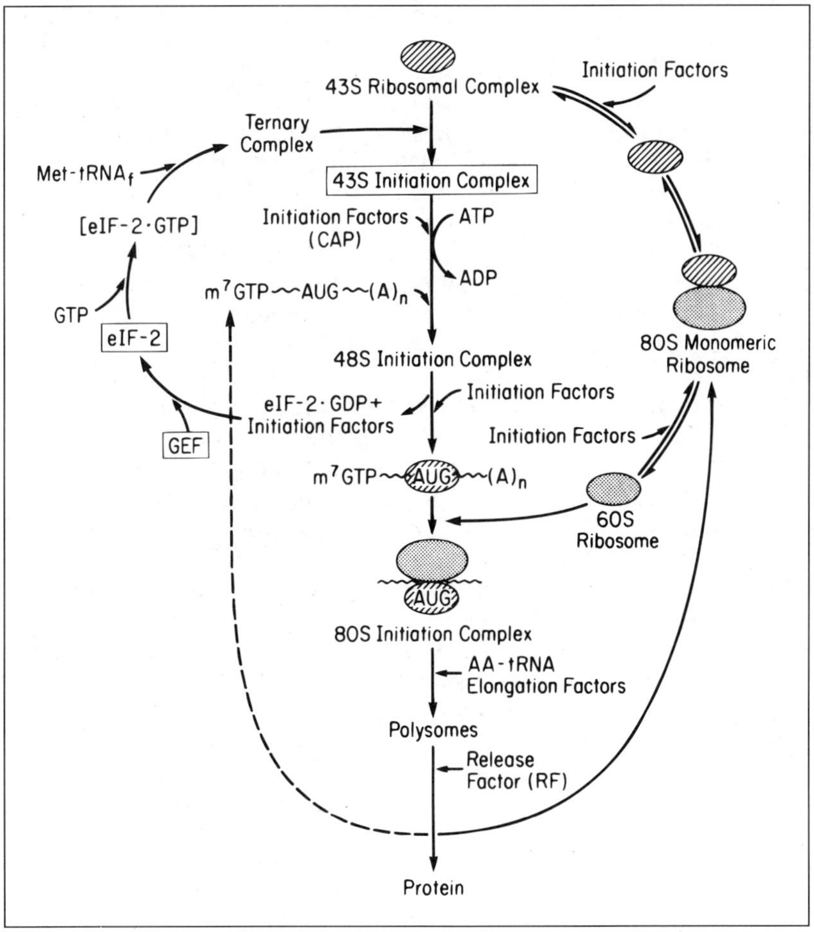

Figure 6-4. An outline of the principal steps involved in the initiation, elongation, and termination of protein synthesis, showing the major sites of action of the various protein factors (initiation, elongation, and termination). (From VM Pain. Initiation of protein synthesis in mammalian cells. *Biochem J* 235:625, 1986.)

hormonal factors are intimately involved in the molecular signaling of dietary changes [17,18]. However, changes in tissue amino acid levels appear to be of importance in achieving a regulatory influence and, in consequence, appear to be involved in a so-called anabolic drive [19]. Additionally, translational regulation of specific mRNAs can be achieved by reversible RNA/protein interactions in the 5′-untranslated region of mRNA; regulation of the iron storage protein ferritin in response to iron levels is an elegant example of this mechanism [20].

With respect to specific transcripts, there are a wide variety of control mechanisms involved in their particular regulation and function; the poly-A tail at the 3′-terminus of most mRNAs influences both mRNA stability and translational efficiency. A general way to regulate the synthesis of specific proteins may involve the binding of *trans*-acting proteins to special *cis*-acting regions of an mRNA molecule. Also, ribosomal frame-shifting and translational read-through of stop codons can also contribute to the regulation of specific gene expression, especially the reverse transcriptase gene in retroviruses [12].

Elongation and Termination

The elongation phase is a process that adds one amino acid residue to the C-terminal end of the nascent polypeptide chain per each turn of the cycle. This phase involves the participation of four promotional proteins, called elongation factors, which have been purified and whose cDNAs have been cloned and sequenced (see Figure 6-4) [12]. The process involves four major steps: (1) binding of aminoacyl-tRNA to the A site of the ribosome, catalyzed by eEF-1α or 2; (2) GTP hydrolysis and ejection of eEF-1α·GDP; (3) formation of the peptide bond, catalyzed by the peptidyl transferase center in the 60S ribosomal subunit; and (4) translocation, promoted by eEF-2. Energy is expended during each cycle of polypeptide chain elongation; one high-energy pyrophosphate bond in GTP was earlier thought to be cleaved at both the binding and translocation steps, and two additional high-energy bonds of ATP are hydrolyzed in the synthesis of the aminoacyl-tRNA that is used in the process. However, it has been proposed recently that two GTP molecules may be hydrolyzed to achieve a binding of aminoacyl-tRNA to the A site of the mRNA-bound ribosomes [21,22], and so it may be that five rather than four high-energy phosphate bonds are used in the synthesis of each peptide bond. This has possible significance for assessment of the energy cost of in vivo protein synthesis and the interrelations between energy and protein metabolism in the surgical patient, as discussed below.

The termination phase, in contrast to the elongation and initiation phases, appears to be relatively simple. When a termination codon is positioned in the A site of the ribosome, a release factor (eRF) promotes cleavage of the completed peptidyl-tRNA, releasing the nascent protein (see Figure 6-4).

Posttranslational Phase

The process of polypeptide synthesis, as outlined above, is limited to the incorporation of the common 20 amino acids; however, chemical analysis of proteins for their constituent amino acids often reveals many more than these 20 amino acids. It is impossible to propose a precise number of amino acids and their derivatives actually present in proteins in the biosphere, but the number may be quite high: as many as 800 to 1000 amino acids in nature, although not all of these are found as protein-bound amino acids. Furthermore, the final polypeptide produced may differ from that specified by the gene through modifications of the number of peptide bonds. Shortening of the polypeptide chain by proteolytic cleavage may occur, or, in other cases, lengthening of the chain by addition of amino acids to the C- or N-terminal ends. All these reactions are relevant when considering the molecular and cellular aspects of protein and amino acid metabolism.

The secondary, or derived, amino acids found in proteins arise by chemical modification of the primary amino acid during or after its gene-specified insertion into the polypeptide. This process is looked on as the *posttranslational phase,* and, together with the highly specific processes by which proteins are folded and delivered to their sites of function, it represents additional essential steps in the synthesis and positioning of protein in all living cells.

The posttranslational modifications of most proteins may be classified into one of three major categories: (1) modifications that involve peptide bond cleavage and formation; (2) modifications that involve amino (N·) or carboxyl (C –) terminal amino acids; and (3) modifications that involve specific amino acid side-chain moieties (Table 6-4). This topic has been reviewed in detail by others [23–25], but it is worth reiterating the point made by Rucker and McGee [25] that posttranslational events often carry the same significance for functional protein production as do the transcriptional and translational events that are responsible for the synthesis of proteins in the first instance.

Protein Degradation

The breakdown of tissue and organ proteins is an extensive, continuous, and regulated process that, along with protein synthesis, determines the qual-

Table 6-4. Selected Examples of Various Types of Posttranslational Modifications of Proteins

Modification	Process	Function
Amino acid side chains	Acylations	Compartmentalization
	Methylations	Regulatory signaling
	Desmosine isomers	Crosslinking
	Carboxylation	Metal binding sites
Peptide bond cleavage and formation	Prepeptide and propeptide cleavage	Enzyme activation
	Ubiquitin-dependent cleavage	Protein degradation
N- and C-terminal amino acids	C-terminal amidation and phosphorylation	Activation of peptide hormones

Source: Based on RB Rucker, C McGee. Chemical modifications of proteins in vivo: Selected examples important to cellular regulation. *J Nutr* 123:977, 1993.

itative and quantitative nature of cellular protein. Before turning toward a more physiologic and whole-body context below, it is relevant to review the underlying molecular and cellular features of protein degradation.

In mammalian cells, there are separate lysosomal and nonlysosomal mechanisms that are involved in different aspects of protein degradation (Figure 6-5) [26]. As summarized by Ciechanover and Schwartz [27], proteins that enter the cell from the extracellular milieu (such as receptor-mediated endocytosed and pinocytosed proteins) are degraded in lysosomes. Lysosomal degradation of intracellular proteins occurs mostly under stressed conditions, such as in starvation [28]. This process is activated by glucocorticoids [29] and suppressed by insulin [28] and by a dietary protein deficiency in skeletal muscle [30]. Nonlysosomal mechanisms are probably responsible for the selective turnover of intracellular proteins that occurs under basal metabolic conditions and for many of the changes that occur in response to diet and hormones.

Thus, the proteolytic system that degrades the bulk of cell proteins, including the rapid elimination of abnormal proteins and short-lived regulatory polypeptides, is nonlysosomal and ATP-dependent. An initial step in the hydrolysis of many such proteins is a "marking" reaction involving their covalent conjugation by the 76-residue polypeptide, ubiquitin. In this ubiquitin proteolytic pathway [27,31,32], the carboxyl terminus of ubiquitin becomes attached by an isopeptide bond to ϵ-amino groups on lysine residues of the protein substrate. Much of the selectivity for proteolysis resides in this conjugation step. It is thought to be rate-limiting, and it requires ATP, at least three enzymes, and, for certain polypeptides, a transfer RNA-dependent modification. Figure 6-6 shows a possible sequence of events in the conjugation and degradation of protein via this system.

Linkage of the polypeptide to a chain of ubiquitins marks the polypeptide for rapid hydrolysis by a large proteolytic complex, the proteasome (approximately 700 kDa). These are high molecular mass cylindrical particles that contain at least five distinct types of catalytic components; they are capable of degrading proteins to small peptides [26,33,34], in both ubiquitin-dependent and ubi-

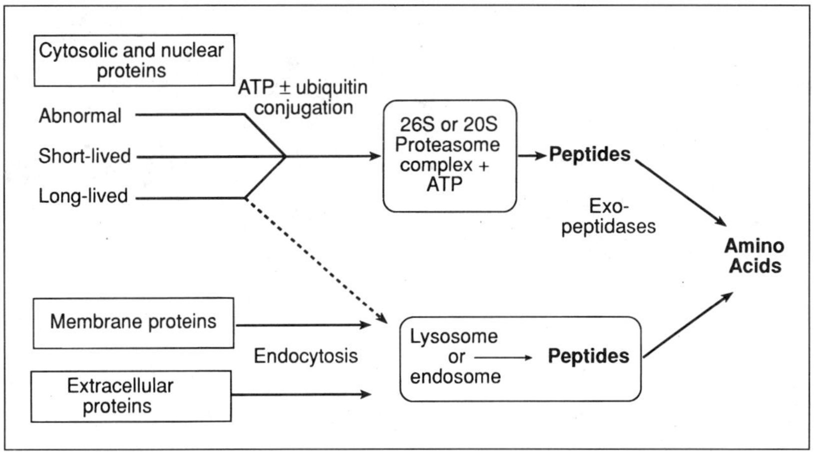

Figure 6-5. Major pathways of protein degradation in eukaryotic cells. (Adapted from AL Goldberg and KL Rock. Proteolysis, proteasomes, and antigen presentation. *Nature* 357:375, 1992.)

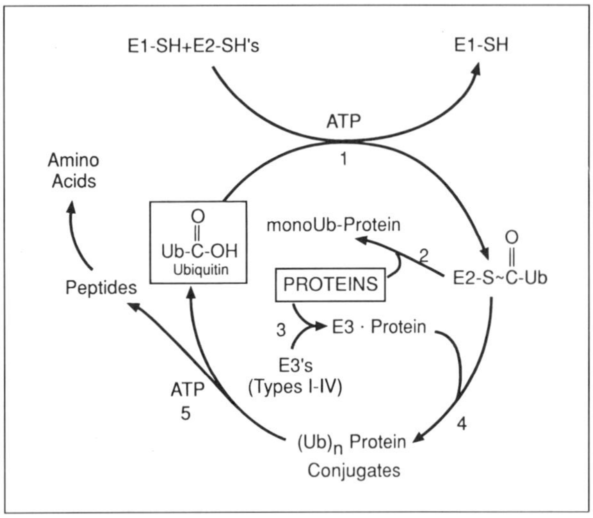

Figure 6-6. A scheme illustrating a possible sequence of events responsible for the ubiquitin-dependent conjugation and degradation of proteins. Activation begins with step 1; step 2 involves formation of monoubiquinated conjugates by E2; E3 (ubiquitin-protein ligase)-protein complex is formed in step 3; conjugation of the protein substrate with multiple molecules of ubiquitin occurs in step 4; and then step 5 involves the ATP-dependent breakdown to peptides and free amino acids. E1 = ubiquitin-activating enzyme; E2 = ubiquitin carrier protein; E3 = ubiquitin-protein ligase-protein complex. (From A Ciechanover and AL Schwartz. The ubiquitin-mediated proteolytic pathway: Mechanisms of recognition of the proteolytic substrate and involvement in the degradation of native cellular proteins. *FASEB J* 8:182, 1994.)

quitin-independent nonlysosomal pathways of protein breakdown. They are found in all eukaryotic cells and tissues and are usually present in the nucleus [35] and in the cytoplasm. The diversity of eukaryotic proteasome localization and subunit composition, as well as the presence of RNA in only a small proportion of particles, suggests the possible existence of subpopulations of proteasomes, with differing functions. Additional details about the organization and functions of proteasomes were discussed by Rivett [33].

Amino Acid Transport

As outlined by Souba and Pacitti [36], the net uptake or release of amino acids is determined by several interacting parameters, including (1) the mass-action gradients of the substrate across the plasma membrane of cells; (2) the activities of the various transport systems that regulate the transport of the amino acid in and out of the cell; (3) the rate at which the substrate is synthesized and degraded within the cell; and (4) the concentrations of competing substrates and their affinities for the transporter and for intracellular enzymes (Figure 6-7). Recent advances in the cloning of genes for some of the transport proteins have added impetus to the study of the role of membrane transport in the regulation of substrate utilization. Coupled with newer tracer techniques and models for exploring interorgan metabolic acid flow [37–39], the transport of amino acids is now receiving increased research attention.

With respect to the membrane transport of amino acids, the major systems responsible for amino acid transport in mammalian cells have been determined largely by inhibition and kinetic studies, and these systems are summarized in Table 6-5 [40]. Most cells express the transport systems, known as A, ASC, and L. However, different cell types have different complements of additional transport systems, and these are likely required for serving the specific physiologic and metabolic functions of different cells. In reference to the amino acid nutrition of the surgical patient, discussed below are some of the advances in the understanding of the regulation of transport at the transcriptional and translational levels and of the role of transport systems under differing pathophysiologic conditions, including stress (surgery, physical trauma, shock, sepsis) and insulin deficiency (diabetes).

Enhancement or reduction in the activity of

Figure 6-7. Some of the major factors determining the uptake and release of amino acids by cells. (From WW Souba and AJ Pacitti. How amino acids get into cells: Mechanisms, models, menus and mediators. *JPEN* 16:569, 1992.)

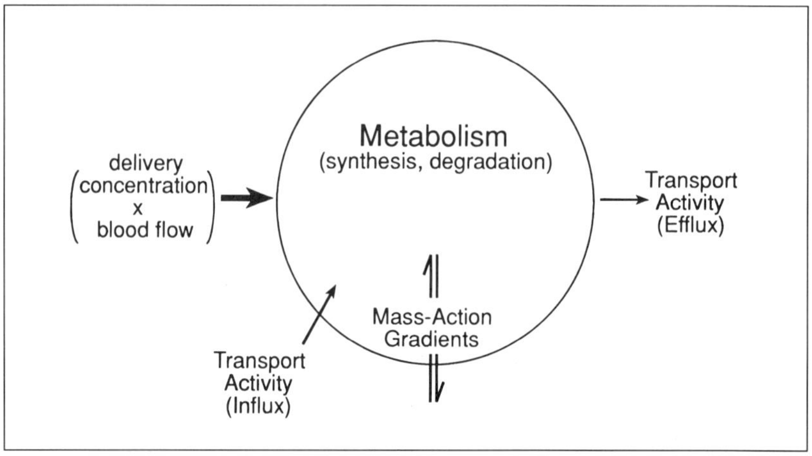

Table 6-5. Some Major Amino Acid Transport Systems in Mammalian Cells

System	Specificity
Na^+-dependent transport systems	
A	Small alphatic amino acids methyl-AlB (W)
ASC	Small alphatic amino acids not methyl-AlB (W)
N	Glutamine, histidine, asparagine
Gly	Glycine, sarcosine (L)
B°	Broad specificity, most neutral amino acids (L)
B	Broad specificity, most neutral amino acids (I)
$B^{\circ+}$	Broad specificity, most neutral acids and basic amino acids
X_{AG-}	Glutamate, asparate (W)
β	β-alanine, taurine (W)
Na^+-independent systems	
L	Mainly branched-chain and amino acids (W)
y^+	Lysine, histidine, arginine (W)
$b^{\circ+}$	Neutral and basicamino acids
x_c^-	Glutamate, cystine

W, L, and I indicate distribution. W = sidespread; L = liver; I = intestine.

Source: Abstracted from JD McGivan, M Pastor-Anglada. Regulatory and molecular aspects of mammalian amino acid transport. *Biochem J* 299:321, 1994.

specific transporters has now been demonstrated for a wide variety of cell types and conditions, and the mechanisms responsible for these changes in transport activity are being elucidated. For example, depletion of amino acid intracellular pools is thought to result in the release of the system A transporter from *trans*-inhibition [41]. Furthermore, the up-regulation of system A transport appears to be the result of increased gene expression of either the transporter protein itself or of a transporter-associated regulatory component; down-regulation caused by amino acid refeeding of cells could perhaps be the result of a repressor protein, make up a part of a mixture of proteins that functionally form an amino acid responsive signaling pathway [42]. It seems likely that with the identification of specific carrier proteins and the cloning of their genes, it will become possible to understand not only the regulation of amino acid transport but also determine in unequivocal terms its quantitative significance in amino acid homeostasis in vivo. For example, we could imagine either overexpressing specific transporters or lowering their activity, using antisense techniques, so that it might be possible to establish their in vivo roles in the utilization of amino acids, especially under the clinical conditions surrounding surgery.

In this latter context, a variety of models are available for the study of amino acid uptake; these were reviewed by Souba and Pacitti [36]. They include (1) measures of regional perfusion, (2) cultured cells, (3) membrane vesicles, and (4) in vivo flux measurements. Although this latter approach does not measure the intrinsic activity of specific membrane carriers of interest or the contributions to transport that the various cells in a tissue make to the overall status of tissue amino acid transport, improved techniques for assessing the in vivo kinetics of amino acid transport and their physiologic significance are emerging. Hence, two important advances should be mentioned.

1. Using a three-compartmental model of leg muscle amino acid kinetics based on use of stable isotope tracers, arteriovenous catheterization, blood flow measurements, and muscle biopsies, Wolfe and Biolo and associates [43–45] have made important headway on an understanding of the relationships between amino acid transmembrane transport and organ protein kinetics in vivo. Thus, they have shown that insulin in healthy human subjects promoted muscle anabolism, primarily by stimulating protein synthesis, and that this was independent of any major effect on transmembrane transport [45]. Models of this kind, perhaps with further adaptations and refinements, offer exciting opportunities for evaluating the quantitative roles of transport, protein synthesis breakdown and amino acid catabolism and, particularly, their interrelationships in the economy of whole-body nitrogen metabolism, especially in the surgical patient.
2. With respect to metabolic regulation, including amino acid transport, a recently recognized pa-

rameter is that of cell volume. Thus, Hausinger and colleagues [46] suggested, particularly in relation to the hepatocyte, that cellular hydration can change within minutes under the influence of hormones and nutrients. They propose that modulation of cell volume within a narrow range acts as a potent signal that modifies cellular metabolism and gene expression. In this context, system A transport is increased by hypertonic shock in a renal epithelial cell line [47], and a proposed mechanism involves an osmotically sensitive gene that codes for a regulatory protein that is able to interact with and activate the A-system transporter (Figure 6-8). These are significant developments, and it will be important now to assess the in vivo or physiologic significance of the osmotic regulation of protein and amino acid metabolism at the level of the gene [48] and at posttranscriptional levels. In particular, it is a challenge to now assess whether this mechanism applies to tissues such as skeletal muscle, whose amino acid and protein balance is so vulnerable to the stress of sepsis and trauma.

Basics in Relation to Protein and Amino Acid Metabolism In Vivo

To illustrate the importance of the above-mentioned molecular and cellular aspects of protein and amino acid metabolism, it might be useful to consider some examples of how this information relates to a more physiologic and pathophysiologic context.

First, does the supply of amino acids regulate protein synthesis or gene expression in eukaryotic cells? Of course, changes in amino acid supply in vivo can modulate protein synthesis via complex endocrine or neural processes rather than via a direct control of transcriptional or translational events. However, Kilberg and colleagues [42] offered a working hypothesis for amino acid–dependent regulation of gene expression, and their view is depicted in Figure 6-9. They propose that a protein transcription factor (regulatory protein) is synthesized in response to starvation, which may enhance the translation of the gene transcript or the synthesis of its corresponding $mRNA_{reg}$. Although much work remains to identify the actual molecular steps by which the cellular concentration of amino acids can regulate the selective expression of genes, the increased availability of genetic and cellular techniques and approaches such as those described by Kilberg and colleagues [42] offer new and exciting opportunities for study of the molecular and cellular basis of mammalian protein metabolism and nutrition.

Second, changes in the rate of breakdown of muscle proteins in response to fasting or in response to growth regulators have been recognized for a long time [49]. However, the rational and effective manipulation of these rates, with particular reference to the care of hospitalized, catabolic patients, requires an understanding of the intracellular mechanisms by which this proteolysis occurs. As reviewed above, lysosomal and nonlysosomal ATP-dependent mechanisms are responsible for the specific and coordinated regulation of

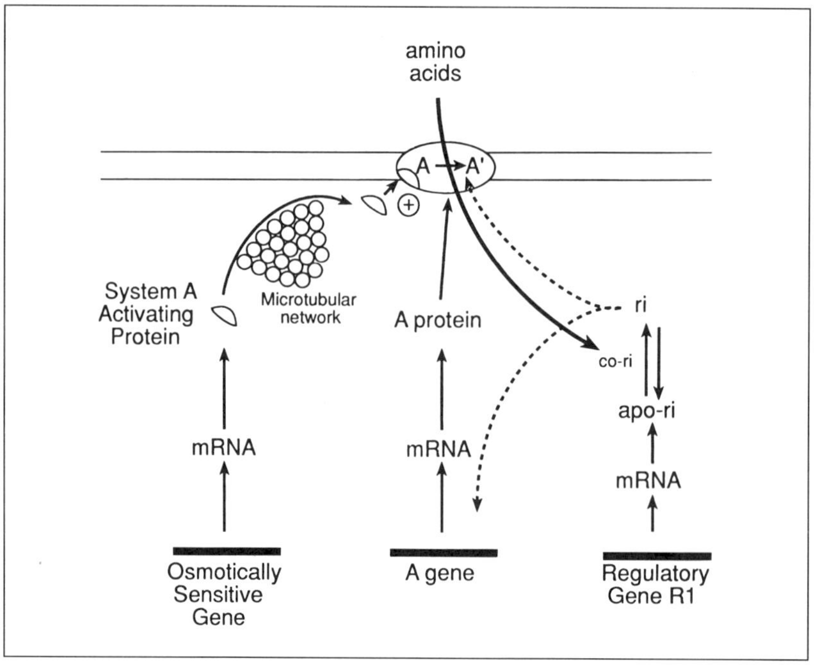

Figure 6-8. A model proposed by Ruiz-Montasell et al. [47] for the regulation of system A activity in osmotically stressed cells. R1 = regulatory gene coding for a regulatory protein, a repressor inactivator that is inactive (apo-ri) in the absence of amino acids. (From B Ruiz-Montasell et al. Evidence for a regulatory protein involved in the increased activity of System A for neutral amino acid transport in osmotically stressed mammalian cells. *Proc Natl Acad Sci USA* 91:9569, 1994.)

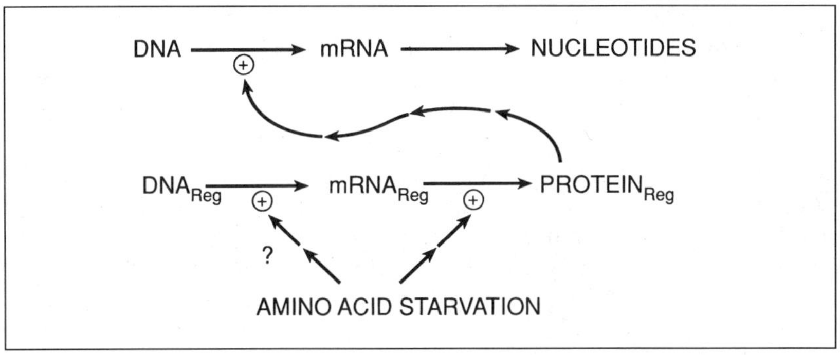

Figure 6-9. A model proposed by Kilberg et al. [42] for the general control by amino acids of gene expression on mammalian cells. The pathway of regulation involves a putative regulatory protein (Reg) that is synthesized in response to amino acid starvation. Although the synthesis of a single regulator is shown, the multiple arrows are meant to acknowledge that the starvation response is probably a cascade of events that collectively represent an amino acid signaling pathway. (From MS Kilberg et al. Amino acid-regulated gene expression in eukaryotic cells. *FASEB J* 8:13, 1994.)

protein breakdown, and so it is of interest to know how diet and hormones affect the ubiquitin-dependent proteolytic system, for example. Recently, Wing and Banville [50] showed that the skeletal muscle levels of the mRNA of ubiquitin-conjugating enzyme (E2; see Figure 6-6 and ubiquitin carrier protein) increase with fasting and return to normal with refeeding in rats. It was also found that insulin lowered the levels of this transcript when tested with myotubes in culture. Because these changes parallel the rates of proteolysis, it appears that a mechanism underlying the effect of dietary protein-energy adequacy or a hormone (insulin) on muscle protein breakdown involves the regulation of expression of a gene involved in the ubiquitin-dependent system. Advances of this kind will assist in the development of effective approaches for attenuating the loss of body protein content in various clinical states, including trauma. In Chapter 3, Hasselgren points out that sepsis in rats increases the levels of ubiquitin mRNA in muscle RNA extracts.

The third example concerns the energy dependency of protein and amino acid metabolism. From the earlier discussion, it is clear that both protein synthesis and degradation are energy-dependent processes and that the utilization of ATP and GTP occurs at multiple sites and in the context of various reactions. Table 6-6 lists some of the major processes that are known to be dependent on a source of ATP or GTP [51]. In addition to the now well-established role of these high-energy intermediates in the initiation and elongation of polypeptide synthesis and in their subsequent breakdown, there has been a further elaboration of the mechanisms responsible for the regulation of cellular processes, such as protein folding and aggregation [52], intracellular trafficking of newly synthesized proteins [53], the transport of proteins across membranes [54,55], including the import of proteins into mitochondria [56] (more than 95% of the mitochondrial proteins are encoded by nuclear genes), and the transduction of signals from outside of cells to their appropriate intracellular sites [57,58]. All involve the participation of energy in the form of ATP or GTP (or cAMP or cyclic guanosine monophosphate) through a series of complex protein interactions and second messenger cascades. Together with the transcription of DNA, splicing of pre-mRNA, peptide chain initiation, the attachment of an amino acid to its cognate tRNA followed by peptide-chain elongation, and the energy required for tissue protein degradation, these complex and interacting processes then will account for and, in part, explain, the molecular and cellular basis for the energy needs for protein maintenance and growth. A challenging problem that we face is how to estimate the energy costs of these processes in vivo. Neverthe-

Table 6-6. Some Energy-Dependent Processes Associated with Protein Turnover and Amino Acid Homeostasis

Protein turnover
Formation of initiation complex
Peptide bond synthesis
Protein degradation
Ubiquitin-dependent
Ubiquitin-independent
Autophagic degradation (sequestration, lysosomal proton pump)
RNA turnover
rRNA; tRNA
pre-mRNA splicing (spliceosome) and mRNA
Amino acid transport
Regulation and integrity
Reversible phosphorylation; enzymes, factors
GTP-GDP exchange proteins (signal transduction)
Second messengers (phosphatidyl inositol system)
Ion pumps and channels
ATP-dependent heat shock protein (folding)
Protein translocation
Nitrogen metabolism
Glutamate-glutamine cycle
Glucose-alanine cycle
Urea synthesis

Source: VR Young. Nutrient interactions with reference to amino acid and protein metabolism in nonruminants; particular emphasis on protein-energy relations in man. *Z Ernahrungswiss* 30:239, 1991.

less, these energy-requiring processes underlie the relationships between protein and energy metabolism in the intact host and the intimate associations between energy intake, protein intake, and overall body nitrogen balance in health and in disease. This topic has been reviewed by us elsewhere [59,60] and so will only be touched on later when we consider body protein turnover in relation to whole-body energy expenditure.

A final example of interest in surgical metabolism and nutrition relates to the posttranslational modifications of protein. First, the methylation of histidine residues occurs within actin and myosin, which are two major fibrillar proteins in skeletal muscle. In 1973, Young and associates [61] proposed use of measurement of 3-methylhistidine (3MH) excretion as an in vivo index of muscle protein breakdown [62]. This suggestion stimulated a great deal of investigation, both in clinical and animal studies, and a recent line of investigation concerns measurement of stable isotopically labeled 3MH by gas chromatography/mass spectrometry [63] and tracer-based estimates of 3MH production [64,65]. This new technique offers great potential for improving an understanding of the in vivo regulation of muscle protein degradation, and it will be interesting to follow the further validation and development of this approach in patients under different pathophysiologic states.

Second, methylated derivatives of arginine occur in muscle proteins [66], and they are excreted in urine [67]. These amino acids have received increased attention recently. In particular, it has been shown that $N^G N^G$-dimethyl-L-arginine is the dominant form of methylarginine synthesized by human endothelial cells and produced in quantities that might affect nitric oxide (NO) on production [68]. Furthermore, the blood level of methylarginines is raised in patients with chronic renal failure [69]. Nitric oxide, a free radical, is a ubiquitous intracellular and intercellular messenger with multiple physiologic and pharmacologic functions [70,71]. More information is needed on the mechanisms determining the intracellular and extracellular levels of these methylated arginines. It will also be important to determine whether these amino acids have any direct or indirect implications for the control of protein or amino acid metabolism, given the plurality of NO function and the fact that there is enhanced NO synthesis in stressed and surgical patients (see Chapter 3).

Amino Acid Oxidation

As shown in Figure 6-1, the process of amino acid oxidation plays an important role in determining body protein amino acid homeostasis. Thus, there is a profound reduction in the rate of oxidation of specific indispensable amino acids when animals are given diets that are low in these amino acids [72,73]. Furthermore, oxidation remains at these reduced levels until approximately the intake level of the amino acid that is necessary to meet the needs for maximum growth is exceeded. Similarly, studies in humans [72] reveal that low intakes of protein or of specific indispensable amino acids bring about an efficient conservation of amino acids, due in large part to a reduced rate of amino acid catabolism. Conversely, high intakes of amino acids raise tissue amino acid levels and increase their rates of oxidation.

The conservation of amino acids when their supply is low occurs in association with a decline in tissue amino acid concentrations [74], and this directly affects the rate of amino acid oxidation. The likely reason for this is that the Michaelis constants (Km's) for the various amino acid degrading enzymes are relatively high [73,75,76] and so they are rarely saturated within the physiologic range of plasma and tissue amino acid concentrations. In contrast, the Km's of aminoacyl-tRNA synthetases are low [73], and they would be expected to be functioning at relatively high rates and their tRNAs essentially fully charged, even when amino acid intakes are low. The net effect of the kinetic properties of these various enzymes would be to more effectively channel into the pathway of protein synthesis. Thus, the efficiency of dietary and endogenous amino acid retention would increase as the intake level is reduced and concomitantly, the oxidation of amino acids would decline. Conversely, high amino acid intakes would reduce the efficiency of amino acid retention as a result of enhanced oxidative catabolism.

It follows, then, that the reduction in amino acid oxidation at low amino acid intakes would parallel changes in plasma amino acid concentrations. This has been shown to occur in adult humans given diets that are low in leucine or in lysine, for example [72,74,77]. Because plasma and tissue amino acid concentrations are highly labile and promptly affected by acute changes in protein and amino acid intake, rates of amino acid oxidation would be expected to change rapidly in response to a dietary change. This is illustrated in Figure 6-10, which shows how the daily pattern of leucine oxidation changes according to the pattern of meal ingestion in healthy adult subjects [78] as well as being affected by the level of leucine intake [compare references 78 and 79]. Thus, substrate availability is an important factor in determining the rate of amino acid oxidation, as

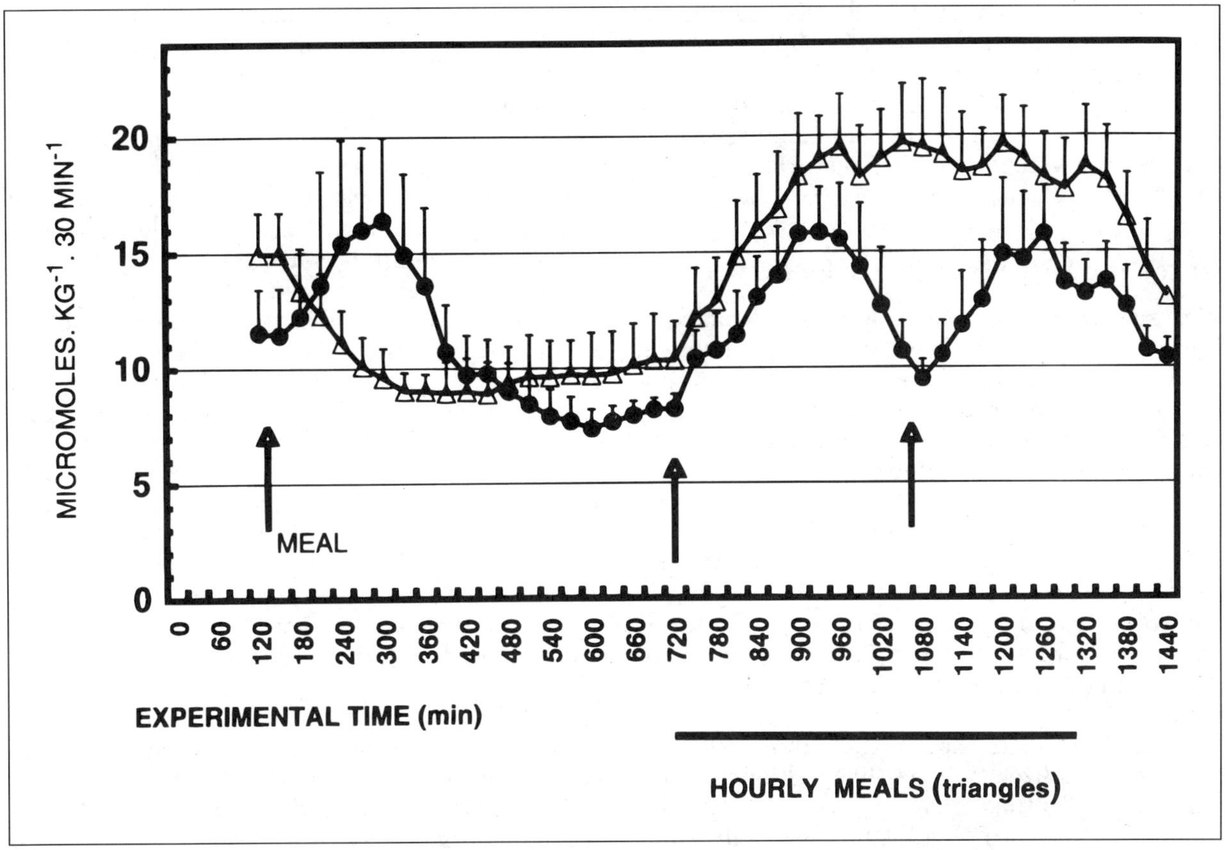

Figure 6-10. A comparison of changes in the rate of leucine oxidation throughout a 24-hour period in young adult subjects receiving a generous dietary leucine intake, given either in the form of small hourly meals over a 10-hour period or as three discrete meals. (From AE El-Khoury et al. Validation of the tracer-balance concept with reference to leucine: 24h intravenous tracer studies with L-[1-^{13}C] leucine and [^{15}N,^{15}N] urea. *Am J Clin Nutr* 59:1000, 1994; AE El-Khoury et al. The 24h pattern and rate of leucine oxidation, with particular reference to tracer estimates of leucine requirements in healthy adults. *Am J Clin Nutr* 59:1012, 1994; and unpublished MIT data.)

predicted from the foregoing discussion of Km's. Furthermore, for generous protein intakes, it now appears that there is a significant prandial rate of oxidation of amino acids, and this may account for about one-half of the daily oxygen consumption by the liver; on this basis, it has been suggested that *gluconeogenesis* from amino acids is to be regarded as a normal prandial process [80].

The status of amino acid oxidation is also determined by the level and properties of tissue enzymes, and these are affected by alterations in protein and amino acid intakes as well as by hormones and cytokines. Involved are allosteric mechanisms, alterations in the amount of enzyme protein, and changes in the proportion of the enzyme in its active and inactive forms. An example of the latter mechanism is the regulation of activity of the second enzyme in the pathway of branched-chain amino acid catabolism; branched-chain keto-acid dehydrogenase (BCKAD) [81]. Here, the activity of BCKAD is regulated by phosphorylation (inactive) and dephosphorylation (active) of the α-subunit of the EI component of the complex, via the BCKAD kinase. This latter enzyme is inhibited by ketoleucine and, to a lesser extent, by the ketoanalogues of isoleucine and valine. Hence, at low leucine intakes, the kinase will be active, giving rise to a reduced activation of BCKAD and, in consequence, a low rate of leucine oxidation. Further, it has been proposed that cytokine-mediated activation of BCKAD may contribute to accelerated branched-chain amino acid oxidation in sepsis [82], and this may also apply to physical trauma.

In summary, amino acid oxidation changes rapidly in response to an altered amino acid intake, and changes in substrate availability appear to be a primary regulatory factor. The amino acid–degrading enzymes are also affected, with alterations in their specific activity as well as the amount of enzyme when protein and amino acid intakes are changed [73] or when the hormonal/

peptide factor milieu is altered. The net effect of these factors is conservation of amino acids and nitrogen, when intake is low and, conversely, higher rates of loss of amino acid nitrogen and carbon when their intakes are abundant or when the prevailing conditions are disturbed by catabolic/stress signals.

Urea Cycle Enzymes and Urea Production

With reference to the major processes depicted in Figure 6-1, the urea cycle enzymes and production of urea should be viewed as a distal pathway involved in the removal of amino nitrogen and for contributing to an adjustment nitrogen loss to nitrogen intake under various conditions. As discussed by Cohen [83], the enzymes of urea biosynthesis associate as a metabolic pathway for conversion of potentially toxic ammonia [84] and removal of excess amino acids via their oxidation and transfer of the nitrogen to arginine and ultimately urea, when the supply of protein or amino acids is high because of variations in the exogenous intake.

The enzymes of the ornithine-urea cycle are compartmentalized in the liver (Figure 6-11) [83,85], and detailed studies of their physical and chemical properties have been described. Additionally, some of these enzymes are abundant in the mitochondria of the intestinal mucosa and in the extramitochondrial fraction in the kidney. The classic studies by Schimke [86] showed that metabolic adaptation to differing consumption levels of protein is associated with changes in the activities of urea cycle enzymes in the liver; these changes were found to be the result of differences in the content of specific protein rather than of changes in their specific activities. The mechanism underlying these alterations in the urea cycle enzyme levels now appears to reside at a pretranslational level [87] for all the enzymes and is largely coordinate. In addition, Das and Waterlow [88] showed that the activity in liver argininosuccinate synthetase was reduced in parallel with the decline in urinary nitrogen output when rats received a low protein diet. However, this parallelism does not necessarily mean that there is a simple cause-and-effect relationship, because the in vitro capacity of the rate-limiting enzyme, argininosuccinate synthetase, in liver of rats given a low protein diet is still, apparently, in considerable excess of the activity that is theoretically needed to handle the flow of nitrogen through the urea cycle. From the standpoint of whole-body N balance, however, it is still not clear whether the process of urea production might "drive" the elimination of amino acids when they are consumed in excess of needs or whether the urea production rate merely accommodates to an increased supply, or transfer, with subsequent removal of amino nitrogen when its supply is high, relative to its use in anabolic pathways.

As discussed above, altered intakes of indispensable amino acids result in changes in rates of amino acid oxidation, and the output of nitrogen in urine also is modulated when the intake of protein shifts from one level to another. Thus, it would be reasonable to predict a parallel change in urea production throughout a relatively wide range of change in the level of dietary nitrogen intake, above and below requirement levels. However, Jackson [89] has reported that in normal adults there is no demonstrable association between urea production and dietary intake over an adequate range of intakes in excess of about 35 g protein/d. He has suggested that the relationship between urea excretion and nitrogen intake does not arise, necessarily, through urea production alone.

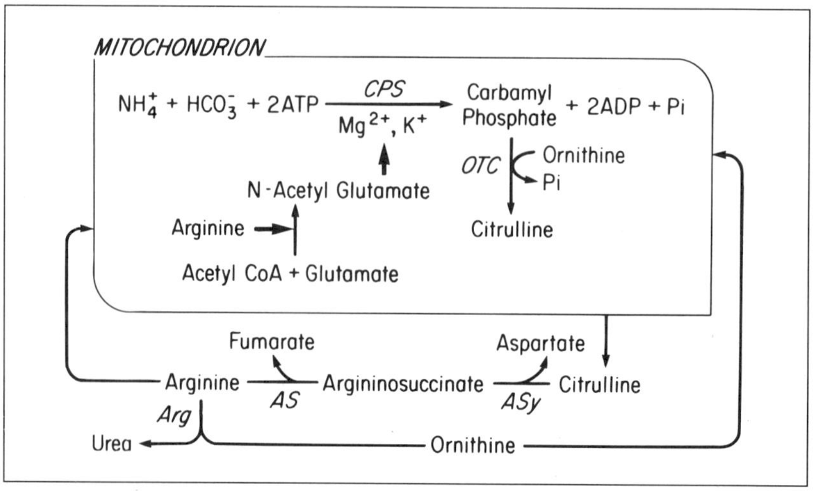

Figure 6-11. The urea cycle enzymes and their distribution within the liver. CPS = carbamyl phosphate synthetase; OTC = ornithine transcarbamylase; ASy = argininosuccinic synthetase; AS = argininosuccinase; Arg = arginase. (From PP Cohen. Regulation of the Ornithine-Urea Cycle Enzymes. In JC Waterlow, JML Stephen (eds), *Nitrogen Metabolism in Man.* London: Applied Science, 1981. P 215.)

Rather, his view is that there is a protein-intake-level–dependent, "salvaging" of urea nitrogen, via intestinal hydrolysis of urea, that is made available to the host as *indispensable* and *dispensable* amino acids in functionally significant amounts. These various conclusions require confirmation, and they are somewhat speculative because the direct evidence currently available does not support this hypothesis [90,91]. Indeed, the physiologic role and importance of urea-nitrogen salvaging in body nitrogen homeostasis is still a matter of uncertainty, but perhaps this process might serve as a mechanism for conserving nitrogen when intakes are very much below physiologic needs. Furthermore, the quantitative role of this process and pathway of urea metabolism in the nitrogen economy of the surgical patient is at present unknown, but it appears that urea-nitrogen recycling may be diminished in children with burn injuries, leading to the suggestion that this could account, in part, for the catabolic nitrogen loss under these conditions [92]. However, we do not believe that there is yet sufficient evidence to warrant a firm conclusion in this context.

An Integration of These Processes and Major Systems

Within the body as a whole, the various biochemical and physiologic processes discussed so far are integrated, and together with results of in vivo studies of various kinds, it is now possible to present a general picture of in vivo protein and amino acid metabolism, as given in Figure 6-12 [93]. This picture is intended to convey the fact that there is a cooperative participation of different organs such as the intestines, liver, kidney, and muscle in determining the fate of the free amino acids that enter the body pools, from either exogenous or endogenous sources.

The fluxes, or rates of transport of specific amino acids within the body, as estimated from plasma tracer kinetics, have been measured in healthy humans, as summarized by Bier (Table 6-7) [93]. However, Christensen [95] reminds us that these fluxes of amino acids are not just simply a consequence of an indiscriminate and intermittent inflow of amino acids arising from protein-containing meals (or from breakdown of endogenous

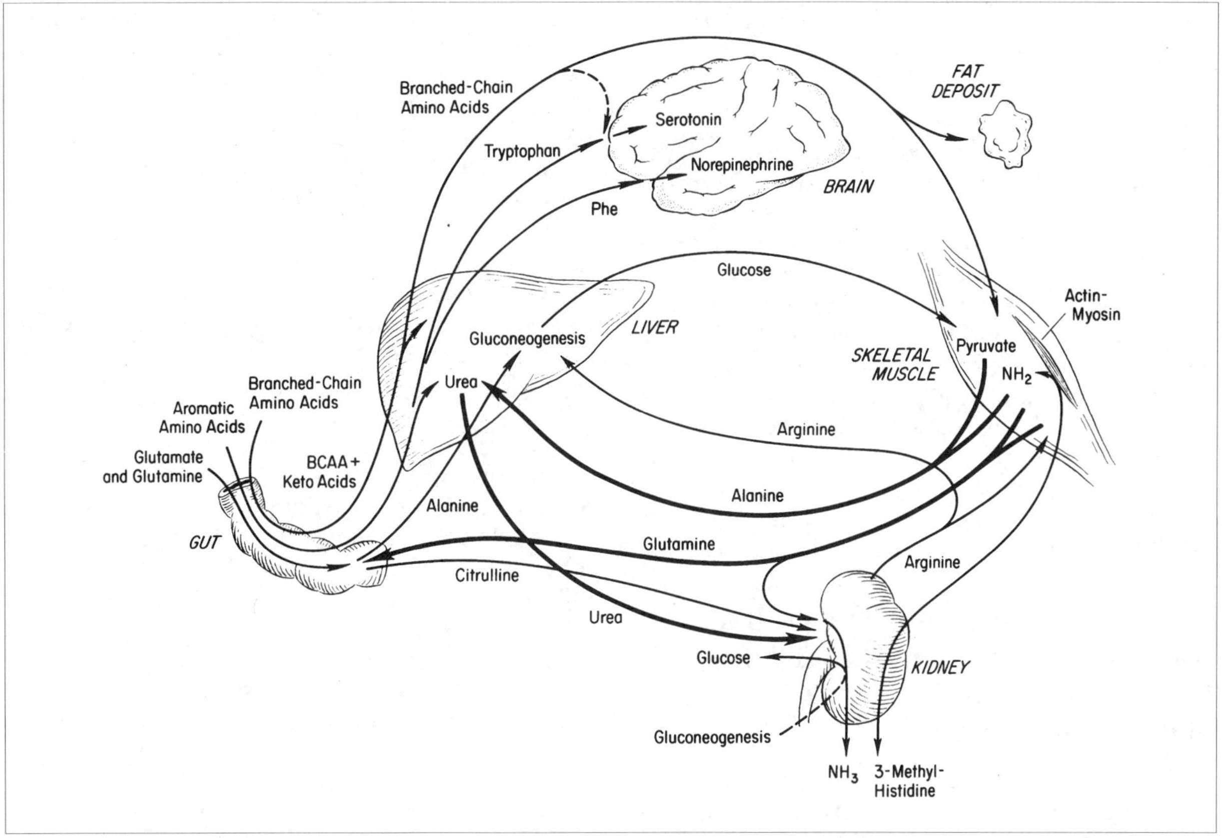

Figure 6-12. Major pathways of transport and fate of selective amino acids between and within organs. (Adapted from HN Munro. Metabolic Basis of Nutritional Care in Liver and Kidney Disease. In RW Winger, HL Green (eds), *Nurtritional Support of the Seriously Ill Patient.* New York: Academic, 1983. P 93.)

Table 6-7. A Summary of Representative and Approximate Plasma Amino Acid Turnover Rates in Healthy Adults

Amino Acid	Flux (μmol kg^{-1} h^{-1})
Indispensable	
Leucine	80–120
Lysine	80–100
Valine	60–85
Threonine	50–70
Isoleucine	60–80
Phenylalanine	30–50
Methionine	20–25
Conditionally indispensable	
Glutamine	250–350
Arginine	60–70
Proline	60–80
Tyrosine	35–45
Cysteine	40–50
Dispensable	
Glutamate	60–100
Glycine	200–250
Alanine	250–350

Source: Adapted from DM Bier. Intrinsically difficult problems: The kinetics of body proteins and amino acids in man. *Diabetes Metab Rev* 5:111, 1989.

proteins), but they are regulated at specific organ sites and by various mechanisms. Indeed, we submit that the quantitative significance of these fluxes, together with an understanding of the in vivo mechanisms and points of control of specific amino acid metabolism in patients under different nutritional and pathophysiologic conditions, is necessary if we are to establish the metabolic basis of the requirements for protein and amino acids in healthy and sick patients. Hence, we should consider briefly some of the methods for measuring whole-body protein turnover and amino acid fluxes before assessing how nutrition and stress affect these aspects of human protein metabolism.

Methods for Measuring Whole-Body Protein Turnover and Amino Acid Fluxes: Particular Reference to Stable Isotope Studies

In recent years, stable isotope tracer techniques have been used extensively to estimate amino acid fluxes and protein kinetics at the whole-body level and in individual tissues and organs. These have been reviewed in detail by Waterlow and colleagues [96–98] and by others [99–101]. The different tracer approaches have been classified generally into one of two major categories: (1) those involving use of ^{15}N and measurement of the label in end products of nitrogen metabolism (*end-product methods*) and (2) those involving administration of specifically labeled amino acids and measurement of the tracer in body fluids, such as plasma or urine. Measurement may also be made of the appearance of the label in metabolic products of the amino acid, such as in expired air or in a more proximal metabolite, such as tyrosine, in the case of a labeled phenylalanine tracer [102,103], or α-ketoisocaproate where labeled leucine is the tracer of choice [104]. This second approach has been termed the plasma or precursor method [97], particularly when applied in investigations and estimations of whole-body protein turnover. The approach may further be regarded as a *substrate-specific method,* when the major focus of interest is on the metabolism of a specific amino acid, in contrast to the case where a labeled amino acid, such as leucine, is used as an index of the overall status of amino acid and whole-body protein kinetics [105].

The determination of the isotopic content of the biologic matrices of interest (e.g., blood, urine, expired air, tissue protein) is achieved most often by mass spectrometric techniques, although other analytical approaches, including nuclear magnetic resonance and emission spectroscopy, may also be used [106] in studies of tissue and whole-body amino acid turnover in vivo. A review of the details of the specific analytical methodology is outside the scope of this chapter, but the reader is referred to valuable discussions by others [107,108] for more complete information on this topic. A general discussion about the principles and application of these two general approaches follows.

End-Product Methods

The principle behind the ^{15}N-product approaches for measurement of protein (nitrogen) turnover in the whole body is depicted in Figure 6-13 [109]; it involves administration of a ^{15}N-labeled precursor (often ^{15}N-glycine) and measurement of the appearance of the isotope in urinary urea, ammonia, or total nitrogen [97,98]. In its simplest form the metabolic nitrogen pool is depicted as a single homogenous pool into which nitrogen enters from protein breakdown and from the diet. Nitrogen leaves via protein synthesis and by pathways of nitrogen excretion. This concept was first proposed by Sprinson and Rittenberg [110] and then later expanded by Picou and Taylor-Roberts [111], who described a one-pool model of whole-body nitrogen metabolism, involving the continuous administration of a ^{15}N-labeled substrate over a

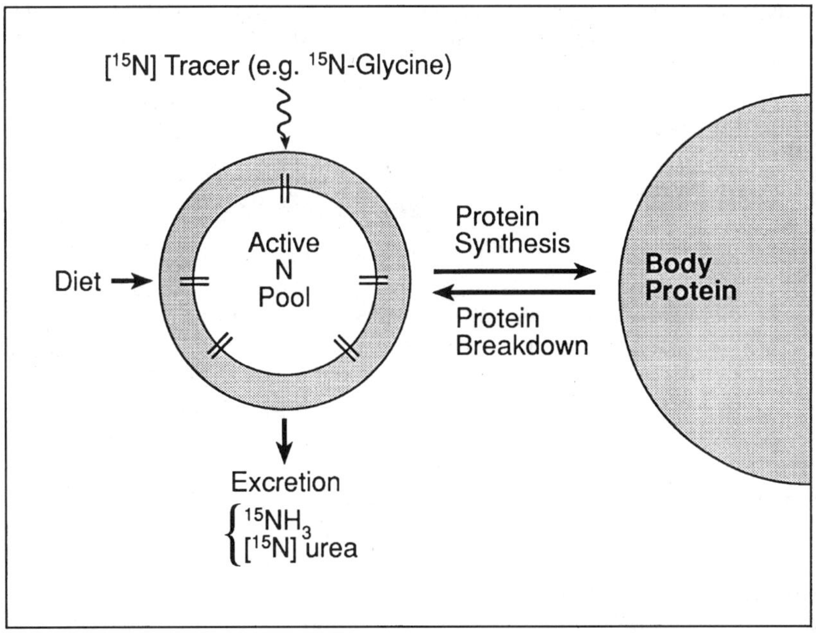

Figure 6-13. General model used to estimate whole-body nitrogen kinetics. The double lines in the active amino acid N pool are meant to signify nitrogen exchange and metabolic reactions that are not included directly in the processes of protein synthesis and breakdown. (Adapted from DM Bier et al. Interpretation of Amino Acid Kinetic Studies in the Context of Whole-Body Protein Metabolism. In JS Garrow, D Halliday (eds), *Substrate and Energy Metabolism in Man.* London: Libbey, 1985. P 27.)

prolonged period. Their model, or modifications of it, has been used extensively by many investigators during the intervening years [97,98,100].

With regard to the application of this model, a number of different procedures of isotope administration have been followed. One involves a continuous or frequent administration of the ^{15}N-labeled amino acid with measurement of the enrichment of the label in the major end products of nitrogen metabolism before and after achievement of an isotopic plateau. Interpretation of the ^{15}N isotopic data, for purposes of estimating body nitrogen flux and rates of body protein synthesis and breakdown, involves a number of basic and simplifying assumptions, and these have been discussed elsewhere [109,111,112]; they are summarized in Table 6-8. Another procedure in using a ^{15}N end-product approach is to give a single bolus administration of the ^{15}N-labeled precursor, either by vein or by the gut, and to measure the ^{15}N-excretion at frequent times or in a relatively few consecutive and complete urine samples, to determine the cumulative excretion of the label [113].

Table 6-8. Assumptions of the ^{15}N-Glycine End-Product Method for Estimating Whole-Body Protein Turnover

^{15}N is biologically indistinguishable from ^{14}N.
^{15}N-glycine is administered as a true "weightless" tracer.
The system is in steady state.
There is a single metabolic nitrogen pool.
The tracer is uniformly distributed within the nitrogen pool.
Glycine nitrogen is a valid tracer for total amino acid nitrogen.
Tracer is not diluted significantly by nitrogen other than diet or protein nitrogen.
Glycine nitrogen does not give rise to quantitatively significant products other than protein or end products.
The proportion of glycine nitrogen to total nitrogen entering end products is equal to the fraction of glycine nitrogen to total nitrogen entering protein.

Source: From DM Bier, DE Matthews, VR Young. Interpretation of Amino Acid Kinetic Studies in the Context of Whole-Body Protein Metabolism. In JS Garrow, D Halliday (eds), *Substrate and Energy Metabolism in Man.* London: Libbey, 1985. P 27.

The isotopic data generated from ^{15}N-labeled tracer administration may be evaluated using a compartmental modeling approach or by applying a stochastic model in which the overall flow of nitrogen in and out of the metabolic pool is of interest, rather than the movement of nitrogen within and among the intermediate pools. As Waterlow [97] pointed out, the stochastic method gives less information than does the compartmental modeling approach, but it is obtained more easily; this might be an advantage in studies dealing with protein and amino acid turnover that are conducted under the demanding experimental conditions that characterize many clinical settings. Additional details, problems, and limitations of this approach have been discussed by us elsewhere [113]. In summary, however, there has been generally good agreement between estimates of whole-body protein turnover as determined by either the continuous ^{15}N-glycine infusion approach and the so-called single-dose procedure and between estimates made from ^{15}N end-product methods and those obtained by application of precursor methods [97].

Still to be answered is the question "What is the appropriate ^{15}N end-product protocol?" A precise answer is still somewhat unclear, because it would appear to depend on the specific purposes and conditions of the study. However, on the basis of the evidence, it seems to us that ^{15}N-glycine represents a reasonable choice of tracer and that, for more precise estimates of the rates of body protein synthesis and breakdown, a continuous (or frequently repeated) ^{15}N dosing administration might be preferable, although the single ^{15}N-glycine dose procedure is convenient. This procedure can be repeated at frequent intervals during a dietary regimen, for example, in studies of host adaptation or adjustment, or during recovery from a pathologic insult such as trauma or after surgery. Also, there is still no clear-cut answer concerning which end product to measure. For the single-dose method, it appears prudent to measure ^{15}N output in both urea and ammonia in a complete 9- to 12-hr urine test. This provides an opportunity to further evaluate the differences in estimates of protein dynamics when based on these two major end products of nitrogen metabolism. A further refinement involves measurement of the retention of ^{15}N in the body urea pool between isotope administration and the completion of urine collection, especially where studies involve a single dose of glycine. The dose of ^{15}N-glycine should not be too large, otherwise the estimates of nitrogen flux may be too low [98].

Precursor, Plasma, or Substrate-Specific Methods

Under this general category of methods, a tracer-labeled amino acid is administered, most often by continuous intravenous infusion, and it is often immediately preceded by a priming dose to help achieve a rapid approach to isotopic plateau equilibrium within the sampled compartment. In human studies, the latter is most often the venous blood circulation, although urine could be sampled as a means of the noninvasive determination of the isotopic enrichment in the free amino acid pool [114]. Alternative procedures within this class include giving the isotope tracer by bolus intravenous injection, oral administration, or both, where simultaneous doses of different specific labeled tracers of an amino acid are used.

The basic features of the precursor procedure are depicted in Figure 6-14, where enrichment of the tracer is measured in the plasma and, if appropriate, the appearance of the label in expired carbon dioxide is also monitored. Using simple

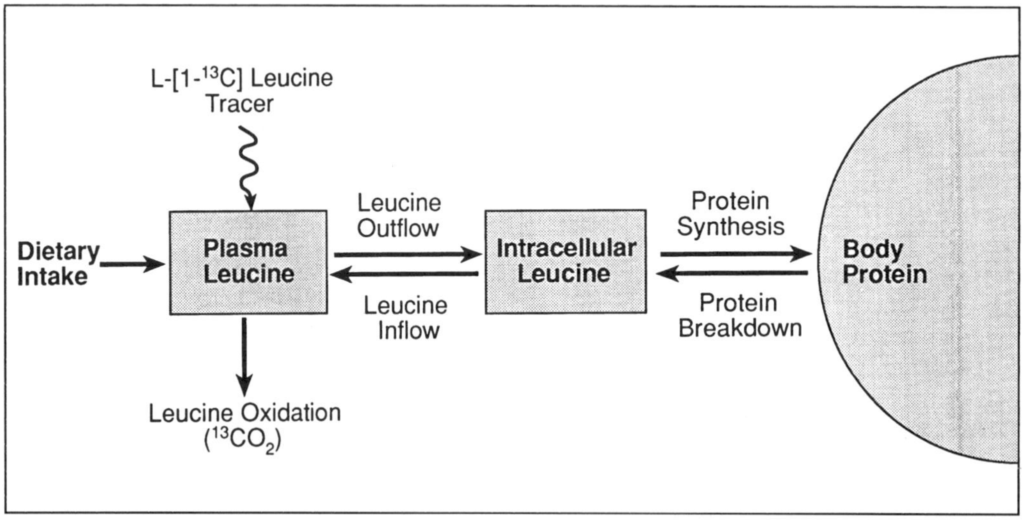

Leucine Flux = Leucine Oxidation + Leucine Outflow for Protein Synthesis = Leucine Intake + Leucine Inflow from Protein Breakdown

Figure 6-14. Simplified model of the so-called precursor method for estimating amino acid inflow to the plasma compartment from proteolysis and outflow from this compartment for protein synthesis, using a representative [1-^{13}C] labeled amino acid tracer, such as leucine. (Taken from DM Bier et al. Interpretation of Amino Acid Kinetic Studies in the Context of Whole-Body Protein Metabolism. In JS Garrow, D Halliday (eds), *Substrate and Energy Metabolism in Man.* London: Libbey, 1985. P27.)

dilution principles, the flux of the amino acid in the sampled compartment can be determined. Under steady-state metabolic and isotopic conditions, when a nutritionally indispensable amino acid is used as a tracer, estimates can be made of the rate of disappearance of the tracer via nonoxidative metabolism (assumed to be a measure of protein synthesis, provided the intake and oxidation rate of the amino acid are also known and estimated). The most extensively used tracer to date in studies of whole-body protein turnover in humans has been L-[1-^{13}C]leucine, given as a primed continuous infusion, with measurement of either plasma ^{13}C-leucine or preferably of ^{13}C-ketoisocaproate as an index of the intracellular enrichment of the tracer. For many investigations, the choice of ^{13}C-leucine as the tracer for quantifying whole-body protein dynamics would appear to be quite reasonable [105]. Nevertheless, for any new physiologic or pathologic condition, caution must be exercised when first attempting to estimate whole-body protein dynamics by use of a single amino acid tracer.

A number of issues ought to be considered when using the plasma or precursor approach for measurement of amino acid fluxes and for estimation of whole-body protein dynamics. Table 6-9 [115] lists some of the major questions faced when attempting to estimate the whole-body amino acid flux and rate of protein synthesis. Some answers to these questions are given elsewhere [115], so a further detailed discussion of them should be unnecessary. However, a particularly important problem is that of determining isotopic enrichment of the precursor of interest to estimate either whole-body amino acid flux or the rate of protein synthesis or the rate of synthesis in its various regions. Because in most clinical investigations it would be difficult or unethical to sample the tissue or organ pools of interest, the problem might be overcome, at least in part, by measuring in blood the enrichment of a metabolite derived from the intracellular metabolism of the tracer that is in rapid equilibrium with the extracellular compartment. In this context, Matthews and colleagues [104] proposed that the transamination product of leucine, α-ketoisocaproate (KIC), would predict intracellular leucine labeling. Subsequent studies have generally supported the value of this approach [116]. A current research challenge is to identify and investigate other blood-borne intracellular markers of the enrichment of specific amino acid tracers and their metabolic products, such as lysine, phenylalanine, threonine, and methionine. For example, α-amino adipic acid may be a useful probe of the intracellular (hepatic) lysine enrichment [117], and the extent of labeling of an amino acid in apolipoprotein B-100 of very low density lipoprotein is gaining use as an index of isotope enrichment of the hepatic amino acid pool [118].

The "Flooding Dose" Technique

Mention should be made of the "flooding dose" method, which Garlick and colleagues used successfully in earlier experimental animals and more recently adapted the procedure to apply with stable isotopes and determine rates of synthesis of muscle proteins and albumin in humans [100]. The approach involves giving the label (such as [1-^{13}C]leucine or [$^{2}H_5$]phenylalanine) together with a large amount of unlabeled amino acid to create a similar isotopic enrichment in the extracellular and intracellular compartments, including the pool supplying amino acids for tRNA charging.

Table 6-9. Some Issues and Questions Related to Choice of Precursor or Plasma Approach for Measurement of Amino Fluxes and Whole-Body Protein Turnover

1. What model and why?
   a. For whole-body protein turnover.
   b. For measurement of organ (regional) protein and amino acid metabolism.
   c. For study of specific amino acid metabolism; its conversions and interconversions and metabolic fate.
   d. For studying the carbon and/or nitrogen moiety and/or functional groups of the molecule.
2. What is the isotopic enrichment of the precursor amino acid pool(s) for accurate measurement of whole-body flux and oxidation rates?
3. What are the appropriate amounts of tracer and length of infusion period; is there a problem with recycling of label?
4. Are infusion and sampling sites important? Which are best?
5. For measurement of components of flux, what is the retention of $^{13}CO_2$?

Source: VR Young. Techniques in Measuring Protein Turnover: In Vivo Techniques. In KS Nair (ed), *Protein Metabolism in Diabetes Mellitus.* London: Smith-Gordon, 1992. P 47.

The idea and approach are highly attractive, particularly because the method involves a relatively brief study period for any one experimental subject and therefore might be applicable in various complex clinical settings. Estimates of albumin synthesis obtained by this method seem to be in general agreement with those derived from the constant tracer infusion approach, but serious concern has been raised about the appropriateness of the technique for estimating synthesis rates of muscle proteins [119,120]. However, published estimated rates of muscle protein synthesis (both within and between laboratories) vary considerably, for biologic as well as experimental reasons, and further critical studies of this procedure are necessary before the utility of the flooding dose method has been sufficiently evaluated for possible widespread application in clinical studies. However, the flooding dose is suited to measurements made on tissues that can be taken during surgery. Table 6-10 summarizes rates of protein synthesis in adult tissues based on [1-^{13}C]leucine and [$^{2}H_5$]phenylalanine as tracers.

Table 6-10. Rates of Protein Synthesis Measured by the Flooding Dose Technique with [1-^{13}C]Leucine or [$^{2}H_5$]Phenylalanine in Various Tissues of Adult Humans

Tissue	Protein Synthesis (% d^{-1}) ($\pm$ SEM)
Skeletal muscle	1.95 ± 0.12
Heart (atrium)	5.2 ± 0.8
Lymphocytes	6.2 ± 0.4
Colon (mucosa)	9.4 ± 1.2
Liver	20.7 ± 1.9
Esophagus	29.5 ± 2.0
Stomach (antrum)	42.9 + 5.0
Stomach (fundus)	44.5 + 10.3

Source: From PJ Garlick, MA McNurlan. Isotopic Methods for Studying Protein Turnover. In NCR Räiha (ed), *Protein Metabolism During Infancy.* New York: Raven, 1994. P 29.

Some Quantitative Aspects of Protein Turnover and Amino Acid Metabolism

So far we have discussed some of the mechanisms of protein synthesis and degradation, amino acid transport, and oxidation, and the methods that might be used in humans to estimate their whole body and organ rates have been mentioned briefly. Next, we will consider the quantitative aspects of the rates of some of these processes, first with reference to whole-body protein turnover.

Protein Turnover

Protein synthesis rates are high in the newborn and, per unit of body weight, these rates decline with progressive growth and development (Table 6-11) [121]. Three points emerge from the data summarized here. First, the higher rate of protein synthesis in the young [121,122], as compared with that for the adult, is not only related to the net protein deposition that occurs during growth, but there is also a high rate of total protein turnover (synthesis and breakdown), possibly related in part to tissue remodeling. Hence, protein *synthesis* in the premature infant is about twice as high as in the preschool child and approximately three or four times as high as in the adult. Second, at all ages the rates of whole-body protein synthesis and breakdown are considerably greater than

Table 6-11. Comparison of Whole-Body Protein Synthesis Rates With Dietary Protein Allowances at Different Ages

Age Group	Protein Synthesis (A)*	Protein Allowance (B)*	Ratio A/B
Infant (premature)	11.3, 14	~3	4.3
Newborn	6.7	1.85	3.6
Child (15 months)	6.3	1.3	4.8
Child (2–8 years)	3.9	1.1	3.5
Adolescent (~13 years)	~5	1.0	–5
Young adult (~20 years)	~4.0	0.75	~5.3
Elderly (~70 years)	~3.5	0.75	4.7

*Measured in g protein·$kg^{-1}d^{-1}$.

Source: From VR Young et al. The Biochemistry and Physiology of Protein and Amino Acid Metabolism with Reference to Protein Nutrition. In NCR Räiha (ed), *Protein Metabolism During Infancy.* New York: Raven, 1994. P 1.

the intakes of dietary protein apparently necessary to meet the needs for maintenance or for the support of growth (see Table 6-11). It follows, therefore, that there is an extensive reutilization within the body of the amino acids entering tissue pools during the course of protein breakdown. Third, there is a general relationship between the age- and developmental-associated changes in protein turnover and the dietary protein needs for each specific age group. This implies to us that when rates of synthesis and breakdown of body proteins change in response to various stimuli, such as infection and trauma, the dietary requirement for nitrogen and specific amino acids intakes will change. This prediction is consistent with the observed increased total nitrogen needs of the injured patient [123], and the importance of protein synthesis and turnover as determinants of the dietary requirement for indispensable amino acids has been discussed previously [77]. Again, therefore, a higher turnover and oxidation rate would inevitably mean a higher requirement for the specific amino acid. Indeed, as summarized in Table 6-12, rates of turnover (or flux) of the indispensable amino acids, together with proline and arginine in patients with burn injuries, for example, are generally much higher than the flux values summarized earlier in Table 6-7 for healthy adults. Furthermore, the measured oxidation rates in burn patients generally exceed those for healthy controls who have been studied in the postabsorptive state. To put these flux data into a further perspective, a leucine flux of 190 μmol $kg^{-1}d^{-1}$ (see Table 6-12) is equivalent to a turnover of 7.3 g protein $kg^{-1}d^{-1}$. In contrast, a healthy adult experiences a turnover of approximately 4 g protein $kg^{-1}d^{-1}$. Similarly, the lysine flux given in Table 6-12 is equivalent to a turnover of about 7 g protein $kg^{-1}d^{-1}$, confirming the presence of much higher rates of protein synthesis and breakdown in this stressful state.

Of metabolic and nutritional interest is the relationship between the resting metabolic rate and the rate of whole-body protein turnover. As summarized in Table 6-13 and based on an interspecies survey, it can be estimated that about 15 to 20 kJ (4–5 kcal) of basal energy expenditure is associated with each gram of whole-body protein synthesis. On this basis, amino acid transport and peptide synthesis alone appear to account for at

Table 6-12. A Summary of Some Estimates of Plasma Amino Acid Kinetics and Oxidation Rates in Burn Patients

Amino Acid	Flux	Oxidation Rate (μmol $kg^{-1}h^{-1}$)	Reference
Leucine	~190	~30	124
Valine	~187	not measured	125
Lysine	~156	not measured	125
Phenylalanine	~71	~15	126
Methionine	~54	~9	127
Proline	~137	~29	128
Arginine	~110	not measured	124

Table 6-13. Whole-Body Protein Turnover in Relation to Resting Metabolic Rate in Adults of Mammalian and Avian Species

Species	Weight (kg)	Protein Turnover ($g{\cdot}kg^{-1}d^{-1}$) [A]	Metabolic Rate ($kJ{\cdot}kg^{-1}d^{-1}$) [B]	Ratio B/A
Mouse	0.04	43.5	760	11
Rat	0.35	22.0	364	17
Rabbit	3.6	9.2	192	20
Wallaby (pamma)	4.2	7.5	163	21
Sheep	63	5.6	96	17
Man	70	4.6	107	23
Cow	575	3.0	60	20
Birds (chickens)	1.4	27	439	16

Source: From VR Young, Y-M Yu, NK Fukagawa. Energy and Protein Turnover. In J Kinney, HN Tucker (eds), *Energy Metabolism: Tissue Determinants and Cellular Corollaries.* New York: Raven, 1992. P 439.

least 20% of basal metabolism. It follows then that major changes in body protein turnover caused, for example, by severe infection or major trauma could not only affect the protein and amino acid requirements but also the status of body energy expenditure and requirements. From the available data, it would be reasonable to conclude that the increased rate of protein turnover in adult burn patients [124–128] accounts for at least about 20% of their increased metabolic rate, relative to that in healthy controls.

It follows from the above that both the levels of protein as well as energy intake can affect body nitrogen balance. Indeed, the available data reveal that the effects of these nutritional factors are interdependent, and their interactions can be complex. It was pointed out some years ago by Calloway and Spector [129] that the level of caloric intake, whether above or below requirements, determines the changes in nitrogen balance that can be achieved by an increase in nitrogen intake. Furthermore, the level of nitrogen intake determines the quantitative effect of energy intake on nitrogen balance [130] (Figure 6-15). The existence of separate protein and energy-dependent phases on nitrogen balance or protein accretion has been demonstrated in both humans and experimental animals, and a recognition of these relationships and interactions is necessary for the design of diets that are efficient in terms of promoting protein retention, while achieving a desirable body and tissue composition in stressed patients.

In quantitative terms, for human subjects, excess energy intake at adequate levels of nitrogen intake causes a retention of approximately 1 to 2 mg nitrogen per kcal in healthy subjects [59], but at limiting or low nitrogen intakes this response is markedly attenuated [130]. At lower energy intakes, within the submaintenance range, the impact of changes in energy intake on N balance is greater; for normal humans it appears that at very low energy intakes the relationship between changes in energy intake and nitrogen balance is approximately 8 mg N $kcal^{-1}$, with the relationship "breaking" at a total energy intake of about 1400 kcal daily [113]. This also applies for depleted, postabsorptive hospitalized patients [59] in whom a value of 7.5 mg N/kcal has been found for energy intakes up to about 15 kcal/kg body weight/d (Figure 6-16). A complete metabolic explanation for this difference in the energy intake–nitrogen balance relationship below and then above maintenance energy intakes is difficult to present, but it is of possible interest that the breakpoint in the energy intake–nitrogen retention relationship referred to above occurs at an energy level approxi-

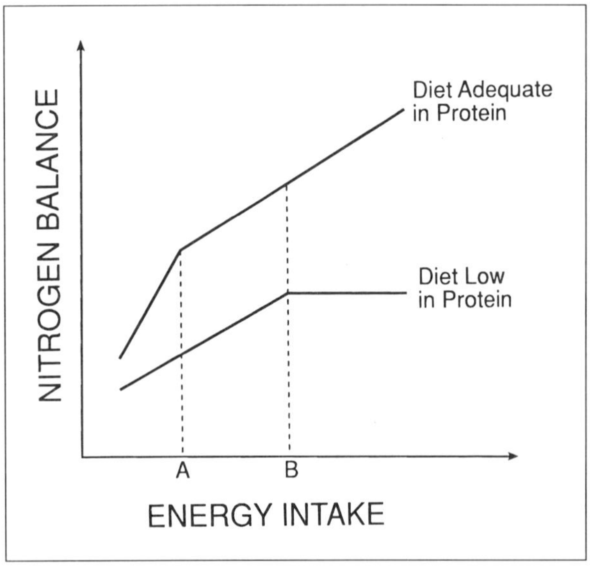

Figure 6-15. Relationship of N balance and energy intake with diets of different protein levels. Between energy intake A (low) and B (higher) the two lines are parallel. (From HN Munro. General Aspects of the Regulation of Protein Metabolism by Diet and by Hormones. In HN Munro, JB Allison (eds), *Mammalian Protein Metabolism.* Vol 1. New York: Academic, 1964. P 381.)

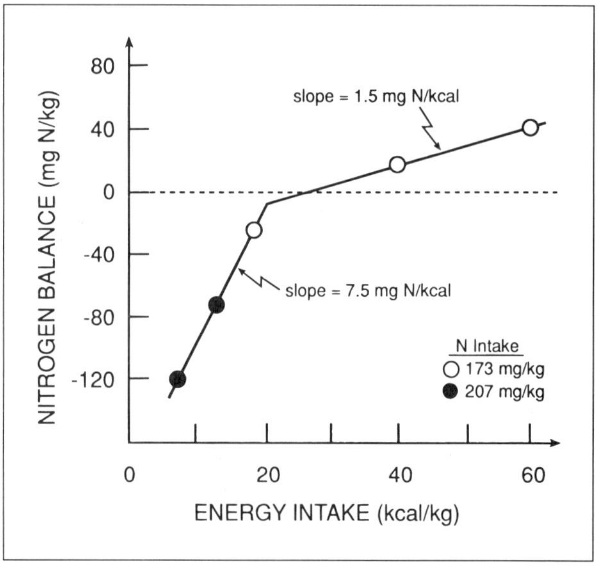

Figure 6-16. Relation between N balance and energy intake in postabsorptive and depleted patients. (Adapted from VR Young, Y-M Yu, NK Fukagawa. Whole Body Energy and Nitrogen (Protein) Relationships. In J Kinney, HN Tucker (eds), *Energy Metabolism: Tissue Determinants and Cellular Corollaries.* New York: Raven, 1992. P 139; DH Elwyn. Nutritional requirements of adult surgical patients. *Crit Care Med* 8:9, 1980; DH Elwyn et al. Changes in nitrogen balance of depleted patients with increasing infusions of glucose. *Am J Clin Nutr* 32:1597, 1979; DH Elwyn et al. Protein and energy sparing of glucose added in hypocaloric amounts to peripheral solutions of amino acids. *Metabolism* 27:325, 1988.)

mately equivalent to a glucose intake of approximately 3 mg $kg^{-1}min^{-1}$. Because this corresponds to about the rate of exogenous glucose administration that maximally suppresses endogenous glucose production in the human adult [134], the change in the energy intake–nitrogen retention relationship shown in Figure 6-16 presumably relates to the fate of gluconeogenic precursors (including amino acids) used for maintenance of body glucose homeostasis when the preformed glucose supply is low.

Amino Acid Kinetics

Arginine Metabolism

It is not feasible to review here in detail the broad topic of amino acid kinetics, so we will illustrate an application of the tracer methods discussed above in studies carried out in young adult humans and in burn trauma patients, with reference to plasma arginine kinetics. These studies are useful in that they expose the complexity and coordination of amino acid metabolism in the human host.

As already noted, the five urea cycle enzymes act in concert to form arginine and urea from ornithine, ammonia, and carbon dioxide. The cycle is complete within the normal liver, and this is the major organ responsible for exerting a major functional capacity for net urea synthesis. However, it has been known for a number of years that urea cycle enzyme activity is present in tissues and organs other than the liver; indeed, the intestine and kidney each function in the extrahepatic synthesis of arginine [135]. Based on biochemical and physiologic studies, it appears that the intestine is capable of synthesizing ornithine and citrulline, and the kidney then converts the citrulline to arginine. This endogenous synthesis plays a critical role in the support of the growth needs in the rat [136] and citrulline availability to the kidney appears to be an important factor in determining the rate of extrahepatic arginine synthesis [137]. With reference to human nutrition, it may also be of interest to point out that the amount of citrulline converted to arginine by this organ is reduced in patients with chronic renal insufficiency (CRI) [138]. Although the nutritional significance of the lower synthesis of arginine by the kidney in these patients is not clear, it might be speculated that it would increase the risk of a cellular arginine inadequacy in times of high demand, such as after infection or trauma and during repletion from an earlier catabolic state.

Our scheme is based on a modification of Brusilow and Horwich [135]. Figure 6-17 depicts a cooperation between the intestine, kidney, and liver in relation to the formation and fate of arginine. Because the skeletal musculature is an important endogenous source of plasma glutamine, which in turn may serve as a major precursor for ornithine and citrulline synthesis by the intestine, this organ is also included in this picture of interorgan aspects of arginine metabolism. On this basis, it would not be unreasonable to speculate that the integrity of the interorgan and metabolic interrelations, as shown here, would be affected, or compromised, by various pathophysiologic states.

From this scheme, it might be construed that tissue arginine needs could be met in various ways: (1) via dietary arginine that escapes metabolism in the liver; (2) via the de novo synthesis of arginine that can occur in the liver and possibly the intestine, because of the presence of ornithine transcarbamylase; (3) via conversion of citrulline, which occurs in the kidneys, and (4) by taking up circulatory endogenous arginine released by the kidneys. An important question is the contribution made by these various sources for meeting tissue arginine requirements and the quantitative extent to which dietary arginine might substitute for, or down-regulate, the net supply of arginine arising via the metabolic conversions depicted in Figure 6-17.

These issues have been explored recently, in our laboratories, using specifically labeled, stable-isotope tracers of arginine, citrulline, and ornithine to determine plasma arginine, ornithine, and citrulline fluxes [139–144]. A number of important observations have emerged from these studies, and the results are summarized in Table 6-14. First, the measured plasma flux of arginine is much lower than might have been expected for the whole-body flux of the guanidino moiety for the amino acid. It can be estimated that the sum of the whole-body (plasma?) arginine flux contributed by protein breakdown and the turnover of the guanidino moiety via the urea cycle would amount to $\geq$ 350 μmol $kg^{-1}hr^{-1}$, for subjects consuming an adequate diet. **This is far higher than the plasma arginine flux shown in Table 6-14.** In our study [142], urea production amounted to about 350 μmol $kg^{-1}hr^{-1}$, and so the expected whole-body flux of the guanidino moiety in this case would have been considerably greater than the value of 350. It seems that the intravenous arginine tracer and therefore plasma arginine fail to exchange extensively with the arginine pool that is continually being formed and hydrolyzed via the hepatic urea cycle enzymes. Indeed, considerable biochemical evidence indicates a tight

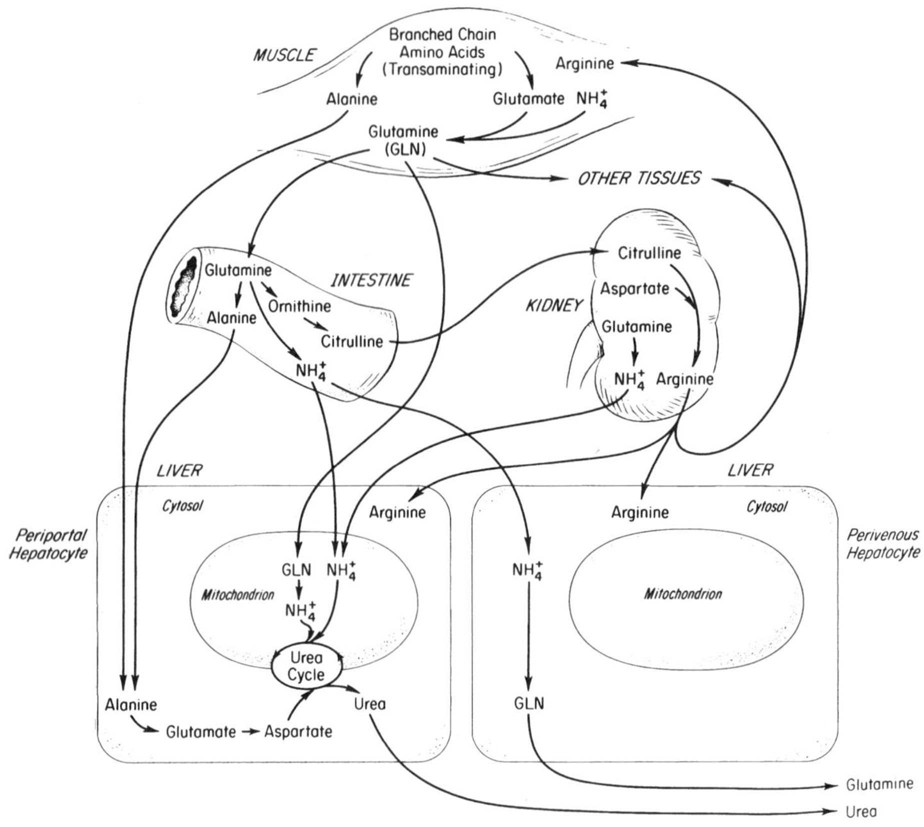

Figure 6-17. Scheme to depict the major organs, cellular specificity within the liver, and some of the interactions among amino acids involved in arginine metabolism in vivo. (Modified from SW Brusilow, AL Horwith. Urea Cycle Enzymes. In CR Scriver et al. [eds], *The Metabolic Basis of Inherited Disease.* New York: McGraw-Hill, 1989. P 629.)

channeling of intermediates between the interacting enzymes of the urea cycle [145,146]. Additionally, there also appears to be a channeling of arginyl-tRNA in the liver cell [147], with the suggestion being that one arginyl-tRNA pool is used for protein synthesis, and the other pool is involved in the arginylation of proteins, which serves as a signal for ubiquitin-dependent protein degradation.

The intracellular compartmentation of arginine metabolism within the liver, as revealed by various biochemical studies, and further exposed by these various tracer studies in humans, is of considerable, functional significance; evidently it allows a maintenance of arginine homeostasis while permitting formation of significant quantities of urea in the liver without draining the cytosolic arginine compartment that is required for protein synthesis or without depleting the plasma pool of arginine that is used to meet the amino acid needs in extrahepatic tissues and organs. Without such a metabolic and structural compartmentation, the daily requirement for arginine, furnished either by way of the diet or by way of endogenous synthesis, would be very high or metabolically demanding. Parenthetically, there is now extensive evidence that cellular metabolism is largely spatially organized (as for arginine), and this is on a scale much smaller than that of the well-known organelles. The benefits of this are efficient substrate transfer, protection of labile intermediates, and improved coordination [148–151]. In addition to an intracellular compartmentation of arginine metabolism, there is also a functional specialization of different hepatocyte populations and regions within the liver [152,153]; urea synthesis occurs largely in the periportal compartment, which is thought to provide an effective means for adjusting ammonia flux into either urea or glutamine formation, according to the metabolic needs of the organism [153]. Hence, there is a distinct interorgan, intraorgan, and intracellular compartmentation of arginine metabolism, adding both complexity and detail to an understanding of the regulation and control of amino acid metabolism in vivo. Because this organization of metabo-

Table 6-14. A Summary of Studies on the Kinetics of Plasma Arginine, Ornithine, Citrulline, and Urea Appearance (Production) in Fed, Healthy, Adult Humans Given Adequate or Arginine-Free Diets for 7 Days

Parameter	Adequate	Arginine-Free	Reference
Arginine flux	73 ± 14	48 ± 9*	140
Ornithine flux	37 ± 4	23 ± 3*	143
Citrulline flux	8 ± 3	10 ± 3	140
Arginine → ornithine	25 ± 5	10 ± 1*	143
Ornithine oxidation	14.4 ± 1.7	7.8 ± 0.7*	143
Ornithine → citrulline	3.7 ± 0.8	2.6 ± 0.1	143
Citrulline → arginine	5.2 ± 2.2	5.7 ± 1.3	140
Urea production	342 ± 57	351 ± 58	142

All values are mean ± SD; μmol $kg^{-1}hr^{-1}$.
*Significantly different from adequate.

lism would not be entirely evident from in vitro and/or cellular studies, we must stress the importance of accumulating relevant and reliable data on amino acid metabolism from the in vivo and clinical setting. This, of course, often presents complex and difficult issues, especially with respect to control of experimental conditions.

Second, from the summary in Table 6-14, it can be seen that when subjects consumed an arginine-free diet for 7 days, the citrulline flux and apparent rate of conversion citrulline-to-arginine were unaffected, suggesting that the net rate of de novo arginine synthesis was low and remained largely unaltered by acute changes in the adequacy of arginine intake. However, its degradation rate was reduced as indicated by the decline in the conversion of arginine to ornithine and in ornithine oxidation when arginine intake was restricted [143]. On the basis of these various findings, Castillo and co-workers [140] developed a scheme that might help to explain, in metabolic/regulatory terms, why arginine is required (conditionally indispensable) under various pathologic conditions. Specifically, they have proposed (Figure 6-18) that whole-body arginine homeostasis is achieved, in healthy adults, principally via a regulation in the rate of arginine degradation, rather than via changes in the net rate of new

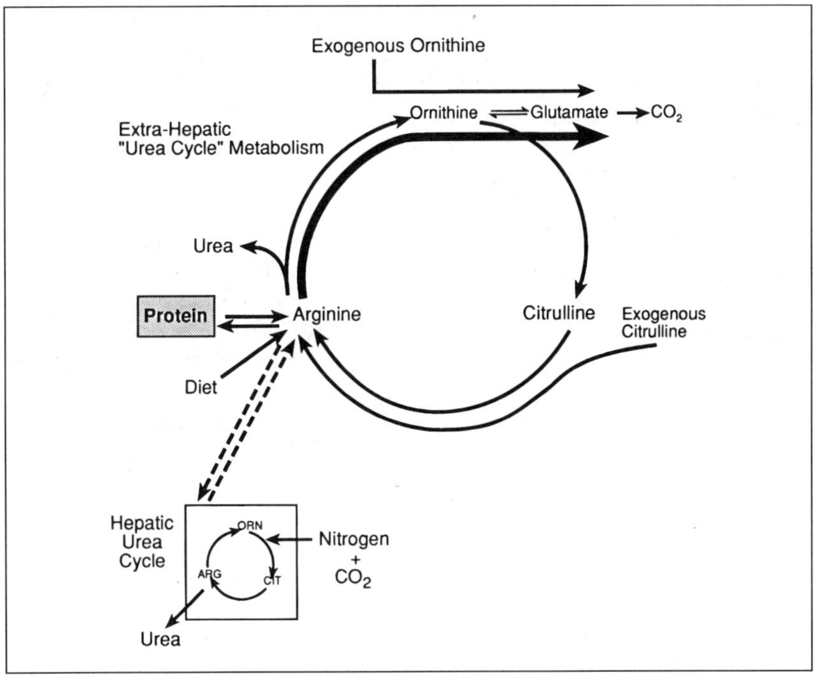

Figure 6-18. A schematic view of the relationships between the metabolism of extrahepatic urea cycle arginine and its precursors, ornithine and citrulline. It is proposed that, in adult humans, arginine homeostasis is achieved via alterations in the dietary intake level and the rate of arginine catabolism via ornithine and glutamate formation. The net synthesis of arginine, via conversion of ornithine to citrulline (in intestine) and of the citrulline to arginine (in kidney) is assumed to be less influenced by a regulatory control. Dotted lines indicate compartmentation between hepatic urea cycle and extrahepatic activity of urea cycle intermediates. (From L Castillo et al. Plasma arginine and citrulline kinetics in adults given adequate and arginine-free diets. *Proc Natl Acad Sci USA* 90:7749, 1993.)

arginine formation (from ornithine and citrulline, and especially in extrahepatic tissues) [140]. This proposition would predict, therefore, that those conditions that greatly increase the metabolic demand for arginine, such as major trauma [154] or during marked catch-up growth and repletion [155–157], may precipitate an inadequacy of arginine at the cellular level, unless an adequate or increased supply of arginine or citrulline from exogenous (enteral or parenteral) sources is available. Table 6-15 summarizes results for plasma arginine, leucine, urea, and citrulline kinetics obtained from two tracer studies in severely burned adults [154; unpublished data]. It might be noted that the higher arginine flux occurs in association with a higher leucine flux and oxidation rate of leucine in these patients, relative to healthy controls, whereas the citrulline flux and conversion of citrulline to arginine are not consistently higher than are the rates in controls (see Table 6-14). These data imply that a higher intake of arginine would be necessary to maintain nitrogen homeostasis and promote recovery under these catabolic conditions. They also reveal that (1) the increased turnover of arginine is the result of the increase in whole-body protein turnover and not the result of higher rates of net arginine synthesis and (2) the relationship between the arginine flux and urea production rate is within the apparent normal range, suggesting that the plasma/hepatic intracellular compartmentation, as discussed above, is probably intact in the burned host. A similar concept to that which we have elaborated for the conditional essentiality of arginine was proposed in 1953 by Arnstein and Neuberger [158], who concluded, from studies in rats, that the constant level of glycine in tissues is maintained by regulation of the rate of degradation of glycine and not by variations in its rate of synthesis. Studies of this kind are adding to our understanding of the metabolic basis for the conditional essentiality of various amino acids in human subjects. A more extensive discussion of this aspect of amino acid nutrition has been given elsewhere [159].

Table 6-15. Plasma Leucine, Arginine, Citrulline, and Urea Kinetics in Severely Burned Adults

Parameter	Value (μmol kg^{-1} hr^{-1})
Leucine flux	199
Leucine oxidation	35
Arginine flux	105
Citrulline flux	8
Citrulline → arginine	3.7
Arginine/leucine flux ratio	0.56
Arginine flux/urea appearance ratio	0.28

Source: From Y-M Yu et al. Plasma arginine and leucine kinetics and urea production rates in burn patients. *Metabolism,* in press; and unpublished data from the authors' laboratories.

Channeling of Amino Acid Metabolism

In vivo tracer studies in human subjects, such as those described above, on the metabolism of the major urea cycle intermediates of arginine, ornithine, and citrulline, have further highlighted not only the significance and complexity of the interorgan and intraorgan compartmentalization of amino acid metabolism, but also the phenomenon of metabolite channeling. Ovadi and Srere [151] define the latter as "a process in which pathway intermediates are transferred from one enzyme to another without complete equilibration with the surrounding medium—it includes processes resulting from either segregation or microcompartmentation of metabolites or direct transfer mechanisms." We alluded above to the importance of the heterogeneity (zonal heterogeneity) of metabolism in the liver, particularly with reference to glutamine, ammonia, and urea metabolism, and its functional implications [152,153]. Two examples from recent studies might be used to expand slightly on the experimental and physiologic significance of metabolite channeling.

First, we mentioned that there are two forms of arginyl-tRNA in rat liver cells [147]: a complex form providing arginyl-tRNA for protein synthesis and a free form that provides arginyl-tRNA for the NH_2-terminal arginine modification of proteins. In subsequent studies, Deutscher and co-workers [160,161] suggested that protein synthesis is channeled, i.e., that the amino acyl-tRNA intermediate is directly transferred among the various components of the protein synthetic apparatus and does not dissociate into the cell fluid. The intracellular location, structural organization, and nature of the complexes involved require further elucidation. However, these insights into metabolic organization have implications for physiology and regulation of amino acid homeostasis, and they also complicate interpretation of in vivo tracer studies of the kinetics of amino acid incorporation into proteins and the quantitative estimates of protein synthesis in vivo.

Second, from recent results of a series of continuous infusion of ^{13}C-phenylalanine tracer studies, lasting for 24 hr in human subjects [162,163], it appears that in spite of the lack of supporting biochemical evidence [164] that the enzymes phenylalanine hydroxylase and tyrosine aminotransferase are located in tight, inaccessible, or multiple compartments. At the very least, the recent human tracer data indicate the need to look at this in vivo issue far more carefully, particularly because it was earlier, difficult-to-interpret tracer data that gave impetus to the study and understanding of metabolite channeling. Metabolite channeling may indeed have nutritional implications because this type of metabolic organization or channeling might explain why phenylalanine alone may not be the most effective way of providing both phenylalanine and tyrosine needs of the rapidly growing pig when receiving nutrients via total parenteral nutrition [165,166]. The implications of this phenomenon for amino acid homeostasis and the nutrition of parenterally nourished hospitalized patients are intriguing and important to evaluate.

Splanchnic Fate and Uptake/Distribution in Various Organs

Quantitative Removal. Another form of channeling to consider in relation to the metabolic uptake and utilization of amino acids is that created by giving nutrients orally or by vein. It is, of course, well appreciated that the splanchnic region plays a major role in the regulation of whole-body amino acid metabolism and that it selectively modifies the pattern of absorbed amino acids subsequently presented to the peripheral circulation [37–39].

The quantitative extent to which the splanchnic tissues account for the disposal of specific endogenous and dietary amino acids in man has not yet been adequately defined. However, it presumably depends not only on the particular amino acid but also on factors such as the metabolic state of the host, the route of amino acid delivery, and the composition and form of the meals or nutritional support. For example, at generous intakes of dietary leucine, mean splanchnic uptake of the amino acid has been reported to range from about less than 10% to about 25% [167–171], based on tracer studies. Relatively few data exist for most other amino acids. For phenylalanine, the tracer-derived value appears to be higher than that for leucine, or about 30% to 58% [162,171,172]. For arginine, the estimates appear to be about 30% to 34% [141], and for tyrosine, they are about 45% [162]. Most of the glutamate leaving the gastrointestinal tract appears to disappear within the splanchnic region [173]. From in vivo tracer studies of methionine and cysteine kinetics [174], it appears that much of dietary cystine is probably removed during its first pass within the splanchnic region. This also seems to be the case in the pig, where quantitative removal of dietary cystine occurs within the intestinal wall [175]. A more extensive, quantitative determination of the relative organ and metabolic fates of specific amino acids in various patient populations would clearly help to define the profile of amino acids that would be most effective for use in the parenteral and enteral nutritional support of surgical patients.

Proteins, Peptides, and Amino Acids. A related issue that should be mentioned here concerns the relative nutritional value and metabolic fate of intact proteins versus small peptides and free amino acids for meeting host requirements. Briefly, protein hydrolysis in the proximal digestive tract leads to the release of a mixture of free amino acids and small peptides in the intestinal lumen, which are then transported by the enterocyte. Peptides are largely hydrolyzed into their constituent amino acids within the enterocyte; it is largely the free amino acids that appear in the portal blood draining the gastrointestinal tract. There is evidence that the peptide transport systems are distinct from those for the free amino acids, and this accounts for differences in the efficiency and speed of absorption of small peptides or free amino acids after intestinal infusion (see Chapter 2). Thus, an area of continuing interest in relation to protein/amino acid metabolism and nutrition of the surgical patient is the qualitative nature of the nitrogen intake in relation to digestion/absorption and to the subsequent utilization of amino acids. This topic was considered in an excellent recent review by Grimble [176], in which he discusses the metabolism of peptides and advances in applications of peptide metabolism to clinical nutrition. Nevertheless, a recent study reported by Collin-Vidal and co-workers [177] is relevant. These investigators studied normal adult subjects during feeding. Their volunteers were given, by continuous nasogastric infusion, a protein- or a peptide-based diet. Leucine kinetics (oral ^{13}C-leucine and intravenous [$^{2}H_2$]leucine) were measured during three consecutive periods: carbohydrates and lipids alone, whole casein, and oligopeptides. It was concluded that the response of leucine kinetics to feeding was modified by the molecular form of nitrogen intake, with the oligopeptides inducing a higher oxidation and protein synthesis and a lesser inhibition of protein breakdown than the intact protein. A limitation of this study was the high test level of leucine intake and the fact that their subjects were in marked positive leucine balance. Therefore, the applicability of these findings to more limiting nutrient intakes is uncertain. Furthermore, clinical studies have not consistently demonstrated advantages for achieving nitrogen balance by use of proteins versus peptides or free amino acids [178,179]. Nevertheless, kinetic/metabolic studies of the kind conducted by Collin-Vidal are desirable, and now that food proteins have been intrinsically labeled with ^{13}C-leucine [180], it seems quite likely that this area of nutritional investigation will intensify, to the nutritional advantage of the surgical patient.

Nutritional Aspects of Proteins and Amino Acids

The preceding analysis of the biochemical, regulatory, and physiologic aspects of protein and amino acid metabolism permits us to now turn to the nutritional requirements for dietary protein, which consist of two components: (1) a usable source of nitrogen (nonspecific nitrogen [NSN]), which may be supplied as a specific amino acid or nitrogen compound or as a mixture of dispensable (nonessential) amino acids, and (2) the indispensable amino acids, (essential) amino acids, and, under certain conditions, the "conditionally essential" or "conditionally indispensable" amino acids. These classes of amino acids are listed in Table 6-16 [181]. The conceptual organization of these classes differs from the classification proposed by Rose and colleagues [182] based on their classic nitrogen balance studies about 40 years ago. The human being requires nine indispensable amino acids under all conditions. In contrast, the chick has specific needs for 13 amino acids.

Nonspecific Nitrogen and the Conditionally Indispensable Amino Acids

As we have reviewed [159], studies in the growing rat, chick, human infant, and human adult have revealed the importance of an adequate level and appropriate dietary source of nonspecific nitrogen for maintenance of an adequate state of body protein balance and nutriture. Indispensable amino acids alone, even when supplied in excess of their physiologic requirements, do not maintain either adequate growth or maintenance. Furthermore, in human studies, the nutritional value of diets that supply low amounts of total nitrogen, or diets containing predominantly the indispensable amino acids, are improved when nonspecific nitrogen is added [183]. In addition to the nitrogen from the indispensable amino acids, there is a requirement for a sufficient intake of nonspecific nitrogen. This need can be met effectively from dispensable amino acids or from utilizable nitrogen sources other than an excessive intake of only the indispensable amino acids. The precise proportion of the total nitrogen requirement that is associated with the nonspecific nitrogen component is not known because there remains, particularly for adults, uncertainties and controversy about the quantitative needs for the indispensable amino acid component of the total protein requirement. Furthermore, the question should be raised as to whether, and to what extent, the chemical source(s) of the nonspecific nitrogen component is important in reference to its efficient use for meeting total "protein" (nitrogen) and amino acid needs. For healthy adults, at least, the chemical pattern of the nonspecific nitrogen sources can be quite simple (a mixture of glycine and diammonium citrate, for example). The 1965 FAO/WHO [184] expert group on protein requirements concluded that the healthy human body is able to use most "nonessential" nitrogen compounds with

Table 6-16. The Changing View of the Classification of Amino Acids in Human Nutrition

Indispensable (Essential)		Conditionally Indispensable	Dispensable (Nonessential)	
1954[a]	Present[b]	Present[b]	1954[a]	Present[b]
Valine	Valine	Glycine	Glycine	
Isoleucine	Isoleucine	Cysteine	Cystine	
Leucine	Leucine	Glutamine	Glutamic acid	Glutamic acid
Lysine	Lysine	Tyrosine	Tyrosine	
Methionine	Methionine	Proline	Proline	
Phenylalanine	Phenylalanine	Arginine	Arginine	
Threonine	Threonine	Taurine	Alanine	Alanine
Tryptophan	Tryptophan		Serine	Serine
	Histidine		Aspartic acid	Aspartic acid
			Histidine	Asparagine
			Hydroxyproline	
			Citrulline	

[a]Based on the "final classification" discussed by Rose and colleagues [182].
[b]Our current interpretation.

equal efficiency. This seems to be less the case for the surgical or stressed patient, as discussed in more detail elsewhere in this volume (see Chapters 3 and 7).

Notwithstanding, the dispensable amino acid nitrogen component is quantitatively significant in the nutrition of human subjects, as suggested by the following. (1) With usual diets, the dispensable (and conditionally indispensable) amino acids account for approximately 50% of total amino acid intake in the human adult (Table 6-17). (2) Munro [2] surveyed the concentration of essential and nonessential amino acids in liver and skeletal muscle of various mammalian species, and Table 6-17 presents his analysis. It can be seen that the contents of the dispensable amino acids exceed those for the indispensable amino acids by about fivefold. (3) It can be calculated that at least about 50% of the net turnover of body "protein" or nitrogen is accounted for by the dispensable amino acids (Table 6-18). Hence, these amino acids contribute in a major way to the intake, processing, turnover, and loss of nitrogen from the body. (4) Based on the summary of amino acid fluxes given earlier (see Table 6-7), it is evident that for some of the so-called dispensable amino acids, such as glycine and alanine, their plasma fluxes are very high relative to their concentrations in protein, indicating substantial de novo synthesis. For others, such as proline and arginine, their fluxes correspond closer to their concentrations in proteins, indicating much lower rates of de novo synthesis than for the dispensable group of amino acids. This suggests that the amino acids such as glycine and alanine, for example, are synthesized at rates in considerable excess of the needs for protein synthesis. It seems unlikely that a dietary supply of these amino acids would be necessary, except under the most extreme of conditions, to ensure maintenance of protein synthesis and tissue pro-

Table 6-17. Intake, Tissue Content, and Net Turnover of Indispensable and Dispensable Amino Acids in the Human Adult

	Amino Acids/70 kg body weight		
Source of Amino Acid	Total (g)	Indispensable (g)	Dispensable (g)
Diet			
"Minimum" needs	56	6	50
Usual diet	90	45	65
Absorbed (and secreted gut proteins)	150	75	75
Free amino acid pools			
Plasma	0.7	0.2	0.5
Tissues	70	10	60
Daily body protein turnover	300	150	150

Source: Data provided by the late Professor HN Munro.

Table 6-18. Postabsorptive Concentration and Total Tissue Content of Five Essential and Five Nonessential Amino Acids in Mammalian Liver and Muscle

		Tissue Concentrations (μmol/g)				Total tissue content of essential amino acids (μmol/kg body weight)		
		Essential amino acids[a]		Nonessential amino acids[b]				
Species	Body weight (kg)	Liver	Muscle	Liver	Muscle	Liver	Muscle	Daily requirement of essential amino acids (μmol/kg body weight)
Mouse	0.03	1.17	1.12	6.6	5.5	62	500	7000
Rat	0.2	0.8	0.76	4.2	4	34	340	4000
Rabbit	2	1.35	0.6	3.9	4	41	270	2200
Dog	30	0.77	0.74	2.6	2.9	15	330	1200

[a]Combined concentrations of isoleucine, leucine, phenylalanine, threonine, and valine.

[b]Combined concentrations of alanine, aspartic acid, glutamic acid, glycine, and serine.

Source: From HN Munro. Evolution of Protein Metabolism in Mammals. In HN Munro (ed), *Mammalian Protein Metabolism,* vol 3. New York: Academic, 1959. P 133.

tein content. On the other hand, the relatively low flux rates of arginine and proline might be taken to imply that there will be situations in which their de novo rates of synthesis are too low to meet enhanced metabolic demands. As we have already discussed above for arginine, under conditions of a major increase in metabolic demands an exogenous supply definitely would be required in the absence of a sufficient change in de novo synthesis, otherwise body protein balance and function would be compromised.

Because we have recently considered in some detail various specific amino acids in relation to nonspecific nitrogen, the reader may wish to consult a recent review for an account of the metabolic characteristics, and nutritional significance, of arginine, proline, glycine, and glutamine [159]. These amino acids are discussed elsewhere in this volume, especially in Chapters 12 and 14, but brief mention is made here of cysteine, before we turn finally to the issue of requirements for protein and the indispensable amino acids. This amino acid is beginning to occupy more of our own research effort, and also of relevance is that the level of cystine (and tyrosine) in parenteral amino acid solutions is most often quite low because of its relative insolubility.

The metabolic and nutritional interrelationships between the nutritionally significant S-amino acids (methionine, cysteine, cystine, taurine) have been reviewed in considerable detail by others [185–189]. However, there are three issues that are particularly important relevant to a consideration of the nutrition of the surgical patient: the impact of dietary cystine on the requirement for methionine; the capacity of exogenous methionine to meet the requirements for cysteine under various pathophysiologic conditions; and the involvement of cysteine in the synthesis of physiologically significant S-containing compounds, particularly of taurine and glutathione.

Cysteine is synthesized by mammals from methionine, and its subsequent metabolism is complex (Figure 6-19) [186,187]. It follows, from the scheme presented here, that a portion of the total requirement for sulfur amino acids could be met by dietary cystine. This has indeed been shown using various animal species, and the percentage of the total sulfur amino acid requirement (methionine and cystine) of the chick, rat, and pig that can be supplied by cystine has been estimated to be about 50% [188,189]. There are comparable, but less complete and more highly variable, data available for humans; methionine is the indispensable S-amino acid in human nutrition [190,191], with cystine being considered as a conditionally indispensable [192] or both conditionally indispensable and acquired indispensable [193] amino acid. According to Rose and Wixom [190], a major portion (80% to 89%) of the dietary need for the total sulfur amino acids in adult humans could be met with cystine. Nevertheless, from recent tracer studies with stable isotopically labeled methionine and cysteine, we [174] have not been able to definitively state the extent to which, or how, cyst(e)ine spares the dietary requirement for methionine in the nutrition of healthy humans. The status of knowledge about these relationships in

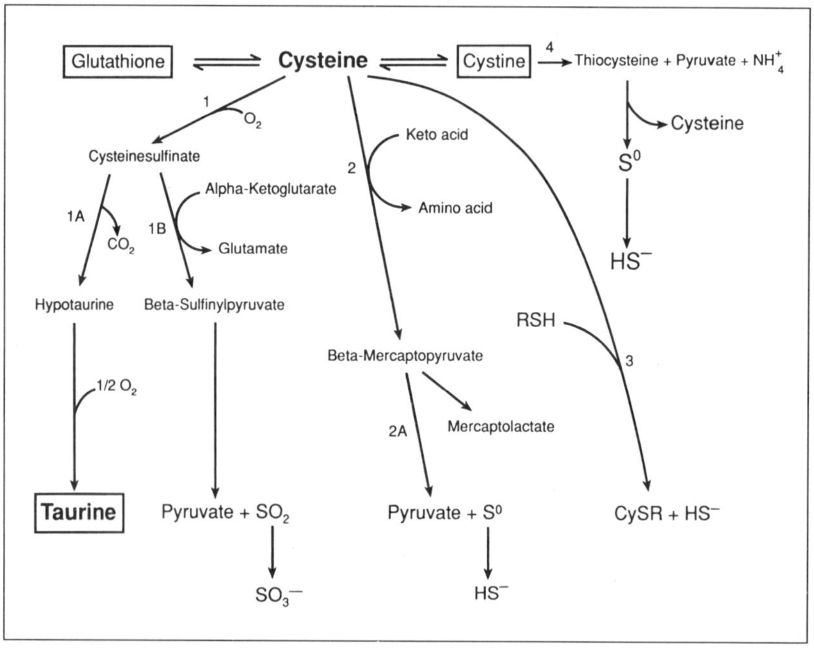

Figure 6-19. Pathways of cyst(e)ine catabolism in mammalian cells. Enzymes that catalyze the numbered reactions are (1) cysteine dioxygenase, (1A) cysteine sulfonate decarboxylase, (1B) aspartate amino transferase, (2) amino transferase(s), (2A) microptopyruvate sulfurtransferase, (3) cystathionine beta-transferase, and (4) gamma-cystathionase (cyst[e]ine desulfydrase). (From MH Stipanuk et al. Catabolism of cyst(e)ine by rat renal cortical tubules. *J Nutr* 120:450, 1990.)

trauma, sepsis, and other pathophysiologic states is even less satisfactory.

With regard to the indispensable and conditionally indispensable amino acids, it should be also mentioned that (1) cysteine synthesis from methionine is limited, even in the healthy adult, when cyst(e)ine free nutritional regimens are provided parenterally [194]; and (2) it has become evident that cysteine synthesis may not always occur at a rate commensurate with meeting tissue needs [195,196]. It is, therefore, more appropriately classified as a conditionally indispensable amino acid. This argument ought to be underscored because cysteine appears to be a superior substrate for glutathione synthesis [197] and also for taurine [198,199] formation as compared with methionine as a precursor. This is meant to emphasize that it is an inadequate concept to simply regard methionine as a sufficient and sole source of sulfur for purposes of maintaining methionine, cyst(e)ine, glutathione, and taurine homeostasis. The evidence indicates that cyst(e)ine or a utilizable derivative of cystine (such as n-acetylcysteine) is also probably required, especially under conditions of severe stress, as in burn injury, where turnover and utilization of all these metabolites is substantially increased relative to normal metabolic conditions.

A particularly important and nutritionally relevant area that has not yet received sufficient attention by those with a primary interest in human and clinical nutrition is the association between cystine and glutathione, which is the most prevalent cellular thiol and the most abundant low molecular weight peptide present in cells [200–202]. It functions in catalysis, metabolism, and transport; it participates in reactions involving the synthesis of proteins and nucleic acids and in those that detoxify free radicals and peroxides. Reduced glutathione (GSH) protects cells from toxic effects of reactive oxygen compounds, and it is an important component of the system that uses reduced pyridine nucleotide to provide the cell with its reducing properties. It is also exported in the plasma to various cells and organs, with the liver being the major site of its formation and release into the blood circulation [203,204]. It functions in the interorgan and intraorgan transfer of cysteine, in the protection of all membranes, and as part of a pathway for membrane transport of cyst(e)ine and probably other amino acids. There is much interest in the potential clinical benefit to be derived from modulating and/or maintaining GSH levels to protect against oxidative damage, toxic compounds, and cellular injury resulting from radiation, physical trauma, and chemotherapy.

The synthesis of this tripeptide (L-y-glutamyl-L-cysteinyl-glycine) occurs intracellularly from its constituent amino acids, together with its degradation, via the reactions of the γ-glutamyl cycle (Figure 6-20). The *availability of cysteine* is considered to be the rate-limiting step of glutathione synthesis [205], and the control point in GSH synthesis appears to be the γ-glutamyl cysteine synthetase reaction, which is subject to feedback regulation by glutathione [200,201]. It has recently been shown that burn injury in rats markedly reduces mitochondrial GSH levels in liver and in several peripheral tissues, including brain, heart, and skeletal muscle [206]. These findings may have important therapeutic implications in increasing antioxidative defenses to limit oxidative stress injury in hypermetabolic patients. Further aspects of the nutritional interrelationships between cystine and glutathione are discussed in detail elsewhere [159,205]. Additional comment on this intriguing aspect of amino acid nutrition and metabolism can be deferred, except to say that it is now reasonably well established that in burn injury sepsis, and immunologic disease, the immune system produces active oxygen species, contributing to the oxidative injury of host tissues. Glutathione (GSH) is a major compound involved in limiting chemically induced and immune-system induced injury to cells and tissues. Cysteine availability is the rate-limiting step in GSH synthesis, and its intake is often low in severely catabolic patients. Methionine is thought not to be highly effective as a precursor of cysteine for GSH synthesis. The potential for improving therapeutic procedures in the case of catabolic trauma patients should be realized from a better understanding of the status and regulation of GSH metabolism, particularly the regulatory significance of dietary cyst(e)ine.

Total Protein Requirement

It follows from a consideration of the underlying metabolic aspects of the needs for nitrogen and for the specific indispensable amino acids that the starting point for estimating total protein needs has been, in most studies, the measurement of the amount of dietary nitrogen needed for zero body nitrogen balance in adults. For determination of the needs for specific indispensable amino acids, the approach has often been the same, but more recently it has been based on a direct measurement of rates of irreversible oxidation of these amino acids [207]. In the cases of the growing infant and child during pregnancy and lactation and with repletion there will be an additional requirement associated with the net deposition of

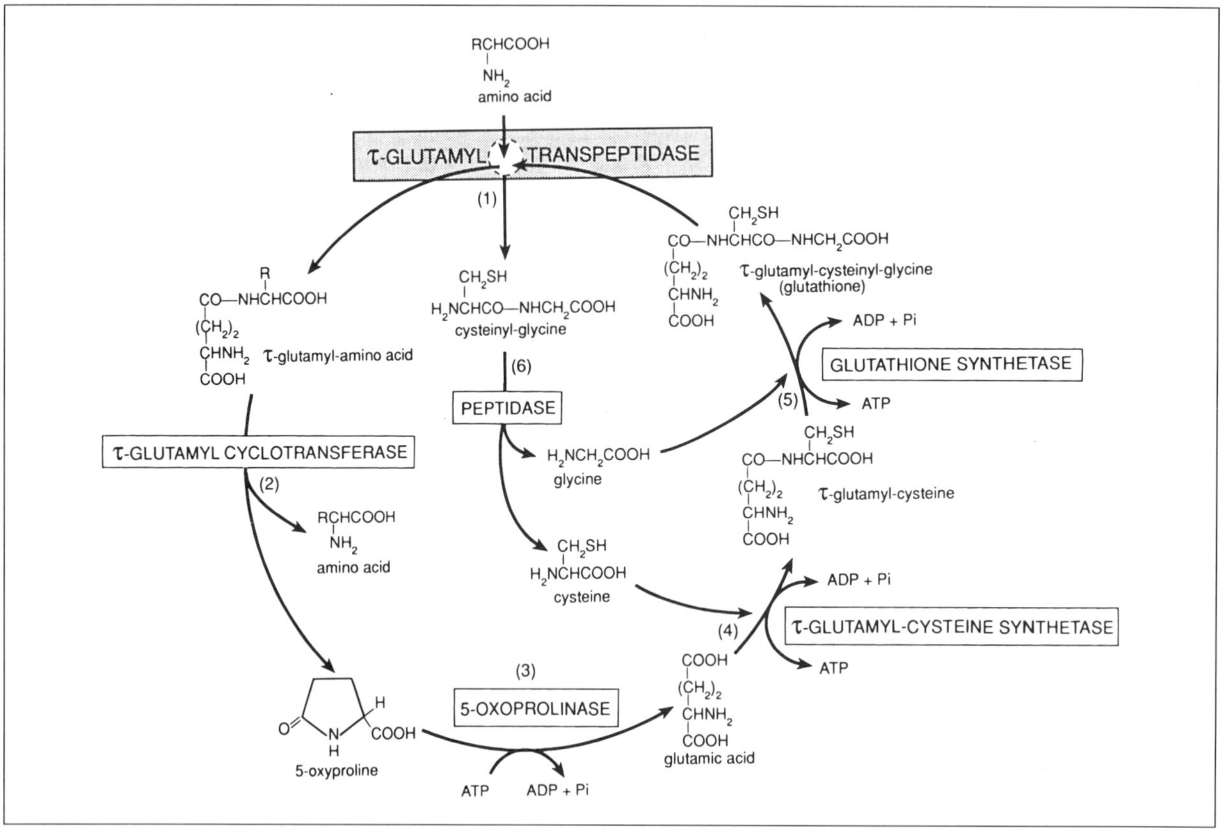

Figure 6-20. The gamma-glutamyl cycle. (From A Meister, A Larsson. Glutathione Synthetase Deficiency and Other Disorders of the Gamma-Glutamyl Cycle. In CR Scriver et al. (eds), *The Metabolic Basis of Inherited Disease.* New York: McGraw-Hill, 1989.)

protein in new tissue and that caused by secretion of milk. Thus, the FAO/WHO/UNU Expert Consultation defined the dietary need for protein as follows [208]: "The protein requirement of an individual is defined as the lowest level of dietary protein intake that will balance the losses from the body in persons maintaining energy balance at modest levels of physical activity. In children and pregnant or lactating women, the protein requirement is taken to include the needs associated with the deposition of tissues or the secretion of milk at rates consistent with good health."

Most estimates of human protein and amino acid requirements have been obtained directly or indirectly from measurements of nitrogen balance, and the use and application of the nitrogen balance technique for this purpose have been discussed in detail in the 1985 FAO/WHO/UNU report [208]. However, it also should be noted that the nitrogen balance technique has serious technical and interpretative limitations [209,210], and so it should not serve as an entirely secure or sufficient basis for establishing the protein and amino acid needs of human subjects.

Because the 1985 report of the FAO/WHO/UNU Consultation [208] provides an extensive discussion of the approaches taken to arrive at estimates of the mean requirements for protein in various age and physiologic groups, we merely present here a summary of the safe protein intakes for infants and young children, together with those for adults, lactating, and pregnant women, as proposed by the FAO/WHO/UNU group. These estimates are given in Table 6-19. It is likely that the needs of surgical patients differ from and exceed those of healthy adults. Hence, the values given in Table 6-19 can only be regarded as a basis from which to begin an evaluation of how disease and stress, including surgery, affects the needs for dietary protein. Unfortunately, the quantitative needs for protein (total nitrogen) in the surgical patient or in those who are sick and who have significant disease can only be crudely approximated. There has been very little headway made on this aspect of protein nutrition since Munro and Young [211] gave their recommendations in 1980; we provide a summary in Table 6-20.

Table 6-19. 1985 FAO/WHO/UNU Safe Protein Intakes for Selected Age Groups and Physiologic States

Group	Age	Safe protein level* ($g \cdot kg^{-1}\ d^{-1}$)
Infants	0.3–0.5 yr	1.47
	0.75–1.0 yr	1.15
Children	3–4 yr	1.09
	9–10 yr	
Adolescents	13–14 yr (girls)	0.94
	13–14 yr (boys)	0.97
Young adults	19+ yr	0.75
Elderly		0.75
Women		
Pregnant	2nd trimester	+ 6 g daily
	3rd trimester	+11 g daily
Lactating	0–6 mo	~+16 g daily
	6–12 mo	~+11 g daily

*Values are for proteins as provided by hen's egg, cow's milk, meat, fish.
Source: Data from FAO/WHO/UNU. Energy and protein requirements: Report of a joint FAO/WHO/UNU expert consultation. Technical Report Series, no. 724, 1985.

Table 6-20. Protein Requirements in Specific Diseases

1. Normal adult
   a. For N equilibrium: 0.6 g/kg raised to 0.8 g/kg by protein quality correction (80%)
   b. Customary intake: 1–2 g/kg
2. Metabolic response to severe injury and burning
   a. Acute phase: 2 + g/kg + cals
   b. Convalescence: 2 + g/kg
3. Malabsorption and gastrointestinal diseases
   a. Malabsorption syndrome: 1 g/kg
   b. Ulcerative colitis: 1–1.4 g/kg[a]
   c. Ileocecostomy: 1–1.4 g/kg[a]
4. Liver disease
   a. Acute hepatic encephalopathy: very low[b]
   b. Recovered encephalopathy: 1–1.5 g/kg
   c. Chronic encephalopathy: 0.5 g/kg[b]
5. Renal disease
   a. Uremia: 0.5 g/kg[b]
   b. Nephrosis: 1–1.4 g/kg[a]
6. Malignant disease
   a. Inreased protein and energy

[a]In each condition losses of proteins can double minimal requirements.

[b]Intake restricted on clinical grounds.

Source: From HN Munro, VR Young. Protein and Amino Acid Requirements. In AN Exton-Smith, FI Caird (eds), *Metabolic and Nutritional Disorders of the Elderly.* Bristol: Wright, 1980. P 13.

Requirements for Indispensable Amino Acids

It is possible to slightly modify the foregoing definition for the requirements for protein (nitrogen) so that the dietary need for a specific, indispensable amino acid might be defined as the lowest level of intake that achieves nitrogen balance or that balances the irreversible oxidative loss of the amino acid, without requiring major changes in protein turnover, where there is energy balance with a modest level of physical activity. Again, in infants, children, and pregnant and lactating women, the requirements for the amino acid will also include that amount of the amino acid needed for net protein deposition and the secretion of milk proteins. We have argued above that trauma and sepsis will also significantly raise the requirements for these amino acids.

The requirements for the specific indispensable (essential) amino acid have been assessed by the 1985 FAO/WHO/UNU Expert Group [208]. Except for some new data for the preschool child group, based on studies carried out by Torun, Viteri, and co-workers in Guatemala [212,213], the values given in the 1985 international group report [208] are similar to those published by FAO/WHO in 1973 [214]. Table 6-21 gives, therefore, the most recent, internationally authoritative, statement concerning the amino acid requirements in various age groups.

From a comparison of the requirements for total protein among the various age groups (see Table 6-19), there is a marked but greater decrease in indispensable amino acid needs when expressed per unit of body weight between infancy and the time adulthood is reached. Thus, there is a lower requirement for the indispensable amino acids when expressed per unit of the total need for protein in the adult as compared to that for the infant or preschool child.

Table 6-21. 1985 FAO/WHO/UNU Estimates of Amino Acid Requirements at Different Ages (mg/kg/d)

Amino Acid	Infants (3–4 mo)	Children (2 yr)	School Boys (10–12 yr)	Adults
Histidine	28	Unknown	Unknown	(8–12)
Isoleucine	70	31	28	10
Leucine	161	73	44	14
Lysine	103	64	55	12
Methionine and cystine	58	27	22	13
Phenylalanine and tyrosine	125	69	22	14
Threonine	87	37	28	7
Tryptophan	17	12.5	3.3	3.5
Valine	93	38	25	10
Total	714	352	216	84
Total per g protein*	434	320	222	111

*Total mg per g crude protein, and based on all amino acids minus histidine.

Source: FAO/WHO/UNU. Energy and protein requirements: Report of a joint FAO/WHO/UNU expert consultation. *Technical Report Series,* no. 724, 1985.

Our laboratories have been actively concerned with a reassessment of current international amino acid requirement values and patterns for practical application in human nutrition. This research has grown out of our interest in the kinetics and quantitative aspects of human amino acid metabolism and interest in evaluating the impact of severe stress, including physical trauma, on the needs for the indispensable amino acids. We have proposed a tentative new amino acid requirement pattern (MIT pattern) (Table 6-22) [215–217] for adults that differs markedly from that proposed for this age group by the FAO/WHO/UNU group (FAO pattern). However, as shown in this table, the MIT pattern is generally similar to that for the preschool child (2–5 years) amino acid requirement pattern [208,218]. The MIT proposal is based on data generated from ^{13}C-labeled amino acid tracer studies and from a consideration of the amino acid composition of body mixed proteins [217]. If this newly proposed pattern (mg amino acid per g protein) proves to be a better, quantitative approximation of adult human amino acid requirements than the 1985 amino acid pattern proposed by FAO/WHO/UNU [208], then it will have a significant impact on the evaluation of dietary protein quality in human nutrition. Furthermore, this argument has important implications for an assessment of the quantitative impact of disease and trauma on the requirements for indispensable amino acids. Unfortunately, the security of current estimates of the quantitative needs for

Table 6-22. New, Tentative Amino Acid Requirement Estimates for the Human Adult and the Corresponding Amino Acid Requirement Pattern, Compared With Those for the Preschool Child

Amino Acid	Tentative Requirement[a] (mg/kg/d)	Adult Amino-Acid Pattern[b] (mg/g protein)	1985 FAO/WHO/UNU Preschool Child Amino-Acid Pattern[c] (mg/g protein)
Isoleucine	23	35	28
Leucine	40	65	66
Lysine	30	50	58
Total sulfur amino acids (methionine and cystine)	13	25	25
Total aromatic amino acids (phenylalanine and tyrosine)	39	65	63
Threonine	15	25	34
Valine	20	35	35
Tryptophan	6	10	11

[a]Based on Young and colleagues [215,216].

[b]Derived from Young and colleagues [215,216]; rounding to nearest value of 5.

[c]From FAO/WHO/UNU [208].

specific indispensable amino acids in humans, both in health and disease, is in doubt. This issue requires immediate resolution if the most effective means of nutritional support of the surgical patient are to be achieved. In the interim, we suggest that it would be prudent to use the MIT tentative estimates as a basis for determining the amino acid requirements of the hospitalized patient. Additional arguments in support of these new estimates are presented in detail elsewhere [217].

Summary

We attempted to provide an overview of human protein and amino acid metabolism, beginning with a focus at the molecular and cellular levels and then continuing up through the organ and complex whole-body levels. It is hoped that an appreciation for the metabolic basis for the requirements emerges for (1) a utilizable source of nitrogen for synthesis of physiologically significant nitrogen-containing compounds and (2) the nutritionally indispensable and conditionally indispensable amino acids. Perhaps, then, the reader might better understand why disease and trauma alter these requirements. The quantitative aspects of these requirements were also considered in brief and in relation to the needs of healthy subjects. There are essentially no precise protein or amino acid requirement data available for the surgical patient. Nevertheless, they are predicted to be higher than those for individuals who are not sick. However, our specific purpose was to develop a backdrop against which the changes in protein amino acid and nitrogen metabolism, and their nutritional corollaries might be more completely understood under such conditions as trauma, sepsis, and specific organ pathology.

Acknowledgments

The authors' investigations referred to in this chapter have been supported largely by NIH grants (DK15856, DK42101, RR88, and GM02700) and through the generous, continuing support of the Shriners Hospitals for Crippled Children, including the mass spectrometry facility (no. 15843).

References

1. Scrimshaw NS, Young VR. The requirements of human nutrition. *Scientific American* 235:50, 1976.
2. Munro HN. Evolution of Protein Metabolism in Mammals. In HN Munro (ed), *Mammalian Protein Metabolism,* vol. 3. New York: Academic, 1959. P 133.
3. Vickery HB, Schmidt CLA. The history of the discovery of the amino acids. *Chem Rev* 9:169, 1931.
4. Burke RF, Hill KE. Regulation of selenoproteins. *Annu Rev Nutr* 13:65, 1993.
5. Jorpes JE. *Jac Berzelius: His Life and Work.* Uppsala, Sweden: Almquist & Wiksells Boktryckera AB, 1970.
6. Wolfe AP. Xenopus transcription factors: Key molecules in the developmental regulation of differential gene expression. *Biochem J* 278:313, 1991.
7. Rosenthal N. Regulation of gene expression. *N Engl J Med* 331:931, 1994.
8. Papavassiliou AG. Transcription factors. *N Engl J Med* 332:45, 1995.
9. Clark AR, Docherty K. Negative regulation of transcription in eukaryotes. *Biochem J* 296:521, 1993.
10. Manely JL. Messenger RNA polydenylyladiton: A universal modification. *Proc Natl Acad Sci USA* 92:1800, 1995.
11. Rhoads RE. Regulation of eukaryotic protein synthesis by initiation factors. *J Biol Chem* 268:3017, 1993.
12. Hershey JWB. Translational control in mammalian cells. *Annu Rev Biochem* 60:717, 1991.
13. Proud CG. Protein phosphorylation in translational control. *Curr Top Cell Regul* 32:243, 1992.
14. Pain VM. Initiation of protein synthesis in mammalian cells. *Biochem J* 235:625, 1986.
15. Kimball SR, Vary TC, Jefferson LS. Regulation of protein synthesis by insulin. *Annu Rev Physiol* 56:321, 1994.
16. deJong FA, Schreiber G. Messenger RNA levels in plasma proteins in rat liver during protein depletion and refeeding. *J Nutr* 117:1795, 1987.
17. Reeds PJ, Davis TA. Hormonal Regulation of Muscle Protein Synthesis and Degradation. In PJ Buttery, KN Boorman, DB Lindsay (eds), *Control of Fat and Lean Deposition.* Oxford: Butterworth-Heineman, 1992. P 1.
18. Sugden PH, Fuller SJ. Regulation of protein turnover in skeletal and cardiac muscle. *Biochem J* 273:21, 1989.
19. Millward DJ, Rivers JPW. The need for indispensable amino acids: The concept of the anabolic drive. *Diabetes Metab Rev* 5:191, 1989.
20. Melefors O, Hentze MW. Translational regulations by mRNA/protein interactions in eukaryotic cells: Ferritin and beyond. *Bioessays* 15:88, 1993.
21. Weijland A, Parmeggiani A. Toward a model for the interaction between elongation factor Tu and the ribosome. *Science* 259:1311, 1993.
22. Schimmel P. GTP hydrolysis in protein synthesis: Two for Tu? *Science* 259:1264, 1993.
23. Rucker RB, Wold F. Cofactors in and as post-translational protein modifications. *FASEB J* 2:2052, 1988.
24. Krishna RG, Wold F. Post-translational modifications of proteins. *Adv Enzymol Relat Areas Mol Biol* 67:265, 1993.
25. Rucker RB, McGee C. Chemical modifications of proteins in vivo: Selected examples important to cellular regulation. *J Nutr* 123:977, 1993.
26. Goldberg AL, Rock KL. Proteolysis, proteasomes and antigen presentation. *Nature* 357:375, 1992.
27. Ciechanover A, Schwartz AL. The ubiquitin-mediated proteolytic pathway: Mechanisms of recognition of the proteolytic substrate and involvement in the degradation of native cellular proteins. *FASEB J* 8:182, 1994.
28. Mortimore GE. Mechanisms of cellular protein catabolism. *Nutr Rev* 40:1, 1982.
29. Wing SS, Goldberg AL. Glucocorticoids activate the ATP-ubiquitin-dependent proteolytic system in skeletal muscle during fasting. *Am J Physiol* 264:E668, 1993.
30. Tawa NE Jr, Kettlehut IC, Goldberg AL. Dietary protein

deficiency reduces lysosomal and non-lysosomal ATP-dependent proteolysis in muscle. *Am J Physiol* 263:E326, 1992.

31. Rechsteiner M. Natural substrates of the ubiquitin proteolytic pathway. *Cell* 66:615, 1991.
32. Jentsch S. The ubiquitin-conjugation system. *Annu Rev Genet* 26:179, 1992.
33. Rivett AJ. Proteasomes: Multicatalytic proteinase complexes. *Biochem J* 291:1, 1993.
34. Rechsteiner M, Hoffman L, Dubeil W. The multicatalytic and 26S proteases. *J Biol Chem* 268:6065, 1993.
35. Tanaka K, Yoshimura T, Tamura T. Possible mechanism of nuclear translocation of proteasomes. *FEBS Lett* 271:41, 1990.
36. Souba WW, Pacitti AJ. How amino acids get into cells: Mechanisms, models, menus and mediators. *JPEN* 16:569, 1992.
37. Christensen HN. Interorgan amino acid nutrition. *Physiol Rev* 62:1193, 1982.
38. Christensen HN. Role of amino acid transport and counter transport in nutrition and metabolism. *Physiol Rev* 70:43, 1990.
39. Elia M. The interorgan flux of substrates in fed and fasted man, as indicated by arterior-venous balance studies. *Nutr Res Rev* 4:3, 1991.
40. McGivan JD, Pastor-Anglada M. Regulatory and molecular aspects of mammalian amino acid transport. *Biochem J* 299:321, 1994.
41. Fong AD, Handlogten ME, Kilberg MS. Substrate dependent adaptive regulation and transinhibition of System A-mediated amino acid transport: Studies using rat hepatoma plasma membrane vesicles. *Biochim Biophys Acta* 1022:325, 1989.
42. Kilberg MS, Hutson RG, Laine RO. Amino acid-regulated gene expression in eukaryotic cells. *FASEB J* 8:13, 1994.
43. Biolo G, et al. A new model to determine in vivo the relationship between amino acid transmembrane transport and protein kinetics in muscle. *JPEN* 16:305, 1992.
44. Biolo G, et al. Transmembrane transport and intracellular kinetics of amino acids in human skeletal muscle. *Am J Physiol* 268:E75, 1995.
45. Biolo G, Fleming RYD, Wolfe RR. Physiologic hyperinsulinemia stimulates protein synthesis and enhances transport of selected amino acids in human skeletal muscle. *J Clin Invest* 95:811, 1995.
46. Haussinger D, Lang F, Gerok W. Regulation of cell function by the cellular hydration state. *Am J Physiol* 267:E343, 1994.
47. Ruiz-Montasell B, et al. Evidence for a regulatory protein involved in the increased activity of System A for neutral amino acid transport in osmotically stressed mammalian cells. *Proc Natl Acad Sci USA* 91:9569, 1994.
48. Douzou P. Osmotic regulation of gene action. *Proc Natl Acad Sci USA* 91:1657, 1994.
49. Young VR. The Role of Skeletal and Cardiac Muscle in the Regulation of Protein Metabolism. In HN Munro (ed), *Mammalian Protein Metabolism.* vol. 4. New York: Academic, 1970. P 585.
50. Wing SS, Banville D. 14-kDa ubiquitin-conjugating enzyme: Structure of the rat gene and regulation upon fasting and by insulin. *Am J Physiol* 267:E39, 1994.
51. Young VR. Nutrient interactions with reference to amino acid and protein metabolism in nonruminants; particular emphasis on protein-energy relations in man. *Z Ernahrungswiss* 30:239, 1991.
52. Beckman RP, Mizzen LA, Welch WJ. Interaction of Hsp7O with newly synthesized proteins: Implications for protein folding and assembly. *Science* 248:850, 1990.
53. Lingappa YR. Intracellular traffic of newly synthesized proteins: Current understanding and future prospects. *J Clin Invest* 83:739, 1989.
54. Rothman JE, Orci L. Molecular dissection of the secretory pathway. *Nature* 355:409, 1992.
55. Rapoport TA. Protein transport across the ER membrane. *Trends Biochem Sci* 15:355, 1990.
56. Baker KP, Schatz G. Mitochondrial proteins essential for viability mediate protein import into yeast mitochondria. *Nature* 349:205, 1991.
57. Berridge MJ. Inositol triphosphate and diacylglycerol: Two interacting second messengers. *Annu Rev Biochem* 56:159, 1987.
58. Berridge MJ, Mitchell RH (eds). *Inositol Lipids and Transmembrane Signalling.* London: Royal Society, 1988.
59. Young VR, Yu Y-M, Fukagawa NK. Whole Body Energy and Nitrogen (Protein) Relationships. In J Kinney, HN Tucker (eds), *Energy Metabolism: Tissue Determinants and Cellular Corollaries.* New York: Raven, 1992. P 139.
60. Young VR, Yu Y-M, Fukagawa NK. Energy and Protein Turnover. In J Kinney, HN Tucker (eds), *Energy Metabolism: Tissue Determinants and Cellular Corollaries.* New York: Raven, 1992. P 439.
61. Young VR, et al. Potential use of 3-methylhistidine excretion as an index of progressive reduction in muscle protein catabolism during starvation. *Metabolism* 22:1429, 1973.
62. Young VR, Munro HN. N^{τ}-methylhistidine (3-methylhistidine) and muscle protein turnover: An overview. *Fed Proc* 37:2291, 1978.
63. Rathmacher JA, et al. Gas-chromatographic/mass spectrometric analysis of stable isotopes of 3-methylhistidine in biological fluids: Application to plasma kinetics in vivo. *Biol Mass Spec* 21:560, 1992.
64. Rathmacher JA, Link G, Nissen SL. Measurement of 3-methylhistidine production in lambs by using compartmental analysis. *Br J Nutr* 69:743, 1993.
65. Rathmacher JA, Flakoll PJ, Nissen SL. A compartmental model of 3-methylhistidine metabolism in humans. *Am J Physiol,* in press.
66. Paik WK, Kim S. Protein methylation: Chemical, enzymological and biological significance. *Adv Enzymol Relat Areas Mol Biol* 42:227, 1975.
67. Yudkoff M, et al. Urinary excretion of dimethylarginines in premature infants. *Biochem Med* 32:242, 1984.
68. Fickling SA, et al. Synthesis of N^GN^G dimethylarginine by human endothelial cells. *Endothelium* 1:137, 1993.
69. Vallance P, et al. Accumulation of an endogenous inhibitor of nitric oxide synthesis. *Lancet* 339:572, 1992.
70. Moncada S, Palmer RMJ, Higgs EA. Nitric oxide: Physiology, pathophysiology and pharmacology. *Pharmacol Rev* 43:109, 1991.
71. Nathan C. Nitric oxide as a secretory product of mammalian cells. *FASEB J* 6:3051, 1992.
72. Young VR, Marchini JS. Mechanisms and nutritional significance of metabolic responses to altered intakes of protein and amino acids, with reference to nutritional adaptation in humans. *Am J Clin Nutr* 51:270, 1992.
73. Harper AE. Enzymatic Basis for Adaptive Changes in Amino Acid Metabolism. In TG Taylor, NK Jenkins (eds), *Proceedings of the XIII International Congress of Nutrition.* London: Libbey, 1986. P 409.
74. Munro HN. Free Amino Acid Pools and Their Role in

Regulation. In HN Munro (ed), *Mammalian Protein Metabolism,* vol 4. New York: Academic, 1970. P 299.

75. Krebs HA. Some Aspects of the Regulation of Fuel Supply in Omnivorous Animals. In G Weber (ed), *Advances in Enzyme Regulation,* Vol 10. New York: Pergamon, 1972. P 397.
76. Waterlow JC, Fern EB. Free Amino Acid Pools and Their Regulation. In JC Waterlow, JML Stephen (eds), *Nitrogen Metabolism in Man.* London: Applied Science, 1981. P 1.
77. Young VR, et al. Amino Acid Kinetics in Relation to Protein and Amino Acid Requirements: The Primary Importance of Amino Acid Oxidation. In JS Garrow, D Halliday (eds), *Energy and Substrate Metabolism in Man.* London: Libbey, 1985. P 119.
78. El-Khoury AE, et al. Validation of the tracer-balance concept with reference to leucine: 24h intravenous tracer studies with L-[1-^{13}C]leucine and [^{15}N, ^{15}N]urea. *Am J Clin Nutr* 59:1000, 1994.
79. El-Khoury AE, et al. The 24h pattern and rate of leucine oxidation, with particular reference to tracer estimates of leucine requirements in healthy adults. *Am J Clin Nutr* 59:1012, 1994.
80. Jungas RL, Halperin ML, Brosnan JT. Quantitative analysis of amino acid oxidation and related gluconeogenesis in humans. *Physiol Rev* 72:419, 1992.
81. Harper AE, Miller RH, Block KP. Branched-chain amino acid metabolism. *Annu Rev Nutr* 4:409, 1984.
82. Nawali MD, et al. Administration of endotoxin, tumor necrosis factor or interleukin 1 to rats activates skeletal muscle branched-chain α-keto acid dehydrogenase. *J Clin Invest* 85:256, 1990.
83. Cohen PP. Regulation of the Ornithine-Urea Cycle Enzymes. In JC Waterlow, JML Stephen (eds), *Nitrogen Metabolism in Man.* London: Applied Science, 1981. P 215.
84. Souba WW. Interorgan ammonia metabolism in health and disease: A surgeon's view. *JPEN* 11:569, 1987.
85. Meijer AJ, Lamers WH, Chamuleau RAFM. Nitrogen metabolism and ornithine cycle function. *Physiol Rev* 70:701, 1990.
86. Schimke RT. Adaptive characteristics of urea cycle enzymes in the rat. *J Biol Chem* 237:459, 1962.
87. Morris SM Jr. Regulation of enzymes of urea and arginine synthesis. *Annu Rev Nutr* 12:81, 1992.
88. Das TK, Waterlow JC. The rate of adaptation of urea cycle enzymes, aminotransferases and glutamic dehydrogenase to changes in dietary protein intake. *Br J Nutr* 32:353, 1974.
89. Jackson AA. Critique of Protein-Energy Interactions In Vivo: Urea Kinetics. In NS Scrimshaw, B Schürch (eds), *Protein-Energy Interactions.* Lausanne, Switzerland: IDECG, Nestlé Foundation, 1992. P 63.
90. Mitch WE, Lietman PS, Walser M. Effects of oral neomycin and kanamycin in chronic uremic patients: I. Urea metabolism. *Kidney Int* 11:116, 1977.
91. Mitch WE, Walser M. Effects of oral neomycin and kanamycin in chronic uremic patients: II. Nitrogen balance. *Kidney Int* 11:123, 1977.
92. Pattereson BW, et al. Urea nitrogen recycling in burned children. *Proceedings of the American Burn Association.* 27th Annual Meeting, Albuquerque, April 19–22, 1995. P 157.
93. Munro HN. Metabolic Basis of Nutritional Care in Liver and Kidney Disease. In RW Winger, HL Green (eds), *Nutritional Support of the Seriously Ill Patient.* New York: Academic, 1983. P 93.
94. Bier DM. Intrinsically difficult problems: The kinetics of body proteins and amino acids in man. *Diabetes Metab Rev* 5:111, 1989.
95. Christensen HN. Interorgan nutrition: Introductory comments from the chair. *Fed Proc* 45:2165, 1986.
96. Waterlow JD, Garlick BJ, Millward DJ. *Protein Turnover in Mammalian Tissues and in the Whole Body.* Holland: North-Holland, 1978. P 804.
97. Waterlow JC. Protein turnover with special reference to man. *Q J Exp Physiol* 69:409, 1984.
98. Waterlow JC, Golden MHN, Garlick P. Protein turnover in man measured with ^{15}N: Comparison of end products and dose regimens. *Am J Physiol* 235:E165, 1978.
99. Garlick PJ. Protein Turnover in the Whole Animal and Specific Tissues. In A Neuberger, LLM VanDeenen (eds), *Protein Metabolism: Comprehensive Biochemistry,* vol 19B, part 1–152. Amsterdam: Elsevier, 1980. P 77.
100. Garlick PJ, McNurlan MA. Isotopic Methods for Studying Protein Turnover. In NCR Räiha (ed), *Protein Metabolism During Infancy.* New York: Raven, 1994. P 29.
101. Rennie MJ, Halliday D. The use of stable isotope tracers as metabolic probes of whole-body and limb metabolism. *Proc Nutr Soc* 43:189, 1984.
102. Clarke JTR, Bier DM. The conversion of phenylalanine totyrosine in man: Direct measurement by continuous intravenous tracer infusions of L-[ring$^2H_5$phenylalanine and L-[1-^{13}C]tyrosine in the postabsorptive state. *Metabolism* 31:999, 1982.
103. Thompson GN, et al. Rapid measurement of whole body and forearm protein turnover using a [$^2H_5$]phenylalanine model. *Am J Physiol* 256:E631, 1989.
104. Matthews DE, et al. Relationship of plasma leucine and α-ketoisocaproate during a L-[1-^{13}C]leucine infusion in man: A method for measuring human intracellular leucine tracer enrichment. *Metabolism* 31:1105, 1982.
105. Millward DJ, et al. Whole body protein and amino acid turnover: What can be measured with confidence? *Proc Nutr Soc* 50:197, 1991.
106. Matthews DE, Bier DM. Stable isotope methods for nutritional investigation. *Annu Rev Nutr* 3:309, 1983.
107. Halliday D, Read WWC. Mass spectrometric assay of stable isotope enrichment for the estimation of protein turnover in man. *Proc Nutr Soc* 42:321, 1981.
108. Wolfe RR. Radioactive and Stable Isotope Tracers in Medicine. In *Principles and Practice of Kinetic Analysis.* New York: Wiley, 1992.
109. Bier DM, Matthews DE, Young VR. Interpretation of Amino Acid Kinetic Studies in the Context of Whole-Body Protein Metabolism. In JS Garrow, D Halliday (eds), *Substrate and Energy Metabolism in Man.* London: Libbey, 1985. P 27.
110. Sprinson DB, Rittenberg D. The rate of interaction of the amino acids of the diet with the tissue proteins. *J Biol Chem* 180:715, 1949.
111. Picou D, Taylor Roberts T. The measurement of total protein synthesis and catabolism and nitrogen turnover in infants in different nutritional states and receiving different amounts of dietary protein. *Clin Sci* 36:283, 1969.
112. Golden MHN, Jackson AA. Assumption and Errors in the Use of ^{15}N-Excretion Data to Estimate Whole Body Protein Turnover. In JC Waterlow, JML Stephen (eds), *Nitrogen Metabolism in Man.* London: Applied Science, 1981. P 323.
113. Young VR, Yu Y-M, Krempf M. Protein and Amino Acid Turnover Using the Stable Isotopes ^{15}N,^{13}C and ^{2}H as Probes. In R Whitehead, A Prentice (eds), *New Techniques*

in Nutritional Research. San Diego: Academic, 1991. P 17.

114. de Benoist B, et al. The measurement of whole body protein turnover in the preterm infant with intragastric infusion of L-[^{13}C]leucine and sampling of the urinary leucine pool. *Clin Sci* 66:155, 1984.
115. Young VR. Techniques in Measuring Protein Turnover: In Vivo Techniques. In KS Nair (ed), *Protein Metabolism in Diabetes Mellitus.* London: Smith-Gordon, 1992. P 47.
116. El-Khoury AE, et al. Whole body protein synthesis in healthy adult humans: $^{13}CO_2$ technique vs. plasma precursor approach. *Am J Physiol* 268:E174, 1995.
117. Arends J, Bier DM. Labeled amino acid infusion studies of in vivo protein synthesis with stable isotope tracers and gas chromatography-mass spectrometry. *Anal Chim Acta* 247:255, 1991.
118. Reeds PJ, et al. VLDL apolipoprotein B-100, a potential indicator of theisotopic labeling of the hepatic protein synthetic precursor pool in humans: Studies with multiple stable isotopically labeled amino acids. *J Nutr* 122:457, 1992.
119. Garlick PJ, et al. Measurements of tissue protein synthesis rates in vivo: A critical analysis of contrasting methods. *Am J Physiol* 266:E287, 1994.
120. Rennie MJ, Smith K, Watt PW. Measurement of human tissue protein synthesis: An optimal approach. *Am J Physiol* 266:E298, 1994.
121. Young VR, et al. The Biochemistry and Physiology of Protein and Amino Acid Metabolism with Reference to Protein Nutrition. In NCR Räiha (ed), *Protein Metabolism During Infancy.* New York: Raven, 1994. P 1.
122. Von Goudoever JB, et al. Whole body protein turnover in premature appropriate for gestational age and small for gestational age infants: Comparison of [^{15}N]glycine and [1-^{13}C]leucine administered simultaneously. *Pediatr Res* 37:381, 1995.
123. Kinney JM, Elwyn DH. Protein metabolism and injury. *Annu Rev Nutr* 3:433, 1983.
124. Yu Y-M, et al. Relationships among arginine, citrulline, ornithine and leucine kinetics in adult burn patients. *Am J Clin Nutr,* in press.
125. Jahoor F, et al. Dynamics of the protein metabolic response to burn injury. *Metabolism* 37:330, 1988.
126. Yu Y-M, et al. Increased requirement of tyrosine for burn patients: A kinetic study of aromatic amino acid metabolism. *Proceedings of the 23rd Annual Meeting of the American Burn Association,* 23rd Annual Meeting, Baltimore, 1991. P 78.
127. Yu Y-M, Burke JF, Young VR. A kinetic study of L-$^{2}H_3$-methyl-1-^{13}C-methionine in patients with severe burn injury. *J Trauma* 35:1, 1993.
128. Jaksic T, et al. Proline metabolism in adult male burn patients and healthy controls. *Am J Clin Nutr* 54:408, 1991.
129. Calloway DH, Spector H. Nitrogen balance as related to caloric and protein intake in active young men. *Am J Clin Nutr* 2:405, 1954.
130. Munro HN. General Aspects of the Regulation of Protein Metabolism by Diet and by Hormones. In HN Munro, JB Allison (eds), *Mammalian Protein Metabolism.* vol. 1. New York: Academic, 1964. P 381.
131. Elwyn DH. Nutritional requirements of adult surgical patients. *Crit Care Med* 8:9, 1980.
132. Elwyn DH, et al. Changes in nitrogen balance of depleted patients with increasing infusions of glucose. *Am J Clin Nutr* 32:1597, 1979.
133. Elwyn DH, et al. Protein and energy sparing of glucose added in hypocaloric amounts to peripheral solutions of amino acids. *Metabolism* 27:325, 1988.
134. Robert JJ, et al. Quantitative aspects of glucose production and metabolism in healthy elderly subjects. *Diabetes* 31:203, 1982.
135. Brusilow SW, Horwich AL. Urea Cycle Enzymes. In CR Scriver et al (eds), *The Metabolic Basis of Inherited Disease.* New York: McGraw-Hill, 1989. P 629.
136. Hoogenrood N, et al. Inhibition of intestinal citrulline synthesis causes severe growth retardation in rats. *Am J Physiol* 249:G792, 1985.
137. Dhanakoti SN, et al. Renal arginine synthesis: Studies in vitro and in vivo. *Am J Physiol* 259:E437, 1990.
138. Tiziannelo A, et al. Renal metabolism of amino acids and ammonia in subjects with normal renal function and in patients with chronic renal insufficiency. *J Clin Invest* 65:1162, 1980.
139. Castillo L, et al. Splanchnic metabolism of dietary arginine in relation to nitric oxide synthesis in normal adult man. *Proc Natl Acad Sci USA* 90:193, 1993.
140. Castillo L, et al. Plasma arginine and citrulline kinetics in adults given adequate and arginine-free diets. *Proc Natl Acad Sci USA* 90:7749, 1993.
141. Castillo L, et al. Dietary arginine uptake by the splanchnic region in adult humans. *Am J Physiol* 265:E532, 1993.
142. Castillo L, et al. Plasma arginine kinetics in adult man: Response to an arginine-free diet. *Metabolism* 43:114, 1994.
143. Castillo L, et al. The plasma flux and oxidation rate of ornithine adaptively decline with restricted arginine intake. *Proc Natl Acad Sci USA* 91:6393, 1994.
144. Castillo L, et al. Plasma arginine, citrulline and ornithine kinetics in adults, with observations on nitric oxide synthesis. *Am J Physiol* 268:E360, 1995.
145. Cheung C-W, et al. Channeling of urea cycle intermediates in situ in permeabilized hepatocytes. *J Biol Chem* 264:4038, 1987.
146. Cohen NS, Cheung C-W, Raijman L. Channeling of extramitochondrial ornithine to matrix ornithine transcarbamylase. *J Biol Chem* 262:203, 1987.
147. Sivram P, Deutscher MP. Existence of two forms of liver arginyl-tRNA for protein synthesis. *Proc Natl Acad Sci USA* 87:3665, 1990.
148. Srere PA. Complexes of sequential metabolic enzymes. *Annu Rev Biochem* 56:89, 1987.
149. Srere PA, Ovadi J. Enzyme-enzyme interactions and their metabolic role. *FEBS Lett* 268:360, 1990.
150. Savageau MA. Metabolic channeling: Implications for regulation of metabolism for quantitative description of reactions in vivo. *J Theor Biol* 152:85, 1991.
151. Ovadi J, Srere PA. Channel your energies. *Trends Biochem Sci* 17:445, 1992.
152. Jungermann K, Katz N. Functional specialization of different hepatocyte populations. *Physiol Rev* 69:708, 1989.
153. Haussinger D. Nitrogen metabolism in liver: Structural and functional organization and physiological relevance. *Biochem J* 267:281, 1990.
154. Yu Y-M, et al. Plasma arginine and leucine kinetics and urea production rates in burn patients. *Metabolism* 44:659, 1995.
155. Zieve I. Conditional deficiencies of ornithine or arginine. *J Am Coll Nutr* 5:167, 1986.
156. Visek WJ. Arginine and disease states. *J Nutr* 115:532, 1985.

157. Visek WJ. Arginine needs, physiological state and usual diets: A reevaluation. *J Nutr* 116:36, 1986.

158. Arnstein HRV, Neuberger A. The synthesis of glycine and serine by the rat. *Biochem J* 55:271, 1953.

159. Young VR, El-Khoury AE. The Notion of the Nutritional Essentiality of Amino Acids, Revisited, With a Note on the Indispensable Amino Acid Requirements in Adults. In L Cynober (ed), *Amino Acid Metabolism and Therapy in Health and Nutritional Disease.* Boca Raton: CRC, 1995. P 267.

160. Negrutskii BS, Deutscher MP. Channeling of amino acyl-tRNA for protein synthesis in vivo. *Proc Natl Acad Sci USA* 88:4991, 1991.

161. Negrutskii BS, Deutscher MP. A sequestered pool of amino acyl-tRNA in mammalian cells. *Proc Natl Acad Sci USA* 89:3601, 1992.

162. Sánchez M, et al. Phenylalanine kinetics and tyrosine kinetics in young men throughout a continuous 24 h period at a low phenylalanine intake. *Am J Clin Nutr* 61:555, 1995.

163. Sánchez M, et al. 24 hour intravenous and oral studies with L-[1-^{13}C]phenylalanine and L-[3,3,$^{2}H_2$] tyrosine at a generous phenylalanine, tyrosine-devoid intake in adults. *Am J Clin Nutr,* in review, 1995.

164. Kaufman S. The phenylalanine hydroxylating system. *Adv Enzymol Relat Areas Mol Biol* 67:77, 1993.

165. Wykes LJ, House JD, Ball PB. Amino acid profile and aromatic amino acid concentration in total parenteral nutrition: Effect on growth, protein metabolism and aromatic amino acid metabolism in the neonatal pig. *Clin Sci* 87:75, 1994.

166. Wykes LJ, et al. Aromatic amino acid metabolism of neonatal pigs receiving TPN: Effect of tyrosine precursors. *Am J Physiol* 267:E672, 1994.

167. Cortiella J, et al. Leucine kinetics at graded intakes in young men: Quantitative fate of dietary leucine. *Am J Clin Nutr* 48:998, 1988.

168. Hoerr RA, et al. Leucine kinetics from [$^{2}H_3$]$^-$ and [^{13}C]leucine infused simultaneously by gut and vein. *Am J Physiol* 260:E111, 1991.

169. Hoerr RA, et al. Effects of protein restriction and acute refeeding on leucine and lysine kinetics in young men. *Am J Physiol* 264:E567, 1993.

170. Horber FH, Haymond MW. Human growth hormone prevents the protein metabolic side-effects of predisone in humans. *J Clin Invest* 86:265, 1990.

171. Biolo G, et al. Leucine and phenylalanine kinetics during mixed meal digestion: A multiple tracer approach. *Am J Physiol* 262:E455, 1992.

172. Matthews DE, Marano MA, Campbell RG. Splanchnic bed utilization of leucine and phenylalanine in humans. *Am J Physiol* 264:E109, 1993.

173. Matthews DE, Marano MA, Campbell RG. Splanchnic bed utilization of glutamine and glutamic acid in humans. *Am J Physiol* 264:E848, 1993.

174. Hiramatsu T, et al. Methionine and cysteine kinetics at different intakes of cystine in healthy adult men. *Am J Clin Nutr* 60:525, 1994.

175. Rerat A, et al. Splanchnic fluxes of amino acids after duodenal infusion of carbohydrate solutions containing free amino acids or oligopeptides in the nonanaesthetized pig. *Br J Nutr* 68:111, 1992.

176. Grimble GK. The significance of peptides in clinical nutrition. *Annu Rev Nutr* 14:419, 1994.

177. Collin-Vidal C, et al. Leucine kinetics are different during feeding and whole protein or oligopeptides. *Am J Physiol* 267:E907, 1994.

178. Moriarity KJ, et al. Relative nutritional value of whole protein, hydrolysed protein and free amino acids in man. *Gut* 26:694, 1985.

179. Ziegler F, et al. Efficiency of enteral nitrogen support in surgical patients: Small peptides vs. non-degraded proteins. *Gut* 31:1277, 1990.

180. Boirie Y, et al. Production of large amounts of [^{13}C]leucine-enriched milk proteins by lactating cows. *J Nutr* 125:92, 1995.

181. Young VR, et al. The Biochemistry and Physiology of Protein and Amino Acid Metabolism With Reference to Protein Nutrition. In NCR Räiha (ed), *Protein Metabolism During Infancy.* New York: Raven, 1994. P 1.

182. Rose WC, Haines WJ, Warner DJ. The amino acid requirements of man: V. The role of lysine, arginine and tryptophan. *J Biol Chem* 206:421, 1954.

183. Kies C. Comparative value of various sources of nonspecific nitrogen for the human. *J Agric Food Chem* 22:190, 1974.

184. FAO/WHO Protein Requirements: Report of a Joint FAO/WHO Expert Group. In *FAO Nutrition Meetings Report Series,* no. 37. Rome: Food and Agriculture Organization of the United Nations, 1965.

185. Mudd SH, Levy HL, Skorby F. Disorders of Transsulfuration. In CR Scriver et al (eds), *The Metabolic Basis of Inherited Disease.* New York: McGraw Hill, 1989. P 693.

186. Stipanuk MH. Metabolism of sulfur-containing amino acids. *Annu Rev Nutr* 6:179, 1986.

187. Stipanuk MH, De LaRosa J, Hirschberger LL. Catabolism of cyst(e)ine by rat renal cortical tubules. *J Nutr* 120:450, 1990.

188. Baker DH. Nutritional and metabolic interrelationships among sulfur compounds in avian nutrition. *Fed Proc* 35:1917, 1976.

189. Smolin LA, Benevenga NJ. Methionine, Homocyst(e)ine, Cyst(e)ine: Metabolic Interrelationships. In M Friedman (ed), *Absorption and Utilization of Amino Acids,* vol 11. Boca Raton: CRC, 1989. P 157.

190. Rose WC, Wixom RL. The amino acid requirements of man: XIII. The sparing effect of cystine on the methionine requirement. *J Biol Chem* 216:763, 1955.

191. Rose WC, et al. The amino acid requirements of man: XI. The threonine and methionine requirements. *J Biol Chem* 215:101, 1955.

192. Chipponi JX, et al. Deficiencies of essential and conditionally essential nutrients. *Am J Clin Nutr* 35:1112, 1982.

193. Laidlaw SA, Kopple JD. Newer concepts of the indispensable amino acids. *Am J Clin Nutr* 46:593, 1987.

194. Stegink LK, Den Besten L. Synthesis of cysteine from methionine in normal adult subjects: Effect of route of alimentation. *Science* 178:514, 1972.

195. Vina J, et al. Impairment of cysteine synthesis from methionine in rats exposed to surgical stress. *Br J Nutr* 68:421, 1990.

196. Grimble RF. Dietary manipulation of the inflammatory response. *Proc Nutr Soc* 51:285, 1992.

197. Stipanuk MH, et al. Cysteine concentration regulates cysteine metabolism to glutathione, sulfate and taurine in rat hepatocytes. *J Nutr* 122:420, 1992.

198. Daniels KM, Stipanuk MH. The effect of dietary cysteine level on cysteine metabolism in rats. *J Nutr* 112:2130, 1982.

199. Stegink LD, Baker GL. Infusion of protein hydrolysates

in the newborn infant: Plasma amino acid co.\centrations. *J Pediatr* 78:595, 1971.

200. Griffith OW, Meister A. Glutathione: Interorgan translocation, turnover and metabolism. *Proc Natl Acad Sci USA* 75:5605, 1979.
201. Meister A, Larsson A. Glutathione Synthetase Deficiency and Other Disorders of the Gamma-Glutamyl Cycle. In CR Scriver, et al (eds), *The Metabolic Basis of Inherited Disease.* New York: McGraw-Hill, 1989.
202. Meister A, Anderson ME. Glutathione. *Annu Rev Biochem* 52:711, 1983.
203. Dolphine D, Poulson R, Avramovid O (eds). *Glutathione: Chemical, Biochemical and Medical Aspects,* parts A & B. New York: Wiley, 1989.
204. Deneke SM, Fanburg BL. Regulation of cellular glutathione. *Am J Physiol* 257:L163, 1989.
205. Taniguchi M, et al. Nutritional Aspects of Glutathione Metabolism and Function. In D Dolphine, R Poulson, O Avramovic (eds), *Glutathione: Chemical, Biochemical and Medical Aspects,* part B. New York: Wiley, 1989.
206. Martensson J, Goodwin CN, Blake R. Mitochondrial glutathione in hypermetabolic rats following burn injury and thyroid hormone administration: Evidence of a selective effect on brain glutathione by burn injury. *Metabolism* 41:273, 1992.
207. Young VR, Bier DM. A kinetic approach for the determination of human amino acid requirements. *Nutr Rev* 45:289, 1987.
208. FAO/WHO/UNU. Energy and protein requirements: Report of a joint FAO/WHO/UNU Expert Consultation. *Technical Report Series,* no. 724, 1985.
209. Hegsted DM. Balance studies. *J Nutr* 106:307, 1978.
210. Young VR. Nitrogen balance studies indicators of human requirements or of adaptive mechanisms. *J Nutr* 116:700, 1986.
211. Munro HN, Young VR. Protein and Amino Acid Requirements. In AN Exton-Smith, FI Caird (eds), *Metabolic and Nutritional Disorders of the Elderly.* Bristol: Wright, 1980. P 13.
212. Pineda O, et al. Protein Quality in Relation to Estimates of Essential Amino Acid Requirements. In CE Bodwell, JS Adkins, DT Hopkins (eds), *Protein Quality in Humans: Assessment and In Vitro Estimation.* Westport: AVI, 1981. P 29.
213. Torun B, et al. Use of Amino Acid Composition Data to Predict Protein Nutritive Value for Children With Specific Reference to New Estimates of Their Essential Amino Acid Requirements. In CE Bodwell, JS Adkins, DT Hopkins (eds), *Protein Quality in Humans: Assessment and In Vitro Estimation.* Westport: AVI, 1981. P 374.
214. FAO/WHO. Energy and Protein Requirements. In *FAO/WHO Nutrition Meetings Report Series,* no. 52. Rome: United Nations Food and Agriculture Organization, 1973.
215. Young VR, Bier DM, Pellett PL. A theoretical basis for increasing current estimates of the amino acid requirements in adult man with experimental support. *Am J Clin Nutr* 50:80, 1989.
216. Young VR, Pellett PL. Current concepts concerning indispensable amino acids needs in adults and their implications for international nutrition planning. *Food Nutr Bull* 12:289, 1990.
217. Young VR, El-Khoury AE. Can amino acid requirements for maintenance in adult humans be approximated from the amino acid composition of body mixed proteins? *Proc Natl Acad Sci USA* 92:300, 1995.
218. FAO/WHO. Protein Quality Evaluation: Report of the Joint FAO/WHO Expert Consultation. *FAO Food and Nutrition Paper,* no. 51. Rome: United Nations Food and Agriculture Organization, 1991.

Selected Readings

The following references are reviews given to direct the reader who is interested in learning in greater detail about areas and topics covered in this chapter, especially human protein and amino acid metabolism.

Garrow JS, Halliday D (eds). *Substrate and Energy Metabolism in Man.* London: Libbey, 1985.

This book contains the papers presented at a symposium concerned with in vivo aspects of both protein and energy metabolism, held at the Clinical Research Center in September 1984. The chapters focus largely on work in humans and include accounts of the potentialities and limitations of stable isotope tracers in clinical research studies, techniques for measuring energy metabolism, hormonal control of substrate and energy metabolism, and the consequences and management of various forms of human malnutrition and endocrine disease. Although published 10 years ago, this book is informative and valuable for those interested in learning more about and investigating the impact of trauma (including surgery) and sepsis on body protein and amino acid metabolism.

Kinney JM, Tucker HN (eds). *Organ Metabolism and Nutrition: Ideas for Future Critical Care.* New York: Raven, 1994.

This book contains the papers and discussions during the second Clintec International Conference held in Amsterdam in May 1993. It is an impressive update of knowledge relevant to organ failure. Included are chapters on substrate kinetics (including amino acids) and catabolic hormones, skeletal and cardiac muscle proteolysis, interorgan exchange of amino acids after trauma, and essential and conditionally essential nutrients in clinical nutrition. This book offers much greater detail on several of the topics we covered briefly in this chapter.

Munro HN, Allison JB (eds). *Mammalian Protein Metabolism,* vols 1 and 2. New York: Academic, 1964; Munro HN (ed). *Mammalian Protein Metabolism,* vol 3. New York: Academic, 1969; Munro HN (ed). *Mammalian Protein Metabolism,* vol 4. New York: Academic, 1970.

This four-volume series remains an exceedingly rich source of information about all aspects of mammalian protein and amino acid metabolism, ranging from the molecular and cellular aspects to the tissue organ and whole-body levels of biological organization. Although the detailed cellular and genetic events of protein metabolism have been elaborated on and greatly expanded since these volumes were first written, the major principles of whole body–amino acid metabolism and nutrition remain largely intact. Munro's ability to integrate diverse areas of inquiry into a conceptual framework of practical, human nutritional relevance is truly remarkable.

Waterlow JC, Garlick PJ, Millward DJ. *Protein Turnover in Mammalian Tissues and in the Whole Body.* Amsterdam: North-Holland, 1978.

This is the first, and remaining, comprehensive discussion of modern studies of protein turnover in the living animal; the book is divided into three parts concerned with processes, methods, and results (turnover rates in the whole animal and whole tissue and the quantitative comparisons of turnover rates under various conditions). This will remain, for some considerable time, an extremely valuable source of information in this field.

Waterlow JC, Stephen JML (eds). *Nitrogen Metabolism in Man.* London: Applied Science, 1981.

Waterlow states in the introduction, ". . . although a great deal is known about the biochemical pathways of amino acid and protein metabolism, our knowledge of the rates at which the various reactions and interconversions occur in the living subject is still very inadequate. We have a reasonably good map, but we do not know much about the flow of traffic along different routes."

The chapters address this subject and also that of protein turnover in the whole animal man. We find it necessary to consult this book frequently. It should be enlightening reading, especially to those who are newly interested in the topic of human nitrogen metabolism.

Wolfe RR. *Radioactive and Stable Isotope Tracers in Biomedicine: Principles and Practice of Kinetic Analysis.* New York: Wiley-Liss, 1992.

This book supplements and extends the information given in the Waterlow reference above. It deals in a comprehensive way with all aspects of tracer usage, from the basic characteristics of isotopic tracers, to compartmental modeling and separate detailed accounts of studies of substrate oxidation, glucose, lipid, urea and amino kinetics, and protein synthesis and breakdown. In view of the emphasis given to in vivo studies of protein and amino acid metabolism in the present chapter, this book is "required reading" for those who wish to delve more deeply into the determination and study of quantitative aspects of human metabolism.

Young VR, Yu Y-M, Fukagawa NK. Energy and Protein Turnover in Energy Metabolism: Tissue Determinants and Cellular Corollaries. In JM Kinney, HN Tucker (eds), *Energy Metabolism: Tissue Determinants and Cellular Corollaries.* New York: Raven, 1992. P 439.

This chapter discusses the relationships between protein turnover and amino acid oxidation and utilization, with emphasis on the effects of disease on energy–protein turnover and the impact of energy source in the nitrogen economy of the body. It is a useful addendum to the present chapter.

7

Carbohydrates

Michael A. Lieberman
John W. Vester

Carbohydrate metabolism is an essential process for life [1,2]. The chemical conversions that allow humans to extract energy from simple sugars have been conserved throughout evolution, from the simplest bacteria to man. Before discussing carbohydrate metabolism in detail, however, there are two important concepts that must be understood. The first of these is the concept of cellular compartmentation, and the second is that of energy generation and storage within biologic systems. Once these concepts have been presented, the pathways of carbohydrate metabolism, including glycolysis, the hexose-monophosphate shunt, the citric acid cycle, fates of pyruvate, and glycogen metabolism, will be discussed in detail.

The Cell Membrane and Energy Metabolism

Overview

All cells contain a series of semipermeable membranes that compartmentalize the intracellular contents. These membranes include an outer or plasma membrane, which protects the cell from its environment, and inner membranes, which allow discrete compartments within the cell to carry out specific functions. In addition to the physical separation of aqueous compartments, membranes contain proteins that perform a number of enzymatic roles. A major role of membrane proteins (mitochondrion in particular) is the generation of a proton gradient across the membrane, which acts as the driving force for energy production and transport of ions and nutrients across the membrane. Additionally, compartmentation allows cells to synthesize and accumulate metabolites so that they are not used by enzymes in other compartments. Additional compartments are specific for metabolite degradation (lysosomes), so that the cytoplasm is protected from intracellular proteases and glycosidases. Because of their diverse functions, membranes and membrane compartmentalization play an important role in the regulation of many metabolic pathways.

Membrane Structure

Membranes are composed of molecules that have both hydrophobic and hydrophilic properties. As seen in Figure 7-1, the primary component of eukaryotic membranes are phospholipids that are molecules with a glycerolphosphate backbone to which long-chain fatty acids are esterified. The hydrophobic tails of the fatty acids face the interior of the membrane, and the charged phosphate-head group of the glycerolphosphate molecule faces the aqueous side of the membrane. Another major component of membranes is cholesterol, also shown in Figure 7-1. Cholesterol enhances the fluidity of the membrane, which allows molecules to flow within the hydrophobic core of the membrane. Protein molecules are also associated with the membrane in either of two configurations. The first is protein association with only the external face of the membranes (known as peripheral proteins), and the second is protein association through an embedding of the protein within the hydrophobic core of the membrane (integral membrane proteins). The peripheral proteins are associated with the membrane through ionic interactions, and they can frequently be removed from the membrane by treatment with salt. The integral membrane proteins require disruption of the phospholipid bilayer for removal, indicating that strong hydrophobic interactions anchor these proteins to the membranes. Although these proteins are deeply embedded within the membranes, they still retain the capacity to move within the plane of the membrane and can associate with other proteins within this environment. Alterations in the lipid component of the membranes will alter the ability of proteins to move within the membrane, which can affect the overall metabolic status of a cell.

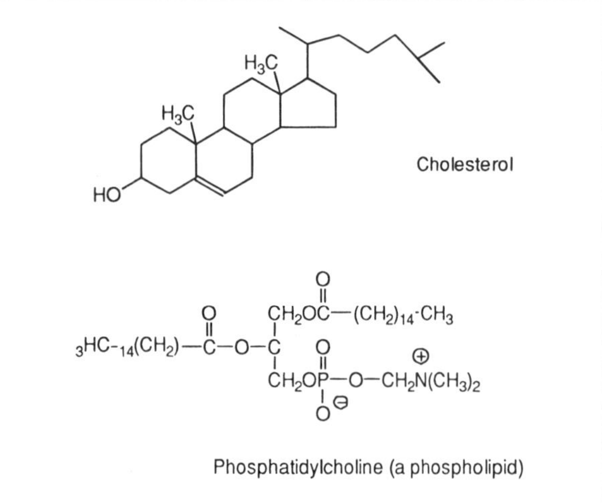

Figure 7-1. The structures of two common membrane components, cholesterol and phosphatidylcholine, a phospholipid.

What Do Membrane Proteins Do?

Membrane proteins perform a number of basic functions. Three major functions are catalyzing the transport of small molecules from one side of the membrane to the other, providing the mechanism for energy production within the mitochondrial membrane, and allowing the cell to communicate with its environment. Because of its structure, membranes separate two aqueous compartments so that the components of each compartment do not mix. This means that the membrane itself is impermeable to many aqueous molecules. However, there is a mechanism to allow for the transport of molecules from one side of the membrane to the other that is mediated by protein molecules within the membrane, such as the sugar and amino acid transport proteins found within intestinal epithelial cells. These proteins allow the intestinal epithelial cells to accumulate amino acids and sugars from the lumen of the small intestine. These cells will then transport the nutrients from the cell via a second distinct transporter located in the membrane on the opposite side of the cell. This second transporter will send the nutrients into the blood and lymph systems so that the nutrients can be used by the rest of the body. Deficiencies in either of the transporters on the intestinal epithelial cells would lead to an inability of the body to properly metabolize and utilize food, which would be a nutritional disaster.

Another example of a transporter is the glucose transport protein, which catalyzes the transfer of glucose from the circulation into cells for either energy production or storage. Insulin is a hormone released by the pancreas when blood glucose levels increase, and one of insulin's many effects is the ability to stimulate glucose uptake by its target tissues. Insulin will stimulate responsive cells to increase the number of glucose transporters within their membrane. Through the expression of an increased number of glucose transporters at the membrane, the cell will be able to transport and metabolize glucose at a rapid rate. The mechanism whereby insulin accomplishes this has been determined [3–5]. Insulin-responsive cells contain a large number of presynthesized glucose transporters within intracellular membranes. Upon insulin binding to the cell, the preformed transporters are mobilized and delivered to the cell surface, where they are now functional and catalyze glucose uptake by the cell. Deficiencies in glucose transport have been associated with diabetes mellitus [6,7].

A third example of a complex transport protein is the sodium-potassium adenosine triphosphatase (ATPase), which exchanges sodium for potassium ions across the cell membrane. The exchange is not 1:1, however, because three sodium ions are transported out of the cell for every two potassium ions transported back in. The proper functioning of this ion pump, which aids in generating an electrical potential across the membrane, is essential for heart function [8,9]. Defects in pump activity (which can occur through the action of certain drugs) will have profound effects on the ability of the cells to respond to nerve impulses and can lead to cardiac arrest.

The three transport systems discussed above allowed for the transfer of small molecules from outside to within the cell. Another class of transporter transfers small molecules between compartments within cells. An example of this type of transporter is the adenine nucleotide translocase in the mitochondrial membrane. This enzyme will exchange adenosine triphosphate (ATP) across the mitochondrial membrane for adenosine diphosphate (ADP) from the cytoplasm. Mitochondria are the energy-generating systems within cells. The energy generated within the mitochondria is stored as ATP, which contains two high-energy bonds (indicating that when these bonds are broken a large amount of energy is released; see below). The reasons why ATP is the energy storage molecule will be discussed shortly. Adenosine diphosphate is a necessary substrate for ATP synthesis, and if mitochondrial ADP levels are depleted, ATP synthesis will stop. To circumvent this problem, the mitochondrial membrane contains the adenine nucleotide translocase activity, which will exchange cytoplasmic ADP for mitochondrial ATP. In this manner, ATP can be used for cytoplasmic and nuclear reactions, and the ADP that is generated in the cytoplasm by the release of energy from ATP (in which ADP is formed as an end product) can be recycled by the mitochondria to form additional ATP.

The second major role of membrane proteins is one of energy generation. There are proteins within the mitochondrial membrane that catalyze the process of oxidative phosphorylation, which couples ATP synthesis with the reduction of oxygen to water. These proteins consist of electron carriers (the electron transport chain) that transfer electrons down their electrochemical gradient, generating energy at discrete steps of the chain. The electrochemical energy generated by the electron transfers is converted to a strictly chemical form of energy, ATP, by another membrane embedded enzyme, the ATP synthase. These processes will be discussed in greater detail shortly.

Compartmentation as a Regulatory Control

One of the primary functions of membranes is that of compartmentation, the separation of aqueous compartments. In this manner, specific functions of the cell are separated, so that opposing reactions do not occur simultaneously. Examples of this are the pathways of fatty acid synthesis and oxidation. The enzymes responsible for synthesizing fatty acids are found in the cytoplasm, yet the enzymes for their degradation reside within the mitochondria. The physical separation of these two enzyme systems enables unique regulatory systems to be used. To be oxidized, the fatty acids must enter the mitochondria, and, because the inner mitochondrial membrane is impermeable to fatty acids, this transport must occur through a specific membrane-associated enzyme transport system. This enzyme system, however, is inhibited by the precursor of fatty acid biosynthesis, malonyl-CoA. Thus, when fatty acids are being synthesized in the cytoplasm and malonyl-CoA levels are high, the transport of fatty acids into the mitochondria is inhibited, and the synthesis of fatty acids will continue unopposed by simultaneous oxidation. Once fatty acid biosynthesis has stopped, however, transport of fatty acids into the mitochondria is not inhibited, and fatty acid oxidation will be favored.

Energy Production: The Mitochondria

The overriding theme to remember while discussing carbohydrate metabolism is that carbohydrates are an excellent energy source. If energy is not required when carbohydrates are available, then the excess carbohydrate will be stored as glycogen, for use in energy production under conditions in which carbohydrate availability is limited. As mentioned above, the mitochondrion is the major site of energy production within the cell, and the measure of available chemical energy is the level of ATP within the cell. The chemical conversion of carbohydrate and oxygen to carbon dioxide and water releases energy. This energy can be given off as heat or it can be conserved within high energy bonds of various metabolites. The cell uses a limited number of reactions to release the energy slowly and in discrete intervals, rather than releasing all the energy in one large step. The conversion of one mole of glucose to six moles of carbon dioxide and water will produce 686,000 calories. How, then, can this energy be conserved through the synthesis of ATP?

The energy is used in the formation of high-energy bonds, and an example of a structure containing two high-energy bonds (ATP) is shown in Figure 7-2. When ATP donates either of its two terminal phosphate groups in reactions, 7.3 kcal/mole of energy is released, which is a considerable sum for biochemical reactions. Therefore, to synthesize ATP from ADP and inorganic phosphate, at least 7.3 kcal of energy per mole is required from the breakdown of carbohydrate. High-energy bonds are also present in other molecules, as shown in Table 7-1. One important molecule to note is creatine phosphate. This is the major energy storage molecule of muscle. Muscle needs to store energy so that contraction can occur on demand. This means that the energy storage molecule needs to be present at high concentration within the muscle. The molecule ATP is frequently used to regulate enzyme activity and, because of its regulatory properties, it would not be a good choice for the stockpiling of high-energy compounds. Thus, the muscle will synthesize creatine phosphate from ATP and use that for energy storage.

Energy production within the mitochondria proceeds by the synthesis of ATP through a process known as oxidative phosphorylation. Oxidative phosphorylation is discussed in more detail later in this chapter, but it is the final step in energy production from the oxidation of glucose to carbon dioxide and water. It is possible to generate 38 molecules of ATP from the total oxidation of one molecule of glucose. Because each high-energy bond in ATP requires 7.3 kcal to produce, 277.4 kcal of energy can be generated and extracted from the oxidation of glucose. This represents a very good efficiency of 40% from the total potential energy contained within glucose (686 kcal). Oxidative phosphorylation requires an intact membrane to function. Without membranes, this high efficiency of energy capture would not occur. Thus, it is reasonable to sequester the enzymes responsible for energy production within the mitochondria so that this process can occur as efficiently as possible. Once the ATP is produced within the mitochondria, a translocase (as discussed above) will export the ATP to the cytoplasm, where the energy can be used to drive metabolic reactions.

Table 7-1. Standard Free Energy Change Upon Hydrolysis of Phosphate Compounds

Phosphate Compound	Free Energy of Hydrolysis (kcal/mole)
Phosphoenolpyruvate	−14.8
1,3-Bisphosphoglycerate	−11.8
Creatine phosphate	−10.3
Acetyl-phosphate	−10.1
ATP	−7.3
Glucose-1-phosphate	−5.0
Fructose-6-phosphate	−3.8
Glucose-6-phosphate	−3.3
3-Phosphoglyceric acid	−2.4
Glycerol-3-phosphate	−2.2

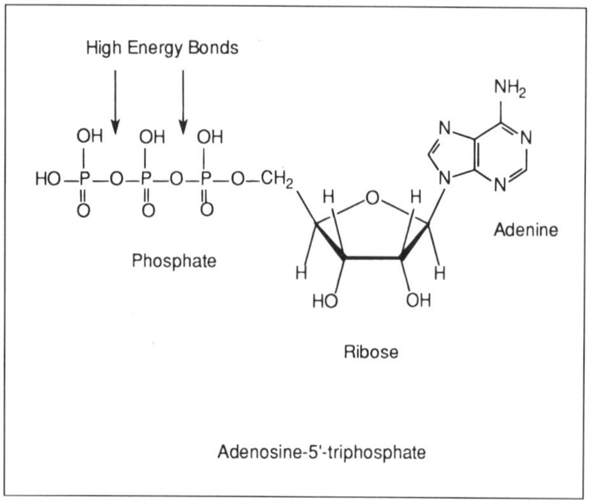

Figure 7-2. The structure of adenosine-5′-triphosphate (ATP), the major energy carrier of the cell. This molecule contains two bonds of high energy, as indicated by the arrows. Hydrolysis of these bonds will release 7.3 kcal of energy.

Membrane Response to the Environment

A final example of the importance of the membrane in regulatory control is that the plasma membrane is the interface between a cell and its environment. As such, it needs to be responsive to alterations in the environment, some of which may require the cell to alter its metabolic functions. An example of this has already been presented, in that the number of glucose transporters on the cell surface increases when insulin is released in response to elevated blood glucose levels. Another example of this type of response is the relationship between the liver and blood glucose levels. One of the liver's functions is to raise blood glucose levels when they become low. The liver therefore needs to be able to sense when blood glucose levels are dropping. This is done through the use of hormonal signals. The pancreas will sense when blood glucose levels are low and will respond by releasing the hormone glucagon. Glucagon will then bind to specific integral membrane proteins on the surface of liver cells. This will transmit a signal to the cytoplasm of the cell that conditions outside of the cell have changed and that the cell now needs to produce glucose for export. All hormones act through such a mechanism, and the effects of hormones on carbohydrate metabolism will be discussed later in this chapter. However, it is important to note that signals can be transmitted across membranes and that the process of interpreting this signal is known as signal transduction.

Summary

Membranes are important in separating cellular compartments. This separation allows different types of reactions to occur within each compartment without interfering with reactions in the other compartments. Many enzymes that are important for metabolism and cell survival are membrane associated, either integrally or peripherally. These proteins not only control the types of reaction that occur in the compartments, but they also regulate which substrates can enter the compartment, through the use of specific transport molecules. The major energy-generating process of the cell occurs through membrane proteins. The major energy carrier within biologic systems is ATP, and carbohydrate oxidation is geared toward the production of ATP from the chemical conversion of carbohydrates to carbon dioxide and water.

Glycolysis

Overview

As discussed above, ATP is the energy "coin of exchange" for the living cell. Although glucose is a remarkable precursor molecule in that it supplies carbon fragments for a vast array of biosynthetic mechanisms, it is quantitatively the major fuel in our diets. If a sedentary man had a 2200-calorie intake, his diet would consist of about 110 g of protein (20% of total calories) and 73 g of fat (30% of total calories); the remaining 50% of the dietary caloric intake would be from carbohydrates. The initial stages of glucose breakdown, once it has entered the cell, begin with two major pathways, glycolysis and the hexose-monophosphate shunt (HMP shunt). The HMP shunt will be considered in the next segment of this chapter; in this section, we will devote our attention to glycolysis.

In the generation of ATP, the ultimate fate of glucose is to be converted to six molecules of CO_2, six molecules of H_2O, and energy in the form of ATP. This total process requires oxidation that consumes six molecules of O_2. All the carbohydrate in the diet, in whatever form, enters into the metabolic machinery of the cell either as glucose itself or as some component of the glycolytic pathway. The process of converting glucose to six molecules of CO_2 and six molecules of H_2O, with the generation of chemical energy as ATP, forms the central core of our understanding of fuel metabolism in the living cell. Its intricacies have been the bane of students of medicine for as long as it has been taught. In actual fact, however, it is easily understood if viewed in its totality. The oxidation of glucose requires that each molecule be converted to two molecules of pyruvate by way of the glycolytic system that takes place in the cytosol. These two molecules of pyruvate are oxidized in the mitochondrion to produce the final net yield of six molecules of CO_2 and H_2O, and ATP.

The process of glycolysis is easier to understand if one remembers that it has three major divisions. The first involves a conversion of the 6-carbon hexose, glucose, into phosphorylated derivatives. The second involves splitting of the phosphorylated 6-carbon chain into two 3-carbon molecules of glyceraldehyde phosphate. The third phase is the conversion of the glyceraldehyde phosphate to pyruvic acid accompanied by the conservation of chemical energy.

The Glycolytic Reactions

Glucose must first enter the cell, and different cell membranes vary in their permeability to the entry of glucose, as has been previously discussed. Once glucose is inside the cell, it must be phosphorylated to begin the first phase of glycolysis because all of the reactions in the glycolytic scheme involve phosphorylated derivatives of 6-carbon and 3-carbon compounds. The phosphorylation of glucose also traps this sugar within the cell because phosphorylated molecules are normally impermeable to membrane travel. Our source of energy for this initial reaction is ATP and we rely on the high-energy content of its terminal phosphate bond to provide the energy that drives the phosphorylation reaction. This reaction is catalyzed by the enzyme hexokinase and requires Mg^{++}, as shown in Figure 7-3. The liver also contains a second enzyme that can phosphorylate glucose, known as glucokinase. Glucokinase is active when glucose concentrations are high, whereas hexokinase is active when glucose concentrations are low. Insulin is a hormone released from the pancreas to indicate an elevation in blood glucose levels. Insulin secretion leads to an induction of glucokinase

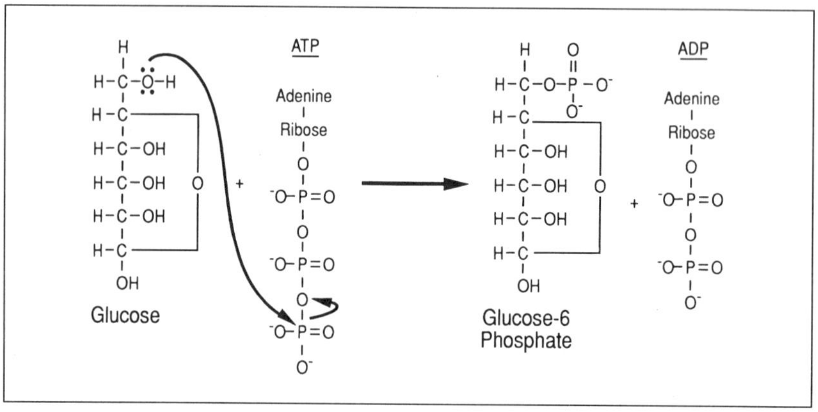

Figure 7-3. The reaction catalyzed by either hexokinase or glucokinase, in which glucose is phosphorylated to form glucose-6-phosphate. Note that this is an irreversible reaction.

gene transcription [10,11], thereby allowing for the synthesis of more enzyme in response to elevated glucose levels in the blood. In this manner, the high glucose levels can be more easily phosphorylated because more enzyme will be produced to handle the load.

The energy content of the terminal bond of ATP is so much higher than the bond of phosphate to glucose that this reaction is essentially thermodynamically irreversible (see Table 7-1). Remember that the goal of glycolysis is to split glucose into two 3-carbon fragments and, in the process, generate a positive yield of chemical energy in the form of molecules of ATP. So far, we have invested one molecule of ATP and our product, glucose-6-phosphate G6P does not have a readily apparent line of cleavage that would make for a symmetrical split. To get ready for this split, we simply isomerize the G6P to fructose-6-phosphate (F6P), as catalyzed by the enzyme phosphohexoisomerase (Figure 7-4).

In contradistinction to the hexokinase reaction, this reaction is readily reversible because of the relatively small change in free energy. This reaction also requires Mg^{++} and is specific for G6P and F6P.

The further reactions in glycolysis necessitate that the derivatives be phosphorylated. This requirement is met by adding another phosphate on the first position of the F6P. This reaction is catalyzed by the key enzyme of the pathway, phosphofructokinase-1 (PFK-1), thus completing the first stage.

As shown in Figure 7-5, the reaction catalyzed by PFK-1 requires a molecule of ATP and magnesium to produce fructose-1,6-bisphosphate. As was the case with hexokinase, the energy considerations are such that this reaction is also essentially irreversible. The enzyme that catalyzes this reaction is PFK-1 because there is a second enzyme, PFK-2, which will phosphorylate F6P to form fructose-2,6-bisphosphate. This compound is not an intermediate in glycolysis but has a very important regulatory role that will be discussed later.

Now that fructose-1,6-bisphosphate has been formed, a line of cleavage is readily apparent, between carbons 3 and 4, and the second stage of glycolysis can begin. Fructose-1,6-bisphosphate is split by the action of aldolase into two triose phosphates, dihydroxyacetone phosphate and glyceraldehyde-3-phosphate (G3P), as shown in Figure 7-6.

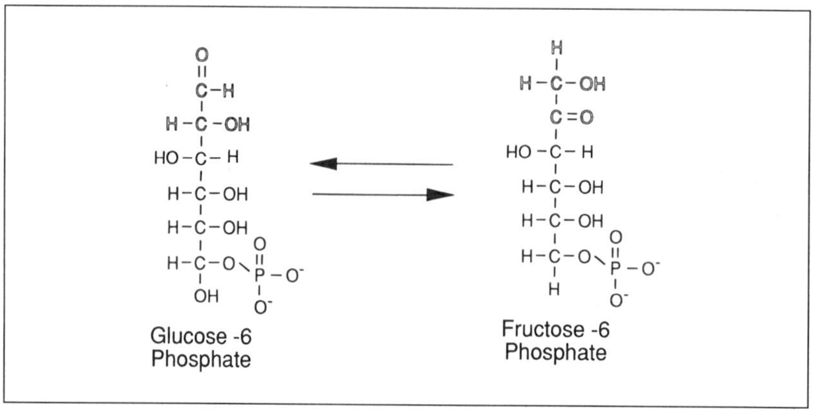

Figure 7-4. The reaction catalyzed by phosphohexoisomerase, in which glucose-6-phosphate is isomerized to fructose-6-phosphate.

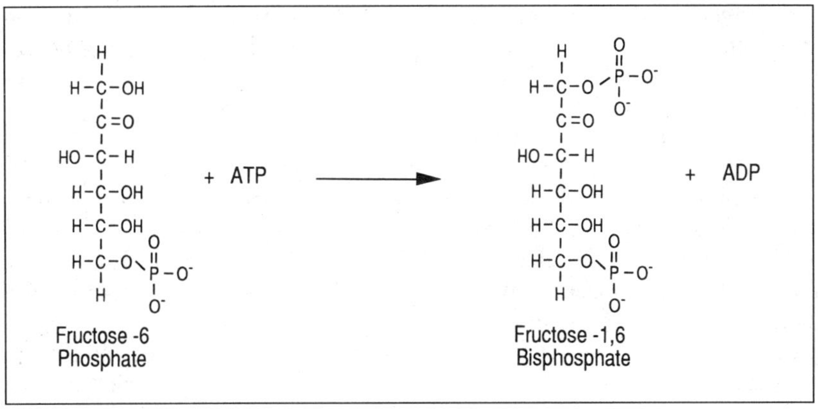

Figure 7-5. The reaction catalyzed by phosphofructokinase-1. This is another phosphorylation reaction generating fructose-1,6-bisphosphate, and is the major regulated step of glycolysis. Note how this reaction is also irreversible, as is the hexokinase reaction.

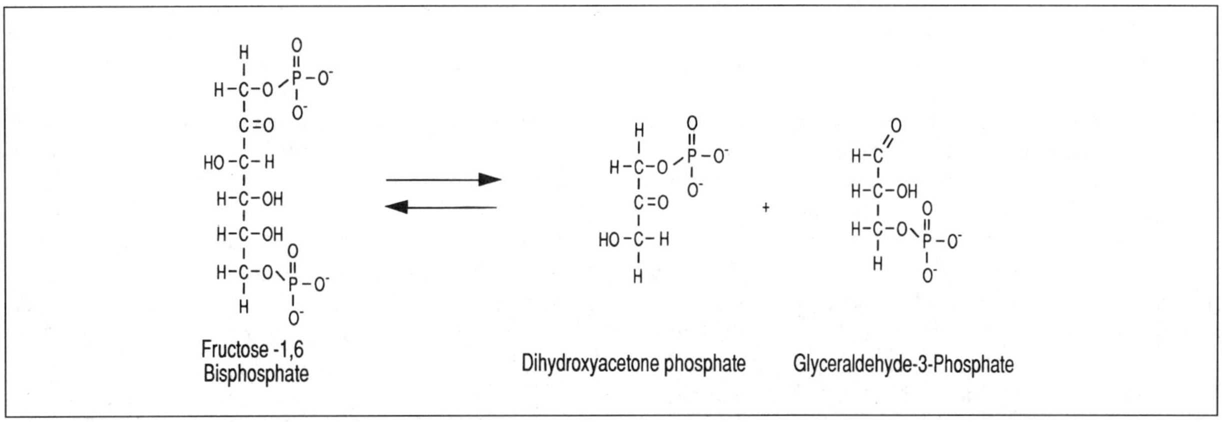

Figure 7-6. The reaction catalyzed by aldolase, in which fructose-1,6-bisphosphate is cleaved to form the isomers glyceraldehyde-3-phosphate and dihydroxyacetone-phosphate.

Glyceraldehyde-3-phosphate is on the mainstream of glycolysis, whereas dihydroxyacetone phosphate is not. A look at the structures of these two triose phosphates (see Figure 7-6) will show that isomerization is an easy matter, and that is indeed what happens. The dihydroxyacetone phosphate is isomerized to G3P, using the enzyme triose-phosphate isomerase, and we now have two molecules of G3P resulting from our split of doubly phosphorylated hexose (Figure 7-7).

Let us stop to reflect for a moment. We have described glycolysis as part of the fuel metabolism of the cell. Implied in such a concept is the end result that a net yield of usable chemical energy will result from any such series of transformations. At this point, we are far from that eventuality. In fact, we are in debt. We have used two molecules of ATP to perform the necessary phosphorylations. Instead of producing a net energy yield, we have produced a net deficit of two ATPs.

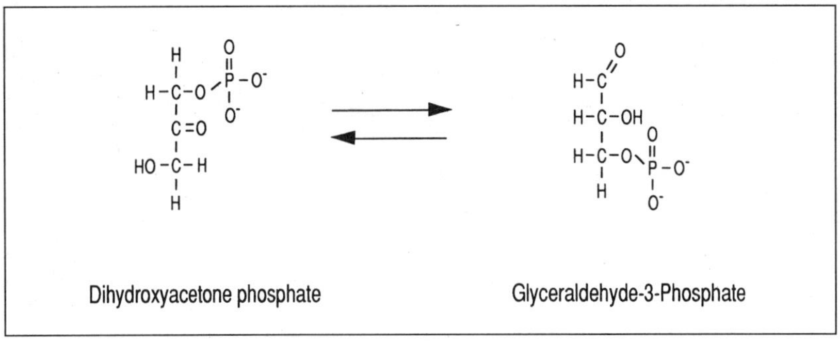

Figure 7-7. The isomerization of glyceraldehyde-3-phosphate and dihydroxyacetone-phosphate as catalyzed by triosephosphate isomerase.

Remember that, in the first stage of glycolysis, we phosphorylated glucose and rearranged its product, G6P, to F6P. In the next stage we added another phosphate to make fructose-1,6-bisphosphate and cleaved it into two triosephosphates that then entered the third stage as G3P.

We now enter the third stage of glycolysis and begin to turn toward a redress of the ATP deficit and to generate a surplus. Glyceraldehyde-3-phosphate is oxidized to 1,3-bisphosphoglycerate by the enzyme G3P dehydrogenase (Figure 7-8). This reaction requires inorganic phosphate and the molecule nicotinamide adenine dinucleotide (NAD^+). NAD^+ is derived from the vitamin niacin and is simply a biochemical electron carrier. It will alternate between its oxidized form (NAD^+) and its reduced form (NADH), depending on whether it is carrying electrons. The electrons carried by NADH are then donated to the mitochondrial electron transport chain to generate ATP via oxidative phosphorylation, which is discussed in more detail later in this chapter. The products of the glyceraldehyde-3-phosphate dehydrogenase reaction are NADH, H^+, and 1,3-bisphosphoglycerate. The aldehyde group of the G3P has been oxidized to form a high-energy phosphoanhydride (see Figure 7-8) in a reaction known as a substrate-level phosphorylation (oxygen is not involved). This type of anhydride, an acyl phosphate, has a very high standard free energy of hydrolysis and can, therefore, be used to react with ADP to produce 3-phosphoglycerate and a molecule of ATP (see Table 7-1 and Figure 7-9) in a reaction catalyzed by phosphoglycerate kinase.

Because these reactions have occurred on both halves of the original glucose, we have now produced two ATPs to balance out the initial investment of two ATPs in the earlier phosphorylation steps. Any further yield of ATP will represent a net gain.

The next reaction converts 3-phosphoglycerate to 2-phosphoglycerate in a Mg^{++}-dependent reaction catalyzed by phosphoglycerate mutase, as shown in Figure 7-10. This reaction sets the stage for the final generation of high-energy phosphate that occurs in glycolysis. This is a dehydration reaction that converts 2-phosphoglycerate to phosphoenolpyruvate. This reaction is catalyzed by the enzyme enolase and is shown in Figure 7-11. The loss of the water molecule from 2-phosphoglycerate causes a redistribution of energy within the product, phosphoenolpyruvate (PEP). The standard free energy change accompanying hydrolysis of the phosphate group of PEP is much greater than that for 2-phosphoglycerate because of the loss of a stabilizing resonance form (see Table 7-1).

The last step in glycolysis is the transfer of

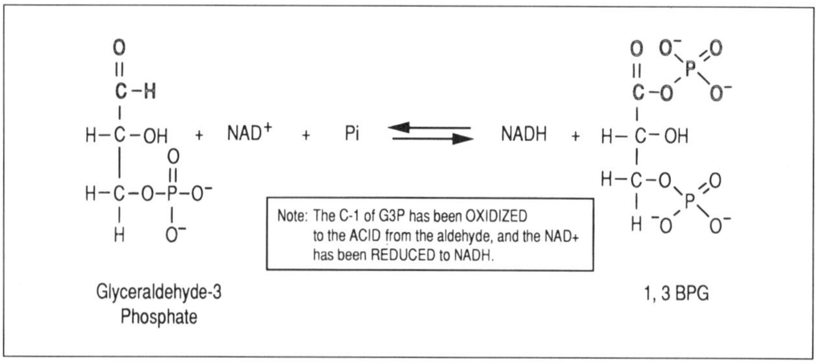

Figure 7-8. The oxidation of glyceraldehyde-3-phosphate to form 1,3-bisphosphoglycerate, as catalyzed by glyceraldehyde-3-phosphate dehydrogenase.

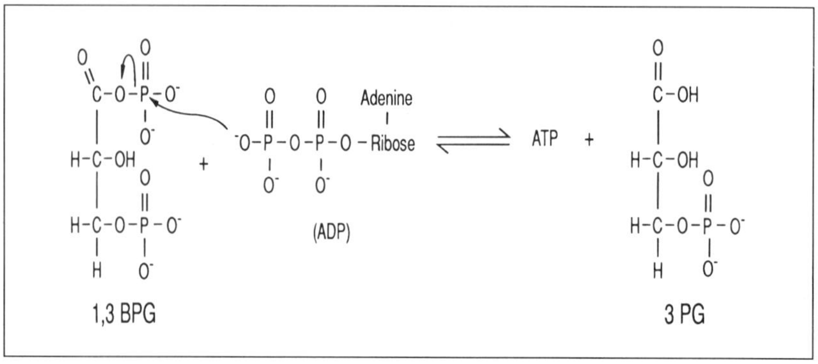

Figure 7-9. The reaction catalyzed by phosphoglycerate kinase, in which ATP is formed from 1,3-bisphosphoglycerate (BPG) and ADP. This is the first reaction in the glycolytic scheme to form ATP, and it is done through a substrate level phosphoryation reaction.

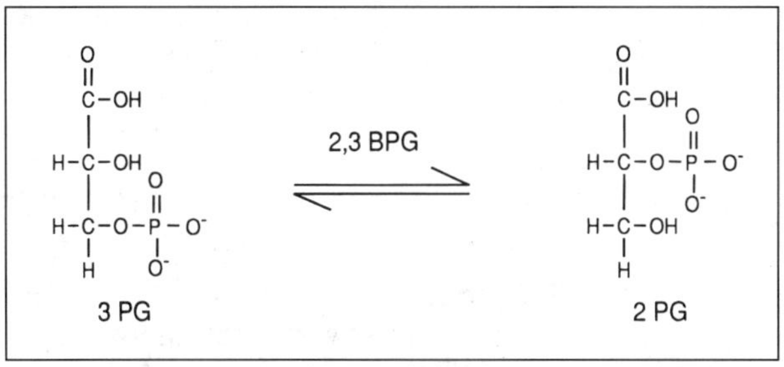

Figure 7-10. The isomerization reaction catalyzed by phosphoglycerate mutase, in which 2-phosphoglycerate is formed from 3-phosphoglycerate, with the requirement of 2,3-bisphosphoglycerate as a co-factor.

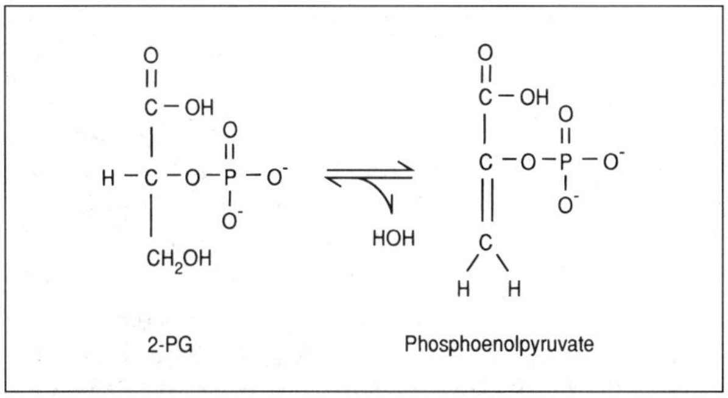

Figure 7-11. The dehydration of 2-phosphoglycerate, to form phosphoenolpyruvate, as catalyzed by enolase. Phosphoenolpyruvate contains a high-energy phosphate bond, as described in the text.

the phosphate group from PEP to ADP catalyzed by the enzyme pyruvate kinase in a reaction that requires both K^+ and either Mg^{++} or Mn^{++}. This reaction is shown in Figure 7-12.

This reaction is another example of a substrate level phosphorylation, which can proceed in the absence of oxygen. The products are pyruvate, in its enol form, and a molecule of ATP. This reaction has a large negative standard free energy change resulting in large part from the spontaneous conversion of the enol form of pyruvate into the keto form that predominates at neutral pH. This isomerization is also shown in Figure 7-12.

The pyruvate kinase step is a very important site of regulation as will be seen later. In addition, this reaction generates two more molecules of ATP because each of the two PEP molecules that arose from the original glucose generates a molecule of ATP. Now, finally, the ATP balance has become positive. Remember, we invested one ATP at the hexokinase reaction and another at the PFK-1 reaction. We then generated two ATP molecules at the phosphoglycerate kinase step and two at the pyruvate kinase step.

There is one final aspect of glycolysis that requires inclusion. The reader will remember the reaction whereby we oxidized G3P, adding a phosphate, to produce 1,3-bisphosphoglycerate. A necessary substrate for that reaction was NAD^+, and it was reduced to NADH + H^+. This reaction occurs in the cytosol, and the total amount of NAD^+ plus NADH in the cytosol remains fairly constant. If all of the cytoplasmic NAD^+ is converted to NADH, then glycolysis will stop because of a lack of substrate (NAD^+) for the G3P dehydrogenase step. If the flow of glucose to pyruvate is to continue, a means of regenerating NAD^+ must be found. When we consider the mitochondrion and the final steps in the conversion of pyruvate to CO_2 and water, it will become apparent how this is done in the intact, oxygenated cell. However, some cells do not have mitochondria (the red blood

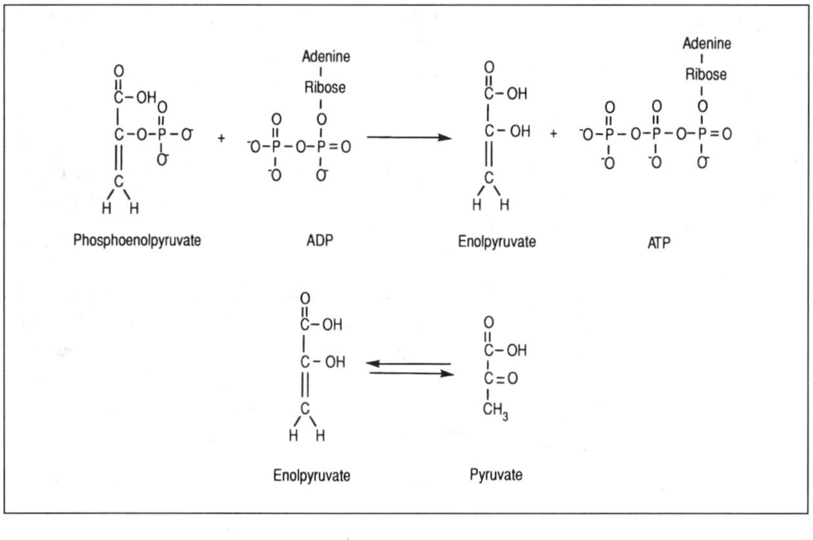

Figure 7-12. The reaction catalyzed by pyruvate kinase. This is the second reaction in glycolysis in which ATP is produced, and the other product of the reaction is pyruvate.

cell), and other cells are sometimes subjected to varying degrees of relative or absolute hypoxia, rendering these mitochondrial functions diminished or absent. Under these circumstances, the pyruvate is converted to lactate in the cytoplasm by the enzyme lactate dehydrogenase. This conversion requires NADH and produces NAD^+, and it is shown in Figure 7-13.

Lactate is essentially an end product. It can only enter a metabolic sequence by being reconverted to pyruvate. In states of excessive pyruvate, the conversion to lactate is favored, and this end product of glycolysis leaves the cell as such. When it does this, it leaves as lactic acid. Accumulation of lactic acid inside the cell can rapidly lead to intracellular acidosis, which impairs function and, ultimately, structure. On the other hand, when it leaves the cell, it places a burden on the acid-base buffering mechanism of the blood that must be dealt with. Rapid accumulation of lactic acid in the bloodstream is the principal reason for the extreme degrees of metabolic acidosis seen in hypoxic states.

This method of disposition of pyruvate with its accompanying regeneration of NAD^+ allows glycolysis to proceed when there is no mode of aerobic disposition of pyruvate or regeneration of NAD^+. Because it can proceed in the absence of oxygen, it is termed anaerobic glycolysis. It must be remembered that the energy yield of glycolysis alone is very small when compared to the total possible energy yield available from the aerobic cellular conversion of one molecule of glucose to CO_2 and H_2O. In anaerobic glycolysis, the production of two molecules of lactic acid from each molecule of glucose results in a net production of two molecules of ATP, or 14.6 kcal. This is far from the potential realization of 277 kilocalories of which an intact, fully oxygenated cell is capable. Thus, anaerobic glycolysis makes it possible for the cell to supply a small amount of net energy from glucose oxidation but it is, by comparison, an inefficient process. Although this process may be inherently low in its high-energy phosphate yield, it is nonetheless the mechanism that makes it possible for the most rapid generation of ATP when circumstances require a rapid formation of energy (i.e., in a 100-m sprint).

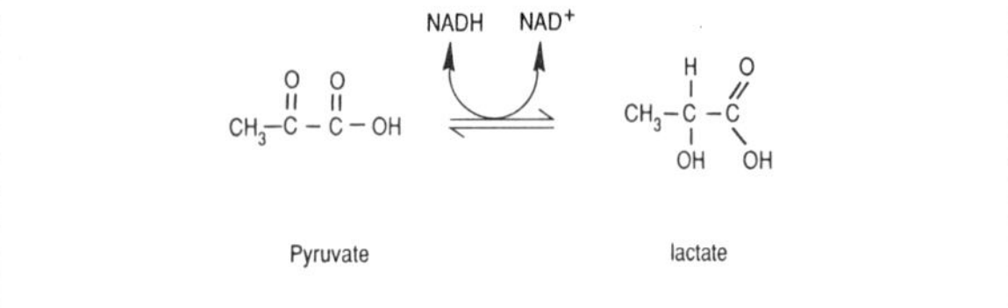

Figure 7-13. The reaction catalyzed by lactate dehydrogenase. This reaction is favored in the absence of oxygen and when NAD^+ levels are low.

Regulation of Glycolysis

The reactions catalyzed by hexokinase, PFK-1, and pyruvate kinase are irreversible and are key regulatory points. The irreversibility means that we will have to provide a different type of reaction to bypass this step when we are involved in gluconeogenesis, the process of synthesizing glucose from pyruvate. The regulatory functions of these enzymes are of very great importance. To maintain homeostasis, there must be a mechanism whereby passage of glucose through the glycolytic system is accelerated when energy supplies are low and inhibited when they are high. Thus, high ATP levels are, of course, indicators that energy supplies are high, and ATP inhibits PFK-1 activity by binding to an allosteric site and lowering the affinity of the enzyme for its other substrate, F6P. ATP also inhibits the activity of pyruvate kinase. When ATP is being used faster than it is made, the levels of ADP and AMP rise and act allosterically to relieve ATP inhibition. Inhibition of PFK-1 by ATP has another effect. Fructose-6-phosphate accumulates and, through the action of phosphohexoisomerase, produces elevated levels of G6P. The high levels of G6P produced inhibit hexokinase activity and further dampen the carbon flow through the glycolytic scheme. Thus, through an inhibition of the three-key regulated enzymes of glycolysis by high energy, flow through glycolysis can be virtually halted.

There is yet another important inhibitor of PFK-1: citrate. This ionized form of citric acid is a key intermediate in the aerobic oxidation of pyruvate and it, too, serves as an allosteric regulator of PFK-1. If flow through the glycolytic system is at such a rate that citrate concentrations rise, citrate will increase the inhibitory effect of ATP and further reduce the flow of glucose through glycolysis.

There is yet another significant allosteric regulator of PFK-1: fructose-2,6-bisphosphate. Fructose-2,6-bisphosphate is formed from F6P by the enzyme PFK-2 and is the most potent activator of PFK-1. PFK-2 will respond to hormonal signals, in particular glucagon and insulin. The concentration of fructose-2,6-bisphosphate in liver decreases in response to glucagon, the net result being a decreased activation of PFK-1. Because fructose-2,6-bisphosphate is the most potent activator of PFK-1, this action of glucagon will result in a reduced glycolytic flux, and an enhanced ability to synthesize glucose in the liver. These regulatory points will be discussed again later in the chapter, when the regulation of all pathways involved in carbohydrate metabolism is integrated.

Louis Pasteur noted during the 19th century that glucose consumption was markedly increased in yeast extracts in the absence of oxygen as compared to the presence of oxygen. This difference in oxygen consumption was called the *Pasteur effect*. Since Pasteur's time, this effect has been demonstrated also in bacterial and muscle systems. We can now understand the molecular basis for the Pasteur effect. Glycolysis produces ATP rapidly, but at a low rate (only two ATP per glucose molecule). Glucose metabolism in the presence of oxygen has the potential for generating 38 molecules of ATP per glucose molecule (see below). Because the cell wants to maintain a high level of ATP, glucose consumption will be greater in the absence of oxygen than in its presence because of the inefficient nature of ATP production under those conditions.

Summary

Glycolysis is the process whereby carbohydrate is converted to pyruvate (or lactate) and through which two molecules each of ATP and NADH are generated. The ATP produced can be used as energy, and the NADH generated can also give rise to energy through oxidative phosphorylation. The pyruvate produced can be used either for other biosynthetic pathways or can itself be further oxidized to carbon dioxide and water, generating substantial energy in the process. All carbohydrate, ingested in whatever form, is initially metabolized through the reactions of glycolysis. There are three irreversible steps in glycolysis, those catalyzed by hexokinase, PFK-1, and pyruvate kinase. These are the regulated steps of glycolysis, which will be discussed in more detail later in this chapter.

The Hexose-Monophosphate Shunt: An Alternative to Glycolysis

Overview

The purpose of the hexose-monophosphate (HMP) shunt pathway is to provide an alternative means of glucose oxidation, with the end products being reduced nicotinamide adenine dinucleotide phosphate (NADP) (NADPH) and the five-carbon sugar ribose. $NADP^+$ is a phosphorylated derivative of NAD^+, which is used primarily for oxidation-reduction reactions which occur in biosynthetic pathways. Ribose is required for the biosynthesis of nucleotides, which are necessary for the activation of vitamins, carbohydrates, and lipid groups, and are also the building blocks of the nucleic acids (DNA and RNA). In metabolism, NADPH is used as a source of reducing power for many biosynthetic pathways. Thus, glucose oxidation via the HMP shunt will allow a cell to prepare for biosynthesis during periods of rapid growth and division.

The Reactions of the HMP Shunt

The enzymes of the HMP shunt, which are located in the cytoplasm of all cells, can be divided into two groups. One group catalyzes reactions classified as oxidative reactions, and the other group catalyzes nonoxidative reactions. The oxidative reactions generate NADPH and ribulose-5-phosphate (Ru5P), an isomer of ribose-5-phosphate (R5P), starting with G6P. The nonoxidative reactions allow the conversion of Ru5P to both F6P and G3P, two intermediates of the glycolytic pathway. By use of these nonoxidative reactions, substrates in the HMP shunt and glycolysis can be linked.

Our discussion will begin with G6P (generated in glycolysis by the hexokinase step) and the oxidative reactions of the HMP shunt. There are two enzymes required for the oxidative reactions, G6P dehydrogenase and 6-phosphogluconate dehydrogenase. The first reaction, shown in Figure 7-14, is the conversion of G6P to 6-phosphogluconic acid. This reaction oxidizes carbon number 1 of G6P from an aldehyde to an acid group. This reaction also reduces $NADP^+$ to generate NADPH. The 6-phosphogluconic acid is then decarboxylated (losing carbon 1) and reduced at carbon 3, to form Ru5P and another molecule of NADPH (see Figure 7-14). These first two oxidative steps are irreversible, and the first oxidation step (that catalyzed by G6P dehydrogenase) represents the regulated step of the pathway. The enzyme is regulated by the ratio of $NADP^+$ to NADPH. When the levels of cytoplasmic $NADP^+$ are high, the enzyme is active (to increase cellular NADPH levels). If the ratio is low, then the enzyme is inactive. Additionally, the rate at which the gene for G6P dehydrogenase is transcribed is also regulated. NADPH is required for the biosynthesis of fatty acids. Under conditions in which the body is producing fatty acids over an extended period of time, the levels of G6P dehydrogenase within the cell will increase (by increased production of the mRNA coding for the enzyme) so that adequate amounts of NADPH will be available for the production of fatty acids [12,13].

Once the Ru5P has been produced by the oxidative steps of the HMP shunt pathway, it can be metabolized in a number of different ways, depending on the needs of the cell. The first case to consider is when the cell requires only NADPH,

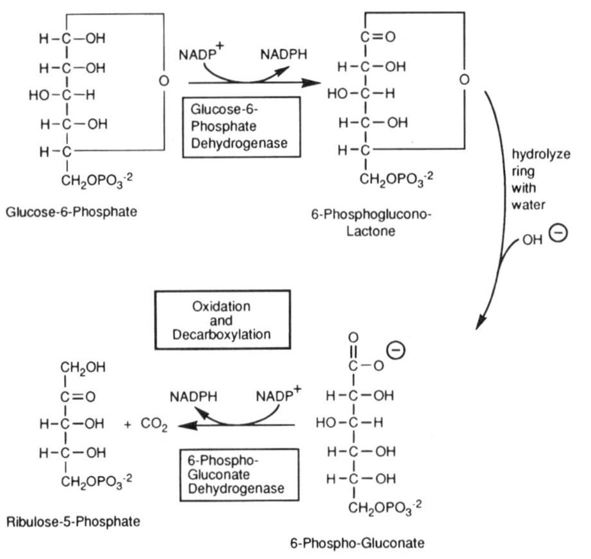

Figure 7-14. The oxidative reactions of the HMP shunt. The enzyme catalyzing the first reaction, glucose-6-phosphate dehydrogenase, is the regulated step of the pathway.

not R5P. A condition under which this might occur is when fatty acid biosynthesis (which requires NADPH) is occurring at a rapid rate, and DNA synthesis is not occurring. Under such conditions, the Ru5P produced will be used to regenerate glucose, which will yield a net equation of:

$$G6P + 12\ NADP^{+} \rightarrow 6\ CO_2 + 12\ NADPH + Pi.$$

This is shown schematically in Figure 7-15. (Pi represents inorganic phosphate.) For this to occur, a series of carbon transfers between sugars is initiated. The enzymes that accomplish this are *transketolase* and *transaldolase*. Transketolase, which requires the cofactor thiamine pyrophosphate (vitamin B1), transfers two carbon units between sugars, whereas transaldolase transfers three carbon units between sugars. Ru5P is not a substrate for either transketolase or transaldolase. For these enzymes to function, Ru5P is either isomerized to R5P or epimerized at the 3-carbon position to xylulose-5-phosphate (Xu5P) (see Figure 7-15). Both transketolase and transaldolase will accept carbon units from a ketose sugar (one with the carbonyl at the 2-carbon position), and both enzymes will donate these carbons to an aldose sugar (one with the carbonyl group at the 1-carbon position). Thus, transketolase will catalyze the movement of two carbons from Xu5P to R5P, forming G3P and sedoheptulose-7-phosphate (Se7P) (see Figure 7-15). Transaldolase will then use these sugars as substrates and transfer three carbons from Se7P to G3P, forming F6P and

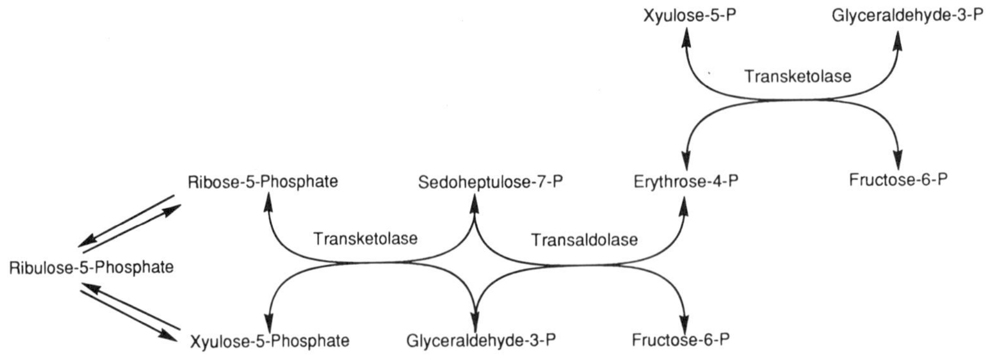

Figure 7-15. An outline of the reactions required to regenerate glucose-6-phosphate from ribulose-5-phosphate. The reactions terminate with either fructose-6-phosphate or glyceraldehyde-3-phosphate, both of which can be used to produce glucose-6-phosphate, as will be described later under gluconeogenesis.

erythrose-4-phosphate (E4P). Transketolase will then complete this series of reactions by transferring two carbons from another molecule of Xu5P to E4P to produce G3P and F6P. The net result of these nonoxidative steps is that three 5-carbon sugars have been converted to two 6-carbon sugars (F6P) and one 3-carbon sugar (G3P). Both F6P and G3P can be used to produce glucose via gluconeogenesis (see below). In this manner, the carbons from Ru5P can be used to regenerate G6P, so that the end result of this series of reactions is the generation of NADPH at the expense of glucose, with the formation of carbon dioxide.

As a result of its requirement for thiamine as a cofactor, transketolase activity can be used as a measure of the thiamine nutritional status of an individual. If thiamine levels are decreased, the addition of vitamin B1 to an extract of erythrocytes will potentiate transketolase activity in a test tube. Such a stimulation of transketolase activity would indicate a thiamine deficiency, whereas individuals without a deficiency would display the same levels of transketolase activity in the presence or absence of exogenous thiamine.

An alternative direction for the HMP shunt is when the cell requires equal amounts of R5P and NADPH. This might occur when a cell is preparing to divide, and it requires the R5P for DNA synthesis and the NADPH for amino acid and protein biosynthesis. *If this were the case, then only the oxidative steps of the HMP shunt will be used, and the overall equation of glucose oxidation can be given by*

$$G6P + 2\ NADP^+ \rightarrow CO_2 + Ru5P + 2\ NADPH$$

The Ru5P formed can be isomerized to R5P, which will be used for nucleotide biosynthesis to allow replication of the cellular DNA.

A third alternative direction for the HMP shunt is to direct the reactions to produce R5P without accumulating NADPH. This might occur when nucleotide biosynthesis is required in the absence of other biosynthetic pathways. *Under these conditions, only the nonoxidative steps of the pathway will be used.* The overall equation for this pathway is

$$5\ G6P + ATP \rightarrow 6\ R5P + ADP$$

To initiate this pathway, G6P is converted to F6P and G3P through steps of the glycolytic pathway. Transketolase will use both F6P and G3P as substrates to produce E4P and Xu5P (Figure 7-16). A second molecule of F6P can then react with E4P, in a reaction catalyzed by transaldolase, to produce G3P and Se7P. Transketolase can then use these substrates to produce Xu5P and R5P. In this manner, the oxidative steps are bypassed, and 5-carbon sugars are produced from 6-carbon sugars.

The final variation of this pathway represents the condition in which the cell is carrying out a large number of biosynthetic reactions, such as in periods of rapid growth or in repair of damaged tissues, such as repair after injury by burns. Under these conditions, the cell requires both NADPH and carbon skeletons for biosynthesis, which can be provided by pyruvate. Therefore, G6P will be metabolized through the oxidative portion of the shunt, which will produce the NADPH, and the Ru5P that is produced will be metabolized to pyruvate, which can act as a precursor for various metabolic pathways. These reactions are shown schematically in Figure 7-17. To do this, the reactions of both the HMP shunt and glycolysis will be utilized. The overall equation for this series of reactions is:

$$3\ G6P + 6\ NADP^+ + 5\ NAD^+ + 5\ Pi + 8\ ADP \rightarrow 5\ pyruvate + 3\ CO_2 + 6\ NADPH + 5\ NADH + 8\ ATP + 2\ H_2O + 8\ H^+$$

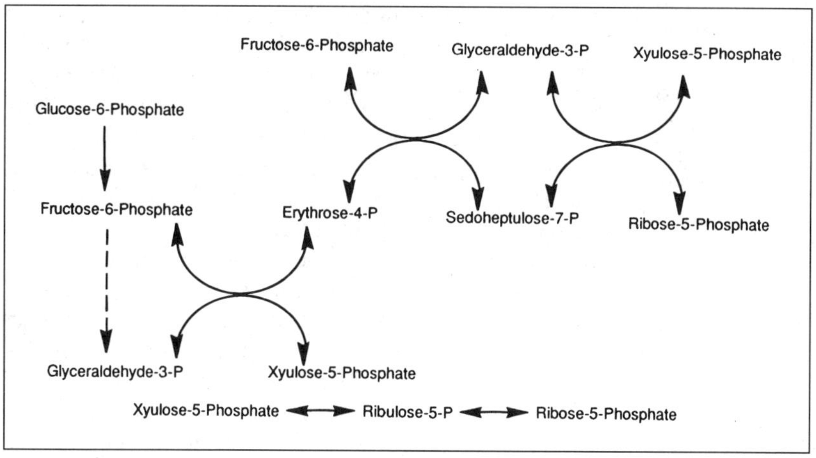

Figure 7-16. Summary of the reactions required when the oxidative steps of the HMP shunt are bypassed and ribose-5-phosphate is produced from glucose-6-phosphate.

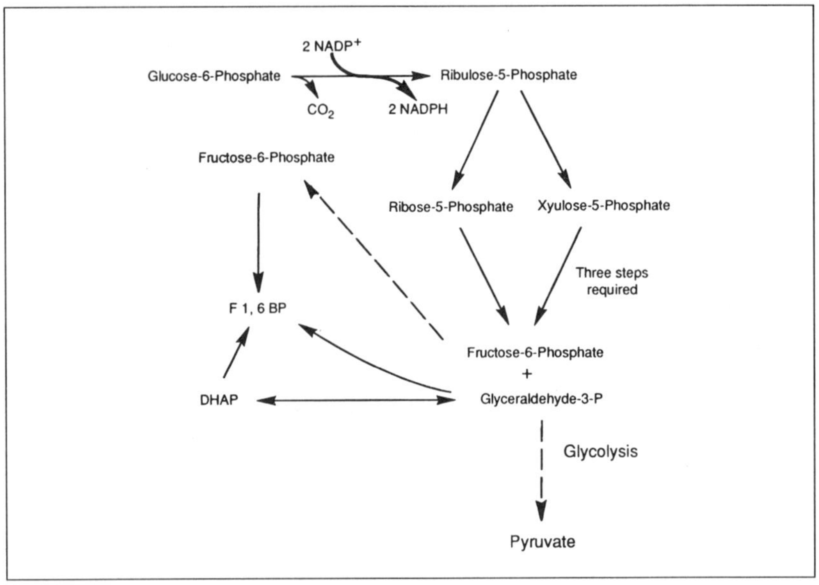

Figure 7-17. Summary of the reactions required to produce both NADPH and pyruvate, using a combination of the reactions of both the HMP shunt and glycolysis.

The NADH and ATP in this equation are derived from the glycolytic pathway, because the 5-carbon sugars are converted to pyruvate through a combination of the actions of transketolase, transaldolase, and glycolysis.

Lack of G6P dehydrogenase activity, which is thought to lead to protection against malaria, is found in persons of Mediterranean or African descent. Under normal conditions, this enzyme defect leads to no pathologic consequence, but in the presence of drugs that are also strong oxidizing agents, individuals with G6P dehydrogenase deficiency exhibit hemolytic anemia because NADPH is required to protect the red cell membrane from being oxidized by blood-borne agents. The agent in the membrane that actually does the protecting is the tripeptide glutathione. Glutathione consists of glutamyl-cysteinyl-glycine, and two molecules of glutathione can be oxidized, forming a disulfide linkage between the two cysteine residues, generating oxidized glutathione. Reduced glutathione, which is present in the membrane, will be preferentially oxidized by blood-borne oxidizing agents instead of proteins within the red cell membrane. This generates oxidized glutathione in the red cell membrane. Then, NADPH is required to regenerate reduced glutathione from the oxidized subunits. Thus, in the absence of the major enzyme that produces NADPH, the red cell membrane is more susceptible to oxidant attack, with the result being premature hemolysis and anemia.

Summary

The HMP shunt pathway provides for the production of NADPH and 5-carbon sugars that are required for nucleotide biosynthesis. The pathway can flow in a variety of directions, depending on the needs of the cell. To function, the pathway requires vitamin B1, and defects in the key regulatory step of the pathway (G6P dehydrogenase deficiency) can lead to hemolytic anemia under conditions of oxidative stress.

Fates of Pyruvate and ATP Yield

Overview

Pyruvate, which is formed from glycolysis, has a number of fates. One is conversion to lactate, which occurs in the absence of oxygen and allows glycolysis to continue at a rapid rate. A second potential fate is the conversion of pyruvate to acetyl-CoA, which is the precursor for fat and cholesterol biosynthesis as well as a substrate for energy production within the mitochondria. The conversion of pyruvate to acetyl-CoA is a key step, because once it has been taken the acetyl-CoA cannot be used as a substrate in the synthesis of glucose. The carbons of acetyl-CoA are committed to either fat or energy production. Because various tissues of the body (the brain in particular) require a constant supply of glucose, the loss of potential gluconeogenic precursors is not taken lightly. Thus, the conversion of pyruvate to acetyl-CoA is highly regulated and will only occur under conditions in which energy levels are high. A third potential fate of pyruvate are reactions known as the anaplerotic (refilling) reactions in which intermediates of the Krebs cycle, also called the tricarboxylic acid (TCA) cycle, are replenished by reactions using pyruvate as a substrate. TCA cycle intermediates are important precursors for amino acid metabolism and can become depleted during active periods of biosynthesis. The anaplerotic reactions allow the replenishment of the cycle intermediates, so that the cycle can be maintained at a constant rate.

Lactate Formation

We have already discussed the formation of lactate earlier in this chapter. Remember that lactate formation occurs to allow the cell to replenish the level of cytoplasmic NAD^+ that is required for the G3P dehydrogenase reaction to proceed. This will occur under conditions of strenuous exercise, in which muscle glycolysis is providing all the energy needed for muscle contraction under limiting amounts of oxygen. For glycolysis to continue at a rapid pace, the NAD^+ concentration needs to be held constant, and for this to occur lactate dehydrogenase will convert pyruvate to lactate. The lactate produced in the muscle is then sent to the liver via the bloodstream, where it is reconverted to glucose and sent back to the muscle for further use in glycolysis.

Formation of Acetyl-CoA: The Tricarboxylic Acid Cycle

Whereas glycolysis represents the most rapid means of producing ATP, only two molecules of ATP are produced per glucose molecule taken through the pathway. The pyruvate produced from glycolysis, however, can be totally oxidized to carbon dioxide and water, with a net yield of 38 ATP molecules per glucose molecule. Because this pathway requires oxygen, and many more steps, it is not as rapid as glycolysis, but it is the major energy-producing pathway of cells. The substrate for this energy-producing pathway is not pyruvate, but rather acetyl-CoA. Pyruvate is converted to acetyl-CoA in one step, as will be outlined further below. This major energy-producing pathway, the TCA cycle (also known as the Krebs cycle and the citric acid cycle), is found sequestered within the mitochondria. The cycle, shown in Figure 7-18, will oxidize acetyl-CoA to carbon dioxide with the generation of one high-energy bond (GTP), three molecules of NADH, and one molecule of another reduced electron carrier, flavin adenine dinucleotide ($FADH_2$). Energy can be obtained from reduced electron carriers by oxidative

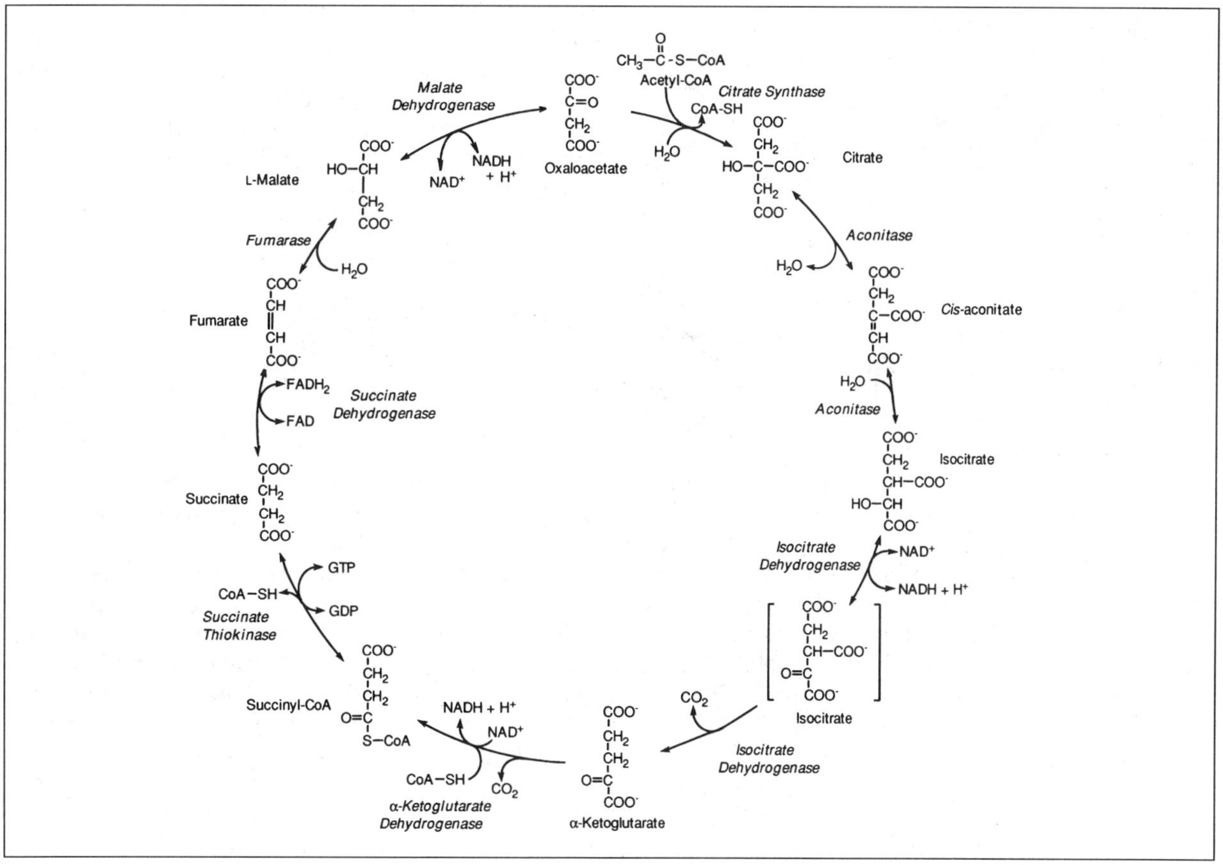

Figure 7-18. The TCA cycle, also known as the Krebs tricarboxylic acid cycle, and the citric acid cycle.

phosphorylation (see below), which requires oxygen. For each molecule of acetyl-CoA that is oxidized through the cycle, ultimately 12 molecules of ATP can be obtained.

The conversion of pyruvate into acetyl-CoA is a very important process. Once pyruvate has been converted into acetyl-CoA, the carbons of acetyl-CoA cannot be used for the net synthesis of glucose. They can be used, however, either for the synthesis of fatty acids for energy storage or for energy production by oxidation through the TCA cycle. The enzyme that converts pyruvate into acetyl-CoA is pyruvate dehydrogenase, a mitochondrial enzyme. Pyruvate, which is generated in the cytoplasm by glycolysis, must enter the mitochondria to be oxidized. The enzymes for both the oxidation of acetyl-CoA (via the TCA cycle) and fatty acids (which yields as a product acetyl-CoA) are found within the mitochondria. Upon oxidation of the acetyl-CoA by the TCA cycle, the potential energy from the oxidation is stored in two distinct electron carriers, NADH and $FADH_2$. These electrons are eventually donated to molecular oxygen to form water. The transfer of electrons to oxygen is an energetically favorable process, with the release of energy at distinct points along the transfer chain. The released energy is harvested and stored through the formation of ATP, in a set of reactions known collectively as oxidative phosphorylation.

The reaction catalyzed by pyruvate dehydrogenase is shown in Figure 7-19. The enzyme consists of three subunits—a decarboxylase, a transacetylase, and a dehydrogenase—and also requires five different co-factors; thiamine pyrophosphate (derived from vitamin B1), lipoic acid, NAD^+ (derived from niacin), $FADH_2$ (derived from riboflavin), and CoA (derived from phosphopantothenic acid). This complex reaction is also tightly regulated, so that when energy levels are high (as indicated by high levels of ATP, NADH, or acetyl-CoA), the reaction rate is decreased. Once acetyl-CoA is formed by this oxidative decarboxylation, it will then be oxidized by the TCA cycle (see Figure 7-18).

The major role of the TCA cycle is to oxidize acetyl-CoA to carbon dioxide. When this occurs, the eight electrons associated with the carbons in acetyl-CoA are lost and are transferred to the electron carriers NADH and $FADH_2$. Note that in the cycle there are three steps at which NADH is produced: the isocitrate dehydrogenase step, the α-ketoglutarate dehydrogenase step, and the malate dehydrogenase step. The $FADH_2$ is produced at the succinate dehydrogenase step. Also note that there are two reactions in which carbon dioxide is released. Those steps are the ones catalyzed by isocitrate dehydrogenase and α-ketoglutarate

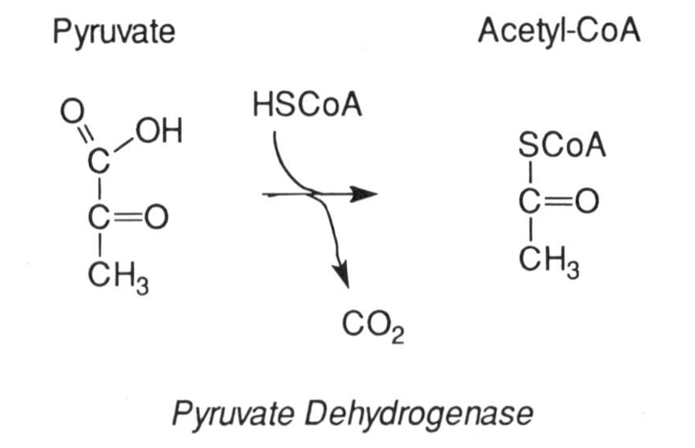

Figure 7-19. The reaction catalyzed by pyruvate dehydrogenase, in which acetyl-CoA is formed from pyruvate in an oxidative decarboxylation reaction.

dehydrogenase. The net reaction catalyzed by the TCA cycle is:

$$\text{Acetyl-CoA} + \text{GDP} + 3\ \text{NAD}^+ + \text{FAD} + \text{Pi} \rightarrow 2\ \text{CO}_2 + \text{GTP} + \text{CoA} + 3\ \text{NADH} + \text{FADH}_2$$

None of the cycle intermediates is created or lost by passage of acetyl-CoA through the cycle. Because of the loss of two molecules of carbon dioxide, there is no net synthesis of oxaloacetate by acetyl-CoA. Since oxaloacetate is the precursor required for gluconeogenesis (as is discussed in the next section), it follows that there can be no net synthesis of glucose from acetyl-CoA. As fatty acid degradation yields entirely acetyl-CoA, there is no net synthesis of glucose from fat, which has important implications for the management and nutritional care of trauma patients.

Oxidative Phosphorylation

The TCA cycle itself is not the pathway that produces large amounts of ATP. The energy obtained by the oxidations of the cycle are stored in the reduced electron carriers generated by the cycle. To gain energy from these carriers, these electrons are donated to specific enzymes within the inner mitochondrial membrane that have a higher affinity for the electrons than the carriers. Because of this higher affinity for the electrons, energy is released during the transfer as a more stable intermediate is formed. The ultimate electron acceptor is oxygen, which will become reduced to form water. As shown in Figure 7-20, the electron transfer chain consists of four complexes. Complex I will accept electrons from NADH. The electrons are passed between various carriers within complex I before transfer to coenzyme Q, which is a lipid soluble vitamin (ubiquinone) found within the mitochondrial membrane. Coenzyme Q ac-

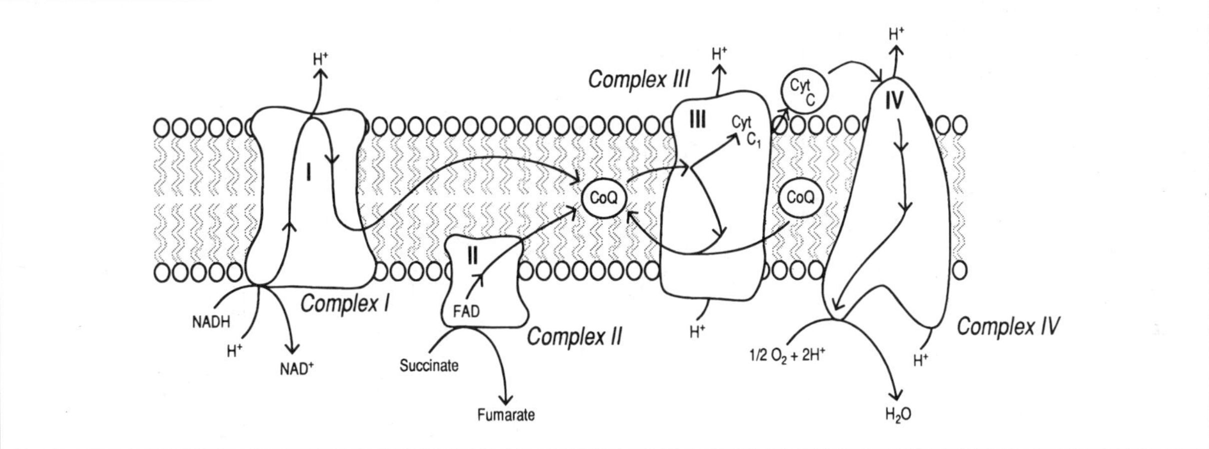

Figure 7-20. The mitochondrial electron transfer chain, with the four major complexes shown.

cepts electrons from both complex I and complex II (which accepts electrons from $FADH_2$) and will transfer them to complex III. At complex III the electrons are eventually shunted to cytochrome C, which donates the electrons to complex IV. Complex IV then accumulates electrons until sufficient electrons are available to reduce oxygen to water (four electrons for one molecule of oxygen).

The energy obtained by these favorable electron transfers is maintained by the establishment of a proton gradient across the inner mitochondrial membrane, with the matrix of the mitochondria having an alkaline pH as compared with the outside, and a net negative charge as compared with outside the membrane (diagramed in Figure 7-20 by the extrusion of protons across the membrane). As electrons flow along complexes I, III, and IV, protons are ejected from the matrix into the intermembrane space. Because the inner mitochondrial membrane is impermeable to protons, a proton motive force (PMF) is generated across the membrane. The PMF consists of two components, a ΔpH term, and a $\Delta\Psi$ term, which refers to the electrical difference across the membrane. As a result of this proton gradient being established across the membrane, the entry of protons into the mitochondria is an energetically favorable reaction, because the proton is traveling down its electrochemical gradient to enter the matrix. The synthesis of ATP is coupled to the inward flow of protons, as shown in Figure 7-21. The enzyme responsible for synthesizing ATP, the ATP synthase, contains a proton pore, through which protons can enter the matrix of the mitochondria. By traveling through this pore, the energy obtained by the inward movement of protons is coupled to ATP synthesis and net ATP is produced. The elucidation of the role of the proton gradient in energy production was the insight of Peter Mitchell, who was awarded the Nobel Prize in Medicine for this radical theory.

Phosphorylation (ATP synthesis) is normally coupled to respiration (oxygen consumption); if ATP synthesis is blocked and there is no route for the re-entry of protons into the matrix of the mitochondria, then respiration will cease. This is because it will shortly become very difficult for the electron transfer chain to eject protons because the magnitude of the proton gradient will be too great. Because it will become energetically unfavorable to eject protons in the face of a large gradient and proton ejection is coupled to electron flow, electron flow will stop, which will also stop oxygen consumption. Uncouplers are drugs that can uncouple oxygen consumption from ATP synthesis. These drugs work by allowing the membrane to become permeable to protons, thereby destroying the PMF. If the PMF is destroyed, ATP synthesis will not occur, although electron transport and oxygen consumption will actually increase in an attempt to regenerate the PMF.

What happens to the ATP that is produced within the mitochondria? The ATP can be exported to the cytoplasm through the adenine nucleotide translocase that will export ATP and bring in ADP. This ensures that there is an adequate supply of ADP within the mitochondria for continued ATP synthesis and that ATP can get out into the cytoplasm where it is needed for many of the reactions already discussed.

The Anaplerotic (Refilling) Reactions

In addition to being converted to either lactate or acetyl-CoA, pyruvate can also be used to regenerate intermediates of the TCA cycle. The TCA cycle

Figure 7-21. The mitochondrial ATP synthase, the enzyme that synthesizes ATP in response to a proton gradient.

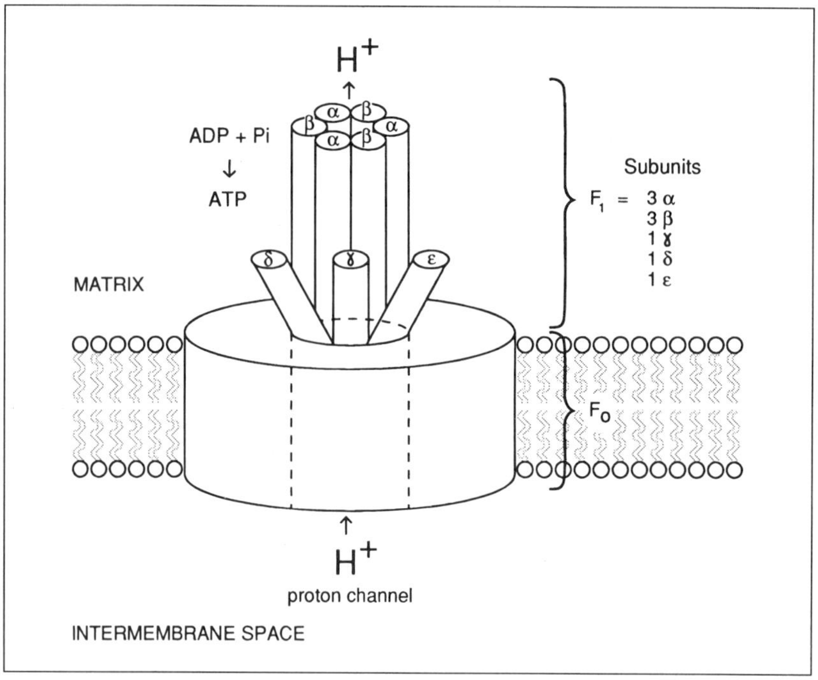

provides a central point in the metabolic scheme. Many amino acids can be synthesized from intermediates of the cycle, as can purines and pyrimidines. If this occurs at a high rate, then the TCA cycle will slow down as a result of a depletion of cycle intermediates. To prevent this from occurring, replenishing reactions (known as the anaplerotic reactions) are used to replace missing components from the cycle. These reactions are shown in Figure 7-22. Pyruvate carboxylase, a mitochondrial enzyme, will catalyze the formation of oxaloacetate through the carboxylation of pyruvate. Malic enzyme will also convert pyruvate into a TCA cycle intermediate, in this case malate. Malate can be converted to oxaloacetate in one step by malate dehydrogenase. This is important because oxaloacetate is a major precursor for glucose synthesis (gluconeogenesis), as will be discussed shortly. These anaplerotic reactions are controlled so that when the rate of operation of the TCA cycle is reduced because of a lack of intermediates, the anaplerotic reactions will be activated to replenish them. The net result is that the concentration of TCA cycle intermediates do not vary much with time and remain relatively constant.

Figure 7-22. The anaplerotic reactions, in which pyruvate can be used to replenish intermediates of the TCA cycle.

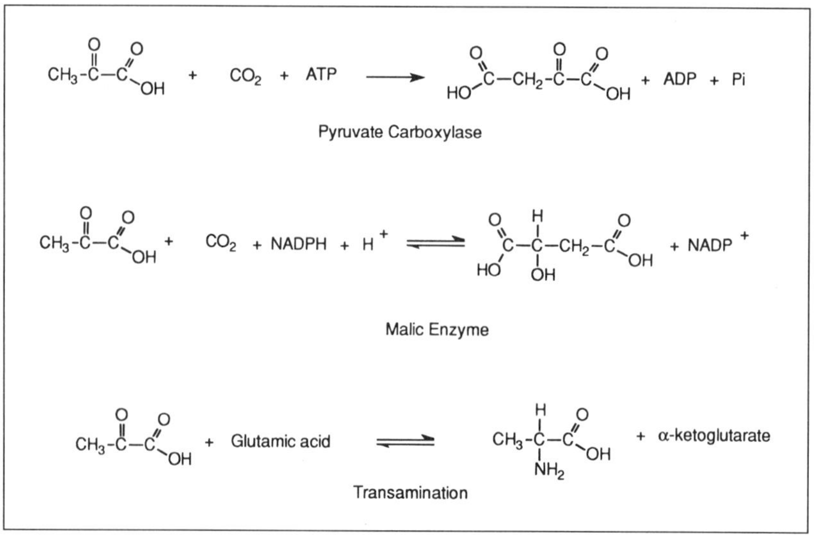

Formation of Alanine

A final potential fate for pyruvate is its ability to form alanine in one step via a transamination reaction (see Figure 7-22). This pathway is often used by muscle when amino acid degradation is occurring at a rapid rate. When amino acids are degraded, there is a problem with the proper disposal of the amino acid nitrogen. The muscle, under such conditions, will generate pyruvate via glycolysis and then transfer amino groups to pyruvate to form alanine, which will be released into the bloodstream for travel back to the liver. The liver will then remove the amino group and safely detoxify the ammonia produced via the urea cycle and use the carbons of pyruvate to regenerate glucose for use by other tissues.

Summary

Once formed, pyruvate can be converted to either lactate (anaerobic conditions, primarily in muscle), acetyl-CoA (for energy generation by the TCA cycle or energy storage via the synthesis of fatty acids), oxaloacetate (gluconeogenesis or to replenish depleted TCA cycle intermediates), malate (anaplerotic), or alanine (muscle protein degradation). The fate of pyruvate depends on the needs of the cell and tissues at the time of its formation. Clearly, pyruvate occupies a central role in metabolism, and its formation and utilization are carefully regulated.

Gluconeogenesis

Overview

Gluconeogenesis is the process of synthesizing glucose from pyruvate or lactate and is accomplished primarily in the liver when blood glucose levels are low. The steps of gluconeogenesis are similar to glycolysis, except for bypassing the three irreversible reactions of glycolysis. Four new reactions are required, two of which are anaplerotic reactions. Gluconeogenesis and glycolysis are reciprocally regulated; both pathways are not active at the same time.

Reactions of Gluconeogenesis

Glycolysis is the set of reactions whereby glucose, taken up from the bloodstream, is converted to pyruvate. Some tissues, such as the brain and nervous system, the kidney medulla, testes, erythrocytes, and embryonic tissues, require glucose from the blood as their sole or major fuel source. For this reason, the blood glucose level must be maintained within very narrow limits regardless of whether glucose or glucose precursors are obtained from the diet. Gluconeogenesis is the mechanism whereby the body generates glucose from nonhexose precursors when glucose is being used and not supplied from exogenous sources. Lactate and pyruvate are primary sources of carbons for gluconeogenesis; they are produced in the body by tissues undergoing glycolysis. Rapidly contracting muscles produce lactate and a lesser amount of pyruvate that diffuse into the circulating blood. The erythrocytes, having no mitochondria, also convert all the glucose they take up into lactate and release the excess lactate into the bloodstream. Thus, pyruvate and lactate from these tissues is available for glucose synthesis by the liver and kidney.

Disposing of lactate is made possible by converting it to pyruvate by the action of lactate dehydrogenase. It must be remembered that lactate itself is a metabolic dead end. For lactate to be metabolized, it must first be converted to pyruvate. Tissues with a high oxidative capacity, such as red muscle fibers and heart, do convert some lactate extracted from the circulating blood to pyruvate that is then further oxidized in mitochondria in the usual way.

Unfortunately, only part of the lactate in the circulating blood can be burned in this fashion. The remainder is reconverted to glucose. This is accomplished primarily by two organs, the liver and the kidney. The total amount of glucose formed from lactate in the kidney is about one-tenth that formed in the liver because of the much smaller mass of the kidneys. The process of converting circulating lactate and pyruvate to free glucose is known as gluconeogenesis. Thus, there is a cycle in which glucose is converted to lactate in skeletal muscles and erythrocytes by glycolysis, and the lactate produced is converted back to glucose in the liver and kidneys by the gluconeogenic pathway. This cycle is known as the Cori cycle, named for the Nobel Laureates who first described it, Carl F. Cori and Gerti T. Cori.

Gluconeogenesis, it must be emphasized, is not simply the reversal of glycolysis. Glycolysis is irreversible in that there are three reaction sequences that are essentially irreversible because of thermodynamic considerations. These irreversible reactions are those catalyzed by hexokinase, PFK-1, and pyruvate kinase. For glucose to be synthesized from lactate, pyruvate, or both, there must be reactions that bypass these irreversible glycolytic steps. At the outset the entry of lactate and pyruvate into gluconeogenesis must meet two essential requirements: (1) the pyruvate kinase reaction must be bypassed and (2) provision must be made for an abundant supply of cytosolic NADH + H^+, to reverse the G3P dehydrogenase reaction.

When lactate enters the cell for use as fuel or in gluconeogenesis, it is first converted to pyruvate by reversal of the lactate dehydrogenase reaction (see Figure 7-13). This yields pyruvate and NADH in the cytosol. The pyruvate then enters the mitochondria where it is converted to phosphoenolpyruvate by two steps that bypass the irreversible pyruvate kinase reaction. The first step is the pyruvate carboxylase reaction (already seen in Figure 7-22 as one of the anaplerotic reactions), which has two stages. First, CO_2 from bicarbonate is bound to a coenzyme, the vitamin biotin, which activates the CO_2. The energy for this activation is supplied by ATP. Next, the activated carboxyl group is transferred from carboxybiotin to pyruvate to form oxaloacetate, as shown in Figure 7-23. Biotin is a key vitamin required for virtually all carboxylation reactions in metabolism, and it is an essential nutrient that must be supplied in the diet. Mammals are not capable of synthesizing this vitamin.

The pyruvate carboxylase reaction is a key control point. The enzyme is totally inactive unless acetyl-CoA is bound to it. It must be emphasized that acetyl-CoA is not a reactant in this process, but it is necessary that it be bound to the enzyme for the enzyme to be activated. The allosteric activation of pyruvate carboxylase by acetyl-CoA works in the following manner. When there is a high level of acetyl-CoA in the mitochondria it is a signal for the need of more oxaloacetate. The activation of pyruvate carboxylase makes possible the formation of more oxaloacetate from pyruvate. Remember that the other enzyme that can use pyruvate as a substrate, pyruvate dehydrogenase, is inhibited by high levels of acetyl-CoA. Thus, when acetyl-CoA levels are high, pyruvate will preferentially form oxaloacetate instead of more acetyl-CoA. If there is also a surplus of ATP, the oxaloacetate produced from pyruvate will be diverted to gluconeogenesis. If, on the other hand, there is a deficiency of ATP, the oxaloacetate will enter the TCA cycle upon condensing with some of the abundant acetyl-CoA that turned on the pyruvate carboxylase reaction. The oxaloacetate that was derived originally from lactate is converted directly to PEP by a mitochondrial form of the enzyme PEP carboxykinase, as shown in Figure 7-24.

The mitochondrial form of PEP carboxykinase is encoded by nuclear genes separate from those for cytosolic PEP carboxykinase. This reaction requires the participation of guanosine triphosphate (GTP), and the end products are PEP, CO_2, and guanosine diphosphate (GDP). PEP is then transported out of the mitochondria and continues up the gluconeogenic path, using the reversible enzymes of glycolysis. This is the pathway of choice starting with lactate, because the reversal of the lactate dehydrogenase reaction in the cytoplasm to generate pyruvate yields sufficient cytoplasmic NADH for the reversal of the G3P dehydrogenase step in gluconeogenesis.

If pyruvate is the starting material, the path

Figure 7-23. The pyruvate carboxylase reaction, the first reaction required to bypass the irreversible reaction catalyzed by pyruvate kinase.

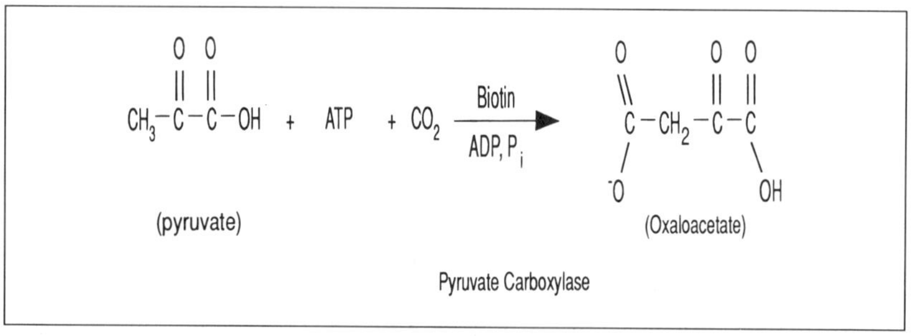

Figure 7-24. The reaction catalyzed by PEP carboxykinase, which is the second reaction required to bypass the pyruvate kinase step.

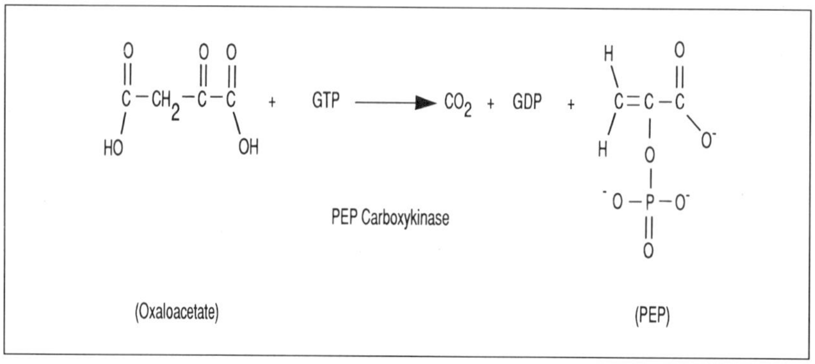

is somewhat different. Pyruvate taken up by the cell can be transported from the cytosol to the mitochondria as such. Once in the mitochondria, the pyruvate is converted to oxaloacetate by pyruvate carboxylase. Note, however, that there has been no opportunity to replenish the cytoplasmic NADH levels when pyruvate has been the starting material. The oxaloacetate that is formed in the mitochondria from pyruvate cannot diffuse out of it. The oxaloacetate can be converted to PEP, and the PEP transported into the cytoplasm, but this would not be productive because of the lack of NADH in the cytoplasm. To solve this problem, the oxaloacetate is converted to malate within the mitochondria using the NADH-linked mitochondrial malate dehydrogenase. The malate produced within the mitochondria can then diffuse across the mitochondrial membrane into the cytoplasm. The malate within the cytosol is reoxidized to oxaloacetate by an NAD^+-linked cytoplasmic malate dehydrogenase. This is the step that will regenerate NADH within the cytoplasm, which is needed for gluconeogenesis to continue. Cytoplasmic PEP carboxykinase, which is very similar to mitochondrial PEP carboxykinase, will then convert the cytoplasmic oxaloacetate to PEP, with the requirement of GTP. Carbon dioxide and GDP are also formed in the course of this reaction.

Gluconeogenesis then continues by using the reversible glycolytic reactions. This can take the sequence up to fructose-1,6-bisphosphate. The next step in the glycolytic sequence which must be bypassed is that catalyzed by PFK-1. The generation of F6P from fructose-1,6-bisphosphate is catalyzed by an Mg^{2+}-dependent fructose-1,6-bisphosphatase that yields F6P and Pi. This is also a regulated enzyme, and its regulation is reciprocal to that of PFK-1. The activators of PFK-1 inhibit fructose-1,6-bisphosphatase, whereas the inhibitors of PFK-1 activate the phosphatase. This type of regulation ensures that both pathways will not be active at the same time and prevents the occurrence of futile cycles. The final irreversible step, at hexokinase, is circumvented by a microsomal enzyme, glucose-6-phosphatase. This enzyme hydrolyzes the phosphate at carbon 6 to produce free glucose and Pi. Keep in mind that only liver and kidney possess this last enzyme. Accordingly, only liver and kidney are capable of producing free glucose from lactate and pyruvate.

It is worthy of note that amino acids are also capable of serving as substrates for gluconeogenesis. Only leucine and lysine are totally unable to furnish carbon for net glucose synthesis. Of the others alanine and glutamate are quantitatively the most important. Both of these amino acids must have their amino groups removed by transamination before entering into gluconeogenesis. Alanine becomes pyruvate (see Figure 7-22) and follows the pathway just discussed. Glutamate becomes α-ketoglutarate and enters the citric acid cycle. Even-numbered fatty acids cannot serve as substrates for the net synthesis of glucose. The oxidation of such fatty acids produces acetyl-CoA as an end product, and for every molecule of acetyl-CoA that enters the TCA cycle, two molecules of CO_2 are produced. Thus, the net synthesis of glucose cannot occur from the oxidation of fatty acids. When fat is mobilized from lipid depots by the action of triacylglycerol lipase, glycerol is released into the circulation as well as fatty acids. The glycerol can be used in gluconeogenesis because it can be phosphorylated by glycerol kinase (only in the liver), and the resulting glycerol-3-phosphate is oxidized to dihydroxyacetone phosphate. Triosephosphate isomerase converts this substance to G3P, which can be oxidized by glycolysis or used as a precursor for glucose synthesis through the pathway of gluconeogenesis.

Summary

To produce glucose from other metabolic intermediates, the three irreversible steps of glycolysis need to be bypassed. There are four enzymes required to do this. Pyruvate carboxylase and PEP carboxykinase are used to bypass the pyruvate kinase step, fructose-1,6-bisphosphatase is used to bypass the PFK-1 step, and G6P is used to bypass the hexokinase step. The other seven steps of glycolysis are reversible reactions, and those enzymes are also used by the gluconeogenic pathway. A rate-limiting factor for glucose synthesis is the availability of NADH within the cytoplasm, such that 1,3-bisphosphoglycerate can be converted into G3P. The NADH is provided either by cytosolic lactate dehydrogenase (if lactate is the gluconeogenic precursor) or cytosolic malate dehydrogenase (if pyruvate is the gluconeogenic precursor). As long as adequate substrate and NADH are available, the gluconeogenic pathway will be active when the glycolytic pathway is inhibited.

Glycogen Metabolism

Overview

Reflect for a moment on the extraordinary flexibility of the fuel economy of human beings. We can meet our energy requirements by the usual three meals a day, by frequent small snacks, or by no food intake at all, and often for long periods of time. We are capable of meeting wide ranges of demand for energy. We are capable of going rapidly from complete rest to maximal physical exertion with the fuel supply seldom limiting. Glycogen is the fuel depot that is first called on when fuel demands of any sort arise. There may be a need for free glucose to enter the bloodstream to maintain its level when there is no exogenous intake. The fuel depot that meets this need is liver glycogen. There also may be a need for extremely rapid generation of ATP in muscles when they are called on to increase abruptly their rate of activity by 100-fold or 1000-fold. The fuel supply to meet this need is muscle glycogen. The manner in which glycogen is produced and degraded and how these pathways are regulated are the main topics to be discussed in this section.

What Is Glycogen?

Glycogen, the storage form of glucose that can be readily mobilized, is a high molecular weight polymer of glucose arranged in linear arrays, connected to each other to form a branching system of glucose residues. These glucose residues in chains are linked by α-1,4-glycosidic bonds. The branches that are necessary are created by α-1,6-glycosidic bonds and they occur, on the average, about once in 10 residues. This structure is shown in Figure 7-25. Glycogen is a storage polysaccharide, and it is deposited into the cytosol of cells as granules with diameters ranging from 100 to 400 angstroms. These granules contain not only the glycogen itself but the enzymes that carry out its synthesis and degradation and some of the enzymes that regulate these reactions.

Reactions of Glycogen Synthesis

Glucose-6-phosphate is the starting point for the synthesis of glycogen. Glucose-6-phosphate can be derived from free glucose in the liver by action of the enzymes hexokinase or glucokinase. In muscle, the enzyme involved is hexokinase. The formation of G6P in the liver from glucose ingested during a meal, however, takes a more roundabout path to glycogen. It is first taken up by erythrocytes in the bloodstream and converted to lactate glycolytically. This lactate is then released by the red cells and taken up by the liver and converted to G6P through gluconeogenesis.

We have previously alluded to the fact that G6P can be degraded by glycolysis, can enter into the hexose monophosphate shunt or can be converted into free glucose in liver and kidney by the action of glucose-6-phosphatase. Entry into glycogen synthesis is yet another possible fate for G6P. When glycogen stores are low and glucose is available, G6P is diverted into restoration of glycogen stores. The first step is a conversion of G6P to glucose-1-phosphate (G1P) through the action of phosphoglucomutase, a reversible reaction.

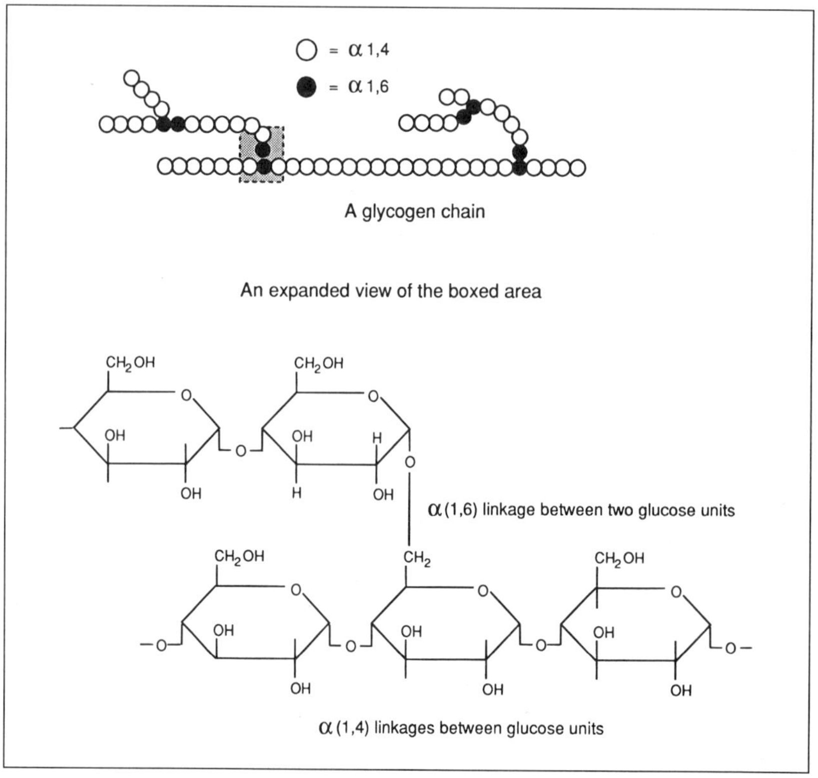

Figure 7-25. The structure of glycogen, consisting of glucose moieties linked in either of two configurations, (α-1,4) and (α-1,6).

Glucose-1-phosphate then reacts with uridine triphosphate to form an activated form of glucose, uridine diphosphate glucose (UDP-glucose). The enzyme that catalyzes this reaction is UDP-glucose pyrophosphorylase and is shown in Figure 7-26. This reaction is readily reversible but is pushed in the direction of the formation of UDP-glucose by the action of an inorganic pyrophosphatase that rapidly hydrolyzes the pyrophosphate formed, preventing reversal of the foregoing reaction. This reaction introduces us to a key mechanism for activation of many different sugars in the cell, i.e., by conversion to a UDP derivative according to the general reaction

Sugar-phosphate + UTP → UDP-Sugar + pyrophosphate

Once UDP-glucose has been formed, the activated glucosyl unit is transferred to the hydroxyl group at a C-4 terminus of glycogen to form an α-1,4-glycosidic linkage. This reaction is catalyzed by the enzyme glycogen synthase and is shown in Figure 7-27. Glycogen synthase requires, as a primer, an α-1-4-polyglucose chain or branch having at least four glucose residues.

After a number of glucosyl residues are joined in α-1,4 linkage by glycogen synthase, a branch is created by the breaking of an α-1,4 link and the formation of an α-1,6 link. This branching enzyme, glycosyl-4:6-transferase, catalyzes the transfer of a segment of a glycogen chain onto the C-6 hydroxyl of a neighboring chain, as shown in Figure 7-28. The enzyme moves a block of seven α-1,4-residues from a chain of at least 11 residues in

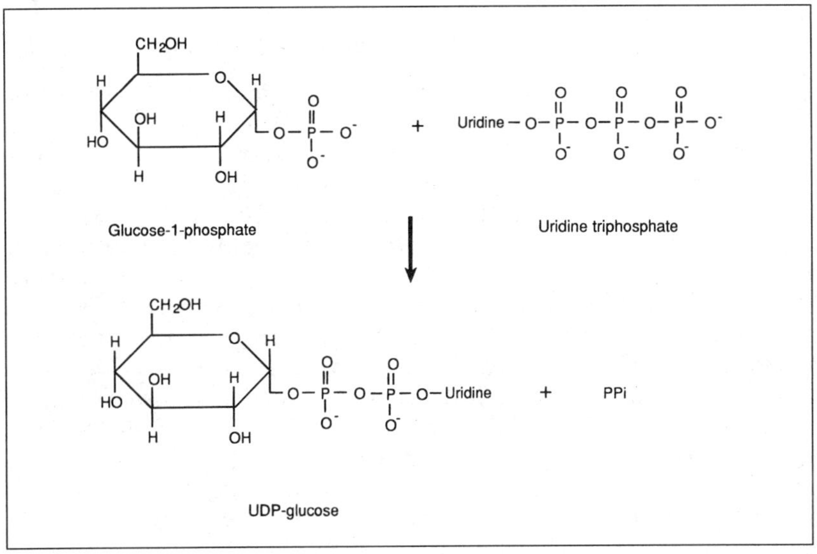

Figure 7-26. The synthesis of UDP-glucose, as catalyzed by UDP-glucose pyrophosphorylase. This activated glucose group is then used to add to an existing glycogen chain.

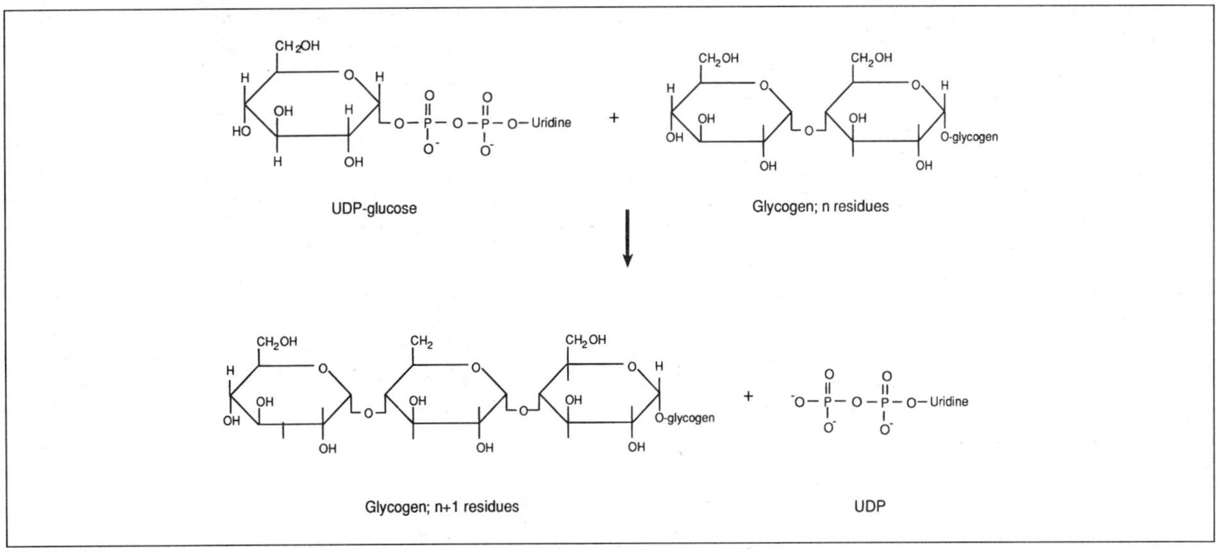

Figure 7-27. The reaction catalyzed by glycogen synthase.

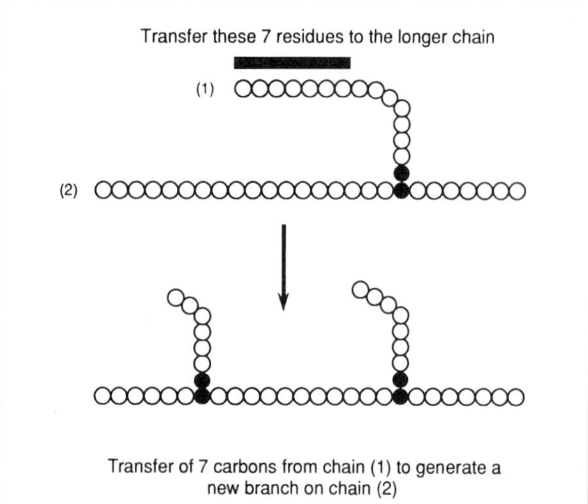

Figure 7-28. The activity of the branching enzyme (glycosyl-4,6-transferase), in which new branch points are created on an existing glycogen chain.

length and transfers it to another segment of the glycogen chain at a point at least four residues removed from the nearest branch, as shown in Figure 7-28.

Branching is important because it increases the solubility of glycogen and creates a large number of nonreducing terminal residues. It is from these nonreducing ends that glycogen is elongated as above. It is also from these nonreducing ends that glucose may be mobilized by the action of glycogen phosphorylase. The more branches there are, the larger the number of nonreducing terminal residues that are the sites of addition of glycosyl moieties. Thus, the branching enzyme increases the potential rate of both glycogen synthesis and glycogen degradation.

Several points about glycogen in the total body economy need to be made here. First, there is an energy cost for laying down glycogen. Because of the need for UTP to activate glucose as UDP-glucose, there is an expenditure of two high-energy phosphate bonds for every glucosyl moiety converted to glycogen. Thus, glycogen is formed in times of plentiful supply of exogenous fuel in the form of food. In the well-fed state the concentration of glycogen in the liver is higher than in muscle. The maximum concentration of glycogen in the liver is in the neighborhood of 400 mmol of glucosyl residues (65 g dry weight) per kilogram. Considering that the liver of the 70-kg man weighs about 1.6 kg, the total liver store of glycogen is 0.6 mol of glucosyl residues. Glycogen concentration in muscle ranges widely; usually it is about 85 mmol per kilogram of muscle tissue. After an hour or two of heavy work, the muscle content of glycogen can fall to as low as 1 mmol per kilogram. After muscle has been depleted in this fashion, several subsequent days of a high-carbohydrate diet can raise the level to as high as 300 mmol of glucosyl residues per kilogram of muscle. Long-distance runners have discovered this fact independently, and part of the routine preparation for a marathon race is several days of high-carbohydrate feeding immediately preceding the contest. In the ordinary state of things, however, the 70-kg man with 28 kg of skeletal muscle will have 2.4 mol of glucosyl residues as glycogen in muscle. The preceding statements underline the fact that glycogen synthesis, and as we shall see later, glycogen breakdown, are controlled processes. The major site of regulation of glycogen synthesis is the reaction catalyzed by glycogen synthase.

Enzymes of Glycogen Degradation

In the breakdown of glycogen, the main reaction is the phosphorolysis of the α-1,4-glucosidic bonds, by Pi, to form G1P. This primary reaction, which is the main site of control of glycogen breakdown, cleaves the terminal α-1,4-glucosidic bond at the nonreducing end of a glycogen chain to produce one molecule of G1P and a glycogen chain shortened by one residue. In vitro, this reaction is freely reversible, and, at equilibrium, the ratio of Pi to G1P is about 3:5. In vivo, the concentration of Pi is about 30-fold greater than the concentration of G1P; therefore, the reaction always proceeds in the direction of G1P. Although the Coris were able to demonstrate synthesis of glycogen by simple reversibility of the phosphorylase reaction in vitro, such a synthetic pathway does not take place in the intact body. Two other bits of information emphasize the fact that the phosphorolysis reaction, in vivo, must proceed in the direction of glycogen degradation. Hormones, to be discussed later, that lead to an increase in phosphorylase activity always elicit glycogen breakdown, not synthesis, and patients with McArdle's disease, who lack muscle phosphorylase entirely, are able to synthesize muscle glycogen.

Glucose residues can be successively removed by phosphorolysis in the manner just described. This proceeds until the reaction approaches a branch point in the glycogen residue. Phosphorolysis will only attack α-1,4-bonds that are at least four residues removed from an α-1,6-branch. If there is no debranching activity, glycogen will be completely sheared by phosphorylase to four residue stubs, and the product is called limit dextrin. For further degradation to continue, a second enzyme, amylo-1,6-glucosidase, catalyzes two successive reactions. First, it acts as a glucosyl transferase reminiscent of the branching enzyme that functions during glycogen synthesis. This enzyme transfers three glucosyl residues from a branch onto a chain terminus to lengthen it. When this enzyme acts on limit dextrin, for example, it will remove three residues of the four-residue stub and add it to another four-residue stub. The second stub is now seven residues long and can be attacked again by phosphorylase. The single residue remaining on carbon 6 at the branch is now hydrolyzed to yield free glucose, not G1P. This enzyme, then, has removed the single-branch residue to expose another straight chain of α-1,4-linked residues down to the next branch, so that phosphorylase can act once again. This action of the debranching enzyme is shown in Figure 7-29. The sequence of glycogen degradation by the action of glycogen phosphorylase and amylo-1,6-glucosidase acting in concert produces a continuous stripping of glucosyl residues. Those produced by phosphorylase are in the form of G1P, and those released by the glucosidase are as free glucose. The degree of branching is such that 11 to 14 molecules of G1P are formed for each molecule of free glucose released. The G1P is converted to G6P by the action of phosphoglucomutase, at no energy cost. The other 10% or so of glucosyl moieties that arose from cleavage at branch points to produce free glucose must be phosphorylated and will cost a molecule of ATP for each free glucose converted to G6P.

It is worth noting, at this point, that two co-factors are necessary for these reactions to take place. Pyridoxal phosphate (vitamin B6) is an essential co-factor in the glycogen phosphorylase reaction; its phosphate group acts as a general acid catalyst, promoting attack by Pi on a glycosidic bond. The enzyme phosphoglucomutase requires glucose-1,6-bisphosphate as a co-factor.

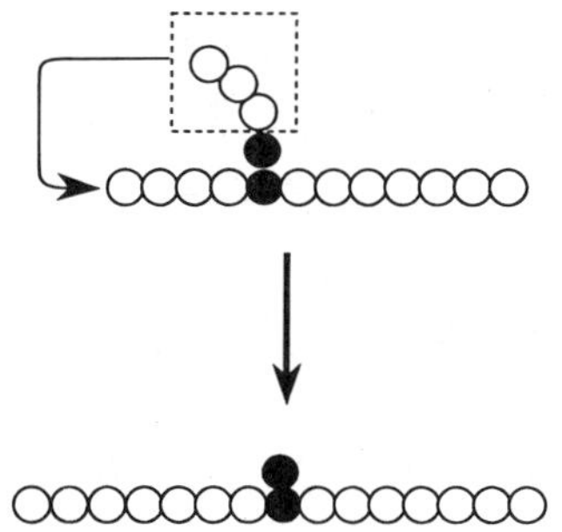

Figure 7-29. The activity of the debranching enzyme (amylo-1,6-glucosidase), which catalyzes two separate reactions, as described in the text.

In any event, the G6P produced by glycogen degradation is now available to the cellular engine. In muscle, this is used to provide a quick burst of energy via glycolysis for sudden activity before sufficient oxygen is available for the aerobic generation of ATP. In liver and kidney, the enzyme glucose-6-phosphatase can produce free glucose to bolster the blood glucose level in times of fasting.

Regulation of Glycogen Metabolism and Hormonal Control of Glycogen Degradation

The processes of synthesis and degradation of glycogen must be tightly and smoothly regulated to meet the demands of body economy. Glycogen must be laid down when the glucose supply is plentiful, such as during absorption from a meal, and when demands for energy are low. When a cell has laid down the maximum amount of glycogen appropriate to its structure and function, the process must be shut off. On the other hand, both muscle and liver must be able to respond to the demands for quick energy, in the case of muscle, or free glucose supply, in the case of liver, for regulation of blood glucose levels. Any stimulus that initiates glycogen synthesis must be able to shut off glycogen degradation at the same time, or a futile cycle, wastefully expending ATP, will be set in motion. The main control points for this regulation are the enzymes glycogen synthase and glycogen phosphorylase, described previously. The changes in activity of these two enzymes are affected allosterically and also by hormonal action. For the most part, these changes in activity of these two enzymes result from their existence in both active and inactive conformations. For example, phosphorylase-a is the active conformation of phosphorylase, and phosphorylase-b is the inactive form of phosphorylase.

Let us first review the mechanism whereby a hormonal stimulus results in conformational changes in these two enzymes. When epinephrine is released into the bloodstream by the adrenal gland when an animal is suddenly confronted by a situation that requires vigorous muscular activity, it binds to the muscle cell membranes and sets in motion a complex set of events that results in the phosphorylation of serine residues on both of these enzymes. This process activates muscle phosphorylase by means of a reaction cascade that involves cyclic AMP (cAMP) and provides a high degree of amplification of the epinephrine signal.

The cascade for the activation of phosphorylase is shown in Figure 7-30.

The binding of epinephrine to the plasma membrane of a muscle cell activates the enzyme adenylate cyclase. This enzyme catalyzes an intramolecular rearrangement of ATP to produce cAMP and pyrophosphate, as shown in Figure 7-31. Cyclic AMP then binds with a cAMP-dependent protein kinase. This enzyme catalyzes an ATP-dependent phosphorylation of phosphorylase-b kinase, which is the enzyme that will activate phosphorylase-b and convert it to phosphorylase-a. This phosphorylase-b kinase is in a relatively inactive form but, by the process of being phosphorylated in this ATP-dependent reaction, it becomes the active form of phosphorylase-b kinase (see Figure 7-30). It must be remembered that phosphorylase itself exists in two forms. Phosphorylase-b is the less active form, and it is converted by the now active phosphorylase-b kinase in another ATP-dependent reaction to the phosphorylated, active phosphorylase-a. This fully active phosphorylase-a now catalyzes the degradation of glycogen by acting at the 1,4-bonds of glycogen as described previously.

Once this cascade is turned on by epinephrine, how is it turned off when the epinephrine stimulus disappears? When the epinephrine stimulus is removed, adenylate cyclase is no longer activated, and the formation of cAMP shuts down. The cAMP

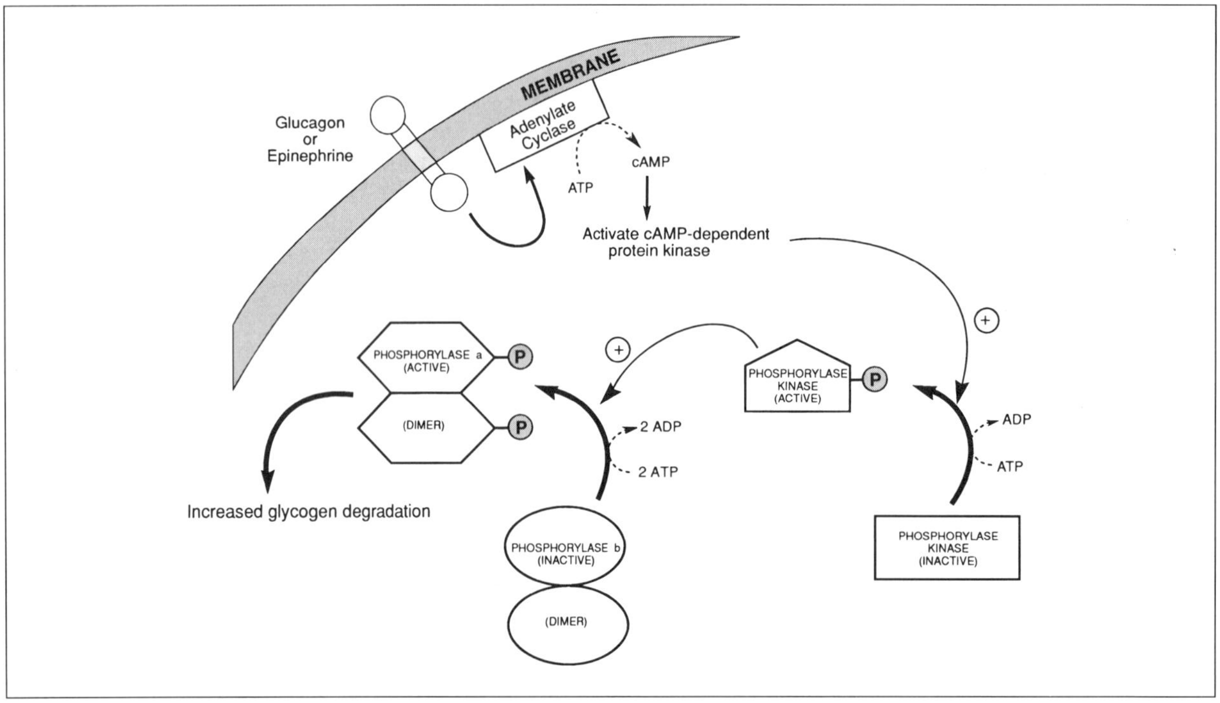

Figure 7-30. The cAMP cascade, in which a hormonal signal triggers the synthesis of cAMP, which in turn activates a protein kinase, which in turn activates phosphorylase-b kinase, which in turn phosphorylates and activates phosphorylase-b, converting it to phosphorylase-a, which enables glycogen degradation to occur.

Figure 7-31. The reaction catalyzed by adenylate cyclase, in which ATP is used to form cAMP.

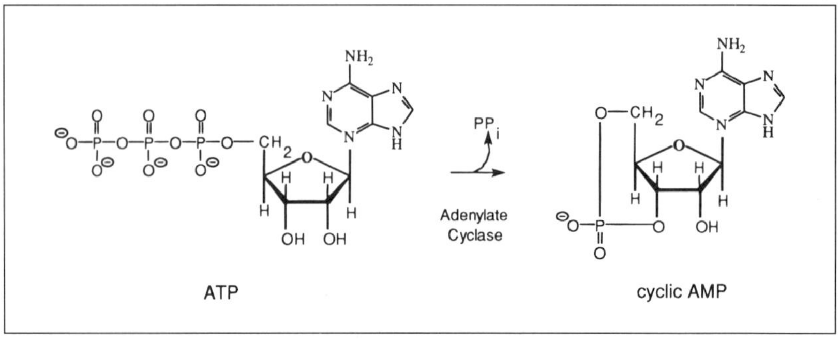

already formed is hydrolyzed by cAMP phosphodiesterase to produce ordinary 5′-AMP. As the intracellular concentration of cAMP falls, the phosphorylase-b kinase loses its phosphate (see below) and is inactivated. Phosphorylase-a also loses its phosphate, and the less active form of phosphorylase, phosphorylase-b, is now predominant.

The phosphate group is removed from these enzymes by a class of enzymes known as phosphatases, which are inactivated by the binding of epinephrine to the plasma membrane of the muscle cell. When the epinephrine stimulus is complete, phosphorylase kinase phosphatase is activated and dephosphorylates the activated, phosphorylated, phosphorylase kinase. In addition, a phosphorylase phosphatase is also activated that dephosphorylates phosphorylase-a, converting it to the relatively inactive phosphorylase-b. Thus, the epinephrine stimulated cascade is shut off as soon as the epinephrine stimulus disappears.

Allosteric Controls of Glycogen Degradation

In muscle, there is a rapid allosteric regulation of phosphorylase-b by ATP and AMP. An increase in concentration in AMP is capable of activating the relatively inactive form of phosphorylase, phosphorylase-b. When ATP is degraded by muscle contraction, the concentration of AMP increases within the cell, thereby activating phosphorylase-b. This stimulation of phosphorylase-b by AMP can be prevented by high concentrations of ATP, which block the AMP binding site. Hence, the activation of phosphorylase-b allosterically requires that the ratio of AMP to ATP rise, and this is what is seen in muscle contraction. Phosphorylase-a is not stimulated by AMP in this fashion, and it is sometimes referred to as the AMP-independent form; phosphorylase-b is called the AMP-dependent form.

A vigorous muscular activity increases the AMP:ATP ratio, very rapidly (in milliseconds) activating phosphorylase-b allosterically. On a longer time scale, seconds to minutes, hormone-triggered phosphorylation of phosphorylase-b converts it to phosphorylase-a that is fully active, as shown in Figure 7-30.

Calcium can also activate glycogen phosphorylase-b in muscle. Calcium is the intracellular signal for muscle contraction and is also an allosteric activator of phosphorylase-b kinase. When the stimulus for muscle contraction produces a transient rise in intracellular calcium levels, it also accelerates conversion of phosphorylase-b to the more active phosphorylase-a. This is because one of the subunits of phosphorylase-b kinase is calmodulin. Calmodulin is a calcium-binding protein that has the ability to either activate or inhibit other proteins it is associated with. Thus, when the calmodulin associated with phosphorylase-b kinase binds calcium, the kinase is partially activated, and it can phosphorylate and activate phosphorylase-b in the absence of a hormonal signal. This activation is transient and still requires activation of the phosphorylation cascade for long-term activation.

Hormonal Controls of Glycogen Synthesis

When the epinephrine stimulus turns on phosphorylase, it must simultaneously turn off glycogen synthase or we would be facing a futile, wasteful cycle. How does the epinephrine stimulus shut off glycogen synthesis at the same time that it turns on glycogen breakdown? Quite simply, the very same series of events results in the phosphorylation of glycogen synthase at the same time that phosphorylase-b is phosphorylated.

Nonphosphorylated glycogen synthase is active and is independent of G6P levels. Hence, the active form of glycogen synthase is called the independent form (I-form). When the epinephrine-stimulated cascade activates protein kinase so that the I-form of glycogen synthase is phosphorylated, the product is the dependent form (D-form). This form is less active and requires high levels of G6P for activity. Therefore, the epinephrine stimulus turned off glycogen synthase activity at the same time that it turned on phosphorylase activity. When the epinephrine stimulus disappears, a glycogen synthase phosphatase dephosphorylates the relatively inactive D-form, converting it to the active I-form that can now promote glycogen synthesis.

Each step in this cascade amplifies the effect of epinephrine. Thus, a minute amount of epinephrine has a very large effect, indeed. It has been estimated that a rise in the concentration of cAMP to 1 μM per kilogram of muscle causes the formation of 25,000 times as much G1P per minute.

When the epinephrine stimulus has been removed and the active I-form of glycogen synthase is synthesizing glycogen in a resting state, how is it that glycogen synthesis shuts down when appropriate amounts of glycogen have been synthesized? This is currently unclear. In the liver, the primary hormonal regulator of glycogen metabolism is glucagon. When this hormone binds to its receptor sites in the plasma membrane of a liver cell, a cascade of events essentially similar to that in muscle results in the conversion of phosphorylase-b to phosphorylase-a, increasing the rate of glycogen breakdown. This same cascade shuts off glycogen synthase in a similar fashion.

Liver Phosphorylase-a as the Glucose Sensor

In liver, glucose is an allosteric regulator of glycogen metabolism, not AMP, as in the muscle. When the concentration of glucose in the blood rises, glucose enters the liver cell and binds to a regulatory site on glycogen phosphorylase-a. This leads to a conformational change that exposes the phosphorylated serine residues to dephosphorylation by phosphorylase-a phosphatase. In this way, glycogen phosphorylase-a acts as the glucose sensor of liver, slowing the breakdown of glycogen whenever the level of blood glucose is high. This is indicated in Figure 7-32.

Summary

Glycogen is a branched-chain polymer consisting entirely of glucose molecules. It is synthesized from an activated glucose moiety, UDP-glucose, and it is stored primarily in the liver and muscle. The pathways of glycogen synthesis and degradation are reciprocally regulated by a hormone-activated amplification cascade mediated by cAMP. The major regulated enzymes are phosphorylase-b kinase, phosphorylase-b, and glycogen synthase. Glycogen synthesis occurs under high-energy conditions for energy storage, whereas glycogen breakdown occurs when energy is required. Liver glycogen is used primarily to maintain blood glucose levels; muscle glycogen is used primarily as a readily available energy source for muscle contraction. Allosteric controls of glycogen-related enzymes are also in effect.

Interconversion of Hexoses

Dietary complex carbohydrates and disaccharides that are digested in the gastrointestinal tract are absorbed as hexoses. Three principal hexoses are metabolized to enter into the glycolytic sequence: fructose, galactose, and mannose.

Fructose comprises a significant portion of the carbohydrate in the human diet. Typically, the daily intake approaches 100 g, both as the free sugar and as part of sucrose. The metabolism of fructose is somewhat different in liver tissue compared with adipose tissue. When dietary fructose is carried to the liver by the bloodstream, it must first be phosphorylated. While liver hexokinase can catalyze this reaction, hexokinase has an affinity for glucose that is 20 times greater than for fructose. Because the glucose levels in the liver approximate that in the bloodstream, the glucose level is quite high at all times, and there is little phosphorylation of fructose by hexokinase. Glucokinase does not phosphorylate fructose. Therefore, the operation of phosphorylating fructose in the liver is carried out by a different enzyme, fructokinase, which is specific for fructose. Once formed, F1P is split into glyceraldehyde and dihydroxyacetone phosphate by F1P aldolase. Glyceraldehyde is then phosphorylated to G3P by a triose kinase and ATP so that it can enter glycolysis as well as the dihydroxyacetone phosphate.

In adipose tissue, the situation is somewhat different. Fructose can enter adipose tissue cells in such a fashion that the level of fructose inside these cells is higher than that of glucose. As a consequence, F6P can be formed by hexokinase activity in adipose tissue and then is metabolized by way of the glycolytic sequence.

Galactose is metabolized differently from fructose. Upon entering the cell, galactokinase and

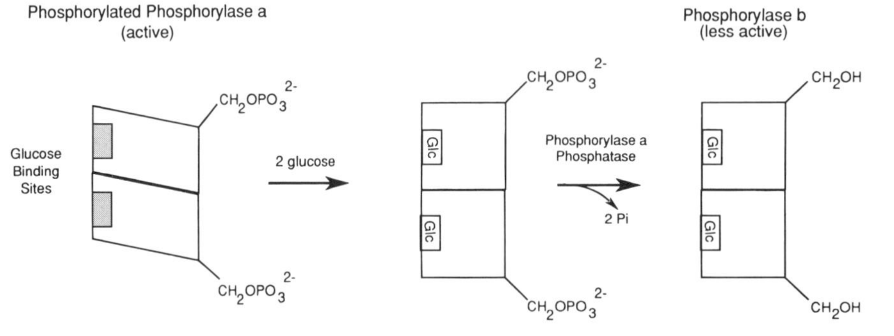

Figure 7-32. The use of phosphorylase-a as the glucose sensor of the liver cell. Note the conformational change that occurs when glucose binds to the enzyme, which allows the phosphate groups to become accessible to a phosphatase.

ATP react with galactose to produce galactose-1-phosphate. Next, galactose-1-phosphate reacts with UDP-glucose in a reaction catalyzed by galactose-1-phosphate uridine transferase, as shown in Figure 7-33. The products of this reaction are UDP-galactose and G1P.

The G1P formed enters glycolysis by way of the phosphoglucomutase catalyzed conversion to G6P. Epimerization of the UDP-galactose at the four-position converts it to UDP-glucose. This UDP-glucose–UDP-galactose interconversion is important. First, when it goes in the direction we have just described, it regenerates UDP-glucose to react with another molecule of galactose-1-phosphate. In the other direction, this epimerization converts UDP-glucose to UDP-galactose, which is essential for the synthesis of galactosyl residues in complex polysaccharides and glycoproteins if the amount of galactose in the diet is inadequate to meet these needs.

The disease galactosemia is caused by an inherited deficiency of galactose-1-phosphate uridine transferase. This disease is treated by the exclusion of galactose from the diet. Because the epimerase is present, patients with galactosemia can meet their requirements for galactosyl residues from UDP-glucose even though galactose is excluded from the diet.

Mannose also is produced by the digestion of various dietary polysaccharides and glycoproteins. It can be phosphorylated at C-6 by hexokinase to yield mannose-6-phosphate and ADP. This mannose-6-phosphate is then isomerized by the action of phosphomannose isomerase to yield F6P, an intermediate of glycolysis.

Overall Regulation of Carbohydrate Metabolism

Glycolysis occurs in all cells, and gluconeogenesis occurs predominantly in liver but also in kidney. We must have controls to ensure that G6P formation is in balance with its rate of utilization, on the one hand, and that gluconeogenesis and glycolysis are reciprocally controlled so that they do not operate fully at the same time, producing futile, wasteful cycles. There are intracellular allosteric controls as well as hormonal regulatory forces.

The intracellular allosteric controls operate at three key enzyme levels. The first is hexokinase, which catalyzes the entry of free glucose into the glycolytic pathway. In muscle cells this enzyme has a very high affinity for glucose so that any glucose that enters the muscle cell from the bloodstream is converted to G6P at its maximal rate. Muscle hexokinase is allosterically inhibited by its product, G6P. When the utilization of G6P in glycolysis is low, G6P levels rise, and hexokinase is temporarily and reversibly inhibited. This brings the rate of G6P formation into balance with its rate of utilization. In liver the situation is somewhat different because the predominant form of hexokinase is glucokinase. This glucokinase differs in two respects from hexokinase. First, its affinity for glucose is much less than that of hexokinase; therefore, its action is dependent upon the concentration of free glucose in the liver cell, which is in equilibrium with that in the bloodstream. When glucose concentration in the blood is high, such as after carbohydrate intake, excess blood glucose is transported into the liver cells where

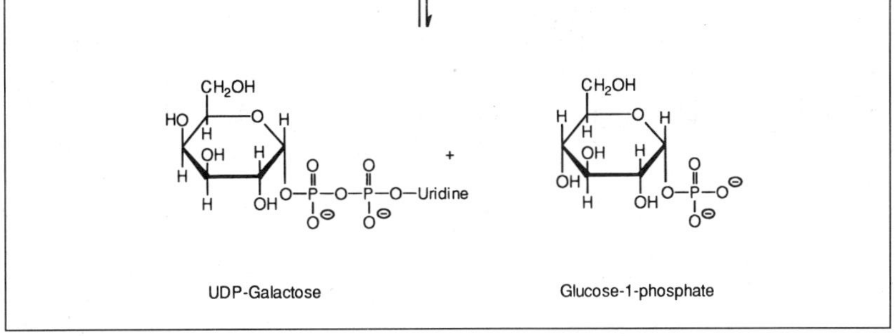

Figure 7-33. The reaction catalyzed by galactose-1-phosphate uridine transferase, to form UDP-galactose.

glucokinase can convert it to G6P because of the high concentration of the glucose. Also, glucokinase is not inhibited by G6P but by F6P. Fructose-6-phosphate is always in equilibrium with G6P because of the enzyme phosphohexoisomerase. Accordingly, when the level of F6P is high, it will partially inhibit glucokinase. This partial inhibition of glucokinase by F6P is mediated by a regulator protein. This regulator protein also has an affinity for F1P, and the F1P can compete with the F6P and cancel its inhibitory effect on glucokinase. Fructose-1-phosphate is only present in the liver when fructose is ingested and then phosphorylated at the 1 position by fructokinase. Thus, ingested fructose can stimulate the phosphorylation of glucose in the liver because of the ability of F1P to limit the inhibitory effect of F6P on glucokinase.

Another important control point of carbohydrate metabolism is pyruvate kinase. When the concentrations of ATP in a cell are high, the flow through the glycolytic sequence must be damped. You will remember that pyruvate kinase catalyzes the reaction between PEP and ADP to produce pyruvate and ATP. When ATP levels in the cell are already high, the affinity of pyruvate kinase for PEP is decreased, slowing the pyruvate kinase catalyzed reaction rate. When other fuels are present in high abundance, this enzyme can also be inhibited. Acetyl-CoA and long-chain fatty acids are both important fuels for the TCA cycle. Because the TCA cycle is a major source of energy for ATP production, the dependence on glycolysis for the production of ATP is decreased. It is for this reason that pyruvate kinase is also inhibited by rising intracellular concentrations of acetyl-CoA and long-chain fatty acids.

Glucose-6-phosphate, once formed, can flow into glycolysis, enter into glycogen synthesis, or pass into the hexose monophosphate shunt. The irreversible reaction catalyzed by PFK-1 is the step that commits a cell to the passage of glucose through glycolysis. This enzyme, then, is a very important control point, and it has several regulatory sites where allosteric activators or inactivators can bind. Remember that ATP levels in the cell are key in regulation. When these levels of ATP are high, they signal that the cell is producing ATP faster than it is consuming it. Accordingly, ATP inhibits PFK-1 by binding to an allosteric site and lowering the affinity of the enzyme for its other substrate, F6P. If the consumption of ATP is at such a rate that it exceeds its production, ADP and AMP levels rise in concentration. These two nucleotides act allosterically, then, to relieve the inhibition by ATP and allow the enzyme to function at a greater rate. These effects combine to produce higher enzyme activity when F6P, ADP, or AMP levels build up and lower activity when ATP accumulates. Citrate is a key intermediate in the oxidation of pyruvate in the TCA cycle, and it also serves as an allosteric inhibitor of PFK-1. When citrate concentrations are high, they signal that glycolysis should decrease, and they do so by increasing the inhibitory effect of ATP.

The most significant allosteric regulator of PFK-1 is fructose-2,6-bisphosphate. This substance is a regulator in the liver, and it strongly activates PFK-1. This will accelerate glycolysis. Fructose-2,6-bisphosphate will also inhibit gluconeogenesis by inhibiting the enzyme fructose-1,6-bisphosphatase. This is the enzyme that makes it possible for the gluconeogenesis system to bypass PFK-1, an irreversible step. The cellular concentration of fructose-2,6-bisphosphate is set by the relative rates of its formation and breakdown. It must be remembered that this substance is not a metabolic intermediate in the true sense but is primarily a regulator. It is formed by phosphorylation of F6P in a reaction requiring ATP and catalyzed by PFK-2. This substance is broken down by the enzyme fructose-2,6-bisphosphatase (FBPase-2). These reactions are shown in Figure 7-34.

Although both are part of a single bifunctional protein, PFK-2 and FBPase-2 are two distinct enzymatic activities. Remember that high levels of fructose-2,6-bisphosphate will activate PFK-1 and stimulate glycolysis. These high levels also inhibit fructose bisphosphatase-1 and slow gluconeogenesis. Glucagon is the hormonal signal for turning on gluconeogenesis and turning off glycolysis. As blood glucose levels drop, glucagon is released from the pancreas and binds to the hepatocyte. This stimulates adenylate cyclase and the cAMP cascade that we discussed previously. Cyclic AMP, now formed in increasing amounts, stimulates a cAMP-dependent protein kinase that transfers a phosphate group from ATP to this bifunctional protein (PFK-2/FBPase-2). This phosphorylation enhances the FBPase-2 activity and inhibits PFK-2. It is in this fashion that glucagon lowers the cellular level of fructose-2,6-bisphosphate, thereby inhibiting glycolysis and stimulating gluconeogenesis. The result, of course, is the production of more glucose by gluconeogenesis, enabling the liver to fulfill its role of replenishing blood glucose supplies. This regulation only occurs in the liver; the muscle isozyme of PFK-2 lacks the serine residues that are phosphorylated by the cAMP-dependent protein kinase, and as such it is not regulated hormonally [14,15].

The role of insulin as a hormonal regulator cannot be overlooked. The intracellular mechanism whereby insulin has its effects are not as

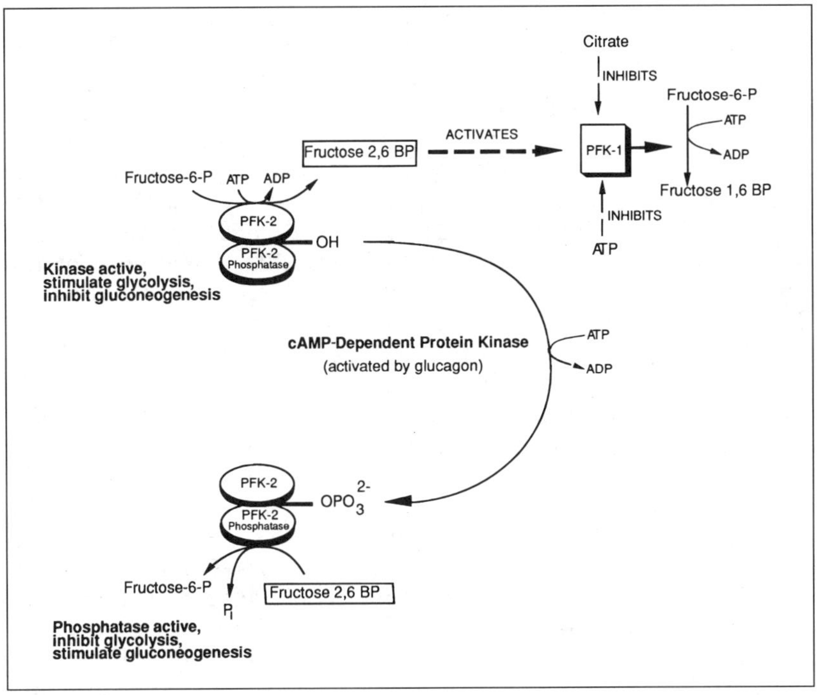

Figure 7-34. Regulation of PFK-2 by the cAMP-dependent protein kinase. Under conditions in which cAMP levels are high, PFK-2 is inhibited, and the rate of glycolysis is slowed in the liver. Muscle PFK-2 is not affected in this manner because the serine residue that is phosphorylated by the cAMP-dependent protein kinase is absent from the muscle isozyme.

clearly worked out as they are for glucagon and epinephrine. For all intents and purposes, insulin acts in a fashion opposite to that of glucagon. In the liver, it inhibits gluconeogenesis and activates glycogen synthesis while inhibiting glycolysis. In muscle and adipose tissue, when insulin binds to the cell membrane it increases the rate of entry of glucose into the cell.

Alterations in Carbohydrate Metabolism During Trauma

Individuals under stress, such as those recovering from trauma (surgery or burn injuries), display an altered carbohydrate metabolic profile compared with nontraumatized individuals. A major difference is that the trauma patient becomes desensitized to insulin, becoming hyperglycemic [16]. The basis for this insulin resistance is unknown. Because there are many hormonal signals released in response to injury, the interplay between the various mediators may either impair insulin release from the pancreas or render circulating insulin ineffective. In either event, the insulin resistance results in a high rate of hepatic gluconeogenesis, even when extraneous glucose is provided. Additionally, in burn patients, glucose is preferentially metabolized through anaerobic glycolysis [17], and this results in excess lactate being produced. The lactate produced is taken up by the liver and converted within the liver to glucose, which exacerbates the already excessive level of gluconeogenesis. Because of these problems, appropriate parenteral nutrition is difficult. One would like to supplement calories without elevating glucose concentrations and perhaps also to reduce the gluconeogenic output. A number of strategies have been attempted to overcome this problem.

One manner in which this problem can be approached is by lipid supplementation of the diet. Because lipid cannot be converted into glucose, such supplementation will not prevent gluconeogenesis from continuing (remember that the brain will still require a continual supply of glucose). However, lipid supplementation will reduce the levels of circulating glucose by the very fact that the lipid is replacing glucose as an energy source in the diet. Thus, lipid supplementation may help to reduce the hyperglycemia, even though gluconeogenesis is continuing. Paradoxically, fat metabolism appears to be continuously active in these patients, even though they are hyperglycemic. Whether lipid metabolism continues normally or in accelerated fashion in sepsis is still a matter of controversy, and conflicting data are present. It may be that in moderate sepsis, fat continues to be used. In severe sepsis, however, fat is not equivalently utilized (but perhaps no source of energy is utilized in the premortem patient). Because the cells in the body have become insulin resistant, the adipose tissue is only responding to released glucagon, which activates the fat metabolism pathway. This is to provide fats for energy metabolism, because glucose metabolism is impaired. To truly understand why these altered metabolic profiles are observed, one needs to obtain a better understanding at the molecular level of the effect of the released hormones after trauma on the pancreatic β-cell and the mode of release of insulin. It is currently believed that the pancreatic β-cell glucokinase is involved in the switching mechanism regulating glucose sensing and insulin secretion [18,19]. Once the mechanism of that process is better understood, it may be possible to more rationally design a proper diet for the trauma patient.

There is another strategy to override the altered regulation of gluconeogenesis, and that is through the administration of sugar alcohols, such as sorbitol and xylitol. The structures of these sugars are shown in Figure 7-35. Alcohol sugars contain an alcohol at the 1- or 2-carbon position of the sugar instead of a carboxylic acid group. The metabolic pathways of these two sugars are similar. The first step for both sugars is the oxidation of the hydroxyl on carbon 2. When this occurs for sorbitol, fructose is generated. When it occurs on xylitol, xylulose is generated. Both fructose and xylulose are then phosphorylated, producing F6P and Xu5P. Fructose-6-phosphate is an intermediate in glycolysis, and it is further metabolized through the glycolytic pathway. Xylulose-5-phosphate is metabolized via the nonoxidative reactions of the HMP shunt pathway, leading to both F6P and G3P. These are also intermediates of glycolysis, and further metabolism occurs through this pathway. The presence of these sugars does not alter blood insulin levels, so that, if the insulin glucagon ratio were low, addition of either sugar alcohol would not change that ratio, and gluconeogenesis would still be active. However, it has been demonstrated that xylitol administration can reduce hepatic glucose production by a factor of two through an unknown mechanism [20]. Thus, xylitol infusion may prove to be effective in reducing hepatic gluconeogenesis and sparing protein catabolism to provide substrates for the glucose being produced. On the other hand, this effect of xylitol on hepatic gluconeogenesis may be injurious. In the early Australian experience of the 1960s, administration of large amounts of xylitol led to approximately 30 deaths from hepatic failure. The use of sorbitol as a nutritional aid has a drawback not found with xylitol. Sorbitol is directly metabolized to fructose, which is then phosphorylated by fructokinase to form F1P. There are individuals in the population, at a frequency of 1 in 21,000, who lack fructose-1-aldolase and are hence fructose intolerant. If compromised with an excess fructose load, these individuals can die. Because the frequency of this disorder is so high in the general population and because most people exhibiting this disorder do not know they have it, there is a significant risk of patient morbidity through use of sorbitol as a nutritional supplement [21].

Another agent that has been used in the past for caloric supplementation is alcohol (ethanol). Alcohol is a convenient source of calories, but its use presents two major drawbacks. First, alcohol is a lipid, not a carbohydrate. Ethanol is metabolized to acetyl-CoA, as shown in Figure 7-36, and the carbons of acetyl-CoA cannot be used for the

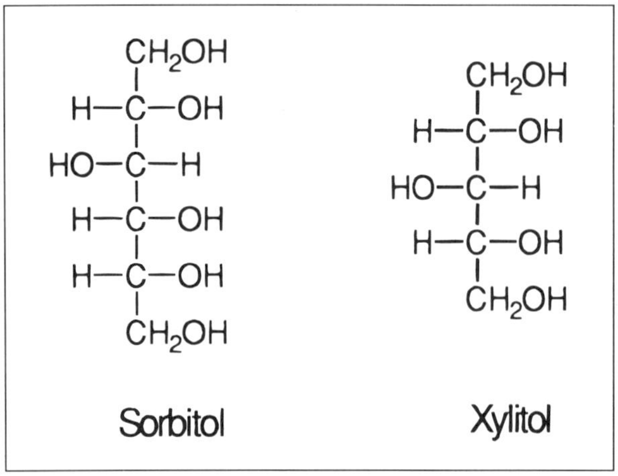

Figure 7-35. The structures of sorbitol and xylitol, two alcohol sugars used for nutritional supplementation of the surgical patient.

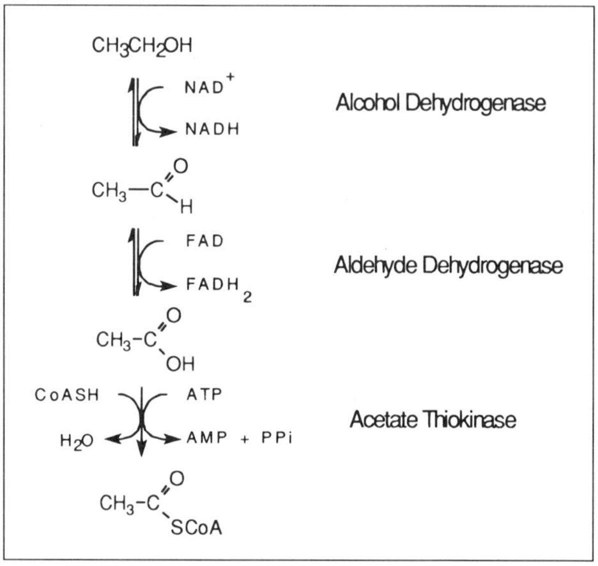

Figure 7-36. The metabolism of ethanol to acetyl-CoA. This is the only pathway for ethanol metabolism, and because acetyl-CoA cannot be used to produce glucose, ethanol also cannot be used to produce net glucose. Also note how the conversion of ethanol to acetyl-CoA requires NAD^+, as described in the text.

production of glucose. Thus, gluconeogenesis will continue unless alcohol is also supplemented with carbohydrate. Because hepatic gluconeogenesis is already excessive in these patients, the provision of nonglucogenic substrates may only exacerbate the high level of glucose being produced by the liver. High levels of alcohol, however, can reduce the rate of gluconeogenesis. Alcohol metabolism requires NAD^+, and it is possible for NAD^+ levels to decrease if alcohol is given in excess. This would lead to an increased intracellular $NADH/NAD^+$ ratio, which would shift the equilibrium conditions for all reactions that use this co-factor pair toward the production of NAD^+. This means that if pyruvate were made available for gluconeogenesis, it would preferentially be shifted to lactate production to regenerate NAD^+. Similarly, any oxaloacetate produced by pyruvate carboxylase would be shifted to malate formation, again to regenerate NAD^+. Thus, alcohol utilization, if moderate, may help to reduce the rate of gluconeogenesis by reducing the concentration of co-factors required for the production of gluconeogenic precursors. Carbohydrate supplementation would still be required for the brain to function properly, however.

The second major drawback of alcohol utilization is that the primary product of alcohol metabolism, acetaldehyde, is toxic, suggesting that alcohol supplementation should be used in moderation.

All the knowledge to date concerning nutritional support of trauma patients has been obtained without a detailed knowledge of the molecular events that regulate carbohydrate and lipid metabolism. As the preceding discussion implies, metabolism is not a "dead" subject, but instead is still confronting scientists and physicians with many new and exciting questions. With the many recent findings concerning the intracellular mechanism of insulin signaling [22–24], it should now be possible to attempt a molecular approach toward understanding the basis of insulin resistance in trauma patients, an understanding of which will aid in their nutritional support and therapy. Such studies are an important goal for the future.

Summary

In this chapter, we have seen how carbohydrates are metabolized to form either energy, in the form of ATP, or glycogen, to use as an energy store. The pathways required for energy production include glycolysis, in some cases the HMP shunt, glycogen degradation, and the TCA cycle. The pathways for energy storage include gluconeogenesis and glycogen synthesis. These pathways are regulated both hormonally and allosterically, and the overriding theme is that opposing pathways are never operative at the same time. Thus, reciprocal regulation ensures that biosynthetic pathways are inoperative, while degradative pathways are needed to preserve energy. It is also apparent that different organs are regulated differently because of their specific functions. The liver maintains blood glucose levels at a fairly constant level. It can do so by "sensing" the blood glucose levels with phosphorylase-a. Muscle phosphorylase-a does not respond to glucose; however, when energy levels are low in the muscle, AMP can partially activate phosphorylase-b, a mechanism which is not operative in the liver. Thus, tissue specific regulation also plays an important role. A thorough understanding of carbohydrate metabolism is necessary to fully understand total body metabolism and to aid in the generation of innovative nutritional treatment for the surgical patient.

References

1. Lehninger AL, Nelson DL, Cox MM. *Principles of Biochemistry,* 2nd edition. New York: Worth, 1993. Of particular interest are Chapters 11,14,15,18,19, and 22.
2. Zubay G. *Biochemistry,* 3rd edition. Dubuque, IA: Wm. C. Brown, 1993. Of particular interest are Chapters 6,12,13,14,15,21, and 24.

   References 1 and 2 are excellent biochemistry textbooks that provide many interesting details about carbohydrate metabolism.
3. Barnard RJ, Youngren JF. Regulation of glucose transport in skeletal muscle. *FASEB J* 6:3244, 1992.
4. Cushman SW, Wardzala LJ. Potential mechanism of action on glucose transport in the isolated rat adipose cell. *J Biol Chem* 255:4758, 1980.
5. Suzuki K, Kono T. Evidence that insulin causes translocation of glucose transport activity to the plasma membrane from an intracellular storage site. *Proc Natl Acad Sci USA* 77:2542, 1980.

   References 3, 4, and 5 discuss the mobilization of existing glucose transporters in response to insulin, particularly in muscle and adipose tissue.
6. Klip A, Marette A, Dimitrakoudis D, et al. Effect of diabetes on glucoregulation: From glucose transporters to glucose metabolism in vivo. *Diabetes Care* 15:1747, 1992.
7. Kahn BB. Alterations in glucose transporter expression and function in diabetes: Mechanisms for insulin resistance. *J Cell Biochem* 48:122, 1992.

   References 6 and 7 bring together problems in glucose transport with diabetes.
8. Smith TW. Digitalis: Mechanism of action and clinical use. *N Engl J Med* 318:358, 1988.
9. Norgaard A, Kjoldsen K. Human myocardial Na,K-pumps in relation to heart disease. *J Appl Cardiol* 4:239, 1989.

   References 8 and 9 provide more information concerning the role of the sodium, potassium ATPase in heart function.
10. Iynedjian PB, Gjinouci A, Renold AE. Stimulation by insulin of glucokinase gene in liver of diabetic rats. *J Biol Chem* 263:740, 1988.

11. Magnuson MA, Andreone TL, Printz RL, et al. Rat glucokinase gene: Structure and regulation by insulin. *Proc Natl Acad Sci USA* 86:4838, 1989.

References 10 and 11 provide more information concerning the regulation of glucokinase gene transcription by insulin.

12. Prostke CR, Fritz RS, Kletzien RF. Nutritional regulation of hepatic glucose-6-phosphate dehydrogenase: Transient activation of transcription. *Biochem J* 258:295, 1989.

13. Kletzien RF, Prostko CR, Stumpe DJ, et al. Molecular cloning of DNA sequences complementary to rat liver glucose-6-phosphate dehydrogenase mRNA: Nutritional regulation of mRNA levels. *J Biol Chem* 260:5621, 1985.

References 12 and 13 provide more information on the regulation of glucose-6-phosphate dehydrogenase activity at the gene level.

14. Kitamura K, Ujeda K, Kangawa K, et al. Purification and characterization of rat skeletal muscle fructose-6-phosphate, 2 kinase:fructose-2,6 bisphosphatase. *J Biol Chem* 264:9799, 1989.

15. Darville MI, Crepin KM, Hue L, et al. 5′-flanking sequence and structure of a gene encoding rat 6-phosphofructo-2-kinase/fructose-2,6-bisphosphatase. *Proc Natl Acad Sci USA* 86:6545, 1989.

References 14 and 15 provide more information on the different isozymes of PFK-2 and why the muscle form is refractory to phosphorylation controls.

16. Baue AE. Nutrition and metabolism in sepsis and multisystem organ failure. *Surg Clin North Am* 71:549, 1991.

17. Tredgett EE, Yu YM. The metabolic effects of thermal injury. *World J Surg* 16:68, 1992.

18. Vionnet N, Stoffel M, Takeda J, et al. Nonsense mutation in the glucokinase gene causes early-onset non-insulin-dependent diabetes mellitus. *Nature* 356:721, 1992.

19. Stoffel M, Froguel P, Takeda J, et al. Human glucokinase gene: Isolation, characterization, and identification of two missense mutations linked to early-onset non-insulin-dependent (type 2) diabetes mellitus. *Proc Natl Acad Sci USA* 89:7698, 1992.

References 18 and 19 provide more information concerning the role of glucokinase in insulin signaling and noninsulin dependent diabetes mellitus.

20. Schricker T, Kugler B, Trager K, et al. Effects of xylitol on carbohydrate and protein metabolism after trauma and during sepsis. *Nutr Hosp* 8:471, 1993.

21. Keller U. Zuckerersatzstoffe Fructose und Sorbit: ein unnotiges riskio in der parenteralen ernahrung (The sugar substitutes fructose and sorbitol: An unnecessary risk in parenteral nutrition). *Schweiz Med Wochenschr* 119:101, 1989.

22. Rose DW, Saltiel AR, Majumdar M, et al. Insulin receptor substrate 1 is required for insulin-mediated mitogenic signal transduction. *Proc Natl Acad Sci USA* 91:797, 1994.

23. White MF, Kahn CR. The insulin signaling system. *J Biol Chem* 269:1, 1994.

24. Skolnik EY, Batzer A, Li N, et al. The function of GRB2 in linking the insulin receptor to Ras signaling pathways. *Science* 260:1953, 1993.

References 22, 23, and 24 indicate an intracellular signaling pathway for the insulin receptor.

8

Plasma Lipoproteins and Intravenous Lipid Emulsions

Yvon A. Carpentier
Denis Y. Dubois
Richard J. Deckelbaum

This chapter aims to provide basic information related to plasma lipoproteins and intravenous lipid emulsions as a guide to clinicians selecting optimal nutritional support for different types of patients. The first part summarizes current knowledge on the structure, composition, and intravascular metabolism of plasma lipoproteins. We have focused on those aspects that are more directly relevant to the metabolic care of patients receiving parenteral nutrition. This offers a basis for the second part on intravenous lipid emulsions, which reviews similarities and differences as well as their interactions with plasma lipoproteins. To foster communication between the lipidologist and the clinician, we have tried to include, where relevant, speculative hypotheses and matters of controversy. It is our hope that this introduction to the intravascular metabolism of lipoproteins and emulsions will further open new areas for basic research and clinical investigations.

Structure and Composition of Lipoproteins

Core Lipid Model

Packaging of all lipoprotein constituents into discrete micellar particles generally follows simple physical guidelines, that is, in solubilizing hydrophobic lipids in an aqueous solution, the size and structure of the particles will relate to the ratio of relatively apolar core components (triglycerides and cholesteryl esters) to the emulsifying surface components (phospholipids, free cholesterol, and apolipoproteins). However, changes in the composition of the constituents may affect their physical properties and the equilibrium between surface and core components.

Individual Lipoproteins

In this chapter, we will use the classification of lipoprotein classes in relation to their density and divide them into triglyceride-rich lipoproteins (chylomicrons and very-low-density lipoproteins [VLDLs]), intermediate-density lipoproteins (IDLs), and cholesterol-rich lipoproteins (low-density lipoproteins [LDLs] and high-density lipoproteins [HDLs]). Occasionally, we will refer to lipoproteins by their apolipoprotein content; e.g., Lp A-I for lipoproteins containing only apolipoprotein A-I.

Triglyceride-Rich Lipoproteins

Chylomicrons. Chylomicrons are the largest lipoproteins (> 80 nm in diameter). They are synthesized by small intestinal mucosal cells after reesterification of absorbed dietary fatty acids into triglycerides and are secreted into intestinal lymphatics [1]. About 90% of the core mass is triglycerides, the remainder being made up of cholesteryl esters and some fat-soluble vitamins. The major apolipoproteins (apo) of the secreted particles are apo B-48, A-I, and A-IV; however, after entering the plasma via the thoracic duct, they acquire apo E and Cs (including apo C-II, which activates lipoprotein lipase), which are transferred from HDL [2]. Chylomicrons are normally found in the plasma after a fat-containing meal. They can be separated from other plasma lipoproteins by ultracentrifugation for only a few minutes at native plasma density. An abnormal accumulation of chylomicrons is observed in type I and V hyperlipoproteinemia.

Chylomicron remnants are produced after hydrolysis of chylomicron triglycerides by lipoprotein lipase at the endothelium wall of extrahepatic tissues. They become enriched with cholesteryl esters, which are transferred from LDL and HDL via cholesteryl ester transfer protein (CETP) [3]. Their particle size ranges from 25 to 80 nm in diameter. These particles are principally removed by the liver through endocytosis as discussed later. They accumulate in the plasma of patients with hepatic lipase deficiency, liver diseases, and abnormal apo E or when apo E is masked or displaced.

Very-Low-Density Lipoproteins. Very-low-density lipoproteins are released principally from the liver and carry more than 90% of plasma triglycerides in the fasting state [1]. During fasting, the intestine releases little amounts of small chylomicrons, similar to VLDL in size. VLDL triglycerides are derived from endogenous fatty acids brought to the liver from peripheral tissues or produced in the liver itself and from exogenous fatty acids present in the triglyceride moiety of chylomicron remnants. Although VLDLs and chylomicrons share many metabolic properties, they vary in the origin of the transported triglycerides and in apolipoprotein content. The apolipoproteins in VLDLs are mainly apo B-100, C, and E. As chylomicrons, VLDLs are lipolyzed by lipoprotein lipase in peripheral tissues so that they are transformed into denser and partially triglyceride-depleted particles, which have accumulated cholesteryl esters mainly by transfer from HDL [3].

Separated in the ultracentrifuge (at density <1.006 g/ml), VLDLs represent a heterogenous population varying in size (30–80 nm diameter) and containing several subfractions. Large VLDLs ($VLDL_1$, S_f 60–400) are rich in triglycerides and apo E [4]. Smaller VLDLs, $VLDL_3$ (S_f 20–60) [5], contain more cholesterol and no apo E. These particles have a different metabolic fate (see later discussion).

Intermediate-Density Lipoproteins

Intermediate-density lipoproteins, which are separated at the density range of 1.006 to 1.019 g/ml, represent an intermediate step in VLDL catabolism [6]. They are found only in low concentrations in normal subjects. An abnormal accumulation of IDL may be observed when the lipolytic transformation of $VLDL_3$ into LDL or the uptake of $VLDL_1$-derived particles by hepatocytes (as observed in type III hyperlipoproteinemia) are impaired.

Cholesterol-Rich Lipoproteins

Low-Density Lipoproteins. Low-density lipoproteins are isolated at a density range of 1.019 to 1.063 g/ml. They usually carry about 60% to 70% of total plasma cholesterol, mainly as cholesteryl esters, which are delivered to tissues where LDLs are taken up and catabolized via at least two different pathways: intact LDLs (normally about 80% of LDL) are cleared from plasma through binding to the ubiquitary LDL (or apo B,E) receptor (see later discussion) [7], whereas the remainder are catabolized through the "scavenger pathway" (a panel of receptors other than the classic LDL receptor) [8]. In plasma from normal subjects, LDL has a fairly long half-life (3.5 days).

Recently, the potential for protein and lipid components of LDL to undergo peroxidation has drawn enormous attention because these modified particles are recognized by the scavenger receptors, which are abundant on macrophages present in the arterial wall. The uptake of oxidized LDL is cytotoxic for macrophages and can transform them into "foam cells." This process is suggested to play a key role in the primary and subsequent development steps of the atherosclerotic lesion [8].

Oxidation of LDL is initiated by the peroxidation of polyunsaturated fatty acids contained in phospholipids and cholesteryl esters. Rapid alterations of apo B structure have also been characterized [9]. Small and dense LDL particles are considered to be more sensitive to oxidative damage than normal-sized LDL.

Most individuals have another definable lipoprotein subpopulation in the higher LDL density fraction. This fraction contains, in addition to apo B, another large apolipoprotein called apo(a) and is designated as Lp(a). Its plasma concentration is genetically determined [10].

High-Density Lipoproteins. High-density lipoproteins originate from four possible sources: (1) they may be directly secreted by the liver; (2) they may be formed in the plasma compartment after lipolysis of chylomicrons and release of surface remnants (phospholipids and some apolipoproteins); (3) a smaller fraction of HDL is produced as nascent particles directly released from the intestine; (4) they may originate from direct assembly of free apolipoproteins (mainly apo A-I and E) and phospholipids in interstitial fluids [6]. In the circulation, nascent HDLs are quickly transformed into larger, mature HDLs by enrichment with free cholesterol that is subsequently esterified and incorporated in the lipoprotein core. These processes will be detailed later.

HDLs are classically isolated by ultracentrifugation at a density range of 1.063 to 1.210 g/ml. A number of HDL subpopulations have been described that differ by particle size, composition, and metabolic properties. Two major HDL subfractions, HDL_2 (d = 1.063–1.125 g/ml) and HDL_3 (d = 1.125–1.210 g/ml), are separated by ultracentrifugation. However, greater heterogeneity of HDL is shown by combining ultracentrifugation and electrophoresis. This method separates at least two subspecies of HDL_2 and three of HDL_3. Mature HDLs contain about 50% protein, two thirds of which is apo A-I; one fifth, apo A-II; and the remainder, apo C, E, A-IV, and D. The lipid moiety is made up mostly of phospholipids and cholesteryl esters, but small amounts of free cholesterol and triglycerides are also present. Both apo A-I and A-II are found in HDL_2 and HDL_3, but some particles found in these fractions contain only apo A-I (LpA-I), whereas others contain both apo A-I and A-II (LpA-I:A-II). These particles have distinct metabolic fates, e.g., LpA-I are suggested to be more efficient in reverse cholesterol transport (see later discussion). Some apolipoproteins (mostly apo C and E) may to some extent be exchanged back and forth between HDL and triglyceride-rich lipoproteins. In fasting conditions, most of these apolipoproteins are found in HDLs, which appear to act as reservoirs for apo Cs and E [2].

HDLs are the site of cholesterol esterification in plasma by the enzyme lecithin:cholesterol acyltransferase (LCAT). They also largely contribute to neutral lipid exchanges with other lipoproteins. In this latter process, HDLs act mostly as acceptors of triglycerides and donors of cholesteryl esters. HDLs are largely involved in so-called reverse cholesterol transport, a process by which excess cholesterol is carried from peripheral tissues to the liver to be excreted into bile [1].

Lipoprotein-X (Lp-X)

In addition to the classic lipoprotein classes, another lipoprotein particle, lipoprotein-X (Lp-X), which is not normally present in plasma, deserves comment. Although Lp-X has a flotation density within the LDL range, it differs by its lipid and protein composition and by the fact that it moves in the opposite direction during electrophoresis. It can also be separated from LDL by zonal ultracentrifugation [11]. This abnormal lipoprotein is characterized by an unusually high proportion of phospholipids and free cholesterol and by a low protein content. It contains no apo B, but some apo C and E, and albumin.

Lipoprotein-X is found in the plasma of patients with biliary obstruction [12] and familial LCAT deficiency [13] and has also been observed in neonates [14], adults [15], dogs [16], and rats [17] receiving total parenteral nutrition (TPN) supplemented with fat emulsions. During TPN, the particle arises from phospholipid particles present in large amounts in some 10% emulsions and co-infused with the triglyceride-rich particles. These phospholipids have a great affinity for attracting free cholesterol from the surface of endogenous lipoproteins or from cell membranes to form a lipoprotein particle that is slowly cleared from the plasma [15,17]. The formation and metabolism of Lp-X is discussed later.

Apolipoproteins

Apolipoproteins (or apoproteins) make up the protein moiety of the plasma lipoproteins. In addition to their strong affinity for binding lipids and for contributing to the varying structural properties of different lipoprotein subclasses, they play an essential role in regulating the metabolism of lipoprotein particles via interactions with key enzymes and receptors. Recently, the use of transgenic animals expressing human genes of different apoproteins is providing great promise in better understanding their role. The major properties and functions of individual apolipoproteins are summarized in Table 8-1.

The A, C, and E apolipoproteins have been shown to have regions of amino-acid-forming amphipathic helices [18]. These regions are particularly suited for emulsifying lipids by acting as amphipathic molecules with nonpolar hydrophobic amino acids on one side and polar water-soluble amino acids on the opposite side.

Apolipoproteins A-I and A-II. Apolipoproteins A-I and A-II are the major apolipoproteins of HDLs and account for 65% and 20% of total HDL protein, respectively. Normal plasma values are 120 to 180 mg/dl for apo A-I and 30 to 50 mg/dl for apo A-II. High-density lipoproteins contain 90% and 95% of plasma A-I and A-II, respectively. Apo A-I plays an essential role in the process by which excess cholesterol is removed from peripheral tissues and transported to the liver. During this process, apo A-I acts as a ligand, allowing HDLs to interact with cell surfaces [19,20] and to promote exchanges of cholesterol between cells and HDLs. In most peripheral tissues, net flux of cholesterol is from cell to small HDL_3 particles, whereas in the liver net flux of cholesterol is from large HDL (HDL_2) to cells. Apo A-I is also the major activator of LCAT, a plasma enzyme interacting with phosphatidylcholine and free cholesterol to form lysophosphatidylcholine and cholesteryl esters [21]. The latter are not soluble in water, so the LCAT reaction allows the esterified form of cholesterol to be kept packed in the core of the HDL particles while being transported to the liver [22]. As detailed in the following section, cholesteryl esters may later be transferred to apo B–containing lipoproteins under the action of CETP. Thus, apo A-I plays an essential role in the antiatherogenic "reverse cholesterol transport." Although apo A-I is largely produced in the liver, substantial amounts are synthesized in the intestine and secreted into chylomicrons during the postprandial phase and into intestinal HDL during fasting.

Table 8-1. Human Plasma Apolipoproteins

Apolipoprotein	Molecular Weight (kDa)	Function
A-I	28.3	Activates LCAT Promotes reverse cholesterol transport
A-II	17	Promotes the formation of large HDL Activates hepatic lipase
A-IV	46	Activates LCAT Promotes reverse cholesterol transport Facilitates LPL activation by apo C-II
B-100	549	Structural protein of VLDL and LDL Ligand for LDL receptor
B-48	265	Structural protein of chylomicron
C-I	6.5	Activates LCAT Inhibits phospholipase A_2 Modulates the clearance of remnants
C-II	8.8	Activates lipoprotein lipase Modulates the clearance of remnants
C-III	8.9	Inhibitor of lipoprotein lipase Modulates the clearance of remnants
D	32	Binds small hydrophobic molecules Involved in repair of tissues
E	34	Important for the clearance of remnants Binds E and LDL receptors Involved in growth and regeneration of nervous tissue
SAA	11–14	Acute-phase protein Interferes with LCAT activity Might redirect HDL to cells expressing SAA receptors Amyloidogenic
H	43–54	Inhibits intrinsic pathway of coagulation
J	70	Protects cell membranes from toxic components Inhibits cytolytic reaction of complement Binds to immunoglobulins

Most apo A-I is transferred to the HDL density range during peripheral lipolysis of chylomicrons [23].

Apo A-II behaves as an antagonist of the recognition of apo A-I by cellular binding sites, at least in adipose cells; hence, HDL particles containing both apo A-I and A-II may be poor candidates for promoting cellular cholesterol efflux [24,25] and may diminish the antiatherogenic properties of apo A-I. This is confirmed by studies in transgenic mice overexpressing human apo A-I and A-II and maintained on an atherogenic diet. After a few weeks, apo A-I/A-II transgenic animals developed significant atherosclerotic lesions, whereas only small lesions were found in the apo A-I mice [26]. However, in HDL metabolism, apo A-II is involved in the transformation of small HDL into large particles [27] and also acts as an activator of hepatic lipase [28]. Apo D_2 or D_2-peptide [29] is the monomeric form of apo A-II [30]. Apo A-II is essentially synthesized in the liver and is not present in native chylomicrons.

Apolipoprotein A-IV. Apo A-IV is synthesized in the intestine and secreted largely in chylomicrons. During postprandial lipolysis, apo A-IV is transferred to HDL particles where it is assumed to replace apo Cs transferred to chylomicrons [31]. This may explain why, in fasting plasma, most A-IV is bound to apo A-I–containing particles [32]. However, apo A-IV may also be found in the lipoprotein-poor (d>1.21 g/ml) plasma fraction, where it is bound to apo A-I and lipids [33]. Apo A-IV has been suggested to play several metabolic roles, such as activating LCAT [34] and promoting reverse cholesterol transport [35,36]. Normal plasma values of apo A-IV are 10 to 15 mg/dl.

Apolipoprotein B. Apo B makes up more than 90% of LDL proteins and 45% of VLDL proteins. Apo B is found in two forms, apo B-100 and apo B-48. Apo B-100 is synthesized in the liver and secreted in VLDL; it remains in VLDL during peripheral lipolysis of triglycerides and is transferred intact to VLDL's catabolic product, LDL [1]. VLDLs, IDLs, and LDLs contain one apo B-100 molecule per particle [2], so that immunologic determination of apo B in selected lipoprotein fractions precisely reflects the number of apo B-100–containing particles. Apo B-48 is formed in the intestinal mucosa, where a stop codon prevents synthesis of full apo B-100 [37]. Apo B-48 is secreted on chylomicrons. In plasma from fasting, normal individuals, apo B-100 makes up all (or almost all) of apo B. Apo B-100 is a major regulator of cholesterol metabolism, being recognized by cellular LDL (or B,E) receptor in a variety of tissues and leading to plasma cholesterol disposal [38]. Although VLDL contains apo B-100, it is not recognized by the LDL receptor, likely because apo B is not in the appropriate conformation on VLDL [39]. Chylomicron does not bind the LDL receptor, which does not recognize apo B-48 [40]. Normal values of plasma apo B concentration are 50 to 120 mg/dl.

C Apolipoproteins. The C apolipoproteins are relatively small in terms of molecular weight and can be separated into discrete proteins. Apo C-I is mostly found in the HDL particles from fasting normal plasma, but substantial amounts of apo C-I are also included in the VLDL fraction [1]. It contributes about 2% to 3% of HDL proteins and 6% to 10% of VLDL proteins. Apo C-I (mainly, but also apo C-III) may modulate the uptake of lipoprotein remnants by masking and/or displacing apo E and by preventing apo E linkage to its cellular binding sites [41]. Apo C-I is capable of activating LCAT [21] and inhibiting phospholipase A_2 [42]. It is synthesized by the liver and by the adrenal glands [43]. Normal plasma apo C-I concentrations are 4 to 10 mg/dl.

Apo C-II is an activator for lipoprotein lipase [44]. Separate regions of the molecule are involved in binding to phospholipids, to lipoprotein lipase, and in activation of the bound lipase. Familial apo C-II deficiency results in severe hypertriglyceridemia [45]. Apo C-II contributes approximately 6% to 8% to total VLDL protein and 1% to 2% to HDL protein. In plasma of fasting normal individuals, 50% to 80% of apo C-II is in the HDL fraction, whereas postprandially (or during lipid infusions), apo C-II is largely transferred to the triglyceride-rich fraction, allowing lipoprotein lipase to hydrolyze triglycerides [1]. Apo C-II is synthesized in the liver [43]. Normal plasma values for apo C-II are 2 to 5 mg/dl.

Approximately 60% of apo C-III circulates with HDL, and 25% circulates with VLDL in normal fasting individuals [1]. Apo C-III makes up to 30% of VLDL total protein content and approximately 3% to 5% of total HDL proteins. A role for apo C-III in modulating apo C-II activity by inhibiting lipoprotein lipase [46] has been suggested by in vitro experiments and seems to be confirmed in vivo [47,48]. Moreover, the use of transgenic mice overexpressing the apo C-III gene has shown that apo C-III inhibits the hepatic uptake of triglyceride-rich particles [49]. Apo C-III is synthesized in the liver [43]. Normal plasma values for apo C-III are 5 to 15 mg/dl.

Thus, apo Cs play a key role in the metabolism of triglyceride-rich lipoproteins by modulating both peripheral triglyceride hydrolysis and remnant uptake. In this respect, recent reports have emphasized the importance of the exchangeable pool of these apolipoproteins that appears to be depleted in hypertriglyceridemic patients [50].

Apolipoprotein D. Apo D is found mainly in small HDL particles. Its role in cholesterol metabolism is still controversial. Apo D seems to act as a carrier for small lipid molecules between plasma HDL and cells (e.g., in nervous tissue) that are not directly exposed to HDL from the bloodstream [51]. Indeed, local accumulation of apo D has been observed at sites of injury to peripheral nerves [52]. Apo D may also play a role in the local distribution of steroid molecules in tissues where steroidogenesis is active (adrenals, ovary, testis) and in hormone-sensitive tissues such as mammary or prostatic tissues [53].

Apolipoprotein E. Apo E is present mainly in HDL, but it is also in VLDL of fasting normolipidemic subjects. During the postprandial phase, chylomicrons acquire apo E from other lipoproteins. Further enrichment of chylomicron remnants with apo E secreted by hepatocytes has been suggested to occur in the space of Disse of the liver [40]. Apo E may be indispensable for the clearance of chylomicron and large VLDL remnants from plasma by serving as a ligand for binding these particles to hepatic receptors such as the LDL receptor and to other chylomicron remnant receptors such as the LDL receptor-related protein [54,55]. Indeed, the apo E "knock-out" mouse develops atherosclerosis spontaneously and more rapidly on atherogenic diets, the major plasma alteration being markedly elevated levels of remnant particles [56,57]. In contrast, transfection of rat hepatoma cells with the human apo E gene induces human apo E secretion and leads to an enhanced binding and intracellular uptake of remnants [58]. In addition, infusion of apo E in hyperlipidemic animals was efficient in accelerating plasma lipoprotein clearance and reducing cholesterol levels [59,60].

Recently, it was suggested that apo E may also facilitate the non-receptor-mediated cellular uptake of VLDL-size and IDL-size particles [61]. In addition to its role in enhancing particle uptake, apo E has additional effects on modulating the cellular metabolism of both triglycerides and cholesterol esters by promoting hydrolysis rather than accumulation [62]. Polymorphism of apo E has a genetic basis, apo E being inherited at a single locus with three common alleles termed 2, 3, and 4. These are related to the three major isoforms of apo E, designated apo E-2, E-3 (the most common form), and E-4, respectively, which are differentiated on the basis of cysteine and arginine contents. Their ability to bind hepatic receptors widely differs: apo E-4 shows the higher affinity, whereas apo E-2 has the lower affinity and is the most common form associated with type III hyperlipoproteinemia [63,64]. Isoforms influence the distribution of apo E between the classes of lipoprotein: apo E-3 displays a preference for HDL, and apo E-4 for VLDL [65]. Apo E is synthesized in a wide variety of tissues, including liver, brain, intestine, kidney, and stimulated macrophages, and appears to be involved in the repair response to tissue injury [64]. Normal plasma apo E concentrations are 4 to 11 mg/dl.

Apolipoprotein SAA. Apo SAA (serum amyloid A protein) is normally found at low concentrations (about 0.1 mg/dl) in plasma. It is synthesized principally by the liver, but some is also produced by heart, lung, spleen, intestine, and kidney. It shows strong similarities with tissue amyloid A protein (protein AA) found in deposits of amyloid substance in various tissues [66]. Protein AA is produced by proteolytic cleavage of some apo SAA isoforms circulating in plasma [67], and amyloid deposits are formed in the presence of other factors such as the "amyloid enhancing factor" [68]. Apo SAA behaves as an acute-phase protein with plasma levels that can increase up to 1000 times after inflammatory stimulation. Apo SAA is associated essentially with HDL particles [66] and may interfere with cholesterol esterification by LCAT [69]. In an animal model of inflammation, catabolism of SAA-rich HDL components is increased; this may be partly the result of increased uptake by up-regulation of some receptor expression [70]. Indeed, specific SAA binding sites have been suggested on macrophages, and the presence of SAA might preferentially direct HDL to macrophages and other reticuloendothelial cells that are able to engulf cholesterol and lipid debris during inflammation. Thus, SAA-rich HDL interaction with these cells may prevent excess intracellular cholesterol accumulation [71]. Apo SAA may also be found in LDL and VLDL fractions [72,73]. In addition, small amounts of apo SAA circulate in the plasma unbound to lipoproteins. Note that C-reactive protein (CRP), another major acute-phase protein, may also interact with triglyceride-rich and apo B–containing lipoproteins [73].

Apolipoprotein H. Apo H [74] or β_2-glycoprotein I exists in plasma in a free form or associated with triglyceride-rich particles or HDL [75,76]. It inhibits the intrinsic pathway of coagulation by interfering with the activation of Hageman factor [76]. Apo H is synthesized in the liver [77].

Apolipoprotein J. Apo J [78] or SP 40,40 [79] or clusterin [80] is associated with small HDL particles. It may play a role in modulating immune reactions. Indeed, it may bind immunoglobulins [80], inhibit cytolytic reaction of complement C5b-9 complex [81], and protect cell membranes by inactivating toxic agents and by regulating access to cell membrane [82]. Apo J is secreted by a wide variety of tissues [81]. Other minor apolipoproteins have been described (apo F, apo G), but their role remains unknown.

Changes of Apolipoproteins During Lipid Infusions

Lipemia induced by lipid infusion shows similarities to postprandial lipemia. Apolipoproteins that appear to play a crucial role in the intravascular metabolism of chylomicrons, by influencing triglyceride hydrolysis (apo Cs) or by modulating binding to, and uptake of, remnants by hepatocytes or macrophages (apo E), are also efficiently transferred from HDL to emulsion particles. In contrast, apo B remains on the original VLDL, IDL, and LDL lipoproteins without being exchanged; because this structural apolipoprotein cannot be acquired by emulsion particles, antibodies directed toward apo B can be used as a means for separating endogenous lipoproteins from exogenous particles in a given density range.

However, differences between postprandial lipemia and emulsion-induced lipemia need to be stressed. Intestinal chylomicrons carry apolipoproteins B-48, A-IV, and A-I. After entering the bloodstream, chylomicrons acquire apo Cs and E from HDL, whereas apo A-IV is transferred to HDL. During peripheral triglyceride hydrolysis, apo A-I–phospholipid complexes are shed from chylomicrons to form new HDL particles in the circulation. Whether this process occurs with emulsion particles and is influenced by their composition remains to be determined. Low apo A-I levels in patients receiving parenteral nutrition with lipids could be the result of the absence of chylomicron production by the intestine and also of accelerated apo A-I clearance, as recently suggested [83].

Metabolism of Plasma Lipoproteins

Although lipoprotein classes with definite composition and physical properties can be isolated from plasma, individual lipid and apolipoprotein constituents and even whole lipoprotein particles are continually undergoing dynamic interactions with other particles as well as with membranes of adjacent cells.

Transport and delivery of lipids are performed via interactions of lipoprotein particles with enzymes and lipid transfer proteins that circulate in or are present in close proximity to the plasma compartment. In addition to the delivery or removal of lipid molecules (or their hydrolytic products) to and from tissues, such interactions result in several effects: formation of lipid molecules in the plasma; transfer and exchange of lipid and protein molecules between lipoprotein particles; and interconversion of lipoprotein families. They involve the participation of lipoprotein lipase, hepatic lipase, and LCAT as well as of specific lipid transfer proteins, such as CETP and different cell receptors.

Because triglycerides represent the major lipid molecules transported both in lipoproteins (100–150 g/d) and in artificial emulsions used in parenteral nutrition, we wish to describe more extensively the complex chain of events related to the intravascular metabolism of triglyceride-rich particles. Other aspects related more to the metabolism of cholesterol and cholesterol-rich lipoproteins will be briefly reviewed.

Interaction of Triglyceride-Rich Lipoproteins With Endothelial Lipases

After its synthesis in parenchymal cells, lipoprotein lipase is transported to the luminal surface of capillary endothelial cells [84]. Evidence for lipoprotein lipase synthesis has been found in adipose tissue, skeletal and cardiac muscles, lung, lactating mammary gland, spleen, ovary, macrophages, and kidney as well as in many areas of the brain and spinal cord [85,86]. The enzyme is anchored at some distance from the endothelium, probably to different types of endothelial cell surface proteins such as heparan sulfate proteoglycans and a specific heparin-sensitive binding protein [87]. The rates of synthesis and release from producing cells, which are under hormonal control, determine the amount of lipoprotein lipase present at the endothelial sites. In addition, the activity of lipoprotein lipase varies in different tissues according to nutritional and hormonal conditions. For example, starvation increases lipoprotein lipase activity in muscle and decreases it in the adipose tissue, whereas the fed state induces the opposite response.

Lipoprotein lipase binds rapidly and avidly to lipid-water interfaces, such as the phospholipid surface of lipoproteins (and emulsion particles) as well as to phospholipid liposomes. The interaction with lipoproteins may be facilitated by electrostatic interactions between the positive charges on apolipoproteins B and E and the negative charges on heparan sulfate [44]. Both chylomicron and VLDL carry not only the substrate molecules (triglycerides and phospholipids) but also apo C-

II, which binds to lipoprotein lipase and activates the enzyme, possibly by bringing it into an optimal orientation with the lipoprotein particle at the lipid-water interface.

In addition to the orientation of its active site, the activity of lipoprotein lipase is governed by its affinity for molecular species and the relative concentration of substrate present in the surface layer of a particle. The enzyme has a low degree of chemical substrate specificity and hydrolyzes (although at different rates) long-, medium-, and short-chain triglycerides, diglycerides and monoglycerides, and long- and short-chain acyl phosphatidylcholine. For example, medium-chain triglycerides are hydrolyzed at a much higher rate than long-chain triglycerides [88], whereas the rate of phosphatidylcholine hydrolysis represents only a small percentage of that for triglyceride hydrolysis. As soon as the lipoproteins and the enzyme interact with each other, hydrolysis of triglycerides begins at the sn-1 and sn-3 positions and results in the formation of fatty acids and sn-2 monoglycerides. Probably most of the monoglycerides but only a proportion of fatty acids are then taken up by the adjacent tissues, and the remaining fatty acids are released into the circulation as free fatty acids (Figure 8-1). Lipoprotein lipase activity is strongly inhibited by long-chain fatty acids, as shown by the need of a fatty acid acceptor (generally albumin) for the reaction to proceed with long-chain triglycerides. This inhibition may control the action of lipoprotein lipase in vivo and prevent generation of fatty acids to exceed the capacity of tissue assimilation [89]. The same triglyceride-rich particle undergoes a number of lipolytic events at different endothelial sites. Partially hydrolyzed particles are smaller and denser than the original lipoproteins and must undergo a series of structural rearrangements, consisting essentially of a physicochemical adjustment of the surface layer to the decreasing core size of the particles by deletion of lipids and apolipoproteins from the surface.

Large-sized chylomicrons and VLDLs appear to interact predominantly with lipoprotein lipase at the endothelial sites of extrahepatic tissues (e.g., heart, skeletal muscles, lungs, adipose tissues). Smaller remnant particles seem to be directed toward the liver, probably because of the preferential loss of apo C-II during remnant formation [90]. In the liver, further hydrolysis of triglycerides by hepatic lipase occurs, and apo E-rich, apo C-poor particles are taken up and catabolized by hepatocytes [41,90]. Recently, bone marrow was identified as another tissue playing a very active role in the removal of triglycerides transported by chylomicron remnants [40]. In addition to acting on particles at different stages of their intravascular metabolism, important differences of hydrolytic activity have been shown in vitro between lipoprotein lipase and hepatic lipase with respect to different fatty acids contained in chylomicron triglycerides [91]. These lipases, which share a common ancestral gene [92], are suggested to play a complementary role in the metabolic channeling of selected fatty acids to different tissues.

The important role of lipoprotein lipase in the metabolism of triglyceride-rich particles is demonstrated by the clinical manifestations associated with the absence of either lipoprotein lipase or apo C-II. Patients with these conditions accumulate chylomicrons and VLDL in their plasma. Triglyceride levels can reach 50 to 100 mmol/L (4000–9000 mg/dl), and recurrent attacks of pancreatitis are common and may be fatal. However, hypertriglyceridemia can also result from the accumulation of remnant particles that are not

Figure 8-1. Binding of a triglyceride (TG)-rich particle to lipoprotein lipase enzymes (small spheres) attached to endothelial heparan sulfate proteoglycans. ALB = albumin; FA = fatty acid; FFA = free fatty acid. (From YA Carpentier. Intravascular metabolism of fat emulsions: The Arvid Wretlind Lecture, ESPEN 1988. *Clin Nutr* 8:115, 1989.)

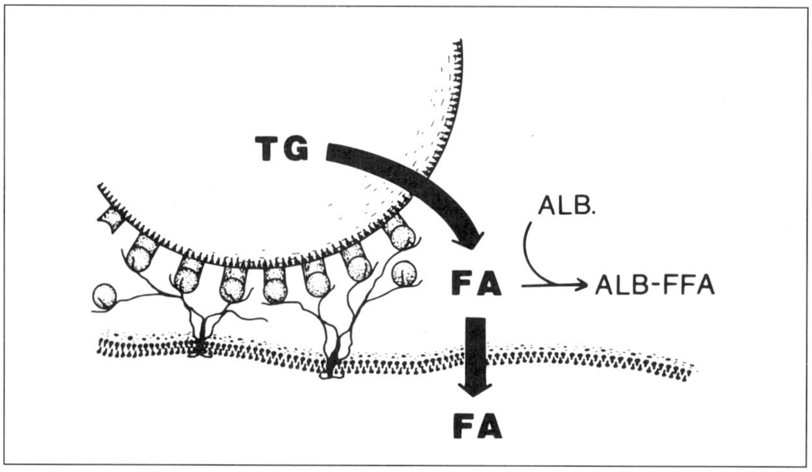

properly cleared by the liver. This type III hyperlipidemia is receiving increased attention because of the well-recognized atherogenic properties of postprandial remnants [93].

Apart from its role as a key enzyme in the hydrolysis of circulating triglycerides, lipoprotein lipase was more recently found to cooperate with apo E in facilitating the binding of remnant particles to hepatic receptors [94]. In addition, evidence is accumulating that lipoprotein lipase may also potentiate the binding to cells of lipid emulsions [95] as well as of different lipoproteins, thereby enhancing the cellular uptake of these particles via a pathway not involving classic lipoprotein receptors.

Infusion of lipid emulsions at relatively high rates markedly increases the usually quite low concentration of circulating lipoprotein lipase [96]. An association between this phenomenon and the rise of plasma free fatty acids suggests that those fatty acids that are not immediately assimilated by the adjacent tissues can exert an inhibitory effect on lipoprotein lipase as well as disrupt its binding to the endothelium, releasing some enzyme into the circulation, presumably bound to remnant particles [96] (Figure 8-2).

Administration of heparin induces the release of lipoprotein lipase (and also hepatic lipase) from its attachment to the endothelial wall into the circulation. It is transiently accompanied by a more rapid hydrolysis of plasma triglycerides, but also by a substantial increase of plasma free fatty acid level, which may become a matter of concern. Plasma "post–heparin lipase activity" is supposed to represent the total amount of lipoprotein lipase and hepatic lipase present at the endothelial surface and therefore is thought to closely reflect the physiologically active compartment. Both enzymes can be further separated by selective procedures. However, this measure of in vitro lipolytic activity cannot be directly used to predict the capability of a given subject to clear circulating triglycerides. The rise of plasma free fatty acids that follows the administration of heparin can be avoided by using synthetic short-chain heparin derivatives that have no effect on the release and activation of endothelial lipases.

Intravascular Lipid Exchanges Between Lipoproteins

These reactions involve exchanges of cholesteryl esters, triglycerides, and phospholipids between lipoproteins. They are mediated by CETP, a glycoprotein that is present or active in only some species (e.g., humans, rabbits, monkeys) [3]. Another phospholipid transfer protein, which has no effect on the exchange of neutral lipids, enhances the transfer of phospholipids from the surface of other lipoproteins or from phospholipid vesicles to HDL [3,97].

Incubation of LDLs or HDLs with VLDLs (or lipid emulsions) and CETP-containing plasma results in a substantial replacement of the LDL (and HDL) cholesteryl ester content by triglycerides [98,99]. A similar type of LDL (poor in cholesteryl esters and relatively rich in triglycerides) is found in the plasma of patients with familial hypertriglyceridemia [100]. Incubation of such triglyceride-enriched LDL with lipoprotein lipase or hepatic lipase causes hydrolysis of 60% to 70% of the transferred triglycerides and the remodeling of LDL into smaller and denser particles [98]. Neutral lipid exchange reactions induce changes in HDL that are similar to those described for LDL, resulting initially in the formation of large triglyceride-enriched cholesteryl ester–depleted HDL_2 particles. Subsequent hydrolysis of the triglycerides accumulated in HDL_2 particles by lipoprotein lipase and hepatic lipase increases the rate of catabolism of these particles, resulting in a reduced pool of HDL_2 [101], and leads to the accelerated

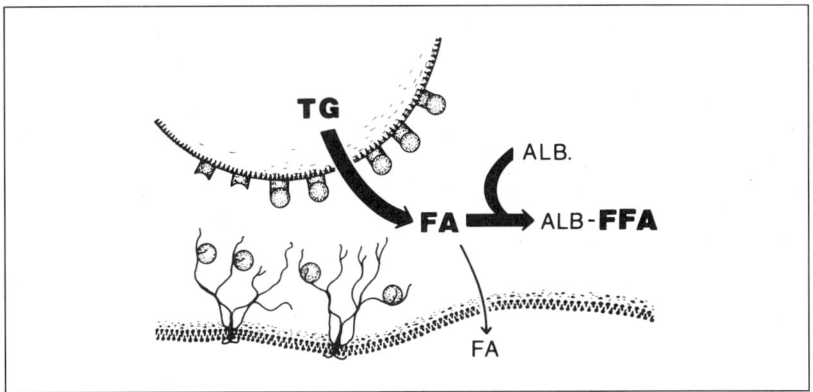

Figure 8-2. Dissociation of lipoprotein lipase from its endothelial binding. In this condition, local production of fatty acids (FA) from triglyceride (TG) hydrolysis exceeds the capacity of assimilation by tissue. These fatty acids inhibit the activity of the lipase but also interfere with its binding to endothelial proteoglycans. Increased plasma free fatty acid (FFA) level is induced by spillage from endothelial hydrolysis and by triglyceride hydrolysis into the circulation. ALB = albumin. (From YA Carpentier. Intravascular metabolism of fat emulsions: The Arvid Wretlind Lecture, ESPEN 1988. *Clin Nutr* 8:115, 1989.)

formation of a small-size and dense subpopulation of HDL_3 that is also present in the plasma of hypertriglyceridemic patients [100]. Of interest, these abnormalities revert toward normal when the patients are treated with triglyceride-lowering drugs.

In these exchange reactions, triglyceride-rich lipoproteins serve as donors for triglycerides and acceptors of cholesteryl esters, whereas HDLs (and LDLs) behave as acceptors for triglycerides and donors of cholesteryl esters (Figure 8-3). Lipid exchanges mediated by CETP are stimulated by accumulation of triglycerides in chylomicrons or VLDL or their remnants, as observed during postprandial or pathologic hypertriglyceridemias [102]. Recent data suggest that CETP mass is rate limiting for cholesteryl ester transfer in hypertriglyceridemic patients, whereas VLDL concentration regulates it in normal subjects [103].

Exchanges of neutral lipids mediated by CETP have attracted a great deal of attention in the field of atherosclerosis, mainly from the observation that animals lacking CETP are not prone to develop atherosclerosis, but that acquisition of CETP activity in transgenic animals induces the disease [104]. This aspect of lipoprotein metabolism is also particularly relevant to lipid infusions in parenteral nutrition because emulsion particles can substitute for triglyceride-rich lipoproteins in these reactions. In this respect, emulsions have been used to study in vitro and in vivo the influence of triglyceride fatty acid composition on the exchange processes [105].

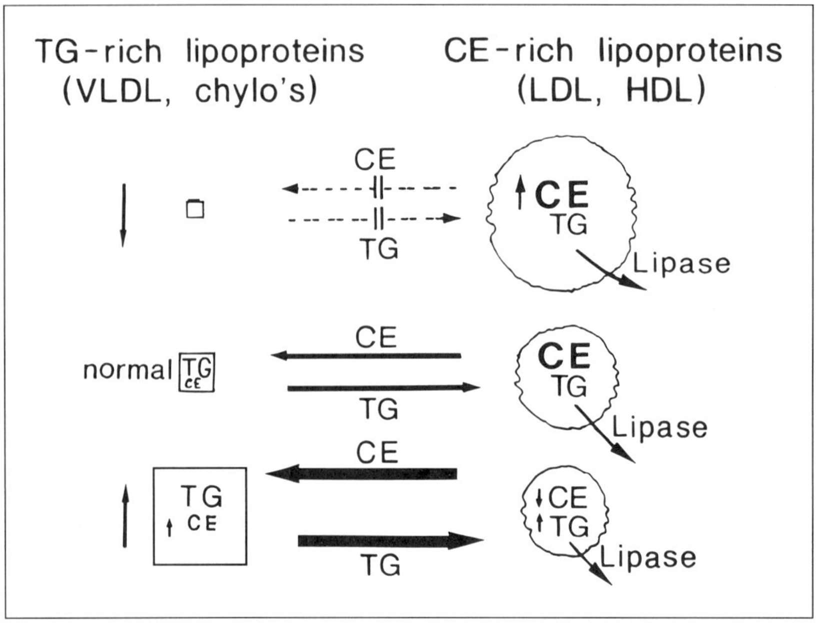

Figure 8-3. The role of neutral lipid exchange processes and lipolysis in modeling human plasma lipoproteins. The scheme depicts three situations in which relative sizes of the triglyceride (*left*) and those of the cholesteryl ester (CE)-rich lipoprotein (*right*) pools vary. Under normal conditions (*middle*), cholesteryl esters that accumulate in low-density lipoprotein (LDL) or high-density lipoprotein (HDL) transfer to the triglyceride (TG)-rich lipoprotein pool, with concomitant transfer of triglycerides to LDL or HDL. The LDL and HDL triglycerides are hydrolyzed by lipases, resulting in LDL and HDL composition and structure as defined in normal subjects. In the top panel, the triglyceride-rich particle pool is almost absent or very small compared with that of the cholesteryl ester lipoproteins. Under these conditions, there is no or relatively little ability to transfer cholesteryl esters out of HDL or LDL, producing abnormally large particles enriched in cholesteryl esters. In the bottom panel, the triglyceride-rich lipoprotein pool is large relative to that of the cholesteryl ester-rich lipoproteins, for example during lipid infusion. With a large triglyceride-rich pool for accepting cholesteryl esters and transferring triglycerides, neutral lipid exchange increases, and LDL and HDL are depleted of cholesteryl esters and acquire triglycerides. Under most conditions, most but not all acquired triglyceride is hydrolyzed in LDL and HDL. Therefore, the sizes of LDL and HDL decrease as they are depleted of cholesteryl ester and acquire triglyceride. VLDL = very low-density lipoprotein; chylo = chylomicron. (From RJ Deckelbaum. Coupled lipid transfer and lipolysis in intravascular processing-remodeling of apoprotein B containing lipoproteins. In K Lippel (ed), *Proceedings of the Workshop on Lipoprotein Heterogeneity*. Washington, DC: National Institutes of Health, Publication No. 87-2616, 1987, p. 57.)

Chylomicron Metabolism

Chylomicrons are synthesized in intestinal absorptive cells as large, triglyceride-rich particles and are secreted into intestinal lymphatics before being released into the circulation from the thoracic duct. In the lymphatics, but mainly in the bloodstream, chylomicrons undergo important compositional changes. They acquire substantial amounts of apo Cs and apo E from HDL and lose phospholipids. In normolipidemic subjects, the half-life of chylomicron triglycerides in the circulation is probably less than 10 to 15 minutes. Triglycerides present in chylomicrons are largely hydrolyzed at the endothelial site of extrahepatic tissues by lipoprotein lipase, a process regulated by apo C-II present on the chylomicron particle. The amount of endothelium-bound lipoprotein lipase is not rate-limiting in healthy individuals [106]. Hydrolysis of triglycerides decreases the lipoprotein core size and is associated with the deletion of surface constituents, namely apo Cs, apo A-I, apo A-IV, phospholipids, and free cholesterol. Other constituents, such as apo B-48 and apo E, appear to remain at the surface of the shrinking particle [6].

The efficiency of chylomicron triglyceride hydrolysis also depends on the action of another group of proteins, the basic proteins (BP)-I (or acylation stimulating protein [ASP]), BP-II, and BP-III. These proteins facilitate the penetration of fatty acids into extrahepatic tissues (e.g., adipocytes, fibroblasts) by stimulating their acylation in the cells [107]. In vitro studies suggest the activity of these proteins to be altered in some common forms of hyperlipidemia (familial combined hyperlipidemia, syndrome X) where an increased number of small and dense $VLDL_3$ are produced by the liver [108]. Decreased BP-I activity together with insulin resistance may result in an impaired uptake of fatty acids by peripheral cells. As previously mentioned, such local accumulation of fatty acids at the endothelial site stops triglyceride hydrolysis at an early stage and releases in the circulation high amounts of free fatty acids together with large remnants loaded with triglycerides and cholesteryl esters (Figure 8-4).

Thus, during its short life in the circulation, chylomicron composition is markedly modified to transform the originally triglyceride-rich particle (with apo-48, A-I, and Cs as major apolipoproteins), into a cholesteryl ester–rich remnant (containing mainly apo-48 and apo E) [6]. In normal conditions, as much as 80% of chylomicron triglycerides may be delivered to extrahepatic tissues, and only 20% or less to the liver. In contrast, cholesteryl esters are delivered mainly (>90%) to the liver. This metabolic scheme accounts for the channeling of chylomicron lipids to different organs: triglycerides to peripheral tissues for storage or utilization, and cholesterol (free and esterified) to the liver. The cholesterol molecules can be reutilized for VLDL formation or excreted into the bile as cholesterol or bile acids [6]. That the liver plays a major role in chylomicron remnant removal is demonstrated by the fact that remnants accumulate in the plasma of hepatectomized animals. These remnants are probably processed by hepatic lipase before binding and uptake [109].

In the sinusoidal spaces of the liver, the chylomicron remnants may be exposed to high concentrations of apo E secreted by hepatocytes. This may facilitate remnant binding to hepatic recep-

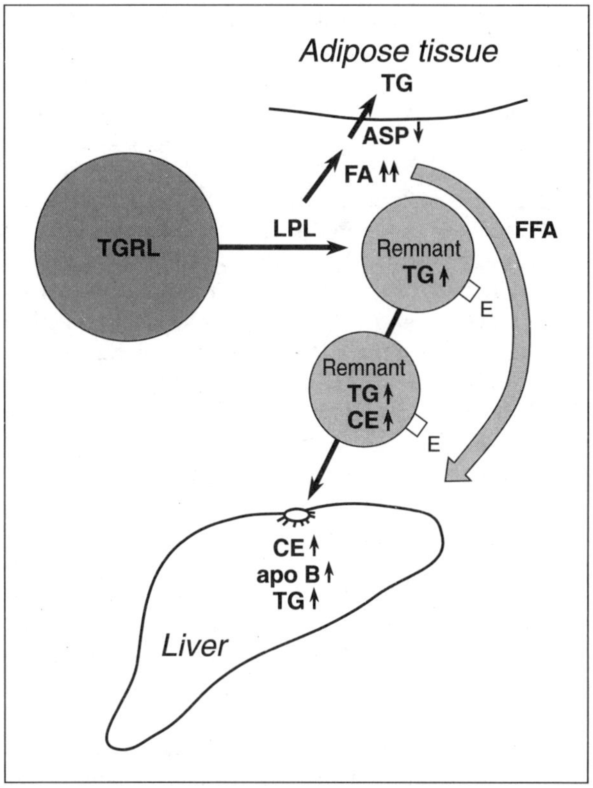

Figure 8-4. Relationship between peripheral lipolysis of triglyceride-rich particles (TGRL) and delivery of fatty acids (FA) to the liver. In normal conditions, FAs released at the endothelial site by the action of lipoprotein lipase (LPL) are largely taken up by peripheral (namely adipose) tissues. Acylation stimulating protein (ASP) stimulates FA reesterification into triglycerides (TG) and increases FA assimilation by adipose tissue. When tissue response to ASP is reduced, high amounts of FA are present at the endothelial site. This leads to the release of abnormally TG-enriched remnants into the circulation that acquire substantial amounts of cholesteryl esters (CEs) by exchange from other lipoproteins. In addition, a large proportion of FAs are released into the circulation and increase the plasma pool of nonesterified FA (FFA). Massive delivery to the liver of FA (as FFA and as TGFA in remnants) stimulates the production of CE, apolipoprotein (apo) B and TG.

tors [110]. Studies in animals have suggested a role for hepatic LDL receptors in the binding of chylomicron remnants [109], but their potential role in humans is still controversial [111]. The presence of apo E on the lipoprotein remnants is essential for their removal, suggesting that a binding site recognizing apo E must be present on the surface of the hepatocyte. A protein that may correspond to the "chylomicron remnant" receptor [110,112] has been isolated from hepatocytes as well as other cells. This receptor, which contains an assembly of four LDL receptor molecules, has been named the LDL receptor–related protein (LRP). In vitro, LRP acts as a clearance receptor for multiple ligands, namely apo E [113], α_2-macroglobulin [114], lipoprotein lipase [94], tissue-type plasminogen activator (t-PA) [115], and urokinase-bound complexes [116]. Although other roles of LRP in vivo have not been precisely determined yet [55], recent studies in transgenic mice [117,118] provide convincing evidence that LRP (in addition to the LDL receptor) is indeed the other hepatic receptor for apo E–mediated uptake of remnants [119].

Elimination of remnants is a much slower process than extrahepatic triglyceride hydrolysis. For example, an oral intake of 70 g of fat leads to prolonged persistence of chylomicron remnants in the plasma, possibly because of a saturation of hepatic uptake [106]. This also offers a likely explanation for the relatively slow elimination of infused lipids when measured after a prolonged infusion, in contrast to the fast triglyceride clearance during the first minutes after a bolus injection (see later discussion).

Metabolism of VLDL, VLDL Remnant, and LDL

The VLDL particles secreted by the liver contain triglycerides and variable amounts of cholesteryl esters in their core. The assembly and secretion of VLDL particles in the liver requires apo B-100 synthesis in conjunction with formation of surface and core lipids. Synthesis of triglycerides depends on the flux of precursor fatty acids (free fatty acids and remnant triglycerides) to the liver and on hepatic lipogenesis. It is regulated by hormones such as insulin [120]. Cholesterol may come from a dietary source or be synthesized in response to a fatty acid load. Apo B production may be stimulated by increasing cholesterol input [121] or cholesteryl ester synthesis [122]. In vitro, oleic acid protects nascent apo B from early degradation, leading to increased net apo B formation. In contrast, eicosapentaenoic acid (EPA) inhibits apo B secretion, and ω-3 fatty acids (EPA and docosahexaenoic acid [DHA]) interfere with lipoprotein packaging into nascent VLDL [123]. Clearly, the flux of fatty acids and cholesterol to the liver acts as a stimulus that can induce increased VLDL formation, although the composition of the VLDL varies depending on the particular primary stimulus [121].

Insulin regulates VLDL lipoprotein production by the liver in two steps. During the early postprandial period, insulin stimulates fatty acid esterification into triglycerides while net apo B-100 production and VLDL secretion are inhibited. At a later stage, when the insulin level falls, apo B-100 degradation stops, and the amount of stored triglycerides dictates the movement of VLDL components into assembly and secretory pathways [123]. Chronic insulin treatment induces insulin resistance and overproduction of VLDL apo B and triglycerides. In vitro studies have shown glucagon and prostaglandins (PGE_2 and PGD_2) to inhibit VLDL secretion [123].

The liver secretes large VLDLs ($VLDL_1$, S_f 60–400) rich in triglycerides and apo E [4]. The lipolyzed $VLDL_1$-derived particles are quickly removed from circulation, mainly by hepatocytes through binding of apo E to cellular receptors, so that few $VLDL_1$ particles are transformed into LDL. Although small amounts of $VLDL_1$ are produced in normal subjects, they are largely secreted in type IV hypertriglyceridemia [5]. Livers of normal subjects produce mainly smaller $VLDL_3$ particles (S_f 20–60) that, being relatively cholesterol-rich and apo E-poor, are quickly transformed into LDL under the action of lipases [5]. In familial combined (or hyper apo B) hyperlipidemia, an increased number of very dense, cholesterol-enriched (and strongly atherogenic) $VLDL_3$ particles are produced by the liver [122].

The intravascular metabolism of native VLDL follows closely that of chylomicrons, at least during the initial steps of the lipolytic process. When released into the circulation, apo Cs and E are transferred from HDL to VLDL, and VLDLs begin their series of interactions with lipoprotein lipase (delivering triglyceride fatty acids to extrahepatic tissues) and undergo a rearrangement of their surface coat. Particles at various stages of lipolysis are found in the plasma, and no less than four intravascular compartments are necessary for adequate simulation of VLDL-apo B kinetics. During lipolysis, apo Cs are transferred back to HDL; some 80% of the phospholipids and free cholesterol present in large-sized VLDL are removed during this process, the major part being transferred to HDL, and also to LDL. However, all apo B-100 and most apo E remain at the surface of the lipolyzed particles, where their relative concentration increases by approximately threefold and twofold, respectively. With continuation of the lipolytic process, the particles become smaller and denser. Like chylomicrons, VLDLs continually exchange neutral lipids with HDLs and LDLs; via this process, they acquire cholesteryl ester, which becomes the major core lipid constituent.

Remnants of VLDL (IDLs) are particles that contain approximately equal amounts of triglycerides and cholesteryl esters and have become heavier than plasma density (1.006–1.019 g/ml). As mentioned, most remnants from large $VLDL_1$ particles are rich in apo E and are degraded primarily via cell-mediated receptor pathways in the liver, whereas remnants derived from apo E-poor $VLDL_3$ particles mainly escape cell uptake and are converted to LDL [6]. In healthy humans, at least 50% of VLDL particles are thought to yield LDLs, which, lacking apo E, are slowly taken up by the liver (~75%) and other tissues (~25%). This occurs for approximately 70% to 80% via an interaction of a receptor-binding domain on apo 100 (between amino acid residues 3000–3500) with the LDL receptor and for approximately 20% to 30% via other receptors or nonreceptor pathways. LRP does not interact efficiently with LDL particles. After binding to the LDL receptor, the receptor-LDL complex is internalized in endosomes that fuse with primary lysosomes to form secondary lysosomes. Lysosomal enzymes degrade apo B into amino acids and hydrolyze LDL cholesteryl esters to free cholesterol and fatty acids. Cholesterol derived from LDL acts as a feedback inhibitor for cell 3-hydroxy-3-methylglutaryl coenzyme A (HMG CoA) reductase activity (which is regulatory for new cell cholesterol synthesis) and also for expression of new LDL receptors. Individuals with genetic abnormalities leading to low receptor–apo B-100 interaction (either from decreased ability to produce normal receptor number or from defective receptors or abnormal apo B) show decreased LDL clearance and increased cholesterol production, resulting in severe hypercholesterolemia [7]. Low-density lipoproteins have a much longer half-life in plasma (3.5 d) than do chylomicrons or VLDL remnants (minutes to hours), so that the number of LDL particles in plasma greatly exceeds that of their precursors [124].

Compelling evidence suggests that LDLs can be oxidized in the arterial wall and that this is likely to play a major role in atherogenesis [125–127]. In this process, LDLs infiltrating the subendothelial space are attacked by reactive oxygen species released by macrophages, smooth muscle cells, or endothelial cells.

Oxidative modifications of LDL affect both the lipid moiety (formation of oxidized lipid derivatives) and surface proteins, mainly apo B-100. Such alterations may mask the apo B binding site to the LDL receptor and create new sites recognized by "scavenger" receptors present on macrophages. Uptake of oxidized LDL by macrophages through this "scavenger" pathway does not exert feedback inhibition on endogenous cholesterol synthesis and on LDL receptor expression at the cell surface. This leads to massive cholesterol accumulation within the macrophages, transforming them into "foam cells" that are found in the arterial wall at the early stages of the fatty streak lesion. Foam cell formation induces a local inflammatory reaction via secretion of mediators such as interleukin-1, growth factors (inducing proliferation of smooth muscle cells), and adhesion molecules on endothelial surface (recruiting circulating monocytes and immobilizing them as macrophages within the atheromatous lesion). Accumulation of macrophages amplifies the rate of LDL oxidation. Oxidized LDLs are chemoattractive and induce procoagulant activity for monocytes [128]. In addition, oxidized LDLs can inactivate production of endothelial-derived relaxing factor (EDRF or nitric oxide) [129]. Of considerable interest, the liver also appears to play an important role in the removal of these modified LDLs (and their oxidized components), primarily by receptors on Kupffer cells [119]. Antioxidants such as α-tocopherol are effective in improving LDL resistance to oxidation [130]. Their use has been associated with a reduced incidence and progression of atherosclerotic lesions.

Lipid and lipoprotein oxidation is likely to occur in several conditions seen in surgical patients (e.g., ischemia-reperfusion, extracorporeal circulation, organ transplantation, severe sepsis) [131], but clinical consequences are still to be evaluated. In parenteral nutrition, emulsion-induced hypertriglyceridemia modifies LDLs' size and composition, making them more susceptible to peroxidative damage. This may be largely amplified by the infusion of emulsions rich in polyunsaturated fatty acids and relatively depleted in α-tocopherol.

High-Density Lipoproteins

High-density lipoproteins have long been recognized as the major agents involved in the reverse cholesterol transport, a mechanism through which excess cholesterol is removed from peripheral tissues to be delivered to the liver and to tissues showing active genesis of steroids (e.g., adrenals and gonads). It is widely believed that reverse cholesterol transport is antiatherogenic and, possibly as important, that this process represents the only means for cholesterol elimination from cells, thereby regulating cell-membrane homeostasis and normal cell function [132].

Different mechanisms have been described for cholesterol efflux from cells. After HDL binding to cell surface [132], cholesterol may passively diffuse from cell membranes to acceptor apolipoproteins and lipoproteins [133]; alternatively, HDL may be internalized in the cell before being resecreted after cholesterol enrichment (retroendocytosis) [134]. Binding of HDL to the cell surface may involve either transient linkage to specific lipid domains on cell membrane [135] or binding to protein receptors [136]. Binding of HDL to protein receptors may promote cholesterol translocation from intracellular pools to plasma membrane, from which it is transferred to the extracellular HDL acceptor. The apolipoprotein composition of HDL may influence cellular cholesterol efflux. In vitro, apo A-I, A-II, and A-IV are capable of promoting cholesterol efflux [137]; however, at least in some tissues, LpA-I particles (lacking apo A-II) appear to be more efficient than LpA-I:A-II particles [24].

In the vascular compartment, portions of chylomicron and VLDL surface (including phospholipids, free cholesterol, apo A-I, A-IV, and Cs) are released during extrahepatic lipolysis to form new HDL particles [138]. Cholesterol esterification by HDL-associated LCAT (and transfer of cholesteryl esters in particle core) drives the influx of further free cholesterol into HDL from other lipoproteins and cell membranes (e.g., erythrocytes, endothelial cells). In humans, CETP activity-mediated exchanges with triglyceride-rich lipoproteins leads to the formation of large, partially cholesteryl ester–depleted, triglyceride-enriched HDL. Thus, the combined action of LCAT and CETP converts small and dense HDL_3 into large, less dense HDL_2. HDL_2-triglycerides may then be hydrolyzed by hepatic lipase [139]. Phospholipase activity of hepatic lipase remodels surface lipids [140] with a loss of apo A-I, which may be recycled to form new small discoidal HDL [132,141] or directly catabolized in the liver or the kidney [138].

Thus, there is a cycle through which HDL_3 particles become enlarged by influx of lipids (phospholipids, free cholesterol) and LCAT action. This is followed by transfer of cholesteryl esters and acquisition of triglycerides (CETP activity) leading to the formation of large HDL_2. Finally, triglyceride and phospholipid hydrolysis by hepatic lipase reconverts HDL_2 into HDL_3. This final step is accompanied by hepatic removal of cholesterol and loss of apo A-I.

In the reverse transport process, cholesterol removed from peripheral tissues may be delivered to the liver directly from HDL or after CETP-mediated transfer to other lipoproteins (chylomicron, VLDL, and LDL). Two putative HDL receptors have been recently isolated from a neoplastic line of hepatocytes [142]. Cholesterol transferred to the liver may be excreted in the bile or used for assembly of new lipoproteins.

The protective effect of HDL against the development of atherosclerosis lies not only in the removal of excess cholesterol from arterial walls, but also in their antioxidant properties. Indeed, HDLs were recently found to protect LDLs from peroxidation by inhibiting neutrophil degradation and superoxide O_2^- production [143] and by scavenging free radicals produced in vivo by various phagocytic cells [144]. In addition, paraoxonase, an HDL-associated enzyme, inhibits the generation of lipid peroxides in LDL [145]. Finally, HDL may have a specific affinity for selectively and rapidly removing oxidized lipids from the arterial wall and delivering them to the liver [146]. Such strong antioxidant properties may apply in sites other than the arterial wall and suggest HDL to play a role in conditions other than atherosclerosis. In this respect, HDL levels are often markedly (but transiently) reduced in acute-phase conditions (e.g., trauma, burns, sepsis), suggesting interactions between HDL and the immune and hematologic systems. Acquisition of apo SAA (produced in high amounts in acute conditions) may direct HDL to sites of injury or infection to deliver lipid components for tissue repair and rapidly proliferating immune cells. Trapping by HDL of superoxide anion O_2^- may prevent its reaction with nitric oxide and maintain vessel relaxation [147]. Antithrombotic properties of HDL may also result from the regulating effect of HDL–apo A-I on prostacyclin (PGI_2) catabolism, indirectly affecting platelet aggregation [148]. Furthermore, apo H (β_2-glycoprotein I), a potent inhibitor of the intrinsic pathway of coagulation, and the "lipoprotein-associated coagulation inhibitor" (LACI) or "extrinsic pathway inhibitor" (EPI) are (at least partly) bound to HDL [76,149]. During bacterial infections, the formation of HDL-endotoxin complexes has long been recognized as an important means of neutralizing agent toxicity [150]. Antiviral properties of HDL have been reported in herpes simplex virus and human immunodeficiency virus (HIV), namely via inhibition by HDL–apo A-I of cell penetration, intracellular replication, and syncytium formation [151]. HDLs are capable of inhibiting the cytolytic activity of complement [82,152], and of binding immunoglobulins through an interaction with apo J [80].

These protective properties of HDL against infection, inflammation, and thrombosis represent promising areas of investigation and may certainly be relevant to the metabolic care of many patients receiving parenteral nutrition, a condition usually associated with low HDL (and apo A-I) levels. In addition to bypassing the intestinal mucosa, it is plausible that some intravenous nutrients may cause increased catabolism of HDL components. [*Editor's Note:* The current thinking in general is that lipid emulsions, especially when given in excess, increase the incidence of infection. The mechanisms given are vague, such as interference with the reticuloendothelial systems. Future research similar to that outlined in this paragraph would be highly useful.]

Structure and Composition of Lipid Emulsions

The role of plasma lipoproteins is to serve as vehicles for transport of water-insoluble lipids (triglycerides, cholesterol, and vitamins) from sites of synthesis and absorption to sites of utilization and storage. Similarly, lipid emulsions provide triglyceride fatty acids to different tissues. Particles forming these emulsions have been designed on the model of an endogenous triglyceride-rich lipoprotein, the chylomicron [153]. These emulsions contain a core made essentially of triglycerides (with some tocopherols, vitamin K, and esterified phytosterols) stabilized by a surface layer of phospholipids (with some free cholesterol and phytosterols). Their diameter, like chylomicrons, generally ranges between 100 and 500 nm, with a mean value of 200 to 350 nm. However, there are significant differences in lipid composition between emulsion particles and endogenous chylomicrons [154]. In contrast to chylomicrons, for example, practically no cholesteryl ester molecules are dissolved in the triglyceride core of artificial particles; only little amounts of free cholesterol (and other vegetable sterols) and no apoproteins are present on their surface. The relative phospholipid content of emulsions exceeds that of chylomicrons, this difference being particularly marked in most 10% preparations. As an example, 10%, 20%, and 30% Intralipid preparations contain the same amount of phospholipid emulsifier (1.2 g/100 ml) to stabilize 10, 20, and 30 g of triglycerides, respectively. In fact, lipid emulsions contain two different particle populations that can be separated by short-term ultracentrifugation in saline (or passage through sepharose columns). One population consists of triglyceride-rich particles (resembling chylomicrons) that float at plasma density, and the other consists of phospholipid-rich particles resembling liposomes (mean particle diameter, 80–100 nm) that are isolated in the aqueous infranatant [155]. Ultracentrifugation of 10% Intralipid separates one third of phospholipids as surface component and two thirds as liposomal particles; in contrast, two thirds of phospholipids contained in the 20% emulsion are surface components of the triglyceride-rich particles, and only one third are present as liposomal particles. Thus, at equal triglyceride intake, 10% Intralipid provides twofold more phospholipids but four times more liposomes than 20% Intralipid [156], and three times more phospholipids and eight to ten times more liposomes than does 30% Intralipid [155]. [*Editor's Note:* This little-appreciated fact should be emphasized.] As discussed later, liposomal phospholipids can interfere at different steps of lipid and lipoprotein metabolism, and they can also modify the lipid composition of cell membranes.

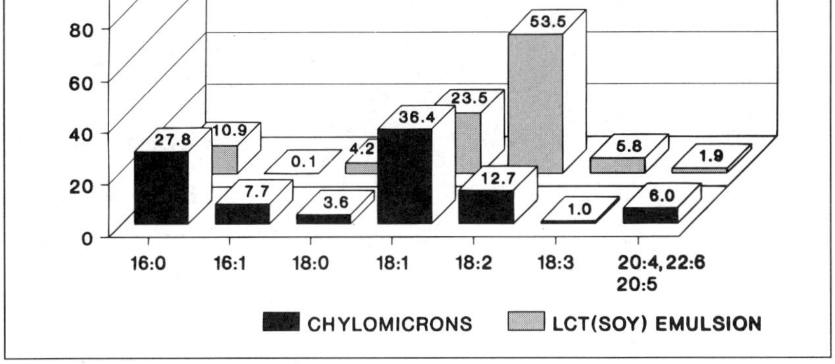

Figure 8-5. Fatty acid pattern of triglyceride fatty acids present in the chylomicron (average values) and in a long-chain triglyceride, soybean-based emulsion (LCT [soy]). (From YA Carpentier. Intravascular metabolism of fat emulsions: The Arvid Wretlind Lecture, ESPEN 1988. *Clin Nutr* 8:115, 1989.)

In addition, substantial differences in the lipid composition exist between the different preparations currently available or at different stages of evaluation. Until recently, lipid emulsions were made of soybean or safflower oil (or a mixture of both) and contained exclusively long-chain triglycerides (LCT). Since 1984, an emulsion has been marketed in Europe with a 50%-50% (w:w) blend of medium-chain triglycerides (MCT) and LCT in the particle core (Figure 8-5). Emulsions supplemented with fish oil–containing ω-3 fatty acids, emulsions derived from olive oil, and preparations made with structured triglycerides (containing both long- and medium-chain fatty acids on the same glycerol backbone) are currently under evaluation.

In most available preparations, egg phosphatides are used as emulsifiers to stabilize the triglyceride content. However, differences in the proportion of phospholipid subcomponents that can be found between the emulsifiers used by different manufacturers (and even between preparations manufactured by the same company) may also influence the metabolism of lipid components.

It is also important to point out the marked differences of fatty acid composition between the triglyceride and phospholipid components of the emulsion. As expected, triglycerides derived from vegetable oils (soybean, safflower, olive) are very rich in C18 monounsaturated or polyunsaturated fatty acids, with a preeminence of the ω-6 series, whereas egg-yolk–derived phospholipids contain a majority of saturated fatty acids.

We propose to review the intravascular processes involved in the metabolism of both types of emulsion particles and to stress the potential influence of the composition of lipid constituents on selected steps (Figure 8-6).

Metabolism of Lipid Emulsions

Metabolism of Triglyceride-Rich Emulsion Particles

The major steps governing the intravascular metabolism of these particles closely resemble those described above for the chylomicron. For example, lipoprotein lipase is most likely the major lipase

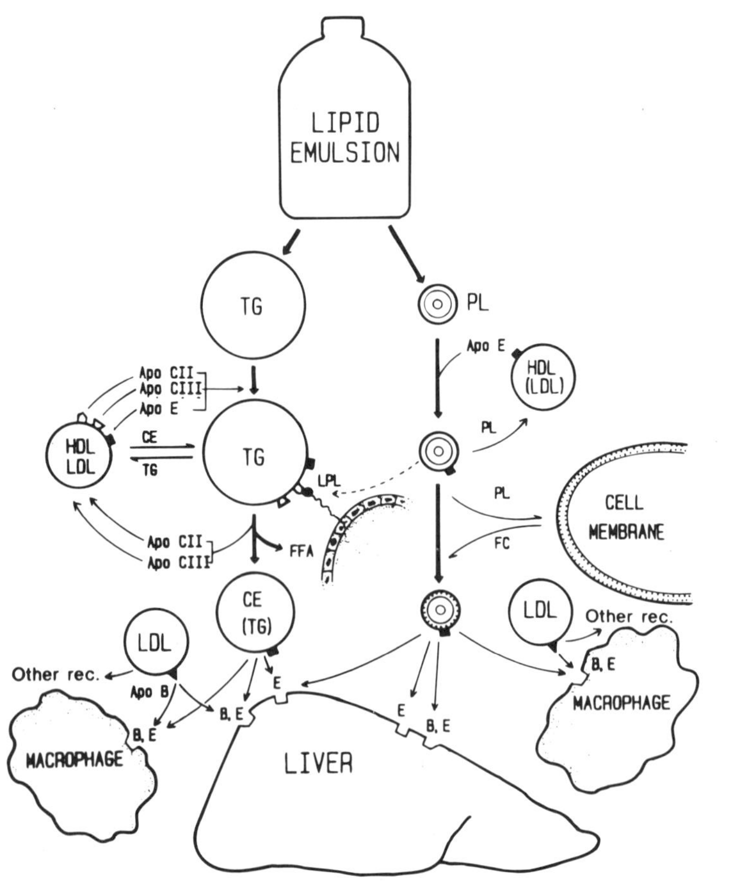

Figure 8-6. Intravascular metabolism of both triglyceride (TG)-rich and phospholipid (PL)-rich particles present in a lipid emulsion. The four key steps previously outlined for the metabolism of endogenous chylomicrons are represented for the triglyceride-rich emulsion particles. On the right side, the formation of phospholipid-free cholesterol (FC) complexes having acquired apolipoprotein (Apo) E is represented, as is the competitive effect of liposomes for lipoprotein lipase. In the lower part, we have speculated on the potential competition of exogenous remnants among themselves and with endogenous lipoproteins for binding to the low-density lipoprotein (LDL) B,E receptor and the chylomicron remnant E receptor, at the site of different tissues. HDL = high-density lipoprotein; FFA = free fatty acid. (From YA Carpentier. Intravascular metabolism of fat emulsions: The Arvid Wretlind Lecture, ESPEN 1988. *Clin Nutr* 8:115, 1989.)

responsible for emulsion triglyceride hydrolysis at the endothelial wall, and the kinetics expressing plasma triglyceride clearance after injection of chylomicrons or emulsions show striking similarities [157].

Acquisition of Apoproteins

Acquisition of selected apoproteins is a key step in the regulation of emulsion triglyceride metabolism. A rapid and substantial transfer of apo Cs and apo E can be demonstrated during in vitro incubation of emulsion particles with a purified fraction of HDL [158]. By contrast, almost no transfer of apo A-I and A-II is detected.

During six-hour infusions of Intralipid in normal subjects, the transfer of apoproteins C-II, C-III, and E from a large HDL reservoir to the d < 1.006 g/ml fraction (containing the vast majority of exogenous triglyceride-rich particles) was directly related to the plasma concentration of triglycerides induced by lipid infusion [159]. At triglyceride levels of 1000 mg/dl, more than 90% of plasma apo C-II, 80% to 85% of apo C-III, and 60% to 70% of apo E were found in the plasma emulsion fraction, and the relative proportion of apoproteins was similar to that of circulating chylomicrons. Again, transfer of apoprotein A-I, A-II, and B was not significant. Recent data suggest that apo A-IV also transfers between HDL and triglyceride-rich particles.

Except for rare cases of congenital deficiency or major urinary losses, decreased availability of apo C-II is unlikely to become a limiting factor for extrahepatic hydrolysis of circulating triglycerides, because only minimal amounts are needed to activate lipoprotein lipase [160]. In contrast, adding apo E to triglyceride-rich particles of different size ranges increases their endocytosis by various types of cells in vitro [61].

The composition of both triglycerides and phospholipids can certainly affect the physical properties of the surface layer and is likely to influence the acquisition of apoproteins by emulsion particles. However, this factor and its potential consequences on the intravascular metabolism of lipid emulsions have not yet been investigated in depth.

Triglyceride Hydrolysis

Hydrolysis of exogenous triglycerides is regulated by endogenous factors as well as by the lipid composition of the emulsion. Hydrolysis of emulsion triglycerides at endothelial sites of extrahepatic tissues depends not only on the availability of active lipoprotein lipase and on the size of exchangeable pools of apo Cs, but also on the capability for underlying tissues to directly assimilate released fatty acids [96] and on plasma albumin to bind the fraction of fatty acids spilled into the circulation as free (or nonesterified) fatty acids. The second step consists of hydrolysis of triglycerides remaining in remnant particles after peripheral lipolysis by lipoprotein lipase. This takes place mainly in the liver, either by the action of hepatic lipase at the endothelial sites or within the hepatocytes after cell uptake of whole remnant particles. This latter process appears to be regulated by ligands such as apo E and lipoprotein lipase present on emulsion remnants [94], but also by proteoglycans and remnant receptors on cell membranes [55]. This process of remnant removal is probably not restricted to hepatocytes. As discussed later, some triglycerides leave the emulsion particles to be transferred to endogenous LDL and HDL, but this fraction is quite small in comparison to that undergoing hydrolysis.

The fatty acid composition of emulsion triglycerides markedly influences their hydrolysis by lipoprotein lipase. Experimental preparations containing only MCT are hydrolyzed much faster than pure LCT emulsions; this is related to the higher degree of MCT solubility at the emulsion surface [88]. When both MCT and LCT are included within the same emulsion particles, MCTs are hydrolyzed at a considerably faster rate than are LCTs, and the remnant particles become progressively enriched with LCT [161]. Redgrave and coauthors have studied in the rat the influence on triglyceride hydrolysis of different arrangements of saturated and unsaturated long-chain acyl chains on the glycerol backbone [162] and have emphasized the particular role for the fatty acid in the sn-2 position [163]. Such information should be particularly relevant when considering the design of new types of structured triglycerides containing, for example, both medium-chain fatty acids and long-chain fatty acids on the same glycerol backbone.

Emulsions containing different types of triglycerides have been tested in man. In most instances, triglycerides from emulsions containing a mixture of MCT and LCT were cleared quite faster than those containing exclusively LCT. Recent data suggest that this is not only the result of a faster peripheral hydrolysis by lipoprotein lipase, but also of a prompt removal of remnant particles and their constituents [164]. In vitro, these emulsions containing both MCT and LCT within the same particle are hydrolyzed faster than a corresponding mixture of MCT and LCT emulsions, but this difference is attenuated in plasma-like conditions [165].

As discussed later, the amount of phospholipids relative to triglycerides can influence the hydrolysis of emulsion triglycerides. This effect is particularly striking in premature infants who more rapidly clear emulsions with a relatively low phospholipid:triglyceride ratio (e.g., 20% emulsions or 10% emulsions with a reduced phospholipid content) than regular 10% emulsions [156,166]. The composition of phospholipid emulsifier can also substantially affect triglyceride hydrolysis, as shown by comparing preparations with soy vs. egg-derived phosphatides or with different proportions of phospholipid fractions [167]. In addition, our group reported that subtle differences in the phosphatidylethanolamine:phosphatidylcholine ratio of egg-derived phospholipid emulsifier can substantially influence the metabolism of emulsions with a similar triglyceride composition [168].

Intravascular Neutral Lipid Exchanges

Similar to triglyceride-rich lipoproteins, emulsion particles can serve as donors of triglycerides and acceptors of cholesteryl esters during CETP-mediated exchanges of neutral lipids with cholesterol-rich lipoproteins [98]. In vitro and in vivo studies have confirmed that plasma triglyceride levels are a major determinant of cholesteryl ester transfer in human plasma [169]. Still, other factors (e.g., free fatty acids and phospholipids) may influence this process [3]. It is of interest that no change in CETP mass was found during lipid infusion.

Emulsions containing MCTs appear to transfer more triglycerides and to accept fewer cholesteryl esters than pure LCT preparations. In fact, spontaneous transfer of MCT occurs even in the absence of CETP and without reciprocal transfer of cholesteryl esters [105]. Again, this is probably associated with the higher solubility of MCT in phospholipids. As a result, remnants formed after extrahepatic lipolysis of MCT-containing emulsions contain far fewer cholesteryl esters than do those derived from LCT particles [166].

Metabolism of Emulsion Phospholipid-Rich Particles

Phospholipids and free cholesterol increase in plasma during lipid infusion in preterm infants and likely in adults as well. However, an association between these changes and the excessive amounts of phospholipid-rich liposomes present in 10% emulsions has not been clearly recognized until recently [166,170]. The limited content of cholesterol in lipid emulsions can account for only a fraction of plasma-free cholesterol rise. The major part originates from other body sources and is absorbed into the plasma compartment by phospholipids until a 1:1 molar ratio is reached between both lipids. This forms free cholesterol–phospholipid complexes that bind to albumin and acquire different apoproteins present in the circulation, namely, apoproteins E, A-I, and possibly Cs and A-IV. These complexes show similarities to Lp-X found in the plasma of cholestatic patients with respect to density and composition [14,15]. They can be isolated by zonal ultracentrifugation in a subfraction located between IDL and LDL populations.

Phospholipid liposomes have been suggested to have a potential for removing cholesterol from atherosclerotic plaques [16,171]. This would be helpful only if the resulting free cholesterol-phospholipid complexes were promptly and efficiently eliminated by the liver and cholesterol excreted in the bile. However, it is unlikely that such cholesterol removal would be so selective; indeed, it was shown that the membrane of cells in contact with the circulation such as erythrocytes was depleted of free cholesterol during infusions of phospholipid-rich emulsions [172]. In addition, Lp-X-like particles have a rather long half-life and interfere with the binding of LDL particles to their specific B,E receptors. This may induce accumulation of LDL, which might then be directed to non-receptor mediated pathways. As mentioned earlier, liposomal complexes may interfere with the hydrolysis of infused triglycerides, probably by competing with the triglyceride-rich particles for binding to endothelial lipoprotein lipase. This effect has been demonstrated in vitro [173] and also in vivo under conditions of limited availability of lipoprotein lipase, e.g., in premature infants receiving lipid-containing parenteral nutrition [166] or in adult subjects infused at high rate [169]. Under such conditions, preparations with a high phospholipid:triglyceride ratio (e.g., most 10% emulsions) induce a higher and sustained rise not only of phospholipids and free cholesterol, but also of plasma triglycerides. Of interest, accumulation of phospholipids in the liver has been reported after prolonged administration of parenteral emulsions [174]. The high content of phosphatidylcholine in the emulsifier has been suggested to represent an appreciable supply of choline [175], but other metabolic considerations suggest limiting phospholipid intake [176].

Other Components of Lipid Emulsions

In addition to triglycerides and phospholipids, lipid emulsions also contain liposoluble vitamins present in vegetable oils as well as free cholesterol and vegetable sterols or phytosterols. Soybean-derived emulsions contain relatively large amounts of tocopherols, but many more γ- and δ-

tocopherols (~92%) than natural vitamin E or α-tocopherol (~8%) [177,178]. γ-tocopherol is a less potent antioxidative agent than α-tocopherol. Both agents are not widely distributed to extrahepatic tissues during peripheral triglyceride lipolysis and remain largely in the remnant particle to be taken up by the liver [179]. At this point, α-tocopherol is selectively recognized by a hepatic protein and is repackaged into newly secreted VLDL, and γ-tocopherol is eliminated in the bile [180]. In addition, α-tocopherol may be exchanged between plasma lipoproteins. During infusion of soy-derived emulsion, α-tocopherol is transferred from LDL and HDL to emulsion particles. LDL and HDL depletion of vitamin E may be prevented only if α-tocopherol content is raised in the emulsion [181].

Depletion of α-tocopherol in LDL and HDL may become a matter of concern because vitamin E is perhaps the most active agent protecting lipoproteins and cell membranes from lipid peroxidative damage caused by free radicals [182]. Indeed, patients receiving long-term parenteral nutrition with Intralipid usually have low α-tocopherol levels and are more prone to oxidative alteration of ω-3 and ω-6 fatty acids, as measured by high elimination rates of ethane and pentane in the expired air [183,184]. Such increase of pentane excretion during lipid infusion corresponds to oxidation of linoleate, present in high concentrations in soy- and safflower-based emulsions, and results from an imbalance between the large intake of polyunsaturated fatty acids compared with that of antioxidants [185]. Furthermore, several authors have recently expressed concern that peroxidative products were generated within lipid emulsions derived from soybean oil and that this was superimposed on the low α-tocopherol status to cause severe side effects in preterm infants, particularly when they receive oxygen or ultraviolet therapy [186–188].

The presence of different plant sterols in both surface and core moieties of emulsions has recently raised concern [189]. Some of these plant sterols, which are either not absorbed or are absorbed only in tiny amounts by the intestine in normal conditions, may interfere with the metabolism of cholesterol [190]. Plasma accumulation of several phytosterols as well as of sitostanol and cholestanol has been observed during parenteral nutrition with lipid emulsions and was associated with cholestatic liver disease and thrombocytopenia.

As recently noted, the vitamin K content of lipid emulsion substantially varies between the available preparations in relation to the source of vegetable oils used [191]. This content is relatively high in soy-derived emulsions and may influence the response to coumarin-based anticoagulants.

Methods for Studying the Metabolism of Lipid Emulsions

It has been assumed that the rate of triglyceride elimination from emulsion particles is an important determinant of emulsion metabolism. However, studies under different conditions of feeding vs. fasting states clearly show an enhancement of plasma clearance, but a reduction of lipid oxidation, in relation to insulin level. This was particularly striking in patients studied after an overnight fast and again during infusion of large glucose loads [192].

Most experiments on human subjects are performed after an overnight fast, a condition characterized by a progressive and continuous increase in the rate of fat mobilization from adipose stores together with enhanced fat oxidation and ketone production. We have shown that plasma free fatty acids and ketones as well as lipid oxidation could be stabilized at low levels within a period of 3 hours by a combined infusion of glucose and amino acids; these parameters remained stable for at least another 6 hours, allowing evaluation of the metabolism of exogenous lipids with minimal interference from the endogenous depots [193]. In addition, the rates of glucose and amino acid infusion required to obtain this effect closely reproduced the condition of patients receiving parenteral nutrition.

Triglyceride elimination is usually measured by following the decay of triglyceride concentration during a short period of time after a bolus injection of exogenous lipids [157]. The slope is divided into a zero order kinetic segment characterized by the maximal elimination rate coefficient, k1, and a first order kinetic segment corresponding to the fractional removal rate coefficient, k2. This method has several limitations [194]. It mainly measures the elimination of triglycerides from newly infused particles, which is much faster than that from partially lipolyzed particles. The assumption is generally made that the process takes place within the vascular compartment, which does not take into account the possibility for emulsion particles to be distributed outside plasma (into one or several compartments) or sequestered at selected intravascular sites. Emulsion particles may displace intravascular endogenous lipids from capillary beds and release them into plasma. Also, exogenous particles have the potential for competing with endogenous lipoproteins for extrahepatic and hepatic lipolytic sites, thus impeding catabolism and increasing plasma concentration of the latter. Finally, released fatty acids may stimulate intracellular triglyceride re-esterification and formation of new endogenous lipoproteins [195].

Infusing, at the same constant rate, emulsions differing in the composition of their lipid constituents generally induces different changes of plasma lipids and indicates which preparation is associated with a faster elimination of exogenous triglycerides (or phospholipids). However, when attempting to determine the role of lipid composition on the properties of different triglyceride-rich emulsion particles (with respect, for example, to neutral lipid exchanges or release of free fatty acids and lipoprotein lipase in the circulation), it is essential to compare similar plasma concentrations of exogenous particles.

Therefore, it seemed important to develop an experimental model where plasma triglyceride concentration would be quickly raised at a predetermined level and maintained constant for several hours. This is obtained by regularly adjusting the infusion rate of (any) lipid emulsion in subjects receiving a combined infusion of glucose and amino acids, as described above [196]. Maintaining such a steady state offers substantial advantages over the previous models. It is reasonable to assume that if infused triglycerides were to be distributed into several compartments, an equilibrium of fluxes between these compartments would occur during the test period. If so, triglyceride removal, which equals the amount infused, represents hydrolysis plus remnant particle clearance. Still, secretion of endogenous triglyceride-rich lipoproteins in response to lipid infusions is not taken into account.

The first applications of this test have demonstrated an enhanced sensitivity in measuring plasma triglyceride elimination compared with previous tests; indeed, differences of elimination rate between various emulsions were larger, and interindividual variability (even between carefully selected normal subjects) was greater than expected from measurements of plasma triglyceride decay after a bolus injection [164]. In contrast to other tests, information from the clamp may be used for recommending a range of infusion rates that will not lead to massive accumulation of infused lipids in most patients receiving parenteral nutrition. The clamp may be particularly useful to ascertain emulsion elimination rate in patients known to present impaired clearance, e.g., those with renal failure [197].

Refined analyses of lipoprotein fractions and of fatty acid pattern in plasma lipids as well as indirect calorimetry measurements may be performed during the hypertriglyceridemic clamp. The association of selected parameters provides a powerful tool for understanding how much the composition of emulsion components influences the metabolism of triglyceride-rich particles, their interaction with other plasma lipoproteins, and lipid contribution to total body energy consumption. In view of the renewed interest for postprandial lipoproteins in lipidology, the hypertriglyceridemic clamp offers an alternative to the oral fat load for studying particular features of chylomicron metabolism in patients [198,199].

Including Lipid Emulsions in Parenteral Nutrition Regimens: Current Status and Future Perspectives

Lipid emulsions are used to provide a large amount of energy within a limited volume, but also as a source of essential fatty acids. From a practical viewpoint, lipid emulsions are isotonic to plasma and can be infused in peripheral veins. Of interest, lipid infusions were reported to prolong the patency of peripheral venous access because of a putative protective role on the endothelium [200,201]. They can also be used in various "all-in-one" preparations, but the stability of emulsions in specific mixtures has to be carefully assessed before routine clinical use.

In addition to triglycerides, the emulsions also supply glycerol (some present in concentrations of 2.25–2.5 g/dl and some released by triglyceride hydrolysis) that is expected to be rapidly converted to glucose in the liver and kidneys. Triglyceride fatty acids represent an efficient source of energy for many tissues of the body. Their oxidation is associated with a lower respiratory quotient ($\sim$0.7) than that of glucose (1.0). Although oxidation of ^{13}C-octanoate was found to be markedly higher (and faster) than that of palmitate (or oleate) [202], including MCTs in a lipid mixture appears to slow long-chain fatty acid oxidation and does not markedly enhance total body fat oxidation [203 and unpublished personal data]. Also, the concept that medium-chain fatty acids do not require carnitine coupling before crossing the mitochondrial membrane is well known [204]; this may apply in hepatocytes, but probably not in extrahepatic tissue [205]. Still, hepatic β-oxidation of medium-chain fatty acids produces relatively large amounts of ketone bodies, which represent an excellent fuel for several kinds of tissues including brain, intestinal mucosa, and lymphocytes. For example, maintenance of moderate ketosis with a 70:30 MCT:LCT emulsion was reported to help control seizures in a 5-year-old child [206].

Of further interest, infusion of medium-chain fatty acids either in triglyceride mixtures or in structured triglycerides leads to much lower rates of fatty acid recycling in adipose tissues than are observed with LCTs [207]. Use of lipid emulsions in parenteral nutrition allows a decrease in the concomitant intake of glucose calories and a reduction in many complications associated with large glucose loads in critically ill patients. These classically cited side effects include hyperglycemia with glucosuria and serum hyperosmolarity, high production of carbon dioxide and pulmonary hyperventilation, increased catecholamine release, excessive glycogen and fat deposition in the liver, and hypophosphatemia. In addition, problems consecutive to abnormal protein glycosylation and to enhanced peroxidative reactions should be more carefully considered [208].

Fat deposition in the liver is markedly reduced by lipid-containing vs. glucose-based parenteral nutrition. Although it was primarily related to the supply of essential fatty acids [209], this effect is at least as marked with medium-chain fatty acids containing emulsions [210].

The lower levels of circulating insulin in lipid-containing (vs. glucose-based) parenteral nutrition are associated with a lesser inhibition of fat mobilization from endogenous adipose stores and of branched-chain amino acid release from muscles, the latter being suggested to improve portasystemic encephalopathy [211]. [*Editor's Note:* On the other hand, the traditional view, as seemingly confirmed by meta-analysis (see Chapter 24), is that mixtures enriched with branched-chain amino acids work best when supplied with glucose.]

In contrast to glucose, high plasma levels of emulsion components (triglycerides and phospholipids) are not thought to be directly associated with severe clinical side effects, with a notable exception for acute pancreatitis [212] if plasma triglycerides were to exceed 1000 mg/dL as commonly observed in patients with type V hyperlipoproteinemia [213,214]. Until recently, little attention was paid to the rate of lipid infusion and the associated changes of plasma lipids. In fact, plasma concentration of plasma lipids is not currently monitored in clinical practice, and proper elimination of infused emulsion is often evaluated by checking whether blood samples drawn at 4 or 6 h after cessation of infusion no longer show opalescent (milky) plasma.

However, the vast majority of side effects attributed to lipid emulsions have been observed when excessive infusion rates were used, as recently reviewed [215,216]. The concept that infusions at a rate exceeding the lipolytic capacity of endothelial lipases result in a direct accumulation of triglycerides in the reticuloendothelial system has often been advocated [217]. However, other factors associated with high-rate lipid infusions could be more directly involved in the development of side effects, e.g., fatty acid toxicity, peroxidative damage, and eicosanoid imbalance.

The toxicity of free fatty acids (unbound to albumin) is well established, and a marked rise of plasma free fatty acids remains a matter of serious concern, especially in patients with low plasma albumin or high bilirubin levels. Of interest, co-infusion of glucose increases free fatty acid removal so that excessively high levels (> 1.5 mmol/L) are usually not observed except in the case of heparin administration [218]. Note also that infusions of MCT-containing emulsions at a similar rate induce higher rises of plasma free fatty acids than infusions of pure LCT.

Changes of lipid composition in endogenous lipoproteins are correlated with the level of hypertriglyceridemia, as shown by several experiments using a single infusion in normal subjects [154]. In this respect, it is interesting to note that MCT-containing emulsions affect HDL cholesterol levels markedly less than do pure LCT emulsions, as confirmed in patients on long-term parenteral nutrition [219]. Also, the potential for remnants formed during the extrahepatic metabolism of triglyceride-rich particles to compete with α_2-macroglobulin for the same hepatic (LRP) receptor may be implied in the enhanced liver toxicity of tumor necrosis factor in animals fed parenterally [220]. This aspect may prove to be particularly important in severely septic patients as well as in those with impaired liver function.

In contrast to these negative aspects of emulsion-induced hypertriglyceridemia, the concept that the cytokine-induced production of triglycerides in sepsis (together with a delayed removal) is a positive response [221] has led some authors to suggest that, similarly to VLDL and chylomicrons, emulsion particles may have a protective role in binding and neutralizing endotoxins [222]. However, one should keep in mind that HDLs are particularly active in this mechanism [223] and that their level is negatively affected by increasing triglyceride concentration.

Emulsion phospholipids are cleared less efficiently than are the triglycerides and can progressively accumulate in association with free cholesterol, especially during infusions of emulsions with a high phospholipid:triglyceride ratio (w:w > 0.06). Apart from impeding triglyceride elimination during infusion at a rate close to saturation of the lipolytic processes, modification of the phospholipid:cholesterol ratio in red blood cell

(RBC) membranes has been associated with diminished oxygen diffusion capacity [224].

Soybean- and safflower-derived emulsions provide large amounts of essential fatty acids (mainly of the ω-6 family), and their use prevents or corrects clinical symptoms of essential ω-6 fatty acid deficiency. However, several issues need to be addressed: (1) the optimal proportion of essential vs. nonessential fatty acids in lipid preparations; (2) the balance between ω-6 and ω-3 fatty acid supply; (3) the need for providing long-chain polyunsaturated fatty acids (rather than exclusively carbon 18 precursors) in selected patients; and (4) the amount of antioxidants relative to the content of polyunsaturated fatty acids.

To address the first points, we have measured the fatty acid pattern of RBC membranes in a group of patients with inflammatory bowel disease (IBD) who were randomly crossed-over to receive home parenteral nutrition (HPN) with a 20% soy-derived LCT and a 20% MCT/LCT emulsion for two consecutive periods of three months [225]. The fatty acid pattern of RBC phospholipids was modified after 3 months of HPN only with LCT. Changes consisted of an enrichment in linoleate (18:2 ω-6) and a relative depletion in arachidonate (20:4 ω-6) as well as in docosohexaenoate (22:6 ω-3). Both arachidonate:linoleate and ω-3:ω-6 fatty acid ratios decreased below control values. In contrast, HPN with MCT/LCT (which supplies only half of carbon 18 essential fatty acids provided by the LCT emulsion) did not change the fatty acid pattern of RBC phospholipids and even corrected the pattern in those patients infused with LCT during the first period. Thus, the use of a mixed MCT/LCT emulsion (at a dose of 1.5 g triacylglycerols/kg/d) can largely prevent the changes of fatty acid pattern associated with the excessive amount of linoleate supplied by similar loads of soybean- and safflower-derived emulsions. Other observations in preterm infants [226] and experimental studies in dogs [227] showed that accumulation of linoleate in plasma and several tissue phospholipids occurred within a rather short period of time (< 7 d). This decreased content of long-chain polyunsaturated fatty acids has raised serious concern about the suitability of soybean emulsions in premature infants where arachidonate and docosohexaenoate are known to play key roles in growth and maturation of the central nervous system and the retina, respectively [228]. Of interest, these fatty acids have been included in recent formulas. The possibility of providing a more immediate precursor (γ-linolenic; C18:3 ω-6) to arachidonate formation and to include ω-3 long-chain fatty acids in lipid emulsions is currently under active investigation. Indeed, such preparations would not only affect the fatty acid composition of various cell membranes, but could also offer a means of modulating the inflammatory and thrombotic reactions via their impact on eicosanoid balance [229,230]. This opens a new area where the use of lipids is considered not because of their metabolic effects, but for their potential role as pharmacologic agents or "nutraceuticals" [231]. The number of publications reporting the advantages of such preparations in animal experiments is rapidly expanding. Although promising, these reports still require confirmation of beneficial effects in humans, and namely in patients.

Another interesting approach consists of mixing fatty acids with long and medium chains on the same glycerol molecule to produce structured triglycerides. Two different types of such structured lipids are currently developed. In one group, the position of specific fatty acids on the glycerol backbone can be predetermined, and the emulsion contains essentially one type of triglyceride molecule, e.g., MLM. In the other group, reesterification of fatty acids is left to proceed at random, which leads to the formation of several triglyceride molecules (e.g., LLM, MML, LML, MLM, LLL, MMM) to be included in emulsion particles. From a theoretical viewpoint, structured triglycerides should provide a means of better targeting the delivery of specific fatty acids to extrahepatic tissues or liver; however, preliminary studies in animals have not demonstrated a major difference from the use of mixed emulsions [232]. Similarly, the first studies in human reported a good tolerance over a few days, but these emulsions have not been tested to demonstrate an advantage over control emulsions containing a mixture of the same fatty acids [233].

Finally, lipid emulsions have been used for several years as vehicles for carrying lipid-soluble drugs such as propofol. One can easily foresee important developments in this field, for instance, the use of artificial lipid preparations (with specific particle sizes) to supply required amounts of liposoluble vitamins (and other agents) to patients with severe lipid intestinal malabsorption.

Conclusions

In recent years, a consensus has been reached concerning the advantages of including lipid emulsions as a regular component of parenteral nutrition. There is good evidence that side effects, although uncommonly observed, are generally associated with fast lipid infusions [215]; hence, we recommend infusion rates less than 0.10 g triglycerides/kg/hr in hospital patients and 0.15 g/kg/hr in home patients receiving cyclic parenteral nutrition. Although there is only indirect evidence that abnormalities associated with the use of 10% emulsions may be deleterious, those preparations are progressively replaced by more concentrated emulsions.

Current soybean- and safflower-derived preparations appear to supply carbon 18 polyunsaturated fatty acids largely in excess of the present recommendations for dietary fatty acid intake (i.e., 30% saturated, 30% to 36% monounsaturated, and 20% to 30% polyunsaturated) [234], and there is a growing concern about the potential for ω-6 polyunsaturated fatty acids to enhance the production of inflammatory and procoagulant derivatives, to modify cell membrane fatty acid pattern, and to stimulate free radical production. Other preparations in which a substantial proportion of soy oil has been replaced by other sources of nonessential fatty acids, such as MCTs, have currently been used in Europe during recent years with no report of clinically relevant side effects. Several new emulsions are currently undergoing experimental evaluation. Some preparations contain only LCTs, derived mainly from olive oil or fish oil or else are supplemented with γ-linolenate. Emulsions made of structured triglycerides are also presently assessed. Whatever the fatty acid composition, a strong priority should be given to include adequate amounts of antioxidants to prevent in vitro and in vivo occurrence of peroxidative damage.

As for most components included in parenteral regimens [235], it is our responsibility to recognize that the composition of presently available lipid emulsions can and should be optimized to better fit the specific requirements of different types of patients. Information obtained from the evaluation of recent and future emulsions should allow relevant advances in this exciting field.

References

1. Gotto AM Jr, Pownall HJ, Havel RJ. Introduction to the plasma lipoproteins. *Methods Enzymol* 128:3, 1986.
2. Havel R, Kane JP, Kashyap MD. Interchange of plasma lipoproteins between chylomicrons and high density lipoproteins during alimentary lipemia in man. *J Clin Invest* 52:32, 1973.
3. Tall AR. Plasma lipid transfer protein. *J Lipid Res* 27:361, 1986.
4. Havel RJ, et al. Structural and Functional Heterogeneity of Triglyceride-Rich Lipoprotein. In O Stein, S Eisenberg, Y Stein (eds), *Atherosclerosis IX. Proceedings of the Ninth International Symposium on Atherosclerosis.* Tel Aviv: R&L Creative Communications, 1992. P 13.
5. Eisenberg S. Lipoprotein abnormalities in hypertriglyceridemia: Significance in atherosclerosis. *Am Heart J* 113:555, 1987.
6. Eisenberg S. High density lipoprotein metabolism. *J Lipid Res* 25:1017, 1984.
7. Brown MS, Goldstein JL. Receptor-mediated control of cholesterol metabolism. *Science* 181:150, 1976.
8. Witztum JL, Steinberg D. Role of oxidized low density lipoprotein in atherogenesis. *J Clin Invest* 88:1785, 1991.
9. Jurgens GHF, et al. Modification of human serum low density lipoprotein by oxidation: Characterization and pathophysiological implications. *Chem Phys Lipids* 45:315, 1987.
10. Hemhold M, et al. Contribution of the apo[a] phenotype to plasma Lp[a] concentrations shows considerable ethnic variations. *J Lipid Res* 32:1919, 1991.
11. Danielsson B, Johansson BG, Petersson BG. Separation of lipoprotein X and beta-lipoprotein by zonal centrifugation or hydroxyapatite chromatography. *Clin Chim Acta* 47:365, 1973.
12. Seidel D, et al. A lipoprotein characterizing obstructive jaundice: II. Isolation and partial characterization of the protein moieties of low density lipoproteins. *J Clin Invest* 49:2396, 1970.
13. Glomset JA, Norum KR, Gjone E. Familial Lecithin: Cholesterol Acyltransferase Deficiency. In JB Stanbury, et al. (eds), *The Metabolic Basis of Inherited Disease,* 5th ed. New York: McGraw-Hill, 1983. P 643.
14. Griffin E, et al. Appearance and characterization of lipoprotein X during continuous Intralipid infusions in the neonate. *J Clin Invest* 64:1703, 1979.
15. Untracht S. Alterations of serum lipoproteins resulting from total parenteral nutrition with Intralipid. *Biochim Biophys Acta* 711:176, 1982.
16. Williams KJ, Scanu AM. Uptake of endogenous cholesterol by a synthetic lipoprotein. *Biochim Biophys Acta* 875:183, 1986.
17. Innis SM, Boyd M. Cholesterol and bile acid synthesis during total parenteral nutrition with and without lipid emulsion in the rat. *Am J Clin Nutr* 38:95, 1983.
18. Atkinson D. Apolipoprotein structure: Crystals and models. *Curr Opin Struct Biol* 2:482, 1992.
19. Rifici VA, Eder HA. A hepatocyte receptor for high-density lipoproteins specific for apolipoprotein A-I. *J Biol Chem* 259:13814, 1984.
20. Graham DL, Oram JF. Identification and characterization of a high density lipoprotein-binding protein in cell membrane by ligand blotting. *J Biol Chem* 262:7439, 1987.
21. Soutar AK, et al. Effect of the human plasma apolipoproteins and phosphatidylcholine acyl donor on the activity of lecithin:cholesterol acyltransferase. *Biochemistry* 14: 3057, 1975.
22. Fielding CJ. Reverse cholesterol transport. *Curr Opin Lipidol* 2:376, 1991.
23. Tall AR, Small DM. Plasma high-density lipoproteins. *N Engl J Med* 299:1232, 1978.
24. Barbaras R, et al. Cholesterol efflux from culture adipose cells is mediated by LpA-I. *Biochim Biophys Res Comm* 142:63, 1987.
25. Fruchart J, Ailhaud G, Bard JM. Heterogeneity of high density lipoprotein particles. *Circulation* 87:22, 1993.
26. Schultz JR, et al. Protein composition determines the antiatherogenic properties of HDL in transgenic mice. *Nature* 365:762, 1993.
27. Calabresi L, et al. Apolipoprotein A-II modulates HDL remodeling in plasma. *Biochim Biophys Acta* 1124:195, 1992.
28. Mowri H-O, et al. Different reactivities of high density $lipoprotein_2$ subfractions with hepatic lipase. *J Lipid Res* 33:1269, 1992.

29. Kostner GM. Apolipoproteins and lipoproteins of human plasma: Significance in health and in disease. *Adv Lipid Res* 20:1, 1983.

30. Dubois DY. *Contribution à l'étude du métabolisme des HDL chez l'être humain: Mise en évidence de fonctions spécifiques des HDL en dehors du Reverse Cholesterol Transport.* PhD Thesis, Faculty of Medicine, Free University of Brussels, 1993. P 29.

31. Goldberg IJ, et al. Lipoprotein apo C-II activation of lipoprotein lipase: Modulation by apolipoprotein A-IV. *J Biol Chem* 265:4266, 1990.

32. Lagrost L, et al. Evidence for high density lipoproteins as the major apolipoprotein A-IV containing fraction in normal human serum. *J Lipid Res* 30:1525, 1989.

33. Malmendier CL, et al. In vivo metabolism of apolipoprotein A-IV and A-I associated with high density lipoprotein in normolipidemic subjects. *J Lipid Res* 32:801, 1991.

34. Lagrost L, et al. Correlation between apolipoprotein A-IV and triglyceride concentrations in human sera. *J Lipid Res* 30:701, 1989.

35. Steinmetz A, et al. Human apolipoprotein A-IV binds to apolipoprotein A-I/A-II receptor sites and promotes cholesterol efflux from adipose cells. *J Biol Chem* 265:7859, 1990.

36. Ghiselli G, et al. Identification of a detergent-solubilized plasma membrane protein from rat liver recognizing apolipoprotein A-IV. *Biochim Biophys Acta* 1044:173, 1990.

37. Scott J. Regulation of the biosynthesis of apolipoproteins B100 and apolipoprotein B48. *Curr Opin Lipidol* 1:96, 1990.

38. Goldstein JL, Brown MS. The low-density lipoprotein pathway and its relation to atherosclerosis. *Annu Rev Biochem* 46:897, 1977.

39. Gianturco SH, et al. Apolipoprotein E mediates uptake of S_f 100–400 hyperlipoproteinemic very low density lipoproteins by the low density L receptor pathway in non human fibroblasts. *J Biol Chem* 258:4526, 1983.

40. Mahley RW, Hussain MM. Chylomicron and chylomicron remnants catabolism. *Curr Opin Lipidol* 2:170, 1991.

41. Weisgraber KH, et al. Apolipoprotein C-I modulated interaction of apolipoprotein E with β-migrating very low density lipoproteins (β-VLDL) and inhibits binding of β-VLDL to low density lipoprotein-related protein. *J Biol Chem* 265:22453, 1990.

42. Poensgen J. Apolipoprotein C-I inhibits the hydrolysis by phospholipase A2 of phospholipids in liposomes and cell membranes. *Biochim Biophys Acta* 1042:188, 1990.

43. Zannis VI, Cladaras C, Zanni EE. Apolipoprotein and lipoprotein synthesis and modifications. *Curr Opin Lipidol* 2:149, 1991.

44. Olivecrona T, Bengtsson-Olivecrona G. Lipoprotein Lipase from Milk: The Model Enzyme in Lipoprotein Lipase Research. In J Borensztajn (ed), *Lipoprotein Lipase.* Chicago: Evener, 1987. P 15.

45. Breckenridge WC, et al. Hypertriglyceridemia associated with deficiency of apolipoprotein C-II. *N Engl J Med* 298:1265, 1978.

46. Brown WV, Baginsky ML. Inhibition of lipoprotein lipase by an apoprotein of human very low density lipoprotein. *Biochim Biophys Res Comm* 46:375, 1972.

47. Malmendier CL, et al. In vivo metabolism of apolipoproteins C-II and C-III in normal and hypertriglyceridemic subjects. *Adv Exp Med Biol* 243:299, 1988.

48. Ito Y, et al. Hypertriglyceridemia as a result of human apo C-III gene expression in transgenic mice. *Science* 249:790, 1990.

49. Aalto-Setälä K, et al. Mechanism of hypertriglyceridemia in human apolipoprotein (apo) CIII transgenic mice: Diminished very low density lipoprotein fractional catabolic rate associated with increased apo CIII and reduced apo E on the particles. *J Clin Invest* 90:1889, 1992.

50. Tornoci L, et al. Abnormal activation of lipoprotein lipase by nonequilibrating pools of apolipoproteins C-II: Further evidence for the presence of nonequilibrating pools of apolipoproteins C-II and C-III in plasma lipoproteins. *J Lipid Res* 34:1793, 1993.

51. Provost PR, et al. Molecular characterization and differential mRNA tissue distribution of rabbit apolipoprotein D. *J Lipid Res* 31:2057, 1990.

52. Boyles JK, Notterpek LM, Anderson LJ. Accumulation of apolipoproteins in the regeneration and remyelinating mammalian peripheral nerve: Identification of apolipoprotein D, apolipoprotein A-IV, apolipoprotein E, and apolipoprotein A-I. *J Biol Chem* 265:17805, 1990.

53. Sánchez LM, et al. Identification of the major components in breast secretions from women with benign and malignant breast diseases. *Cancer Res* 52:95, 1992.

54. Bradley WA, Gianturco SH. Lipoprotein receptors. *Curr Opin Lipidol* 1:216, 1990.

55. Van Berkel TJC, et al. Lipoprotein receptors and atherogenic receptor-mediated mechanisms. *Curr Opin Lipidol* 5:331, 1994.

56. Plump AS, et al. Severe hypercholesterolemia and atherosclerosis in apolipoprotein E-deficient mice created by homologous recombination in ES cells. *Cell* 71:343, 1992.

57. Zhang SH, et al. Spontaneous hypercholesterolemia and arterial lesions in mice lacking apolipoprotein E. *Science* 258:468, 1992.

58. Ji ZS, et al. Secretion-capture role for apoprotein E in remnant lipoprotein metabolism involving cell surface heparan sulfate proteoglycans. *J Biol Chem* 269:2764, 1994.

59. Mahley RW, et al. Intravenous infusion of apolipoprotein E accelerates clearance of plasma lipoproteins in rabbits. *J Clin Invest* 83:2125, 1989.

60. Yamada N, et al. Increased clearance of plasma cholesterol after injection of apolipoprotein E into Watanabe heritable hyperlipidemic rabbits. *Proc Natl Acad Sci USA* 86:665, 1989.

61. Granot E, et al. Effects of particle size on cell uptake of model triglyceride-rich particles with and without apoprotein E. *Biochemistry* 33:15190, 1994.

62. Schwiegelshohn B, et al. Effects of apoprotein E on intracellular metabolism of model triglyceride-rich particles are distinct from effects on cell particle uptake. *J Biol Chem* 270:1761, 1995.

63. Bury J, et al. Apolipoprotein E quantified by enzyme-linked immunosorbent assay. *Clin Chem* 32:265, 1986.

64. Mahley R. Apolipoprotein E: Cholesterol transport protein with expanding role in cell biology. *Science* 240:622, 1988.

65. Weisgraber KH, Pitas RE, Mahley RW. Lipoproteins, Neurobiology, and Alzheimer's Disease: Structure and Formation of Apolipoprotein E. *Curr Opin Struct Biol* 4:507, 1994.

66. Eriksen N, Benditt EP. Serum Amyloid A (Apo SAA) and lipoproteins. *Methods Enzymol* 128:311, 1986.

67. Tape C, et al. Direct evidence for circulating apoSAA as the precursor of tissue AA amyloid deposits. *Scand J Immunol* 28:317, 1988.

68. Hol PR, et al. Amyloid-enhancing factor (AEF) in the pathogenesis of AA-amyloidosis in the hamster. *Virchows Arch [B]* 52:273, 1986.

69. Steinmetz A, et al. Influence of serum amyloid A on cholesterol esterification in human plasma. *Biochim Biophys Acta* 1006:173, 1989.

70. Tape C, Kisilevsky R. Apolipoprotein A-I and Apolipoprotein SAA half-lives during acute inflammation and amyloidogenesis. *Biochim Biophys Acta* 1043:295, 1990.

71. Kisilevsky R, Subrahmanyan L. Serum amyloid A changes high density lipoproteins cellular affinity: A clue to serum amyloid A's principal function. *Lab Invest* 66:778, 1992.

72. Bekaert ED, et al. Alterations in lipoprotein density classes in infantile visceral leishmaniasis: Presence of apo SAA. *Eur J Clin Invest* 22:190, 1992.

73. Cabana VG, Siegel JN, Sabesin SM. Effects of the acute phase response on the concentration and density distribution of plasma lipids and apolipoproteins. *J Lipid Res* 30:39, 1989.

74. Lee NS, Brewer HB Jr, Osborne JC Jr. β_2-glycoprotein I: Molecular properties of an unusual apolipoprotein, apolipoprotein H. *J Biol Chem* 258:4765, 1983.

75. Polz E, Wurm H, Kostner GM. Investigations on β_2-glycoprotein I in the rat: Isolation from serum and demonstration in lipoprotein density fractions. *Int J Biochem* 11:265, 1980.

76. Henry ML, Everson B, Ratnoff OD. Inhibition of the activation of Hageman factor (factor XII) by β_2-glycoprotein I. *J Lab Clin Med* 111:519, 1988.

77. Reid KBM, Day AJ. Structure-functions relationships of the complement components. *Immunol Today* 10:177, 1989.

78. de Silva HV, et al. Apolipoprotein J: Structure and tissue distribution. *Biochemistry* 29:5380, 1990.

79. Murphy BF, et al. SP-40,40 a newly identified normal human serum protein found in the SC5b-9 complex of complement and in the immune deposits in glomerulonephritis. *J Clin Invest* 81:1858, 1988.

80. Wilson MR, Easterbrook-Smith SB. Clusterin binds by a multivalent mechanism to the Fc and Fab regions of IgG. *Biochim Biophys Acta* 1159:319, 1992.

81. Schmitz G, Williamson E. High-density lipoprotein metabolism, reverse cholesterol transport and membrane protection. *Curr Opin Lipidol* 2:177, 1991.

82. Jordan-Starck TC, et al. Apolipoprotein J: A membrane policeman? *Curr Opin Lipidol* 3:75, 1992.

83. Hajri T, et al. Total parenteral nutrition and plasma lipoproteins in the rat: Evidence for accelerated clearance of apo-A-I-rich HDL. *Biochim Biophys Acta* 1166:84, 1993.

84. Olivecrona T, Bengtsson-Olivecrona G. Lipases involved in lipoprotein metabolism. *Curr Opin Lipidol* 1:116, 1990.

85. Eckel RH. Lipoprotein lipase: A multifunctional enzyme relevant to common metabolic diseases. *N Engl J Med* 320:1060, 1989.

86. Bessesen DH, et al. Spinal cord of the rat contains more lipoprotein lipase than other brain regions. *J Lipid Res* 34:229, 1993.

87. Stins MF, et al. Specificity of lipoprotein lipase binding to endothelial cells. *J Lipid Res* 34:1853, 1993.

88. Deckelbaum RJ, et al. Medium-chain versus long-chain triacylglycerol emulsion hydrolysis by lipoprotein lipase and hepatic lipase: Implications for the mechanisms of lipase action. *Biochemistry* 29:1136, 1990.

89. Olivecrona T, Bengtsson-Olivecrona G. Lipoprotein Lipase and Hepatic Lipase. In G Schettler, AJR Habenicht (eds), *Handbook of Experimental Pharmacology,* vol 109: *Principles and Treatment of Lipoprotein Disorders.* Heidelberg: Springer-Verlag, 1993.

90. Windler E, Havel RJ. Inhibitory effects of C apolipoproteins from rats and humans on the hepatic uptake of triglyceride-rich lipoproteins and their remnants by the perfused rat liver. *J Lipid Res* 26:556, 1985.

91. Melin T, et al. Hydrolysis of chylomicron polyenoic fatty acid esters with lipoprotein lipase and hepatic lipase. *Biochim Biophys Acta* 1075:259, 1991.

92. Komaromy MC, Schotz MC. Cloning of rat hepatic lipase cDNA: Evidence for a lipase gene family. *Proc Natl Acad Sci USA* 84:1526, 1987.

93. Zilversmit DB. Atherogenesis: A postprandial phenomenon. *Circulation* 60:473, 1979.

94. Beisigel U, Weber W, Bengtsson-Olivecrona G. Lipoprotein lipase enhances the binding of chylomicrons to low density lipoprotein receptor-related protein. *Proc Natl Acad Sci USA* 88:8342, 1991.

95. Rumsey SC, et al. Lipoprotein lipase-mediated uptake and degradation of low density lipoproteins by fibroblasts and macrophages. *J Clin Invest* 90:1504, 1992.

96. Peterson J, et al. Fatty acid control of lipoprotein lipase: A link between energy metabolism and lipid transport. *Proc Natl Acad Sci USA* 87:909, 1990.

97. Jauhiainen M, et al. Human plasma phospholipid transfer protein causes high density lipoprotein conversion. *J Biol Chem* 268:4032, 1993.

98. Granot E, et al. Core modification of human low density lipoprotein by artificial triglyceride emulsion. *Biochim Biophys Acta* 833:308, 1985.

99. Deckelbaum RJ, et al. Conversion of human plasma high density lipoprotein-2 to high density lipoprotein-3: Roles of neutral lipid exchange and lipase. *J Biol Chem* 261:5201, 1986.

100. Eisenberg S, et al. Abnormalities in very low, low and high density lipoproteins in hypertriglyceridemia. *J Clin Invest* 74:470, 1984.

101. Le N-A, Ginsberg HN. Heterogeneity of apolipoprotein A-I turnover in subjects with reduced concentrations of plasma high density lipoprotein cholesterol. *Metabolism* 37:614, 1988.

102. Lechleitner M, Miesenböck G, Patsch JR. HDL cholesterol, triglycerides and coronary heart disease. *Curr Opin Lipidol* 1:330, 1990.

103. Mann CJ, et al. Mechanisms of plasma cholesteryl ester transfer in hypertriglyceridemia. *J Clin Invest* 88:2059, 1991.

104. Marotti KR, et al. Severe atherosclerosis in transgenic mice expressing simian cholesteryl ester transfer protein. *Nature* 364:73, 1993.

105. Richelle M, Deckelbaum RJ, Carpentier YA. Long chain vs. medium chain triacylglycerol intravenous emulsions in lipid exchange processes with human plasma low density lipoprotein. *Biochemistry* 33:4872, 1994.

106. Berr F. Characterization of chylomicron clearance by retinyl palmitate label in normal humans. *J Lipid Res* 33:915, 1992.

107. Sniderman A, Baldo A, Cianflone K. The potential role of acylation stimulating protein as a determinant of plasma triglyceride clearance and intracellular triglyceride synthesis. *Curr Opin Lipidol* 3:202, 1992.

108. Kwiterovitch PO Jr, Motevalli M, Miller M. The effect of three serum basic proteins on the mass of lipids in normal and hyperapoB fibroblasts. *Arteriosclerosis Thromb* 14:1, 1994.

109. Havel RJ. Postprandial hyperlipidemia and remnant lipoproteins. *Curr Opin Lipidol* 5:102, 1994.

110. Brown MS, et al. The low-density lipoprotein receptor-related protein: Double agent or decoy? *Curr Opin Lipidol* 2:65, 1991.

111. Rubinsztein DC, et al. Chylomicron remnant clearance from the plasma is normal in FH homozygotes with defined receptor defects. *J Clin Invest* 86:1306, 1992.

112. Kowal RC, et al. Low density lipoprotein receptor-related protein mediates uptake of cholesteryl esters derived from apoprotein E-enriched lipoproteins. *Proc Natl Acad Sci USA* 86:5810, 1989.

113. Beisiegel U, et al. The LDL-receptor-related protein, LRP, is an apolipoprotein E-binding protein. *Nature* 341:162, 1989.

114. Strickland DK, et al. Sequence identity between the α_2-macroglobulin receptor and low density lipoprotein receptor-related protein suggests that this molecule is a multifunctional receptor. *J Biol Chem* 265:17401, 1990.

115. Bu G, et al. Low density lipoprotein receptor-related protein/α_2-macroglobulin receptor is an hepatic receptor for tissue-type plasminogen activator. *Proc Natl Acad Sci USA* 89:7427, 1992.

116. Nykjaer A, et al. Purified α_2-macroglobulin receptor/LDL receptor-related protein binds urokinase-plasminogen activator inhibitor type-1 complex: Evidence that α_2-macroglobulin receptor mediates cellular degradation of urokinase receptor bound complexes. *J Biol Chem* 267:14543, 1992.

117. Ishibashi S, et al. The two-receptor model of lipoprotein clearance: Tests of the hypothesis in "knockout" mice lacking the low density lipoprotein receptor, apolipoprotein E, or both proteins. *Proc Natl Acad Sci USA* 91:4431, 1994.

118. Willnow TE, et al. Inhibition of hepatic chylomicron remnant uptake by gene transfer of a receptor antagonist. *Science* 246:1471, 1994.

119. Gianturco SH, Bradley WA. Atherosclerosis: Cell biology and lipoproteins. *Curr Opin Lipidol* 5:313, 1994.

120. Chait A, Albers JJ, Brunzell JD. Very low density lipoprotein overproduction in genetic forms of hypertriglyceridaemia. *Eur J Clin Invest* 10:17, 1980.

121. Fungwe TV, et al. Regulation of hepatic secretion of very low density lipoprotein by dietary cholesterol. *J Lipid Res* 33:179, 1992.

122. Sniderman A, et al. From familial combined hyperlipidemia to hyperapoB: Unravelling the overproduction of hepatic apolipoprotein B. *Curr Opin Lipidol* 3:137, 1992.

123. Sparks JD, Sparks CE. Hormonal regulation of lipoprotein assembly and secretion. *Curr Opin Lipidol* 4:177, 1993.

124. Havel RJ. Triglyceride-rich lipoproteins and atherosclerosis: New perspectives. *Am J Clin Nutr* 59:795, 1994.

125. Steinberg D. Modified forms of low-density lipoprotein and atherosclerosis. *J Intern Med* 233:227, 1993.

126. Chait A, Heinecke JW. Lipoprotein modification: Cellular mechanisms. *Curr Opin Lipidol* 5:365, 1994.

127. Parthasarathy S, Santanam N. Mechanisms of oxidation, antioxidants, and atherosclerosis. *Curr Opin Lipidol* 5:371, 1994.

128. Li ZF, et al. Oxidized LDL induce procoagulant activity in human monocytes. *Clin Nutr* 13(Suppl 1):31, 1994.

129. Chin JH, Azhar S, Hoffman BB. Inactivation of endothelial derived relaxing factor by oxidized lipoproteins. *J Clin Invest* 89:10, 1992.

130. Harats D, et al. Fish oil ingestion in smokers and nonsmokers enhances peroxidation of plasma lipoproteins. *Atherosclerosis* 90:127, 1991.

131. Siderova VS, et al. Intravascular metabolism of different fatty acids during lipid infusion in man. *Clin Nutr* 12:329, 1993.

132. Barter P. High-density lipoproteins and reverse cholesterol transport. *Curr Opin Lipidol* 4:210, 1993.

133. Phillips MC, et al. Mechanisms of cholesterol efflux from cells. *Atherosclerosis* 36:409, 1980.

134. Schmitz G, et al. Interaction of high density lipoproteins with cholesteryl esters-laden macrophages: Biochemical and morphological characterization of cell surface receptor binding, endocytosis and resecretion of high density lipoproteins by macrophages. *EMBO J* 4:613, 1985.

135. Rothblat GH, et al. Apolipoproteins, membrane cholesterol domains, and regulation of cholesterol efflux. *J Lipid Res* 33:1091, 1992.

136. Oram JF. Cholesterol trafficking in cells. *Curr Opin Lipidol* 1:416, 1990.

137. Hara H, et al. Alpha-helical requirements for free apolipoproteins to generate HDL and induce cellular lipid efflux. *Lipids* 27:302, 1992.

138. Tall AR. Plasma high density lipoproteins: Metabolism and relationship to atherogenesis. *J Clin Invest* 86:379, 1990.

139. Warwick G, Packard CJ, Sheperd J. Plasma lipid measurement. *Curr Opin Lipidol* 1:500, 1990.

140. Collet X, et al. Behaviour of phospholipase-modified HDL towards cultured hepatocytes: I. Enhanced transfers of HDL sterols and apoproteins. *Biochim Biophys Acta* 1043:301, 1990.

141. Clay MA, et al. Cholesteryl ester transfer protein and hepatic lipase activity promote shedding of apo A-I from HDL and subsequent formation of discoidal HDL. *Biochim Biophys Acta* 1124:52, 1992.

142. Barbaras R, et al. Specific binding of free apolipoprotein A-I to a high-affinity binding site on Hep G2 cells: Characterization of two high-density sites. *Biochemistry* 33:2335, 1994.

143. Blackburn WD Jr, et al. Apolipoprotein A-I decreases neutrophil degradation and superoxide production. *J Lipid Res* 32:1911, 1991.

144. Chander R, Kapoor NK. High density lipoprotein is a scavenger of superoxide anions. *Biochem Pharmacol* 40:1663, 1990.

145. Macknens MI, et al. Protection of low-density lipoprotein against oxidative modification by high-density lipoprotein-associated paraoxonase. *Atherosclerosis* 104:129, 1993.

146. Sattler W, Stocker R. Greater selective uptake by Hep G2 cells of high-density lipoprotein cholesteryl ester hydroperoxides than of unoxidized cholesteryl esters. *Biochem J* 294:771, 1993.

147. Halliwell B. Free radicals and antioxidants: A personal view. *Nutr Rev* 52:253, 1994.

148. Aoyama T, et al. Prostaglandin I_2 half-life regulated by high density lipoprotein is decreased in acute myocardiac infarction and instable angina pectoris. *Circulation* 81:1784, 1990.

149. Novotny WF, et al. Purification and properties of heparin releasable lipoprotein-associated coagulation inhibitor. *Blood* 78:394, 1991.

150. Ulevitch RJ, Johnston AR, Weinstein DB. New function for high density lipoproteins: Isolation and characterization of a bacterial lipopolysaccharide-high density lipoprotein complex formed in rabbit plasma. *J Clin Invest* 67:827, 1981.

151. Srinivas RV, et al. Inhibition of virus-induced cell fusion

by apolipoprotein A-I and its amphipathic peptide analogs. *J Cell Biochem* 45:224, 1991.

152. Packman CH, Rosenfeld SI, Leddy P. High-density lipoproteins and their apolipoproteins inhibit activity of complement: Studies on the nature of the inhibitory moieties. *Biochim Biophys Acta* 812:107, 1985.
153. Wretlind A. Development of fat emulsions. *JPEN* 5:230, 1981.
154. Carpentier YA. Intravascular metabolism of fat emulsions: The Arvid Wretlind Lecture, ESPEN 1988. *Clin Nutr* 8:115, 1989.
155. Férézou J, et al. Lipid composition and structure of commercial parenteral emulsions. *Biochim Biophys Acta* 1213:149, 1993.
156. Haumont D, et al. Parenteral nutrition with 20% compared to 10% Intralipid is associated with lower plasma lipid concentrations and only minor changes in plasma lipoproteins in LBW infants. *J Pediatr* 115:787, 1989.
157. Hallberg D. Elimination of exogenous lipids from the blood stream: An experimental methodological and clinical study in dog and man. *Acta Physiol Scand* 65(Suppl 254):1, 1965.
158. Richelle M, et al. In vitro exchanges of lipids and apoproteins between HDL and exogenous fat. *Clin Nutr* 5:55, 1986.
159. Bury J, et al. Influence of an intravenous fat emulsion on the concentration and distribution of plasma apolipoproteins in man. *Clin Nutr* 5:116, 1986.
160. Iriyama K, et al. Apolipoprotein C-II modifications associated with an infusion of artificial lipid particles. *JPEN* 12:60, 1988.
161. Dahlan W. Intravenous Infusion of Triacylglycerol-Phospholipid Complexes in Man: Effects on Fatty Acid Pattern of Plasma and on Erythrocyte Membrane Lipid Composition. PhD Thesis, Free University of Brussels, 1989.
162. Mortimer BC, et al. Effects of triacylglycerol-saturated acyl chain on the clearance of chylomicron-like emulsions from the plasma of the rat. *Biochim Biophys Acta* 1211:171, 1994.
163. Redgrave TG, Kodali DR, Small DM. The effect of triacyl-sn-glycerol structure on the metabolism of chylomicrons and triacylglycerol-rich emulsions in the rat. *J Biol Chem* 263:5118, 1988.
164. Richelle M. Influence of intravenous lipid emulsions on cholesterol homeostasis. *Clin Nutr* 11:49, 1992.
165. Sato N, et al. Hydrolysis of mixed lipid emulsions containing medium chain and long chain triacylglycerol with lipoprotein lipase in plasma-like media. *JPEN* 18:112, 1994.
166. Haumont D, et al. Effect of liposomal content of lipid emulsions on plasma lipids in low birth weight infants receiving parenteral nutrition. *J Pediatr* 121:759, 1992.
167. Redgrave TG, et al. Effects of sphingomyelin and phosphatidylcholine acyl chains on the clearance of triacylglycerols from plasma: Studies with lipid emulsions in rats. *Biochim Biophys Acta* 1126:65, 1992.
168. Richelle M, et al. Phosphatidyl ethanolamine (PE) content of emulsifiers can influence intravascular metabolism of fat emulsions. *Clin Nutr* 7:76, 1988.
169. Carpentier YA, et al. Phospholipid excess of fat emulsion slows triglyceride removal and increases lipoprotein remodelling. *Arteriosclerosis* 7:541A, 1987.
170. Roulet M, et al. Effects of intravenously infused egg phospholipids on lipid and lipoprotein metabolism in postoperative trauma. *JPEN* 17:107, 1993.
171. Williams KJ, et al. Low density receptor independent hepatic uptake of a synthetic, cholesterol-scavenging lipoprotein: Implications for the treatment of receptor deficient atherosclerosis. *Proc Natl Acad Sci USA* 85:242, 1988.
172. Dahlan W, et al. Modification of erythrocyte membrane lipid composition induced by a single intravenous infusion of phospholipid-triacylglycerol emulsions in man. *Clin Nutr* 11:255, 1992.
173. Rojas C, Olivecrona T, Bengtsson-Olivecrona G. Comparison of the action of lipoprotein lipase on triacylglycerols and phospholipids when presented in mixed liposomes or in emulsion droplets. *Eur J Biochem* 197:315, 1991.
174. Degott C, et al. Liver phospholipidosis induced by parenteral nutrition: Histologic, histochemical, and ultrastructural investigations. *Gastroenterology* 95:183, 1988.
175. Zeisel SH. Phosphatidylcholine: The Unappreciated Nutrient in Total Parenteral Nutrition. In JM Kinney, HN Tucker (eds), *Organ Metabolism and Nutrition: Ideas for Future Critical Care.* New York: Raven, 1993. P 331.
176. Carpentier YA, et al. Exogenous Lipids and Hepatic Function. In JM Kinney, HN Tucker (eds), *Organ Metabolism and Nutrition: Ideas for Future Critical Care.* New York: Raven, 1993. P 349.
177. Henton DH, Merritt RJ, Hack S. Vitamin E measurements in patients receiving intravenous lipid emulsions. *JPEN* 16:133, 1992.
178. Stephen AC, et al. Vitamin E status of patients receiving long-term parenteral nutrition: Is vitamin E supplementation adequate? *JPEN* 15:647, 1991.
179. Kayden HJ, Traber MG. Absorption, lipoprotein transport and regulation of plasma concentrations of vitamin E in humans. *J Lipid Res* 34:343,1993.
180. Traber MG, Kayden HJ. Preferential incorporation of α-tocopherol vs γ-tocopherol in human lipoproteins. *Am J Clin Nutr* 49:517, 1989.
181. Traber MG, et al. Alterations in plasma alpha- and gamma-tocopherol concentrations in response to intravenous infusion of lipid emulsions in humans. *Metabolism* 42:701, 1993.
182. Burton GW, Joyce A, Ingold KU. First proof that vitamin E is major lipid-soluble, chain-breaking antioxidant in human blood plasma. *Lancet* 2:327, 1982.
183. Lemoyne M, et al. Plasma vitamin E and selenium and breath pentane in home parenteral nutrition patients. *Am J Clin Nutr* 48:1310, 1988.
184. Wispe J, Bell F, Roberts R. Assessment of lipid peroxidation in newborn infants and rabbits by measurement of expired ethane and pentane: Influence of parenteral lipid infusion. *Pediatr Res* 19:374, 1985.
185. Van Gossum A, et al. Increased lipid peroxidation after lipid emulsion as measured by breath pentane output. *Am J Clin Nutr* 48:1394, 1988.
186. Pitkanen O, Hallmann M, Andersson S. Generation of free radicals in lipid emulsion used in parenteral nutrition. *Pediatr Res* 29:56, 1991.
187. Helbock HJ, Motchnik PA, Ames BN. Toxic hydroperoxides in intravenous lipid emulsions used in preterm infants. *Pediatrics* 91:83, 1993.
188. Kljuchnikov S, et al. Haemolysis in adult and neonatal erythrocytes caused by autoxidation of lipid emulsion (Intralipid). *Acta Paediatr* 82:348, 1993.
189. Clayton PT, et al. Phytosterolemia in children with parenteral nutrition-associated cholestatic liver disease. *Gastroenterology* 105:1806, 1993.
190. Salen G, et al. Sitosterolemia. *J Lipid Res* 33:945, 1992.

191. Lennon C, et al. The vitamin K content of intravenous lipid emulsions. *JPEN* 17:142, 1993.

192. Carpentier YA, et al. Relationship between rates of clearance and oxidation of ^{14}C-Intralipid in surgical patients. *Surg Forum* 30:72, 1979.

193. Carpentier YA, et al. Stabilization of plasma substrate concentrations: A model for conducting metabolic studies. *Clin Nutr* 9:313, 1990.

194. Robin AP, et al. Plasma clearance of fat emulsion in trauma and sepsis: Use of three-stage lipid clearance test. *JPEN* 4:505, 1980.

195. Dubois DY, et al. Stimulation of endogenous triglyceride (TG)-rich lipoprotein release during infusion of lipid emulsions in man. *Clin Nutr* 13(Suppl):1, 1994.

196. Carpentier YA, et al. Hypertriglyceridaemia clamp: A new model for studying lipid metabolism. *Clin Nutr* 9(Suppl):1, 1990.

197. Druml W, et al. Fat elimination in acute renal failure: Long-chain vs. medium-chain triglycerides. *Am J Clin Nutr* 55:468, 1992.

198. Redgrave TG, et al. Clearance from plasma of triacylglycerol and cholesteryl ester after intravenous injection of chylomicron-like lipid emulsions in rats and man. *Biochem J* 290:843, 1993.

199. Sehayek E, Eisenberg S. The role of native apolipoprotein B-containing lipoproteins in atherosclerosis: Cellular mechanisms. *Curr Opin Lipidol* 5:350, 1994.

200. Pineault M, et al. Beneficial effect of coinfusing a lipid emulsion on venous patency. *JPEN* 13:637, 1989.

201. Phelps SJ, Cochran EB. Effect of the continuous administration of fat emulsion on the infiltration of intravenous lines in infants receiving peripheral parenteral nutrition solutions. *JPEN* 13:628, 1989.

202. Paust H, Rating D, Helge H. Measurement of fatty acid oxidation in premature newborn with the ^{13}C-triolein breath test. *Clin Nutr* 3:89, 1984.

203. Cotter R, et al. Competitive effects of long-chain-triglyceride emulsion on the metabolism of medium-chain-triglyceride emulsions. *Am J Clin Nutr* 50:794, 1989.

204. Bach AC, Babayan VK. Medium-chain triglycerides: An update. *Am J Clin Nutr* 36:950, 1982.

205. Rössle C, et al. Medium chain triglycerides induce alterations in carnitine metabolism. *Am J Physiol* 258:E944, 1990.

206. Rosenthal E, Weissman B, Kyllonen K. Use of parenteral medium-chain triglyceride emulsion for maintaining seizure control in a 5-year-old girl with intractable diarrhea. *JPEN* 14:543, 1990.

207. Drews D, Schluter MD, Stein TP. Glycerol kinetics with parenteral lipid emulsions (long-chain triglycerides, medium-chain triglycerides, and structured lipids) in rats. *Metabolism* 42:743, 1993.

208. Kawamura M, Heinecke JW, Chait A. Pathophysiological concentrations of low density lipoprotein by a superoxide-dependent pathway. *J Clin Invest* 94:771, 1994.

209. Jeejeebhoy KN, et al. Total parenteral nutrition at home: Studies in patients surviving 4 months to 5 years. *Gastroenterology* 71:943, 1976.

210. Baldermann H, et al. Changes of hepatic morphology during parenteral nutrition with lipid emulsions containing LCT or MCT/LCT quantified by ultrasound. *JPEN* 15:601, 1991.

211. Glynn MJ, et al. High lipid parenteral nutrition improves portasystemic encephalopathy. *JPEN* 12:457, 1988.

212. Lashner B, Kirsner J, Hanaver S. Acute pancreatitis associated with high-concentration lipid emulsion during total parenteral nutrition for Crohn's disease. *Gastroenterology* 90:1039, 1986.

213. Frederickson DS, Lees RS. Familial Hyperlipoproteinemia. In JB Stanbury, JB Wyngarden, DS Frederickson (eds), *The Metabolic Basis of Inherited Disease,* 2nd ed. New York: McGraw-Hill, 1966. P 423.

214. Greenberger N. Pancreatitis and hyperlipidemia. *N Engl J Med* 289:586, 1973.

215. Miles JM. Intravenous fat emulsions in nutritional support. *Curr Opin Gastroenterol* 7:306, 1991.

216. Carpentier YA, et al. Lipid Metabolism in Parenteral Nutrition. In JL Rombeau, MD Caldwell (eds), *Clinical Nutrition: Parenteral Nutrition,* 2nd ed. Philadelphia: Saunders, 1993. P 35.

217. Seidner DL, et al. Effects of long-chain triglyceride emulsions on reticuloendothelial system function in humans. *JPEN* 13:614, 1989.

218. Zoban P, et al. Influence of intravenously administered Intralipid on free fatty acid concentration and albumin binding capacity to bilirubin in newborn infants. *Czech Med* 12:68, 1989.

219. Richelle M, et al. Plasma lipoprotein pattern during long-term home parenteral nutrition with two different lipid emulsions. *JPEN* 17:432, 1993.

220. Matsui J, et al. Nutritional, hepatic, and metabolic effects of cachectin/tumor necrosis factor in rats receiving total parenteral nutrition. *Gastroenterology* 104:235, 1993.

221. Harris HW, et al. Human very low density lipoproteins and chylomicrons can protect against endotoxin-induced death in mice. *J Clin Invest* 86:696, 1990.

222. Jarstrand C, Rasool O. Intralipid decreases the bacterial lipopolysaccharide induced release of oxygen radicals and lysozyme from human neutrophils. *Scand J Infect Dis* 23:481, 1991.

223. Ulevitch RJ, Tobias PS, Mathison JC. Regulation of the host response to bacterial lipopolysaccharides. *Fed Proc* 43:2755, 1984.

224. Bagdade JD, Ways PO. Erythrocyte membrane lipid composition in exogenous and endogenous hypertriglyceridemia. *J Lab Clin Med* 75:53, 1970.

225. Dahlan W, et al. Effects of essential fatty acid contents of lipid emulsions on erythrocyte polyunsaturated fatty acid composition in patients on long-term parenteral nutrition. *Clin Nutr* 11:262, 1992.

226. Haumont D, et al. Modifications of surfactant phospholipid pattern in premature infants treated with Curosurf: Clinical and dietary correlations. *Biol Neonate* 61(Suppl 1):37, 1992.

227. Simoens C, et al. Manipulation of tissue fatty acid profile by i.v. lipids in dogs. *Clin Nutr* 14:177, 1995.

228. Morgan JB, Kovar IZ. The low birth weight infant and parenteral nutrition. *Nutr Res Rev* 5:115, 1992.

229. Karlstad MD, et al. Effects of intravenous lipid emulsions enriched with γ-linolenic acid on plasma ω-6 fatty acids and prostaglandin biosynthesis after burn and endotoxin injury in rats. *Crit Care Med* 21:1740, 1993.

230. Carpentier YA. Lipid Emulsions. In P Fürst (ed), *New Strategies in Clinical Nutrition.* Munich: W Zuckschwerdt, *Klinische Ernährung* 33:52, 1993.

231. Blackburn GL, Mascioli EA. Designer lipids as a nutraceutical. *Crit Care Med* 21:1632, 1993.

232. Hultin M, et al. Metabolism of emulsions containing medium and long chain triglycerides or interesterified triglycerides. *J Lipid Res* 35:1850, 1994.

233. Sandstrom R, et al. Structured triglycerides to postoperative patients: A safety and tolerance study. *JPEN* 17:153, 1993.

234. Report of Panel: Dietary reference values for food energy and nutrients for the United Kingdom. London: HMSO, Cmd DH RMSS 41, 1991.

235. Wilmore DW, Carpentier YA (eds). *Metabolic Support of the Critically Ill Patient,* vol 17. New York: Springer, 1993.

Selected Readings

Blackburn WD Jr, et al. Apolipoprotein A-I decreases neutrophil degradation and superoxide production. *J Lipid Res* 32:1911, 1991.

Apo A-I may play an important role during the inflammatory response by reducing IgG-mediated neutrophil degranulation and superoxide production. The authors suggest that apo A-I should be first displaced from HDL, possibly by serum amyloid A during the acute phase, before it could exert its anti-inflammatory effect on the nearby cells.

Hajri T, et al. Total parenteral nutrition and plasma lipoproteins in the rat: Evidence for accelerated clearance of apo-A-I-rich HDL. *Biochim Biophys Acta* 1166:84, 1993.

Infusion of Intralipid 20% decreases apo A-I concentration in the rat, mainly because of faster uptake of HDL_3 by the liver.

Pitkanen O, Hallmann M, Andersson S. Generation of free radicals in lipid emulsion used in parenteral nutrition. *Pediatr Res* 29:56, 1991.

An increased pentane excretion in expired breath was demonstrated in infants infused with Intralipid. In vitro peroxidation of Intralipid is shown to induce hemolysis. The authors suggest that adverse effects of parenteral Intralipid infusion are partially caused by lipid peroxidation.

Rumsey SC, et al. Lipoprotein lipase-mediated uptake and degradation of low density lipoproteins by fibroblasts and macrophages. *J Clin Invest* 90:1504, 1992.

Lipoprotein lipase is able to mediate binding, internalization, and degradation of LDL or apolipoprotein-free triglyceride emulsions in fibroblasts or macrophages via a pathway not involving the LDL receptor. The authors suggest that this pathway may be involved in lipoprotein-lipase synthesizing cells.

Steinberg D. Modified forms of low-density lipoprotein and atherosclerosis. *J Intern Med* 233:227, 1993.

This excellent review discusses the mechanisms and pathophysiologic implications of LDL oxidative modifications.

9

Vitamins

Harry L. Greene
Robert A. Burns

In 1987, a commercial shortage of multivitamins for parenteral use resulted in the omission of vitamins from the total parenteral nutrition (TPN) mixture for several patients unable to consume oral feedings. This catastrophe resulted in several deaths of infants and adults due to vitamin deficiency. Three points can be addressed from this unfortunate experience: (1) The average time to develop clinical signs of deficiency was 3 weeks in adults and 2 weeks in children; (2) the dominant vitamin causing the deficiency was thiamine, presumably due to the continued high intake of carbohydrate energy; and (3) the predominate presenting symptoms were severe lactic acidosis, followed in 8 to 24 hours by congestive heart failure, and death within 2 days if thiamine treatment was not initiated.

The usual classification of vitamins pertains to their relative solubility. The fat-soluble group—A, D, E, and K—are more soluble in organic solvents, whereas the B-complex group and vitamin C are water-soluble. This general separation on the basis of solubility is useful not just for purposes of noting gross physical properties, but also as a reminder that the fat-soluble vitamins are absorbed, transported, and stored for longer times and in a manner generally similar to fats. Most water-soluble vitamins share the fate of other solutes more compatible with an aqueous, physiologic medium, including a lesser tendency to be retained for long times in the body and a greater loss by way of urinary excretion. Additionally, a general functional difference also exists since the water-soluble vitamins function as coenzymes for a number of important enzymatic reactions in mammals as well as microorganisms [1]. By contrast, the fat-soluble vitamins generally do not function as coenzymes and are rarely utilized for metabolic functions in microorganisms.

Vitamins Essential to Humans

Table 9-1 lists the 13 vitamins and vitameric groups known to be essential to humans. For 11 of these, there are well-discerned levels of requirements that have led to recommended daily dietary allowances (RDA) in the United States; for two (biotin and pantothenic acid), there is somewhat less information on which to base allowances and thus only "estimated safe and adequate daily dietary intakes" have been published.

A number of compounds that are similar to vitamins in that they also are cofactors for important enzymatic reactions include carnitine, choline, inositol, lipoic acid, para-aminobenzoic acid, pteridines, and ubiquinone. They are not considered vitamins because they are normally synthesized; however, they are present in a large number of foods, and there is some evidence that certain chronic conditions may interfere with the normal capacity for endogenous synthesis. Because of the possibility of depletion of these compounds during chronic illness or immaturity, some authors refer to them as "conditionally essential nutrients."

General Comments

The water-soluble vitamins include thiamine (B_1), riboflavin (B_2), niacin (B_3, nicotinic acid, or nicotinamide), pyridoxine (B_6), folate, vitamin B_{12} (cyanocobalamin), pantothenic acid, and biotin (see Table 9-1). Each of these vitamins acts as a cofactor for a variety of biochemical reactions. Compared to the fat-soluble vitamins A, D, and E, water-soluble vitamins may be more easily depleted because of the shorter half-life of 2 to 4 weeks and the normal rate of catabolism. Frequent dietary intake is necessary to avoid deficiency. During low or marginal intakes, deficiencies may not occur unless there is a coexisting condition such as a hypermetabolic state (severe injury, infection, pregnancy, hyperthyroidism), malabsorption, or rapid rates of growth. Thus, signs and symptoms of vitamin deficiency may become clinically overt only with increased requirements superimposed on borderline intakes.

The greater need for vitamins with ample (rather than deficient) intakes of energy and protein may promote overt vitamin deficiency. For example, if all vitamins are omitted from total parenteral nutrition, which supplies all energy requirements as carbohydrate, there is an increased need for thiamine, relative to other vitamins, due to the high carbohydrate intake. Thus, the first signs of acute beriberi with heart failure may occur within 14 to 24 days rather than the expected 2 to 3 months based on the findings from individuals with low carbohydrate intake.

Several members of the vitamin B complex are utilized in the metabolism of a common substrate. Therefore, a deficiency of one vitamin will affect utilization of another. For example, oxidation of ketoacids involves nicotinamide-adenine dinucleotide (NAD) derived from niacin, thiamine, and coenzyme A (which contains pantothenate). In addition, because several vitamins are common to single foods, dietary deficiency of one vitamin is commonly associated with deficiencies of other vitamins. Thus, the classic clinical manifestations of a single vitamin deficiency is generally not seen except with unusual diets, specific disease, or with chronic intake of drugs that interfere with absorption or metabolism of a vitamin.

Several clinical states related to abnormal vitamin metabolism have been observed. These include a number of inborn errors of metabolism that may respond to pharmacologic doses of vitamins and certain conditions resulting in inadequate vitamin intake or increased vitamin requirements [2]. A discussion of these conditions is outside the scope of this chapter.

Conditions That May Increase Vitamin Needs

Liver Disease

Most vitamin deficiencies seen in liver disease are ascribed to fat-soluble vitamins, particularly vitamin A. However, patients with chronic liver disease may also have low circulating levels of pyridoxine (vitamin B_6) and pyridoxal-5-phosphate (PLP), thiamine pyrophosphate (vitamin B_1), and riboflavin (vitamin B_2). This may represent a combination of reduced intake, decreased absorption, increased metabolism, and reduced conservation. Supplemental pyridoxine as well as other water-soluble vitamins is recommended.

Pregnancy

Pregnancy increases the requirements for many vitamins. In particular, the recommended intake of folate is increased from 180 μg/day to 400 μg/day due to its role in preventing neural tube defects. The recommended intake of vitamin A is not increased during pregnancy, but an increased

Table 9-1. Recommended Dietary Allowances of Fat-Soluble and Water-Soluble Vitamins[a]

Category and Age (years)	Fat-Soluble Vitamins				Water-Soluble Vitamins								
	Vitamin A (μg R.E.)[b]	Vitamin D (μg)[c]	Vitamin E (mg α-T.E.)[d]	Vitamin K (μg)	Vitamin C (mg)	Thiamine (mg)	Riboflavin (mg)	Niacin (mg N.E.)[e]	Vitamin B_6 (mg)	Folacin (μg)	Vitamin B_{12} (μg)	Biotin (pg)[f]	Pantothenic Acid (mg)[g]
Infants													
0–0.5	375	7.5	3	5	30	0.3	0.4	5	0.3	25	0.3	10	2
0.5–1.0	375	10	4	10	35	0.4	0.5	6	0.6	35	0.5	15	3
Children													
1–3	400	10	6	15	40	0.7	0.8	9	1.0	50	0.7	20	3
4–6	500	10	7	20	45	0.9	1.1	12	1.1	75	1.0	25	3–4
7–10	700	10	7	30	45	1.0	1.2	13	1.4	100	1.4	30	4–5
Males													
11–14	1000	10	10	45	50	1.3	1.5	17	1.7	150	2.0	30–100	4–7
15–18	1000	10	10	65	60	1.5	1.8	20	2.0	200	2.0	30–100	4–7
19–24	1000	10	10	70	60	1.5	1.7	19	2.0	200	2.0	30–100	4–7
25–50	1000	5	10	80	60	1.5	1.7	19	2.0	200	2.0	30–100	4–7
51+	1000	5	10	80	60	1.2	1.4	15	2.0	200	2.0	30–100	4–7
Females													
11–14	800	10	8	45	50	1.1	1.3	15	1.4	150	2.0	30–100	4–7
15–18	800	10	8	55	60	1.1	1.3	15	1.5	180	2.0	30–100	4–7
19–24	800	10	8	60	60	1.1	1.3	15	1.6	180	2.0	30–100	4–7
25–50	800	5	8	65	60	1.1	1.3	15	1.6	180	2.0	30–100	4–7
51+	800	5	8	65	60	1.0	1.2	13	1.6	180	2.0	30–100	4–7

[a]Allowances are expressed as average daily recommended intakes.

[b]1 Retinol equivalent (R.E.) = 1 μg all-*trans* retinol or 3.33 IU vitamin A. 1 μg R.E. = 6 μg of all-*trans* β-carotene or 12 μg of other provitamin A carotenoids.

[c]Cholecalciferol. 1 μg cholecalciferol = 40 IU vitamin D.

[d]1 α-tocopherol equivalent (α-T.E.) = 1 mg d-α-tocopherol (RRR-α-tocopherol) or 1.49 IU vitamin E. 1 mg α-T.E. = 0.74 mg all-*rac*-α-tocopherol (synthetic vitamin E).

[e]1 niacin equivalent (N.E.) = 1 mg niacin or 60 mg tryptophan.

[f]For biotin and pantothenate, information is presented as Estimated Safe and Adequate Daily Dietary Intakes because there is insufficient information to establish a recommended allowance.

Source: Adapted with permission from Recommended Dietary Allowances (10th ed.). Copyright 1989 by the National Academy of Sciences. Courtesy of the National Academy Press, Washington, DC.

intake (1300 μg R.E. vs. 800 μg R.E.) is recommended during lactation. The recommended allowances of many other vitamins are also increased during lactation.

Drugs

Agents such as isonicotinic acid hydrazide (INH), cycloserine, hydralazine, and penicillamine increase pyridoxine requirements. With chronic intake of these agents, B_6 deficiency may occur. Sulfasalazine (Azulfidine) interferes with folate absorption and chronic use of amitriptyline, chlorpromazine, and imipramine may interfere with riboflavin metabolism. Other pharmacologic agents, including antibiotics, have known and unknown effects on the status, absorption, and/or metabolism of vitamins or vitamin cofactors. Known effects are discussed under specific vitamins. The most commonly consumed agent resulting in both impaired absorption and metabolism of thiamine and riboflavin is *ethanol.*

Hypermetabolism

Severe trauma, burns, and chronic or acute infection are often associated with an increased excretion of several of the B vitamins. The degree to which supplemental vitamins are needed in extreme exercise has not been clearly defined, although increased excretion of several water-soluble vitamins occurs in marathon runners.

Total Parenteral Nutrition

Many patients are treated with parenteral nutrition for brief or prolonged periods. Intravenous multivitamins are therefore added to the nutrient solutions daily or at weekly intervals. Table 9-2 lists the suggested daily intakes for all age groups who require parenteral nutrition.

Thiamine

Thiamine (vitamin B_1, aneurine) is stable on heating to 100°C in the dry form and in aqueous

Table 9-2. Suggested Intakes of Parenteral Vitamins in Infants and Children

Vitamin	Adults: Dose/Day	Term Infants and Children: Dose/Day[a]	Preterm Infants: Dose/Kg Body Weight (Maximum not to exceed term infant dose)	
			Current Suggestions[b]	Best Estimate for New Formulation
Lipid-soluble				
A (μg R.E.)	990	700	280	500
E (mg α-T.E.)	10	7	2.8	2.8
K (μg)[c]	0[c]	200	80	80
D (μg)	5	10	4	4
Water-soluble				
Ascorbic acid (mg)	100	80	32	25
Thiamin (mg)	3	1.2	0.48	0.35
Riboflavin (mg)[d]	3.6	1.4	0.56	0.15
Pyridoxine (mg)[e]	4	1.0	0.4	0.18
Niacin (mg)[f]	40	17	6.8	6.8
Pantothenate (mg)[g]	15	5	2.0	2.0
Biotin (μg)	60	20	8.0	6.0
Folate (μg)	400	140	56	56
Vitamin B_{12} (μg)	5	1.0	0.4	0.3

[a]These guidelines for term infants and children are identical to those of the AMA (NAG). MVI-Pediatric (Astra) meets these guidelines. Recent data indicate that 1 μg (40 IU)·kg^{-1}·d^{-1} of vitamin D (maximum of 10 μg (400 IU)/day) is adequate for term and preterm infants (Koo et al., *J Parent Enteral Nutr* 11:172, 1987). The higher dose of 4 μg (160 IU)·kg^{-1}·d^{-1} has not been associated with complications and maintains blood levels within the reference range for term infants fed orally. This dosage, therefore, appears acceptable until further studies using the lower dose formulation indicates its superiority.

[b]These represent a practical guide (40% of the currently available single dose vial MVI-Pediatric (Astra) formulation per kg body weight), which will provide adequate levels of vitamins D, E, and K but low levels of retinol and excess levels of most of the B vitamins. The maximum daily dose is one single dose vial for any infant.

[c]Vitamin K is not present in MVI-12 (Astra) although all other vitamins listed under "Adults" are present as listed in a single vial of MVI-12.

[d]As phosphate.

[e]As hydrochloride.

[f]As nicotinamide.

[g]As dexpanthenol.

solution, provided the pH is kept below 5.5. Sterilization of solutions at physiologic pH results in destruction of thiamine. Some destruction also occurs in the presence of alkaline drugs, such as sodium phenobarbital, or by the tannins found in wine and tea.

Thiamine is absorbed both actively at low doses and passively at higher doses. It is dependent on the sodium ion for active absorption [3]. Active absorption can be inhibited by ethanol and, unless higher doses are administered, the usually physiologic dose is insufficient to maintain normal levels with chronic alcohol consumption.

Cocarboxylase (thiamine pyrophosphate), the phosphorylated, active form of thiamine, is an integral component of two general enzymatic sequences: (1) decarboxylation of α-ketoglutaric and branched-chain α-ketoacids, and (2) transketolase reactions involving a direct pathway for metabolism of glucose. Although less than 10% of glucose is utilized in the transketolase pathway, it is the only way the body can produce ribose for RNA synthesis.

Dietary sources of thiamine are numerous and include rice husks, cereal grains, yeast, liver, eggs, milk, green leaves, and roots. Human milk is relatively low in thiamine (16 μg/ml) compared to cow's milk, which contains 42 μg/ml. Freezing foods results in little loss.

Deficiency

Thiamine deficiency, or beriberi, occurs in adults when the level of intake drops below 1 mg/day. The biologic half-life of ^{14}C-labeled thiamine is 9 to 18 days, and deficiency symptoms usually develop within 2 to 3 months on a thiamine-deficient diet [4] unless large amounts of carbohydrate are consumed as with TPN; in this case acute cardiac beriberi may develop within 3 weeks. Deficiency may result among individuals who subsist largely on rice, wheat, or corn, or among those unable to obtain thiamine-containing foods. A combination of low intake plus increased requirements (increased growth, lactation, heavy physical labor with primarily carbohydrate energy, and conditions giving rise to increased catabolic states) may also cause symptomatic thiamine deficiency. In the United States, beriberi is most commonly associated with alcoholism. Ethanol inhibits the active transport of thiamine [5]. Passive transport of thiamine continues, however, and larger doses of thiamine should prevent thiamine deficiency under these conditions. Certain foods, such as shellfish and raw carp or herring, contain thiamine-destroying enzymes (thiaminases) that may decrease the thiamine content of food by as much as 50%. If a diet containing these foods is already low in thiamine and is continued for a sufficient period of time, thiamine deficiency may result.

Permanent neurologic symptoms of beriberi may not occur for several months after tissue levels of thiamine are depleted because of the slow degeneration of affected nervous tissue. Reactions involving decarboxylation of α-ketoacids are more affected, and accumulation of pyruvate, lactate, α-ketoglutarate, and glutamate occur in the serum and urine before neurologic symptoms develop.

Clinical Features of Deficiency

There are three classic forms of beriberi: dry, wet, and acute. The dry and wet (edematous) forms are different manifestations of a polyneuritis. The pathogenesis of the edema in wet beriberi is unclear. Infantile beriberi may be more subtle than that found in adults. Children may present with a polyneuritis (pseudomeningitic type), cardiopathy, and/or aphonia. The disease may be slowly progressive or wax and wane. When left untreated, the disease may result in death after a few weeks in the infantile form or years in the adult form, where the diet may not be totally devoid of thiamine. As mentioned earlier, patients given TPN without added vitamins develop acute myocardiopathy within 2 to 3 weeks and die within 48 hours of presentation if untreated.

Thiamine deficiency should be suspected whenever there is starvation and/or malnutrition or when the patient's diet consists primarily of refined rice, wheat, or corn coupled with shellfish, raw carp, or raw herring. The differential diagnosis should also include chronic poisoning (arsenic, triorthocresol phosphate, γ-hexochlorobenzene, etc.), infection, porphyria, mononeuritis complex, Guillain-Barré syndrome, pernicious anemia, and pellagra. A number of clinical states may result in congestive heart failure in children. However, with associated lactic and pyruvic acidemia congestive heart failure (cardiomyopathy) or a burning sensory neuropathy, the diagnosis strongly favors beriberi. Recent findings in Thailand and other developing countries using polished rice as a dietary stable have linked sudden unexplained death in field laborers to thiamine deficiency. Reports from Cuba suggest a similar condition among its workers.

Diagnosis of Deficiency

The diagnosis of thiamine deficiency may be confirmed by measuring erythrocyte transketolase activity, blood thiamine concentration, 24-hour urinary thiamine excretion, or by computing the urinary thiamine-to-creatine ratio from a single urine sample. If erythrocyte transketolase activity increases by 20% or more with the addition of thiamine, thiamine deficiency must be considered. However, transketolase activity may be abnormal in acute febrile states.

Treatment of Deficiency

Treatment of beriberi with thiamine usually leads to resolution of neurologic symptoms within 24 hours, cardiac symptoms in 24 to 48 hours, and edema in 48 to 72 hours. Motor weakness, however, may require 1 to 3 months before being completely resolved. Occasionally, treatment will apparently be progressing satisfactorily when the patient will die suddenly in congestive heart failure. The precise reason for this phenomenon is unclear, but it may be related to inadequate treatment or severe degeneration of cardiac muscles.

Treating children with mild beriberi with an oral dose of 5 mg thiamine per day is usually satisfactory. Severely ill children should receive 10 mg intravenously twice daily. Adults with mild beriberi respond to 10 mg orally three times daily or, in severe cases, to 25 mg intravenously twice daily. In the management of fulminate heart disease, 100 mg thiamine hydrochloride plus vigorous treatment of congestive heart failure is necessary [1].

Toxicity

Doses of 500 mg given intravenously to thiamine-deficient individuals have been well tolerated. In mice, the LD_{50} is 3 g/kg orally. Rapid, intravenous injection of 50 mg/kg thiamine in dogs causes respiratory paralysis, hypotension, bradycardia, and vasodilation. However, if adequate ventilation is maintained, these effects are transient. In rare instances, 100 mg thiamine or less has caused an anaphylactic-type reaction [6]. Hypersensitivity has also been demonstrated by passive transfer. The nature of this toxicity or so-called thiamine shock is not understood.

Riboflavin

Riboflavin (vitamin B_2) is water-soluble, is yellow or orange-yellow in color, and shows a characteristic green fluorescence under ultraviolet (UV) radiation. It is relatively stable in the dry state and in the dark at acid pH is resistant to heat and oxidation. However, it deteriorates rapidly in an alkaline solution, a reaction accelerated by visible or UV light. It is present in all cells only as functioning compounds and not as stored material. The liver (with 16 μg/g) and kidney (with 25 μg/g) usually contain more than other tissues, which average about 2.3 μg/g of tissue.

Riboflavin is absorbed in the small intestine by a site-specific, saturable, specialized transport process. In the liver it is transformed by riboflavin kinase (flavokinase) and adenosine triphosphate (ATP) into flavin mononucleotide (FMN), a reaction that may also occur in intestinal epithelium. FMN is further phosphorylated by flavinadenine dinucleotide (FAD) pyrophosphorylase and ATP in the liver to form FAD. Both FAD and FMN serve as cofactors for several enzymes, the majority of which are oxidases [7].

Flavoproteins are relatively unstable, especially when tissue protein is depleted by physiologic stress, dietary deficiency, or disease. Under these conditions, increased levels of riboflavin are excreted in the urine.

Dietary sources of riboflavin are milk products, eggs, meat, fruits, and green leafy vegetables. It is not destroyed by ordinary cooking unless alkali is added, although prolonged exposure to sunlight may degrade it. Intravenous preparations of riboflavin usually contain it in its more stable phosphorylated form (FMN); however, it is rapidly dephosphorylated upon administration.

Deficiency

Riboflavin deficiency may occur from inadequate intake or malabsorption. In adults, 3 to 8 months may be required before deficiency symptoms appear. In infants and children, dietary deficiency, which is most common in spring and summer, may lead to symptoms within 1 to 2 months. During pregnancy and the rapid growth of children, there is an increased need for riboflavin. Similarly, acute and chronic infection or trauma may increase excretion and therefore increase riboflavin requirements. Structural similarities between riboflavin and amitriptyline, imipramine, and chlorpromazine have been noted. When taking these drugs on a chronic basis, tissue depletion of flavins, increased urinary riboflavin excretion, and reduced erythrocyte glutathione reductase activity have been noted [8]. Riboflavin absorption is decreased in hepatitis, cirrhosis, and probenecid treatment.

Clinical Features of Deficiency

Clinical features are manifest by photophobia, a burning ocular sensation, dim vision, and sore mouth and tongue. Nonspecific symptoms of anorexia, weight loss, weakness, headache, dizziness, and confusion may precede overt symptoms of stomatitis, pharyngitis, glossitis, seborrheic dermatitis, normochromic normocytic anemia, and corneal vascularization. Skin lesions may improve and recur irregularly. Late complications of ariboflavinosis are unusual with prompt therapy. Corneal opacities usually resolve with additional vitamin A, which often increases the rate of response. Rarely, evidence of brain damage may persist in infants.

Diagnosis of Deficiency

Diagnosis should be considered with a history of dietary deficiency and clinical manifestations. The diagnosis can be confirmed by a decreased 24-hour urinary excretion of riboflavin for adults (< 50 μg/24-hr). Increased erythrocyte glutathione reductase activity of more than 20% with the addition of FAD (activity coefficient of 1.20) is also indicative of riboflavin deficiency [9]. This latter test is particularly useful in diagnosing deficient riboflavin intake before development of overt disease. High-performance liquid chromatography (HPLC), with fluorescent detection, has been used to measure riboflavin in plasma and its active cofactors in red cells; detection of plasma riboflavin concentrations below 10 ng/ml suggest inadequate riboflavin intake.

Treatment of Deficiency

Children may be successfully treated orally with 1 mg riboflavin three times daily for several weeks, and infants usually respond to 0.5 mg twice daily. Increased strength and sense of well-being usually occurs within 24 hours. Often, therapeutic doses of vitamin A will improve the corneal lesions more rapidly. If oral administration is precluded, intramuscular or intravenous injection of a similar amount of multiple-vitamin preparation may be necessary three times daily until oral administration is possible.

In animals, large doses of riboflavin have prevented the toxicity associated with boric acid poisoning. Riboflavin appears to bind boric acid. The riboflavin-boric acid complex is stable and excreted in the urine. Massive riboflavinuria, a condition known to occur after accidental poisoning in humans, occurs after administration of boric acid to animals. These observations raise the possibility that pharmacologic doses of riboflavin may be therapeutically useful in boric acid poisoning in humans [10].

Toxicity

Riboflavin toxicity has not been clearly demonstrated in humans. Large doses of riboflavin (600 mg/kg body weight) given intraperitoneally caused riboflavin crystals to develop in the renal collecting system of experimental animals. No other pathology was observed. Even with large doses of riboflavin, tissue levels of riboflavin and of the flavin coenzymes were not substantially increased, suggesting there is a limit above which riboflavin cannot be increased. Preterm infants have shown more than a 100-fold increase in plasma riboflavin with little change in red cell riboflavin and FAD content [11]. Riboflavin may enhance the reduction of serum bilirubin in newborns receiving phototherapy. In vitro studies indicate that riboflavin in the presence of light alters the DNA structure of HeLa cells. These results imply a carcinogenic potential when large doses of riboflavin are given in conjunction with phototherapy. Although no actual toxicity has been demonstrated in term gestation infants, the administration of pharmacologic amounts of the vitamin to preterm infants requiring phototherapy is associated with increased urinary products of lipid peroxidation (TBARS). These findings suggest that some toxicity may exist from pharmacologic doses when given to preterm infants [12].

Niacin

Nicotinic acid and nicotinamide are both referred to as niacin (vitamin B_3). Biosynthesis of this vitamin occurs in almost all organisms, but in humans the conversion ratio of tryptophan to nicotinic acid is only about 60 to 1, making it possible for large amounts of tryptophan to meet niacin requirements. Niacin is absorbed in the proximal small bowel and incorporated into nicotinamide adenine dinucleotide (NAD) and nicotinamide adenine dinucleotide phosphate (NADP). These two compounds are coenzymes for oxidation-reduction reactions (including synthesis of high-energy phosphate compounds, glycolysis, pyruvate metabolism, pentose biosynthesis, glycerol, and fatty acid metabolism), for obtaining energy from protein, and in excision-repair mechanisms of DNA.

Dietary sources of niacin include liver, yeast, white meat, poultry, peanuts, and legumes; some niacin is present in potatoes, vegetables, and wheat. Because of their high tryptophan content, milk and eggs are also good sources of niacin. Roasting of coffee converts trigonelline to nicotinic acid so that one cup of coffee may contain 1 to 2 mg of nicotinic acid. Niacin is stable in boiling water but is incompatible with sodium nitrite, the substance used to maintain normal meat coloring. An excess of dietary leucine, which is found, for example, in corn, interferes with conversion of tryptophan to niacin and accounts for the high prevalence of niacin deficiency in individuals who subsist almost entirely on corn. Nicotinic acid is not totally absent in corn, but it is present in an unavailable form (niacytin). When corn is lime-treated, however, as is the practice when making tortillas in Central America, or when sweet corn is roasted, for example, by the Hopi Indians of Arizona, the niacin is made available.

Deficiency

Niacin deficiency leads to pellagra, named after the pathognomonic skin changes that result: *pelle,* skin; *agro,* rough. Pellagra is prone to occur in individuals subsisting predominantly on corn, corn products, or millet (sorghum) because of the high leucine content. Pellagra resulting from millet ingestion can be reversed by isoleucine. In the United States, pellagra may be seen in alcoholics or, rarely, in food faddists during pregnancy. By and large, pellagra occurs in low-income groups and in patients with anorexia or gastrointestinal disease associated with severe malabsorption. Because vitamin B_6 is required for transformation of tryptophan to niacin, pellagra is occasionally seen in individuals treated with isonicotine hydrazine (INH) who develop B_6 deficiency. It is also common in patients with malignant carcinoid tumors, and in infants with Hartnup disease, an inborn error of tryptophan metabolism.

Clinical Features of Deficiency

Clinical features of niacin deficiency are chronic, relapsing, and popularly characterized by three (or four) Ds: dermatitis, diarrhea, dementia, and, if untreated, death. The cutaneous lesions, usually noted first, appear as an erythema resembling sunburn on those parts of the body exposed to sunlight, heat, and other forms of mild trauma. These areas are erythematous and infiltrated, and they itch and burn. More acute cases may progress to vesiculation, ulceration, and secondary infection. Classically, the erythema progresses to roughening and keratosis with scaling. In most cases, a brownish pigmentation develops and, in the process of healing, peels off, leaving pink skin underneath. Oral lesions with angular stomatitis are often present but may reflect associated vitamin deficiencies. The rectum and anus are often inflamed as well, with an extension to the small bowel to produce varying degrees of villus effacement and infiltration. This involvement accounts for the diarrhea and malabsorption frequently accompanying the dermatitis. Daily dietary intakes of less than 7.5 mg niacin without tryptophan have been associated with the development of pellagra.

Although neurologic manifestations may appear without skin manifestations, they usually follow development of skin lesions. Neurologic signs may be mild to moderate, presenting with some weakness, malaise, anxiety, and/or short attention span, or, when severe, with delirium. In most chronic forms, amentia, posterolateral cord degeneration, and peripheral nerve lesions are present. Only in the most severe and chronic cases do the neurologic lesions persist after adequate treatment with niacin [13].

Diagnosis of Deficiency

Diagnosis may be suspected by a history of inadequate diet, isonicotine hydrazine treatment, or chronic ethanol ingestion when the typical skin lesions, diarrhea, and mental symptoms are present. Determination of urinary excretion of niacin or one of its products (N^1-methylnicotinamide) is most helpful in confirmation of the clinical impression.

Normal excretion of N^1-methylnicotinamide is usually between 4 and 6 mg/day, and values less than 3 mg/day suggest deficient niacin intake; in pellagra, urinary N^1-methylnicotinamide is 0.5 to 0.8 mg/day. With a niacin intake of 5.5 mg/day, urinary niacin excretion was between 0.5 and 1 mg/day. One study showed that the pyridone derivative of N^1-methylnicotinamide was not excreted unless niacin intake was sufficient [1]. However, measurement of this compound is difficult, and few laboratories are equipped to determine it on a routine basis.

Treatment of Deficiency

Treatment of pellagra is usually more effective with oral niacin than with parenteral administration because blood levels remain elevated longer following oral treatment. The usual daily dose is about 10 times the recommended dietary intake or about 50 to 100 mg for adults. Nicotinamide is usually preferred over nicotinic acid because it avoids certain unpleasant side effects (flushing, tachycardia, etc.) seen with large doses of nicotinic acid. Parenteral therapy may be preferable when gastrointestinal absorption is deficient, and a dose of 25 mg five times a day is recommended. In infants, 50 to 100 mg nicotinamide can be dissolved in the daily milk allotment. Parenteral nicotinamide may also be given at 5 mg three to five times a day. Prevention of pellagra can be achieved by eating an adequate protein diet containing tryptophan and foods containing niacin.

Toxicity

Pharmacologic doses of nicotinic acid (not nicotinamide) have been used to treat patients with types II, IV, and V hyperlipoproteinemia. The dose is generally 1.5 to 3 g, but may be as much as 9 g/day. Abnormal liver function tests or insulin resistance may develop, but these resolve when the dose is decreased. A typical cystoid macular edema with loss of central vision has been the most potentially serious toxic manifestation. However, vision improved and the macular edema resolved with discontinuation of nicotinic acid. Nicotinic acid, but not nicotinamide, will cause dilatation of skin capillaries, a reaction most severe with systemic injection. The severe flushing seen with large doses of nicotinic acid may be improved by pretreatment with salicylates.

Pyridoxine

Pyridoxine (vitamin B_6) occurs in nature as three closely related compounds: pyridoxine, most abundant in plants, and pyridoxal and pyridoxamine, which predominate in animal tissues. All three forms, and their respective phosphates, can be interconverted to the enzymatically active form, PLP. They, and their phosphate derivatives, are all water-soluble, stable to air and light, and relatively resistant to heat.

The active form, PLP, acts as a coenzyme for a number of biologically important reactions mostly involving nitrogen metabolism. These reactions include transamination, decarboxylation, racemization, amine oxidation (monoamine oxidase and diamine oxidase), aldol reactions, and desulfhydration. Synthetases, phosphorylase b kinase, and phosphorylase phosphatase are also B_6-requiring enzymes. Approximately one-half the B_6 content of the body can be accounted for in the phosphorylase of skeletal muscle [14].

Pyridoxine is actively absorbed almost completely from the upper gastrointestinal tract. Little or none is absorbed from that produced by microorganisms in the colon.

Most ordinary diets contain adequate levels of B_6. Excellent sources are liver, vegetables, fruits, whole-grain cereals, and meats. Milling of wheat may reduce B_6 content by 80% to 90%, and cooking frozen vegetables may reduce the B_6 content by 25%.

Deficiency

Pyridoxine deficiency, due to an inadequate intake of B_6, generally occurs only with deficiencies of other B vitamins. Although specific pyridoxine deficiency is rare in the United States, in the early 1950s, a formula containing only 60 μg/l vitamin B_6 (one-third to one-half the recommended dose) was inadvertently given to a number of infants. After several weeks, symptoms of hyperactivity, hyperacusis, and convulsive seizures developed. Symptoms were aggravated by increases in protein intake and corrected by 5 to 10 mg pyridoxine. These observations suggest that a decreased B_6 intake could produce symptoms primarily manifest by abnormal central nervous system (CNS) function. One possible explanation for this disturbance is the lowering of CNS levels of α-aminobutyric acid in B_6 deficiency, which may decrease the irritability threshold of the brain [15].

Pyridoxine deficiency in the United States most commonly occurs in individuals who are genetically "slow-inactivators" of INH, a potent antagonist of B_6. These individuals are particularly susceptible to developing a B_6-responsive peripheral neuropathy. In addition, INH may precipitate a B_6-responsive anemia. Contraceptive steroids, penicillamine, hydrazine (used in rocket fuels), and hydralazine (an antihypertensive agent) may precipitate B_6 deficiency [15].

Clinical Features of Deficiency

Although deficient adults may present initially with a peripheral neuritis, children, who seem to be resistant to developing neuritis, may present with diarrhea instead. Other clinical features are nonspecific and include insomnia, weakness, mental depression, cheilosis, stomatitis, nasolabial seborrhea, and dermatitis. Later symptoms usually include peripheral neuropathy and convulsive seizures.

Diagnosis of Deficiency

Diagnosis may be difficult in areas of the world where malnutrition is not endemic. It should be considered in infants with convulsive disorders, microcytic hypochromic anemias unresponsive to iron, poor nutrition, severe catabolic states, and in persons with anorexia nervosa or food faddism. The diagnosis in adults may be confirmed by several laboratory methods [16]. Urinary excretion of 4-pyridoxic acid less than 0.2 mg or pyridoxine less than 10 μg/mg creatinine indicates deficiency in adults. Accepted values for children have not been determined. Indirect evaluation of pyridoxine status can be assessed by determining the glutamic-pyruvic or glutamic-oxaloacetic transaminase activities in red cells with or without preincubation with PLP. Increased activity of greater than 20% with PLP preincubation suggests pyridoxine deficiency. Urinary excretion of xanthurenic acid of greater than 50 mg and kynurenic acid greater than 30 mg following an L-tryptophan load (50 mg/kg to a maximum of 2 g) may also be used to determine pyridoxine status. Increased xanthurenic acid excretion is seen in children with leukemia, infection, diabetes, porphyria, and other illnesses. As a result, urinary excretion of tryptophan metabolites should not be used as the sole determinant of B_6 status. Newer methods of pyridoxine measurement in blood by HPLC have not defined clear-cut levels at which deficiency is established, although plasma PLP concentrations below 10 mg/mL would support the clinical impression of deficiency.

Treatment of Deficiency

Treatment is generally the same as that outlined under the treatment of the various pyridoxine dependency syndromes. A convulsive disorder and other symptoms of B_6 deficiency in infants are usually promptly relieved by administration of 10 mg pyridoxine intravenously with an oral dose of 10 mg daily for 1 to 2 weeks or until the clinical manifestations of the illness have been corrected.

Other therapeutic uses of vitamin B_6 have included the treatment of anemia, cardiac decompensation, the side effects of radiation therapy, skin grafting, isoniazid toxicity, atherosclerosis, and alcoholism. In general, there does not appear to be any specific requirement for B_6 other than the prevention of pyridoxine deficiency, ameliorating various dependency syndromes, and as an adjunct to INH therapy. Oral pyridoxal in doses of 50 to 100 mg three times weekly reportedly aids in moderating vomiting during pregnancy. However, these reports have not been confirmed in controlled studies. Pyridoxine has been used in some patients with hereditary or primarily acquired sideroblastic anemia (sideroachrestic anemia). Some responded to relatively small doses (0.5 to 1.0 mg/day), whereas others required much larger doses. These conditions must be distinguished from pyridoxine-responsive anemia.

Toxicity

Toxicity in humans has been seen with 1000 to 2700 times the RDA (2 to 6 g/day) being used for treatment of carpal tunnel syndrome. These patients developed a peripheral neuropathy similar to that seen with B_6 deficiency. The synthetic analogue, desoxypyridoxine, is highly poisonous.

Pantothenic Acid

Pantothenic acid (vitamin B_5) is an unstable, pale yellow, viscous oil that is difficult to purify. It is easily destroyed by acids, bases, and heat and is commercially available as the water-soluble calcium salt. Pantothenate is absorbed in the proximal small intestine; in the liver it becomes an integral part of coenzyme A. Coenzyme A plays a fundamental role in many metabolic reactions. Its active form, acetylcoenzyme A, is involved primarily in the Krebs cycle, the transfer of two-carbon units, and the synthesis of fats, steroids, and porphyrins. Pantothenate is found in virtually all naturally occurring foods.

Deficiency

As an isolated entity, pantothenate deficiency rarely occurs. The deficiency may occur under extreme circumstances, for example, famine, prolonged anorectic illness, imprisonment during wartime, or alcoholism. Deficiency of pantothenate probably only exists with other vitamin deficiencies to which the symptoms may be ascribed. Isolated deficiency of pantothenate has been experimentally produced in humans on a "pantothenate-free" diet together with a pantothenic acid antagonist, ω-methylpantothenic acid [17,18].

Clinical Features of Deficiency

Clinical features of experimental pantothenate deficiency consist of apathy, lethargy, irritability, depression, insomnia, burning paresthesia, numbness, muscle cramping, incoordination, and occasional vomiting and diarrhea. Fatigue, headache, and weakness are the most persistent and annoying symptoms. Evidence that humans suffer from naturally occurring pantothenate deficiency is primarily suggestive. The "burning foot" syndrome observed in Japanese war prisoners was reported to respond to administration of pantothenic acid [19]. No evidence of pantothenate deficiency has been presented in infants and young children.

Diagnosis of Deficiency

Diagnosis is based on symptoms produced during experimental studies. These symptoms, plus a blood pantothenate level of less than 100 μg/1 dl, is suggestive of a deficient intake. Urinary excretion of pantothenate normally ranges between 0.78 and 7.4 mg/day, and deficiency is suggestive with urinary levels less than 0.7 mg/24-hr.

Toxicity

Toxicity has not been demonstrated, even with daily doses of 50 to 100 mg/day for a month. A single dose of 100 mg intravenously had no apparent toxic effect.

Biotin

Biotin is a coenzyme for carbon dioxide fixation (carboxylation reactions). Six such reactions have been found to require biotin as an essential cofactor in mammals: acetyl coenzyme A carboxylase, β-methylcrotonyl-CoA carboxylase, propionyl-CoA carboxylase, geraniol-CoA carboxylase, and pyruvate carboxylase. Avidin, a specific protein in egg albumin in vivo, markedly inhibits each of these enzymes because of its great affinity for biotin. Overt biotin deficiency may not occur naturally because gastrointestinal bacteria produce biotin.

Dietary biotin sources include liver, egg yolk, milk, yeast extracts, and meat. Nuts, chocolate, and some vegetables (especially cauliflower) have lesser amounts present. Cereals are relatively poor sources.

Deficiency

Biotin deficiency can be produced experimentally after long-term feeding with a biotin-deficient diet in conjunction with either large doses of antibiotics to destroy gastrointestinal flora or large amounts of raw avidin. Biotin deficiency has been observed in individuals who consume large numbers of raw eggs (rich in avidin) for several months. The avidin in raw eggs that binds biotin is not hydrolyzed by gastrointestinal enzymes and thus prevents biotin absorption. Cooking of eggs destroys avidin. Before biotin was routinely added to TPN solutions, several children developed biotin deficiency with the typical skin and biochemical changes seen in adults [20]. Biotin deficiency has also been described in children receiving long-term treatment with TPN with no source of biotin.

Clinical Features of Deficiency

Clinical features of biotin deficiency include a fine, nonpruritic dermatitis; after 5 weeks, lassitude, muscular pain, and hypesthesias appear. After 10 weeks, anorexia, nausea, anemia, and hypercholesterolemia develop. In infants, the skin rash is a seborrheic dermatitis and resembles Leiners disease. The rash is characterized by scaling of inflamed skin, particularly on the cheeks and neck, in the gluteal region, and sometimes around the umbilicus and groin.

Diagnosis of Deficiency

Diagnosis is difficult because it is seldom suspected clinically. The symptoms are relatively nonspecific, and definitive laboratory tests are usually unavailable. An assay of blood and urine may reveal biotin deficiency. Whole blood biotin levels usually range between 820 and 2700 pg/ml and urinary excretion of biotin between 14 and 100 μg/day [21].

Treatment of Deficiency

A parenteral biotin dose of 200 μg daily for 2 to 5 days effectively treated deficiency secondary to the ingestion of raw egg whites. Oral administration of 2 to 5 mg daily for 2 to 3 weeks is recommended for mild cases.

Toxicity

Toxicity to biotin has not been described.

Vitamin C

Most animals synthesize ascorbate from glucose via glucuronic acid and gluconic acid. Humans and other primates, the guinea pig, the elephant, the red-breasted bulbul bird, and the fruit-eating bat, however, do not synthesize vitamin C.

Vitamin C appears to function primarily in the capacity of a strong reducing agent or in reactions involved in electron transport within biologic systems. Although it appears to have multiple functions in humans, its specific biochemistry is not clearly defined. Its most striking property is its capacity for reversible oxidation-reduction.

Ascorbic acid is absorbed in the upper small intestine. An average dietary intake of 50 to 150 mg/day maintains a plasma level of about 1.2 mg/1 dl. The renal threshold of ascorbate is about 1.4 mg/1 dl. Vitamin C appears unchanged in the urine or as the sulfate when the renal threshold is exceeded. It is metabolized to 2,3-diketogluconic acid and oxylate, both of which are excreted in urine.

Dietary sources of vitamin C include raw liver, fruits, and vegetables. Much of the vitamin C in foods may be lost in cooking and storage because both heat and oxidation destroy it. Ascorbate is relatively stable in canned and frozen foods.

Deficiency

Vitamin C deficiency is manifest by formation of abnormal collagen fibers. After proline is inserted into a precollagen protein unit by the cellular ribosomes, ascorbate and oxygen are necessary for hydroxylation of carbo-4 proline to form normal collagen. The enzyme collagen proline hydroxylase catalyzes this reaction. Ascorbate also is involved in the hydroxylation of other compounds, such as norepinephrine, tryptophan, and certain steroids. All hydroxylations presumably involve ascorbate-dependent electron-transfer mechanisms at the microsomal level. Other reactions involving ascorbate include the oxidation of phenylalanine and tyrosine, hydroxylation of tryptophan, utilization of iron, conversion of folic to folinic acid, maintenance of normal activity of serum complement, and conversion of cholesterol to bile acids. Ascorbate also spares or protects several of the B vitamins including B_1, B_2, folate, and pantothenate. However, ascorbate will destroy vitamin B_{12} in serum [22].

Prolonged vitamin C deficiency results in scurvy. The more common associations leading to scurvy are food faddism, alcoholism, famine, or other reasons for marginal subsistence such as deficiencies suffered by prisoners of war. Infantile scurvy has occurred most commonly in infants fed exclusively cow's milk for the first 6 to 12 months of life. At present, most commercial distributors in the United States supplement their milk with vitamin C, making scurvy uncommon in this country. However, losses of vitamin C may increase substantially following severe trauma, and more than the usual recommended doses of vitamin C may be necessary to facilitate healing of extensive burns.

Clinical Features of Deficiency

In infancy, clinical features of scurvy (Barlows disease) occur between 8 and 13 months of age and begin with anorexia, intermittent diarrhea, failure to gain weight, pallor, irritability, apathy, and increased susceptibility to infection. As the illness progresses, long-bone tenderness and failure of spontaneous leg movement may occur. Hemorrhage under the periosteum of long bones, mucus membranes, and skin is common. Advanced stages of scurvy are characterized by hematuria, hematemesis, bloody diarrhea, epistaxis, ecchymosis of the eyelids, and proptosis from orbital hemorrhage.

The scorbutic infant is often febrile with tachycardia and tachypnea out of proportion to the degree of fever. A rounded type of costochondral beading (scorbutic rosary) may be confused with rickets. This phenomenon is due to costochondral separation that causes the sternum to sink slightly inward, leaving a sharp edge on the rib side of the junction.

Radiographic changes are seen at the cartilage shaft junction and appear earliest at sites of most active growth, for example, sternal ends of ribs, distal femur, proximal humerus, both ends of tibia and fibula, and distal radius and ulna [23]. There is broadening of the zone of divisional calcification at the epiphyseal end of the shaft causing a thickened white line (of Fraenkel) that results from accumulation of calcified cartilage. If there is a zone of rarefaction under the white line at the metaphysis, the x-ray is said to be diagnostic of scurvy. The cortex of the bone is thinned, giving a ground glass appearance and causing the white line to be more prominent. After several days of treatment with ascorbate, areas of subperiosteal hemorrhage become clearly outlined by bone formation in the periphery. The zone of rarefaction, called the scurvy line, gradually becomes filled with normal bone trabeculae, which form a dense shadow that fuses with the epiphyseal line. Following a year of treatment, normal bone architecture is usually restored.

The radiographic features of copper deficiency may be identical to those features resulting from ascorbate deficiency because both ascorbate and copper are required for mature collagen formation. The use of total parenteral feedings without copper supplements has caused an increase in the prevalence of copper deficiency during infancy, which may be confused radiographically with the scurvy of ascorbate deficiency.

Diagnosis of Deficiency

Diagnosis can be made by the presence of characteristic physical findings and a history of dietary inadequacy of vitamin C. Roentgenograms of the bones may be diagnostic in infantile scurvy. Low plasma ascorbate may not be diagnostic because the level may be near zero for as long as three months before scurvy develops. The vitamin C content of leukocytes may be a valuable aid in diagnosis. However, levels may be depressed by tetracycline, which lowers leukocyte ascorbate content and increases urinary losses. Long-term hemodialysis, chronic inflammatory diseases, heavy cigarette smoking, and contraceptive steroids are also associated with low serum ascorbate levels. Serum levels of less than 0.10 mg/1 dl are considered deficient, and a level of 0.20 mg/1 dl is generally considered the lower limit of normal.

Treatment of Deficiency

Treatment is often dramatic, with improvement in appetite and disposition within 24 to 48 hours. Tenderness of extremities, fever, and hemorrhagic phenomena disappear within a few days. The usual treatment dose for infantile scurvy is 25 mg four times daily (usually given with feedings) for 4 to 5 days, then decreased to 25 mg twice daily until complete healing occurs. Prevention of scurvy in areas where milk is not fortified with vitamin C can be accomplished by administering 1 to 2 oz of orange or tomato juice or an intake of 25 mg of vitamin C daily. Although limes have relatively small amounts of vitamin C, when taken in sufficient quantity they are also effective in prevention. In controlled trials, pharmacologic doses of vitamin C have failed to prevent upper respiratory infections. However, a relationship has been demonstrated between the level of dietary ascorbate and strength of wound healing. Because of the decrease in plasma ascorbate following severe trauma or surgical procedures, it has been suggested that the daily dose of vitamin C be increased from the recommended adult intake of 60 mg to between 100 and 300 mg. Because vitamin C is a cofactor in the in vitro reaction of homogentisic acid oxidase, it is conceivable that pharmacologic doses could be of benefit in the treatment of homogentisic aciduria (alkaptonuria).

Toxicity

Daily administration of 12 g ascorbate for several months has caused no detrimental effects, although changes in lipid levels may occur. Large doses may cause diarrhea in children and may precipitate hemolysis in individuals with glucose-6-phosphate dehydrogenase deficiency [24]. Large doses of vitamin C can interfere with vitamin B_{12} absorption and metabolism in humans, and this interference may be overcome by supplemental vitamin B_{12} [22]. Healthy adults can become conditioned to high doses of ascorbate (0.5 to 1.6 g/day) over a 2-week period, resulting in a lower-than-normal serum and leukocyte ascorbate level on returning to a normal vitamin C intake.

Because ascorbate is an acidifying agent, large doses may be contraindicated in gout, renal tubular acidosis, cirrhosis, paroxysmal nocturnal hemoglobinuria, and other conditions aggravated by acid loading [25].

Vitamin B_{12}

The generic term vitamin B_{12} refers to a group of physiologically active substances chemically classified as cobalamins or corrinoids. Cobalamins differ in the nature of additional side groups bound to cobalt. Examples are methyl (methylcobalamin), 5′-deoxyadenosyl (deoxyadenosylcobalamin), hydroxyl (hydroxocobalamin), H_2O (aquocobalamin), and cyanide (cyanocobalamin). Cyanocobalamin is a stable compound that forms dark red needlelike crystals; it is the reference compound for measuring serum cobalamin concentration. Less stable serum cobalamins may be converted to this compound for quantitation. The predominant physiologic form of cobalamin in serum is methylcobalamin, whereas that in cytosol is 5′-deoxyadenosylcobalamin. It is recommended that the term vitamin B_{12} be used as the generic descriptor for all corrinoids exhibiting qualitatively the biologic activity of cyanocobalamin [26].

Vitamin B_{12} is a coenzyme for two physiologically important functions in humans: (1) the synthesis of methionine, which requires methylcobalamine, and (2) the conversion of methylmalonic acid to succinic acid, which requires 5′-deoxyadenosylcobalamin.

To provide a matrix for B_{12} absorption, a complex is formed with intrinsic factor (IF) secreted from gastric parietal cells. When the vitamin B_{12}-IF complex reaches the distal ileum, it is bound by special receptors on the surface of mucosal epithelial cells and then enters the cells. Within the mucosal epithelial cells, the vitamin B_{12}-IF complex is dissociated, and the vitamin then passes into the plasma of the mucosal capillaries and next to the portal vein. Almost all of the vitamin B_{12} is taken up by hepatocytes as the portal blood passes through the liver. It is stored within the liver and released as needed into the plasma. If the quantity of vitamin B_{12} exceeds the capacity of hepatocyte receptors, most of the excess is excreted by the kidneys. Normally, approximately 1 mg of vitamin B_{12} is stored in the liver, a quantity equivalent to meet the daily metabolic needs for 2000 days. It is for this reason that when the dietary supply of vitamin B_{12} is interrupted or mechanisms of absorption are impaired, vitamin B_{12} deficiency does not become evident for five years or more.

Three classes of vitamin B_{12} transport proteins are found in humans: (1) IF, which occurs only in gastric juice, (2) transcobalamin II (TC II), which is found in plasma and other body fluids, and (3) cobalophilin or R proteins, which are ubiquitous. The most important transport protein in plasma is TC II [27]. It transports vitamin B_{12} to receptors on cell membranes throughout the body. The TC II-vitamin B_{12} complex enters the cell by pinocytosis. Lysosomal proteolysis degrades TC II and releases the vitamin B_{12}. Unbound vitamin B_{12} can also enter the tissue cells, but the process is much less efficient.

The only significant dietary sources of vitamin B_{12} are meats, milk or milk products, and eggs. Because vitamin B_{12} can be stored in significant amounts and it is conserved through reabsorption from that secreted in bile, vegetarians are able to receive only intermittent small amounts of the vitamin without becoming deficient.

Deficiency

Deficiency of vitamin B_{12} causes serious and often irreversible neurologic disorders such as burning pain or loss of sensation in the extremities, weakness, spasticity and paralysis, confusion, disorientation, and dementia. This condition has been given the name subacute combined degeneration of the spinal cord. Neurologic symptoms may occur without any discernible hematologic changes in the blood. The classic morphologic changes in the blood, in approximate order of appearance, are hypersegmentation of neutrophils, macrocytosis, anemia, leukopenia, and thrombocytopenia, with megaloblastic changes in bone marrow accompanying the peripheral blood changes. Approximately one-third of patients who have vitamin B_{12} deficiency and who respond to cobalamin therapy are not anemic and do not have macrocytosis of RBCs. Serum vitamin B_{12} is not always decreased in cobalamin deficiency, and low serum levels of vitamin B_{12} may result from various mechanisms. Assays of methylmalonic acid or homocysteine are more sensitive for detection of vitamin B_{12} deficiency than is measurement of serum vitamin B_{12}. Among the causes of vitamin B_{12} deficiency are lack of IF secretion by the stomach and intestinal malabsorption. In the absence of IF (pernicious anemia), vitamin B_{12} cannot be absorbed from food. Pernicious anemia most commonly occurs in young black women or in middle-aged to elderly whites. Pernicious anemia may also occur in children due to either failure of IF secretion or secretion of biologically inactive IF.

Diagnosis of Deficiency

Diagnosis of pernicious anemia usually requires demonstration of IF blocking antibody in serum, inability to absorb vitamin B_{12} when administered orally (in the Schilling test) without exogenous IF, and absorption of vitamin B_{12} when exogenous IF is given. Absence of IF also follows total gastrectomy, which is usually performed for gastric carcinoma. However, few such patients survive long enough to develop vitamin B_{12} deficiency. Vitamin B_{12} deficiency may also occur many years after partial gastrectomy (usually performed for peptic ulcer disease).

Intestinal malabsorption of vitamin B_{12} may be caused by gastrectomy or ileal resection, with an inverse relationship between the length of ileum resected and the absorption of vitamin B_{12}. Other causes of malabsorption are tropical sprue, inflammatory disease of the small intestine, and intestinal stasis with overgrowth of colonic bacteria, which consume the vitamin B_{12} ingested by the host. In very rare cases, infestation of the small intestine by the fish tapeworm *Diphyllobothrium latum* can consume intestinal vitamin B_{12} and thus cause systemic vitamin B_{12} deficiency. Because ample quantities of vitamin B_{12} are present in all types of meat, milk, cheese, eggs, and other sources of animal protein, only the most extreme form of vegetarianism (veganism), in which all animal products are excluded from the diet, can lead to vitamin B_{12} deficiency—and then only after decades of nutritional impoverishment. In fact, most vegans do not develop signs or symptoms of vitamin B_{12} deficiency. Another cause of vitamin B_{12} malabsorption is failure to extract cobalamin from food. Some patients fail to absorb cobalamin bound to food, while absorption of non-food-bound cobalamin in the Schilling test is unimpaired. This is particularly a problem in patients with compromised gastric status or early in the course of development of pernicious anemia.

Treatment of Deficiency

When vitamin B_{12} deficiency is the result of inadequate absorption, a single injection of 100 μg or more of vitamin B_{12} (cyanocobalamin) produces a complete therapeutic remission in any patient whose deficiency is not complicated by unrelated systemic disease or other factors. The remission is sustained for life by monthly injections of 100 μg of vitamin B_{12}. It is important to inform the patient who has permanent gastric or ileal damage that monthly injections of vitamin B_{12} must be continued for life.

For simultaneous differential diagnosis and therapy, patients should be treated with an injection of 1 μg of vitamin B_{12} daily for 10 days after a control period of a few days to establish the constancy of the reticulocyte level and the elimination of dietary sources. Initial therapy with doses of vitamin B_{12} greater than 1 μg daily is desirable when the vitamin B_{12} deficiency is complicated by other debilitating illness such as infection, hepatic disease, uremia, coma, severe disorientation, or marked neurologic damage. In such patients, 30 μg or more of vitamin B_{12} is given daily parenterally for 5 to 10 days. Daily parenteral doses larger than 30 μg have no proven therapeutic advantage, and much of the excess is rapidly excreted in the urine.

Vitamin B_{12} can also be administrated in a nasal gel, facilitating self-administration. Preliminary data indicate that nasal B_{12} is more effectively absorbed than oral B_{12} in normal individuals, that it is effective in counteracting intestinal B_{12} malabsorption, and that it can be used to treat B_{12}-deficient patients.

Hydroxocobalamin and other depot preparations of vitamin B_{12} may be retained longer at the site of injection and in serum, but this possible slight therapeutic advantage over cyanocobalamin does not warrant their greater cost; they also may have undesirable side effects. More detailed discussion of vitamin B_{12} preparations, routes of administration, dosage, and therapeutic responses may be found elsewhere [28].

Ten different inherited metabolic defects that impair the pathways of vitamin B_{12} transport or metabolism have been identified. Three affect absorption and transport; the remaining seven affect cellular utilization and coenzyme production. The three former defects manifest themselves in infancy or early childhood as developmental delay with megaloblastic anemia and usually respond favorably to periodic injections of the vitamin. The remaining seven defects result in manifestations that depend on whether the enzyme requiring either adenosylcobalamin or methylcobalamin is affected or whether the formation of both forms of B_{12} are affected. Two defects involve utilization of adenosylcobalamin and result in methylmalonic acidemia and respond most favorably to pharmacologic supplements of cyano- or hydroxocobalamin. Two defects result from methylcobalamin synthesis and cause homocystinuria with hypomethiominemia. These children have developmental delay, failure to thrive, and megaloblastic anemia; they usually respond to pharmacologic doses of vitamin B_{12}. Three defects lead to impaired synthesis of both adenosylcobalamin and methylcobalamin. The children have both methylmalonic acidemia and homocystinuria, have severe developmental delay, and respond less favorably to pharmacologic doses of vitamin B_{12}.

Toxicity

Vitamin B_{12} is generally felt to be nontoxic, even in doses that exceed the adult human requirement by 10,000 fold. A rare allergic reaction has been reported, possibly due to impurities in an unusual preparation of crystalline cyanocobalamin. Hydroxocobalamin injections and injections of various depot preparations of cyanocobalamin have been associated with the appearance of antibody to plasma vitamin B_{12}-binding protein. Although the significance of this antibody is not yet clear, such preparations offer no clear advantage over cyanocobalamin to warrant their use, especially in view of their greater cost and the pain on injection of some of the depot preparations. The pharmaceutical preparation cyanocobalamin is not metabolically active in humans. Tissue enzymes remove the cyanide to make the cobalamin active. The rare infant who is born with a congenital lack of this cyanide-removing mechanism can be harmed, of course, by cyanocobalamin, which serves in that case as an antimetabolite of vitamin B_{12}.

Folic Acid

Folate and folic acid are general terms for a family of compounds related to pteroic acid. Pteroic acid is composed of a pteridine ring joined to a *p*-aminobenzoic acid residue. When pteroic acid is conjugated with one molecule of L-glutamic acid, pterolyglutamic acid (PteGlu) is formed. It can be reduced to dihydrofolic acid (7,8 H_2PteGlu or FH_2) or to tetrahydrofolate 5,6,7,8 H_4PteGlu or FH_4). Only the reduced forms are biologically active. Although various forms of folic acid are normally present in human serum and other body fluids, the principal form is N^5-methyltetrahydrofolate. It is slowly oxidized in alkaline solution, but this can be reversed by adding ascorbic acid. It is relatively stable in acid solutions but unstable when exposed to light. Multiple forms of folic acid occur with substitutions of functional groups such as methyl, formyl, methylene, hydroxymethyl, and others at various nitrogen atoms in the pteroic acid residue. These forms of folate serve to transfer single carbon units.

Folate coenzymes are essential for the transfer of single carbon units, the major reactions being conversion of serine to glycine, catabolism of histidine, and synthesis of thymidylate, methionine, and purine. Different folates are involved in these reactions depending on the chemical state of the single carbon fragments transferred, as illustrated in Table 9-3.

Other folate derivatives have multiple glutamic acid residues (H_4PteGlu$_n$), when *n*, the number of glutamate residues, may be one to seven. Recent studies indicate that these folate polyglutamates are the preferred substrates and active coenzyme forms in one-carbon metabolism [29].

Polyglutamate forms of folate present in food are first converted to monoglutamates, by pteroylpolyglutamate hydrolase, in the intestinal mucosa. After cellular uptake, most of the folate is reduced and methylated and enters the circulation as N^5-methyltetrahydrofolate. Dietary sources provide approximately 500 μg of folate per day.

Table 9-3. Folate Coenzymes and Major Reactions

Reaction	Folate Coenzyme
Serine/glycine metabolism	N^5, N^{10}-Methylene FH_4
Histidine catabolism	N^5-Formimino FH_4
Thymidylate synthesis	N^5, N^{10}-Methylene FH_4
Methionine synthesis	N^5-Methyl FH_4
Purine synthesis	N^5, N^{10}-Methyenyl FH_4 N^{10}-Formyl FH_4

Body stores of folate range from 5 to 10 mg, of which approximately half is in the liver. Interruption of absorption of folate may therefore result in deficiency within a few months because about 50 μg/day are lost by excretion.

Folic acid and B_{12} metabolism are linked by the reaction that transfers a methyl group from N^5-methyltetrahydrofolate to cobalamin. In cases of cobalamin deficiency, folate is "trapped" as N^5-methyltetrahydrofolate. It is "metabolically dead" in the absence of vitamin B_{12} and cannot be recycled as tetrahydrofolate back into the folate pool to serve as the main one-carbon unit acceptor for many biochemical reactions. Cellular depletion of methylenetetra-hydrofolate eventually ensues, causing a reduction in thymidylic acid synthesis, which in turn results in megaloblastic anemia and neuropathies. This concept is supported by the fact that tetrahydrofolate corrects the megaloblastic anemia in patients with congenital methylmalonic aciduria and homocystinuria, whereas it is not corrected with methyltetrahydrofolate. However, some investigators have suggested that vitamin B_{12} is required for the conversion of folic acid to the formyl form and that formyltetrahydrofolates are the natural substrates for forming folate polyglutamates.

Folate in plasma appears to be distributed in three fractions: free folate, loosely bound, and highly bound folate. Study of the high-affinity serum folate binders was initiated by the discovery of such binders in chronic myeloid leukemia cells and in the serum of the same patients [30].

Most stored folate is present as polyglutamates, which have far greater molecular size and charge than monoglutamates. Transport across cell walls probably requires hydrolysis to monoglutamates, and the enzymes responsible for polyglutamate synthesis and hydrolysis are thus thought to play a major role in folate storage.

Folate is excreted in urine and bile in metabolically active and inactive forms. Urinary excretion of the biologically active material occurs after glomerular filtration of the free fraction and reabsorption of some filtered folate by active transport across the tubular cell wall. About 100 μg of biologically active folate is excreted in the bile daily. Studies with radioactive tracer folates indicate that a large proportion of injected radioactivity is excreted in the bile as a biologically inactive compound that is not a product of cleavage at the 9,10 position, but that has not been well characterized. Alcohol interferes with the folate enterohepatic cycle, believed to be important in the maintenance of serum folate levels. Nearly all alcoholics are in negative balance, and the majority are clinically folate-deficient.

The primary foods containing folate are green leafy vegetables and liver, although folates are present in nearly all natural foods. Unlike vitamin B_{12}, folate is highly susceptible to oxidation: 50% to 94% may be destroyed by protracted cooking and canning.

Deficiency

Folate deficiency has been divided into progressive stages leading to deficient erythropoiesis, secondary to decreased DNA synthesis, and finally clinical manifestations of macrocytic anemia with ovalocytosis.

Clinical Features of Deficiency

The early clinical features of folate deficiency are similar to those of vitamin B_{12} deficiency, namely macrocytic anemia and megaloblastic changes in bone marrow. The order of appearance of morphologic changes in the blood is hypersegmentation of neutrophils, macrocytosis, anemia, leukopenia, and thrombocytopenia. Unlike vitamin B_{12}, however, the progression of folate deficiency does not result in neurologic symptoms unless there is a coincident vitamin B_{12} deficiency. Although folate deficiency does not result in impaired myelination, it is associated with irritability and loss of memory. Other nonspecific features of folate deficiency are fatigue and weight loss. Diarrhea is also occasionally observed in folate deficiency, whereas constipation is more frequent in vitamin B_{12} deficiency.

Diagnosis of Deficiency

One of the early symptoms of folate deficiency is a decrease in serum folate from a normal level of over 5 ng/mL to levels less than 3 ng/mL. As the folate deficiency state is prolonged, erythrocyte folate levels continue to decrease from a normal of over 200 ng/mL to less than 120 ng/mL. Low erythrocyte folate alone is not sufficient to diagnose folate deficiency as it can also occur in vitamin B_{12} deficiency.

Folate deficiency can also be confirmed by an abnormal diagnostic deoxyuridine suppression test that is correctable by the in vitro addition of *folate,* not vitamin B_{12}.

Treatment of Deficiency

For combined differential diagnosis and therapy, the patient is treated with 0.1 mg of folic acid orally daily (if the suspected diagnosis is folate malabsorption). This dosage produces a maximal hematologic response in patients with folate deficiency but does not produce hematologic response in patients with vitamin B_{12} deficiency [28]. As in treated vitamin B_{12} deficiency, treatment of folate deficiency returns subnormal leukocyte and platelet levels to normal within 1 week of the start of therapy, at approximately the time of the reticulocyte peak.

Therapy with doses of folic acid greater than 0.1 mg daily is desirable when the folate deficiency state is complicated by conditions that may suppress hematopoiesis (such as unrelated systemic disease), conditions that increase folate requirement (pregnancy, hypermetabolic states, alcoholism, hemolytic anemia), and conditions that reduce folate absorption. Therapy should then consist of 0.5 to 1 mg daily. There is no evidence that doses greater than 1 mg daily have any greater efficacy; additionally, loss of folate in the urine becomes roughly logarithmic as the amount administered exceeds 1 mg.

Maintenance therapy is normally 0.1 mg of folic acid daily for 1 to 4 months, which then should be discontinued only if the diet contains at least one fresh fruit or fresh vegetable daily. If the daily folate requirement is increased owing to an increased metabolic or cell-turnover rate, the maintenance dose should be 0.2 to 0.5 mg daily.

Toxicity

Several hundred times the RDA for folate has not caused demonstrable clinical or biochemical abnormalities in humans. Excess amounts are secreted into the urine. Although no such effect has been observed in controlled studies using oral doses of 15 mg folic acid daily, experimental and clinical evidence suggests that very high concentrations of folic acid can have a convulsant effect. The convulsant dose in normal rats was shown in one study to be 45 to 125 mg if administered intravenously and 15 to 30 mg if preceded by the induction of focal cortical lesions. Convulsions have been reported in one of eight epileptics given parenteral folic acid under electroencephalographic monitoring. This reaction occurred after the rapid intravenous infusion of 14.4 mg folic acid, which presumably elevated serum folate concentration in the cerebral vessels several times higher than would be the case after folic acid ingestion [31]. Anticonvulsant drugs and folic acid compete with each other for absorption across the intestinal epithelial cells and probably also compete at the brain cell wall [32]. However, despite evidence in uncontrolled studies suggesting increased fit frequency in epileptics given oral therapeutic doses of folic acid, so far no such effect of oral folic acid has been demonstrated in carefully conducted controlled trials.

Oral folic acid supplements of 350 μg daily may reduce zinc absorption when zinc intake is marginal. This interaction may promote zinc depletion and subsequent intrauterine growth retardation during pregnancy.

Vitamin A

The term vitamin A is used as a generic descriptor for retinoids exhibiting qualitatively the biologic activity of retinol. Other naturally occurring retinoids of biologic interest, mainly in the all-*trans* form, include retinal (also termed retinaldehyde), retinoic acid, 3-dehydroretinol (vitamin A_2), retinyl palmitate, retinoyl β-glucuronide, and retinotaurine. The term provitamin A carotenoids is used as a generic descriptor for all carotenoids exhibiting qualitatively the biologic activity of vitamin A.

Vitamin A and the carotenoids are sensitive to oxidation, isomerization, and polymerization when diluted under light in the presence of oxygen. The destruction of these compounds is particularly rapid when they are absorbed as a thin surface film in the presence of light and oxygen.

Preformed vitamin A, present as retinol or fatty acyl esters, and carotenoids in the diet are largely released from protein during proteolysis in the stomach. Retinol in a bile salt-containing micelle is well absorbed (70% to 90%), whereas retinyl esters are less well absorbed. Vitamin A is absorbed by a carrier-mediated process at low concentrations, but mainly by diffusion from the micellar phase at high doses. Carotenoids are not as efficiently absorbed as preformed vitamin A but are more efficiently absorbed when present as the component of a lipid emulsion rather than when in tablet form or in a low lipid matrix. Thus, although β-carotene can be converted to 2 molecules of retinal in enterocytes and hepatocytes, dietary β-carotene is considered to have only one-sixth the vitamin A activity of all-*trans* retinol (see Table 9-1).

Within intestinal cells, newly formed chylomicra contain retinyl ester, primarily as retinyl palmitate [33]. By interaction with cell surface receptors on liver parenchymal cells, retinyl esters are internalized and hydrolyzed to retinol combined with cellular retinol-binding protein (CRBP) in the cytosol of the hepatocyte. For storage, retinol is directly esterified to retinyl palmitate and stored in lipid globules in the hepatocyte or transferred to stellate cells. Under normal physiologic conditions, stellate cells contain 80% to 90% of the stored vitamin A and hepatocytes 10% to 20%. The retinyl ester stored in stellate cells and hepatocytes can be readily hydrolyzed to retinol and mobilized for secretion.

Within the hepatocyte, a precursor of RBP, preapo-RBP is first formed, which is then proteolytically cleaved, with the loss of a peptide, to apo-RBP [34]. All-*trans* retinol combines with apo-RBP in a specific 1:1 molecular complex to form holo-RBP. The latter is transported through the Golgi apparatus and then is secreted into the plasma. Human RBP, a single polypeptide chain with 182 amino acids within the plasma, combines in plasma with transthyretin (prealbumin).

In adults, the total RBP concentration in plasma is 1.9 to 2.4 μmol/L (40 to 50 μg/ml), 80% to 90% of which exists as holo-RBP [34]. In children up to the age of puberty, the total RBP concentration is approximately 50% of the adult level. However, preterm infants tend to have blood levels < 20 μg/ml (0.9 μmol/L).

Holo-RBP interacts primarily with epithelial cell surface receptors where retinol is internalized. Apo-RBP is modified and released and is ultimately catabolized, primarily by the kidney [35]. Because retinol-RBP can also interact with receptor-free lipid membranes [36,37], specific cell surface receptors for holo-RBP are not always required for the uptake of retinol by tissues. Once in the cell, specific binding proteins chaperon their movements. These proteins seem to function as transport agents, as sequestering entities, as coligands in enzymatic transformations, or as coligands for genetic expression.

Functions of vitamin A include vision, cellular differentiation, morphogenesis, and transmembrane transport (in bacteria). Many other complex physiologic processes in animals, such as growth, reproduction, and the immune response, seem to be affected as a result of these cited functions.

The role of vitamin A in vision is well defined. Its role in cell differentiation is more recently investigated. In this capacity, retinol is converted to all-*trans* retinoic acid or 9-*cis* retinoic acid and transported to the nucleus, where it is bound to one or more of the three (α, β, γ) retinoic acid receptors (RAR) [38] or to one or more of the three (α, β, γ) retinoid X receptors (RXR) [39], respectively. In the activation of retinoic acid-responsive genes, the RAR or RXR binds to the response element of the gene to initiate transcription [40]. RXR also serves as a coregulator for the expression of genes responsive to triiodothyronine, to calcitriol, and perhaps to other hormones. In this latter role, RXR forms a heterodimer with the nuclear receptor for other hormones, thereby enhancing its affinity for the response element of the gene. The carboxyl terminal end of these receptors is involved in heterodimer formation. Thus, 9-*cis* retinoic acid seems to play a general role in cell differentiation, whereas all-*trans* retinoic acid has more specific effects.

Good dietary sources of preformed vitamin A are liver, other internal organs, whole eggs, dairy products, and whole small fish, whereas good sources of provitamin A carotenoids are carrots, dark green leafy vegetables, yams, spinach, tomatoes, yellow maize, papayas, ripe mangoes, and oranges. The richest sources of preformed vitamin A are the liver oils of marine fish and of marine mammals, whereas those of carotenoids are red palm oil and carrot oil.

In the United States, multivitamin pills, which usually contain 1500 to 3000 μg R.E. (5000 to 10,000 IU) of vitamin A, are also a major source of vitamin A for approximately 30% of the adult population.

Deficiency

Vitamin A deficiency is a serious nutritional problem among preschool children in southern and southeastern Asia and in parts of Africa and South America. Of an estimated 5 million children who develop xerophthalmia annually, approximately a quarter million become blind and, within one year, half of those children die. The major signs of vitamin A deficiency in preschool children are a history of night blindness, low serum vitamin A values, and a sequence of abnormalities of increasing severity in the conjunctiva and cornea of the eye, generically termed xerophthalmia. Severe irreversible changes in the cornea, which ultimately perforates with loss of the aqueous humor, is called keratomalacia. The corneal involvement seems to result from proteolytic destruction of collagen and other structural proteins following leukocyte infiltration into the corneal stroma. Viral infections, such as measles, exacerbate the process. Skin changes showing follicular hyperkeratosis and phrynoderma are also characteristic, although other nutritional deficiencies produce similar skin disorders.

Diagnosis of Deficiency

Plasma vitamin A concentrations lower than 0.35 μmol/L (<10 μg/dl) as measured by HPLC are indicative of vitamin A deficiency, and those higher than 1.05 μmol/L (>30 μg/dl) are associated with a satisfactory status. Vitamin A concentrations in breast milk that are lower than 0.35 μmol/L (<10 μg/dl) indicate that the nursing child is at risk of vitamin A deficiency [41]. Values higher than 0.7 μmol/L (>20 μg/dl) should provide adequate vitamin A for growth and development. Liver vitamin

A concentrations associated with deficiency are lower than 17.5 nmol (5 μg)/g, those associated with a marginal status are 17.5 to 70 nmol (5 μg to 20 μg)/g, and those associated with an adequate status are higher than 70 nmol (>20 μg)/g.

Relative dose response (RDR) assays have been used for screening both deficient and marginal vitamin A status [42]. The assay measures the change in plasma retinol concentration before and 5 hours after the oral administration of 450 μg to 1000 μg retinyl ester in oil. The RDR value, expressed as a percentage, is the increment in plasma retinol observed divided by the concentration at 5 hours. RDR values higher than 50% are characteristic of deficiency, values between 20% and 50% indicate marginal status, and values lower than 20% indicate adequate status [42].

During vitamin A depletion, goblet cells of the conjunctiva of the eye disappear and epithelial cells become enlarged and keratinized. Conjunctival cells can be absorbed on a piece of filter paper that is pressed against the eye and then can be stained and examined microscopically. The procedure, termed conjunctival impression cytology, indicates deficient and marginal status. The procedure has primarily been used as a screening procedure to detect populations at risk.

Nutrient Interrelationships

Vitamin A status is affected by intakes of protein, fat, iron, zinc, vitamin E, and possibly other nutrients. Indeed, because of the crucial roles of vitamin A in vision, cellular differentiation, morphogenesis, and most other physiologic processes, *any* nutritional imbalance should adversely affect the functions of vitamin A. In zinc deficiency, vitamin A in the plasma decreases but that in the liver rises, the synthesis of proteins and nucleic acids is impaired in most organs, including the eye, and night blindness can ensue. Because of the "zinc finger" structure required for the binding of many nuclear transcription factors to deoxyribonucleic acid (DNA), zinc seems to play a general role in gene expression. Children at high risk of vitamin A deficiency also show low plasma vitamin E levels and low ratios of plasma vitamin E to total lipid. Vitamin A may also interact in various ways with vitamins C, K, and D, calcium, copper, and iodine.

Toxicity

In amounts several times higher than the recommended dietary allowances (RDA), performed vitamin A causes toxicity. Three toxic syndromes exist: acute, chronic, and teratogenic. Acute toxicity is produced by a single extremely large dose of vitamin A (more than 200 mg R.E. (660,000 IU) in adults or 100 mg R.E. (330,000 IU) in children) or by several large doses taken during a short period. Chronic toxicity (>10 times the RDA for several weeks or months) leads to similar clinical disorders. Teratogenic effects, leading to spontaneous abortion, birth defects, and permanent learning disabilities, occur from lower doses (30 to 90 mg R.E. (100,000–300,000 IU) acutely or smaller doses of 7.5 mg R.E. (25,000 IU)/day for several weeks), particularly when taken in early pregnancy [43].

Carotenoids, even when taken in extremely large doses for long periods, are generally nontoxic. One exception is canthaxanthin, which can induce retinopathy when it is ingested in large amounts for long periods [44]. Another exception is apparently in chronic liver disease where excessive carotenoids, like excess vitamin A, may hasten the fibrosis.

In hypervitaminosis A, holo-RBP in the plasma is not markedly elevated, whereas retinyl esters are usually substantially increased.

Pharmacologic Uses

Retinoids and, to a much smaller extent, carotenoids are extensively used in management of abnormalities of the skin as well as certain malignancies.

Skin. Various retinoids, and particularly 13-*cis* retinoic acid, are used to treat acne and other skin disorders. Topical all-*trans* retinoic acid can reduce wrinkling and hyperpigmentation caused by photoaging. Although highly effective, retinoic acid is teratogenic at high doses when given orally and is a skin irritant when applied topically. In general, the most efficacious retinoids are also toxic, but some conjugated forms, such as retinoyl β-glucuronide and hydroxyphenyl retinamide, retain their therapeutic actions with less potential toxicity.

Cancer. Large doses of vitamin A reduce the recurrence of some forms of skin cancer, including mycosis fungoides, but not melanoma. All-*trans* retinoic acid is effective in treating acute promyelocytic leukemia (APL); however, the response is transient. In all responsive patients, a specific gene translocation occurs in which the gene for the retinoic acid receptor RARα is fused with another gene, termed PML. Other malignancies have also been responsive to vitamin A analogues. Carotenoids have been implicated in reducing the oxidative potential of low-density lipoproteins development of cortical cataract and the oxidative stress induced by smoking. Leukoplakia, considered a precancerous condition, responds well to high daily doses of β-carotene or vitamin A analogues in some patients.

Vitamin D

The two forms of vitamin D, ergocalciferol (D_2) and cholecalciferol (D_3), are steroid-derived compounds. D_2 does not occur naturally but is produced by ultraviolet irradiation of ergosterol, which occurs in molds, yeast, and higher plants; the action of light causes ring cleavage to yield an intermediate pre-ergocalciferol (plus lumisterol and other related congeners), which rearranges under thermal conditions to ergocalciferol. Vitamin D_3 does occur in our bodies but similarly derives from irradiation of provitamin D_3 (7-dehydrocholesterol) in skin to produce, via thermal arrangement of pre-cholecalciferol, the natural cholecalciferol. The only chemical difference between the two vitamin and provitamin forms is in the side chain. There are at least 10 compounds known to yield vitamin D-active compounds upon irradiation. Most differ only in the side chain at C-17 of the sterol nucleus, for example, 22,23-dihydroergocalciferol. Vitamin D is generally stable to heat, alkalis, acids, and oxidation.

The awareness that the alarming increase in the incidence of skin cancer is related to chronic exposure to sunlight has led to the recommendation that people should wear sunscreen before going outdoors. The solar radiation that is responsible for causing wrinkles and skin cancer, however, is the same radiation that is responsible for producing previtamin D_3 in the skin. Thus, the application of a sunscreen with a sun protection factor of only 8 can completely prevent the cutaneous production of previtamin D_3. The use of sunscreens by children and young adults should not affect their vitamin D status because it is unlikely that they will always wear a sunscreen before going outdoors. The elderly, however, often are more conscious of their health and apply a sunscreen on their skin before going outdoors. Evidence exists that chronic use of sunscreens by the elderly can decrease circulating concentrations of 25-hydroxyvitamin D (25-OH-D), which is a hallmark for determining vitamin D deficiency.

Metabolism

Vitamin D is efficiently absorbed from the gastrointestinal tract unless there is fat malabsorption due to lack of bile salts, pancreatic insufficiency, or a defect of intestinal mucosal function. When absorbed, the vitamin is bound directly to chylomicrons and transported initially via the lymphatics. To exert its biological activity, vitamin D must be metabolically altered. Much of the prohormone-like vitamin initially supplied to the liver is hydroxylated at the terminal side-chain position to yield 25-hydroxy-D; this process involves molecular oxygen and a pyridine nucleotide-dependent, microsomal, mixed-function oxidase system. The 25-hydroxycholecalciferol, which represents the major metabolite of D_3 in plasma, circulates bound to a vitamin D-binding α-globulin. In kidneys, a second hydroxylation at the 1α-position results from the action of a cytochrome P_{450}-mediated, mixed-function oxidase located on inner mitochondrial membrane. The kidney 1α-hydroxylase is regulated by vitamin D status and by calcium/phosphate levels that are controlled by parathormone (PTH) and calcitonin.

Other aspects of vitamin D metabolism include the ability of the kidney to direct formation of 24,25-dihydroxy-D when calcium and phosphate ion levels are normal. Increased formation of 1α,25-dihydroxy-D occurs when decreased blood Ca (II) leads to parathormone release, cyclic AMP formation, renal loss of phosphate, and stimulation of the 1α-hydroxylase. The 1α,25-dihydroxycholecalciferol formed in the kidney complexes with the vitamin D-binding protein for transfer via blood to target tissues, for example, small intestine and bone. In the intestinal mucosal cell, the hormonally active dihydroxy-D binds to a cytosolic receptor protein (M.W. $\approx$ 45,000) before entering the nucleus and associating with a chromatin receptor. A prime effect is on DNA-dependent RNA polymerase II to mediate synthesis of a specific calcium-binding protein.

Other Biologic Actions

A considerable amount of effort has been directed toward identifying actions of $1,25(OH)_2D$ that are not directly related to maintenance of calcium and phosphorus homeostasis. The impetus for this search resulted from the observation that a variety of tissues that were not related to calcium metabolism possessed nuclear receptors for $1,25(OH)_2D$. Careful analysis has shown that these tissues as well as activated B and T lymphocytes [45] and several cultured normal and tumor cell lines possess high-affinity, low-capacity $1,25(OH)_2D$-receptor-like proteins that are quantitatively similar to the intestinal receptor [46].

The first insight into a noncalcemic action of $1,25(OH)_2D_3$ was suggested when promyeloid leukemic cells that had nuclear receptors for $1,25(OH)_2D_3$ responded to this hormone by differentiating into macrophages [47]. $1,25(OH)_2D_3$ induced in a time- and dose-dependent manner phagocytic activity and expression of cell surface antigens including Fc and C3 receptors and lysozyme activity. Similar studies were done in a human promyelocytic leukemic cell line (HL-60). Cell growth was inhibited by as little as 10^{-9}M of $1,25(OH)_2D_3$ in a dose-dependent manner. $1,25(OH)_2D_3$ was also found to be an effective antiproliferative agent for cultured tumor cells, such as mammary tumor cells and melanoma cells, that possessed its nuclear receptor [48]. The effect of $1,25(OH)_2D_3$ on leukemia cells is reversible. When clones of HL-60 cells that possessed less than 10% of nuclear binding activity for $1,25(OH)_2D_3$ were incubated with $1,25(OH)_2D_3$, little difference in their proliferative activity was apparent. Human studies, however, have been somewhat disappointing since calcium metabolism is also affected by large doses of vitamin D. The use of vitamin D analogues that cause little effect on calcium/phosphorus metabolism, but substantial effect on promyelocyte differentiation, offer new therapeutic potential.

Of interest also are the reports that human epidermal cells had nuclear receptors for $1,25(OH)_2D_3$. $1,25(OH)_2D_3$ inhibited the proliferation and induced terminal differentiation of cultured murine and human keratinocytes in a dose-dependent manner [49]. These laboratory observations have been put to practical use by the development of $1,25(OH)_2D_3$ and its analogues as a safe and effective treatment for the hyperproliferative epidermal disorder psoriasis [50].

Deficiency

Clinical manifestations of rickets include skeletal deformities with bone pain, muscle weakness, failure to grow, hypocalcemia, and hypophosphatemia. The failure to mineralize osteoid tissue at the epiphyseal-diaphyseal junction of bones causes a variety of deformities, for example, craniotabes, enlargement of joints, rachitic rosary at the costochondral junctions, bow legs, and knock-knees. X-ray examination of long bones in rickets shows rarefied shafts and uneven, blurred ends that brighten with vitamin D treatment. Fractures are not uncommon. Laboratory data reveal hypocalcemia, hypophosphatemia, and elevated alkaline phosphatase. The $25\text{-}(OH)D_3$ levels in plasma are reduced to below normal. These features are also seen in osteomalacia, the adult form of vitamin D deficiency.

Human milk is deficient in vitamin D and contains only 0.55 μg (22 IU) per liter, mostly from $25\text{-}(OH)D_3$. Breast-fed infants must receive an additional source of vitamin D unless they have exposure to sunlight sufficient to generate adequate previtamin D_3. Cow's milk and most formulas are enriched to the level of 10 μg (400 IU) per liter. Treatment of rickets should begin with a dose of 100 μg (4000 IU) of vitamin D daily, roughly 10 times the RDA.

Vitamin D-Resistant Rickets

There are several types of vitamin D-resistant rickets (VDRR). One results from familial hypophosphatemia due to a hereditary defect in renal resorption of phosphate associated with low calcium absorption. This disorder can be treated with oral $1,25(OH)_2D_3$ plus phosphate supplements.

Other types are due to abnormalities in the metabolism of vitamin D. In type I disease, the defect is in the activity of the 1-α-hydroxylase in the kidney with resulting elevated levels of $25\text{-}(OH)D_3$ and reduced levels of $1,25(OH)_2D_3$ in plasma. Physiologic doses (0.05 μg/kg) of $1,25(OH)_2D_3$ are curative.

Type II VDRR is due to a defect in the vitamin D receptor (VDR) protein. Children have high levels of $1,25(OH)_2D_3$ in plasma and do not respond to massive doses of vitamin D hormone. Partial management results from high calcium and phosphate intake. Molecular biologic studies of persons with type II VDRR have identified defects in all three parts of the VDR.

Diagnosis

Specific assays for $1,25(OH)_2D$ in serum and plasma have been developed with a competitive receptor binding assay using a nuclear/cytosolic receptor for $1,25(OH)_2D$. After several improvements, the assay now involves the use of a bovine thymus $1,25(OH)_2D$ receptor that recognizes $1,25(OH)_2D_2$ and $1,25(OH)_2D_3$ equally well. A bioassay has also been developed using cultured calvaria. This assay, which is tedious to conduct, measures directly the biologic activity of $1,25(OH)_2D$ in serum.

The half-life of circulating $1,25(OH)_2D$ has been estimated to be between 4 and 6 hours. Normal range of serum values is between 38 and 144 pmol/L (16 and 60 pg/ml). As vitamin D deficiency develops, the body responds by increasing the production and secretion of parathyroid hormone. Parathyroid hormone in turn enhances the 1-hydroxylation of 25-OH-D. Thus, secondary hyperparathyroidism associated with vitamin D deficiency accelerates the conversion of 25-OH-D to $1,25(OH)_2D$. Because the circulating concentration of 25-OH-D is about three orders of magnitude higher than that of $1,25(OH)_2D$, even low levels of 25-OH-D in the blood can provide enough substrate for the formation of $1,25(OH)_2D$. Thus, a patient who is becoming vitamin D deficient will still have enough 25-OH-D substrate for the renal 25-OH-D-1α-hydroxylase. As a result, a patient who has low stores of vitamin D and is becoming vitamin D deficient can have low, normal, or even high circulating concentrations of $1,25(OH)_2D$. Thus, serum $1,25(OH)_2D$ concentrations are of little value in evaluating vitamin D deficiency. In an absolute vitamin D deficiency state, however, $1,25(OH)_2D$ is undetectable in plasma.

The measurement of circulating concentrations of $1,25(OH)_2D$ has been of great value to clinicians for evaluating patients with inherited and acquired disorders of 25-OH-D metabolism. Patients with chronic renal failure, hyperphosphatemia, hypoparathyroidism, pseudohypoparathyroidism, tumor-induced osteomalacia, hypercalcemia of malignancy (in most cases), or vitamin D-dependent rickets type I (an inborn error reducing the conversion of 25-OH-D to $1,25(OH)_2D$) often have low circulating concentrations of $1,25(OH)_2D$. Serum concentrations of $1,25(OH)_2D$ are above normal in some patients with primary hyperparathyroidism; vitamin D-dependent rickets type II (an inborn error in which the recognition of $1,25(OH)_2D$ by target tissue receptors is defective); chronic granulomatous disorders such as sarcoidosis, tuberculosis, and silicosis; and lymphoma. It is now recognized that chronic granulomatous disorders and some lymphomas that activate macrophages and lymphoma cells, respectively, can 1α-hydroxylate 25-OH-D, a process that is inhibited by glucocorticoids.

Toxicity

Vitamin D is the most likely vitamin to cause overt toxic reactions in small multiples of the United States RDA. An epidemic of idiopathic hypercalcemia in infants, with anorexia, vomiting, hypertension, renal insufficiency, and failure to thrive, occurred in England in the 1950s. It was traced to an intake of vitamin D between 50 and 75 μg (2000 and 3000 IU)/day. In adults, dosages of 250 μg (10,000 IU)/day of vitamin D for several months have resulted in marked disturbances in calcium metabolism with hypercalcemia, hyperphosphatemia, hypertension, anorexia, nausea, vomiting, weakness, polyuria, polydypsia, azotemia, nephrolithiasis, ectopic calcification, renal failure, and, in some cases, death.

Vitamin E

Vitamin E occurs naturally only as the stereoisomer of α-tocopherol, formerly known as d-α-tocopherol. The synthetic α-tocopherol, formerly known as dl-α-tocopherol, is designated all-*rac*-α-tocopherol (for all racemic α-tocopherol). Esters of tocopherols are designated as esters (for example, α-tocopherol acetate).

Tocopherols are stable to heat and alkali in the absence of oxygen and are unaffected by acids up to 100°C. They are, however, slowly oxidized by atmospheric oxygen. Oxidation is accelerated by exposure to light, heat, and alkali, and by the presence of iron and copper salts. Because the esters of the free phenolic hydroxyl group are much more stable in the presence of oxygen, tocopherol is usually provided commercially as the acetate ester. The esters, however, cannot function as antioxidants. Absorption of tocopherols depends on factors generally important in lipid digestion and intestinal uptake. Bile salts and pancreatic enzymes are known to be important in the absorption process [41]. The efficiency of the absorption, however, decreases as large amounts of tocopherol are consumed. In normal humans, an average absorption of at least 50% and perhaps as high as 70% can be assumed for dietary levels of α-tocopherol consumption (for example, 0.4 to 1 mg); however, the efficiency falls to less than 10% with pharmacologic doses such as 200 mg.

The malabsorption of fat seen in patients with various forms of steatorrhea results in a parallel malabsorption of tocopherols. Once absorbed, vitamin E isomers are transported with fat predominantly by lymphatic vessels to the venous system and distributed in plasma in association with lipoproteins. No specific carrier protein has been identified. A rapid exchange of plasma tocopherol and erythrocyte tocopherol occurs at the red blood cell membrane. Alpha-tocopherol is taken up by most tissues, including liver, lung, heart, skeletal muscle, and adipose tissue. Contrary to the other tissues, fat accumulates α-tocopherol continuously and can sequester the vitamin. Tocopherol present in adipocytes is not readily available to other tissues and should not be considered as a storage depot [51].

There is widespread agreement that vitamin E functions as a biologic antioxidant to protect cellular membranes from oxidative destruction. Most of the evidence for this function has been obtained not only from in vitro experiments, but also in vivo studies. Moreover, it has been well established that some manifestations of vitamin E deficiency in chicks and rats can be prevented completely by feeding antioxidants [52].

Alpha-tocopherol functions primarily as a free radical scavenger in membranes. Phospholipids in cellular and subcellular membranes contain polyunsaturated fatty acids (PUFA) that are susceptible to peroxidation. Vitamin E is the fat-soluble antioxidant capable of protecting these fatty acids by interrupting free radical reactions that otherwise can cause membrane damage in subcellular organelles. Other antioxidant systems involving enzymes (for example, glutathione peroxidase and superoxide dismutase) can also function in helping the cell control free radical attacks on peroxidizable fatty acids. Thus, the well-known interrelationship between α-tocopherol and selenium has been explained by the fact that glutathione peroxidase is a selenoenzyme.

The importance of free radicals in cellular metabolism has been stimulated in recent years because of concern that adverse effects of environmental toxins are mediated through free radicals, that aging is associated with inadequately controlled free radical reactions, and that carcinogenesis can be triggered by peroxidation [53].

The major role of vitamin E as an antioxidant is to "neutralize" free radicals, which could otherwise initiate the chain reaction, especially in membranes that contain a large proportion of highly unsaturated fatty acids. To be effective, α-tocopherol must be localized in membrane sites susceptible to free radicals.

The tocopherol content of diets shows great variation depending on harvesting, processing, storage, and final food preparation procedures. The major sources of vitamin E consumed by Americans are the vegetable and seed oils, such as corn oil, soybean oil, and safflower oil. Although these common oils, and the less commonly consumed wheat germ, are rich sources of tocopherols, the actual concentration and distribution of vitamin E isomers are quite variable. Animal products are not good sources. Although butter provides very little α-tocopherol, American margarine contains a range from 3.2 to 32.7 mg/100 g and, therefore, can supply a significant amount of vitamin E in the diet. Soybean oil has become particularly prevalent and accounted for 74% of oils and fats used in edible United States products according to a USDA survey in 1982/83. Soybeans contain predominantly γ-tocopherol with lesser amounts of δ-tocopherol and only a relatively small amount of α-tocopherol. As a result of the rather high content of non-α vitamins, soybean oil provides a disproportionately low amount of vitamin E activity in comparison to its concentration of total tocopherols. Other dietary lipid sources such as coconut and fish oils are low in tocopherols. Except for fish oil, however, the concentration of tocopherols increases in proportion to the amount of PUFA present.

Deficiency

The occurrence of vitamin E deficiency of pure dietary origin is rare in developed countries. On the other hand, there are three categories of patients who have been well established as susceptible to vitamin E deficiency: (1) premature infants, (2) patients with gastrointestinal diseases leading to malabsorption, and (3) individuals with abetalipoproteinemia. Also, children with protein-calorie malnutrition have sometimes been noted to show abnormally low levels of circulating tocopherol. A brief description of these conditions is presented below.

First, newborn infants delivered prematurely show evidence of vitamin E deficiency due to several factors, including limited tissue storage at birth, intestinal malabsorption, and rapid growth rates that increase nutrient requirements in general. Also, some infant formula preparations have been marginal to low in α-tocopherol content relative to the amount of PUFA and iron present.

Several investigations of the past decade support the potential benefits of correcting deficiency early in these patients with parenteral or enteral α-tocopherol acetate. The prophylactic value of pharmacologic doses of vitamin E is not warranted, however. The deaths of a number of premature infants treated with an intravenous preparation of vitamin E (E-Ferol) highlights the concern regarding the need to carefully and scientifically elucidate the cause of retinopathy of prematurity and the role of pharmacologic treatment with products containing vitamin E.

The second category of human subjects who manifest vitamin deficiency includes a variety of patients with intestinal malabsorption. This is a very heterogeneous group with a common clinical feature, namely steatorrhea. Vitamin E deficiency has been associated with disturbances affecting nearly every component of the gastrointestinal tract, including the stomach (postgastrectomy syndrome), liver (biliary atresia and cirrhosis), pancreas (cystic fibrosis, chronic pancreatitis, and pancreatic carcinoma), and intestinal mucosa (gluten enteropathy and regional enteritis). Although the degree of tocopherol malabsorption varies in these conditions and in individual patients, it may be concluded in general that if steatorrhea is of sufficient duration and magnitude, vitamin E deficiency is likely to ensue as a consequence of tocopherol malabsorption.

Studies on the possible consequences of vitamin E deficiency in patients with cystic fibrosis and other malabsorption syndromes have focused on erythrocyte stability and the neuromuscular system. Although erythrocyte survival is decreased in vitamin E deficiency, patients with malabsorption are not likely to show clinically evident hemolytic anemia.

The third category of patients consists of those with abetalipoproteinemia and chromic cholestasis. Neuromuscular system involvement is often the first clinical manifestation. The clinical progression of the neurologic disorder in childhood cholestasis includes hyporeflexia at age 18 to 24 months, frank neurologic dysfunction by age 3 to 4 years, and disabling neurologic deficits by 10 years. The characteristic neurologic symptoms improve with vitamin E treatment using the water-soluble tocopherol polyethylene glycol or systemic injections of tocopherol acetate.

Treatment of Deficiency

Premature infants are difficult to treat adequately using oral supplementation because of the necessity of delayed feedings in critically ill babies, the frequent occurrence of early gastrointestinal intolerance, and the presence of prolonged tocopherol malabsorption. The use of intramuscular vitamin E is under investigation. Multivitamin mixtures can be given intravenously to provide α-tocopherol acetate, which is readily hydrolyzed in vivo to an α-tocopherol. Recommendations of 2.7 to 4.0 mg (4 to 6 IU)/kg/day have been made. When enteral feedings are established, the usual oral dose of water-miscible α-tocopherol acetate is 17 mg (25 IU)/day.

Patients with vitamin E deficiency due to simple malabsorption such as cystic fibrosis usually respond to 17 to 34 mg (25 to 50 IU)/day for infants, 34 to 67 mg (50 to 100 IU)/day for children, 67 mg (100 IU)/day for adolescents, and 134 mg (200 IU)/day for adults. On the other hand, patients with biliary atresia or other causes of chronic obstructive biliary disease and patients with abetalipoproteinemia are extremely difficult to treat and often require parenteral vitamin E supplementation. An alternative oral treatment with pharmacologic doses of d-α-tocopheryl polyethylene glycol 1000 succinate (TPGS) has been useful in treatment of these patients. TPGS is available commercially in some health food stores.

Pharmacologic Doses

Evidence that vitamin E supplementation will improve the quality of one's life by reducing the probability of "free radical" damage is growing. It is not surprising, therefore, that a large proportion of the American population takes vitamin E supplements. The usual doses range from 100 to 800 mg/day, although the amount absorbed is far less. Specific disorders that might respond to large doses of vitamin E include ischemic heart disease, intermittent claudication, and pulmonary oxygen toxicity. Results of carefully controlled studies, however, do not support these claims on a consistent basis. Recent preliminary studies suggest that 266 mg (400 IU)/day may be helpful in reducing the risk of plaque formation in hypercholesterolemic individuals, although definitive results have not been reported for large population groups.

Toxicity

Experience over many years and limited studies have indicated no consistent evidence of toxicity when doses of 100 to 800 mg/day are taken orally by adults. Reported toxic effects in adults have included increased bleeding tendency, impaired immune function, decreased levels of vitamin K-dependent clotting factors, and impairment of leukocyte function [54]. Reports of toxicity in infants include the intravenous preparation of E-Ferol, although the toxicity may have been related to non-vitamin E constituents in the formulation. The use of plasma or serum of vitamin E determinations to avoid toxicity is problematic because of a lack of reliable correlation with tissue concentrations. Therefore, a cautious approach is recommended, particularly when tocopherol preparations are administered parenterally.

Vitamin K

Vitamin K refers to a group of menadione derivatives important in normal coagulation. Vitamin K_1 or phytonadione (phylloquinone) is the naturally occurring fat-soluble vitamin that composes the majority of normal dietary intake and represents the commonly used parenteral preparation AquaMEPHYTON (Merck Sharp & Dohme). Vitamin K_2, or menaquinone, is synthesized by intestinal bacteria and has only 60% of the activity of vitamin K_1 [55]. It is also fat-soluble and serves as the major source of vitamin K in infants after absorption in the colon. A synthetic form of the vitamin, referred to as menadione or K_3, is water-soluble, which makes it useful in the treatment of various malabsorptive states. It is commercially available as Synkavite (Roche).

The colonic absorption of vitamin K, which is produced by intestinal bacteria, is the most important source in infancy. As a result, antibiotic treatment, with resulting disruption of normal gut flora, may seriously interfere with vitamin K production and result in symptomatic deficiency in as little as 2 weeks [55]. In contrast, the intestinal source is less important in older children and adults, who rely on upper small intestinal absorption of dietary vitamin K. Absorption of the vitamin requires the presence of both bile acids and pancreatic enzymes. Data from rat gut sacs implicate an energy-requiring, saturable transporter. Dietary PUFA and large doses of vitamin A may interfere with vitamin K absorption. Following absorption, vitamin K is transported by way of chylomicrons to the liver, kidney, skin, heart, and muscle. Placental transport of vitamin K in the rat occurs by facilitated diffusion. Transport by the human placenta appears to be poor based on the increased risk of preterm infants to hemorrhagic disease due to vitamin K deficiency. However, maternal administration of vitamin K late in pregnancy is effective in preventing hemorrhagic disease, indicating intact transfer by the end of gestation [56].

The physiologic role of vitamin K is in the maintenance of normal coagulation by means of its influence on the synthesis of the active forms of the vitamin K-dependent factors II (prothrombin), VII, IX, and X. Vitamin K serves as a cofactor for the γ-carboxylation of glutamic acid residues of the inactive precursor factors. Carboxylation is necessary for the binding of calcium and phospholipid by prothrombin.

Two vitamin K-dependent bone proteins have been discovered in the last 15 years. The first is bone Gla protein (BGP, or osteocalcin) secreted by osteoblasts. The second is the matrix Gla protein (MGP) in bone, dentin, and cartilage. In vitro BGP binds strongly to hydroxyapatite and inhibits its formation. Both properties are lost when the Gla residues are decarboxylated. MGP has different properties and is found in the organic matrix of bone and does not react with hydroxyapatite. Warfarin inhibits the synthesis of both BGP and MGP, but unlike the coagulation proteins synthesized in the liver, vitamin K does not overcome the effect of warfarin on BGP and MGP synthesis [57].

The Conradi-Hunermann teratogenic type of chondrodysplasia punctata may occur in infants born to mothers taking warfarin during the first trimester [58]. This defect appears to result from a deficiency of BGP and MGP during embryogenesis.

Vitamin K is widely distributed in both animal and vegetable foods and varies from less than 22 nmol/L (1 μg/10 dl) in milk to over 8.8 μmol/kg (400 μg/100 g) in spinach, kale, and turnip greens. The concentration of vitamin K in the fasting plasma of healthy persons is less than 1 ng/ml (2.2 nM). Liver usually contains a mixture of phylloquinone and menaquinones that totals between 11 and 89 nmol/kg (5 and 40 ng/g). Both biologic and chemical methods have been used to measure vitamin K in foods. Because vitamin K is light sensitive, precautions must be taken to protect the vitamin during analysis.

Deficiency

Primary vitamin K deficiency is uncommon in healthy adults. Several factors protect adults from a lack of vitamin K. These include (1) widespread distribution of vitamin K in plant and animal tissues, (2) the vitamin K cycle, which conserves the vitamin, and (3) the microbiologic flora of the normal gut that synthesize menaquinones, which can contribute to the requirement for vitamin K. On the other hand, vitamin K deficiency in the breast-fed newborn remains a major worldwide cause of infant morbidity and mortality [59]. In the United States, infants normally receive 0.5 to 1.0 mg vitamin K intramuscularly shortly after birth. The causes of reduced levels of the vitamin K-dependent coagulation factors in adults are largely secondary to disease or drug therapy. Deficiency of vitamin K occurs more rapidly than for the other fat-soluble vitamins because of its relatively short half-life. In children with biliary obstruction, bleeding may occur within two weeks without supplemental parenteral vitamin K. In adults, 60% to 70% of a parenteral dose of vitamin K is cleared in the bile and urine within three days [60].

Clinical Features of Deficiency

In the neonate, deficiency is manifest as hemorrhagic disease of the newborn, with spontaneous bleeding into the skin, gastrointestinal tract, lungs, and CNS posing potentially life-threatening problems. High-risk settings include the breast-fed infant because of the low vitamin K content of human milk, the infant of the malnourished mother because of poor placental transfer, and the home-delivered infant who does not receive prophylactic vitamin K at birth.

Infants of mothers on hydantoin anticonvulsants should have prophylactic vitamin K because diphenylhydantoin is an antagonist to vitamin K. Neonatal complications such as diarrhea, malabsorption, cystic fibrosis, idiopathic cholestasis, atresia of the bile duct, and prolonged parenteral nutrition are all indications for intramuscular or intravenous vitamin K administration to infants.

Assessment of vitamin K sufficiency is most readily accomplished by the measurement of the one-stage prothrombin time. Factor VII activity is actually a more sensitive indicator of marginal deficiency [55], declining before a prolongation of prothrombin time is detectable. Recently, HPLC measurement of plasma vitamin K levels has become possible but is not widely employed.

Treatment of Deficiency

Dietary deficiency of vitamin K becomes manifest more quickly in patients following surgery and in debilitated patients with or without antibiotics.

In protein-calorie malnutrition, amino acid deprivation may cause hypoprothrombinemia that is not responsive to vitamin K but that does respond to protein feeding. Because the secretion of bile salts is essential for the absorption of fats and fat-soluble vitamins, it is not surprising that biliary obstruction was early identified as a cause of vitamin K deficiency. All patients with obstructive jaundice should receive parenteral vitamin K_1 (11 μmol/day, or 5 mg/day) for three days prior to surgery. The synthetic water-soluble vitamin K_3 (Synkavite) may be given orally at 1 to 5 mg/day. Children's dose is 1 mg/day. A similar treatment protocol may be used with malabsorption syndromes.

Patients with parenchymal liver disease may have hypoprothrombinemia and an elevation in plasma descarboxyprothrombin. They are unable to utilize vitamin K in the biosynthesis of vitamin K-dependent clotting factors, usually as a result of destruction of the rough reticulum in the hepatocyte. Patients with liver disease should be challenged with vitamin K to determine the extent of the blockade of prothrombin synthesis. There is no need, however, to give repetitive high doses of vitamin K if the patient is refractory to a single intravenous dose of 22 μmol (10 mg) of vitamin K.

Various drugs, including the 4-hydroxycoumarins, salicylates, certain broad-spectrum antibiotics, and vitamins A and E in pharmacologic doses, will antagonize the action of vitamin K.

Toxicity

Naturally occurring, fat-soluble vitamin K_1 is generally nontoxic, although the rapid intravenous infusion of large doses (>1 mg/kg) may result in an anaphylactic reaction. In contrast, synthetic vitamin K_3 is relatively more toxic to the newborn infant, especially the preterm infant, and its use is not recommended in the neonatal period. Doses as low as 5 mg of synthetic vitamin K (Synkavite) may produce hemolysis, hyperbilirubinemia, and kernicterus, particularly in preterm infants, although the toxicity is generally dose-related [60].

References

1. Herman RH, Stifel FB, Greene HL. Vitamins. In Dietschy JM (ed), *Disorders of the Gastrointestinal Tract, Disorders of the Liver, Nutritional Disorders,* Vol. I. New York: Grune & Stratton, 1976. P 364.
2. Scriver CR, et al. (eds). *The Metabolic Basis of Inherited Disease* (6th ed.). New York: McGraw-Hill, 1989. P 3008.
3. Rindi G, Ventura V. Thiamine intestinal transport. *Phys Rev* 52:821, 1963.
4. Drenick EJ, Joven CB, Swendseid ME. Occurrence of acute Wernicke's encephalopathy during prolonged starvation for the treatment of obesity. *N Engl J Med* 274:937, 1966.
5. Hoyumpa AM Jr, et al. Intestinal thiamine transport: Effect of chronic ethanol administration in rats. *Am J Clin Nutr* 31:938, 1978.
6. Tetreault AF, Beck IA. Anaphylactic shock following intramuscular thiamine chloride. *Ann Intern Med* 45:134, 1956.
7. Rivlin RS. Riboflavin metabolism. *N Engl J Med* 283:463, 1970.
8. Pinto J, Haung YP, Rivlin RS. Inhibition of riboflavin metabolism rat tissues by chlorpromazine, imipramine, and amitriptyline. *J Clin Invest* 67:1500, 1981.
9. Tillotson JA, Baker EM. An enzymatic measurement of the riboflavin status in man. *Am J Clin Nutr* 25:425, 1972.
10. Rivlin RS, et al. Increased excretion of riboflavin due to boric acid intoxication. *Clin Res* 24:424A, 1978.
11. Baeckert PA, et al. Vitamin concentrations in very low birth weight infants given vitamins intravenously in a lipid emulsion: Measurement of vitamins A, D, and E and riboflavin. *J Pediatr* 113:1057, 1988.
12. Greene HL, et al. Guidelines for the use of vitamins, trace elements, calcium, magnesium, and phosphorus in infants and children receiving total parenteral nutrition: Report of the Subcommittee on Pediatric Parenteral Nutrient Requirements from the Committee on Clinical Practice Issues of the American Society for Clinical Nutrition. *Am J Clin Nutr* 48:1324, 1988.
13. Jolliffe N, et al. Nicotinic acid deficiency encephalopathy. *JAMA* 114:304, 1940.
14. Sebrell WM Jr, Harris RS (eds). *The Vitamins,* Vol. 2. New York: Academic, 1968. P 1.
15. Kelsall MA. Clinical pyridoxine deficiency. *Ann NY Acad Sci* 166:1, 1969.
16. Sauberlich HE, et al. Biochemical assessment of the nutritional status of vitamin B_6 in the human. *Am J Clin Nutr* 25:629, 1972.
17. Bean WB, Hodges RE. Pantothenic acid deficiency induced in human subjects. *Proc Soc Exp Biol Med* 86:693, 1954.
18. Hodges ER, Ohlson MA, Bean WB. Pantothenic acid deficiency in man. *J Clin Invest* 37:1642, 1958.
19. Glusman M. Syndrome of "burning feet" (nutritional melalgia) as manifestation of nutritional deficiency. *Am J Med* 3:211, 1947.
20. Mock DM, et al. Biotin deficiency: An unusual complication of parenteral alimentation. *N Engl J Med* 304:820, 1981.
21. Baker H, et al. A new assay method for biotin in blood, serum, urine and tissues. *Ann Biochem* 3:31, 1962.
22. Herbert V, Jacob E. Destruction of vitamin B_{12} by ascorbic acid. *JAMA* 230:241, 1974.
23. Hood J, Burns CA, Hodges RE. Sjögren's syndrome in scurvy. *N Engl J Med* 282:1120, 1970.
24. Campbell GD, Steinberg MH, Bower JD. Ascorbic acid-induced hemolysis in G-6 PD deficiency. *Ann Intern Med* 82:810, 1975.
25. Rhead WJ, Schrauzer GN. Risks of long-term ascorbic acid overdosage. *Nutr Rev* 29:262, 1971.
26. Herbert V. Vitamin B_{12} and folate metabolism. In Gibson

AJ, Smoak WM, Weinstein MB (eds), *B_{12} and Folate Analysis with Radionuclides in Hematopoietic and Gastrointestinal Investigations with Radionuclides.* Springfield, IL: Thomas, 1972. P 8.

27. Herbert V. Recommended dietary intakes (RDI) of vitamin B_{12} in humans. *Am J Clin Nutr* 45:671, 1987.
28. Herbert V. Current concepts in therapy—megaloblastic anemia (concluded). *N Engl J Med* 268:201,368, 1963.
29. Ratnam M, Freisheim JH. Proteins involved in the transport of folates and antifolates by normal and neoplastic cells. In Picciano MF, Stokstad ERL, Gregory JF III (eds), *Folic Acid Metabolism in Health and Disease.* New York: Wiley-Liss, 1990. P 91.
30. Rothenberg SP. A macromolecular factor in some leukemic cells which binds folic acid. *Proc Soc Exp Biol Med* 133:428, 1970.
31. Colman N, Herbert V. Folate metabolism in brain. In Kumar S (ed), *Biochemistry of Brain.* Oxford: Pergamon, 1979. P 127.
32. Colman N, Herbert V. Folates and the nervous system. In Blakey RL (ed), *Folates and Pterins,* vol. 3. New York: Wiley, 1986. P 339.
33. Goodman DS. Biosynthesis, absorption and hepatic metabolism of retinol. In Spron MB, Roberts AB, Goodman DS (eds), *The Retinoids,* vol. 2. New York: Academic, 1984. P 1.
34. Blaner WS. Retinoid-binding protein: The serum transport protein for vitamin A. *Endocrinol Rev* 10:308, 1989.
35. Hendriks HFJ, et al. Distributions of retinoids, retinoid-binding proteins and related parameters in different types of liver cells isolated from young and old rats. *Eur J Biochem* 171:237, 1988.
36. Noy N, Xu ZJ. Interactions of retinol with binding proteins: Implications for the mechanism of uptake by cells. *Biochemistry* 29:3878, 1991.
37. Noy N, Xu ZJ. Kinetic parameters of the interactions of retinol with lipid bilayers. *Biochemistry* 29:3883, 1991.
38. Giguere V, et al. Identification of a receptor for the morphogen retinoic acid. *Nature* 330:624, 1987.
39. Levin AA, et al. 9-Cis retinoic acid stereoisomer binds and activates the nuclear receptor RXRA. *Nature* 355:359, 1992.
40. Yu VC, et al. RXR Beta: A coregulator that enhances binding of retinoic acid, thyroid-hormone, and vitamin D receptors to their cognate response elements. *Cell* 67:1251, 1991.
41. Farrell PM, Machlin LJ. Human health and disease. In Machlin LJ (ed), *Vitamin E, A Comprehensive Treatise.* New York: Dekker, 1980. P 520.
42. Underwood BA, Olson JA (eds). *A Brief Guide to Current Methods of Assessing Vitamin A Status.* Washington, DC: International Vitamin A Consultative Group, International Life Science Institute, Nutrition Foundation, 1994.
43. Hathcock JN, et al. Evaluation of vitamin A toxicity. *Am J Clin Nutr* 52:183, 1990.
44. Daicker B, et al. Canthaxanthin retinopathy: An investigation by light and electron-microscopy and physicochemical analysis. *Graefes Arch Clin Exp Ophthalmol* 225:189, 1987.
45. Bhalla AK, et al. Specific high-affinity receptors for 1,25-dihydroxy vitamin-D_3 in human peripheral-blood mononuclear cells presence in monocytes and induction in lymphocytes-T following activation. *J Clin Endocrinol Metab* 57:1308, 1983.
46. Holick MF. Vitamin D: Biosynthesis, metabolism, and mode of action. In DeGroot LJ (ed), *Endocrinology,* Vol. 2. New York: Grune & Stratton, 1989. P 902.
47. Abe E, et al. Differentiation of mouse myeloid-leukemia cells induced by 1-alpha,25-dihydroxyvitamin D_3. *Proc Natl Acad Sci USA* 78:4990, 1981.
48. Eisman JA. 1,25-Dihydroxyvitamin D3 receptor and role of 1,25-dihydroxyvitamin D3 in human cancer cells in vitamin D. In Kumar R (ed), *Vitamin D: Basic and Clinical Aspects.* Boston: Martinus Nijhoff, 1984.
49. Smith EL, Walworth ND, Holick MF. Effect of 1-alpha, 25-dihydroxyvitamin D3 on the morphologic and biochemical differentiation of cultured human epidermal keratinocytes grown in serum-free conditions. *J Invest Dermatol* 86:709, 1988.
50. Holick MF. Will 1,25 dihydroxy vitamin D_3, MC903, and their analogs herald a new pharmacologic era for the treatment of psoriasis? *Arch Dermatol* 125:1692, 1989.
51. Bieri JG. Kinetics of tissue alpha-tocopherol depletion and repletion. *Ann NY Acad Sci* 203:181, 1972.
52. Hoekstra WG. Biochemical function of selenium and its relation to vitamin E. *Fed Proc* 34:2083, 1975.
53. Pryor WA. Free-radical biology: Xenobiotics, cancer, and aging. *Ann NY Acad Sci* 393:1, 1982.
54. Bell EF. Upper limit of vitamin E in infant formulas. *J Nutr* 119:1829, 1989.
55. Olson RE, et al. Vitamin K-dependent carboxylase. In Johnson BC (ed). *Post-Translational Covalent Modifications of Proteins.* New York: Academic, 1983. P 295.
56. Traverso HP, Hauschka PV, Gallup PM. Vitamin K-dependent gamma carboxyglutamic acid formation by mouse renal adenocarcinoma cells. *Calcif Tissue Int* 30:73, 1980.
57. Motohara K, Endo F, Matsuda L. Effect of vitamin K administration on acarboxy-prothrombin (PIVKA-II) levels in newborns. *Lancet* 2:242, 1985.
58. Warkany J. Warfarin embryopathy. *Am J Dis Child* 129:287, 1975.
59. Lane PA, Hathaway WE. Vitamin K in infancy. *J Pediatr* 106:351, 1985.
60. Shearer MJ, et al. Plasma vitamin K_1 in mothers and their newborn babies. *Lancet* 2:460, 1982.

Selected Readings

American Medical Association, Department of Foods and Nutrition. Multivitamin preparations for parenteral use: A statement by the Nutrition Advisory Group. *J Parent Enteral Nutr* 3:258, 1979.

This is the journal publication from the panel of experts who met in 1972 to establish the first set of recommendations for intravenous vitamins for all age groups. These recommendations received regulatory approval and were published in the *Federal Register* 37(145):15027, 1972.

Greene HL, et al. Guidelines for use of vitamins, trace elements, calcium, magnesium and phosphorus in infants and children receiving total parenteral nutrition. *Am J Clin Nutr* 48:1324, 1988.

A literature review with guidelines from an expert panel on the intravenous use of multiple vitamins. Recommendations for children remained the same as published in the 1972 *Federal Register,* but new guidelines are given for preterm infants.

National Research Council, Food and Nutrition Board. *Recommended Dietary Allowances* (10th ed.). Washington, DC: National Academy Press, 1989.

This 10th edition reflects the current state of knowledge regarding the Recommended Dietary Allowances for all known nutrients, by population group segmented by age and physiologic status. Recommendations for vitamins are summarized in Table 9-1. The panel establishing these recommendations recognized that for some nutrients under certain conditions higher intakes may be optimal, but that there is insufficient information to establish optima. Note that the U.S. Recommended Daily Allowances (US RDAs) used for food labeling are based on the generally higher levels in the 7th (1968) edition of the Recommended Dietary Allowances.

Scriver CR, et al. (eds). *The Metabolic Basis of Inherited Disease* (6th ed.). New York: McGraw-Hill, 1989. P 3008.

Discusses biochemical mechanisms by which symptoms of certain inborn errors of metabolism may be improved by therapy with pharmacologic doses of vitamins.

Shils M, Olson J, Shike M (eds). *Modern Nutrition in Health and Disease* (8th ed.). Philadelphia: Lea & Febiger, 1993. P 1657.

This text provides an in-depth review of each of the vitamins with an emphasis on recent findings related to vitamin metabolism. The chapters focus substantially on the relationship of the newer findings to clinical application.

10

Essential Trace Metals: Deficiencies and Requirements

Khursheed N. Jeejeebhoy
Wei-Kuen Cheong

The human body contains elements at concentrations of less than 50 mg/kg that are called trace elements; those of biologic importance are called essential elements. In the natural diet, trace metals are taken in association with macronutrients. Their deficiency usually becomes obvious when intake of a specific element is limited in the face of an adequate intake of other nutrients. Therefore, it was in the use of total parenteral nutrition (TPN), where it is possible to create a single element deficiency, that trace metal deficiency became apparent in the human. Measurements and indices relating to functional trace metal status of the body remain imperfect [1]. As such, rational administration during TPN is as much a matter of clinical judgment as it is a science. It should be recognized that the following factors modify the availability and dose of trace elements:

1. Amino acid and electrolyte solutions often contain significant amounts of trace metals as contaminants, which vary between manufacturers and between lots. Zinc, copper, chromium, iron, and manganese are documented contaminants. Stable plasma protein solutions (SPPS), that is, all products containing proteins from plasma, also contain significant amounts of trace elements.
2. The constituents of the nutrient solution itself modify the biologic availability of the metal.

3. The nutrient solution constituents may also modify the body losses of an element, for example, amino acid infusion increases urinary zinc and copper.
4. The bioavailability and pharmacokinetics of different compounds of the same trace element may differ significantly, for example, manganese and selenium in their different forms.

Iron

Physiologic Considerations

Total body iron (approximately 54 to 90 mmol) may be divided conceptually into two physiologic compartments: functional iron and storage iron. Total body iron is composed of heme (65%), reticuloendothelial stores (30%), ferroproteins (myoglobin, cytochrome system) as bone marrow ferritin and hemosiderin (5%), and serum iron (less than 0.1%). Available iron reserves amount to 18 mmol in males and 5 to 9 mmol in females. Losses are estimated at 4 to 9 μmol/day in feces (largely as exfoliated enterocytes), 4 μmol/day in urine, small amounts in bile, and variable amounts in sweat. Destruction of red blood cells releases about 0.5 mmol of iron per day, all of which is virtually salvaged. Daily loss in the adult male is estimated to be about 18 μmol. Menstruation increases losses by 9 to 14 μmol/day or more. Theoretically, therefore, there are sufficient iron stores to last between 1 and 3 years in a patient with normal stores. Additional blood loss, bile, or small intestinal drainage and inflammatory exudates may increase iron loss and deplete iron stores further.

Because of the absence of a physiologically controlled mechanism for iron excretion, iron stores are controlled by changes in gastrointestinal absorption. Excess iron ingested is trapped as ferritin in the enterocyte and is subsequently lost with enterocyte shedding. Iron is present in food in two major forms: 10% as heme and 90% as nonheme compounds, with 30% to 40% of heme iron being absorbed. Absorption occurs directly as the porphyrin complex, independent of gastric pH, intestinal factors, and total body iron status. In contrast, non-heme iron undergoes variable absorption between 3% and 8% with a ceiling of about 20%. Absorption is modified by total body iron status, gastric pH, and other luminal factors.

Absorption of iron occurs largely from the duodenum. Short-bowel patients therefore can potentially maintain significant iron absorption if the duodenum is intact. Patients with 40 to 100 cm of healthy small bowel appear capable of maintaining positive iron balance at an oral intake of 150 to 300 μmol of iron per day [2]. Many drugs interact with iron to form complexes that impede absorption of both moieties. Manganese, nickel, zinc, and cobalt share part of the iron absorptive mechanism. Trace elements such as zinc therefore can reduce iron absorption if given in large amounts. Copper deficiency reduces absorption. Ascorbic acid, organic acids, iron deficiency, hypoxia, and anemia increase absorption. However, iron absorption is not increased in hemolytic disorders except for thalassemia major, sideroblastic anemia, and pyruvate kinase deficiency.

Transport of iron occurs as transferrin. When all transferrin sites are saturated because of iron overload, nonspecific binding of iron to albumin occurs. Free iron is toxic.

Deficiency Symptoms

Iron aids oxygen transport as an essential constituent of porphyrin-based compounds such as hemoglobin and myoglobin. While anemia is the most important manifestation of iron deficiency, various nonhematologic sequelae of iron depletion have been proposed. These include epithelial abnormalities (accounting for angular stomatitis, esophageal webbing, gastric atrophy, and chronic gastritis), muscle and brain dysfunction, immunologic sequelae, and body temperature derangements.

Indices of Body Status

The best indicator of iron status is the actual assay of iron stores in bone marrow. Histologic evaluation of bone marrow for stainable hemosiderin is less quantitative. Ferritin in plasma is a good reflection of iron stores. However, being an acute-phase protein, its serum level increases in response to inflammation. Levels are also increased in liver disease and after iron-dextran injections. In the absence of inflammation, serum concentrations of 1 μg/L of ferritin corresponds to 2.5 μmol/kg body weight (BW) of iron store [3]. Serum ferritin of less than 12 μg/L in the absence of inflammation or less than 50 μg/L in the presence of inflammation suggests iron deficiency.

Transferrin levels are dependent on nutritional status. Malnutrition would be expected to depress transferrin levels and falsely elevate the iron/TIBC (TIBC = Total Iron Binding Capacity) ratio. Transferrin saturation determines the iron flow to tissues. Saturation levels (iron/TIBC ratios) of below 16% imply suboptimal iron supply. Serum iron levels undergo changes quite independent of body iron status. During acute infection and after surgical trauma, serum iron falls as a result of iron uptake by cells of the reticuloendothelial system. Interleukin-1 and other cytokines cause iron redistribution in sepsis and trauma.

Requirements

Considering the daily estimated losses, males require 17.9 μmol/day and females 35.8 μmol/day of elemental iron to maintain balance in the absence of additional losses. These amounts also appear to be the minimal requirements in patients on long-term TPN. Iron deficiency anemia may also result from functional abnormalities in iron utilization resulting from copper deficiency, reduced macrophage transfer in the presence of inflammation, and reduced transferrin levels. Supplementation with parenteral iron would not improve anemia in these patients. Where supplementation is deemed necessary, iron may be administered safely as a dilute solution of iron-dextran (high molar mass complex of ferric hydroxide and dextran) in TPN where added iron-dextran has been shown to be stable [4].

Toxicity and Therapeutic Window

The effect of iron on the immune system and the susceptibility to infection remains unclear. The induction of hypoferremia by interleukin-1 may represent an important host defense mechanism against bacterial proliferation and invasion. Therefore, on theoretic grounds, parenteral iron therapy may increase susceptibility to infection, and some studies support this possibility. However, other studies do not demonstrate an increase in infection rates [5].

Zinc

Physiologic Considerations

Zinc is the second most abundant of all the trace elements, after iron. Total body stores range between 22 and 35 mmol, 99% of which are intracellular, mainly in the liver, kidneys, and muscle, and only 1% in serum. While zinc is an integral part of over 200 metalloenzymes, it is especially important because it is a part of nucleic acid and protein synthesizing systems. It is a constituent of thymidine kinase and nucleoside phosphorylase and is important for polysome conformation during protein synthesis [6].

Twenty to thirty percent of orally ingested zinc is absorbed by the small intestine, but colonic absorption is minimal. Absorption involves binding to an acceptor with subsequent internalization into enterocytes where a variable amount is bound to a metallothioneine and subsequently lost when the enterocyte is shed. High body zinc levels stimulate metallothioneine synthesis and therefore self-regulate absorption. Phytates, phosphates, copper, iron, lead, and calcium in the diet inhibit gastrointestinal absorption. Pregnancy, corticosteroids, endotoxins, and leukocyte endogenous mediators (LEM) enhance absorption. Excretion is mainly in bile and pancreatic juices and less is lost in urine and sweat. Urinary losses are usually less than 10 μmol/day but may increase during stress [7] and in patients with liver disease. [*Editor's Note:* In situations where proteolysis is pronounced, urinary losses may chronically exceed 20 μmol/day, resulting in total body zinc depletion. Patients with chronic diarrhea are also at risk for zinc deficiency.]

Deficiency Symptoms

Clinical zinc deficiency was first described by Prasad et al. [8] in individuals who were geophagic. They failed to grow and mature sexually. Zinc replacement induced growth and sexual maturation. Later, zinc deficiency was seen in patients receiving TPN with purified macronutrients. In this situation, anabolism increased zinc requirements without providing this trace element in sufficient quantities. These patients developed a syndrome similar to acrodermatitis enteropathica within 5 to 10 weeks of starting TPN [9].

Predominant features of TPN-induced zinc deficiency are acrodermatitis with skin lesions involving the face and hands, and impaired immunity with increased susceptibility to infection. The features are similar to those seen in a genetically transmitted, autosomal recessive condition called acrodermatitis enteropathica. In this condition, zinc absorption is impaired, and the resulting deficiency causes skin lesions and immune deficiency that lead to death from infections and wasting. The patients present with stomatitis, scaly or vesicobullous pustular rash around the eyes, the oral, anal, and genital areas, and over articular prominences. There is erythema of the palms and soles, paronychia, diarrhea, alopecia, growth retardation, and predisposition to infections. It is of interest that cutaneous manifestations of essential fatty acid deficiency are aggravated by concomitant deficiency of zinc.

An immune deficiency due to zinc deficiency is characterized by reduced cell-mediated immunity, lymphopenia, and altered CD4/CD8 ratio caused by a fall in thymulin levels [10].

Indices of Body Status

Serum zinc is a poor index of total body zinc status because it is predominantly intracellular and there is poor correlation between muscle (60% total body zinc) and serum levels. Serum levels of zinc are dependent on serum albumin levels and on factors causing an intracellular shift, such as TPN-induced anabolism, pregnancy, oral contraceptives, sepsis, and corticosteroid therapy. However, Baer and King have attempted to use a combination of plasma and urine zinc to identify depletion. They identify minimal deficiency as urinary zinc of less than 2.3 μmol/day and severe deficiency as, in addition to reduced urine output, plasma levels that fall to less than 3.8 μmol/L [11]. Hair and erythrocyte zinc levels at the best reflect long-term changes in zinc status. They are poor indices of current zinc status in acute/subacute illnesses because of the slow turnover of zinc at these sites. Furthermore, zinc deficiency arrests hair growth; therefore, the zinc level in the remaining hair is normal and is not representative of the zinc status. Zinc levels in lymphocytes, granulocytes, platelets, and muscle biopsies may be more reflective of tissue deficiency. Serum levels of thymulin, a zinc-containing thymic hormone, may be another assay by which to ascertain zinc status. Alkaline phosphatase activity in neutrophils and serum may be useful. A specific, sensitive, and easily available test does not exist at present, and the assessment of zinc status requires an integrated appreciation of the underlying clinical circumstances and laboratory tests.

Requirements

Patients likely to have zinc deficiency include alcoholics and those with Crohn's disease, chronic malabsorption syndrome, chronic liver disease, and malignancies. In addition, treatment with drugs such as penicillamine or chlorothiazide may increase zinc losses. Increased zinc losses have been observed in septic patients and those with burns and with nephrotic syndrome. Increased needs occur in children during growth spurts and in pregnant and lactating women.

Patients with 40 to 100 cm of healthy small bowel appear capable of maintaining satisfactory gastrointestinal zinc absorption and a positive zinc balance on 145 to 203 μmol/day of dietary zinc [2]. Wolman et al. [7] found that zinc balance may be achieved by intravenous supplementation of 46 μmol/day of elemental zinc in patients without additional losses. In other studies, 76 μmol/day of intravenous elemental zinc maintained plasma zinc levels comparable with controls. The American Medical Association [12] recommends 38 μmol/day of zinc in stable patients, but recommends that the intake be increased by 187 μmol/L of zinc of small intestinal fluid loss via fistula or duodenojejunocolostomy and 261 μmol of zinc/L of stool or ileostomy output.

Toxicity and Therapeutic Window

Zinc toxicity has been described after the intake of about 3.4 mmol of elemental zinc. Pharmacologically administered doses between 1.5 and 4.6 mmol of elemental zinc inhibit intestinal absorption of copper, inducing hypochromic microcytic anemia and leucopenia. Rapid infusion of 153 μmol of zinc over an hour resulted in transient flushing, blurred vision, and sweating. Administration of 352 μmol of zinc/L of TPN mixture produced asymptomatic hyperamylasemia.

Copper

Physiologic Considerations

Copper is the third most abundant trace element in the body, after iron and zinc. Total copper content in the healthy human body is about 1.3 to 3.1 mmol, largely intracellular. About 70% is found in the liver and brain; the rest is found in the heart, kidneys, spleen, muscle, and bone. Ninety percent of blood copper is tightly bound to ceruloplasmin, a nonexchangeable, nontransport form of copper. The rest is loosely bound to albumin and amino acids (histidine, threonine, glutamine), which represent the vehicles for transport of copper to tissues.

Thirty to fifty percent of dietary copper is absorbed in the upper gastrointestinal tract. Absorbed copper is then transported via the portal system to the liver, where a part of it is incorporated into ceruloplasmin, another part released into the circulation, and the rest excreted in the bile. Zinc inhibits copper absorption by promoting intestinal metallothioneine synthesis. Copper is bound to metallothioneine and is lost with enterocyte shedding. Zinc therefore has been used therapeutically in the treatment of Wilson's disease. Absorption is also inhibited by dietary phytates, iron, ascorbic acid, and cadmium. It is enhanced by copper deficiency.

Copper homeostasis is maintained by the liver, and the major route of copper excretion is in the bile where 8 to 58 μmol/day are excreted with taurodeoxycholate. There is no enterohepatic recirculation. Urinary losses are minimal, about 0.47 to 0.94 μmol/day, but this increases nearly four- to nine-fold in critically ill patients. Infusion of amino acids during TPN increases urinary copper loss. Loss of copper in sweat is variable and averages 1.6 to 9.2 μmol/day.

Deficiency Symptoms

Copper is a constituent, or is associated with the activity, of a number of proteins and enzymes. These include ceruloplasmin, lysyl oxidase (involved in elastin and collagen synthesis), cytochrome oxidase (mitochondrial energy metabolism), Zn-Cu superoxide dismutase (free radical scavenging), tyrosinase (melanin synthesis), ferroxidase (iron metabolism), monoamine oxidase, and dopamine β-hydroxylase (catecholamine metabolism) [13]. The clinical features of copper deficiency are correlated with the functions of the two major copper-dependent proteins: ceruloplasmin and lysyl oxidase. The most common manifestation of copper deficiency is hematologic. Patients develop a microcytic, hypochromic anemia with pancytopenia, refractory to iron supplementation. The bone marrow is hypocellular, contains iron, and there is cytoplasmic and nuclear vacuolizations of the erythroid and myeloid series. Serum iron is low in the initial stages of deficiency but rises spontaneously later in the clinical course with no improvement in hematologic indices [14]. Because cell iron is in the ferrous form, it has to be oxidized to ferric iron by ceruloplasmin before it can be bound to transferrin for transport to marrow or tissues. Copper deficiency therefore leads to a functional failure of iron transfer and utilization [15]. Leucopenia is another feature that is more commonly encountered in infants [14]. The cause of pancytopenia is not clear, but it may be partly linked to the development of an antineutrophil antibody [16].

Lysyl oxidase performs oxidative deamination of peptidyl lysine residues. The resultant product, α-aminoadipic acid d-semialdehyde (allysine), is required for the formation of cross-linkages in collagen and elastin. Copper deficiency therefore leads to defective collagen and elastin structures. Abnormalities are noted in the bones of infants and not of adults. Bony anomalies are reminiscent of scorbutic bone disease, including diffuse osteoporosis, delayed bone age, widened cupped metaphyses with beaks and fractures, subperiosteal hematoma, ossifications in the shafts of long bones, and diaphyseal fractures [17]. Weakness of vascular structures with resultant aneurysms secondary to elastin abnormalities have been described in animals rendered copper-deficient.

Abnormalities of catecholamine metabolism in association with dopamine β-hydroxylase deficiency have also been proposed as a potential consequence of copper deficiency.

Copper also appears to be essential for normal function and structure of the central nervous system, taste sensation, and pigmentation. An association with psychiatric abnormalities has also been suggested. Menkes disease is a sex-linked recessive inborn error of copper absorption and cellular copper metabolism. Patients have excessive intestinal and kidney accumulation of copper but low brain and liver copper levels. Neurologic disease has not been described as a feature of nutritional copper deficiency, but it is a feature of Menkes disease [18]. Manifestations include growth retardation, steely kinky hair (defective disulfide bonding in keratin), skin depigmentation (tyrosinase deficiency), hypotonia, and focal cerebral and cerebellar degeneration secondary to neuronal demyelination. Patients have seizures, diffuse arterial aneurysms, and skeletal demineralization. Anemia and neutropenia are not features. Ceruloplasmin is low. The disease starts in the first few months of life and death usually occurs by 2 years of age.

Cases of copper deficiency occurring during TPN have been reported [19]. Within a week of administering copper to deficient patients, the pancytopenia resolves. Radiologic osseous abnormalities, however, take months to resolve [20].

Indices of Body Status

Serum copper is an insensitive indicator of body copper status for many reasons. As serum copper is largely in the form of ceruloplasmin, its concentrations bear a close relationship to factors that alter the level of this protein. Hepatic dysfunction, protein caloric malnutrition, and nephrosis with increased urinary protein losses all depress ceruloplasmin and hence serum total copper levels. Ceruloplasmin is also an acute-phase reactant. Serum levels may be elevated during stress states, for example, in patients with lymphomas, leukemias and other forms of cancer, in users of oral contraceptives, in patients following myocardial infarctions, and in those with acute chronic infections or active Crohn's disease. Serum copper in patients with cancer may represent a "tumor marker" and, in this situation, cannot be used as an index of requirements during nutritional support. Despite negative copper balances, serum copper may remain normal because liver stores are released to maintain normal serum levels.

Hair copper is not a reliable index of deficiency because of copper contamination from substances applied during hair dressing. Zn-Cu superoxide dismutase of erythrocytes may be a more sensitive monitor of copper status.

Requirements

Risk factors for the development of copper deficiency include inadequate stores due to prematurity, chronic malabsorption, excessive losses from diarrhea, fistulas, especially biliary-enteric and biliary-cutaneous fistulas, a proximal stoma, exudative enteropathy, long-term use of chelating agents, high-dose oral zinc ingestion, and burns.

Dietary requirements of copper amount to 0.47 μmol/kg/day in a normal adult [21]. Deficiency states have not been reported in patients ingesting 31.5 to 63 μmol/day. Patients with 40 to 100 cm of healthy small bowel appear capable of maintaining a positive copper balance at oral intakes between 8.6 and 42.2 μmol/day of copper (average = 25.4 μmol/day) [2].

Copper given at 15.7 μmol/day has been shown to maintain serum copper levels in the upper range of normal controls, while falling serum copper levels have been documented in patients receiving only 3.1 μmol/day of copper in TPN. Under normal circumstances, copper losses through the intestines amount to 3.1 μmol/day [22]. Shike et al. [22] recommend that in the absence of diarrhea, parenteral administration of 4.7 μmol/day is sufficient to meet requirements. Diarrhea (>300 g/day), high-output stomas, the presence of enterocutaneous, biliary-enteric or biliary-cutaneous fistulas, and increased nasogastric suction may be expected to elevate copper losses to 4.7 to 5.5 μmol/day. In these patients, copper content in TPN should be increased to between 6.3 and 7.9 μmol/day [22].

In stressed patients, urinary copper excretion rises to a mean of 4 μmol/day, and adrenocortical insufficiency reduces urinary copper losses. Therefore, in critically ill patients, a higher intake of copper, 7.9 μmol/day, has been recommended. Patients with evidence of liver dysfunction (increased serum bilirubin, alkaline phosphatase) experience reduced copper losses through the gastrointestinal tract because of diminished biliary copper excretion. As intravenous copper infusion does not result in increased urinary excretion, copper given in excess of requirements is retained. Therefore, in the presence of abnormal liver function, only 1.6 μmol/day should be given. This reduction is less important during short-term TPN but is crucial in patients on long-term TPN [22]. It should also be noted that TPN solutions may contain significant amounts of copper as contaminants. This is of particular importance in patients on long-term parenteral nutrition in the presence of liver function abnormalities. Copper content should be carefully evaluated and controlled in these circumstances. On the basis of studies, 15.7 μmol/day for 2 weeks followed by 7.9 μmol/day is recommended for repletion therapy [12].

Toxicity and Therapeutic Window

As an element, copper is more toxic than zinc. While the manifestations of acute copper intoxication have been described, clinical manifestations of chronic toxicity are less well defined. The only well-studied clinical model remains that of Wilson's disease. Sequestration of copper in hepatic lysosomes protects against toxicity, until this mechanism is overwhelmed. Subsequent accumulation of copper in the cytosol of hepatocytes leads to hepatitis and eventually cirrhosis. Hemolysis may occur. Accumulation, particularly in renal tubules, cornea, and brain, results in damage. The best indicator of copper overload is the measurement of copper in a liver biopsy. The neurotoxic effects of copper may be related to its role in inhibition of carbohydrate metabolism in the brain.

Chromium

Physiologic Considerations

Total body chromium content in health has been reported to be about 115 μmol. From autopsy studies, its concentration has been demonstrated to decline with age [23]. This may contribute to the increased incidence of glucose intolerance seen in the older age groups [24]. In animal models, chromium has been demonstrated to promote insulin action in peripheral tissues, improve lipogenesis, glycogenesis, and amino acid transport [25]. It is not found in any metalloprotein in man, but its existence in the form of a glucose tolerance factor (a complex of chromium, nicotinic acid, and amino acids) plays a crucial role in the action of both endogenous and exogenous insulin.

Only about 1% to 3% of orally ingested inorganic chromium and about 10% to 25% of organic sources is absorbed. Gastrointestinal absorption is inhibited by zinc and phytate. Excretion is mainly renal. Glucose loading, hyperglycemia, and trauma enhance urinary loss. Smaller amounts are lost in stools.

Deficiency Symptoms

Chromium deficiency leads first to insulin resistance and hypersecretion following glucose loads. This progresses to frank glucose intolerance and disturbances in lipid metabolism. In the course of long-term TPN, the onset of previously undocumented glucose intolerance in the absence of a precipitant (for example, infection), peripheral neuropathy, ataxia, and progressive weight loss despite increasing caloric load should suggest the possibility of chromium deficiency. Concomitantly, lipids become the major metabolic substrate, respiratory quotient (RQ) falls, and serum free fatty acid rises [26].

Indices of Body Status

Serum chromium levels are technically difficult to measure, and wide variations of "normal" serum levels are seen in different laboratories. Plasma chromium falls in deficiency states but also in acute illness. Its level is increased by insulin injections and glucose loads [27]. The best index of chromium deficiency is the correction of biochemical and clinical abnormalities with a therapeutic trial of chromium supplementation at 3.8 to 4.8 μmol/day. However, despite reversal of glucose intolerance, serum chromium levels may remain unchanged and in fact may remain below normal levels, again reflecting the insensitivity of serum chromium as a yardstick of functional body chromium status. Serial intravenous glucose tolerance test before and after chromium supplementation is a proposed functional test.

Requirements

Chromium needs during TPN are unclear. Adults receiving 0.12 μmol/day have demonstrated clinical deficiency, and requirements of 0.19 to 0.38 μmol/day have been suggested [26]. Total chromium losses in healthy subjects amount to 0.11 to 0.19 μmol/day; this can increase to 0.37 μmol/day in diabetics. Because of the glucose loading, the application of TPN significantly increases urinary chromium losses in healthy patients. Losses as high as 2.8 μmol/day have been reported.

Contaminant chromium levels in TPN stock solutions vary greatly. Amino acid solutions, particularly those high in phosphate and phosphate salt additives, are major contributors of chromium. Lipid emulsions would also be a major contributor if high-percentage lipid formulations are used. Together, these components would constitute 85% to 90% of the chromium contaminant in TPN solutions, amounting up to about 0.15 μmol/day of chromium for a low-lipid formulation and 0.2 μmol/day for a high-lipid formulation. The chromium content may vary from 0.046 to 0.2 μmol/day between stocks of TPN solutions.

Toxicity and Therapeutic Window

There is no documented adverse reaction to parenteral chromium, although chromium toxicity in industrial settings is well known. Elemental chromium as the chloride salt was administered at 3.8 to 4.8 μmol/day for 14 days to correct a deficiency state, without untoward effects.

Manganese

Physiologic Considerations

The human body contains 0.22 to 0.36 mmol of manganese, mainly within the brain, kidney, pancreas, liver, and bone. It is found largely within mitochondria as Mn-superoxide dismutase [28]. About 3% to 4% of ingested manganese is absorbed. Homeostasis is maintained largely via excretory mechanisms rather than control of absorption, although absorption is enhanced by low intakes and depressed when intakes are high. It is excreted in bile. Smaller amounts are excreted in pancreatic juices and through the intestinal wall. Enterohepatic recirculation is negligible (less than 1%). There is negligible urinary excretion.

Deficiency Symptoms

Manganese is a component of two metalloenzymes, Mn-superoxide dismutase and pyruvate carboxylase, but it remains unclear if it is essential in humans on TPN. No report of deficiency symptoms have been published except for a suggestion that concomitant manganese administration was required to correct a vitamin K-resistant prolonged prothrombin time. This patient was fed a manganese-free diet and developed a prolonged prothrombin time after 17 weeks. The addition of a carbohydrate moiety to convert preprothrombin to prothrombin is thought to be manganese-dependent [29]. Defective hair and nail growth, transient dermatitis, pronounced decline of cholesterol level in blood, and changes in hair color have also been observed as possible effects of manganese deprivation [30].

Manganese is an essential component of mitochondria Mn-superoxide dismutase, which catalyzes the dismutation of superoxide free radicals to hydrogen peroxide and water, thus protecting the cells from superoxide-induced tissue damage. This enzyme is distinct from cytosolic superoxide dismutase, which contains copper and zinc. Cytosolic Cu-Zn superoxide dismutase is sensitive to cyanide; mitochondrial Mn-superoxide dismutase is not. In animals, manganese is important for the action of glycosyltransferases, which are involved in the synthesis of glycosaminoglycans and glycoproteins. Manganese-deficient animals manifest cartilage abnormalities, abnormal carbohydrate and lipid metabolism, neurologic anomalies, and ultrastructural changes in various organs. Teratogenicity during gestation has been documented in manganese-deficient animals; however, no human case has been documented to date. This observation may become of importance in the administration of TPN to pregnant women.

Indices of Body Status

Manganese circulates in serum bound to transferrin. It is not known if serum or whole blood manganese correlates with whole body manganese status, although excess intake probably results in elevated levels [31]. Plasma manganese levels reflect the amount of manganese administered in TPN [32]. Mn-superoxide dismutase activity can be measured only in tissue samples rich in mitochondria. As such, the measurement of this enzyme cannot be used routinely in clinical practice.

Requirements

Enteral requirements of manganese are believed to range from 22.8 to 54.6 μmol/day. Patients with oral intakes of less than 36.4 μmol/day do not appear to show any adverse effects [33]. With an estimated 3% to 4% absorption, this equates to only 14.7 μmol/day or less of manganese. Requirements during TPN have not been established in humans. Doses of 0.18 to 1.8 μmol/day maintained serum manganese levels comparable to normal controls [32], while those on home TPN receiving 36.4 μmol/day had elevated levels of whole blood manganese [34]. Manganese should be provided with caution to patients with cholestasis because of anticipated impaired excretion. Catabolic states and increased gastrointestinal fluid losses are thought not to contribute to increased losses or requirements. Manganese contamination of TPN formulations has been estimated to range between 0.15 to 0.4 μmol/bag of TPN. Amino acid solutions are the major contributors, although manganese is also found in dextrose, lipid, electrolyte, and vitamin preparations.

Toxicity and Therapeutic Window

The symptoms associated with chronic manganese poisoning are well described [35], occurring largely in those exposed to mining, steel work, voltaic cell, bleaching, and electrowelding industries. Manganese toxicity results in symptoms resembling Parkinson's disease (gait disturbance, bradykinesia, tremor, dystonia, weakness, rigidity, choreoathetoid movements) in addition to emotional and psychiatric abnormalities and impotence. Histologically, increased astroglial reaction is noted in the basal ganglia [35].

It has been reported recently that patients on long-term parenteral nutrition have T1-weighted hyperintensity in the medial region of the globus pallidus on magnetic resonance imaging (MRI). Manganese accumulation with subsequent neuronal damage has been suggested as a possible cause for this finding [36]. These patients received 27.3 to 36.4 μmol/day of manganese. While the significance is yet unknown, it clearly indicates the need for further investigations into whether the dose and molecular form of manganese administered in TPN is excessive and requires revision.

Molybdenum

Physiologic Considerations

The liver and kidneys have the highest molybdenum concentrations. Molybdenum is easily absorbed and is excreted in the urine. Urine excretion is enhanced by increased sulfate intake or when endogenous sulfate production increases. A high molybdenum diet enhances urinary copper excretion.

Deficiency Symptoms

Molybdenum is an essential component of xanthine oxidase (conversion of hypoxanthine to xanthine to uric acid), sulfite oxidase (conversion of sulfite to sulfate; essential for metabolism of sulphur in amino acids such as cystine and methionine to sulphate for excretion), and aldehyde oxidase. To date, only one case of deficiency has been documented [37]. Deficiency was associated with intolerance of sulphur-containing amino acids, manifesting as tachycardia, tachypnoea, night blindness, central scotoma, irritability, headache, vomiting, progressive disorientation, and coma. The patient had biochemical evidence of hypermethioninemia and hypouricemia. Urinary inorganic sulphate excretion was markedly decreased, and there was hypouricosuria with concomitant increase in urinary hypoxanthine and xanthine. These were all corrected with the addition of ammonium molybdate at 300 μ/day (1.86 μmol molybdenum/day).

Indices of Body Status

Measurements of serum and urinary molybdenum are technically difficult.

Requirements

Requirements are not known, but balance studies suggest that 0.5 to 1.0 μmol/day of molybdenum may be required. In addition, Crohn's patients lose 6.3 μmol/day of molybdenum in stools. TPN solutions may contain molybdenum as a contaminant, and this has been estimated to range from 0.05 to 0.16 μmol/L of amino acid solutions [37].

Toxicity and Therapeutic Window

At very high oral doses, molybdenum can cause hyperuricemia and increased ceruloplasmin.

Selenium

Physiologic Considerations

Selenium is interrelated with other antioxidants such as vitamin E. Deficiency of one can be partially corrected by giving the other. To understand the need for these two micronutrients, it is necessary to examine the alternative means by which oxygen is reduced in biologic systems. Normally, the enzyme cytochrome oxidase accepts electrons from cytochrome *c* at the end exposed to the cytosol and discharges them by reacting with $4H^+$ to form water [38]. The alternative path involves the monovalent addition of electrons to form superoxide [39]. The superoxide, if left unaltered, disproportionates to H_2O_2 and oxygen. The H_2O_2 hydrogen can also react by the Haber-Weiss [40] reaction with superoxide to form hydroxyl ions. Thus, in the absence of appropriate controls, a number of reactive peroxide and hydroxyl radicals can form and damage the cell. In well-nourished cells, superoxide dismutase (SOD) disproportionates superoxide to H_2O_2, and the peroxide so formed is reduced by glutathione peroxidase (GSHpx) to water.

$$O_2 \xrightarrow{e^-} O_2^- \xrightarrow{e^-} O_2^{2-}$$

$$O_2^- + H_2O_2 \rightarrow O_2 + OH^- + OH^+$$

$$O_2^- + H^+ \xrightarrow{SOD} H_2O_2 \xrightarrow{GSHpx} H_2O$$

Glutathione peroxidase is an enzyme made up of four subunits, each containing selenocysteine as an integral part of the molecule [41]. In association with superoxide dismutase, it controls the levels of superoxide and peroxide in the cell. This in turn affects lipid peroxidation of polyunsaturated fatty acids in cell membranes. Vitamin E is another line of defense and controls the formation of hydroperoxides in the fatty acid residues of phospholipids, a process that depends on the antioxidant role of the vitamin and also involves its entering into a structural relation with membrane phospholipids [42]. Finally, any lipid hydroperoxides may be reduced by glutathione peroxidase to hydroxyacids.

Biologic reactions that produce superoxide are: (1) enzyme reactions such as those involving xanthine oxidase; (2) metabolic pathways such as the hexose monophosphate shunt and oxidative reactions mediated by cytochrome P_{450}; (3) interaction of dioxygen with the electron transport chain in the mitochondria; and (4) phagocytosis, where a burst of oxidative metabolism is associated with generation of NADPH by the hexose monophosphate shunt, which in turn is used by NADPH oxidase to generate superoxide. The excess superoxide is controlled by superoxide dismutase and glutathione peroxidase. Hence, it is not surprising that bacterial killing is affected by selenium deficiency. In addition, some antineoplastic agents such as bleomycin produce superoxide. Thus, a number of different pathophysiologic situations and metabolic states can increase superoxide evolution and the need for protection by vitamin E and glutathione peroxidase.

Selenium is incorporated into tissue proteins as selenocysteine. The incorporation of selenium into an amino acid occurs in a unique tRNA and into protein through specific codons in the mRNA. Protein catabolism releases toxic selenocysteine that is rapidly hydrolyzed by selenocysteine β-lyase, and free selenium is released.

Selenium is present in high concentrations in seafood (tuna), meat, and onions, and in all cells of the body. The liver, kidneys, and pancreas have the highest concentrations; cardiac muscle is a close fourth. These levels are responsive to dietary intake. In blood, selenium is present in plasma and red cells. In tissues, selenium occurs as a part of glutathione peroxidase or as seleno-substituted sulphur-containing amino acids.

Selenium in inorganic and organic form is absorbed in the duodenum and carried in the plasma to tissues. Absorption is very efficient and amounts to between 76% and 100% of an oral dose. It is excreted in the feces, urine, and breath. In human studies with orally ingested selenite, 14% to 20% was excreted during the first week in the urine and 33% to 58% in stool over 3 weeks. The half-life was found to have a slow component of 96 to 144 days.

Absorbed selenium is initially bound to albumin and also, after being processed by red cells, circulates in association with β-lipoprotein. It is taken up by tissues and incorporated into proteins and glutathione peroxidase. Selenium is excreted in both feces and urine. Fecal excretion varies between 57% and 61% and urinary excretion between 29% and 43% of total losses.

Deficiency Symptoms

Patients receiving parenteral nutrition without added selenium may develop selenium deficiency with associated muscle pains; cardiomyopathy has also been described in two patients receiving long-term TPN [43–45]. Between 60 and 120 μg/day of selenite has been given to patients on home parenteral nutrition (HPN) without toxic effects and have succeeded in maintaining levels of plasma selenium.

Indices of Body Status

Plasma selenium and glutathione peroxidase levels are sensitive to selenium intake [46] and can be used to assess the need for this element. However, in functional terms, selenium and vitamin E are interrelated, and it has not been determined how much the supply of one conditions the need for the other in humans.

Requirements

The dietary intake of selenium varies from a low of 0.23 to 0.33 μmol/day in New Zealand to a high of 1.9 to 2.8 μmol/day in Canada. Garlic contains substantial amounts of the element. Human metabolic studies would suggest a minimum intake of 0.25 μmol/day, and in studies from China, 0.38 μmol/day was considered to constitute a minimal intake. In North American volunteers, the requirements have been estimated to be 0.68 μmol/day. The RDA is defined as 0.011 μmol/kg/day. This allowance should be increased by 0.12 and 0.24 μmol/day in pregnant and lactating women. Abnormal losses of selenium from wounds and pus may be as high as 130 μg/L, and fistula fluids contain 100 to 380 μg/L in patients living in a low-selenium diet area (for example, New Zealand). Similar data are not available for other parts of the world. Such losses should increase requirements in patients with wounds and fistula drainage.

Toxicity and Therapeutic Window

Selenium is as toxic as arsenic. Large doses can cause nausea, vomiting, and diarrhea. Bleeding from the gastrointestinal tract as well as loss of hair have been reported. We have administered 120 μg/day to HPN patients for years without the development of high selenium levels in plasma or clinical toxicity.

References

1. Versieck J, Cornelis R. Normal levels of trace elements in human blood plasma. *Anal Chim Acta* 116:217, 1980.
2. Engels LGJ, van den Hamer CJA, von Tongeren JHM. Iron, zinc and copper balance in short bowel patients on oral nutrition. *Am J Clin Nutr* 40:1038, 1984.
3. Finch CA, Hubers H. Perspectives in iron metabolism. *N Engl J Med* 306:1520, 1982.
4. Kwong KW, Tsallas G. Dilute iron dextran formulation for addition to parenteral nutrient solutions. *Am J Hosp Pharm* 37:206, 1980.
5. Barr LH, Dunn GD, Brennan MF. Essential fatty acid deficiency during total parenteral nutrition. *Ann Surg* 193:304, 1981.
6. Vallee BL, Falchuk KH. Zinc and gene expression. *R Soc Lond Proc* (Series B) 294:185, 1981.
7. Wolman SL, et al. Zinc in total parenteral nutrition: Requirements and metabolic effects. *Gastroenterology* 76:458, 1979.
8. Prasad AS, Halsted JA, Nadimi M. Syndrome of iron deficiency anaemia, hepatosplenomegaly, hypogonadism, dwarfism, and geophagia. *Am J Med* 31:532, 1961.
9. Kay RG, et al. A syndrome of acute zinc deficiency during total parenteral alimentation in man. *Ann Surg* 183:331, 1976.
10. Prasad AS, et al. Serum thymulin in human zinc deficiency. *J Clin Invest* 82:1202, 1988.
11. Baer MT, King JC. Tissue zinc levels and zinc excretion during experimental zinc depletion in young men. *Am J Clin Nutr* 39:556, 1984.
12. American Medical Association, Working Conference on Parenteral Trace Elements II. Section on clinical nutrition. *Bull NY Acad Med* 60:115, 1984.
13. Mason KE. A conspectus of research on copper metabolism and requirements of man. *J Nutr* 109:1979, 1979.
14. Ruocco L, et al. Severe pancytopenia due to copper deficiency. Case report. *Acta Haematol* 76:224, 1986.
15. Golden MHN. Trace elements in human nutrition. *Hum Nutr: Clin Nutr* 36C:185, 1982.
16. Higuchi S, et al. Anti-neutrophil antibodies in patients with nutritional copper deficiency. *Eur J Paediatr* 150:327, 1991.
17. Velin P, Dupont D, Daoud A. Nutritional copper deficiency: Apropos of a case. *Annales De Pediatrie* 36:269, 1989.
18. Danks DM, et al. Menkes' kinky hair syndrome. An inherited defect in copper absorption with widespread effects. *Pediatrics* 50:188, 1972.
19. Karpel JT, Peden VH. Copper deficiency in long-term parenteral nutrition. *J Pediatr* 80:32, 1972.
20. Fujita M, et al. Copper deficiency during total parenteral nutrition: Clinical analysis of three cases. *JPEN* 13:421, 1989.
21. World Health Organisation Expert Committee on Trace Elements in Human Nutrition. Trace elements in human nutrition (Report of WHO Expert Committee, Geneva, April 9–17, 1973). Technical Report Series—World Health Organization, 532, 1973.
22. Shike M, et al. Copper metabolism and requirements in total parenteral nutrition. *Gastroenterology* 81:290, 1981.
23. Schroeder HA, Nason AP, Tipton IH. Chromium deficiency as a factor in atherosclerosis. *J Chronic Dis* 23:123, 1970.
24. Offenbacher EG, et al. Metabolic chromium balances in men. *Am J Clin Nutr* 44:77, 1986.
25. Roginski EE, Mertz W. Effects of chromium (III) supplementation on glucose and amino acid metabolism in rats fed a low protein diet. *J Nutr* 97:525, 1969.
26. Jeejeebhoy KN, et al. Chromium efficiency, glucose intolerance, and neuropathy reversed by chromium supplementation in a patient receiving long-term total parenteral nutrition. *Am J Clin Nutr* 30:531, 1977.
27. Glinsmann WH, Feldman FJ, Mertz W. Plasma chromium after glucose administration. *Science* 152:1243, 1966.
28. Cotzias GC. Manganese in health and disease. *Physiol Rev* 38:503, 1958.

29. Doisy EA Jr. Trace substances in environmental health. University of Missouri Conference on Trace Substances in Environmental Health. In Hemphill DD (ed), *Trace Substances in Environmental Health,* Vol. 6. Missouri, Columbia, 1972. P 193.
30. Friedman BJ, et al. Manganese balance and clinical observations in young men fed a manganese-deficient diet. *J Nutr* 117:133, 1987.
31. Mena I, et al. Chronic manganese poisoning. *Neurology* 19:1000, 1969.
32. Shike M, et al. Manganese status in long-term home TPN patients [Abstract]. *Clin Res* 34:804A, 1986.
33. Guthrie BE, Robinson MF. Daily intakes of manganese, copper, zinc and cadmium by New Zealand women. *Br J Nutr* 38:55, 1977.
34. Jeejeebhoy KN, et al. Total parenteral nutrition at home: Studies in patients surviving 4 months to 5 years. *Gastroenterology* 71:943, 1976.
35. Yamada M, et al. Chronic manganese poisoning: A neuropathological study with determination of manganese distribution in the brain. *Acta Neuropathol* (Berlin) 70:273, 1986.
36. Mirowitz SA, Westrich TJ, Hirsch JD. Hyperintense basal ganglia on T1-weighted images in patients receiving parenteral nutrition. *Radiology* 181:117, 1991.
37. Abumrad NN, et al. Amino acid intolerance during prolonged total parenteral nutrition reversed by molybdate therapy. *Am J Clin Nutr* 34:2551, 1981.
38. Chance B, Sies H, Boveris A. Hydroperoxide metabolism in mammalian organs. *Physiol Rev* 59:527, 1979.
39. Hill HAO. The superoxide ion and the toxicity of molecular oxygen. In Fraustro da Silva JRR, Williams JRP (eds), *New Trends in Bioinorganic Chemistry* London: Academic, 1978. P 173.
40. Haber F, Weiss J. The catalytic decomposition of hydrogen peroxide by iron salts. *Philos Trans R Soc Lond A* 147:332, 1934.
41. Rotruck JT, et al. Selenium: Biochemical role as a component of glutathione peroxidase. *Science* 179:588, 1973.
42. Diplock AT, Lucy JA. The biochemical modes of action of vitamin E and selenium: A hypothesis. *FEBS Lett* 29:205, 1973.
43. Lane HW, Dudrick S, Warren DC. Blood selenium levels and glutathione peroxidase activities in university students and chronic intravenous hyperalimentation subjects. *Proc Soc Exp Biol Med* 167:383, 1981.
44. Fleming CR, et al. Selenium deficiency and fatal cardiomyopathy in a patient on home parenteral nutrition. *Gastroenterology* 83:689, 1982.
45. Johnson RA, et al. An occidental case of cardiomyopathy and selenium deficiency. *N Engl J Med* 304:1210, 1981.
46. Underwood EJ. Selenium. In *Trace Elements in Human and Animal Nutrition* (4th ed). New York: Academic, 1977. P 302.

Selected Readings

American Medical Association, Working Conference on Parenteral Trace Elements II. Section on clinical nutrition. *Bull NY Acad Med* 60:115, 1984.

This is an important consensus document about trace element requirements in parenteral nutrition.

Finch CA, Hubers H. Perspectives in iron metabolism. *N Engl J Med* 306:1520, 1982.

This is an excellent review of iron metabolism and requirements in health and disease.

Fleming CR, et al. Selenium deficiency and fatal cardiomyopathy in a patient on home parenteral nutrition. *Gastroenterology* 83:689, 1982.

This report points out that selenium deficiency occurs in patients on parenteral nutrition and may even be fatal if prolonged.

Prasad AS, et al. Serum thymulin in human zinc deficiency. *J Clin Invest* 82:1202, 1988.

This important paper points out the profound effects even of marginal zinc deficiency on immunity.

Wolman SL, et al. Zinc in total parenteral nutrition: requirements and metabolic effects. *Gastroenterology* 76:458, 1979.

This paper shows that in the presence of gastrointestinal losses such as diarrhea and fistula drainage, zinc requirements are markedly elevated. Increased zinc supplementation in this situation improves the metabolism of other nutrients.

11

Two Dozen Syndromes: Pattern Recognition in Diagnosis and Treatment of Fluid and Electrolyte Disorders

Francis D. Moore

Back to Normal Cellular Function

Cellular metabolism, the process of life, is conducted in a salty, protein-rich body fluid. One component of this fluid lies within the cells themselves. Another portion circulates freely outside of cells; is pumped through the blood vessels and capillaries; appears in the interstitial fluid, lymphatics, and gut; is rapidly replenished by oral intake; and serves as the secretory and excretory pathway of kidneys, lungs, liver, and bowel.

Whatever disorders arise in these intracellular and extracellular fluids, the ultimate message of damage or benefit is to be found in cellular function itself.

Homeostasis is the sum of bodily activities and inborn regulators by which these solute concentrations and solvent volumes are maintained to support normal cellular function. The inborn regulators—the physiologic feedback system—are the central issue in patient care: One must understand what the patient is doing for himself or herself before effective assistance can be provided. Autoregulation and feedback loop regulators operate throughout this system. Their function or malfunction may be as important as the disease state or the external cause of the disorder. Fluid and electrolyte concentrations, pools, and volumes are interrelated and cross-connected through membrane boundaries; each acts directly on the other. The physician encounters these complex disorders in repetitive "patterns" or "syndromes." It is easier to understand and treat them if we learn to identify and recognize them by their distinct patterns. Pattern recognition is the basis of effective fluid and electrolyte management. [*Author's Note:* The value of pattern recognition and the use of identified patterns of fluid/electrolyte change as the basis for patient care was first explored in Moore FD. Common patterns of water and electrolyte change in injury, surgery, and disease. *N Engl J Med* 258:277, 1958. This concept was then applied to certain aspects of burn treatment (Moore FD. Burns: An annotated outline for practical treatment. *Med Clin North Am* 36:1201, 1962), and in a textbook of surgical management (Moore FD. *Metabolic Care of the Surgical Patient.* Philadelphia: Saunders, 1959). This pattern-chemistry was updated and the method further expanded in the Rhoads-Hardy text (Rhoads JE, Hardy JM. *Textbook of Surgery.* Philadelphia: Lippincott, 1975), and it is here again brought up-to-date with several additional patterns observed in patients receiving parenteral nutrition.]

Complicated descriptions of the total system have been erected, often multivariate structures involving exponential and logarithmic functions. Such mathematical models have their appeal, providing chemical and teleologic insight, but they are a poor guide for the clinician. The sailor lost at sea searches for a few buoys or lighthouses to guide him home safely, even though he may be intellectually fascinated by the total interaction of forces that determine wind, ocean currents, and the formation of beaches, reefs, and shoals.

It is the purpose of this chapter to identify and describe 24 syndromes of disorder in body fluids: the volume of body water, body composition, electrolyte concentration, and acid-base change.

TWENTY-FOUR SYNDROMES: A GUIDE TO CHAPTER 11

Introductory Tables

Useful Expressions and First Approximations (Table 11-1)
Equations for Compositional Relationships (Table 11-2)
Useful Expressions and First Approximations in Acid-Base Homeostasis (Table 11-3)
Normal Values (Table 11-4)

Fifteen Disorders of Body Water, Salts, and Protein: Fluid Volumes and Tonicity

Syndrome 1. Hypovolemia (Table 11-5)
Syndrome 2. Plasma Loss Hypovolemia (Table 11-6)
Syndrome 3. Hypoproteinemia
Syndrome 4. Hypervolemia (Table 11-7)
Syndrome 5. Polycythemia (Table 11-8)
Syndrome 6. Desalting Water Loss (Table 11-9)
Syndrome 7. Oversalting: Extracellular Fluid Excess (Table 11-10)
Syndrome 8. Desiccation-Dehydration (Table 11-11)
Syndrome 9. Overhydration-Hypotonicity (Table 11-12)
Syndrome 10. Solute-Loading Hypertonicity (Table 11-13)
Syndrome 11. Hypokalemia (Table 11-14)
Syndrome 12. Hyperkalemia (Table 11-15)
Syndrome 13. Hypochloremia
Syndrome 14. Hyperchloremia (Table 11-16)
Syndrome 15. The Normal Postoperative Patient (Table 11-17)

Three Syndromes Related to Starvation and Intravenous Feeding

Syndrome 16. Cellular Steal
Syndrome 17. Parenteral Nutrition Overload
- 17-I. Fluid Overload
- 17-II. Hyperosmolar Nonketotic Hyperglycemic Coma in TPN (Table 11-18)
- 17-III. Hyperphosphatemia in TPN
- 17-IV. Hypercalcemia in TPN
- 17-V. The Satiety Syndrome in TPN
- 17-VI. Amino Acid Overload in TPN
- 17-VII. Acid-Base Distortion in TPN

Syndrome 18. Insulin Anomalies in TPN
- 18-I. Weaning Syndrome (Lingering Hyperinsulinemia) and Digestive Inhibition Before Weaning
- 18-II. Flask Insulin Hypoglycemia
- 18-III. Latent Diabetes and Post-Traumatic Pseudodiabetes in TPN

Six Syndromes of Disordered Acid-Base Homeostasis

Syndrome 19. Acute Hypercapnia (Table 11-19)
Syndrome 20. Chronic Hypercapnia (Table 11-19)
Syndrome 21. Acute Hypocapnia (Table 11-20)

Body Composition

In normal body fluid composition, concentration is held constant, whereas size (total volume) is variable. The total mass of a solute is, in turn, the product of the volume of the solution multiplied by the concentration of the solute. Many clinical problems in the understanding of body fluid disorders and their treatment arise from confusion between total volume and total mass and from the failure to appreciate the tremendous compositional differences among various patients, even though their ideal concentration parameters are identical.

The term *body composition* has been given to the study of these phenomena, relating mass and concentration in the body and identifying the total of body cells, fluids, and salts in a meaningful way. Body composition is the study of the total mass and volume of body components in relation to body size, body configuration, age, sex, disease, and concentration changes.

An understanding of the patterns of disordered body fluid chemistry requires an adequate systematic knowledge of physiologic chemistry and body composition. This chapter does not provide such background knowledge, but assumes it in the reader. The Selected Readings section at the end of this chapter includes summaries that provide a useful background review.

Addition or Subtraction?

Is the patient suffering from loss or gain? From deficit or plethora? Often obvious, this question should always be asked. Subtraction disorders include desalting water loss, various forms of dehydration, plasma volume deficit, and selective deficit of certain ions. But even here the balance between loss and gain is extremely important. A low hematocrit may mean the loss of red cells, but it also means an absolute increase in plasma volume.

Addition disorders, excesses in body fluid components, sometimes arise from disease as in liver failure, heart failure, or renal failure. Quite frequently, in an age of intravenous therapy, excesses result from overzealous treatment. An overabundance of body fluid and salt can embarrass the circulation and become lethal; overtransfusion of blood and plasma can produce all the chamber-pressure alterations of congestive heart failure.

The balance of loss and gain will determine the most rational treatment. A low serum sodium concentration, for example, should often be treated by withholding water or by a water diuresis, rather than by the careless administration of huge amounts of sodium salts, which can overload the circulation, producing cerebral and pulmonary edema. What appears superficially to be a deficit of salt may, in such instances, actually be an overload of water. The question of whether the disorder is *addition* or *subtraction* is thus always important, and sometimes subtle as well.

Homeostatic Feedback Regulators

Land-dwelling vertebrates spend their lives fighting off acidosis and dehydration. The excretion of acid and conservation of body water are, in a sense, the most primitive life-maintaining systems of those organisms that have removed themselves from the watery buffers of the ocean.

In the past 75 years it has become evident that the human body contains an elaborate system of interlocking regulators that, sensing a disorder, then guide the body back to normal in a cybernetic fashion, a feedback loop.

When the body senses a disorder, for example, desalting water loss, there is an elaborate homeostatic regulator system that within moments, or hours at the most, results in the conservation of water and salt. These feedback loops regularly involve three components: a sensor (often vascular muscle walls or special sense organs in them), a central arc (usually neuroendocrine), and an effector arm (respiratory, excretory, or circulatory).

The physician should perceive the state of these homeostatic regulators and determine by appropriate tests whether they are providing a feedback that is normal and corrective. If the inborn regulators are operating normally, it is a good portent indicating favorable outcome by simple treatment. If, owing to disease, the feedback regulator loop cannot operate normally, treatment becomes more complicated. Guides to progress must involve measures of the homeostatic regulators as well as the disorder itself. Examples to follow will make this point more clear.

In some cases, the disorder itself results from a primary malfunction of the homeostatic feedback mechanism. The simplest example is the unlimited diuresis seen in certain forms of kidney disease. A huge and unregulated loss of urine results in severe dehydration through the very organ whose normal function is to conserve water.

Four homeostatic regulatory mechanisms or feedback loops are preeminent in regulation of fluid and electrolyte, body water, salt, and acid.

Osmolar Regulation

Total osmolality is not to be confused with colloid osmotic pressure, the latter being a biologic property exhibited when any system of membranes is facing a solute to which the membranes are poorly permeable. Total osmotic pressure is a colligative property of all solutions based on the number of molecules dissolved. Colloid osmotic pressure is a biologic property regulated in human plasma by the concentration of albumin. Total osmotic pressure is approximately linear with sodium concentration in plasma water. Depressed osmolality of extracellular fluid (hypotonicity) has as its normal response a brisk free water clearance. Upward departure from the normal of 300 ± 10 mOsm/L is referred to as hypertonicity and is associated, in normal renal function, with a urine of increased osmolality and negative free water clearance.

The calculation of total body solute is a useful model for calculating water deficits or excesses, based on the assumption of osmotic equilibrium throughout body water. The total body solute is the product of total plasma tonicity (either calculated from electrolyte concentrations, or measured as osmolality) and total body water (Table 11-1). In most acute illness in previously healthy people, the crystalloid and "unaccounted" tonicity is trivial and need not be taken into the calculation. In certain other conditions, as will be made clear, these values may be quite high but will decrease rapidly with treatment; one must be cautious in calculating a water deficit based on total body solute including pathologic crystalloid or "unaccounted" tonicity. In such cases, the measured osmolality should not be used, but rather the sum of sodium and potassium concentrations multiplied by 2 (plus 10) to give total electrolyte solute (as in normal plasma). As a convenient close approximation, normal plasma solute is entered at 300 mOsm/L.

Sodium Homeostasis

By the law of electroneutrality, the sum of cations (e.g., sodium and potassium) is balanced by an equal charge of anions in the plasma, chiefly chloride and bicarbonate. The sum of electrolytes present determines the normal water-holding property of the body. For the extracellular fluid, the predominant and determining ion is sodium. It is, therefore, also water-volume determining. The sodium concentration is regulated by water clearance, aldosterone secretion, and a reciprocal relationship with the plasma potassium concentration. Abnormalities in function of the adrenal glands, the pituitary, the central nervous system, and the kidneys may rob the body of its normal ability to conserve water and/or sodium and maintain a normal sodium mass and concentration. In hypertension, heart disease, and chronic vascular disease, body sodium is chronically elevated as a result of a distortion in the balance of sodium homeostatic regulators.

Volume Regulation

By a variety of subtle mechanisms, the body perceives the total volume of certain fluid components. When blood volume is expanded, diuresis ensues; when the blood volume is low, there is conservation of fluid and salt and an increased rate of synthesis of albumin. The total volume of extracellular fluid is closely guarded by the body, involving sensing mechanisms in the heart, mediastinum, great vessels, renal juxtaglomerular apparatus, and macula densa. Overfilling of the "capacity-sensitive sensors" produces a water diuresis and a salt diuresis. Volume underfilling, often indicated by decreased chamber pressures (i.e., lowered central venous pressure, diastolic pressure of the two ventricles, and a low mean pulmonary artery pressure), is associated with water and salt conservation. The term *chamber pressures* will be used throughout this chapter to indicate either left atrial pressure, pulmonary wedge pressure, pulmonary artery diastolic pressure, right ventricular and diastolic pressure, or central venous pressure. The pressures are interrelated, especially in disorders of body fluid volume regulation.

When these volume-sensing mechanisms are disordered or chronically stressed, as in chronic congestive heart failure, the body metabolism of water and salt is markedly altered, and the normal responses are blunted or distorted and no longer reliable. The perception of this loss of normal feedback loop autoregulation is a vital element in rational treatment.

Acid-Base Regulation

Cellular processes always result in the accumulation of acid waste, while stress, trauma, and the endocrinology of injury paradoxically favor the development of mild alkalosis. Balance between renal excretion of inorganic acids and protons and the pulmonary excretion of carbon dioxide are responsible for normal acid-base regulation. When either of these mechanisms is disordered, acid-base regulation is lost, even though no external stress is introduced into the system.

Table 11-1. Useful Expressions and First Approximations

Terms	
BV	Blood volume
PV	Plasma volume
RV	Red cell volume
LVH	Large vessel hematocrit
BWt	Body weight
Δ BWt	Change in body weight
TBW	Total body water
TBCl	Total body chloride
Total solute	Plasma solute concentration × TBW
ECF	Extracellular fluid
IF	Interstitial fluid
IF/PV	Ratio of interstitial fluid to plasma volume
ECF/PV	Ratio of extracellular fluid to plasma volume
Notations	
Subscript 1	Starting or normal value for term shown (e.g., LVH_1)
Subscript 2	Value observed during disease before treatment (e.g., PV_2)
Subscript 3	Value observed later on or after treatment (e.g., PV_3)
Subscript def	Deficit of the term shown (e.g., PV_{def})
Subscript exc	Excess of the term shown (e.g., TBW_{exc})
(Delta) Δ	Change in the term shown (e.g., Δ PCO_2)
Subscript $[\,]_p$	Plasma concentration
Subscript $[\,]_u$	Urine concentration

BLOOD VOLUME BY HABITUS IN HEALTH

Habitus	*% BWt Males*	*% BWt Females*
Normal	7.0	6.5
Obese	6.0	5.5
Thin	6.5	6.0
Muscular	7.5	7.0

LVH AT SEA LEVEL	Males: 40% to 43% cells (0.40–0.43)	Females: 38% to 41% cells (0.38–0.41)

TOTAL BODY WATER BY HABITUS IN HEALTH

Habitus	*% BWt Males*	*% BWt Females*
Normal	55	48
Obese	48	40
Thin	50	44
Muscular	58	50

EXTRACELLULAR FLUID BY HABITUS IN HEALTH
(Males: 42% of TBW; Females: 43% of TBW)

Habitus	*% BWt Males*	*% BWt Females*
Normal	0.23	0.21
Obese	0.21	0.17
Thin	0.22	0.20
Muscular	0.24	0.22

EXTRACELLULAR FLUID RELATIONSHIPS

ECF = Sum of plasma volume (PV) + interstitial fluid (IF)

$ECF/PV = 6.0 \pm 0.5$

$IF/PV = 5.0 \pm 0.4$

$PV = BV - (LVH \times BV)$

Table 11-2. Equations for Compositional Relationships

Blood Volume	Example (Normal 65 kg Male)
BV = (% BWt) × BWt	BV = 0.7 × 6.5 = 4550 ml
LVH = 0.40 = BV/RV	LVH = 1820/4550 = 0.40
RV = BV × LVH	RV = 4550 × 0.4 = 1820 ml
PV = BV − (BV × LVH)	PV = 4550 − 1820 = 2730 ml
BV = RV + PV	BV = 1820 + 2730 = 4550 ml
Total Body Water	Example (Obese 60 kg Female)
TBW as % BWt = TBW/BWt × 100	23.9/60 × 100 = 39.8%
Total Body Chloride	Example (Muscular 80 kg Male)
TBCl = BWt × ECF/kg × $[Cl]_p$	80 × 0.24 × 103 = 1978 mEq
Plasma Tonicity	
Total plasma tonicity = electrolyte tonicity + crystalloid tonicity	
Electrolyte tonicity = $[Na]_p$ + $[K]_p$ × 2 = (143 + 2) × 2 = 294 mOsm/L	
Crystalloid tonicity = glucose + urea = approximately 6 mOsm/L	
Total plasma tonicity = 294 + 6 = 300 mOsm/L (the figure of 300 is "assumed normal")	
Crystalloid Tonicity	
Glucose (mg/dl) ÷ 18 = glucose (mOsm/L)	
Urea (mg/dl) ÷ 2 = urea N (mg/dl)	
Urea N (mg/dl) ÷ 30 = urea (mOsm/L)	
"Unaccounted" Tonicity	
"Unaccounted" tonicity = total tonicity − (electrolyte tonicity) − (glucose + urea tonicity)	
Total Body Solute	Example (75 kg normal male)
Total body solute = plasma tonicity × TBW	300 × (0.55 × 75) = 12,375 mOsm/L)

Disorders of body fluid and electrolyte may bear one of three relationships to the homeostatic regulators that would ordinarily compensate:

1. Feedback regulators *normal:* the body assists the therapist in restoration to normal.
2. Feedback regulators *abnormal:* the body fails to sense or to activate homeostatic responses.
3. Feedback regulators *at fault:* the disorder is caused, per se, by an abnormality in the regulatory mechanism.

In the description of each syndrome, identification of normal and abnormal homeostatic responses will be included.

Tables 11-1 through 11-4 list helpful terms that are used in some of the mathematical expressions and derivations for the syndromes as well as normal values and some conversion data for pH readings.

Fifteen Disorders of Body Water, Salts, and Protein: Fluid Volumes and Tonicity

Syndrome 1. Hypovolemia

See Table 11-5.

Definition, Terminology, and Related Terms

Hypovolemia is a blood volume that is lower than normal, without reference to hematocrit. Related or confusing terms include *oligemia* (synonymous), *hypotension* (refers to a low blood pressure without respect to cause), *shock* (a clinical picture), *low flow state* (generalized hypoprofusion without respect to cause), and *anemia* (usually used as meaning a low peripheral concentration of red blood cells).

The *hematocrit,* or fractional volume of cells

Table 11-3. Useful Expressions and First Approximations in Acid-Base Homeostasis

Conversion of pH to $[H^+]$ in nM/L

pH $[H^+]$	pH $[H^+]$	pH $[H^+]$	pH $[H^+]$
7.10 = 79	7.32 = 49	7.38 = 42	7.44 = 37
7.15 = 71	7.34 = 48	7.39 = 41	7.46 = 36
7.20 = 63	7.35 = 46	7.40 = 40	7.48 = 34
7.25 = 58	7.36 = 44	7.41 = 39	7.50 = 32
7.30 = 50	7.37 = 43	7.42 = 38	7.60 = 25

Bedside Acid-Base Equation to Check Lab Work

$$[H^+] = \frac{24 \times PCO_2}{HCO_3} = \frac{24 \times 40}{24} = 40 \text{ nM/L} = \text{pH } 7.40$$

Quickie Conversions to Check Lab Work

Pure resp. acidosis: $\Delta\, [H^+] = 0.8\ \Delta\, PCO_2$

Comp resp. acidosis: $\Delta\, [H^+] = 0.3\ \Delta\, PCO_2$

Acute resp. alkalosis: $\Delta\, [H^+] = 0.8\ \Delta\, PCO_2$

Metabolic acidosis (addition): $PCO_2 = 1.1\ \Delta\, [HCO_3^-]$ (PCO_2 in mm Hg, $[HCO_3^-]$ in mEq/L)

Anion Gap (Normal)

Anion gap = $[Na]_p - [Cl]_p = 143 - 103 = 40$ mEq/L

Anion gap + 1.6 = predicted $[HCO_3^-]$

40/1.6 = 25 mEq/L

"Unaccounted" Anion (Abnormal Metabolites)

"Unaccounted" anion = [anion gap/1.6] − $[HCO_3^-]$

Example: $[Na]_p = 145$ mEq/L; $[Cl]_p = 90$ mEq/L; $[HCO_3] = 15$ mEq/L

Then, 55/1.6 − 15 = 19 mEq/L "unaccounted" anion (Ketones? Lactate? Inorganic acids?)

in a blood sample centrifuged to constant meniscus, is a measure of the peripheral concentration of erythrocytes. It is used throughout this account, although the hemoglobin concentration and red cell count are linear functions, save in the presence of disordered red cell synthesis. The *large vessel hematocrit* is the hematocrit as measured on a sample of blood taken from a major vessel, usually a large vein of the arm. The *whole body hematocrit* is a conceptual term to mean the ratio of the entire red blood cell volume to the entire blood volume (i.e., sum of measured PV + RV). Because of axial streaming of red cells in small blood vessels and capillaries, the whole body hematocrit is somewhat lower (0.85X-0.92X) than the large vessel hematocrit. Relationships between the two indicated by the WBH/LVH ratio are interesting and important in some very severe disorders of blood volume (late shock, severe polycythemia), but they do not appear in everyday blood volume measurement and therapy.

Clinical Setting

1. Whole blood loss
2. Plasma loss
3. Desalting water loss
4. Desiccation, dehydration

The symptoms are weakness and faintness, particularly on assuming the erect posture. These mild symptoms progress to those of a severe low flow state, with hypotension, oliguria, and dangerous hypoperfusion of critical organs (brain, heart, and lungs) if the volume loss is severe and continuing.

Addition or Subtraction

Hypovolemia is always a subtraction disorder.

Body Composition and Body Weight

The normal blood volume is about 7% of body weight in males and 6.5% of body weight in females. The term *hypovolemia* refers to a blood

Table 11-4. Normal Values

Datum	Units	Normal	Comments
Body weight	kg change	—	Reliable weight important, very difficult to measure in critically ill
Hematocrit	% cells	Males 40–43 Females 38–41	Spun large vessel venous hematocrit; centrifuge to constant meniscus
Plasma			
Protein	g/dl	6.0–6.5	Marked method variance between hospitals; plasma slightly higher than serum
Tonicity	mOsm/L	290–300	Freezing point methods yield osmolality, not osmolarity
Nonelectrolyte tonicity	mOsm/L	5–10	See Table 11-2
Sodium	mEq/L	141–144	May be measured on either plasma or serum
Chloride	mEq/L	101–104	May be measured on either plasma or serum
Potassium	mEq/L	4.2–4.6	May be measured on either plasma or serum
Whole Blood			
Std. bicarbonate [HCO_3^-]	mEq/L	24–27	CO_2 content of whole blood corrected to standard conditions
Urea N	mg/dl	10–18	—
Blood pH_{art}	units	7.41–7.42	Must be measured on fresh chilled arterial blood
pH_{ven}	units	7.35–7.38	Varies somewhat with sampling site
$PCO_{2\ art}$	mm Hg	40	Not dependent on sampling site
$PCO_{2\ ven}$	mm Hg	43	Depends on sampling site
$PaO_{2\ art}$	mm Hg	70–90	Depends on inhaled gas mixture and shunting
$PVO_{2\ ven}$	mm Hg	30–50	Depends on sampling site
Urine			
Tonicity	mOsm/L	200–1400 300–400	Normal widest range of tonicity in man Characteristic tonicity in renal failure (i.e., isotonic with plasma)
Sodium	mEq/L	0.1–75	The low value shows good tubular function
Potassium	mEq/L	10–100	High potassium values accompany aldosterone effects and metabolic alkalosis (require good tubular function)
pH	units	4.5–6.5	Urine acidification below pH 5.5 not seen in renal failure
Volume	ml/hr	25–100	Three consecutive hours below 15 or over 150 requires explanation

Table 11-5. Hypovolemia (Syndrome 1)

		Major Findings	
	Unit	Typical	Extreme
Hematocrit	% cells	40 → 30	40 → 15
Plasma protein	g/dl	6.5 → 6.0	6.5 → 5.0
Blood urea nitrogen	mg/dl	Normal	15 → 30
Blood volume	% BWt	7.0 → 6.0	7.0 → 4.0
Central venous pressure	cm H_2O	12 → 5	12 → 0

volume approximately 1% of body weight lower than normal, approximately 10% to 15% reduced. In the chronic form, plasma volume gradually rises, owing to transcapillary refill, resulting in a "stabilized posthemorrhagic anemia" with a red cell volume lower than normal, plasma volume restored to values higher than normal, normal blood volume, and low hematocrit.

Abnormalities of Autoregulation

The normal homeostatic regulation of blood volume in hypovolemia is by the inflow of interstitial fluid at the distal end of the capillary, occasioned by lowered venous pressure at the venular end of the capillary. Simple hydrostatic filling, resulting in an increase in the plasma volume, is the normal transcapillary refill of the blood volume. This results in the restoration of the blood volume to normal or near normal by the influx of a plasma-like fluid (interstitial fluid and lymph) with a low protein concentration. At the close of this period of refill there is a low red cell mass, a plasma volume much higher than normal, a blood volume close to or near normal (with the exceptions indicated), and a slightly low protein concentration. There is a low hematocrit.

An additional homeostatic regulator in hypovolemia is the secretion of antidiuretic hormone (stimulated by a volume receptor mechanism) and of aldosterone (stimulated by the juxtaglomerulus-renin-angiotensin-adrenal cortex effector arc). The firing off of these two homeostatic regulators after simple hemorrhage is a classic example of isotonic volume reduction as a stimulator of endocrine change. The result of this combination of hormone effectors is to save water and salt for the body so that the transcapillary refill may arise from an interstitial fluid of normal volume and tonicity. The principal abnormalities of this regulator, whose normal function is to conserve interstitial volume for transcapillary refill, occur in (1) *renal* disease, in which the renal response is abnormal or absent, (2) *adrenal cortical* disease, in which the aldosterone mechanism fails, (3) *central nervous system* disease, in which antidiuretic hormone production is abnormal, and (4) *low flow state,* wherein the loss has been more massive than these regulators can compensate and circulatory anoxia becomes a governing deterioration.

Treatment

The ideal infusion fluid for hypovolemia is fully compatible normal fresh human blood. However, if blood transfusion is to be less than 1000 ml, one should exercise restraint in the use of blood bank blood with its attendant problems. Virus-free plasma or one of its derivatives, or isotonic salt solutions, free of both protein and cells, can be used. If a protein-free, cell-free electrolyte solution is used, approximately 3 times the volume of lost blood must be administered to allow for equilibration throughout the extracellular volume.

Guides to Progress

Restoration of urine volume to normal is the most reliable sign of restoration of blood volume and tissue perfusion to normal. If hypotension has resulted from acute hypovolemia, the restoration of normal systolic blood pressure is an important sign, often confused by the administration of drugs. There are other, more subtle signs of volume restoration, such as the cessation of the transcapillary refill. If blood volume is restored by the use of cell-free solutions, the fall in the hematocrit is even more pronounced; this anemia is due to an expanded plasma volume and persists until red cell resynthesis restores the red cell volume to normal. The primary cellular signs of hypovolemia are to be seen in the kidney; if low flow is severe, all body cells suffer, ultimately including the brain. Almost any index of cellular function demonstrates improvement when severe hypovolemia is returned toward normal. In elderly people or those with cerebrovascular diseases, abnormalities of mental function and of the electrocardiogram indicate cerebral and myocardial responses to the hypoperfusion, and later to the restoration of normal blood volume and tissue perfusion.

One of the chamber pressures, such as central venous pressure, right atrial pressure, pulmonary artery pressure, or pulmonary artery wedge pressure, may profitably be measured in monitoring a patient who has suffered hypovolemia or hypervolemia from any cause. These pressures all tend to be lower than normal in hypovolemia; because the pressures are normally quite low, the initial reading is not as significant as the increase toward normal on restoration of volume to normal.

There is a further important precaution about blood transfusion in late hypovolemia when transcapillary refill has been complete. If at that point the volume of lost blood is transfused, acute hypervolemia will be produced. In the elderly patient or those with congestive heart failure, this can be dangerous. Such an error results from a misreading of the low hematocrit in a stabilized posthemorrhagic patient: The low hematocrit indicates a high plasma volume, not a low blood volume.

Relevant Mathematical Expression

Mathematical expressions serve only as a guide to the appropriate general magnitude of treatment.

In hypovolemia, the red cell volume deficit after stabilization of transcapillary refill in a chronic bleed is given by:

$$RV_{def} = RV_1 - RV_2$$

BV_1 and RV_1 from Table 11-1

$$RV_2 = LVH_2 \times 0.9\ BV_1$$

This assumes refill to 90% of normal BV. For complete refill (bleed has stopped; hematocrit stable):

$$RV_2 = LVH_2 \times BV_1$$

Example: Obese woman, 50 kg, menorrhagia, continuing; hematocrit 18

$$RV_2 = 0.18 \times 0.9\ (0.055 \times 50) = 445\ \text{ml}$$

$$RV_1 = (0.4 \times 0.055 \times 50) = 1100\ \text{ml}$$

$$RV_{def} = 1100 - 445 = 655\ \text{ml red cells}$$

$$RV_{def} = \text{about 3 units of cells}$$

This will restore deficit of oxygen transport capacity but makes no allowance for further bleeding.

Syndrome 2. Plasma Loss Hypovolemia

See Table 11-6.

Definition, Terminology, and Related Terms

Plasma loss hypovolemia refers to a lowering of the blood volume, owing to the loss of plasma or a plasma-like transudate. In this condition the plasma loss so predominates that the loss of red cells is trivial or negligible. A rising hematocrit is therefore inevitable. Plasma loss hypovolemia may progress to hypotension in a severe low-flow state, resulting in death. The elevated hematocrit produces an increase in blood viscosity, which further slows tissue perfusion. Related terms include *third space effect,* a term coined to signify the accumulation of plasma-like fluid in an area of traumatic edema, peritonitis, or in venous thrombosis.

Clinical Setting

1. Thermal burn
2. Acute peritonitis
3. Acute pancreatitis
4. Retroperitoneal edema
5. Mesenteric venous thrombosis
6. Portal thrombosis
7. Peripheral venous obstruction
8. Large surgical dissections

Addition or Subtraction

This is always a subtraction disorder, as fluid is moved out of the plasma volume into a peripheral injured or edematous area; nonetheless, if treatment is instituted to restore the plasma volume to normal, the body gains weight. The increment of total body water and salt produced by treatment renders the net effect that of an addition disorder superimposed on an initial loss of plasma volume.

Body Composition and Body Weight

The normal plasma volume is approximately 4% of body weight in men and 3.6% of body weight in women. Loss of approximately one liter of plasma produces the typical rapidly rising concentration of erythrocytes as measured by hematocrit, red cell count, or hemoglobin concentration. Lesser amounts of plasma loss produce the same change, but it is less readily evident. If the plasma is lost within the body, weight is unchanged thereby. Because therapy consists of infusion of plasma and other fluids into the bloodstream to maintain an effective plasma volume, the situation in treated plasma-losing hypovolemia is one of a rapid gain in weight.

Abnormalities of Autoregulation

The body has no endogenous corrective mechanism for a severe generalized plasma-losing state because the transcapillary refill of the plasma that would ordinarily compensate for hypovolemia is, by the very nature of the pathologic state, impaired or reversed. If the plasma loss occurs in one focal area (a small burn would be an example), transcapillary refill may occur from other undamaged areas of the capillary bed. This is the "parasite" effect of a burn.

The homeostatic regulators readily observed are those of the renal response to hypovolemia: antidiuresis and sodium conservation, with a low urine volume and very low sodium concentration. Some of the lowest urine sodium concentrations—as low as 0.1 mEq/L—are observed in plasma-losing states. The principal abnormality of this renal sodium and water conservation is seen in the diuretic phase of acute nephrosis or in renal or adrenal disease, in which a normal water-sodium conserving renal response cannot occur.

Table 11-6. Plasma Loss Hypovolemia (Syndrome 2)

		Major Findings	
	Unit	Typical	Extreme
Hematocrit	% cells	50 → 55	60 → 70
Plasma protein	g/dl	6.5 → 6.0	6.5 → 5.0
Blood urea nitrogen	mg/dl	Normal	15 → 30
Blood volume	% BWt	7.0 → 6.0	7.0 → 4.0
Central venous pressure	cm H_2O	12 → 5	12 → 0

Laboratory Findings

A rising concentration of red cells in the plasma, usually measured as a rising hematocrit, is the most characteristic finding in plasma-losing states. The magnitude of elevation of the hematocrit is a linear function of the volume of plasma lost. It is therefore possible to formulate a simple mathematical expression to indicate the static deficit, that is, the amount of plasma that must be infused over a short time to restore blood volume to normal. To this amount of rapid infusion must be added the amounts needed to compensate for concomitant losses. Urinary findings have been mentioned previously.

Chamber pressures are reduced, as in any other form of hypovolemia; their rise toward normal is a significant monitor of treatment. Their rise above normal is a sign of overtreatment.

Treatment

Infusion of plasma, various plasma fractions, albumin, and dextran are all effective. In plasma loss the infusion of ionic solutions without protein (for example, saline or Ringer's lactate) lowers the hematocrit and refills the plasma volume if rather large amounts are used (approximately three times the amount of lost plasma). In such a case there is considerable dilution of plasma protein. A few days later, after diuresis of this water and salt, the plasma protein concentration usually returns to normal.

Guides to Progress

As is evident from the foregoing discussion, acute changes in the concentration of red cells (usually measured by hematocrit) are the most sensitive and direct guides to progress, with appropriate changes in renal function and in tissue perfusion. In most acute plasma-losing states—such as burns, pancreatitis, and peritonitis—the pathologic condition itself is limited by treatment or becomes self-limited; the only alternative is death if the loss continues unabated. Severe loss of body water of any variety can produce plasma loss secondarily, for example, those described under *Syndrome 6, Desalting Water Loss.*

Relevant Mathematical Expression

In plasma loss hypovolemia, the plasma volume deficit is given by:

$$PV_{def} = BV_1 - BV_2 \text{ (assuming RV constant)}$$

PV_1, RV_1, and BV_1 from Table 11-1

$$BV_2 = \frac{RV_1}{LVH_2}$$

Example: Muscular man, 80 kg, burn, hematocrit 65

$$BV_1 = 0.075 \times 80 = 6000 \text{ ml}$$

$$RV_1 = 0.43 \times 6000 = 2580 \text{ ml}$$

$$BV_2 = \frac{2580}{0.65} = 3970 \text{ ml}$$

$$\text{Then: } PV_{def} = 6000 - 3970 \text{ ml} = 2030 \text{ ml}$$

If plasma alone is used (or similar substitute), about 2000 ml or 8 units will bring the hematocrit down to 40 to 45. If balanced salt is used, about 8000 ml will be needed for the PV requirement alone; neither ration is in any sense a complete burn budget for skin, respiratory, and urinary losses. Continuing losses must be compensated.

Syndrome 3. Hypoproteinemia

Definition, Terminology, and Related Terms

Hypoproteinemia is a low concentration of proteins in the plasma, without reference to the volume of blood plasma, interstitial fluid, or total body water; it connotes a low colloid osmotic pressure. *Hypoalbuminemia* is essentially synonymous, as is *lowered plasma oncotic* (or *colloid osmotic*) *pressure. Dilutional hypoproteinemia* refers to one of the common causes of hypoproteinemia.

Clinical Setting

1. Overadministration of water and salt
2. Loss of whole protein from the body
3. Liver cell disease with failure of protein synthesis
4. Late starvation especially with overadministration of salt and/or water

Addition or Subtraction

Hypoproteinemia is due to addition of water and salt, masquerading as a subtraction syndrome (lack of albumin) in most cases. Only in advanced liver disease is the net albumin synthesis deficit the primary difficulty. In other instances some plasma or albumin loss has been overbalanced by water and salt administration and/or retention.

Body Composition and Body Weight

Because of the exogenous dilutional component in most cases of hypoproteinemia, body weight gain is a regular feature. As colloid osmotic pressure falls, edema readily forms in subcutaneous tissues and as ascites and hydrothorax. Body weight gain is therefore sometimes its most prominent feature. Diuretic treatment often results in a subsequent weight loss, with restoration of serum protein to normal.

Approximately one-half of the albumin in the

body is outside the plasma volume, circulating in the much larger interstitial fluid volume (including lymph) but at a low concentration. Certain stimuli produce an increased flow of albumin up the thoracic duct from the liver to the great veins of the mediastinum, a sort of internal plasma infusion. One of the stimuli to this albumin influx is hemorrhage.

Abnormalities of Autoregulation

As mentioned, normal urinary excretion of water and salt and normal hepatic synthesis of albumin are the normal homeostatic regulators. Anything interfering with either tends to produce hypoproteinemia.

Serum albumin concentration is measured by a great many different methods, and one must know the hospital norms to ascertain the degree of abnormality. If the laboratory norm is a serum albumin concentration of 5 g/dl, values below 3.5 constitute significant hypoalbuminemia or hypoproteinemia. In the hypoalbuminemia of liver disease, there is characteristically an excess of globulins, both relative and absolute, with a reversal of the normal albumin-globulin ratio.

Treatment

Because the syndrome is often dilutional in part, the use of diuretics that increase the excretion of water and salt is sometimes effective. The administration either of concentrated human albumin or of plasma is rational. Concentrated salt-poor albumin should be reserved for patients in whom additional salt loads will embarrass cardiac function.

Guides to Progress

Rise of serum protein and albumin concentrations to normal are cardinal signs, with diuresis and weight loss where dilution has been prominent.

Syndrome 4. Hypervolemia

See Table 11-7.

Definition, Terminology, and Related Terms

Hypervolemia is a blood volume larger than normal, without reference to the hematocrit. The term *plethora* has been used to indicate a high blood volume, but it connotes any elevated concentration of red cells. *Polycythemia* denotes a hematocrit that is higher than normal. Polycythemia and plethora often coexist with hypervolemia. Terms such as *congestive heart failure* should not be used interchangeably with *hypervolemia,* even though the two may coexist and chamber pressure elevation may develop in both.

Clinical Setting

1. Overinfusion of blood or other parenteral fluids
2. Chronic visceral failure (heart, kidneys, or lungs)

Addition or Subtraction

Hypervolemia is always an addition disorder; the source may be endogenous (as in visceral failure with ordinary oral intake) or exogenous, arising from infusions.

Body Composition and Body Weight

The term *hypervolemia* denotes a blood volume that is more than 15% elevated. That is, it is elevated by approximately 1.0% of body weight, or more. Body weight is usually elevated by an appropriate amount; if chronic visceral failure (heart, liver, lungs, kidneys) plays a role, the extent of weight elevation may be quite remarkable as all body water is expanded.

Abnormalities of Autoregulation

If produced acutely by overtransfusion of blood, hypervolemia results in a prompt plasma dispersal and disposal. This is the exact physiologic reverse of the transcapillary refill observed in hypovolemia. Plasma dispersal and disposal is effected by the selective loss of plasma by ultrafiltration from the capillary, the degradation of excess protein through its normal half-life, with the excretion of the extra water and salt. The result is a slowly rising plasma protein that then returns to normal, a rising hematocrit that remains high, appropriate to the half-life of the healthy red cells infused as they live out their span. The abnormalities of these homeostatic regulators clearly reside in disease of those viscera concerned with plasma

Table 11-7. Hypervolemia (Overtransfusion) (Syndrome 4)

		Major Findings	
	Unit	Typical	Extreme
Hematocrit	% cells	40 → 50	40 → 65
Plasma protein	g/dl	6.5 → 6.8	6.5 → 7.5
Blood volume	% BWt	7.0 → 8.0	7.0 → 10.0

dispersal and disposal: the heart, the liver, and the kidneys. All are essential for the metabolism of excessive blood volume; when they are abnormal, plasma dispersal and disposal are impaired. When there is acute or chronic pulmonary disease or direct injury to the lungs, modest degrees of hypervolemia are much more likely to produce pulmonary edema.

In its acute phase the major *laboratory finding* is elevation of cardiac chamber pressures. Then, as plasma dispersal and disposal proceed, there is a rising concentration of red cells and protein. Of greatest significance are the laboratory findings relative to visceral function. If liver failure is present, hypervolemia is ill-tolerated. In the presence of oliguric renal failure, the renal mechanism for disposal is cut off and hypervolemia is dangerous. In heart failure, even modest degrees of exogenous hypervolemia added to the endogenous overexpansion of body water and salt rapidly produce pulmonary edema. If pulmonary function is embarrassed (particularly likely in primary pulmonary disease, or in injuries such as burns or crush, or chronic congestive heart failure), failing oxygenation and/or carbon dioxide accumulation are laboratory evidence of an uncorrected hypervolemia. Measurements of function of heart, lungs, liver, and kidneys are therefore essential in the management of hypervolemia.

Treatment

When hypervolemia results from overenthusiastic infusion of blood or other fluids, a most important step is often somewhat difficult: stop those infusions! Phlebotomy or direct bleeding is an effective emergency measure. The application of limb tourniquets is, at best, a weak substitute for phlebotomy. When renal failure also exists, hypervolemia (associated with a high volume of intracellular fluid and body water) can be managed, though with difficulty, by pressure filtration dialysis.

Guides to Progress

In most instances of hypervolemia, a reduction of chamber pressures to normal is the primary indicator of a response to treatment. Renal functional changes are an inconstant guide to progress. The chest x-ray film may be valuable if pulmonary edema has been a feature. Phlebotomy and diuretics have very different effects on volume, because diuretics act on all components of body water, particularly the extracellular phase, whereas bleeding operates initially on blood volume alone and, in the presence of chronic disease of liver, kidney, or heart, may be followed by transcapillary refill that is "inappropriate," as if the body intended to maintain a high volume. In some cases the body has become so "accustomed" to a high blood volume that some degree of hypotension and hypoperfusion may be observed if volume is restored to normal. For this reason, phlebotomy and/or diuretics must always be accompanied by careful measure of perfusion of organs, particularly brain and kidneys. Most cases of overtransfusion result from the sudden infusion of large amounts of blood bank blood to meet an unexpected emergency; in banked blood, the red blood cells are frequently approaching their expiration date, and hemolysis may be very prominent. In such a case, the hemolytic component adds greatly to the elevation of bilirubin that so frequently appears in low flow states.

Syndrome 5. Polycythemia

See Table 11-8.

Definition, Terminology, and Related Terms

The term *polycythemia* should be reserved for those states in which there is elevation in hematocrit, regardless of the blood volume; just as *anemia* signifies a low hematocrit without reference to volume. The term *hypervolemia* is not strictly synony-

Table 11-8. Polycythemia (Secondary) (Syndrome 5)

		Major Findings	
	Unit	Typical	Extreme
Hematocrit	% cells	55	80
Plasma protein	g/dl	6.5	7.0
Uric acid	mg/dl	8.5	10.0
Blood volume	% BWt	7.5	12.0
Plasma volume	% BWt	2.0	1.0
Red cell volume	% BWt	5.5	11.0
Arterial oxygen saturation	% sat.	90	75
Reticulocytes	%	5.0	15.0
Central venous pressure	cm H_2O	5–10	20–30

mous because the hematocrit may not be elevated, at least in the early stages. The term *polycythemia vera* denotes an excessive volume of red cells associated with primary disease of the bone marrow. *Secondary polycythemia* denotes the compensatory elevation of red cell mass that occurs in response to a deficit of oxygen transport capacity. Oxygen transport capacity (OTC) is a product of cardiac output times effective oxygen-carrying capacity, including total hemoglobin, the state of the hemoglobin, and location of the oxyhemoglobin association curve. Barring unusual variations in hemoglobin chemistry, it is a simple product of cardiac output times whole blood oxygen-carrying capacity. A term little used in the cardiac or cardiovascular literature, it is of great importance in the management of acutely ill or injured patients.

Clinical Setting

The idiopathic form of polycythemia vera will not be discussed further. With a hematocrit over 55, there is a severe viscosity increase, threatening thrombosis of the mesenteric circulation, the brain, or the limbs.

Secondary polycythemia occurs most commonly in response to congenital heart disease and chronic obstructive pulmonary disease. The former, by left-to-right shunting, deprives the periphery of oxygenated red cells. The latter interferes with oxygenation by loss of ventilation. In both cases there is a reduction in OTC modified, in turn, by the ability of the hemoglobin present to unload oxygen in the tissues. The symptoms of polycythemia are initially those of the underlying disease; the polycythemic component is responsible for the cyanotic appearance, increased blood viscosity, and susceptibility to thrombosis.

Addition or Subtraction

This is an addition disorder due to overproduction of erythrocytes by the marrow, in response to a deficit in OTC.

Body Composition and Body Weight

In mild polycythemia due to chronic obstructive lung disease, the blood volume is normal. In the more severe forms of the disorder, due either to heart or lung disease, the blood volume is elevated. In congenital heart disease (such as tetralogy of Fallot), the blood volume may be as high as 12% of body weight, with a hematocrit of 75% to 80%. Uric acid concentrations in plasma tend to be elevated in the presence of any son of polycythemia, probably a manifestation of an increased turnover rate of red cells. In hyperparathyroidism there is a low plasma phosphate concentration; for this reason, there is a very low value for red cell diphosphoglycerate (2,3-DPG). This produces a left shift of the oxyhemoglobin association curve with a resultant slight but chronic anoxia of perishable tissues, including bone marrow. This, in turn, leads to reticulocytosis and a high red cell production rate. The combination of hyperparathyroidism, polycythemia, and hyperuricemia is, therefore, a rare but interesting syndrome, demonstrating some of these interrelationships.

Abnormalities of Autoregulation

As volume rises with polycythemia, plasma disposal and dispersal are hastened. The plasma volume is therefore low. In extreme cases, with hematocrits as high as 75% and blood volume as high as 10% to 12% of body weight (in congenital heart disease), the plasma volume is diminished to become a small component of the total blood volume. This dispersal of plasma is merely a chronic homeostatic response to the excessive volume of red cells. This increases viscosity and further reduces tissue perfusion. Under ordinary circumstances, an excess of total OTC (red cell concentration multiplied by cardiac output) results in bone marrow inhibition. This is frequently observed following surgical repair of congenital heart disease. There will be a gradual downward restitution of red cell volume to normal by inhibition of marrow erythropoiesis, as cardiac output is restored. In polycythemia secondary to chronic obstructive lung disease, the chronic desaturation constitutes a continuous stimulus to the marrow, and most treatment (other than the fringe benefits from decreased smoking, for example) is unavailing. In cases of chronically depressed inorganic phosphate concentration in the plasma (in hyperparathyroidism and in certain types of hyperalimentation), a left-shifted oxyhemoglobin dissociation curve may be severe enough to constitute a stimulus to increased erythropoiesis, with resultant polycythemia.

Treatment

It may be advisable to carry out preoperative phlebotomy (with or without replacement of the shed blood with plasma) to carry the patient through operation with a lower hematocrit. In such instances, high oxygen concentration in the airway should be used to compensate for the sudden apparent deficit in OTC. If the basic cause of secondary polycythemia remains uncorrected, the polycythemia with its attendant problems of hypervolemia, blood viscosity, hypercoagulability, chronic desaturation, and cyanosis will remain.

Guides to Progress

These are primarily based on hematocrit and viscosity; in some cases of polycythemia vera the platelets are also elevated, contributing further to the hypercoagulable state.

Syndrome 6. Desalting Water Loss

See Table 11-9.

Definition, Terminology, and Related Terms

Desalting water loss is the loss of water and salt from the body at concentrations close to isotonic, regardless of the final concentration of sodium or other salts in the plasma. The term *extracellular fluid deficit* refers to the result. *Third space effect* refers to one of the causes. *Dehydration* is carelessly used to include this syndrome, failing to differentiate it from desiccation-dehydration (see below). *Hyponatremia* and *hypotonicity* refer to a frequent late result of desalting water loss.

Clinical Setting

1. *Extrarenal causes:* loss from the gastrointestinal tract as in fistula, obstruction, vomiting, short-bowel syndrome, typhoid fever, colitis
2. *Renal desalting:* unregulated diuresis in the diuretic phase of recovering acute tubular necrosis; profound osmotic diuresis in diabetes mellitus

Addition or Subtraction

In all instances this is a subtraction disorder.

Body Composition and Body Weight

The normal extracellular fluid volume is approximately 20% of body weight or 12 to 14 liters in 60- to 70-kg adults. Approximately 1 liter of volume, or 8% of the normal extracellular fluid volume, may be considered as tolerable variation in either direction. Losses of more than this produce the symptomatology referred to here. Extracellular fluid deficit is usually partitioned throughout the extracellular fluid and ultimately throughout total body water; the initial reduction is in the entire extracellular fluid; plasma and interstitial fluid are in hydrostatic and ionic equilibrium. Losses of extracellular fluid are therefore represented as plasma volume reduction to the extent of approximately 25% to 30% of the total. The normal ratio of plasma volume to interstitial fluid (PV/IF) is 0.25, and of plasma volume to total extracellular fluid 0.20.

Abnormalities of Autoregulation

Desalting water losses initially produce an isotonic volume reduction, the characteristic renal responses being decreased urine volume with increased urine osmolality and decreased sodium concentration. The principal abnormality of this homeostatic regulator is renal—a failure to implement the feedback loop. In adrenal disease (or in diseases of the central nervous system involving the area above the pituitary), there may be an accentuation of borderline renal insufficiency or diabetes insipidus, impeding the homeostatic regulation. With impaired homeostatic regulation, the task of replacement becomes much more formidable, and much larger volumes are required.

In response to lower tissue pressure (and aldosterone secretion), sodium-free water enters (and is retained in) the bloodstream, largely from cells; this is a weak compensation toward volume restoration and occurs at the expense of sodium concentration, which falls. There is an increased excretion of potassium.

Initially with desalting water loss, the principal *laboratory findings* are in the urinary responses already described. In some instances, abnormalities of renal response are noteworthy (with unregulated diuresis or adrenal impairment): anomalous natriuresis indicates this failure of normal homeostasis.

Approximately one-quarter to one-third of the volume lost (depending on rate) may be considered as coming from the plasma. There is, therefore, a gradual rise in hematocrit, somewhat slower than

Table 11-9. Desalting Water Loss (Syndrome 6)

		Major Findings	
	Unit	Typical	Extreme
Body weight	kg	Fall 1–5	Fall 4–7
Hematocrit	% cells	40 → 45	48 → 55
Plasma protein	g/dl	6.5 → 6.8	6.5 → 8.0
Plasma tonicity	mOsm/L	295 → 270	295 → 250
Plasma sodium	mEq/L	143 → 115	143 → 115
Plasma chloride	mEq/L	103 → 95	103 → 80
Plasma potassium	mEq/L	4.2 → 4.5	4.2 → 6.5
Std. bicarbonate	mEq/L	24 → 20	24 → 15
Blood pH	—	7.42 → 7.30	7.42 → 7.22

that seen in loss of plasma alone. Associated changes in blood viscosity are seen when the hematocrit rises above 50 or 55.

Any addition of sodium-free water adds further to the hyponatremia observed in desalting water loss. The ingress of sodium-free water into the extracellular fluid, diluting the sodium concentration, occurs by three principal routes: mobilization of cell water, oxidation of fat, and the administration of salt-free water by vein. The fall in sodium concentration with desalting water loss is thus primarily dilutional, resulting from the addition of sodium-free water to the system. Only in rare circumstances, such as pancreatic fistulas, is sodium lost from the body in hypertonic concentrations, leading immediately to hyponatremia.

The circulatory effects of decreased effective extracellular fluid volume are hypovolemia, low cardiac output, oliguria, and a low flow state. These are accentuated by hyponatremia. The low sodium concentration in plasma contributes to decreased cardiovascular responsiveness; if the loss from the gastrointestinal tract is primarily alkaline, severe acidosis results (see below). This combination is particularly unfriendly to normal cardiac function, rendering the heart insensitive to digitalis alkaloids, and, in elderly patients, it may prove fatal.

Treatment

The treatment consists of replacement by intravenous infusion of saline liquids. If the disease is long-standing, some protein should be added. If hematocrit is markedly elevated, the early replacement components should be largely plasma (whole plasma or a plasma protein preparation) to rectify the circulatory disorder first. In young people with normal renal function, the use of isotonic sodium chloride solutions is acceptable at the start. Potassium solutions (10 mEq/L) should be added as repletion proceeds. In elderly people, excess sodium chloride results in hyperchloremia, and it is wiser to infuse some sort of a balanced salt solution, such as Ringer's lactate. If sodium concentration is low, a portion of the replacement fluid may consist of hypertonic salt solutions.

Guides to Progress

These consist of restoration of urine output and plasma electrolyte concentrations to normal, reduction of hematocrit, and restoration of normal tissue perfusion.

Relevant Mathematical Expression

In desalting water loss, if the patient has previously been in good health with normal renal function and is now oliguric because of extrarenal loss (diarrhea, intestinal fistula, vomiting), assume that 30% to 40% of ECF volume has been lost. Obtain normal ECF volume from Table 11-1; give 30% to 40% of this volume as a balanced salt solution (i.e., containing both sodium and potassium and chloride together with an organic anion such as bicarbonate or lactate) quite briskly (i.e., in 3 to 5 hours). This *starter* infusion is critical because it will be a guide to further treatment. Response to this initial infusion is more useful than any sort of complex mathematical expression. In this situation plasma electrolyte concentrations are too variable to be a guide.

If blood pressure is low, losses have been more massive (typhoid, salmonella, cholera) and one must assume 50% to 60% of ECF volume has been lost, proceeding as above.

In either case when loss is continuing (as is usually the case due to the continuance of disease), such losses must be measured and appropriate maintenance volumes added to the above.

While abnormalities of blood chemistry are a helpful index they are extremely variable depending on the disease, the presence or absence of blood loss, of severe insensible water loss via lungs (as in hyperventilation and fever), and any treatment previously administered either intravenously or by mouth.

General Rules in Desalting Water Loss

1. If the hematocrit is elevated, it provides an index for the degree of plasma volume deficit. Calculation of this plasma deficit is carried out exactly as in an acute burn (Syndrome 2), and this plasma (or a plasma substitute) should be given very briskly in 3 to 5 hours as initial replacement to restore blood pressure and cardiac output. Then, at least three times this plasma volume loss should be given in the next 3 hours to replace the interstitial fluid losses. Following this, the balanced salt solution may be given more slowly depending on response, with the object of restoring intracellular dehydration.

2. If the plasma sodium concentration is reduced, it suggests dilution of body electrolyte due to prior water intake (by mouth or vein). Hyponatremia may also be observed in certain types of gastrointestinal disease, especially those involving loss of hypertonic body fluids. While rare, this is observed in pancreatic fistula and some cases of cholera. It is here that concentrated salt solutions (3% sodium chloride or equivalent) are most useful and can be life-saving, especially if started in modest quantities (300 to 500 ml in about 45 minutes), taking care to observe the changes in sodium concentration, urine volume, clinical appearance, and always observing the patient closely for pulmonary or cerebral edema.

3. Elevated plasma potassium concentration in desalting water loss is universally due to oliguria. Potassium solution should never be administered intravenously in the face of elevated potassium concentrations in the plasma, no matter how much potassium may be calculated as previously lost. Recall that plasma potassium concentrations and total body stores often move in opposite directions. If there is no renal response (diuresis) with initial saline or plasma therapy as described above and plasma potassium remains elevated, dialysis must be considered as an emergency and the electrocardiogram monitored closely.

4. In all instances of desalting water loss the response to initial treatment dictates subsequent management. If volume restoration proves the key (as it usually does) and diuresis results, very large volumes of saline fluids may be required (up to 8 to 12 liters) over the course of the first two or three days, especially with continuing disease. Once the pattern of loss and replacement is established, the most common error is undertreatment.

Syndrome 7. Oversalting: Extracellular Fluid Excess

See Table 11-10.

Definition, Terminology, and Related Terms

Oversalting with extracellular fluid excess is isotonic expansion of the extracellular fluid volume, regardless of the sodium concentration. *Fluid overload* is a common term more or less synonymous, but less specific. *Hypertonicity* is one occasional result of oversalting. *Congestive heart failure* is one visceral cause of extracellular fluid excess.

Clinical Setting

1. Overadministration of saline fluids
2. Visceral disease of heart, kidneys, or liver

Addition or Subtraction

Oversalting with extracellular fluid excess is an addition disorder; as in the case of hypervolemia, however, the superimposition of visceral failure adds an important endogenous component. When visceral disease is present and severe, extracellular fluid excess can occur spontaneously on the basis of ordinary oral intake with no apparent fluid overload.

Body Composition and Body Weight

Elevated extracellular fluid volumes, approximating 30% of body weight or more, are seen in this disorder. Total body water is elevated, but cell water expansion is rarely, if ever, proportional to the extracellular expansion, particularly in chronic congestive heart failure. In mitral stenosis, for example, extreme cellular wasting accompanies the extracellular excess. Very characteristic disjunctions are therefore seen, with extreme constriction of the total body potassium as a manifestation of the diminished cell mass, on the one hand, together with overexpansion of total body sodium as a manifestation of extracellular fluid excess, on the other. The ratio of total exchangeable sodium to potassium therefore becomes a very meaningful index. In the normal male the Na_e/K_e ratio is slightly below 1.0, and, in the female, slightly more than 1. In disorders of this category, Na_e/K_e ratio is markedly elevated and may be as high as 2.5. The curious reciprocal relationships that exist with these two cations are nowhere better epitomized than in congestive heart failure with a very high Na_e/K_e ratio, while the plasma concentration of sodium is characteristically low and of potassium characteristically high. Concentration and body content are inversely distorted, and to a marked degree.

Abnormalities of Autoregulation

When extracellular fluid expansion is due simply to overtreatment with such solutions as Ringer's

Table 11-10. Oversalting: Extracellular Fluid Excess (Syndrome 7)

		Major Findings	
	Unit	Typical	Extreme
Body weight	kg	Gain 3–4	Gain 5–10
Hematocrit	% cells	32–36	28–32
Plasma protein	g/dl	5.5–6.0	4.5–5.0
Plasma sodium	mEq/L	140–150	140–155
Plasma chloride	mEq/L	103–110	103–115
Plasma potassium	mEq/L	4.5–4.0	4.5–3.5
Std. bicarbonate	mEq/L	24–26	24–26
Central venous pressure	cm H_2O	5–20	29–60

lactate (for example, in treating hemorrhage with huge amounts of isotonic salt solution), a homeostatic regulation in the form of greatly increased urinary output is present and normal. There is a sharp cutoff of secretion of aldosterone and, under most circumstances, of antidiuretic hormone. Experiments in man have demonstrated that, given a choice between maintaining volume and tonicity, the body will sacrifice tonicity. Thus, in some overexpanded body water syndromes, there is an anomalous and continuing high renal excretion of sodium, leading to dangerous degrees of hypotonicity.

If renal function is normal and there has been overadministration of saline fluids, huge urine volumes (5000 to 7000 ml/day) are seen. In the visceral forms of extracellular fluid expansion, particularly when due to disease of the heart, liver, or kidney, the disorder itself is due in part to an abnormality of this homeostatic regulator; there is a pathologic failure of diuresis with retention of fluid and salt. With extracellular fluid overexpansion and a restricted urine sodium concentration (i.e., less than 15 mEq/day), one has clear evidence of this abnormality of homeostasis. Frequent measurements of total urine volume are useful in the critically ill patient; the normal oliguric response to volume reduction has been mentioned several times in the foregoing. Here, normal renal response results in urine volumes over 100 ml/hour for 3 hours or more; such large urine volumes should indicate to the therapist that intravenous infusion rates should be sharply reduced, as long as the rest of the picture indicates good renal function.

In simple isotonic overexpansion of the extracellular fluid, electrolyte *concentrations* are often normal while the protein concentration is low by dilution. The hematocrit is also low by dilution. In more chronic forms, particularly in diseases of heart, lungs, liver, and kidneys, hypotonicity accompanies the volume overexpansion. Plasma sodium concentration and osmolality are therefore depressed. The ingestion or injection of large amounts of water adds to this depression of serum sodium and osmolality. Central venous pressure is usually high.

Treatment

When overadministration of fluids is the cause of the condition, fluid administration must be stopped promptly; this may require very strong steps because of the heavy-handed habits of those in attendance. If renal function shows a normal diuretic response, no other treatment is usually needed. In other instances, if some degree of pulmonary edema has resulted, the use of concentrated human albumin, with sodium-losing diuretic agents, is effective. In the more difficult forms of extracellular fluid overload seen in diseases of heart, liver, and kidney, however, such simple measures will not suffice. The use of digitalis and diuretics in heart disease is beyond the scope of this chapter. The use of diuretics plus concentrated albumin in diseases of liver and lung may be quite effective to combat fluid overload.

Guides to Progress

Lowering of central venous pressure (and other chamber pressures) to normal, gradual tapering off of diuresis if overadministration has been the cause, or the establishment of diuresis in chronic visceral disease—all of these are important guides to progress. A fall in body weight should occur.

Syndrome 8. Desiccation-Dehydration

See Table 11-11.

Definition, Terminology, and Related Terms

Desiccation-dehydration is loss of water from the body, essentially as pure water. The term *dehydration* alone is more appropriately used here than

Table 11-11. Desiccation-Dehydration (Syndrome 8)

		Major Findings	
	Unit	Typical	Extreme
Hematocrit	% cells	50	60
Plasma protein	g/dl	6.5–7.0	7.5–8.0
Plasma tonicity	mOsm/L	320–340	350–370
Plasma nonelectrolyte tonicity	mOsm/L	5	10–20
Plasma sodium	mEq/L	155	175
Plasma chloride	mEq/L	110	120
Plasma potassium	mEq/L	3.5–4.0	5.0–7.0
Std. bicarbonate	mEq/L	25–27	15–20
Blood urea nitrogen	mg/dl	15–20	40–70

for desalting water loss. Here we are dealing with a global body water deficit suffered throughout all compartments of the body, in contrast to desalting water loss that always involves the extracellular fluid first. *Hypernatremia* is a result of desiccation-dehydration, as is *hypertonicity,* yet neither of them is synonymous nor specific. The term *intracellular dehydration* was formerly used to refer to the results of desiccation-dehydration, implying thereby that there must be an increase in intracellular tonicity to match the increase in extracellular tonicity indicated by the hypernatremia. Although this is true, the term is unnecessarily limiting.

Clinical Setting

1. Loss of pure water from the respiratory tract (intubation, dry gas ventilation)
2. Evaporative loss from normal, burned, or injured skin or tissue
3. Castaways in hot, dry atmosphere, desert or ocean
4. Renal desiccation: diabetes insipidus or diseases of distal renal tubular water reabsorption
5. Heat stroke

Addition or Subtraction

Desiccation-dehydration is always a subtraction disorder. One may think of it as the loss of distilled water as vapor or "steam" from the body.

Body Composition and Body Weight

Total body water comprises approximately 50% to 55% of the body weight. Body fat, being anhydrous, constitutes a component of body composition that is not included in body water; the fraction of body weight occupied by water is inversely proportional to the body fat, that is, the degree of obesity. For this reason, very fat people have very low values for total body water and its various divisions. The loss of approximately 10% of normal body water, or approximately 5% of normal body weight (2500 to 4000 ml in a normal individual), is required to produce significant hypertonicity and severe thirst. The loss of body weight is appropriate to the amount of water lost. The body weight change should be followed during rehydration.

Abnormalities of Autoregulation

The principal symptom of desiccation-dehydration is severe thirst. If the individual is conscious, hypertonicity produces an overpowering thirst; the slaking of this thirst by the oral intake of water is the primary homeostatic response. If the individual is unconscious, the complaint of thirst is neither felt nor made, and it is up to the physician to sense it and provide the water.

Desiccation-dehydration produces hypertonicity, the primal stimulus to antidiuretic hormone production and distal renal tubular reabsorption of water. Secretion of small volumes of urine of high osmolality is therefore the principal manifestation of a normal homeostatic response. If this is lacking, as in diabetes insipidus and in water-losing nephritis, it is evident that the lack of this homeostatic regulator is, per se, largely responsible for the disorder itself.

A gradual increase in serum osmolality and sodium concentration is the characteristic *laboratory finding.* The concentration of potassium may not rise at an equal rate; that of chloride usually rises; the bicarbonate is variable. Urinary findings have been mentioned in the foregoing discussion. In general, serum sodium concentrations over 160 mEq/L are very dangerous, and values over 175 mEq/L are rarely compatible with survival. These values would correspond to osmolality of 325 to 375 mOsm/L, depending to some extent on the quantity of nonelectrolyte osmolar solute present. With oliguria, blood urea rises, and therefore in severe dehydration-desiccation (sometimes seen in heat stroke or in poorly conditioned athletes suddenly exercising in hot weather), the accumulated urea makes a real contribution to the elevated osmolality, as does the sugar concentration in diabetic dehydration.

Treatment

The primary treatment of desiccation-dehydration is the administration of water. This can be done by mouth, by gastric tube, or by vein (using 5% dextrose in water). The actual amounts of water required are almost always more than one might expect, particularly because the pathologic condition producing the water loss usually persists for at least a day or two. Body weight, osmolality, and renal function should all be followed with care. It is particularly important to be assured that one is not dealing with some element of solute loading (see Syndrome 10), in which case simple massive rehydration can be very dangerous.

Guides to Progress

Decreased urinary output with beginning diuresis is the key occurrence. If plasma osmolality is elevated over 310 mOsm/L and serum sodium is over 150 to 155 mEq/L, sudden restoration of body water to normal will result in acute cerebral overhydration, with cerebral edema. This is due to the fact that the brain is more permeable to water than it is to salt. With sudden rehydration, therefore, the brain gains water before it loses salt. Cerebral edema can therefore be the result of too-rapid restoration of desiccation-dehydration to normal. Pulmonary edema is likewise a threat if cardiopulmonary function is impaired. Body weight should be followed during rehydration, and rehydration should be initiated at a modest rate.

Relevant Mathematical Expression

In desiccation-dehydration, the total body water deficit is given by:

$$TBW_{def} = TBW_1 - TBW_2$$

TBW_1 from Table 11-1

$$(\text{Total Body Solute})_1 = (\text{Plasma Total Tonicity})_1 \times (TBW)_1$$

$$TBW_2 = \frac{(\text{Total Body Solute})_1}{\text{Observed } (\text{Plasma Electrolyte Tonicity})_2}$$

Example: Normally built 80 kg male thirsting as castaway on a life raft for 4 days. Drank no sea water. Observed plasma tonicity = 340 mOsm/L; no abnormal nonelectrolyte or crystalloid tonicity is present.

TBW_1 (from Table 11-1) $= 80 \times 0.55 = 44.0$ L

Normal Total Body Solute (plasma tonicity normal assumed at 300 mOsm/L) (Table 11-2) $= 300 \times 44 = 13{,}200$ mOsm/L

$$TBW_2 = \frac{(\text{Total Body Solute})_1}{(\text{Plasma Electrolyte Tonicity})_2} = \frac{13{,}200}{340} = 38.83 \text{ L}$$

$$TBW_{def} = TBW_1 - TBW_2 = 44.0 - 38.83 = 5170 \text{ ml}$$

Notes on Treatment

This 5200 ml of electrolyte-free water must be given *and retained* to rectify the desiccation hypertonicity in this patient. It must be given cautiously at first because of the threat of cerebral edema. It would expectably produce a beginning diuresis. Despite the welcome diuresis and the continuing insensible water loss through lungs, the patient's weight should be followed because the final dose of electrolyte-free water will inevitably be much larger than the initial dose required for rectification, as a result of other persisting and concomitant losses. Weight gain is mandatory as evidence of reconstitution of body composition.

In this patient who drank no sea water, there was no added solute; not being in renal failure or a diabetic, there was no abnormal crystalloid tonicity. In some cases of desiccation-dehydration, abnormal crystalloid tonicity such as urea or glucose is present. In those cases the calculated total body solute must be limited to electrolyte tonicity because the urea will be excreted with diuresis and the glucose oxidized. The final total amount of fluid required in two or three days to rectify this situation may be surprising, because of persisting lung and skin losses, especially in patients with high fever or burns. The commonest errors are those of administering the first 2 or 3 liters too rapidly, and therefore administrating inadequate amounts of free water. The brain can take up water faster than it can release electrolyte. The result of a too-rapid fluid load is therefore cerebral edema with convulsions. The overriding habit of giving salt solutions to all sick patients must be opposed vigorously because, in this situation, any additional solute merely slows down recovery. If the patient had consumed sea water, the observed plasma electrolyte osmolality may be as high as 400 mOsm/L (with a sodium concentration, for example, of 180 mEq/L). Again, rectification can only be done with close monitoring and sometimes active control of CSF pressure.

To the calculated water requirement here of 5200 ml must be added appropriate amounts for insensible losses (skin and lung losses) (1000–3000 ml per day). These losses will be on the higher side with fever or concomitant injury and extremely high in burns or hyperthermia (heat stroke).

Potentially lethal desiccation-dehydration can only be managed by massive water infusion with close monitoring or control of CSF pressure. Ingestion of sea water by castaways is an example. The same is true in some cases of heat stroke. In both these situations (sea water toxicity and heat stroke) treatment must tread a very fine line between lethal hypertonicity on the one hand and cerebral edema from overtreatment with water on the other. While the latter is very dangerous, it can be monitored and controlled. Expert neurologic collaboration is essential.

Hyperosmolar coma (see Syndrome 17-II, Table 11-18) is a special example of hypertonicity, bearing many resemblances to desiccation-dehydration, with additional solutes (usually glucose in severe diabetes) rather than water losses the initiating factor. *Solute-loading hypertonicity* (see Syndrome 10, Table 11-13) is also comparable in some respects, with the solute of exogenous origin (as in excessive tube feeding, for example) while in hyperosmolar coma unregulated diabetic hyperglycemia is a major internal "solute load." One must take care to be sure which of these superficially similar hypertonic states is presenting in any individual case.

Syndrome 9. Overhydration-Hypotonicity

See Table 11-12.

Definition, Terminology, and Related Terms

Overhydration-hypotonicity is an abnormally large body water unaccompanied by a proportional increase in body salt or solute. It is the hypotonic analogue of extracellular fluid excess described in Syndrome 7; it is the hypotonic converse of dehydration-desiccation with hypertonicity as described in Syndrome 8. *Hyponatremia* is a related term; although hyponatremia is a characteristic of overhydration with hypotonicity, it is also observed in late desalting water loss. *Water intoxication* is an analogous term for the severe form of overhydration hypotonicity.

Clinical Setting

1. *Overadministration* of water by mouth or vein
2. *Postoperative* patients, particularly sensitive to overadministration of free water or hypotonic fluids
3. Patients with *chronic visceral disease,* particularly that of the heart, who have been on a salt-free diet and taking large amounts of water by mouth

Addition or Subtraction

Overhydration-hypotonicity is usually an addition disorder, and there is associated weight gain. If compounded by concomitant loss of salt (renal or extrarenal), the disorder is a combined one, and with severe degrees of hypotonicity the body weight increase may be less.

Body Composition and Body Weight

In the pure state of overhydration-hypotonicity, total body salt content is normal, but total body water is markedly elevated. The normal elasticity of total body water volume would permit the addition of 2000 to 3000 ml in an adult male with little symptomatic change. Amounts larger than this produce significant hypotonicity. An appropriate weight gain will therefore have occurred. Weight measurement usually can begin only at the time of the diagnosis. Weight loss is to be expected during repair.

Abnormalities of Autoregulation

Increased free water clearance due to complete cessation ("ADH cutoff") of antidiuretic hormone secretion is the normal homeostatic response to the overadministration or overaccumulation of water. This is "beer drinkers diuresis," unloading what has been loaded. In the presence of visceral disease, this homeostatic feedback loop is impaired on either the sensor or the effector side, and one may therefore see overhydration develop primarily because of restricted water excretion. After operations, or when there has been any prior injury or volume reduction, water excretion is impaired by a variety of mechanisms. The postoperative or post-traumatic patient is therefore one in whom water retention regularly occurs. Overhydration-hypotonicity so severe as to justify the term *water intoxication* is readily produced by overzealous administration of salt-free fluid in the postoperative or post-traumatic state. Anomalous increase in sodium excretion due to volume expansion ("aldosterone cutoff") may further complicate the hypotonicity.

A fall in the serum sodium concentration linear with the fall in serum osmolality is the characteristic *laboratory finding.* In overhydration, the sum of sodium and potassium concentrations (mEq/L) multiplied by 2 is almost always exactly equivalent to the serum osmolality (mOsm/L). If water loading has been severe, there may be eleva-

Table 11-12. Overhydration-Hypotonicity (Syndrome 9)

		Major Findings	
	Unit	Typical	Extreme (water intoxication)
Body weight	kg	Gain 1–5	Gain 4–10
Hematocrit	% cells	30–35	25–30
Plasma protein	g/dl	4.0–5.0	3.0–4.0
Plasma tonicity	mOsm/L	260	220
Plasma sodium	mEq/L	120	105
Plasma chloride	mEq/L	80	70
Plasma potassium	mEq/L	4.0	3.5
Std. bicarbonate	mEq/L	25	20
Blood urea nitrogen	mg/dl	8–10	5–8

tion of chamber pressures. Urinary findings are discussed earlier in this section.

Treatment

Cessation of water administration is mandatory. The establishment of a water diuresis is attainable, in some cases, by the use of a solute diuretic such as mannitol. When total body solute is elevated (Syndrome 10), its sudden hydration by the administration of large amounts of water is dangerous because of the production of cerebral or pulmonary edema. We have the exact analogue when total body water is elevated in hypotonicity: Restoration to normal solute concentration by the careless administration of huge amounts of salt solutions is dangerous because of the threat of cerebral and pulmonary edema. By the same token, in overhydration-hypotonicity, the loss of water should be the objective, with loss of weight, rather than mere restoration of salt concentration.

Guides to Progress

Weight loss with restoration of tonicity to normal are the objectives. Serum sodium concentrations above 130 mEq/L are rarely symptomatic, but when they fall to 115 to 120 mEq/L, weakness, lassitude, drowsiness, and hypotension occur. Serum sodium concentrations below 115 mEq/L are dangerous (hypotension, coma) and below 100 mEq/L are rarely compatible with survival.

Relevant Mathematical Expression

In overhydration-hypotonicity, the body water excess is given by:

$$TBW_{exc} = TBW_2 - TBW_1$$

TBW_1 from Table 11-2

$$TBW_2 = \frac{(\text{Total Body Solute})_1}{(\text{Plasma Total Tonicity})_2}$$

$$TBW_{exc} = TBW_2 - TBW_1$$

Example: 65 kg normally built male, stressed by continued infection, given large extra amounts of water as a vehicle for antibiotic administration. Found to have gained some weight, observed to have a plasma sodium concentration of 110 mEq/L and potassium 3.5 mEq/L (electrolyte tonicity = (110 + 3.5) × 2 + 10 = 237 mOsm/L).

$$TBW_1 = 65 \times .55 = 35.75 \text{ L (from Table 11-2)}$$

Total Body Solute (assumed normal) = 35.75 × 300 = 10,725 mOsm/L Total

$$TBW_2 = \frac{10{,}725}{237} = 45.25 \text{ L}$$

$$TBW_{exc} = 45.25 - 35.75 = 9.5 \text{ L}$$

In this patient the observed weight gain (were it to have been measured) would approximate 10 kg. Water balance charts (had they been available) would have shown even greater water overload because insensibility and urine losses have been assisting this patient in avoiding the fix into which his excessive intravenous solutions were placing him.

Treatment here, when little solute has been added, is simply that of withholding water. That is the most important step. It is very difficult to convince others of this necessity. A solute diuretic can also be given. If some extra solute is present as in renal failure (urea), diabetes (glucose), or liver failure (unidentified solutes in modest amount), the amount of water overload is even more excessive. In this situation there is a strong tendency to give concentrated salt solution as a quick way of solving the hypotonicity. In this particular case with little extrarenal loss and no renal disease, such will only retard recovery. In other cases it can be given cautiously (3% NaCl or a concentrated balanced salt solution). [*Editor's Note:* Dr. Moore's caution is appropriate. My experience is that a total deficit should not be replaced immediately or rapidly and indeed is not often required. During the first 24 hours after discovery of one of these syndromes described, to replace or correct approximately one-third the deficit in a patient with reasonable renal function will allow a patient to participate in and complete the correction. Too rapid a correction of hypotonicity may be damaging to the brain, as pointed out repeatedly in this section.]

A more useful aid is giving a solute diuretic (mannitol, low molecular weight dextran), which will hasten free water excretion.

If, because of renal disease the patient is also oliguric, pressure filtration dialysis must be considered.

Syndrome 10. Solute-Loading Hypertonicity

See Table 11-13.

Definition, Terminology, and Related Terms

The term *solute-loading hypertonicity* refers to an elevated plasma osmolality due to the combined action of two pathogenic factors: ingestion of a large amount of osmotically active solute, accompanied by a continued profuse solute diuresis. Although other solutes are important, sodium concentration is always elevated, so that the term *hypernatremia* is sometimes used, though it is nonspecific as to cause. *Tube feeding syndrome* refers to the initial description of this disorder as

Table 11-13. Solute-Loading Hypertonicity (Syndrome 10)

		Major Findings	
	Unit	Typical	Extreme
Hematocrit	% cells	50	55
Plasma protein	g/dl	6.0–6.5	6.0–6.5
Plasma tonicity	mOsm/L	320	370
Plasma nonelectrolyte tonicity	mOsm/L	40	60
Plasma sodium	mEq/L	160	170
Plasma chloride	mEq/L	110	115
Plasma potassium	mEq/L	4.5	6.5
Std. bicarbonate	mEq/L	25	15
Blood urea nitrogen	mg/dl	20–40	60–80
Blood sugar	mg/dl	120	1000
Central venous pressure	cm H_2O	5–15	20–40

a complication of tube feeding of a mix rich in solute, with inadequate water provision, in unconscious patients. *Hyperosmotic nonketotic hyperglycemic coma,* or some variant of that term, is used to describe an extreme form of this disorder accompanied by high blood sugar elevations and anomalously low plasma insulin concentrations. This, also, is usually associated with prolonged enteral or parenteral feeding in unconscious patients. This variant is described separately (Syndrome 17-II).

Clinical Setting

1. *Solutes forced* by mouth or vein for nutrition, with too little water, particularly prone to occur in patients who are semicomatose
2. *Insulin lack* (pancreatectomy, untreated diabetes)
3. *Borderline renal failure* (inadequate distal tubular water reabsorption, or water-losing nephritis)
4. *Coma or head injury,* and in some cases CNS injury salt retention
5. *Tube feeding* in comatose patients

Addition or Subtraction

Solute-loading hypertonicity is due to the addition of large amounts of low molecular weight solutes to the body fluids, with inadequate water, together with the inability to excrete them in a concentrated urine. It is usually a mixture of addition of solutes and subtraction of water.

Body Composition and Body Weight

In desiccation-dehydration with hypertonicity, the total body sodium is normal, water has been subtracted, and sodium concentration is elevated. In solute-loading hypertonicity, there is a large increase in total body solute, including sodium. In some cases total body water may also be high. Body water and salt are therefore at extremely high levels, and weight has been gained. If the body solute is rapidly rehydrated by careless administration of large amounts of water, generalized edema occurs, with cerebral and pulmonary edema that are life-endangering. Sudden massive rehydration of solute-loading hypertonicity is one of the dangerous and immediately lethal errors that can be made in body fluid therapy.

Abnormalities of Autoregulation

In *desiccation-dehydration* with hypertonicity, a normal renal response is extreme oliguria with production of a scanty, highly concentrated rapid elevation of cardiac chamber pressures and urine. A key diagnostic signal that *solute-loading hypertonicity* is developing is the continued production of a high volume of urine (solute diuresis) at a fixed osmolality around 750 mOsm/L. High urine volumes with a rising plasma tonicity are the first clue to the onset of this syndrome.

Any diabetic trend worsens this syndrome. If a patient is on tube feedings or prolonged intravenous alimentation and has undergone pancreatic surgery or has had pancreatitis or borderline diabetes in the past, or is on long-continued cortisone administration, this syndrome should be suspected if hypertonicity is found.* The diagnosis is

*The patient with severe bleeding from the upper gastrointestinal tract (e.g., duodenal ulcer) is frequently treated with large amounts of milky and salty substances by mouth (antacid therapy) with inadequate water. The patient is frequently in and out of coma, cannot complain of thirst, and fails to move his or her bowels. Hypertonicity with severe fecal impaction is a serious complication seen in this circumstance.

established by finding a large amount of nonelectrolyte solute in the plasma, as indicated by the difference between the observed plasma osmolality and the sum of sodium and potassium multiplied by 2. This "osmolar gap," normally trivial, may rise to 20 to 40 mOsm/L in this disorder (see Table 11-2).

A high serum sodium concentration with proportionally higher osmolality, as mentioned, is the cardinal *laboratory finding*. The rise in hematocrit is slow to occur because overwatering and oversalting rather than true water loss are the pathogenic factors. The urinary findings have been mentioned. Calculation of the osmolar gap is helpful.

Treatment

In this syndrome, a rapidly lethal outcome is produced if an attempt is made to rehydrate body solutes suddenly by the administration of large amounts of water. Because total body solute is high, the result of such an effort is merely a massive overhydration and oversalting, with rapid elevation of cardiac chamber pressures and the production of pulmonary and cerebral edema. It is for this reason that treatment should consist of cessation of solute loading, the administration of insulin in some cases (if blood glucose is high), and the cautious administration of water. The key to success is the excretion of solute, as well as the rehydration of residual body salt. If renal failure is present, dialysis is essential to success. If diuretics are used, the urine must be analyzed to be certain that solute is being excreted, rather than a urine of low osmolality, which would only accentuate the defect. (See also Syndrome 8.)

Guides to Progress

Monitoring of body weight, blood and urine chemical values, electrocardiogram, cerebral function, and chamber pressures is essential to safety during rehydration.

Syndrome 11. Hypokalemia

See Table 11-14.

Definition, Terminology, and Related Terms

Hypokalemia signifies a low plasma potassium concentration without reference to total body potassium content. *Hypokalemic alkalosis* and *hypokalemic hypochloremic alkalosis* refer to the frequently accompanying alkalosis and depressed chloride concentration. They are terms that include many cases of hypokalemia. *Potassium deficiency* is a misnomer, because hypokalemia may occur with little or no potassium deficit. By the same token, huge losses of body potassium with cellular wasting may be accompanied by a perfectly normal or high plasma potassium concentration.

Clinical Setting

1. *Loss of acid gastric juice* in duodenal or pyloric obstruction
2. *Loss of acid gastric juice* in the presence of small bowel obstruction; rare cases of bowel foreshortening
3. *Loss of acid gastric juice* in gastric obstruction, exaggerated in the Zollinger-Ellison syndrome
4. *Hyperaldosteronism* due to adrenocortical disease or tumor

Table 11-14. Hypokalemia (with Hypochloremia and Alkalosis) (Syndrome 11)

		Major Findings	
	Unit	Typical	Extreme
Body weight	kg	None	Loss 1–2
Hematocrit	% cells	40	38
Plasma protein	g/dl	6.0–6.5	5.5–6.0
Plasma tonicity	mOsm/L	300–310	280–300
Plasma sodium	mEq/L	143	150
Plasma chloride	mEq/L	80	60
Plasma potassium	mEq/L	2.0–2.5	1.2–1.5
Std. bicarbonate	mEq/L	35	50
Blood urea nitrogen	mg/dl	30	70
Blood pH	—	7.52	7.55
Blood PCO_2	mm Hg	35	45
Blood PaO_2	mm Hg	80–90	75–80

5. *Hyperaldosteronism* due to renal artery stenosis or with other stimuli to excessive renin-angiotensin-aldosterone secretion
6. Chronic administration of *ACTH, cortisone,* or *aldosterone,* particularly if the patient is traumatized or operated on

Addition or Subtraction

Hypokalemia is another combination syndrome due both to addition and subtraction. Loss of potassium plays a role but is not critical; losses as small as 100 mEq may be sufficient. Loss of hydrogen ion, with production of a subtraction alkalosis, is very important. Then, if sodium salts are given by mouth or vein, the syndrome becomes much worse.

Body Composition and Body Weight

Body compositional changes may be negligible; possibly the most important is the reduction in extracellular volume that stimulates aldosterone production; body weight changes are then appropriate to this rather mild extracellular fluid loss.

Potassium exists within body cells in a rather fixed ratio to protein (approximately 3 mEq of potassium per gram of nitrogen). Balanced cellular loss, as in starvation, does not produce noticeable disorders of plasma potassium regulation. In a stressful situation, or with marked secretion of aldosterone or cortisone, potassium is lost from the cell at a high K:N ratio (as high as 15 mEq/g). This "*differential potassium loss*" is the setting for hypokalemia, and as mentioned, it need not be large in magnitude if accompanied by alkalosis. It is characteristic of this syndrome that the plasma sodium concentration is normal or slightly elevated. Again, note the tendency of these two ion concentrations to move in opposite directions.

Abnormalities of Autoregulation

"Alkalosis begets hypokalemia, hypokalemia begets alkalosis, alkalosis is difficult to repair in the presence of potassium deficiency, and hypokalemia is almost impossible to repair in the presence of a continuing alkalosis." This disorder is a disorder of the complex neuro-endocrine-renal feedback loop between potassium metabolism and acid-base homeostasis. This is a complex homeostatic arrangement regulating cation distribution across cellular membranes and the retention or excretion of hydrogen ion. The disorder is threatened if there is excessive loss of hydrogen ion as in vomiting of highly acid gastric juice. This engenders a disorder of one of the body's most delicate homeostatic arrangements. The intracellular potassium concentration is around 150 mEq/L. If extracellular potassium concentration is allowed to approach even one-twentieth of this value (7.5 mEq/L), death results. It is thus clear that the regulation of potassium concentration in the plasma is of extreme importance.

The loss of acid gastric juice, threatening extracellular alkalosis, would ordinarily be accompanied by an alkaline urine designed, as it were, to correct the disorder. With a slight volume reduction, aldosterone is instead secreted. Sodium bicarbonate is reabsorbed, and the "paradoxical aciduria" so characteristic of hypokalemia and alkalosis is produced. This tendency to secrete an acid urine is greatly intensified by operative stress or by anything that increases ACTH or cortisone production, as well as aldosterone. The alkalosis therefore becomes suddenly much worse. Loss of acid gastric juice may occur without any warning, simply through an indwelling gastric tube, by suction. The alkalosis itself causes a sharp reduction in plasma potassium concentration, and thus an "inappropriate positive feedback" is initiated, in which the alkalosis produces loss of acid and potassium in the urine, lowering plasma potassium concentration in a self-perpetuating cycle. As one might predict, this disorder is virtually never observed in oliguric renal failure. This disorder "requires" a normal kidney, responding normally to endocrine influences activated by volume reduction and loss of hydrogen ion.

Plasma potassium concentrations in the region of 2.5 to 3.5 mEq/L are regular *laboratory findings* in this syndrome; levels below 1.5 mEq/L are very dangerous. The plasma sodium concentration is usually normal or slightly elevated. One might expect to find the plasma sodium concentration at about 135 mEq/L; in hypokalemic alkalosis the value is quite regularly approximately 143 to 145 mEq/L. The degree of metabolic alkalosis is indicated by the bicarbonate concentration, which is virtually always over 30 mEq/L and may approximate 40 to 60 mEq/L. The loss of acid gastric juice results in loss of chloride and, therefore, hypochloremia, with plasma chloride concentrations below 90 mEq/L.

The urinary findings are of key importance. Early in the syndrome there is secretion of an acid urine with large amounts of potassium. This is typically the aldosterone-induced urinary change. At the height of this syndrome, renal tubular reabsorption of sodium bicarbonate is almost 100%.

Electrocardiographic changes are characteristic: The heart becomes very sensitive to digitalis effects, and if the patient has previously been digitalized, the occurrence of this syndrome produces digitalis toxicity without alterations in digitalis dosage. Cardiac chamber pressures are normal or low, unless heart failure develops. In any case, cardiac arrhythmias are commonplace in hypokalemic alkalosis.

Treatment

Treatment is the administration of potassium with a hydrogen ion donor, or an anion. The administration of chloride ion has an acidifying effect on the extracellular fluid. For this reason the administration of KCl is standard therapy. The administration of ammonium chloride is another way of adding large amounts of hydrogen ion to the extracellular fluid and, in certain cases, actually brings the plasma potassium concentration toward normal without administration of any potassium. Mixtures of the two are usually administered. When there is volume reduction as indicated by oliguria, some sodium can be administered after the first or second day of treatment. In some instances, the alkalosis is remarkably resistant to therapy; the intravenous administration of 0.1 N HCl is rational and effective.

Guides to Progress

The electrocardiographic changes are quite remarkable and were for some time thought to be a function of the plasma potassium concentration, but alkalosis itself produces similar changes. Nonetheless, electrocardiographic changes are helpful. This is a metabolic alkalosis, yet plasma pH is rarely elevated much above 7.5; restoration to normal occurs with treatment. Restoration of plasma potassium concentration to normal is the principal index of rectification.

Renal artery stenosis, with high values for renin, angiotensin, and aldosterone, produces mild hypokalemic alkalosis along with hypertension. Here, the aldosterone effect has, alone and without any loss of gastric juice or other chemical stimuli, produced hypokalemic alkalosis. As accounted in Syndrome 15 *(The Normal Postoperative Patient),* hemorrhage, stress, and trauma tend to move the patient in the direction of hypokalemic alkalosis.

Syndrome 12. Hyperkalemia

See Table 11-15.

Definition, Terminology, and Related Terms

Hyperkalemia is an elevation of plasma potassium concentration without reference to total body potassium content. The term is appropriate regardless of any other concomitant changes that may be occurring, the most common being acidosis. Few other terms are used for this disorder. As mentioned, renal acidosis is a regular accompaniment, but it is not synonymous. *Potassium toxicity* refers to a hazard of hyperkalemia, but it is not a synonymous physiologic term. *Chloride acidosis* refers to a metabolic acidosis with an elevated chloride concentration; potassium concentration does not always follow, and therefore the term is not a synonym.

Clinical Setting

1. *Renal failure*
2. Overadministration of *potassium salts* with borderline renal function
3. *Very severe injury* (with loss of intracellular potassium) greatly accentuates the rate of potassium rise when renal failure coexists

Addition or Subtraction

This is an addition syndrome, but the addition to extracellular and plasma potassium arises from

Table 11-15. Hyperkalemia (with Renal Failure) (Syndrome 12)

		Major Findings	
	Unit	Typical	Extreme
Body weight	kg	Gain	Gain
Hematocrit	% cells	Variable	Variable
Plasma protein	g/dl	Variable	5.5–6.0
Plasma tonicity	mOsm/L	290	320
Plasma nonelectrolyte tonicity	mOsm/L	40	70
Plasma sodium	mEq/L	120	110
Plasma chloride	mEq/L	105	105
Plasma potassium	mEq/L	7.5	9.0
Std. bicarbonate	mEq/L	10	5
Blood urea nitrogen	mg/dl	70–100	100–200
Blood pH	—	7.25	7.15

within the body, owing to redistribution of potassium from body cells: the disorder is greatly accentuated by the administration of exogenous potassium.

Body Composition and Body Weight

The body compositional change can be quite trivial. A redistribution of potassium sufficient to cause death by hyperkalemia and potassium toxicity can occur with no change in total body potassium. Body weight usually rises, owing to the accumulation of fluid (in renal failure).

Abnormalities of Autoregulation

Potassium is a strong diuretic, excreted both by filtration and by tubular secretion. The absence of normal renal function therefore obliterates the normal homeostatic regulator of serum potassium concentration. Potassium administered to a normal person is distributed largely (98%) within cells, particularly if there is protein synthesis and cellular growth. It is the absence of this normal intracellular potassium-holding aspect of the body cell mass, in stress or after injury, that makes the potassium distribution so abnormal; if renal function were normal, the stress-induced cellular potassium loss would be reflected by increased renal potassium excretion. When a large meat meal is eaten in the course of a normal diet, more potassium is ingested by mouth than is required to cause severe hyperkalemia, were it all to remain in the extracellular phase. The normally rapid distribution, partition, and excretion of potassium is markedly inhibited by severe injury or in renal failure.

Just as *alkalosis* usually accompanies *hypokalemia* and/or potassium deficiency, so also *acidosis* characteristically accompanies *hyperkalemia* and/or potassium excess. Acidosis is also an end result of renal failure because of the loss of the normal renal functional capacity for excretion of metabolic acids. If acidosis is corrected by dialysis, hyperkalemia tends to be more tractable. If large amounts of hydrogen ion are removed from the body, for example, by gastric acid aspiration, hyperkalemia is much less notable even though the amounts of potassium so removed are trivial. Plasma potassium concentrations over 5.5 mEq/L are dangerous; with concentrations over 7.5 mEq/L, severe cardiac arrhythmias and death may suddenly occur. The degree of acidosis is quite impressive in these cases, with pH values around 7.15 to 7.25 in typical renal acidosis with hyperkalemia.

Treatment

The treatment consists of removal of potassium from the extracellular fluid, either by hemodialysis or peritoneal dialysis, or by the use of exchange resins in the gastrointestinal tract; the removal of gastric acid by suction is a mildly effective treatment and is helpful if prolonged.

Guides to Progress

The restoration of potassium concentration downward or toward normal may require dialysis daily. If urine volumes are in the range of 500 to 1500 ml per day, dialysis is less important and other measures may be more effective. Because acidosis is an important component, the restoration of pH toward normal is a sign of progress. Attempts to rectify this acidosis by the administration of large amounts of alkali salts is dangerous. The treatment of renal failure by any sort of infusion of sodium salt rapidly produces pulmonary edema, hypertension, and congestive heart failure.

Electrocardiogram must be monitored closely. A sudden fall in potassium concentration even from a high level will accentuate digitalis effects.

Syndrome 13. Hypochloremia

Definition, Terminology, and Related Terms

Hypochloremia is a lowering of the plasma chloride concentration regardless of other findings. *Hypochloremic alkalosis* describes the frequent accompaniment of extracellular alkalosis, with hypochloremia. *Gastric juice loss hypochloremia* describes the most common cause of hypochloremia in surgical patients. *Metabolic alkalosis* refers to an acid-base disorder that may or may not coexist with hypochloremia.

Clinical Setting

1. Chloride loss through *gastric juice;* vomiting and obstruction
2. Treatment of *gastric obstruction* without chloride
3. *Gastric hypersecretion* (Zollinger-Ellison syndrome or other causes), particularly with outlet obstruction or gastric fistula

Addition or Subtraction

Hypochloremia is always a subtraction disorder.

Body Composition and Body Weight

The total chloride of the body is markedly reduced in hypochloremia, the reduction being linear with the reduction of concentration. This is one situation in body composition and chemistry wherein the plasma concentration changes occur *pari passu* with changes in total body content. As mentioned earlier, hypokalemia regularly accompanies hypochloremia, but the latter may be extremely marked with only minor degrees of hypokalemia if operative stress has been absent, as in gastric obstruction.

Abnormalities of Autoregulation

As the body is depleted of chloride, gastric secretion of hydrochloric acid is diminished. When gastric secretion of hydrochloric acid is maintained at a very high level (e.g., with duodenal ulcer or in disorders such as the Zollinger-Ellison syndrome), the losses become massive. Severe and dangerous degrees of alkalosis can be produced. Hypergastrinemia from any cause, with obstruction, greatly accentuates hypochloremia and alkalosis. One occasionally observes situations in which the bicarbonate concentration (at 60 or 70 mEq/L) is actually higher than the chloride concentration, which has fallen to similar or lower values. In the more typical case, bicarbonate is in the region of 35 mEq/L and chloride approximately 75 to 85 mEq/L.

Renal conservation of chloride does not follow the renin-aldosterone cycle but instead bears on renal acid-base regulation. Because the kidney expends energy to secrete an acid urine, one ordinarily finds only minor amounts of chloride present in the urine during gastric juice loss hypochloremia.

In any case of hypochloremia, the plasma potassium concentration should be watched closely as it will fall rapidly to low levels, given the addition either of a corticosteroid stimulus, of operative stress, or acute volume reduction. The sodium concentration in plasma is normally 135 to 140 mEq/L in hypochloremia.

Treatment

The best treatment is the use of KCl with sodium chloride, the latter in modest amounts. Treatment with sodium bicarbonate or other sodium salts low in chloride such as lactate makes the disorder much worse by further diluting the chloride ion. Only by close monitoring of chloride and bicarbonate concentrations, as well as plasma potassium concentrations and the electrocardiogram, can such patients be brought back to normal. With close attention, however, essentially normal extracellular chemical values can be produced in 36 hours if it should be necessary to operate on a patient with obstructing duodenal ulcer and severe hypochloremia. If gastric juice loss by nasogastric suction is playing a role, one might inquire as to whether such suction must be continued. If the amount of gastric juice is large, one should question the presence of either some gastric secretogogue in the drug mix or the Zollinger-Ellison syndrome. On several occasions the diagnosis of the Zollinger-Ellison syndrome has been rightly suspected on the basis of a severe and intractable hypochloremia.

Guides to Progress

All plasma chemical values are important here. Either arterial or venous pH should be followed. The pH values are normally not very high (7.52, for example). Close monitoring of all components is essential, including chamber pressures (if there is any evidence of cardiopulmonary disease).

As indicated under *Syndrome 11. Hypokalemia,* alkalosis renders the heart very sensitive to digitalis alkaloids and produces cardiac arrhythmias in elderly patients with myocardial ischemia. In the patient with heart disease, particularly if digitalized, close monitoring of cardiovascular function is therefore essential in hypochloremia and alkalosis.

Nasogastric suction has become such a regular part of the surgical armamentarium that it has been easy to forget that in most patients the purpose of such suction is only the removal of swallowed air. Swallowed air constitutes the gas of the gastrointestinal tract; the body can neither absorb nor solubilize the gas, which is mostly nitrogen, and it leads to distention if not expelled as flatus. Most of the fluid removed in routine nasogastric suction can be reinfused into the stomach for absorption lower down, as long as the swallowed air is vented.

Any sort of alkalosis exerts a weak inhibitory effect on the respiratory center; a mild inhibition of ventilation, with a very mild elevation of the carbon dioxide tension in whole blood (PCO_2, 42 to 45 mm Hg), is often seen.

Relevant Mathematical Expression

In hypochloremia, chloride deficit is given by:

$$TBCl_{def} = TBCl_1 - TBCl_2$$

$TBCl_1$ = from Table 11-1 (extracellular fluid volume × normal plasma chloride concentration)

$$TBCl_2 = ECF_1 \times Cl_2$$

Example: Thin male, 70 kg, vomiting from obstructing duodenal ulcer. Plasma chloride 70 mEq/L; plasma sodium 143 mEq/L.

$$TBCl_1 = 70 \times 0.23 \times 103 = 1658 \text{ mEq/L}$$

$$TBCl_2 = 70 \times 0.23 \times 70 = 1127 \text{ mEq/L}$$

$$Cl_{def} = 1658 - 1127 = 531 \text{ mEq/L}$$

Note: Because of the marked tendency to depression of potassium concentration in this type of subtraction alkalosis, the chloride deficit can be made up using potassium chloride, ammonium chloride, and sodium chloride, the last in less abundance because of the tendency toward normal sodium in this disorder. Start slowly and watch progress chemically.

Syndrome 14. Hyperchloremia

See Table 11-16.

Definition, Terminology, and Related Terms

Hyperchloremia is elevation of plasma chloride concentration regardless of other considerations. *Hyperchloremic acidosis* refers to the fact that hyperchloremia is usually accompanied by acidosis. *Renal acidosis* is another term that is sometimes used interchangeably, although renal acidosis can be quite severe without hyperchloremia. *Metabolic acidosis* is not synonymous because it refers to any increase in hydrogen ion concentration that is due to metabolic rather than respiratory factors.

Clinical Setting

1. Administration of *large amounts of chloride* by mouth or by vein, particularly where renal function is poor and an acid urine cannot be excreted
2. Chronic *obstructive uropathy* as with prostate diseases
3. *Acute tubular necrosis in diuresis* may show this change

Addition or Subtraction

Hyperchloremia is an addition syndrome. It is due to the addition of chloride ion when renal tubular function is abnormal and the kidney is unable to secrete an acid urine high in chloride.

Body Composition and Body Weight

Extracellular fluid volume is high and total body chloride elevated. Body weight rises because of the water and salt-loading components.

Abnormalities of Autoregulation

As noted, some element of renal tubular disorder, with inability to excrete titratable acidity and a urine of low pH, is essential to the development of this syndrome. It is the lack of this normal homeostatic response to chloride administration that makes the syndrome most common in older people, particularly older men with prostatic disease. The overadministration of sodium chloride solutions is, in the normal individual, a stimulus to gastric secretion of hydrochloric acid. With hyperchloremia one may therefore find increased gastric secretion, and in patients with a history of duodenal ulcer this can be significant.

Chloride concentrations in the vicinity of 108 to 120 mEq/L are characteristic *laboratory findings*. The acidosis is usually severe, pH being approximately 7.2. Bicarbonate depression is usually a linear function of the chloride elevation. The "anion gap" is here reduced proportionally.

Treatment

The treatment consists of the cessation of chloride administration and the administration of sodium bicarbonate by mouth or by vein. In chronic renal tubular disease, the regular administration of sodium bicarbonate is advisable. Patients with ureterosigmoidostomies or other forms of ureteral diversion that result in abnormal reabsorption of ammonium chloride from the right colon should be given sodium bicarbonate by mouth to avoid hyperchloremic acidosis. Oversalting, hypoproteinemia, and edema result if too much sodium is given.

Guides to Progress

These are restoration of serum chloride, bicarbonate, and pH to normal, and downward adjustment of ventilation to normal, with rise of PCO_2 to normal levels.

Table 11-16. Hyperchloremia (Syndrome 14)

		Major Findings	
	Unit	Typical	Extreme
Body weight	kg	No change	Slight gain
Hematocrit	% cells	40–43	38–40
Plasma protein	g/dl	6.0–6.5	6.0–6.5
Plasma sodium	mEq/L	140	130
Plasma chloride	mEq/L	115	125
Plasma potassium	mEq/L	5.2	6.0
Std. bicarbonate	mEq/L	12	8
Blood pH	—	7.30	7.18
Blood PCO_2	mm Hg	35	25
Blood urea nitrogen	mg/dl	40	75–100

Syndrome 15. The Normal Postoperative Patient

See Table 11-17.

Definition, Terminology, and Related Terms

With unanesthetized trauma or elective surgery of mid-grade severity or greater, there are stimuli to alterations in body fluid and electrolyte metabolism that justify consideration of this as a "syndrome." If managed by even the simplest of means, no manifest disorder need result. *Post-traumatic alkalosis* is a very common disorder after severe injury and is described in Syndrome 22. *Low flow acidosis* is another acid-base disorder seen after injury, when a severe low flow state has supervened (see Syndrome 21). Neither of the foregoing terms is synonymous with the normal postoperative physiology.

Clinical Setting

1. Severe unanesthetized *traumatic injury*
2. Major *operations*
3. Either of the above with unwise *overadministration of alkalinizing fluids*
4. Either of the above with *overadministration of hypotonic fluids*
5. Any one of the above with continued physiologic "*stress factors,*" particularly sepsis, undrained abscesses, severe immobilization, and pain
6. Any of the above with added *cortisone* or *ACTH* administration

Addition or Subtraction

If properly managed, the normal postoperative patient need show no abnormalities of either addition or subtraction.

Body Composition and Body Weight

The normal postoperative patient tends to lose body weight by the oxidation of fat and the hydrolytic destruction of protein, with the excretion of the end products of both (H_2O, carbon dioxide, and nitrogen). This is normal. If there is no weight loss, the patient is being given too much fluid.

Abnormalities of Autoregulation

The normal postoperative patient is under the sway of a variety of endocrine influences, all of which are normal homeostatic regulators: conservation of salt, conservation of water, stimulation of fat oxidation, stimulation of gluconeogenesis from muscle protein, and maintenance of cardiovascular function by increased levels of catecholamines and corticosteroids.

If the patient is well managed, these normal post-traumatic influences quickly pass off (2 to 6 days, depending on the severity of the trauma), and the patient can return to normal intake as needed.

Treatment

For minor grades of trauma, no intravenous infusions need be given, and the patient can weather several hours or a day with little fluid intake and with no challenge to his welfare. If the patient is elderly or has poor renal function, one should not hazard even that degree of dehydration because it can be a setting for renal failure if there is a later complication such as sepsis or a mismatched blood transfusion. It has become customary to provide intravenous fluids to almost all postoperative patients, in some of whom it is not a necessity.

If the patient has been the subject of injury of mid-grade or greater severity (e.g., ruptured spleen, fractured femur, bowel resection, closed cardiac surgery), intravenous infusion should be given to maintain normal hydration. Many of the disorders seen in the postoperative patient result from a wrongly prescribed intravenous regimen, usually excessive water and salt.

"Moderation in all things" seems to describe the management of the postoperative patient bet-

Table 11-17. The Normal Postoperative Patient (Syndrome 15)

		Major Findings	
	Unit	Typical	Overadministration of Fluid
Body weight	kg	Loss 1–2	Gain 1–2
Hematocrit	% cells	35	30
Plasma protein	g/dl	6.5	5.0
Plasma sodium	mEq/L	130	120
Plasma chloride	mEq/L	100	105
Plasma potassium	mEq/L	4.0	2.5
Std. bicarbonate	mEq/L	30	35
Blood pH	—	7.52	7.62

ter than any other single aphorism. If large amounts of water or hypotonic fluids are administered, the antidiuretic hormone activity produces water retention with hypotonicity and, in severe cases, a rapid water intoxication. The same sort of analogous maladjustment results from too much salt, too much glucose, too much fat, too much transfusion, and too many amino acids.

If given nothing by mouth for several days and given infusions without potassium, the patient will show a typical hypokalemia after a few days; this is greatly accentuated by continued nasogastric suction or vomiting.

Therefore, the keynote should be administration of enough water to counterbalance skin and lung losses as well as the secretion of a slightly concentrated urine (in a volume of about 1200 ml/24 hr). This amount of water will total about 1500 to 2000 ml in a normal-sized adult male and somewhat less in the female. The patient should be given an amount of salt required to fill up any "third space effect" from the operative trauma itself and to compensate for a urine sodium excretion of 10 to 50 mEq during the first day. This would correspond to approximately 500 ml of Ringers lactate solution. Finally, if it is anticipated that the patient is to be without oral intake for a few days, he or she should be given 40 to 80 mM of KCl daily.

Moderation in transfusion has already been mentioned. If the patient is to receive only 500 to 1000 ml of blood transfusion, it is advisable for him to be awake before it is given so that he can complain of the early symptoms of a transfusion reaction (itching, restlessness, fever, pain in the back). It may be wise to omit such transfusion completely, realizing that the patient's own albumin synthesis and erythropoiesis will soon compensate for such minor losses. If more blood must be given, one must recall the readiness with which massive blood transfusion produces alkalosis after trauma, through the combination of an aldosterone effect and the oxidation of sodium citrate to sodium bicarbonate (see Syndrome 19).

While the use of antibiotics and vitamins is beyond the scope of this chapter, large volume infusions of fluid to maintain dosage of such drugs is one of the common causes of overwatering and oversalting, as already mentioned. Frequently, to save the patient the discomfort of repeated venipuncture, a "keep open" intravenous needle is left in place. If poorly guarded, this may also result in overinfusion of fluid. The patient care team seems to have the innate tendency to infuse fluids without regard to real daily requirements. In such a situation the use of a heparin lock intravenous catheter may save the patient venipunctures without challenging him with an overinfusion of fluid.

Guides to Progress

Repetitive laboratory determinations after injury have become a costly hospital habit. Prior to operation, or as soon as possible after injury, a simple laboratory profile should be undertaken to assess renal function, the presence or absence of diabetes, and the normal homeostatic relationship of ions and acids. Hematocrit, blood urea nitrogen, blood sugar, sodium, potassium, chloride, bicarbonate—all analyzed on venous blood—should suffice. If normal, they need not be repeated.

On the first postoperative morning a repetition of these measurements is advisable in anyone with severe trauma. If convalescence is normal, such chemical determinations need not be repeated for 48 to 72 hours and, if normal at that time, can be discontinued.

If the patient's condition is more complicated—if he develops infection or has a large dissection area, burn or thrombosis, heart disease, diabetes, or an acid-base disorder—careful planning of the nature and frequency of chemical tests will effect not only an economy of funds but an economy of blood. It is not unusual for patients to lose 350 to 500 ml of blood in the first 10 days if overzealous blood sampling for repetitive chemical determinations is made a habit.

Three Syndromes Related to Starvation and Intravenous Feeding

Syndrome 16. Cellular Steal

Definition, Terminology, and Related Terms

The term *cellular steal* is used to denote a monovalent deficiency, usually of a mineral, an electrolyte, or a vitamin, brought on in a starving patient by the abrupt initiation of cellular anabolism with intravenous macronutrients. As an example, the case of zinc deficiency is described here. *Zinc deficiency* is therefore an analogous term, as are, under other circumstances, *potassium deficiency, phosphate deficiency, monovalent deficiency,* and various *vitamin deficiencies.*

Clinical Setting

The clinical setting is prolonged starvation, followed by macronutrient provision intravenously without one or more key anabolic elementary requirements.

Addition or Subtraction

This might be thought of as a subtraction syndrome because it is the lack of a single element or compound that brings it on. Rather than simple lack, however, it is the *failure to provide the ele-*

ment during a period of cellular anabolism that causes the disorder. It is therefore a syndrome of *addition failure.*

Body Composition and Body Weight

The characteristic situation compositionally is that of prior global weight loss (or "balanced starvation") through the loss of fat and muscle tissue. Then, with the addition of intravenous (or oral) feeding of a highly purified or unbalanced food mixture (an example would be amino acids plus glucose without additives of any sort), cellular anabolism and protein synthesis suddenly recommence. The occurrence of cellular protein synthesis without the essential trace substance lacking "steals" this material from its available concentration in the extracellular fluid. Concentration in plasma abruptly falls, and the signs and symptoms of deficiency develop.

As previously mentioned, deficiency syndromes (for example, zinc deficiency or potassium deficiency) are poorly correlated with the plasma concentration but are more a product of total body stores. Yet this is not always true. The lowering of body stores renders the patient *vulnerable* to the acute fall in plasma concentration which, in turn, produces the acute peripheral symptoms and signs.

In the case of zinc, this element is required for the synthesis of a large number of zinc metalloenzymes. If protein anabolism commences without it, plasma concentration is "robbed" as the only available source of zinc. Thus, while chronic balanced starvation may produce little change in the plasma zinc concentration, and no skin changes of zinc deficiency, it falls drastically with beginning anabolism in its absence. The signs suddenly appear. In hospital care this is most noticeable in patients given hyperalimentation intravenously in which the single element, in this case zinc, is lacking.

Abnormalities of Autoregulation

Autoregulation of the body content of minerals such as zinc, magnesium, manganese, chromium, and cobalt is not well understood. There is a good deal of information on autoregulation of certain electrolytes, such as potassium, sodium, and phosphate. In the monovalent cellular steal syndromes of trace mineral deficiency, abnormalities of autoregulation involve both intracellular and plasma concentrations.

But far more important are the disorders of protein synthesis that result when general anabolism commences in the absence of these trace elements. In the case of zinc there is every reason to believe, as with iron, that when a complex organic molecule containing the element (a zinc metalloenzyme, for example) is broken down, the heavy metal is recycled and can be incorporated into a new molecule being synthesized. It is only when there is a lack of that element in the extracellular fluid, and synthesis has begun, that the deficiency becomes manifest. In the case of zinc, this produces the symptoms of zinc deficiency, which, in the acute form, consist of a papular eruption around the mouth, lips, and tongue, often with secondary staphylococcal infection; loss of hair; and dermatitis of the extremities (acrodermatitis). In growing children, protein synthesis occurring in the absence of zinc produces these manifestations, anabolism being the result of normal growth in the absence of the element, rather than macronutrient-induced growth, as is seen in the treatment of adult starvation.

In the case of the iron example already mentioned, an analogous situation prevails. When acute hemorrhage occurs (i.e., balanced loss of all the components of blood), the initial findings in the peripheral blood or marrow do not suggest deficiency of any element other than a gross reduction in the red cell volume. It is days, weeks, or months later—if red cell synthesis is again begun, but without provision of adequate iron—that the so-called iron deficiency anemia occurs. This is a classic example of the cellular steal syndrome and is accompanied by very low plasma iron concentrations with normal or elevated concentrations of the transport protein.

Treatment

The treatment consists of providing the missing element. The effects are often dramatic and virtually immediate. Of all the nutritional syndromes, monovalent deficiencies of this type are among the most rewarding for their consideration, recognition, and treatment.

Determination of the plasma zinc concentration is not always easy; the same goes for chromium, cobalt, and manganese. Determinations of plasma concentrations of iron, folate, and other elements or compounds notable for monovalent deficiency during intravenous feeding are more straightforward. There is not space here to review all the different treatment modalities that can be used depending on the element missing. In the case of zinc, if a patient has the clinical manifestations of zinc deficiency, zinc should be given intravenously in small doses. It is wise to provide a trace mineral solution containing other trace minerals as well.

Syndrome 17. Parenteral Nutrition Overload

Definition, Terminology, and Related Terms

This is not one but a series of several syndromes of fluid overload or overuse of parenteral nutrition

Table 11-18. Hyperosmolar Nonketotic Hyperglycemic Coma in TPN (Syndrome 17-II)

		Major Findings	
	Unit	Typical	Severe
Hematocrit	% cells	45	55
Plasma protein	g/dl	6.0–6.5	6.5–7.0
Plasma tonicity	mOsm/L	320	390
Plasma nonelectrolyte tonicity	mOsm/L	10	20
Plasma sodium	mEq/L	155	185
Plasma chloride	mEq/L	140	170
Plasma potassium	mEq/L	4.5	6.5
Std. bicarbonate	mEq/L	27	22
Blood urea nitrogen	mg/dl	20–40	80–120
Blood sugar	mg/dl	175	1500
Central venous pressure	cm H_2O	5–15	20–40

solutions. These will be described briefly under several headings.

Syndrome 17-I. Fluid Overload

This is to be compared with Syndrome 7, *Oversalting: Extracellular Fluid Excess* and Syndrome 9, *Overhydration-Hypotonicity.* With TPN solutions,* the exact response of the patient to an overload depends to some extent on his prior condition and the nature of the fluids given. All intravenous nutrition is in a sense a race between *provision* of substrate and *utilization;* if the former prevails, utilization and excretion are unable to keep up, and an overload syndrome of some type results.

Because of the high solute content of TPN solutions, an acute overload readily produces pulmonary edema under almost any circumstance. A persistent high urine volume is a first warning. If a solution is given briskly, an overload will produce pulmonary edema without a marked increase in chamber pressures. The warning signals here are to be found, over the short-term, in a persistently high urine volume (assuming renal function to approximate the normal); consistent urine outputs of greater than 100 ml/hr for three hours or more strongly suggest that the patient is fighting off a fluid overload. Other indices that constitute a warning are anomalous weight gain, fall in hematocrit or protein concentration, and a rise in plasma osmolality (see Syndrome 17-II). The ominous finding in all cases, however, is that of bubbly wet rales at the lung bases and, in many cases, a beginning rise in central venous pressure. If amino acids are given, disorders of mental and CNS function result from overload (see Syndrome 17-VI).

*TPN refers to *total parenteral nutrition.* Whether or not the nutrition is "total" is irrelevant if large amounts of parenteral nutritive substances are given intravenously. TPN is used for brevity.

Syndrome 17-II. Hyperosmolar Nonketotic Hyperglycemic Coma in TPN

See Table 11-18.

This is a highly specific syndrome that can be produced by overload of rich parenteral feeding solutions containing a large amount of low-molecular-weight solute, and particularly large amounts of glucose (as well as by tube feedings). See Table 11-13 for solute-loading hypertonicity, of which this is a remarkable exaggeration. A notable event here is the finding not only of high plasma tonicity (for example, 350 mOsm/L or higher), but excessively high glucose concentrations (as high as 1500 mg/%). From the first description of this syndrome, it was noted that this high blood glucose was not accompanied by an appropriate insulin concentration or degree of ketosis. Excessive urine volumes for several previous days are a characteristic sign of the persistent solute diuresis that underlies the dehydration.

Treatment consists of providing water at modest load rates to provide the kidneys with enough water to float out the excess solute. Beware overtreatment with water. As previously described, overwatering is a hazard in treatment of any form of hypertonicity because of the threat of cerebral edema.

The addition of insulin is essential. The plasma insulin concentration is usually found to be inappropriately low for the degree of hyperglycemia, and yet, there is no permanent damage to the pancreas. It was thought for a time that this indicated a sort of pancreatic exhaustion syndrome, analogous in this sense to pituitary-induced diabetes mellitus. This is an aspect of the syndrome that is still not well understood. After a few days of treatment with insulin, no more insulin is usually required.

If unrecognized, this situation is rapidly fatal. Its persistence, even for 24 hours (once the extreme hypertonicity and hyperglycemia have developed), may be considered to be life-threatening. Its avoidance is clearly a matter of awareness in monitoring, especially checks on the plasma osmolality, plasma sodium concentration, and plasma glucose. The calculation of unaccounted or nonelectrolyte tonicity shows extreme values in this syndrome. Sudden emergence of hyperglycemia in a patient who has previously tolerated TPN well is usually associated with sepsis.

Hyperosmolar coma can also be observed in acute diabetic ketoacidosis without prior solute loading. Here, the administration of insulin and water with control of the diabetic crisis is essential.

Syndrome 17-III. Hyperphosphatemia in TPN

Hyperphosphatemia occurs in TPN when large amounts of phosphorus-containing solutions are given, especially in the presence of borderline renal failure. The most common cause of this is the administration of large amounts of intravenous fat emulsion in the presence of poor renal function. Stabilizing phosphatides in some commercial fat emulsions contain organic phosphorus. As this material is metabolized and hydrolyzed, inorganic phosphate is released to the extracellular fluid, and if renal function is not normal, it produces a rapidly rising phosphate. This can be accompanied by a falling calcium concentration and may be part of the pathogenesis of the pseudohyperparathyroidism mentioned below, because a chronic imbalance of this type should stimulate parathyroid function much as in long-standing uremia. A rising inorganic phosphate concentration far out of proportion to the rise in BUN or creatinine is the clue that this complication of parenteral nutrition is occurring. A high parathormone concentration confuses the diagnosis but does not rule it out.

Syndrome 17-IV. Hypercalcemia in TPN

In the early days of TPN, many patients were reported to have a syndrome closely resembling hyperparathyroidism. In one or two instances, exploration of the parathyroid glands was undertaken or was imminent before the nature of the syndrome was recognized.

This is not necessarily due to the excessive infusion of calcium but is a more subtle complication of TPN, not always well understood. An acutely threatened hyperphosphatemia might be one aspect, as mentioned earlier. Contrariwise, the chronic infusion of a TPN mixture without any phosphorus in it at all would be associated with hypophosphatemia, and this might be accompanied by a high calcium concentration even in the absence of hyperparathormonemia. In some of these instances, elevated levels of parathormone in the blood have been reported.

In any patient receiving TPN who is considered to be suffering from hyperparathyroidism, it is absolutely essential to discontinue all parenteral feeding solutions for at least 7 to 10 days to determine whether or not the patient actually has hyperparathyroidism. There are few situations in human nutrition in which the lack of large amounts of macronutrients for 7 to 10 days is in any way deleterious. As with fluid infusions, the hospital team has become so habituated to using intravenous nutrients that an obsessive-compulsive desire to maintain such infusions is sometimes difficult to combat.

Syndrome 17-V. The Satiety Syndrome in TPN

About 25 years ago, when fat emulsion was first available, some studies were carried out in normal human volunteers in whom normal dietary intake was continued by mouth and a superimposed large supply of calories in the form of fat emulsion was provided. Fever, right upper quadrant pain, and deterioration of liver function were reported. It was thought at that time that this was specific for fatty overload and was pathognomonic of fatty liver.

More recently it has become evident that caloric super-supply far in excess of energy needs, whether as a result of the provision of fat or carbohydrate, can produce right upper quadrant pain and deterioration of liver function (as manifested by a rise in transaminase enzymes and, in some cases, in bilirubin). This can result from overloads of either carbohydrate or fat, but with fat it may well be more common. More recently a case report has suggested that overloads of carbohydrate that are excessive in relation to the provision of protein precursors, such as amino acids, can likewise produce liver functional changes. Too much nutrient intake, or an unbalanced ration will quickly produce the satiety syndrome. One cannot produce or force anabolism by providing nutrients.

The *satiety syndrome* is defined as that of a patient who is being given more caloric supply than is required, and more than can be utilized. This is usually seen with a supracaloric intake of either carbohydrate or fat, or a feeding that is at an excessively high calorie-nitrogen ratio. Liver function deteriorates. If the patient is conscious, right upper quadrant pain is often a feature of this syndrome.

Patients with intravenous feeding for prolonged periods of time are subject to gallstones and the precipitation of sludge and mud in the biliary tract. Presumably part of the mechanism here is the lack of secretion of secretin and cholecystokinin in patients without any food intake by mouth. Right upper quadrant pain can therefore be confusing, signifying either the satiety syndrome or hepatobiliary disease.

It is important to understand that fatty liver is also produced by patients who lose their own body fat at excessively rapid rates of oxidation. An example would be excessive weight loss in small bowel shunt surgery. It has also been reported in ulcerative colitis with rapid weight loss. The mechanism is possibly the inability of the liver adequately to phosphorylate endogenous fat. It is conceivable that there is a kindred mechanism in the satiety syndrome in which fat may be appearing intravenously at a rate more rapid than hepatic metabolism can accommodate it.

Syndrome 17-VI. Amino Acid Overload in TPN

Early in our experience with intravenous feeding, we encountered a few patients who, receiving central vein mixtures involving 2 to 4 liters of amino acid solution per day, showed some abnormalities of emotional or mental function. Often these patients were septic or had been acutely ill in the days preceding and mental aberrations were not unexpected.

More recently it has become evident that patients may be especially sensitive to excess in loading rates of the phenolic and polycyclic amino acids, particularly if sepsis and/or liver function impairment are present.

It is not clear at this time whether all these abnormalities have a single cause. Provision of carbohydrate alone lowers the plasma branched-chain amino acid concentration either in starvation or with the provision of amino acids intravenously. The provision of carbohydrate lowers the concentration of amino acids in patients who have been starving.

Summarizing these aspects, it appears that excessive amounts of amino acid, if not properly metabolized, can produce toxic manifestations, and that this syndrome is most marked in patients with sepsis or liver disease with respect to the phenolic amino acids (tyrosine and tryptophan, and possibly histidine and histamine). The clinical lesson is a simple one: If patients are receiving large amounts of amino acids and have any mental symptoms, sepsis, and/or liver disease, caution should be exercised. The determination of individual amino acids or an amino acid profile in the blood may at times be helpful.

A balanced diet is again emphasized as the surest guide to sound parenteral alimentation. Glucose assists not only in protein synthesis but in the metabolism of amino acids; glucose likewise fosters normal metabolism of fat. If either glucose or fat is given in excess or alone, the situation is harmful. A balance not only in total amounts but in relationships among constituents is essential. "Meat intoxication" can be produced by excess doses of amino acids by peripheral vein as well as by an Eck fistula or liver failure; hyperammonemia is not a feature in most of these cases.

Syndrome 17-VII. Acid-Base Distortion in TPN

Both alkalosis and acidosis (metabolic in both cases) can be made worse by large amounts of parenteral alimentation solutions, including amino acids, particularly when renal function is poor.

The pathogenesis is variable, depending on the clinical background of the patient.

When the loss of gastric juice is partly responsible for the alkalosis (gastric suction with an obstructed duodenal ulcer), the mechanism seems evident enough: With adequate energy and amino acids in good supply, gastric secretion is stimulated and supported at a high level. There may be even some actual stimulation of gastrin by the amino acid mixture. The tube suction is actively maintained. Gastric losses are therefore high and continuing, and alkalosis becomes much worse. Large-scale infusions are also gastric secretogogue in effect. In a sense, this worsening of alkalosis is a byproduct of the "surgery of procrastination," all too common in TPN.

The worsening of metabolic acidosis with multiple amino acids is probably related to borderline renal function (especially in children with some evidence of renal tubular acidosis or in elderly adults who have had obstructive uropathy). In these situations, when global renal function is reduced and the ability of the kidney to secrete a strongly acid urine has been compromised, the infusion of large amounts of amino acids (some of which are infused in the acidic form as the amino acid hydrochloride) has a net acidifying effect on the extracellular phase, much as an equal volume of dilute ammonium chloride.

These syndromes are mentioned here briefly because, in our experience with parenteral alimentation, we have seen worsening of acidosis or of alkalosis on several occasions. Physicians are often mystified as to how a single form of intravenous nourishment can make either acidosis or alkalosis worse, seemingly direct opposites.

Related to this, in the general strategy of surgical care, is the prolonged and inadvisable procrastination of operation itself, which sometimes occurs in patients on hyperalimentation, for whom almost indefinite postponement of needed surgery (e.g., for pancreatic abscess) is encouraged and tolerated because the patient appears to be maintaining "good nutrition." The worst example of alkalosis promoted by intravenous alimentation we have observed was a patient with high-grade outlet obstruction due to chronic duodenal ulcer, being treated on a medical department unit. He was kept in "good nutrition" for several weeks of total parenteral alimentation. His gastric juice outputs were gigantic. A severe gastric juice loss resulted, with typical hypokalemia and hypochloremia (Syndromes 11 and 13). He could be given additional potassium, and this helped somewhat, but the gastric juice volume persisted. The situation suggested that some element in the amino acid-glucose mixture acted as a strong gastric stimulus. This could either be the high load of sodium and chloride itself, which is a mild gastric secretogogue, or the presence of certain amino acids, which may stimulate gastrin production. This was a classic example of a case in which the best nutritional step for the patient was a surgical operation for relief of gastric obstruction, the cessation of all efforts at intravenous feeding, and the initiation of oral diet.

Syndrome 18. Insulin Anomalies in TPN

Syndrome 18-I. Weaning Syndrome (Lingering Hyperinsulinemia) and Digestive Inhibition Before Weaning

The human pancreas has tremendous insulin production capacity. In individuals receiving glucose at concentrations around 5%, the blood sugar is maintained in a normal range and the plasma insulin rarely exceeds 8 mμ/ml. In high-dose glucose infusions (as in central vein alimentation), that is, at glucose concentrations around 20% or higher (up to 80 mμ/ml) and total glucose loads of 500 g/day or more, plasma insulin concentration ranges as high as 35 to 70 mμ/ml.

At these higher rates of glucose infusion with high plasma insulin concentration, the sudden cessation of glucose infusion will be followed by reactive hypoglycemia. In patients with heart disease this can be dangerous. In subjects undergoing surgical operations, it could lead to death if not recognized during anesthesia. The way to avoid this type of weaning syndrome is merely to reduce gradually the concentration of glucose by administering, after the hypoglycemic mixture, an infusion of 5% dextrose for 12 to 24 hours.

The provision of glucose intravenously inhibits gastric peristalsis and gastric secretions. This may be a part of the normal decline in gastric secretion that follows the intestinal phase of digestion and the normal postprandial hyperglycemia. Whatever its origin, the provision of high-calorie macronutrients by vein is inhibitory to gastric function.

Clinical evidence suggests that it is also inhibitory to small bowel motility, though this is less clear cut.

In any event, before the transition can be made from parenteral to oral nutrition, it is essential that the parenteral nutrition be stopped, even for several days or a week, to permit normal gastric responses, whether to the presence of food or to psychological stimuli ("cephalic phase"), to manifest themselves. Although this is not a disorder of water and electrolyte metabolism, it is mentioned here because the undue prolonged continuation of parenteral alimentation may be due to this biofeedback mechanism, whereby the provision of the alimentation itself tends to inhibit its discontinuance.

Syndrome 18-II. Flask Insulin Hypoglycemia

Patients requiring insulin with hyperalimentation (see below) are rare. It is most exceptional (less than 1% of instances) for ordinary hyperalimentation, even with concentrated central vein mixtures, to require concomitant insulin.

In patients with borderline diabetes, with overt diabetes following pancreatectomy, with pancreatitis, or with other diabetes-threatening situations, insulin must be used: Regular, or isophane insulin (NPH) should be given subcutaneously and the blood sugar and urine sugar used to monitor the insulin dose, just as in the treatment of a diabetic patient.

Under no circumstances should the insulin be added directly to the intravenous flask because of the danger of sudden, unintentional discontinuation of the infusion by displacement of the line, occlusion of the line if the patient lies on it, or interruption of the drip for anesthesia or some other purpose, which should be forbidden in any case.

With sudden cessation of an infusion containing both glucose and insulin, the glucose is oxidized within moments, whereas the insulin has a half-life of 6 to 12 hours, depending on the patient and the nature of the insulin used. This will produce an insulin reaction much more certainly and much more severely than the weaning syndrome already mentioned. It is for this reason that insulin should be given subcutaneously (slowly absorbed) and should not be added to the infusion mix.

Syndrome 18-III. Latent Diabetes and Post-Traumatic Pseudodiabetes in TPN

This situation is recognized readily and is far less hazardous than the two syndromes of excessive insulin mentioned previously. The simplest forms of monitoring of parenteral nutrition will uncover hyperglycemia, glycosuria, or polyuria. Any high urine volume of course should be accompanied by studies of urine sugar. In post-traumatic diabetes, for instance after burns *(burn pseudodiabetes),* after certain types of pancreatic resection, even though some pancreas is left behind, in pancreatitis, and in certain forms of trauma, one sees a tendency toward diabetes that mandates the temporary administration of insulin to normalize blood sugar. With a normal pancreas, infusions of high glucose loads produce blood sugars of 110 to 120 mg/dl fairly regularly. This mild hyperglycemia is harmless and is accompanied by an appropriate high level of insulin. If the blood sugar exceeds 150 mg/dl, the patient should be given insulin subcutaneously, with blood and urine sugars monitored as with any mild diabetic. We have seen insulin requirements as high as 40 units per day after severe burns, accentuated by the provision of large amounts of glucose intravenously. Upon recovery, the patient was totally free of any diabetic taint and displayed a normal glucose tolerance curve.

Six Syndromes of Disordered Acid-Base Homeostasis

In many of the foregoing syndromes of disordered body water and salt metabolism, there has been some reflection in acid-base distortion, sometimes a very important feature. In the following six syndromes, disorders of acid-base homeostasis predominate, and the disturbances of other ions or water distribution appear as secondary effects. In some instances, when repetitious description would result, cross-reference is given.

Confusion regarding terminology and mathematical expressions for disordered acid-base balance have led to much misunderstanding. We believe it is important to emphasize the Bronsted schema, namely, that the only acid is hydrogen ion and that bases are substances, such as bicarbonate or hydroxyl ion, that will accept hydrogen ion in buffer linkage. Most of the ionic components of human plasma, in the Bronsted schema, are therefore referred to as cations and anions, and they include sodium, potassium, chloride, certain trace minerals, calcium, phosphorus, and magnesium.

On the mathematical side, it is possible to construct elaborate curvilinear plots or logarithmic analyses of hydrogen ion relationships, traceable in part to the fact that the conventional terminology of pH has been used for so many years and is based on the negative logarithm of the hydrogen ion concentration. We have preferred to continue to use the pH mode of expression rather than the H^+ concentration in most cases because it is so widely adopted and so readily adapted to a wide variety of acid-base disorders. For graphic representation of acid-base disorders, we believe that the simple linear plot of pH against bicarbonate (the pH-bicarbonate diagram), as illustrated in Davenport's book (see Selected Readings at the end of the chapter) is by far the simplest and most useful. Using this, it is possible to discern at a glance the mixture of metabolic and respiratory components and to understand significant departures from expectation. By converting pH to direct hydrogen ion concentration, it is possible also to make simple linear expressions for "pure" respiratory and metabolic acid-base disturbances. Some of these formulations are shown in Table 11-3.

One other preliminary note concerns the *standard bicarbonate.* Because there is no direct analytic method for bicarbonate, it must always be estimated from a direct analysis of the arterial carbon dioxide content, with appropriate corrections for carbon dioxide tension and pH. The result is a figure for bicarbonate referred to as the *standard bicarbonate.* The corrected venous carbon dioxide content can be thus used if performed on whole blood. It is this simple form of expression that we use for bicarbonate, namely the pH and PCO_2 of whole blood measured at two separated pH levels, and appropriately corrected to normal carbon dioxide tension. This sort of correction is evident from the pH-bicarbonate diagram previously mentioned. To depart from this simple terminology by introducing the phrases *base excess* and *negative base excess* (to signify a base deficit) appears to us to be an elaborate and scholastic nicety that only confuses the clinician. Better, by far, to stick with the simple *standard bicarbonate,* understanding its derivation and meaning (Figure 11-1).

Syndrome 19. Acute Hypercapnia

See Table 11-19.

Definition, Terminology, and Related Terms

Acute hypercapnia is an acute elevation of the partial pressure of carbon dioxide in the blood. *Acute hypoventilation* refers to the usual mechanism; *acute respiratory acidosis* is synonymous. *Hypoventilation acidosis* is synonymous.

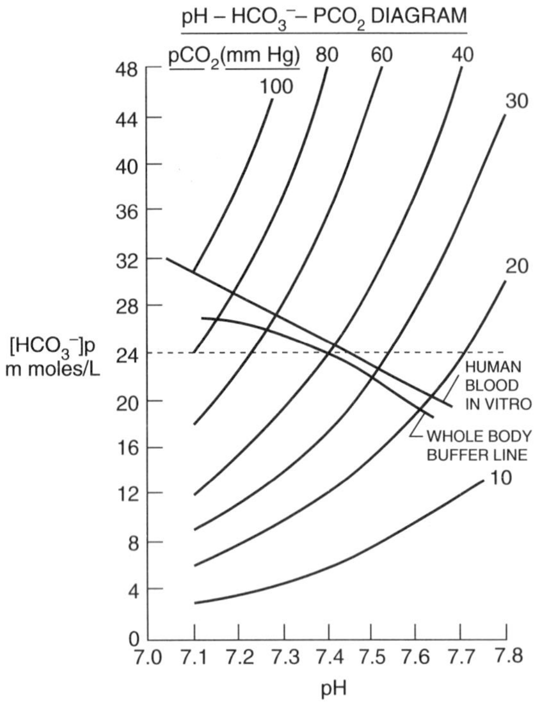

Figure 11-1. The pH bicarbonate diagram as first developed by Davenport. It is the simplest way to analyze acid-base disturbances. Every student should be able to draw one reasonably accurately on a freehand basis. The in vitro blood buffer line shows the change in bicarbonate and pH that would result from a progressive change in carbon dioxide tension if there were no other metabolic, renal, or compensatory mechanisms and if one were dealing with whole blood in a test tube. Actually, the in vivo whole body buffer line is much less steep and is shown as such because blood in the body is in contact with extracellular and cellular buffers, which modulate the change in bicarbonate with alteration in PCO_2. Each student should take one or two clinical examples of acid-base disturbance encountered in the hospital and locate them on this pH bicarbonate diagram. Enter the bicarbonate (sometimes given as the "plasma CO_2"), as best estimated from your lab, and the PCO_2 and calculate the pH. Check it. More complicated curvilinear diagrams are adapted for the use of certain commercial acid-base analytic machinery and are far more difficult to visualize graphically. The terms *base deficit* or *base excess* add little conceptual clarity to the simple expression of pH, bicarbonate, and PCO_2. In complex disorders involving metabolic change (whether primary or compensatory), other anions (lactate, pyruvate, metabolic acids) enter the equation and the findings depart from these standards. Their very departure (direction and magnitude) may indicate the other forces at work.

Clinical Setting

1. *Central:* drug, brain tumor, or brain injury
2. *Nerve conduction or mechanical:* injury in the neck or phrenic nerve areas and/or diaphragm, chest wall, pleural space (pneumo- or hemothorax)
3. *Pulmonary:* acute failure of ventilation due to tracheal stenosis, tracheal impingement, tracheobronchial disease, chronic bronchopulmonary disease with an acute exacerbation, pneumothorax, pulmonary edema, pneumonia

Addition or Subtraction

This is an addition disorder of endogenous source, the carbon dioxide arising from normal metabolism.

Body Composition and Body Weight

There is no acute change in body composition, save for slight increase in total body carbon dioxide. There is no acute change in body weight.

Abnormalities of Autoregulation

This is clearly a disorder due to an abnormality of the prime homeostatic regulator of the partial pressure of carbon dioxide: pulmonary alveolar ventilation. There is no compensation for this save for the excretion of an acid urine and bicarbonate generation. These are such slow and ineffective regulators that they are of little short-term significance. Acute hypercapnia can result from rebreathing or from acute upper respiratory tract obstruction and progress to virtually lethal proportions within minutes.

Elevation of the partial pressure of carbon dioxide in the blood (PCO_2) is the most common and the characteristic *laboratory finding* in this disorder. This is best measured on arterial blood, freshly sampled. However, in acute respiratory acidosis, one should not stand on ceremony for arterial puncture because the venous PCO_2 also is markedly elevated. There is an immediate slight increase in bicarbonate, as shown by the whole-body buffer line, but this has little or no significance in acute hypoventilation.

The concomitant arterial oxygen tension is almost always low, but may not be threatening, depending on the balance between ventilation and perfusion in the pulmonary circulation.

Arterial pH values may fall below 6.95 within 20 to 30 minutes of the onset of rebreathing or acute hypoventilation, with PCO_2 approaching 100 mm Hg. When the onset is less acute, as in pneumothorax, hydrothorax, or early pulmonary edema, the fall in pH is much more gradual, and the arterial oxygen desaturation is due largely to shunting of blood through nonventilated portions of the lung rather than hypoventilation as such.

Treatment

There is only one treatment: adequate ventilation. There is no substitute or alternative treatment. It is beyond the scope of this chapter to deal with the various respiratory steps taken to restore ventilation to normal.

Table 11-19. Hypercapnia (Syndromes 19 and 20)

		Major Findings	
	Unit	Acute	Chronic
Body weight	kg	None	Gain in CHF
Hematocrit	% cells	38–42	45–50
Plasma protein	g/dl	6.0–6.5	7.0
Plasma tonicity	mOsm/L	295–300	295–300
Plasma nonelectrolyte tonicity	mOsm/L	5	5
Plasma sodium	mEq/L	143	150
Plasma chloride	mEq/L	103	80
Std. bicarbonate	mEq/L	29–30	45
Blood urea nitrogen	mg/dl	15	50
Blood PCO_2	mm Hg	85	60
Blood PaO_2	mm Hg	85	70
Blood pH	—	7.05	7.25
Blood oxyhemoglobin dissociation curve	—	Right shift	Left shift

No other form of acidosis lowers the whole blood pH as rapidly or to such profound levels. The principal laboratory guides to progress are therefore a reduction of the partial pressure of carbon dioxide and restoration of pH to normal.

Acute trauma or wounds to the upper airway, bleeding directly into the bronchus, rupture of the bronchus, mediastinal emphysema, and bilateral pneumothorax are all acute traumatic events that demand immediate clearing of the airway by surgical steps, usually including endotracheal intubation or tracheotomy. Details are beyond the scope of this chapter. Very aggressive surgical steps are often required for the prevention or correction of respiratory failure producing severe and often lethal hypercapnia.

Syndrome 20. Chronic Hypercapnia

See Table 11-19.

Definition, Terminology, and Related Terms

Chronic hypercapnia is underventilation with hypercapnia of long-enough duration to permit a compensatory metabolic change to occur. *Chronic respiratory acidosis* is synonymous. *Compensated respiratory acidosis* is, in a sense, a misnomer because the compensation is never complete. *Respiratory acidosis with metabolic alkalosis* is a confusing mixture of terminologies. As long as the hydrogen ion concentration is elevated and the pH lower than normal, this must be referred to as acidosis, even though the metabolic changes that occur are "in the direction of" metabolic alkalosis. *Chronic obstructive pulmonary disease (COPD)* refers to the disease usually at fault.

Clinical Setting

1. Chronic heavy *smoking* habit
2. *Asthma, emphysema,* bronchiectasis on the basis of intrinsic infection
3. Asthma and emphysema on the basis of *allergic* disease
4. Chronic *dust diseases* and other chronic inhalation disorders producing emphysema and respiratory insufficiency

Addition or Subtraction

This is an addition disorder due to the accumulation of carbon dioxide from endogenous sources when pulmonary excretion is inadequate. It is in part compensated by the renal excretion of metabolic acid, a subtraction component. This accounts for the characteristic elevation of bicarbonate concentration and lowering of plasma chloride concentration.

Body Composition and Body Weight

There is no essential change in body weight through chronic obstructive pulmonary disease, per se. As the disease progresses, the sufferer becomes thin and wasted, possibly owing to the sheer effort and energy cost of respiration. Finally, if right heart failure is produced, there is weight gain with edema.

Abnormalities of Autoregulation

As noted in Syndrome 19 *(Acute Hypercapnia),* the homeostatic regulator, pulmonary excretion of carbon dioxide, is itself impaired, accounting for the disorder. In the more chronic form, another homeostatic regulator consists in the renal excretion of urine of low pH and high titratable acidity and containing large amounts of chloride. Thus, the change in the direction of "metabolic alkalosis" may actually lower the hydrogen ion concentration and raise the pH so that there is a restoration toward normal, if not fully to normal. The characteristic chemical signs of this are the low plasma chloride concentration and elevated bicarbonate, and a urine of pH as low as 4.5 if renal tubular function is good.

Once chronic congestive heart failure (cor pulmonale) becomes manifest, the renal excretion of acid becomes less efficient and the acidosis becomes more severe. Any supervening infection, such as bronchopneumonia or transient respiratory infection of the epidemic virus variety, makes the condition much worse and soon fatal.

In acute hypercapnia the PCO_2 may rise to levels of 70 to 120 mm Hg. This is the characteristic *laboratory finding.* In chronic hypercapnia the PCO_2 values rarely exceed 50 or 60 mm Hg. Even those levels are harbingers of extreme illness if some pneumonic infection is superimposed. Bicarbonate values, usually normal in acute hypercapnia, may now exceed 35 to 50 mEq/L. Chloride concentration is usually depressed to the region of 75 to 90 mEq/L. Urine pH is acid.

Treatment

Normalization of ventilation is the ideal. In chronic obstructive lung disease it may be difficult or impossible to achieve. If, in chronic lung disease, superimposed infection or pulmonary edema develops, treatment of the infection may ameliorate the situation, at least temporarily. Anything that interferes with the excretion of an acid urine, such as abnormalities of renal tubular function or renal failure, inhibits the metabolic compensation of chronic hypercapnia and makes the disease much more difficult to treat and much more apt to become lethal. The lethal mechanism is usually cardiac failure, or an acute arrhythmia, or both.

Syndrome 21. Acute Hypocapnia

See Table 11-20.

Definition, Terminology, and Related Terms

Acute hypocapnia is acute hyperventilation, with depression of the carbon dioxide tension in the blood. *Hyperventilation tetany* refers to one occasional end result. Acute *respiratory alkalosis* is a synonymous term.

Clinical Setting

1. *Anxiety* or emotional excitement with hyperventilation
2. *Induced* hyperventilation under anesthesia, or due to an erroneous setting of machine-assisted ventilation
3. With pulmonary *shunting,* a persistent hyperventilation of the perfused segment as seen in post-traumatic pulmonary insufficiency

Addition or Subtraction

This is a subtraction disorder due to excessive removal of carbon dioxide from the blood.

Body Composition and Body Weight

There is no gross change in body composition and no essential change in body weight.

Abnormalities of Autoregulation

With chronic respiratory alkalosis, one would predict some compensatory metabolic changes. There is a decreased renal secretion of acid and a tendency toward a compensatory metabolic acidosis with depression of bicarbonate, but this is a weak response, and it is of more theoretic than clinical

Table 11-20. Acute Hypocapnia (Syndrome 21)

		Major Findings	
	Unit	Typical	Extreme
Body weight	kg	No change	No change
Hematocrit	% cells	38–42	43–46
Plasma protein	g/dl	6.0–6.5	6.5–7.0
Plasma sodium	mEq/L	140	140
Plasma chloride	mEq/L	100	100
Plasma potassium	mEq/L	3.5–4.0	2.5–3.0
Std. bicarbonate	mEq/L	24	15
Blood pH	—	7.65	7.75
Blood PCO_2	mm Hg	25	10
Blood PaO_2	mm Hg	80–90	80–90

interest. Acute hypocapnia can progress to severe degrees of alkalosis with tetany and/or cardiac arrhythmias in short order (minutes or hours).

The blood carbon dioxide tension may fall below 30 mm Hg with great rapidity, this being the characteristic *laboratory finding* of the disease. Levels around 30 to 35 mm Hg are characteristic of most acutely ill patients, particularly those on assisted ventilation. If the PCO_2 falls below 15 mm Hg, alkalosis can become extremely severe (pH over 7.70), and there is a threat of sudden death due to cardiac arrhythmias. Characteristically, potassium is depressed—again an association of the hypokalemia with alkalosis. In acute hypercapnia, whole-blood pH falls directly to low levels with great rapidity. Here, conversely, in hypocapnia, whole-blood pH rises to levels higher than in any other situation and is characteristically highly refractory to treatment; pH values as high as 7.75 have been recorded. If the patient is digitalized, digitalis toxicity can occur without any change in dose or blood level.

Treatment

Normalization (reduction) of ventilation is the only treatment for this disorder. There are many ways of doing this in patients on respiratory assistance. In acute hypocapnia, an essentially respiratory situation, treatment by the infusion of metabolic acids is both unavailing and dangerous.

Alkalosis shifts the oxyhemoglobin dissociation curve to the left without any acute change in synthesis of diphosphoglycerate. This produces an anomalous failure to oxygenate the tissues, even though the hyperventilation would appear to be a sort of "super oxygenation." There is, therefore, a rising concentration of lactate that, in this disorder, may reach levels around 3.0 mM/L, a lesser elevation of lactate than is associated with low-flow acidosis. The anomalous association of lactate accumulation with alkalosis should be noted. If carbon monoxide poisoning is suspected, if the patient has been a heavy smoker or has been in a closed space with a conflagration, or if the patient has been exposed to drugs or industrial toxins, the oxyhemoglobin dissociation curve should be measured. A markedly left-shifted oxyhemoglobin dissociation curve may also be associated with hypophosphatemia and with an anomalous increase in lactate owing to failure of tissue oxygenation. A mild hypocapnia is the tip-off to the compensatory hyperventilation.

Syndrome 22. Post-Traumatic Alkalosis

See Table 11-21.

Definition, Terminology, and Related Terms

Post-traumatic alkalosis is the alkalosis characteristically observed in the severely injured patient, the result of multifactorial pathogenesis, as will be described. *Transfusion alkalosis* refers to one very important component of post-traumatic alkalosis without reference to the remainder of the picture. *Post-traumatic pulmonary insufficiency with hyperventilation* likewise refers to a component. *Acute post-traumatic hyperaldosteronism* refers to a third component. None of these terms is synonymous with the total picture as described here.

Clinical Setting

1. *Severe injury* with adequate resuscitation
2. *Severe injury,* particularly if associated with:
   a. Prolonged *nasogastric suction* with removal of gastric juice

Table 11-21. Post-Traumatic Alkalosis (Syndrome 22)

		Major Findings	
	Unit	Typical	Extreme
Body weight	kg	Gain 1	Gain 3–4
Hematocrit	% cells	37	37
Plasma protein	g/dl	6.0	5.0
Plasma sodium	mEq/L	135	130
Plasma chloride	mEq/L	90	70
Plasma potassium	mEq/L	3.5–4.0	2.5–3.0
Std. bicarbonate	mEq/L	28	32
Blood pH	—	7.55	7.70
Blood PCO_2	mm Hg	30	25
Blood PaO_2	mm Hg	70	60
Blood lactate	mM/L	2.0	4.0

b. Multiple *transfusions* with transfusion alkalosis
c. A prior volume-reduction with a prolonged *aldosterone* effect on the kidney
d. Some *pulmonary shunting* with hyperventilation of perfused segments

Addition or Subtraction

As evidenced from the above, this is a combined syndrome. The addition of sodium citrate in transfusion obviously contributes to the alkalosis, while renal excretion of acid, hyperventilation, and gastric juice loss are all subtraction components in a multifactorial disorder whose net vector is in the alkalotic direction.

Body Composition and Body Weight

As noted in the section on the normal postoperative patient, severe trauma brings in its wake a transiently elevated level of catecholamines in the blood, followed by a gradually rising level of blood glucagon. There is gluconeogenesis at the expense of muscle protein. Fat oxidation is hastened. This net combination produces weight loss, and that is the typical situation during post-traumatic alkalosis. Nonetheless, overinfusion of sodium-rich fluid greatly accentuates the disorder and may obliterate the normal weight loss. After severe trauma patients should be expected to lose some weight; the net deficit in body composition is negligible through the oxidation of this small amount of fat and protein. If the weight loss is obliterated by infusions, it means that too much fluid has been given.

Abnormalities of Autoregulation

As is evident from the foregoing, this disorder, like several other syndromes described herein, is a mixture of pathogenic factors, some of which are the result of the exaggerated operation of normal homeostatic regulators. Post-traumatic hyperaldosteronism is an obvious example here. In general, any stress that tends to produce hypokalemia and alkalosis (e.g., liver disease with hemorrhage and transfusion) is made much worse by the superimposition of the surgical operation because of its greatly increased stimulus to adrenocortical production of aldosterone. Clearly, this should be taken into consideration by the surgeon in the administration of potassium-enriched acidifying solutions such as KCl.

The typical combination of *laboratory findings* in post-traumatic alkalosis on the second or third day is a pH mildly elevated at 7.55; a chloride mildly depressed at 85 mEq/L; and potassium depressed at 2.5 to 3.0 mEq/L. Serum sodium concentration is usually 135 to 138 mEq/L. Oxygenation may be borderline, as indicated by an arterial oxygen tension of 80 mm Hg on room air. There are rapid respiration and hyperventilation of portions of lung normally perfused. The carbon dioxide tension is in the region of 28 to 34 mm Hg, and the urine is acid, containing large amounts of potassium and almost no sodium.

Treatment

The best treatment of post-traumatic alkalosis is merely the continued energetic management of the patient to maintain good tissue perfusion, bearing in mind the factors that will make the alkalosis worse. Gastrointestinal suction should be discontinued as soon as possible. As already mentioned, some of the fluid removed by aspiration can be replaced, as long as the gastrointestinal tract is prevented from accumulating swallowed air. The administration of acidifying solutions such as KCl should be liberal (e.g., 120 to 160 mM per day). If hyperventilation is a persistent component and the patient is on assisted ventilation, it is possible to normalize the carbon dioxide tension. In extreme cases with continued obstinate inability to excrete sodium in an acid potassium-rich urine, the use of aldosterone antagonists is rational but should be done with great care in cardiac patients who have been digitalized. Treatment with HCl is rational if carried out with caution and close monitoring.

Post-traumatic alkalosis in mild form is both common and harmless.

The principal hazard of post-traumatic alkalosis when it is severe lies in the production of cardiac arrhythmias and increased sensitivity to digitalis. Arrhythmias may be sudden and fatal and often come without warning. In addition, there is a tendency to narcosis, sleepiness, and lack of normal cerebral function.

Reduction of bicarbonate and pH to normal with the opening up of urinary excretion of sodium are signs that the post-traumatic alkalosis is abating. Post-traumatic alkalosis of very severe grades can occur after open-heart surgery; as noted several times in the preceding, hypokalemia and alkalosis are especially hazardous in cardiac patients.

Syndrome 23. Base-Loss Acidosis

See Table 11-22.

Definition, Terminology, and Related Terms

Base-loss acidosis is a metabolic acidosis due to a desalting water loss in which the fluid lost from the body has an alkaline pH. Base-loss acidosis is the most common form of subtraction acidosis found in surgical patients.

Table 11-22. Base-Loss Acidosis (Syndrome 23)

		Acute	Chronic	
	Unit	Severe Acute	Poorly Compensated (Pulmonary and Renal Disease)	Well Compensated
Std. bicarbonate	mEq/L	15	10	10
Blood pH	—	7.25	7.16	7.35
Blood PCO_2	mm Hg	35	30	20
Blood PaO_2	mm Hg	80	80	90
Urine pH	—	5.0	6.0	4.5
Urine titratable acidity	—	Low	Low	Very high

Notes: 1. See Table 11-9, *Desalting Water Loss,* for general setting.

2. The acid-base changes depend on the extent of the loss of sodium bicarbonate in gastrointestinal secretions (such as diarrhea), the extent of the ventilatory-respiratory compensation (hypocapnia), and the ability of the kidney to secrete an acid urine. Three groups are discernible: severe acute, poorly compensated, and well compensated.

Clinical Setting

1. *Diarrheal disease* in the infant or adult, including salmonella, typhoid, cholera, ulcerative colitis, Crohn's disease
2. *Pancreatic fistula*
3. *Small bowel fistula*

Addition or Subtraction

This is a subtraction acidosis, pure and simple.

Body Composition and Body Weight

Body composition shows a marked reduction in the total exchangeable sodium; there is loss of weight corresponding to the desalting water loss.

Abnormalities of Autoregulation

The homeostatic regulator called into play here is renal conservation of sodium by both of the mechanisms that stimulate aldosterone: the renin-angiotensin mechanism on the one hand, and ACTH on the other. This conservation mechanism may become chronically active in patients with ileostomies who are constantly in a mild state of hyperaldosteronism.

Though this homeostatic regulator tends to conserve sodium and favor loss of potassium in the urine, it is not particularly effective when the loss of alkaline juices from the body exceeds 1500 ml/day, a common occurrence in diarrheal diseases, intestinal fistulas, pancreatic fistulas, and the like.

The deep respirations so often seen in diabetic acidosis (an addition metabolic acidosis), compensating to some extent for addition of acid by ventilatory loss of carbon dioxide, are rarely seen here and would be of little effectiveness in any event.

In base-loss acidosis, the typical *laboratory finding* is a pH that rarely falls below 7.25. In pure metabolic acidosis this is a dangerously low pH. Bicarbonate falls commensurately to the region of 15 mEq/L. Plasma sodium concentration usually drops, and potassium concentration rises. The "anion gap" or difference between sodium and chloride concentrations will be narrowed to an extent usually proportionate to the fall in bicarbonate.

Treatment

As already indicated, desalting water loss is the ideal setting for the infusion of sodium-rich fluids. In this syndrome, in which acidosis is a complication, the infusion of sodium bicarbonate is uniquely appropriate; sodium lactate also can be used, the lactate being rapidly oxidized to bicarbonate.

It should be noted in passing that metabolic acidosis of the addition type (examples are renal acidosis and diabetic acidosis) should not be treated with sodium bicarbonate save with the most extreme caution because of the danger of oversalting and cardiac failure. In the pure base-loss acidosis, sodium bicarbonate infusion is most appropriate.

Syndrome 24. Low Flow Acidosis

See Table 11-23.

Definition, Terminology, and Related Terms

Low flow acidosis is the lactic acidosis of shock or other low flow states (cardiac arrest). *Lactic acidosis* refers to a chemical state, but without reference to the cause. *Hypoxic acidosis* is a misnomer because ventilatory hypoxia is a weak stimulus to lactate generation. *Hypoperfusion acidosis* and *ischemic acidosis* are synonymous terms. *Shock acidosis* is synonymous; *washout acidosis* refers to an analogous situation arising from the reperfusion of localized ischemic tissue.

Table 11-23. Low Flow Acidosis (Syndrome 24)

		Major Findings	
	Unit	Typical	Extreme
Body weight	kg	Falling	Falling rapidly
Hematocrit	% cells	37	30
Plasma protein	g/dl	5.0	4.5
Plasma tonicity	mOsm/L	280	270
Plasma nonelectrolyte tonicity	mOsm/L	5–10	5–10
Plasma sodium	mEq/L	130	120
Plasma chloride	mEq/L	100	100
Std. bicarbonate	mEq/L	12	8
Blood lactate	mM/L	5	15
Blood urea nitrogen	mg/dl	15–30	70–90
Blood PCO_2	mm Hg	30	25
Blood PaO_2	mm Hg	70	60
Blood pH	—	7.25	7.15
Blood oxyhemoglobin dissociation curve	—	Left shift	Right shift

Clinical Setting

1. *Hypoperfusion of tissues due to shock* and low flow states resulting from trauma
2. *Hypoperfusion of tissues resulting from cardiac damage,* as in myocardial infarction with shock or following cardiac arrest
3. *Other low flow states* associated with trauma to the mediastinum or hemopericardium, and pericardial tamponade
4. *Occlusion of the aorta* or other arteries, sometimes large enough in mass to produce a generalized acidosis, particularly when circulation is restored as a "washout effect"

Addition or Subtraction

This is an addition acidosis due to the accumulation of lactic acid within cells. In this regard it is unique because the acidosis arises within the cells rather than within the extracellular fluid; the changes in blood are therefore but a dim reflection of the primary disorder within the cell.

Body Composition and Body Weight

Changes are not marked in most cases and depend on the underlying cause and the rest of the clinical setting. Low flow states are usually associated with such severe stressful disease that rapid loss of body weight is the rule.

Abnormalities of Autoregulation

It is the intracellular acidosis, dimly perceived as an extracellular pH change and lactate accumulation, that is fundamentally at fault in low flow acidosis. Lactate is itself a harmless anionic intermediary in carbohydrate oxidation. It can be injected in large amounts without harm and is quickly oxidized in most situations. In the lactic acidosis of low flow state, the accumulation of extracellular lactate is a barometer of the extent of hydrogen ion accumulation within cells due to lactic acid. The homeostatic regulator is therefore lactate oxidation, and in low flow states this cannot occur. If flow is returned to normal, lactate oxidation occurs rapidly, but it is noteworthy that patients that have been in a low flow state for a relatively long time may show residual lactate elevations for several days after recovery. Both hydrogen ion and lactate can be excreted by the kidney; in a low flow state renal function is essentially nil, and this pathway is unavailable. Upon return to normal flow, lactate can be burned in many tissues, notably heart and liver; it disappears rapidly. Treatment of patients in a low flow state by infusions of lactate-containing solutions, such as Ringers lactate, does not make the disorder worse because the lactate ion is merely a harmless bystander; it is the hydrogen ion that has been at fault. Ringers lactate solution is buffered to a pH above that of normal blood in the pharmacy before it is used; while providing lactate, it does not present the threat of increasing the acidosis. If its infusion helps the circulation, it may assist in clearing lactate.

Depression of plasma bicarbonate as a linear function of the lactate accumulation and is the typical *laboratory finding* in almost all cases. The lactate accumulates at a more rapid rate than pyruvate, with an elevated lactate-pyruvate ratio, otherwise expressed as an accumulation of excess lactate. These various measurements of lactate and pyruvate are not clinically essential, but they may be helpful and instructive. The blood pH typically is in the region of 7.15 to 7.25. It must be emphasized again that pH values in this range are dangerous when they are of metabolic origin, whereas they are quickly produced and rectified when the cause is purely respiratory. The patient who has been in a low flow state (e.g., shock after trauma and blood loss) and is observed to have a low plasma bicarbonate level with an arterial pH of 7.15 is in severe and dangerous low flow acidosis.

Treatment

The treatment of low flow acidosis is the restoration of tissue perfusion to normal, usually by blood transfusion. There can be no better example of the importance of viewing the patient in his entire perspective than the treatment of this particular form of metabolic acidosis by blood transfusion. Whatever steps are taken to restore flow to normal—and they include many details not covered in this section—the result should be an improvement in perfusion, with diffuse oxidation of lactate. In many instances, syndromes have been described in this chapter wherein surgical steps themselves are essential to the treatment of metabolic disorders. Low flow acidosis is the prototypic example. If this is due to hemorrhage, for example, or undrained sepsis, aggressive surgical steps, including major operation, may be necessary for its rectification. The infusion of sodium bicarbonate must be considered as both dangerous and temporizing. If large amounts are given, pulmonary edema and death will almost surely ensue. In appropriate dosage, it may tide the patient through a difficult phase of low flow acidosis. Most important, however, is the fact that low flow acidosis is rather quickly rectified if tissue perfusion is returned to normal, and it is this, rather than the mere buffering of acid, that should be the objective of treatment.

Restoration of blood flow, urine volume, and tissue perfusion to normal is essential. The pH and plasma bicarbonate concentration are important guides to progress. If lactate itself has been measured, its gradual disappearance and oxidation is a demonstration that metabolic evidences of the low flow state have been oxidized.

Selected Readings

Davenport, HW (ed). *ABC of Acid Base Chemistry: The Elements of Physiological Blood-Gas Chemistry for Medical Students and Physicians.* (6th ed). Chicago: University of Chicago Press, 1974.

Gamble, JL. *Chemical Anatomy, Physiology and Pathology of Extracellular Fluid: A Lecture Syllabus* (6th ed). Cambridge, MA: Harvard University Press, 1967.

12

Glutamine as a Metabolic Intermediate

Steve F. Abcouwer
Barrie P. Bode
*Wiley W. Souba**

Physiologic and Biochemical Importance of Glutamine

Glutamine is a neutral nonessential glycogenic amino acid with an anhydrous molecular weight of 146.1. Unlike most other amino acids, it has two nitrogen side chains: an α-amino group and an amide group. Glutamine is the most abundant amino acid in the blood, present at a concentration of 600 to 800 μM. A high tissue delivery (delivery = blood flow × concentration) and the presence of two nitrogen side chains combine to make glutamine the most important "nitrogen shuttle" in the body, accounting for 30% to 35% of all amino acid nitrogen transported in the blood. In this capacity, glutamine serves as a vehicle of transporting ammonia in a nontoxic form from peripheral tissues to visceral organs where the ammonia can be excreted as ammonium (kidneys) or converted to urea (liver). In fact, it can be estimated that as much as 50% of the nitrogen excreted in the urine (as ammonium or urea) is derived from glutamine.

The circulating concentration of glutamine is maintained at a fairly constant level and is dependent on the relative rates of net glutamine uptake and release by the various organs in the body. Under normal conditions, systemic rates of uptake equal rates of release, so that blood glutamine levels are maintained at approximately 600 μM.

*Supported by NIH grants HL44986 and CA45327, a grant from the American Institute for Cancer Research, and a Career Development Award from the American Cancer Society.

The metabolism of glutamine has been studied in numerous tissues, and its net flux rates across a variety of organs have been measured [1]. Although interspecies differences exist, it is apparent that the small intestine is the principal organ of glutamine uptake in the postabsorptive, basal state [2–7]. In contrast, after a meal, the liver becomes the major glutamine consumer, acting in its capacity as an organ of glutamine homeostasis. The kidneys also exhibit net glutamine uptake in the postabsorptive state, but renal glutamine consumption only becomes appreciable during acidosis [8], when additional circulating glutamine is needed to support renal ammoniagenesis. In contrast, net glutamine release occurs from skeletal muscle and from the lungs [9], both of which have a considerable capacity to synthesize glutamine de novo from glutamate and ammonia. In the rat, whole-body glutamine exchange occurs at the rate of about 1300 nmol/100 g body weight/min. At this rate, daily whole-body exchange exceeds total body glutamine stores several-fold and indicates that de novo glutamine biosynthesis constantly occurs at an appreciable rate. Glutamine consumed in the diet participates in these interorgan relationships and modifies the rate at which the splanchnic bed consumes circulating glutamine.

Glutamine plays an important role in a number of metabolic pathways (Figure 12-1). In 1955, Eagle [10] reviewed the nutritional needs of mammalian cells in culture and emphasized the importance of glutamine as a nutrient. Its importance in nitrogen metabolism was more recently emphasized by Krebs, who stated, "Most amino acids have multiple functions, but glutamine appears to be the most versatile" [11]. Glutamine is found in relatively high concentrations in many mammalian cells where it serves as a major respiratory fuel source; as a nitrogen donor for the biosynthesis of a number of important compounds such as nucleotides, amino sugars, and amino acids; and as the precursor of many amino acids, metabolic intermediates, and macromolecules.

Glutamine has several additional properties that suggest it occupies an important position in normal and pathophysiologic states. Besides its distinction as the most abundant amino acid in the blood, glutamine is usually the most abundant amino acid in the intracellular free amino acid pool (Figure 12-2). [*Editor's Note:* It should be noted that in different rat skeletal muscles, which may be composed of largely one fiber type, the free amino acid concentrations are quite variable. In soleus, glutamic acid levels can approach those of glutamine, whereas in plantaris and gastrocnemius, glycine and glutamine are present in roughly equal concentrations (12)]. Excluding taurine, glutamine can comprise approximately 60% of the amino acid pool in human skeletal muscle, where it is present at a concentration of approximately 20 mmol/L of intracellular water. This level is 30 times higher than the circulating glutamine concentration (0.6 mmol/L), so that a large intracellular/extracellular gradient is established. It has been hypothesized that maintenance of this gradient may be important for muscle to fulfill its role as a glutamine exporter, because glutamine efflux from skeletal muscle may be impaired when the muscle concentrations fall to very low levels such as those observed during sepsis.

Glutamine concentrations in blood and tissues

Figure 12-1. Some pathways of glutamine metabolism and some functions served by glutamine in mammalian cells.

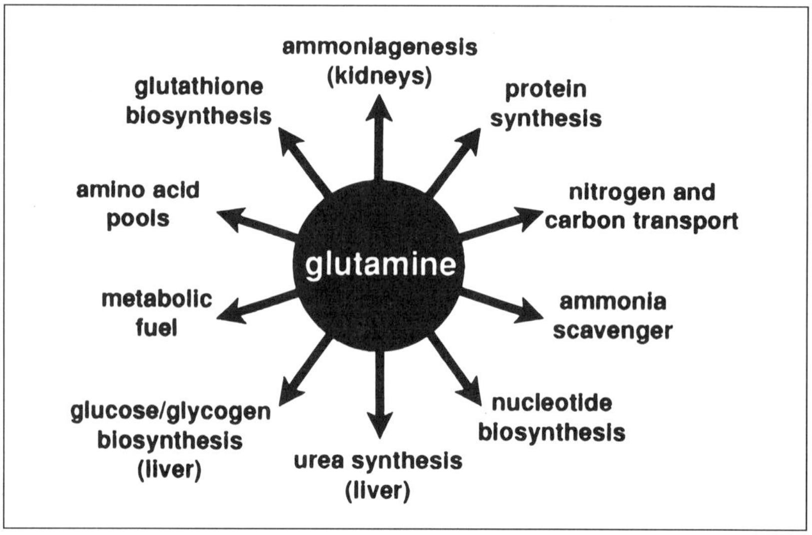

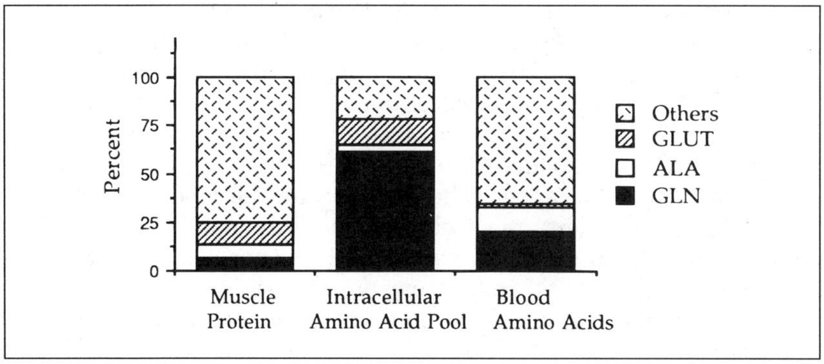

Figure 12-2. Relative concentrations of glutamine in skeletal muscle myofibrillar protein, the intracellular amino acid pool, and in blood. The intracellular:plasma gradient is 30:1. ALA = alanine; GLN = glutamine; GLUT = glutamate. (Modified from Bergstrom J, et al. Intracellular free amino acid concentration in human muscle tissue. *J Appl Physiol* 36:693, 1974; Kominz DR, et al. The amino acid composition of actin, myosin, tropomyosin, and the meromyosins. *Arch Biochem Biophys* 50:48, 1951; Souba WW, Smith RJ, Wilmore DW. Glutamine metabolism by the intestinal tract. *J Parenter Enteral Nutr* 9:608, 1985.)

fall markedly after catabolic stress such as surgery, trauma, and infection [13–15]. The decline in glutamine concentrations caused by these insults exceeds that of all other amino acids in both magnitude and duration. Although the cause for this lengthy depletion is not entirely clear, the return of glutamine concentrations to preinjury levels correlates with the return of a patient's functional capacity. Thus, the glutamine concentration in the convalescent period may be a biochemical marker of return to health and well-being. Consequently, glutamine has become of considerable interest to clinicians and nutritionists, and this interest has stimulated studies that have tested the hypothesis that glutamine is a conditionally essential nutrient [16–19].

Under conditions of health, the assumption that glutamine is not required in the diet is probably valid, although it is difficult to test the hypothesis because glutamine is present in virtually all dietary proteins. Studies evaluating the effects of glutamine-free nutrition have used specially formulated diets that have other characteristics (besides being glutamine-free) that may adversely affect health. For example, enteral studies evaluating the impact of glutamine have used liquid elemental diets that may be fiber-free. Nonetheless, there is growing evidence that, in certain catabolic disease states, glutamine is a conditionally essential amino acid. Most naturally occurring food proteins contain between 4% and 8% of their amino acid residues as glutamine [20], and therefore less than 10 g of dietary glutamine is likely to be consumed daily by the average person. In contrast to this usual dietary availability, recent studies in stressed patients indicate that considerably larger amounts of glutamine (20–40 g/day) may be necessary to maintain glutamine homeostasis after a catabolic insult. Thus, from a nutritional standpoint, glutamine may be thought of as a drug as well as a nutrient.

Transport of Glutamine Across Cell Membranes

Except for the brush border, which takes up glutamine from the gut lumen, the bloodstream is the source of glutamine for all cells. Three fundamental factors determine the exchange (flux) of glutamine (or any amino acid) across an organ: (1) the delivery of the amino acid to the tissue (delivery = flow × arterial concentration); (2) the rate of intracellular synthesis and degradation of the substrate; and (3) the intrinsic activity of cell membrane carriers that transport glutamine into and out of the cell. The transport of extracellular glutamine into the cytoplasm occurs via distinct amino acid transport systems [21]. Each system presumably relates to a discrete integral plasma membrane-bound transporter protein that contains several membrane-spanning domains. The characteristics of specific carrier(s) that mediate glutamine transport across the plasma membrane vary from cell to cell. Most of these are sodium-dependent carriers because they require sodium ions to transport glutamine into the cells.

The Mechanism of Carrier-Mediated Glutamine Transport

The transport of glutamine into the cytoplasm of the cell is an active process that involves binding of the amino acid to an active site on the carrier protein [21–25]. Glutamine can also diffuse into cells, but this component of uptake is a minor pathway at physiologic amino acid concentrations. Distinct glutamine transport systems have been functionally defined on the basis of their amino acid selectivities and physicochemical properties. None of these carriers are specific for glutamine, but rather they transport both glutamine and structurally related amino acids.

In the case of Na^+-activated glutamine transporters (i.e., systems A, ASC, N, B^{o+}), the substrate movement is coupled to the electrochemical gradient established across the cell membrane, largely by the Na^+/K^+ ATPase. The driving forces that energize glutamine transport are provided by the sodium chemical gradient as well as the membrane electrical potential. Extracellular to intracellular transport and accumulation of glutamine is favored when the activator sodium ion binds to the transporter, followed by binding of the glutamine to its active site (Figure 12-3). The transmembrane electrical potential (intracellularly negative) promotes binding of the sodium ion to the carrier, which in turn increases the affinity of the extracellularly oriented co-transporter binding site for the amino acid. Subsequent glutamine attachment forms a sodium/glutamine co-transporter complex. A conformational change of the complex results in delivery of the Na^+ ion and glutamine into the cytoplasm. Co-transport of sodium allows the cell to use this ion's electrochemical driving force to accumulate glutamine in the cytoplasm at levels far above those that would be achieved by equilibrium across the plasma membrane.

In general, the vectorial movement of sodium-independent amino acid transport (into the cell or out of the cell) depends on the relative intracellular and extracellular concentrations of the amino acid [26]. That is, the direction of transport is usually determined by the amino acid gradient. Because of the large glutamine concentration gradient, most glutamine efflux is mediated by Na^+-dependent carriers. However, sodium-independent transport can participate in the concentrative uptake of amino acids under the appropriate conditions. For example, because of its high "exchange" transport properties, the Na^+-independent system L (which can mediate glutamine transport) can accumulate amino acids against a concentration gradient by counter-transport of a second amino acid whose gradient has been established by one or more of the sodium-dependent systems [21].

The activity of the specific cell membrane glutamine transporter refers to its intrinsic ability to bind glutamine and to its capacity to transport it in (or out of) the cell (Figure 12-4). Characterization of carrier-mediated glutamine transport across cell membranes includes determination of

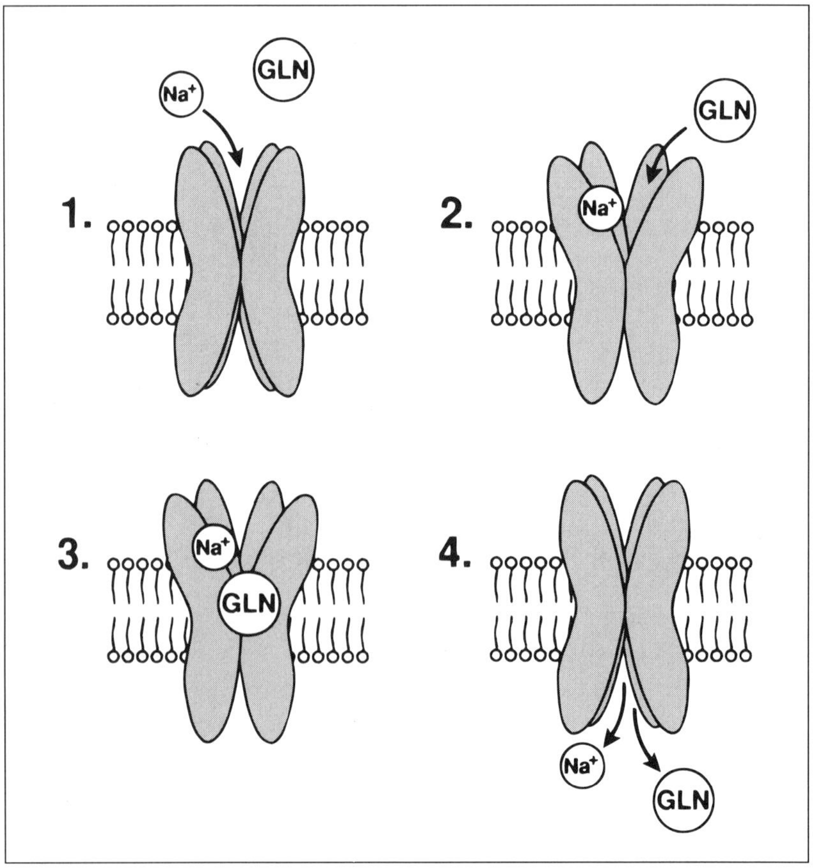

Figure 12-3. Conceptual schematic of a membrane-bound sodium-dependent amino acid carrier. (1) In the "preferred random" binding model, glutamine transport is favored when the activator sodium ion binds preferentially to the transporter. (2) Initial binding of the sodium ion increases the affinity of the extracellularly oriented co-transporter binding site for subsequent glutamine attachment. (3) A sodium/glutamine/co-transporter complex is formed. (4) A conformational change of the complex results in delivery of the sodium ion and glutamine into the cytoplasm of the cell. The translocated sodium ion is transported out of the cell by the Na^+/K^+ ATPase transporter to maintain the electrochemical gradient, while glutamine is metabolized within the cell. (Modified from Stevens BR, Wright EM. Kinetics of the intestinal brush-border proline (Imino) carrier. *J Biol Chem* 262:6546, 1987.)

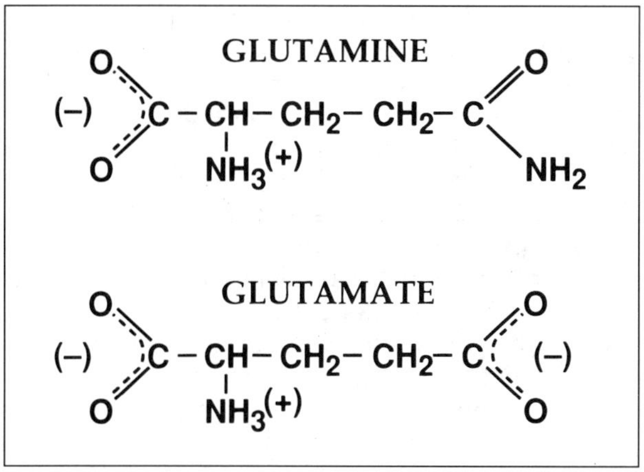

Figure 12-4. Molecular structure of glutamine and glutamate. At physiologic pH, the carboxyl group of glutamine carries a negative charge while the amino group is protonated, resulting in the molecule carrying a net 0 charge (neutral). Note the similarity in structure to glutamate, in which the amide nitrogen has been replaced by a hydroxyl group, conferring to it a negative charge. This apparently minor change accounts for the inability of glutamate to replace glutamine in culture medium and for the transport of these two amino acids across mammalian cell membranes via different transport systems.

the maximal transport velocity (Vmax, expressed in pmoles of glutamine transported/mg of vesicle or cell protein/time) and the Michaelis constant (Km, expressed in μM) of the specific transporter. Vmax reflects the number of functional carriers in the cell membrane, and Km relates to affinity for glutamine. A saturation plot is generated when transport velocity is plotted as a function of glutamine concentration. The Vmax is reached when all of the transport molecules in the plasma membrane are saturated by substrate. Under these conditions, adding more amino acid will not increase the rate of transport. The Vmax, therefore, reflects the number of functional carriers in the plasma membrane. The Km is the concentration of substrate necessary to achieve one-half maximal transport velocity. At the Km, half of the transporters will be bound and, therefore, the Km reflects the affinity of the carrier for glutamine.

Transporter kinetics can also be depicted graphically using an Eadie-Hofstee diagram that plots transport velocity (y-axis) as a function of velocity/substrate concentration (x-axis). A homogeneous population of transporters (i.e., uptake by one system) results in a single straight line plot. In this plot, the y-intercept is the Vmax and the negative slope of the line is the Km. Frequently, an amino acid can gain entry into a cell via two sodium-dependent carriers; in this case nonlinear regression analysis generates two lines with different kinetic parameters. An example of this is the Na^+-dependent transport of glutamine by type II alveolar cells, in which glutamine uptake is mediated by system A and system ASC [27].

In general, the transport activity of a specific carrier can increase or decrease in two principal ways; either the affinity of the transporter for its substrate changes (Km effect) or the number of active transporters in the cell membrane changes (Vmax effect, Vmax = maximal transport velocity). Conceptually, an increase in transporter affinity occurs because the conformation (tertiary structure) of the carrier protein (or possibly an adjacent co-modulator protein) changes such that the substrate binds more easily (more rapidly, more tightly) to its binding site on the transporter. Presumably, such a change would result in more amino acid molecules translocated into the cell in a given period of time for a given substrate concentration below saturating levels. In contrast to a Km effect, an increase in the number of active transporter proteins in the cell membrane often involves de novo protein synthesis, often of the carrier itself. Alternatively, a regulatory protein could be synthesized that activates transporters that are normally repressed. Theoretically, the specific activity of individual transporter molecules might be modulated, such as the case of amino acid–dependent activation of hepatic transport system N [28]. Perhaps through posttranslational modifications, carrier structure could be altered in such a way as to promote or attenuate the conformational shift that results in substrate delivery to the interior of the cell. Although feasible, this mechanism of altering Vmax has not yet been demonstrated. [*Editor's Note:* In general, although changes in Km do occur, one must be cautious, because most changes in transport (as detailed below) are secondary to changes in Vmax or other factors.]

Changes in the extracellular Na^+ concentration generally affect only the Km and not the Vmax. Therefore, changes in membrane permeability to Na^+, changes in the coupling, and changes in potential difference will always affect Km (affinity). The Km and Vmax may be affected together, depending on the exact transport mechanism and the coupling-to-membrane potential difference.

In the intact organ, an increase in glutamine uptake indicates an increase in transport but does not necessarily equate to an increase in plasma membrane transport activity (i.e., an increase in carrier number or in carrier affinity). For example, the carrier may have an enormous capacity to handle an increased delivery in glutamine, and the increased uptake will be caused by an increase in transport by carriers that are normally unbound. A good example is the 10-fold increase in hepatic glutamine consumption observed 12 hours after an endotoxin challenge [29]. Measurement of glutamine transport across the hepatocyte plasma membrane showed no increase in transport kinetic parameters with endotoxin treatment; instead, the marked increase in consumption was the result of a 50% increase in hepatic blood flow, a small increase in the arterial glutamine concentration, and a substantial increase in intracellular glutamine metabolism. Although the amount of glutamine that was transported across the cell membrane was enhanced, this increase was not the result of a change in carrier affinity or number, but rather of the capacity of the carrier to handle the "extra" glutamine load delivered to the liver.

Glutamine Transport Systems

Few of the transporter proteins have been identified or isolated, so investigators have relied on kinetic and competitive-inhibition analyses to define and characterize the individual systems (Table 12-1) [21,23,30,31]. Assignment of system names has been confounded by several factors, including overlapping substrate specificities, lack of unique transportable analogues that define single systems, variations among species, changing conventions for nomenclature, and the failure to date to purify and clone most of the transporter proteins.

Most of the glutamine transport systems described in Table 12-1 are present in the plasma membrane of many different cells. As pointed out earlier, these carriers are not specific for glutamine, but rather transport several amino acids. Unique carriers include the sodium-dependent system N carrier, which to date has been identified only in the hepatocyte plasma membrane [32]. Designated system N because of its selectivity for amino acids with nitrogen-containing side chains (glutamine, histidine, and asparagine), the transporter exhibits characteristics that distinguish it from the other two primary sodium-dependent amino acid transporters (systems A and ASC) present in the rat hepatocyte [31]. Similarly, the liver contains a sodium-independent carrier that also appears to be selective for amino acid amides (glutamine, histidine, and asparagine) and has been named system n. A sodium-dependent transporter in skeletal muscle has been named Nm because of its similarity to hepatic system N [30].

The brush border of the intestinal epithelium may also possess a unique glutamine transporter not found thus far in other tissues, although its substrate profile closely matches that of system ASC with some notable exceptions. The system B carrier (formally NBB, i.e., neutral brush-border carrier) is sodium dependent, transports glutamine and most dipolar amino acids, and is closely related to system Bo^{+} found in blastocysts and oocytes. System B has been found in the brush border of the human Caco-2 intestinal epithelial cell line [33,34], rabbit intestine [35,36], and in human small intestine [37]. After a meal, when the glutamine concentration in the gut lumen is high, the carriers become saturated, and simple passive diffusion may actually exceed carrier-mediated uptake. In response to increased availability of glutamine in the gut lumen, the system B protein (which may bear some similarity to system N) appears to be up-regulated to more effectively accomplish uptake [38]. The absorbed amino acids are transported via the basolateral membrane to the portal blood.

Other well-defined transporters that mediate glutamine transport into cells include system A, which mediates a portion of glutamine transport

Table 12-1. Some Tissues in Which Sodium-Dependent Carrier-Mediated Glutamine Transport Has Been Characterized

Tissue	Transport System	Regulation	Comments
Hepatocytes	N and A	Insulin, glucagon, glucocorticoids, IL-6?	85% of transport is via system N; may be unique to hepatocytes
Pulmonary artery endothelial cells	ASC	Endotoxin, cytokines	Cytokine-stimulated increase in transport takes 8–12 hr
Type II alveolar cells	A and ASC	Unknown	
Fibroblasts	A and ASC	TNF	System A carrier is induced when cells are starved
Small intestinal brush border	B	EGF, γ-IFN	Unique to brush border
Muscle	N^{m}	Glucocorticoids	? Similar to system N in hepatocytes
Human lymphocytes	ASC	Unknown	Increase in Vmax in cells stimulated by concanavalin A

into hepatocytes [31], lymphocytes [39], type II alveolar cells [27], and fibroblasts [40], and system ASC, which mediates glutamine transport by pulmonary endothelial cells [41], fibroblasts [40], and type II alveolar cells [27].

Mitochondrial Glutamine Transport

The transport of glutamine into the mitochondria (where it can be metabolized by glutaminase) has been less extensively studied than has plasma membrane glutamine transport. Attempts have been hampered by the ability to distinguish glutamine transport from its metabolism in intact mitochondria. Mitochondria contain both an outer and inner mitochondrial membrane with an intervening intermembrane space, an anatomic arrangement that has made it difficult to study glutamine transport. Moreover, because of the rapid rate of mitochondrial glutamine breakdown by phosphate-dependent glutaminase, it is impossible to monitor glutamine transport directly. Attempts to use glutaminase inhibitors have been largely unsuccessful because of the lack of specificity of these compounds.

To circumvent this problem, Sastrasinh has developed a method of preparing submitochondrial particles (SMP, membrane vesicles from inner mitochondrial membrane) to study glutamine transport [42]. This preparation results in membranes nearly completely devoid of glutaminase activity, thus allowing transport to be studied independently of metabolism. In contrast to studies with intact organelles, in which the presence of a specific carrier has never been rigorously demonstrated, glutamine transport in SMP has characteristics indicative of carrier-mediated transport. These features include saturation kinetics, trans-stimulation effects, substrate specificity, and the inhibition of glutamine transport by sulfhydryl reagents [Souba et al., unpublished data, 1993]. This methodology will allow further studies to be performed to gain insight into how mitochondrial glutamine transport is regulated during critical illness.

Glutamine Metabolism

Glutamine is an important source of cellular fuel as well as a source of carbon and nitrogen atoms for metabolic intermediates and for macromolecular synthesis (Figure 12-5). Glutamine can provide cellular energy through its partial oxidation to form lactate or its complete oxidation to form carbon dioxide. Glutamine is used for peptide synthesis, as the precursor to other amino acids and metabolic intermediates, and as a nitrogen donor in many pathways, including those leading to purine and pyrimidine nucleotide synthesis and the

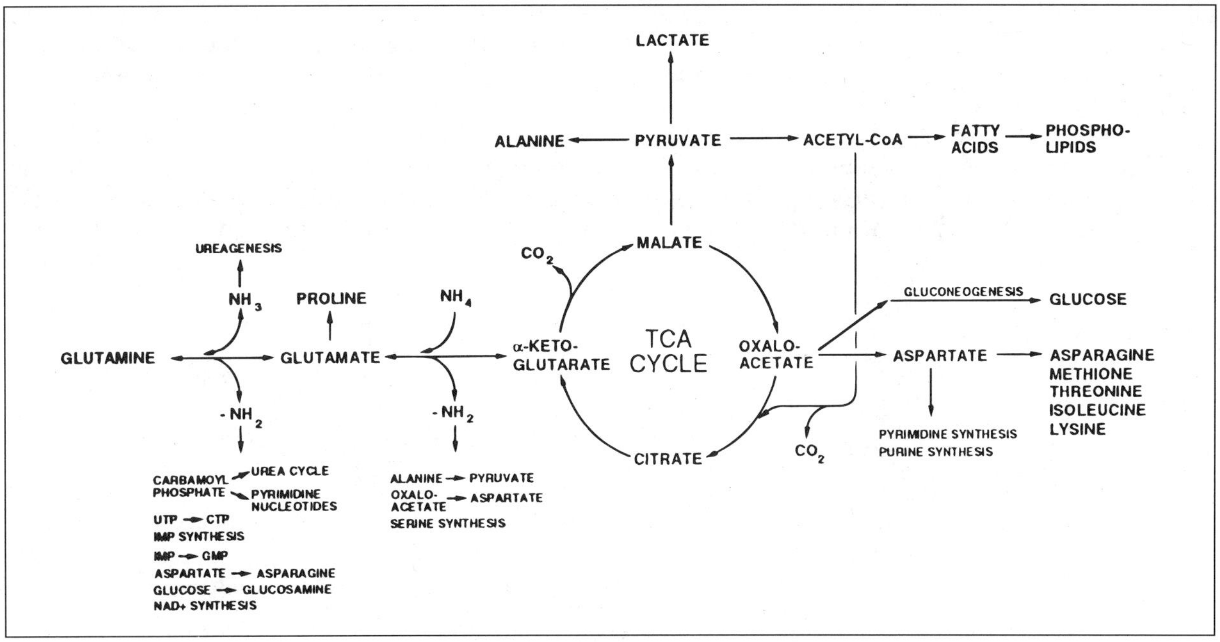

Figure 12-5. Metabolic pathways of glutamine utilization. Besides being utilized in protein synthesis, glutamine is utilized as an amide donor in many synthetic reactions that produce glutamate. Glutamate, formed in these reactions and principally by the hydrolysis of glutamine (forming ammonia), is utilized as an amine donor in many synthesis reactions. By forming α-ketoglutarate from glutamate, the carbon skeleton of glutamine enters the TCA cycle where it serves as fuel and provides many metabolic intermediates.

formation of glucosamine. In the kidneys and liver, the carbon skeleton of glutamine can be utilized for gluconeogenesis during times of starvation. Acetyl groups derived from glutamine can even be utilized in the synthesis of fatty acids. Thus, glutamine does not act simply as a building block in protein synthesis, but rather, glutamine serves many important metabolic and synthetic roles essential for cellular viability.

It is by conversion to glutamate that glutamine serves as a key respiratory fuel, metabolic precursor, and nitrogen donor (Figure 12-6). Glutamate is formed by hydrolysis of glutamine's amide side chain, and when glutamine transfers its amide group to another molecule in various synthetic reactions. Ammonia originating from glutamine via its hydrolysis and the deamination of the resulting glutamate has been found to be the major source of nitrogen used in hepatic ureagenesis [43]. Enzymatic transfer of the glutamine amide group to another molecule occurs in various synthetic reactions. For example, glutamine donates an amide group for the formation of carbamoyl phosphate, which enters the urea cycle or is used in the synthesis of pyrimidine nucleotides. Transamination from glutamine is again used in the synthesis of the pyrimidine nucleotide CTP from UTP. Glutamine contributes two amine groups in reactions leading to the synthesis of the purine nucleotide IMP and donates a third amine group in the conversion of IMP to GMP. It is by inhibition of these aminations that the glutamine analogues azerine and DON interfere with DNA synthesis and exert their antiproliferative effects [44,45]. Glutamine also donates its amide group in the synthesis of asparagine, glucosamine, and nicotinamide adenine dinucleotide (NAD^+). In the form of glutamate, the α-amino group of glutamine also is utilized in several transaminations, including the synthesis of alanine from pyruvate, the synthesis of aspartate from oxaloacetate, and the formation of phosphoserine, which is hydrolyzed to form serine.

Glutamate formed from glutamine can be converted to proline or back into glutamine. Through conversion to glutamate and then to α-ketoglutarate (2-oxoglutarate), the five-carbon backbone of glutamine enters the tricaboxylic acid cycle (TCA cycle, also known as the citric acid cycle or Kreb's cycle). In this way, glutamine serves as a major respiratory fuel source and as the precursor of many important synthetic intermediates. It is through oxaloacetate, a TCA cycle intermediate, that glutamine is converted to glucose in gluconeogenesis. Via the TCA cycle, glutamine can eventually be converted to aspartate or to alanine. Aspartate can be converted to asparagine, methionine, threonine, isoleucine, and lysine. Aspartate serves as a precursor in pyrimidine synthesis and again as an amine donor in purine synthesis. Pyruvate (the precursor of alanine) is produced from malate, a TCA cycle intermediate. Through pyruvate, glutamine can be converted to lactate or to acetyl-CoA. The acetyl group of acetyl-CoA can reenter the TCA cycle, eventually leading to the complete respiratory oxidation of glutamine carbons to carbon dioxide. Acetyl-CoA can also provide glutamine-derived carbon atoms for the synthesis of fatty acids used in the production of phospholipids for cellular membranes.

By entering the TCA cycle, glutamine can serve as the cells' primary respiratory fuel under physiologic conditions [46]. Cultured cells have been shown to convert approximately 30% of catabolized glutamine carbons to carbon dioxide and 15% to lactate, and approximately 20% of the carbons incorporated into macromolecules [46,47]. The amount of energy derived from each gluta-

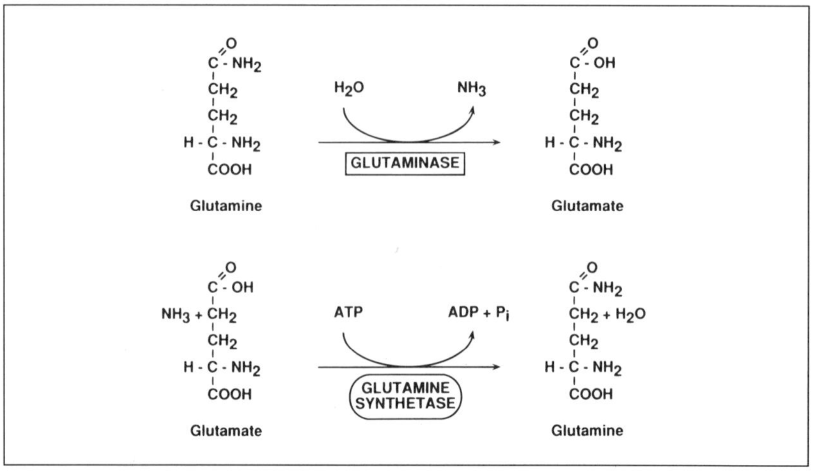

Figure 12-6. Major enzymes of glutamine degradation and synthesis in mammalian cells. Glutaminase catalyzes the hydrolysis of glutamine to glutamate, generating free ammonia. Glutamine synthetase catalyzes the formation of glutamine from glutamate and ammonia, requiring energy derived from the hydrolysis of an ATP molecule.

mine molecule is dependent on the extent of oxidation. Conversion of a glutamine molecule to alanine, aspartate, or lactate produces 9 adenosine triphosphate (ATP) molecules, conversion to pyruvate produces 12 ATPs, conversion to acetyl-CoA produces 15 ATPs, and complete oxidation of glutamine to carbon dioxide produces 24 to 27 ATPs [48]. Thus, the total amount of cellular energy derived from glutamine depends on the extent of oxidation and the rate of glutamine utilization. These factors in turn depend largely on the absolute amounts and relative proportions of glutamine and glucose available as well as the type and proliferative state of the cell [49–54]. Under physiologic conditions, glutamine oxidation can account for as much as a third of the cellular ATP production [55–58], and relative glutamine oxidation increases at lower glucose levels [46,47,59]. Cells can survive and even grow in glucose-free media containing sufficient glutamine and nucleic acid precursors [19,60,61].

Regulation of Glutamine Metabolism

There are two principal intracellular enzymes of glutamine metabolism that regulate the breakdown and synthesis of glutamine [62]. The glutaminase enzyme (GA) catalyzes the hydrolysis of glutamine to glutamate and ammonia, and glutamine synthetase (GS) catalyzes the de novo biosynthesis of glutamine from glutamate and ammonia (see Figure 12-6). Most tissues are either predominantly glutamine consumers and contain relatively high amounts of glutaminase (i.e., gut mucosal cells, lymphocytes, renal tubular cells) or net glutamine producers consistent with their high activity of glutamine synthetase (i.e., skeletal muscle cells, neurons, certain cells in the lung) (Figure 12-7). One exception is the liver, which can behave as either a net glutamine consumer or producer depending on extrahepatic demands [63].

Glutaminase is present in many different types of cells, including intestinal epithelial cells, fibroblasts, lymphocytes, macrophages, renal tubular cells, periportal hepatocytes, endothelial cells, and pancreatic acinar cells [64–72]. Although there appears to be a propensity for replicating cells to contain large quantities of the glutaminase enzyme, relatively quiescent cells such as muscle cells, neurons, and astrocytes also contain glutaminase [73,74]. Phosphate-dependent glutaminase, also known as phosphate-activated glutaminase (PAG), is bound to the inner mitochondrial membrane. As its name implies, it requires inorganic phosphate and also ammonium for activity. Because glutaminase is located in the mitochondria, a separate compartment from the cytoplasm, glutamine must first be transported across the inner mitochondrial membrane before it can be hydrolyzed by glutaminase. Although these are likely to be separate steps, it is possible that transport and metabolism are coupled and that the rapid rate of mitochondrial glutamine transport has made it difficult to distinguish transport from metabolism. Furthermore, mitochondria have two separate membranes (an inner and outer membrane with an intervening intermembrane space), which further complicates kinetics studies of mitochondrial transport. The location of PAG is appropriate because most of the glutamate formed enters the TCA cycle, which operates within the mitochondria.

There appears to be a positive relationship between the rate of glutamine utilization, the activity of phosphate-dependent glutaminase, and the proliferative state of cells. This observation holds for both normal and malignant cells. In both lymphocytes and thymocytes, mitogenic stimulation can induce a large increase in glutamine ca-

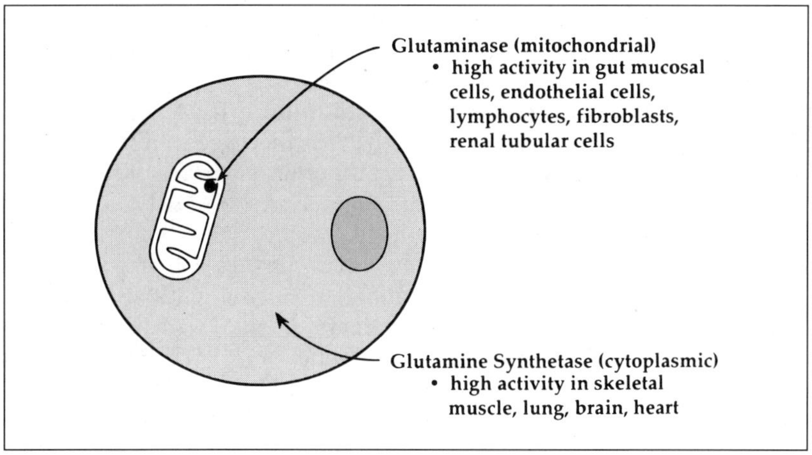

Figure 12-7. Location of glutaminase and glutamine synthetase in mammalian cells and the distribution of their activities. High activities of glutaminase in tissues correspond to cell types with high rates of glutamine utilization whereas high glutamine synthetase activities correspond to tissues that are net glutamine producers.

tabolism [49,50,52]. Thymocytes stimulated to proliferate exhibit as much as an eightfold increase in glutamine utilization, accompanied by a threefold increase in glutaminase activity [50]. Proliferating human diploid fibroblasts, Chinese hamster fibroblasts, bovine pulmonary endothelial cells, and various cell lines exhibit high levels of glutaminolysis [46,58,67,75–78]. An inverse correlation has been observed between glutaminase activity and tumor doubling times [79,80]. The high rate of glutamine utilization in proliferative cells may reflect the cells increased need for energy or for metabolic intermediates and macromolecular precursors [81,82]. However, the mechanism by which proliferative cells obtain their high glutamine utilization rate is not known. It has recently been demonstrated that glutamine, aspartate, and glutamate strongly inhibit glycolysis in Ehrlich ascites tumor cells by inhibiting phosphofructokinase [51]. This effect was dependent on transamination reactions and led to an increased level of cellular ATP. This suggests that increased delivery and transport of glutamine leading to increased glutaminolysis inhibited glycolysis through an increase in the activity of the TCA cycle [51]. This model provides a mechanism by which cells can preferentially use available glutamine; increased hydrolysis of glutamine via glutaminase, resulting from increased amino acid transport and/or enzyme activity, leads to inhibition of glucose oxidation.

Glutamine synthetase is the major enzyme of glutamine biosynthesis and is located in the cytoplasm, although it has been reported to co-localize with the mitochondrial fraction of perivenous hepatocytes [83]. The amidation it catalyzes is energy-dependent, requiring 1 mol of ATP per mole of glutamine synthesized [84]. Under normal conditions, net glutamine synthesis occurs mainly in the liver (primarily in the perivenous hepatocytes), skeletal muscle, brain, and lung, that is, those tissues that produce glutamine for export [9,85–88]. However, considerable GS activity is present in many tissues and, very likely, in nearly all cells [89,90].

Simple, easy-to-learn enzymatic assays have been described [91–100] that allow the investigator to measure the specific activity of each of these enzymes in vitro. Furthermore, in the past several years, the genes (complementary DNAs [cDNA]) for each of these enzymes have been cloned (see Figure 12-7) [101,102], and antibodies to both GA and GS have been produced. These advances have provided us with additional tools to study the regulation of these enzymes and therefore the control of glutamine metabolism at the molecular level.

Influence of Operative Stress on Interorgan Glutamine Flow

The stress of a major operative procedure combined with a general anesthetic is characterized by a fall in circulating and muscle glutamine concentrations postoperatively. Using a hindquarter dog model, Kapadia and colleagues [103] demonstrated that plasma glutamine levels fall by 25% to 30% and that skeletal muscle glutamine concentrations are diminished by as much as 50% within 24 to 48 hours of the stress of a standard laparotomy. The reduction in muscle glutamine concentration results principally from an accelerated release of glutamine, rather than an increase in intramuscular degradation. In surgical patients, the fall in muscle glutamine levels that occurs after surgery is generally transient and inconsequential, although muscle glutamine content may not return to normal for 4 to 6 weeks. This time frame usually corresponds to the period of time when wound healing is maximal and when food intake and ambulation are returning to preinjury levels. Unless the patient develops a complication (such as a wound dehiscence or anastomotic disruption) that initiates further glutamine depletion or precludes food intake for a longer period of time, the hospital stay is usually relatively short.

The accelerated muscle glutamine release that occurs after surgical stress appears to be mediated, in part, by the glucocorticoid hormones, which are secreted by the adrenal glands in increased amounts in stress states. Muhlbacher and colleagues [96] studied muscle glutamine metabolism in chronically catheterized dogs using a hindquarter model. Muscle glutamine efflux was accelerated fourfold in animals receiving dexamethasone. Over a 9-day period, the steroid-treated dogs developed muscle glutamine depletion and negative nitrogen balance. Similar studies in rats [104] have demonstrated that glucocorticoids cause induction of muscle GS. The induction is associated with a marked increase in the level of GS messenger RNA (mRNA). Similarly, dexamethasone causes a striking increase in GS activity [93,105] and mRNA in L6 muscle cells in culture [93]. This increase in mRNA abundance is caused by an enhanced rate of transcription of the gene that occurs as early as 1 hour after incubation of L6 cells with dexamethasone.

The lungs play an important role in regulating glutamine metabolism during catabolic states, and the glucocorticoid hormones also regulate lung glutamine metabolism [91,106]. Sarantos studied dexamethasone-treated rats and demonstrated an increase in both GS activity and mRNA

[107]; this was associated with a twofold increase in lung glutamine release [106]. The location of GS in lung has not been carefully investigated, but both endothelial cells [41,67] and type II alveolar cells [27] play a role in lung glutamine metabolism.

Despite the accelerated release of glutamine by both lung and skeletal muscle that occurs after stress and after steroid administration, circulating levels do not change appreciably, indicating a marked increase in glutamine utilization in other tissues. Studies using a catheterized dog model have demonstrated that glutamine uptake by the gastrointestinal tract in vivo nearly doubles after operative stress [62,108]. Gut glutamine uptake is increased postoperatively despite a fall in the circulating concentration and a reduction in intestinal blood flow, suggesting that an active process for glutamine uptake occurs independent of substrate delivery. This postoperative effect is related to the operative stress itself and not to a decrease in food intake [109].

Further studies showed that gut glutamine uptake more than doubled after the administration of dexamethasone [110]. Glucocorticoids increase the fractional extraction of glutamine from the bloodstream [110] and increase the activity of mucosal glutaminase [111]. A single dose of dexamethasone also increases glutaminase mRNA levels in the jejunal mucosa [112], a response that is time dependent. Teleologically, the purpose of this increased intestinal glutamine extraction is unclear, but it may be designed to support gut glutamine requirements at a time when food intake may be limited because of illness. In addition, glucocorticoids increase glutaminase activity and mRNA in mesenteric lymph nodes [113], suggesting an important role for lymphocytes in glutamine metabolism in stress states. During glucocorticoid treatment, the gut switches from an organ of glucose uptake to one of net release [114], an adaptation that may spare glucose for the wound or for other tissues that are obligate glucose consumers. The increase in gut glutamine utilization also supports intestinal alanine release, which enters gluconeogenic pathways in the liver. Although net hepatic glutamine exchange did not significantly change after surgical stress [108] or after glucocorticoid treatment [110], glutamate consumption by the liver was markedly increased when dexamethasone was given to the healthy dog [110]. In addition, Gebhardt has demonstrated that both dexamethasone and glucagon increase glutamine uptake in primary hepatocyte cultures [115].

The pancreatic hormone glucagon, which is produced in increased amounts after injury, may also regulate glutamine metabolism in the intestine and liver. Geer and colleagues infused glucagon into chronically catheterized dogs that had basal pancreatic secretion "clamped" with somatostatin [116]. Glucagon administration diminished glutamine concentrations by 25% and caused a threefold enhancement in intestinal glutamine uptake and an increase in portal ammonia production. Such a portal profile of low glutamine and high ammonia stimulates hepatic glutamine release in metabolic acidosis, but during hyperglucagonemia, hepatic glutamine uptake was accelerated, most likely from a direct effect of glucagon on system N transport.

Renal glutamine uptake is increased after operative stress [108], an event that again appears to be regulated in large part by the glucocorticoid hormones [110]. An increased renal requirement for glutamine may be necessary postoperatively to support renal ammonia genesis. Adrenalectomized animals exhibit a blunted response to an acid load resulting largely from an impaired ammonium excretion [117]. Chronic exposure to triamcinolone stimulates renal glutamine uptake, which supports ammonia production and bicarbonate generation [118].

In summary, the alterations in interorgan glutamine flow that occur after operative stress appear to be mediated, in part, by the glucocorticoid hormones and by glucagon. Because food intake is often interrupted after operation secondary to ileus or anorexia, the source of glutamine is derived primarily from de novo synthesis in skeletal muscle and in the lungs. The response appears to be designed partially to meet the glutamine requirements of the gut, where it serves as a major source of energy, and of the kidneys, where glutamine is utilized to support ammonia genesis. Glutamine is also consumed by lymphocytes and macrophages as well as by the healing wound. There is a temporary loss of glutamine homeostasis after "surgical stress" resulting from the redirection of glutamine flow as a consequence of the injury response. As a consequence, the blood glutamine level falls, and tissue glutamine depletion develops. Fortunately, in the majority of patients, these alterations are short-lived and have no impact on outcome.

Glutamine Transport and Metabolism During Infection

The alterations in interorgan glutamine flow that occur after severe infection are profound and often of significant duration, depending on the magnitude and severity of the illness. Only when the disease process resolves does glutamine homeostasis return to normal, and this assumes no permanent organ damage was sustained. The changes in organ flux that occur during critical illness may be affected by the prior nutritional status of the patient as well as the presence of other abnormalities such as metabolic acidosis [119]. Nonetheless, many of the adaptive changes in glutamine metabolism that take place are mediated directly or indirectly by glucocorticoid hormones, endotoxin, cytokines, and prostaglandins.

Some of the alterations in interorgan glutamine metabolism that occur during severe infection are similar to those that occur after operative stress, suggesting a common mediator(s). However, during severe infection profound and prolonged glutamine depletion can develop, particularly because major infectious complications often occur in patients who are already malnourished and glutamine depleted (Figure 12-8). For example, muscle glutamine concentrations are generally lower in septic individuals than in postoperative patients [14]. Much like the response to pure operative stress, muscle glutamine release is markedly accelerated during endotoxemia (Figure 12-9).

As a model of sepsis, the administration of a single dose of *Escherichia coli* endotoxin to rats is often used. A moderate dose (7.5–10 mg *E. coli* lipopolysaccharide [LPS] endotoxin), which results in hyperdynamic state (increased cardiac output) and an associated 24-hour mortality of 5% to 10% [120], has been shown to mimic many of the metabolic responses that occur in patients and animals with bacteremia and sepsis. Endotoxin initiates marked changes in interorgan glutamine metabolism, but the responses appear to be primarily mediated by cytokines and the counterregulatory hormones, rather than by LPS itself. The circulating concentration of glutamine reflects the sum of various rates of glutamine uptake and release that occur in the body's organs, and, predictably, blood glutamine concentrations vary depending on the time after LPS administration. There is an early fall in circulating glutamine within 2 to 4 hours of LPS treatment, whereas at the 12-hour time point, the circulating level is slightly but significantly increased [121]. Similarly, the specific rates of net glutamine uptake or release exhibited by the various organs studied also vary as a function of time.

In vivo studies using a hindquarter rat model have demonstrated that endotoxin accelerates muscle glutamine efflux despite a small reduction in hindquarter blood flow. Simultaneously, the activity of glutamine synthetase nearly doubles, preventing the muscle glutamine pool from being completely depleted. This increase in activity is preceded by a threefold to sixfold increase in GS mRNA levels in skeletal muscle. Glutamate extraction by the hindquarter increases in the endotoxin-treated rat [121,122], but apparently the increase in GS expression cannot fully compensate for the accelerated glutamine release by muscle, because glutamine depletion develops.

Lung glutamine release is also accelerated during sepsis [123,124], but the response is temporally different than that for muscle. Within 1 hour of an intravenous bolus of endotoxin, net lung glutamine efflux is increased, but this augmented output is short-lived; these temporal observations

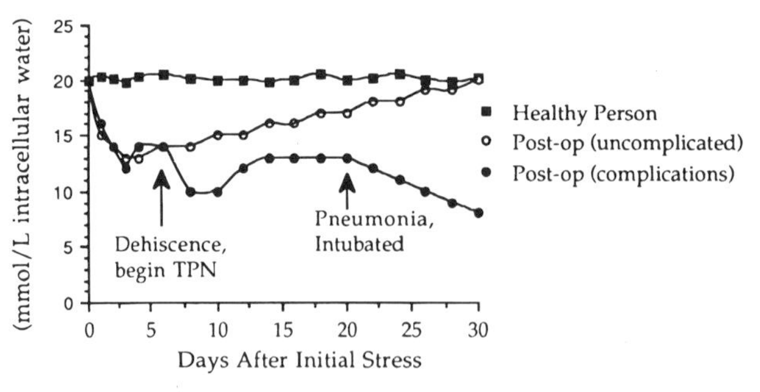

Figure 12-8. Skeletal muscle glutamine concentration in three human beings. The healthy person has a stable concentration that is maintained at about 20 mmol/L of intracellular water. The patient undergoing uncomplicated elective abdominal surgery develops a 35% fall in muscle glutamine concentration over the first three days after operation. Glutamine levels slowly return to normal over the course of four to five weeks. In contrast, the patient who develops a postoperative complication (an additional catabolic stress) will generally become further glutamine depleted. Often such complications preclude the use of enteral nutrition, necessitating the use of parenteral nutrition, which currently does not contain glutamine.

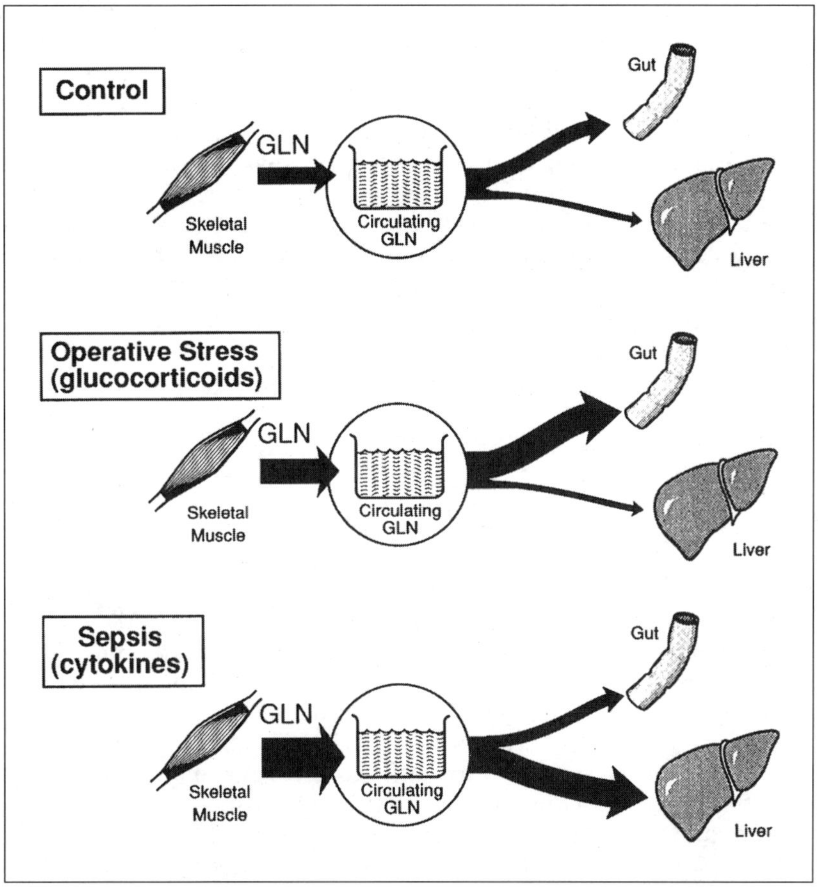

Figure 12-9. Flow of glutamine from skeletal muscle to the splanchnic bed following operative trauma and during severe infection. Many of the alterations in glutamine flux that occur following operative stress are mediated by the glucocorticoid hormones and also by glucagon. In septic states, cytokines also appear to play an important role. Intestinal glutamine uptake increases after surgery, but falls during sepsis when the liver assumes the major role in glutamine consumption. The exchange rates and tissue glutamine levels normalize when the patient recovers.

have been made in rats [123] and in patients [124]. The accelerated release of glutamine from the lungs is limited to the time period directly after the onset of sepsis; the subsequent development of pulmonary edema in rats and adult respiratory distress syndrome (ARDS) in patients resulted in elimination of this augmented response. The apparent reversion to net glutamine balance may be the result of a simultaneous increase in glutamine uptake by pulmonary endothelial cells. Both endotoxin [125] and the cytokines tumor necrosis factor (TNF) and interleukin-1 (IL-1) [126] increase glutamine transport by the lung endothelium, which may account for the whole organ glutamine balance observed at a time when GS levels are increased [123].

A major difference between sepsis and operative stress is the handling of glutamine by the bowel. Gut uptake of circulating glutamine is diminished in septic patients and in endotoxemic rats [127–129], and this is associated with a fall in mucosal glutaminase activity and the development of gram-negative bacteremia [129]. Such relationships are only associations and no cause-and-effect should be inferred, although in other models of bacterial translocation exogenous glutamine has been shown to improve gut barrier function. Glutamine transport across the brush border exhibits a biphasic response to endotoxemia. Early after LPS treatment (4 hr), Na^+-dependent glutamine transport is enhanced [128], a response that may support the increased intestinal protein synthesis that is observed in septic animals [130]. At later time points, endotoxemia decreases glutamine transport across the brush border of endotoxemic rats and septic humans [131]. Likewise, thermally injured rats exhibit a reduced glutamine uptake across the basolateral membrane of the enterocyte [132]. These changes are in contrast to the augmented glutamine uptake that occurs in postoperative and in steroid-treated animals. Interleukin-1 treatment also diminishes intestinal uptake of circulating glutamine [133], whereas lymphocyte glutaminase activity in mesenteric lymph nodes is increased in septic rats [134]. Studies by Brand and colleagues [135,136] have demonstrated that glutamine utilization is 10-fold greater in proliferating lymphocytes as compared with resting cells. Thus, the reduced gut uptake of glutamine that occurs during sepsis may occur primarily in the mucosal cells as opposed to lymphatic tissues, which may actually consume more glutamine during stress states.

Significant changes in renal glutamine metabolism also occur after endotoxin administration. Endotoxin treatment causes the kidneys to change from an organ of slight glutamine uptake to an organ of net glutamine release [137]. This "switch" is associated with a 50% increase in glutamine synthetase activity and a fall in urinary ammonium excretion. These changes take place when there was evidence of renal damage, suggesting that the early renal failure associated with sepsis may impair the kidneys' ability to maintain acid/base homeostasis by altering renal glutamine metabolism. In this in vivo model of endotoxemia, the kidneys contribute net amounts of glutamine to the bloodstream along with skeletal muscle and possibly the lungs.

Despite these dramatic changes in interorgan exchange rates, the blood glutamine level remains fairly constant, particularly in view of the magnitude of exchange rates that simultaneously exist. Under these circumstances, the liver becomes the major glutamine consumer in the body [127], exceeding gut glutamine uptake threefold. Hepatic glutamine uptake increases 10-fold after endotoxin treatment secondary to increases in hepatic blood flow, in intracellular metabolism, and in transhepatocellular membrane transport. Inoue and colleagues [138] examined the effects of endotoxin on glutamine transport activity (system N) in rat hepatic plasma membrane vesicles (HPMVs) from rats treated with *E. coli* endotoxin in vivo. The HPMVs were prepared by differential centrifugation, and the transport of ^{3}H-glutamine (system N) was assayed by a rapid mixing/filtration technique. Endotoxemia resulted in a time-dependent twofold to threefold increase in Na^+-dependent glutamine transport activity in HPMVs secondary to an increase in the transport Vmax, consistent with the appearance of increased numbers of corresponding transporter proteins in the hepatocyte plasma membrane. Maximal increases in transport were observed 4 hours after exposure to endotoxin. This increase in transport activity represents an important mechanism underlying the accelerated hepatic amino acid uptake that occurs during critical illness.

Mediators of the Septic Response

It has been well established that endotoxin stimulates the release of multiple cytokines that regulate metabolic responses via complex interrelationships with one another and with the classic endocrine hormones. Much like endotoxin, treatment of rats with TNF-α, IL-1, or IL-6 causes an increase in glutamine transport in HPMVs within 2 to 4 hours of administering the cytokine (Figure 12-10). Pacitti and co-workers [unpublished data] investigated the activities of Na^+-dependent transport system N in HPMVs prepared from rats treated with TNF in vivo. Although TNF alters sodium uptake, it results in time- and dose-dependent 50% maximal increases in system N activity secondary to an increase in the transport Vmax. Like endotoxin treatment, maximal increases in transport activity are observed 4 hours after exposure to TNF, and activity returns to basal levels within 24 hours. Incubation of HPMVs from normal rats in vitro with TNF does not alter transport activity, indicating that TNF-induced stimulation of glutamine uptake is not an event mediated by a direct action of TNF at the membrane surface (i.e., clustering of membrane proteins, changes in fluidity characteristics). Pretreatment of animals

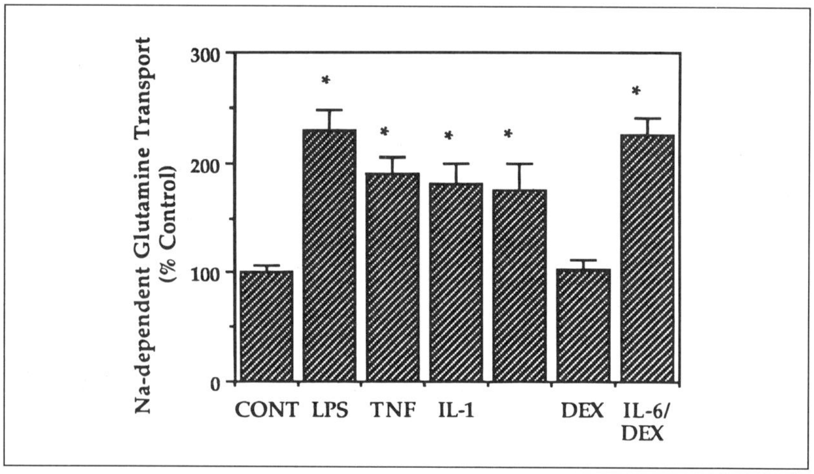

Figure 12-10. Sodium-dependent glutamine transport in hepatocyte plasma membrane vesicles prepared from rats treated with various mediators. Studies with anticytokine antibodies indicate that the LPS-induced increase in transport activity is, in part, cytokine-mediated. CONT = control; DEX = dexamethasone; IL-1 = interleukin-1; IL-6 = interleukin-6; LPS = lipopolysaccharide; TNF = tumor necrosis factor; * = $p < 0.05$ vs. control. (From Souba et al., unpublished observations.)

with the glucocorticoid receptor antagonist RU38486 attenuates the TNF-induced enhancement in transport activity by 50%. These data indicate that the marked increase in system N transport activity stimulated by TNF is mediated, in part, by the glucocorticoid hormones and represents an important mechanism underlying the accelerated hepatic amino acid uptake that occurs during critical illness. Muscle proteolysis, another sepsis-related metabolic alteration induced by TNF, has also been shown to be glucocorticoid mediated [139].

Consistent with these results are studies by Gebhardt [115] that demonstrate that pretreatment of rats with a cyclooxygenase inhibitor or with a glucocorticoid receptor antagonist attenuates the endotoxin-induced increase in system N activity. Inoue and Souba [unpublished data] found that pretreatment of rats with a hamster anti-TNF monoclonal antibody causes an approximately 50% reduction in the up-regulation of hepatic system N caused by injection of endotoxin (Figure 12-11). Anti-TNF administered after LPS has no effect on the induction of hepatic system N, suggesting that TNF functions as a proximal mediator in this response.

In contrast to the in vivo results discussed above, incubation of hepatocytes from normal animals with endotoxin, TNF, or IL-1 does not alter Na^+-dependent amino acid transport indicating that these mediators work through (or with) another mediator(s). Interleukin-6, on the other hand, does increase system N activity by approximately 30% in cultured hepatocytes, a response that is accentuated when dexamethasone is added to the medium [Fischer and Souba, unpublished data]. Administration of IL-6 to rats increases hepatic system N and system A activities by as much as twofold and threefold, respectively, but has no effect on system y^+ [140]. The glucocorticoid alone does not induce hepatic system N, but does induce systems A and y^+. Interestingly, dexamethasone enhances the response of system N to IL-6, whereas it has no synergistic effect on system A.

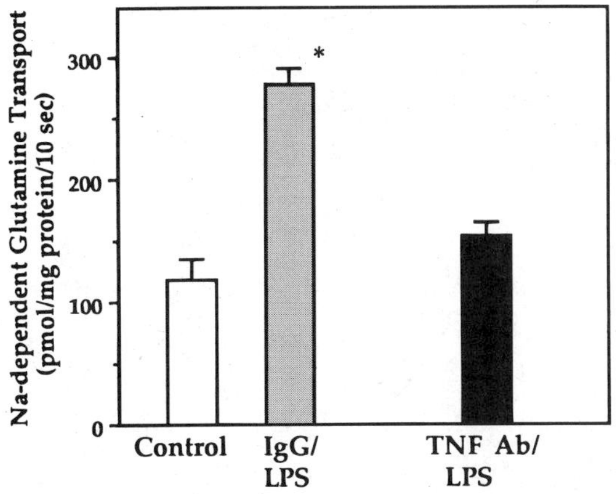

Figure 12-11. Effect of TNF-blocking antibodies on endotoxin induction of rat hepatic glutamine transporter activity. Sodium-dependent glutamine transport was assayed in hepatic plasma membrane vesicles obtained from rats four hours after injection of LPS (7.5 mg/kg BW, ip). Rats received hamster anti-TNF or nonimmune IgG (4 mg, ip) either two hours before or one hour after endotoxin injection. IgG = nonimmune globulin; LPS = lipopolysaccharide; TNF Ab = tumor necrosis factor antibody; * = $p < 0.05$ vs. control.

Previous studies in other cells have shown that endotoxin and cytokines modulate glutamine transport. For example, endotoxin [125], TNF, and IL-1 [126] stimulate glutamine uptake by endothelial cells, whereas high doses of TNF diminish glutamine transport in fibroblasts [40]. In cultured Caco-2 cells, γ-interferon decreases glutamine transport across the brush border, whereas TNF and IL-1 do not alter transport [33]. Here again, we see that the effects of cytokines, whether direct or indirect, are diverse and tissue-specific. This is in keeping with the concept that the body responds to prevailing metabolic pressures to redirect the flow of glutamine during critical illness, and this is often accomplished at the plasma membrane level. For the present, it appears that hepatocytes, lymphocytes, and endothelial cells rank high on the body's list of cells that must have adequate amounts of glutamine after a septic insult. Although sepsis causes marked increases in both net glutamine consumption and in net glutamine production (Figure 12-12), with time, demands outstrip the body's ability to produce glutamine and tissue and plasma levels fall.

What are the consequences of this interorgan glutamine cycle in patients who have chronic sepsis and develop profound glutamine depletion? Consider the individual who develops a breakdown of the gut mucosal barrier from a combination of insults (shock, malnutrition, sepsis, antibiotic therapy, etc.). A central part of the metabolic response to sepsis is mobilization of glutamine stores in an attempt to maintain the blood glutamine level and thereby "nourish" other tissues (Figure 12-13). In skeletal muscle, the intracellular glutamine concentration is a regulator of protein synthesis [141–144] that may further lead to net catabolism. Under these circumstances, glutamine availability may eventually become rate-limiting and result in inadequate amounts of this key substrate for certain cells [145]. Moreover, such critically ill patients often have a gastrointestinal tract that is unusable, and hence they are nourished with total parenteral nutrition that currently does not contain glutamine.

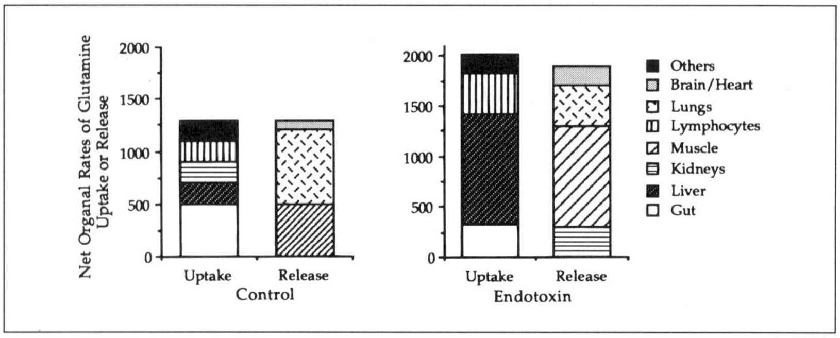

Figure 12-12. Regional contributions to whole-body glutamine exchange rates in the rat. The small intestine is the principal organ of glutamine consumption in the postabsorptive state, with lesser amounts being taken up by the kidneys and the lymphocytes. Skeletal muscle and lung are the major producers of circulating glutamine. During homeostasis, net rates of uptake balance net rates of release and each total approximately 1300 nmol/100 gm BW/min. (Data in part from [6, 8, 9, 19].)

Glutamine Metabolism in the Tumor-Bearing Host

A substantial body of experimental evidence indicates that glutamine is the major respiratory fuel for tumor cells [46,146,147]. Glutamine has been shown to be an unusually good substrate for oxidation by tumor cell mitochondria [148]. Tumor glutaminase activity is relatively high and correlates well with tumor glutamine consumption and growth rates (Figure 12-14) [79,80]. Studies in the late 1950s in rats with large malignancies demonstrated a reduction in plasma and hepatocyte intracellular glutamine concentrations compared with nontumor-bearing controls [149,150]. Simultaneously, tumor utilization is substantial, particularly if the cancer is a rapidly proliferating one. Studies on skeletal muscle glutamine metabolism in rats bearing Walker carcinosarcomas in the thigh demonstrated glutamine uptake by the leg containing the tumor, whereas the contralateral leg demonstrated glutamine release at an accelerated rate [150]. Since these early studies, other investigations have demonstrated the important role of glutamine for the growing tumor [151,152].

The methylcholanthrene-induced sarcoma (MCA tumor) model has probably been most extensively used to investigate interorgan glutamine

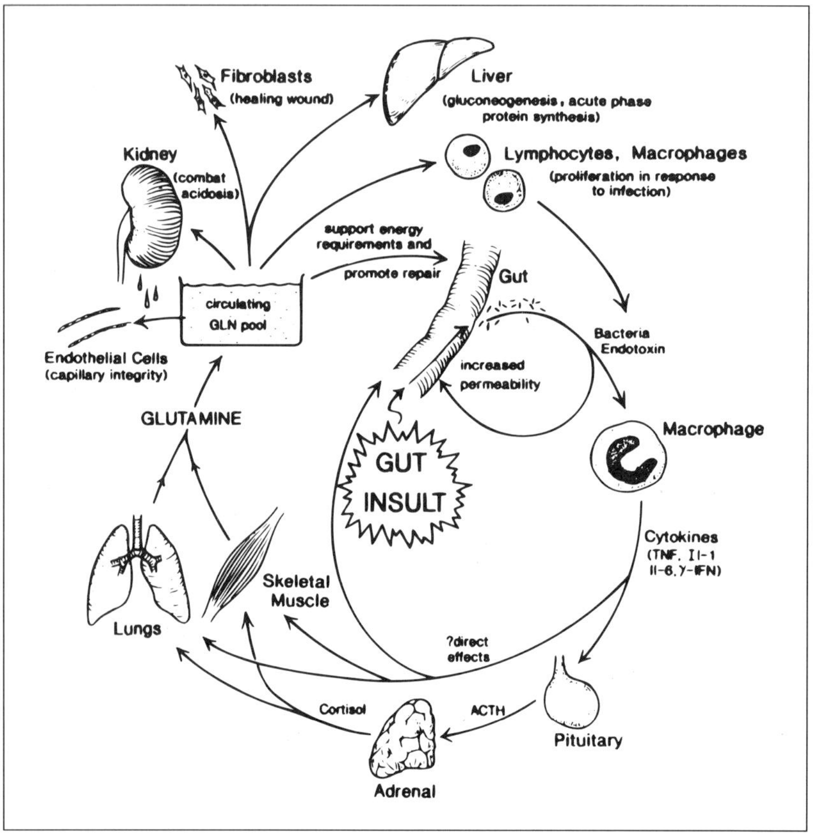

Figure 12-13. The Interorgan Glutamine Cycle can be initiated by any local and/or systemic catabolic insult that redirects the flow of glutamine and results in glutamine depletion. In the case illustrated here, the patient develops a breakdown in the gut mucosal barrier, which causes an increase in bowel permeability and bacterial translocation. Bacteria and endotoxins stimulate macrophages to release cytokines (TNF, IL-1, IL-6), which exert direct effects on glutamine metabolism in various organs and also stimulate release of the counter-regulatory hormones. These mediators work together to mobilize glutamine stores from muscle and to stimulate glutamine production by the lungs. A central goal is to support the increased glutamine requirements in other tissues. It is unclear why organs such as the gut should subserve other tissues, but it is apparent that if the cycle persists, or if the patient is unable to take oral feedings or remains glutamine deficient, a prolonged catabolic state develops.

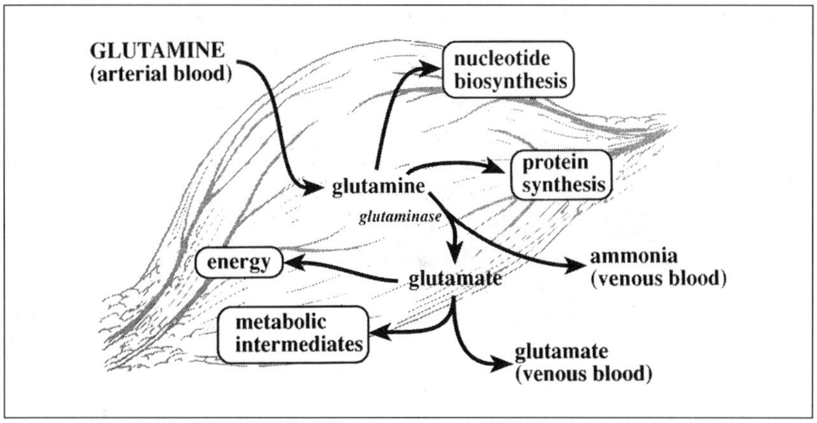

Figure 12-14. Glutamine metabolism in tumor cells. Glutamine is utilized by tumor cells to produce protein, energy, nucleotides, and metabolic intermediates. Tumors exhibit high rates of glutaminolysis results in the production of free ammonia. This can explain the hyperammonemia observed with advanced malignant disease.

metabolism [153–160]. This tumor is locally aggressive but rarely metastasizes, causing death (from inanition) 5 to 6 weeks after tumor implantation, at which time tumor size may account for nearly half of total body weight. The tumor grows most effectively in the Fischer-344 rat and has several advantages over murine models. First, the larger size of the rat makes the technical skills involved in regional flux measurements easier to acquire. Second, the larger organs in the rat often do not require pooling of tissue from several animals to do metabolic studies (e.g., preparation of hepatocyte plasma membrane vesicles). Furthermore, the volume of blood that can be sampled for repeated analysis is greater. Because a portion of the tumor-induced cachexia in this model is the result of a fall in voluntary food intake (tumor-induced anorexia), this must be taken into account when trying to differentiate between derangements in interorgan glutamine metabolism as a consequence of simple starvation as opposed to abnormalities that are secondary to the growing tumor (i.e., elaboration of a circulating factor that alters intermediary metabolism). Therefore, control nontumor-bearing rats should be pair-fed to carcass weight to control for simple starvation effects.

Predictably, both the magnitude and direction of glutamine flow in tumor-bearing rats changes during the course of the disease process. The changes that develop appear to be designed, in part, to maintain the blood glutamine concentration as the tumor grows and utilizes more glutamine. Many of the adaptive changes that occur regionally (i.e., in specific organ beds) result in changes in net glutamine exchange by the organ. In the case of the MCA tumor, the cancer becomes the principal glutamine consumer with time, exceeding glutamine uptake by the intestinal tract [153]. Progressive glutamine depletion invariably develops, particularly in skeletal muscle, and this is associated with cachexia and anorexia. Glutamine extraction by this fast-growing tumor has been quantitated in vivo by measuring blood glutamine levels in afferent and efferent blood vessels that nourish and drain the tumor [155]. The rate at which this tumor can extract glutamine from plasma is impressive and may be as high as 45%, greater than the rate of glutamine extraction for any organ under conditions of health. The tumor thus behaves like a "glutamine trap." The high rates of intracellular glutaminolysis (when the sarcoma is large) are evident by the enormous release of ammonia into the venous effluent [155].

A feature of the host response to the growing cancer is the development of muscle glutamine depletion (Figure 12-15). This depletion is apparent early in the course of the disease process when the animal appears healthy and has a normal appetite. When the tumor comprises about 8% of total body weight, there is a 20% fall in the muscle glutamine concentration, which is associated with

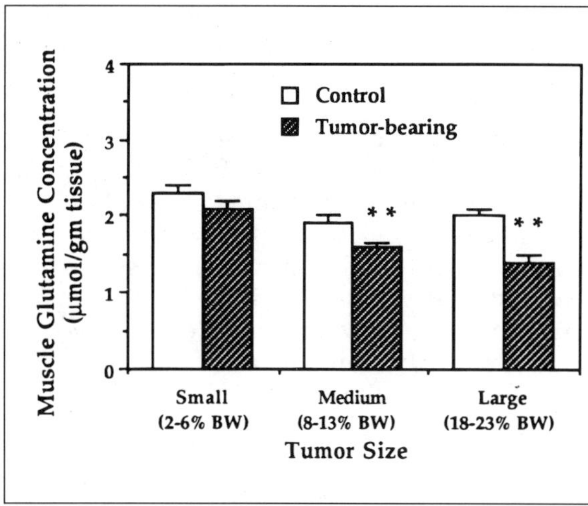

Figure 12-15. Muscle glutamine metabolism in tumor-bearing rats. ** = $p < 0.01$ vs. control.

an increased glutamine efflux from the hindquarter. This efflux is not secondary to an increase in regional blood flow, but instead is the result of a twofold increase in the fractional release rate of glutamine. Simultaneously, the specific activity of the GS enzyme increases, as does the quantity of GS mRNA in muscle [161]. The activity of muscle glutaminase does not increase, consistent with no change in the rate of intracellular glutamine hydrolysis, indicating that the muscle glutamine depletion that develops in cancer is the result of an acceleration in glutamine efflux from the cell. With time, the muscle glutamine depletion that develops becomes severe and late in the course of the disease muscle appears to become "exhausted." This progressive glutamine depletion coincides with the development of cancer cachexia. [*Editor's Note:* Cancer anorexia is a centrally mediated mechanism, and some investigations (162) suggest that alterations in neuropeptide Y (NPY) are important in the pathogenesis of cancer anorexia.]

Although temporally related, the hepatic response to the growing cancer differs from that observed in skeletal muscle. Early in the course of the disease, the liver switches from an organ of glutamine uptake to an organ of net glutamine release [160]. This response appears to be different than that which occurs during acidosis or starvation because portal ammonia levels are unchanged at this early time point [154]. The onset of this switch appears to be the result of a fall in tissue glutaminase activity and a significant increase in intracellular glutamine levels [160]. This increase in hepatic glutamine content coupled with a fall in blood glutamine results in a 68% increase in the intracellular/circulating concentration gradient that may "push" glutamine out of the hepatocyte and into the bloodstream, because non-carrier–mediated glutamine release (i.e., diffusion) is an important mode of glutamine efflux from hepatocytes.

Carrier-mediated glutamine transport out of the hepatocyte is also enhanced in response to a growing tumor (mediated by the Na^+-independent system "n") [Souba et al., unpublished data]. Studies in rats with small tumors (7.5% of body weight) have demonstrated that the Vmax of system n is increased nearly threefold [156]. The Na^+-dependent transport of glutamine (system N), the component primarily responsible for the uptake and accumulation of glutamine by the hepatocyte, was also increased in the tumor-bearing rat, but only by about 25%. This would appear to be inconsistent with the observation of accelerated hepatic glutamine efflux in the tumor-bearing animal, and this clearly can contribute little to favor efflux. One must keep in mind that, in contrast to the in vivo situation described above for Na^+-independent transport, the Na^+-dependent carrier is not operating at maximal capacity but near its Km (approximately 500–600 μM blood glutamine). Thus, it can be seen that the transmembrane flux resulting from a 25% increase in the sodium-dependent Vmax of transport cannot compensate for the near threefold increase in the sodium-independent Vmax of transport favoring efflux. The increase in the quantity of sodium-dependent transporters may be a compensatory response of the liver to conserve its stores of glutamine in the face of the tumor's increasing demand. Thus, the accelerated hepatic glutamine efflux that develops in rats with relatively small tumors seems to be a function of both the mass-action effect of an increased glutamine gradient from liver to blood and an elevation of Na^+-independent glutamine transport activity of the hepatocyte plasma membrane.

As tumor growth proceeds, circulating cytokine levels in the host may be elevated [163], and the response of the liver to the growing tumor may include the synthesis of defense proteins. Warren and associates have shown that hepatic protein synthesis is increased in tumor-bearing animals [164,165]; in this setting the requirement for precursor amino acids will be greater. Accordingly, the liver shifts the activities of its transporters to favor uptake. The increase in system n activity persists, but the activity of the influx carrier system N increases as the tumor grows [166]. This augmentation of system N transport functions to convert the liver to a net glutamine consumer. Simultaneously, the intracellular glutamine concentration falls, minimizing additional glutamine efflux by diffusion. These relative rates reflect the flux measurements that are observed in vivo [Dudrick et al., unpublished data]. Prevailing metabolic pressures at this point in time, when the animal is critically ill, demand that the liver consume glutamine at the expense of the circulating pool. Shortly thereafter (within 1–2 weeks), the animal dies with profound glutamine depletion.

At the same time that changes in muscle and liver glutamine metabolism occur, changes in glutamine utilization take place in the small intestine [157,158,160]. Intestinal glutamine extraction ([arterial glutamine − portal venous glutamine]/[arterial glutamine]) falls as the tumor grows, an alteration that is not solely related to the fall in circulating glutamine that develops. With time, the tumor becomes the major organ of glutamine uptake in the body, "stealing" as much as 50% to 60% of glutamine from the circulating pool. This fall in uptake is associated with a marked fall in mucosal glutaminase activity, the major enzyme of glutamine hydrolysis in the gut [158,159]. Other mucosal enzymes do not appear to be so dramatically affected by the growing cancer. The decrease in gut glutaminase is caused by a reduction in enzyme synthesis rather than a change in enzyme-substrate affinity. It thus appears that one mechanism by which fast-growing tumors that have an absolute requirement for glutamine may diminish gut glutamine utilization is by partial inhibition of intestinal glutaminase biosynthesis.

An interesting response to the growing tumor occurs in the activity of the brush-border glutamine transporter. Salloum and colleagues [157] studied the effects of progressive malignant growth on the activities of several amino acid transport systems in the brush border at various stages of tumor growth (tumor sizes = 7%, 20%, and 29% of total, nontumor body weight). These time points were chosen on the basis of previous studies with this tumor that demonstrated (1) food intake begins to diminish when tumor weight reaches approximately 10% of total body weight; (2) shortly thereafter, when the tumor comprises about 15% of total body weight, visible evidence of the stigmata of cancer cachexia begin to appear; and (3) when the tumor accounts for approximately 30% of total body weight, the animals are moribund. [*Editor's Note:* In our own laboratory, death of the Fischer-344 rat occurs when the tumor is 60 to 70 g. The nontumor carcass weight is approximately 180 to 190 g.] In the study by Salloum [157], control and tumor-bearing rats were pair-fed, and jejunal brush-border membrane vesicles (BBMVs) were used to assay transport, a method that offers several advantages over other approaches. First, transport can be evaluated separately from the influences of other confounding factors such as intracellular metabolism and amino acid–induced trans-stimulation/inhibition. Second, as opposed to isolated enterocytes from tumor-bearing animals, which may lose or fail to display changes in transport activity once placed in culture media, membrane vesicles offer a unique way of avoiding these problems because they are prepared immediately. In addition, it has been shown that transport activity is preserved during preparation of the vesicles, and thus they provide a "snapshot" of in vivo activity.

The rate of glutamine uptake by BBMVs from all tumor-bearing rats was significantly greater than controls, regardless of tumor size. The increase in transport activity was not the result of a change in carrier affinity, but rather of an increase in maximal transport velocity, consistent with an increase in the number of functional transporters in the brush border. In marked contrast, the transport of alanine was diminished in BBMVs from tumor-bearing rats (TBR), whereas glucose and leucine transport activity was unchanged. The results suggest that the up-regulation in brush-border transport that occurs in this tumor model may be specific for glutamine, indicating the high cellular priority and requirement for glutamine. The specific signals involved in controlling these changes in brush-border substrate transport that occur in the tumor-bearing rat are unknown. Regardless of the mechanism(s) involved, it appears that maintenance of glutamine transport activity is a major synthetic priority that is preserved even when severe cachexia is present. Provision of luminal nutrition at a time when glutamine transport activity is increased may provide a biochemical rationale for the use of glutamine-enriched nutrition in certain cancer patients. An important consideration is the effectiveness of glutamine supplementation in providing needed glutamine to these host cells.

Chen and colleagues [161] have studied the effects of progressive tumor growth on renal glutamine metabolism using the MCA tumor model. Rats with subcutaneous sarcomas, or TBR, were studied and compared to sham-implanted pair-fed controls at 2 and 3 weeks after tumor implantation. At 2 weeks (tumor weight = 4% of body weight), arterial glutamine levels were reduced in TBR as compared with controls, but no change in renal glutamine metabolism was observed. At 3 weeks (tumor weight = 19% of body weight), blood glutamine was further depressed and the TBR were acidotic (arterial pH 7.36 in controls vs. 7.31 in TBR, $p < 0.01$). The classic adaptation of elevated renal glutaminase activity and accelerated renal glutamine utilization was not observed in these acidotic tumor-bearing rats. Instead, glutamine synthetase activity increased by 40%, and the kidneys switched to an organ of glutamine balance or slight release. Despite this impairment in renal glutamine metabolism, the kidneys of acidotic tumor-bearing rats were still able to increase HCO_3^- production by 36% and increase urinary NH_3 excretion by 250%. Thus, fast-growing tumors may "block" the kidneys' ability to utilize circulating glutamine to maintain acid/base balance. The kidneys appear to adapt by increasing endogenous glutamine synthesis and/or using other ammonia-generating pathways to help combat the acidosis associated with rapid tumor growth.

The specific mediators that regulate the changes in interorgan glutamine metabolism that occur in the tumor-bearing rat are unknown. However, there is good evidence that cancer cachexia is mediated by circulating factors in plasma. For example, Norton and associates [167] demonstrated that nontumor-bearing rats parabiotically united with methylcholanthrene (MCA)-induced sarcoma-bearing rats developed features of cachexia, consistent with the release of factors by the tumor or by the host in response to the tumor that gained access to the nontumor-bearing animal via the circulatory bridge. Subsequently, Illig and colleagues [168] infused nontumor-bearing rats with plasma from tumor-bearing animals over a 4-day period. Compared with animals receiving control plasma, the rats infused with "tumor-bearing plasma" developed negative nitrogen balance, weight loss, a voluntary decrease in food intake, and a decrease in muscle mass. These data demonstrate that the syndrome of cancer cachexia is likely to be mediated by circulating factors.

Consistent with these studies are preliminary investigations designed to identify specific mechanisms and mediators of the alterations in glutamine metabolism that occur in the tumor-bearing rat. For example, incubation of hepatocytes from normal rats with serum from tumor-bearing rats increases system N activity (sodium-dependent glutamine transport) [165]. In vivo, the augmentation of hepatic system N transport by advanced tumors seems to be mediated in part by tumor necrosis factor, a cytokine released by monocytes and macrophages. Tumor necrosis factor has been implicated in the cachexia that results from advanced tumor burden [169,170]. Injection of rats with TNF-α has been shown to induce hepatic amino acid transport systems [171]. Furthermore, the repeated administration of rabbit antimurine TNF antibodies to rats implanted with the MCA tumors resulted in a 75% inhibition of tumor-induced increase of hepatic system N activity (Figure 12-16). The stimulatory effect of TNF on hepatic system N was also inhibited by the glucocorticoid receptor antagonist RU38486. In contrast, when isolated hepatocytes were treated with TNF in vitro, no effect on glutamine transport was observed [Souba et al., unpublished data]. These data indicate that TNF, which is presumably released by tumor-infiltrating monocytes and macrophages, indirectly mediates the MCA tumor-induced hepatic glutamine transport upregulation and that the pathway of induction requires the presence of glucocorticoid hormones in the host.

Glutamine Nutrition

During catabolic disease states, glutamine homeostasis is threatened; net rates of glutamine utilization exceed net rates of production, leading to a state of marked glutamine depletion. This depletion is most obvious in skeletal muscle, which serves as the major "glutamine bank" in the body. In the long run, this depleted state may have two serious consequences: (1) the morphology and function of tissues that require glutamine (i.e., replicating cells) may exhibit impairments if glutamine availability in the blood becomes rate-limiting; and (2) tissues that store glutamine may suffer if their own stores fall too low. Although there is abundant evidence that glutamine occupies an key position in the maintenance of metabolism, structure, and function in several organs, the exact role that glutamine plays as a dietary supplement in the overall care of patients remains unclear.

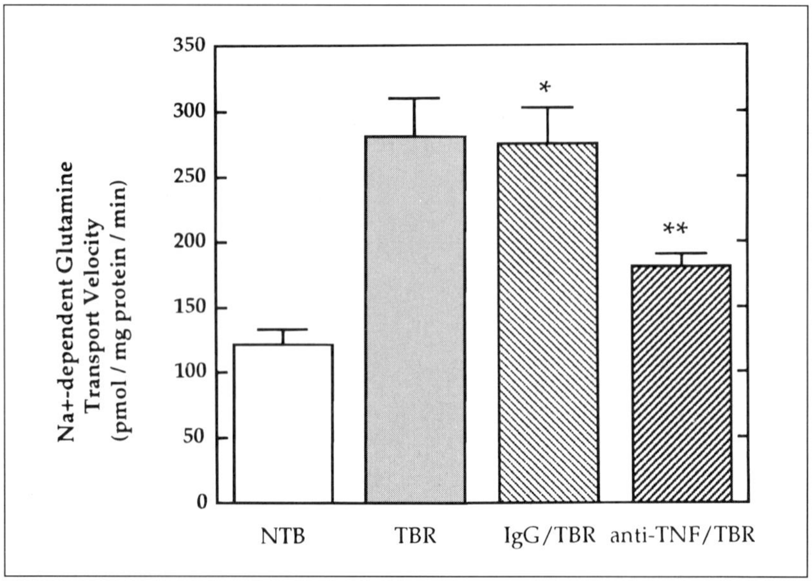

Figure 12-16. Effect of anti-TNF on glutamine transport in tumor-bearing rat. IgG = nonimmune globulin; NTB = nontumor-bearing rat; TBR = tumor-bearing rat; TNF = tumor necrosis factor; * = $p < 0.01$ vs. control; ** = $p < 0.05$ vs. control.

The classification of glutamine as a nonessential or nutritionally dispensable amino acid implies that, in its absence from the diet, it can be synthesized in adequate quantities from other amino acids and precursors. For this reason, and because of glutamines' relative instability and short shelf-life compared with other amino acids, it has not been considered necessary to include glutamine in nutritional formulas. Glutamine has been eliminated from TPN (total parenteral nutrition) solutions and, with few exceptions, glutamine is present in oral and enteral diets only at the relatively low levels characteristic of its concentration in most animal and plant proteins (about 3% to 10% of total amino acids) [17].

Based on our knowledge of the changes in glutamine metabolism that are characteristic of catabolic states, the categorization of glutamine as a nonessential amino acid may be misleading. Under certain circumstances, glutamine may be required in the diet, even though the body has glutamine-synthesizing enzymes in numerous tissues. During such conditions, there appears to be an inability to keep up with the accelerated rate of glutamine consumption. This thinking has led to a number of studies that have examined the impact of glutamine-supplemented diets. In past years, there has been a steady increase in such investigations, and many of these studies indicate that glutamine may be a conditionally essential amino acid during critical illness (Table 12-2). In general, these studies demonstrate that glutamine is not required during states of health, but it appears to be beneficial when glutamine depletion is severe or when cells that have a substantial glutamine requirement under normal circumstances are damaged. These reports also indicate that pharmacologic doses of glutamine are neces-

Table 12-2. Is Glutamine a Conditionally Essential Amino Acid?

Required Effect/Criteria	Evidence/Examples
EFFECTS OF CONDITIONALLY ESSENTIAL NUTRIENT (GLUTAMINE) ABSENCE	
Fall in blood and tissue glutamine concentrations	Tumor-bearing animals [176,177], endotoxin-treated animals [121,175], and catabolic patients [13,14,16,18,205] develop glutamine depletion.
Atrophy or dysfunction of a specific tissue(s)	Rats on glutamine-free TPN develop bacterial translocation, villous atrophy, and a fall in lamina propria lymphocyte populations [52,138,188,190].
	Rats treated with radiation, chemotherapy, or endotoxin develop bacteremia and mucosal damage when no glutamine is provided [194–196,198].
	Muscle protein synthesis is decreased after injury when no glutamine is provided [16,18,175].
EFFECTS OF CONDITIONALLY ESSENTIAL NUTRIENT (GLUTAMINE) REPLETION	
Correct tissue glutamine depletion	Glutamine-enriched diets restore muscle glutamine in tumor-bearing rats [176,177] and in postoperative patients [16,18].
Enhance cellular utilization	Glutamine-enriched TPN increases gut uptake of circulating glutamine [182]; feeding a glutamine diet to rats increases brush-border transport [149,183].
Improvement in tissue morphology and function	Glutamine-enriched TPN increases villous height and decreases bacterial translocation [52,138,184,186, 188,190,204,213] and supports the pancreas [200,201].
	Glutamine-enriched TPN improves gut morphology and protein synthesis in septic rats [199].
	Glutamine-enriched enteral diets improve recovery and enhance mucosal healing after chemotherapy or radiation therapy [66,84,85,193,198].
Improvement in protein economy	Glutamine-enriched TPN increases protein synthesis in skeletal muscle and improves nitrogen balance after operation [16,18].
	Glutamine-enriched enteral diets increase carcass weight in tumor-bearing rats [177].
Improvement in outcome	Glutamine nutrition in bone marrow transplant patients decreases infections and shortens hospital stay [208, 215].

Note: Bracketed numbers correspond with references.

sary to accomplish this benefit, and thus glutamine may be considered a drug as well as a nutrient (nutritional pharmacology).

Glutamine Nutrition and Skeletal Muscle

The marked skeletal muscle glutamine depletion that is characteristic of catabolic states [13,14,121,172] has stimulated several investigators to evaluate the effects of glutamine-enriched diets on muscle glutamine concentrations and protein synthesis. This may be clinically important because a statistically significant correlation between survival in septic patients and the intracellular muscle glutamine concentration has been demonstrated [14]. Kapadia and colleagues [173] demonstrated that a glutamine infusion in the postoperative period could diminish the efflux of glutamine from the hindlimb of the dog. It has also been suggested that the decrease in muscle protein synthesis observed in sepsis and endotoxemia is causally related to decreased intracellular glutamine concentrations [144]. MacLennan and colleagues [174] used the perfused rat hindlimb model to manipulate intramuscular glutamine concentrations and found that a rise in glutamine stimulated protein synthesis. The impact of exogenous glutamine on protein synthesis was greatest at low intramuscular glutamine concentrations, in the range characteristic of critical illness. Similarly, Millward and associates [175] demonstrated that the muscle glutamine concentration is correlated directly with the rate of muscle protein synthesis and the RNA/protein ratio and inversely correlated with the rate of protein degradation. Hammarqvist and associates [16] randomized patients after cholecystectomy to TPN with and without glutamine (approximately 20 g/d). The postoperative fall in skeletal muscle intracellular glutamine was less pronounced in the group receiving glutamine (22% vs. 39%). Simultaneously, the total muscle ribosome concentration did not fall in the glutamine-fed patients, but it fell by 27% in controls. Furthermore, the cumulative nitrogen loss was significantly less in the glutamine group compared with the control group during the study period (2.3 g vs. 8.5 g). Similar results were reported by Stehle and colleagues [18], who used a glutamine dipeptide rather than free glutamine. Together these results suggest that nutritional delivery of glutamine can decrease net muscle glutamine efflux, which in turn helps support muscle protein synthesis. [*Editor's Note:* Although these results are statistically significant, are they biologically significant?]

Austgen and colleagues studied the effects of glutamine-enriched TPN (TPN + glutamine) in tumor-bearing rats [176]. Rats were implanted with the MCA sarcoma and were studied when the tumor comprised less than 5% and less than 10% of carcass weight. The provision of 20% of TPN protein as glutamine produced a significant increase in the arterial glutamine level and maintained the skeletal muscle intracellular glutamine concentration (2.0 ± 0.1 vs. 1.4 ± 0.1 μmol/g). Concurrently, hindquarter glutamine fractional release increased nearly threefold in the TPN + glutamine group. Similar studies by Klimberg and colleagues [177] demonstrated that the provision of glutamine-enriched elemental diets orally to the tumor-bearing rat helps replete muscle glutamine stores. Repletion of glutamine stores in muscle was associated with a rate of hindquarter glutamine release that was similar to that observed in the healthy postabsorptive rat. The glutamine released by the hindquarter in the glutamine-fed animals may have been taken up by the tumor as well as by other tissues, but tumor growth was not stimulated.

Impact of Glutamine Nutrition on the Intestinal Mucosa and on Gut Immune Function

The gut has received the most attention with regard to studies designed to evaluate the impact of glutamine nutrition on a particular tissue. The importance of circulating glutamine for the gut was pointed out by a study in which the enzyme glutaminase (converts glutamine to glutamate) was infused into several animal species [178]. Blood glutamine levels fell to near undetectable levels, and the animals developed diarrhea, mild villous atrophy, mucosal ulcerations, and intestinal necrosis. Other investigators have shown that glutamine may be useful in protecting against aspirin-induced gastric ulcerations [179] and in treating peptic ulcer disease [180].

Glutamine is found in virtually all foods and in many specialized diets provided to hospitalized patients, but it is present in relatively small amounts. Glutamine comprises 3% to 8% of dietary protein [17], and hence enteral feedings may provide as little as 2 to 6 g of glutamine daily, a quantity insufficient to support the requirements of the stressed, depleted individual. In addition, current TPN solutions are glutamine-free, which may in part explain the development of villous atrophy in patients receiving long-term TPN. Hwang et al. [181] demonstrated that glutamine enrichment of TPN solutions resulted in an increase in jejunal mucosal weight and DNA content, and supplementation also significantly attenuated the villous atrophy associated with standard TPN. Klimberg and associates [182] showed that supplementation of standard TPN solutions with glutamine increased gut glutaminase activity and stimulated gut glutamine utilization. Both enteral [38] and parenteral [183] glutamine accelerate transport of glutamine across the jejunal brush border. Others have demonstrated the ability of glutamine-supplemented intravenous or enteral diets to increase villous height and mucosal nitrogen content [184,185] and stimulate intestinal mucosal growth after starvation [186]. Combined therapy with glutamine-supplemented TPN and subcutaneous injections of epidermal growth factor had a synergistic effect on the thickness of the small intestine [187]. Thus, combination therapy with hormones (e.g., growth hormone) or growth factors that act as trophic factors may help preserve the integrity of the intestinal mucosa.

An important observation was made by Alverdy and colleagues, who reported that TPN promotes bacterial translocation from the gut in rats. When rats were allowed to drink the standard TPN solution, the rate of bacterial translocation was significantly reduced but, unlike regular chow diet, the rate of bacterial translocation was not fully abrogated. Subsequent studies by this group [188] showed that glutamine-enriched TPN results in decreased bacterial translocation when compared with standard formulas. This decrease in translocation was associated with a normalization of secretory immunoglobulin A levels and a decrease in bacterial adherence to enterocytes, suggesting that glutamine-supplemented TPN may enhance gut immune function. Glutamine-supplemented TPN also maintained both B-cell and T-cell populations in the lamina propria of the terminal ileum [189]. [*Editor's Note:* An extensive note on translocation is obviously beyond the scope of this chapter. It is important, however, to note that whether glutamine increases or decreases translocation, one should not make the mistake of equating glutamine's effect on translocation of gut bacteria or their products with efficacy as far as villous atrophy or lack of villous atrophy. It is unfortunate that any gut fuel has been associated with increased gut integrity and, it follows, arguing by analogy, a decrease in translocation. This may not be completely correct. Translocation of gut bacteria and their products may in fact be a normal process, and a little translocation may be a good thing. Indeed, there is evidence that provision of glutamine provides energy for the translocation process [190]. It may be that a little translocation is normal, but massive breakdown of the barrier is abnormal. A little translocation may be a normal process involved in immunosurveillance and the development of antibodies to potential invaders.]

Glutamine's effect on translocation cannot be directly equated with efficacy in preventing villous atrophy. However, other investigators have shown that provision of glutamine-supplemented nutritional support may accelerate healing of the intestinal injury that occurs secondary to chemotherapy or radiation therapy. Fox and colleagues [191] showed that the addition of glutamine to an elemental, enteral diet resulted in a significant reduction in the severity of methotrexate-induced enterocolitis, as reflected by improved morphometric parameters in the jejunum and colon. Provision of glutamine reduced endotoxin transmigration from the gut lumen and improved survival. Similar benefits were reported by Jacobs and associates [192], who demonstrated that a glutamine-enriched intravenous diet accelerated healing of the gut mucosa in rats receiving 5-fluorouracil (5-FU). O'Dwyer and colleagues [193] also showed that after 5-FU treatment, rats maintained on glutamine-enriched TPN demonstrated greater mean jejunal villous height and an increase in mucosal DNA content. When glutamine-supplemented TPN was given before the administration of 5-FU, there was even more marked effect on mucosal cellularity and significantly lower mortality than in animals maintained on standard TPN.

Glutamine feeding has been shown to diminish the incidence of bacterial translocation to the mesenteric lymph nodes in an experimental radiation enteritis model [194]. Jejunum from rats receiving the glutamine diet demonstrated increased villous height and number and nearly three times the number of mitoses per crypt [195]. Provision of oral glutamine after abdominal irradiation also supports gut glutamine metabolism and decreases the morbidity and mortality (Table 12-3) associated with abdominal radiation [195]. Administration of a glutamine-enriched oral diet before abdominal radiation was equally effective in exerting a protective effect from radiation [196]. More recent studies suggest that glutamine enhances the transport of methotrexate into malignant cells [Klimberg et al., unpublished data]. Thus, provision of glutamine to patients undergoing abdominal or pelvic irradiation may protect the intestinal mucosa from injury and accelerate healing of radiated bowel and possibly attenuate the long-term sequelae of radiation enteritis.

Glutamine may also be useful in the treatment of diarrhea. Nath and colleagues [197] demonstrated that intestinal sodium absorption in diarrheagenic *E. coli*–infected rabbits can be enhanced by administering enteral glutamine. In a different

Table 12-3. Benefits of Oral Glutamine Provided After Whole Abdominal Radiation in Rats

Diet Provided	Gut GLN Extraction (%)	No. of Animals Surviving for 8 Days	No. of Animals With Culture-Positive MLNs (Day 4)	Jejunal Villous Height (mm)	Jejunal Villous no. (no./cm bowel)
Control	12 ± 7	5/11	8/9	0.29 ± 0.03	79 ± 11
Glutamine	35 ± 8	11/11[a]	2/10[b]	0.54 ± 0.05[a]	101 ± 4[a]

GLN = glutamine; MLNs = mesenteric lymph nodes.

[a]$p < 0.01$.

[b]$p < 0.05$ vs. control.

Source: Modified from VS Klimberg, et al. Oral glutamine accelerates healing of the small intestine and improves outcome after whole abdominal radiation. *Arch Surg* 125:1040, 1990; and WW Souba, et al. Oral glutamine reduces bacterial translocation following abdominal radiation. *J Surg Res* 48:1, 1990.

study, Frankel and colleagues [198] showed that infusion of glutamine into the lumen of transplanted small intestine increased small bowel protein and augmented glucose absorption. A recent study by Yoshida et al. [199] evaluated the combination of TPN and sepsis on intestinal mucosal morphology and protein synthesis. Addition of glutamine to the TPN solution attenuated the endotoxin-induced damage to the jejunum and ileum. Sepsis was associated with an increase in mucosal protein synthesis, and the increase was greatest when supplemental glutamine was supplied.

Impact of Glutamine Nutrition on the Liver and Pancreas

Because glutamine is an important respiratory fuel for the exocrine and endocrine pancreas, Helton and colleagues [200] studied the effects of glutamine-enriched TPN on the exocrine pancreas in laboratory rats with and without a 60% small bowel resection. In both resected and unresected animals, the addition of glutamine significantly increased pancreatic weight, DNA content, and protein content. Glutamine supplementation also increased total pancreatic trypsinogen and lipase content. These beneficial effects of glutamine resulted in pancreatic acinar hyperplasia rather than hypertrophy. These investigators also demonstrated that glutamine supports pancreatic growth and function during elemental enteral feeding [201].

Opara and associates [202] have approached the pancreas from the standpoint of examining the role of glutamine as a regulator of endocrine function. When isolated pancreatic islets were perfused with L-glutamine, basal glucagon output was stimulated, but insulin production was suppressed. This alteration in the portal glucagon/insulin ratio has been shown to influence fatty infiltration in the liver. Infusion of excess carbohydrate calories leads to hepatic steatosis in rats, an event associated with an elevated portal insulin/glucagon molar ratio. Based on these observations, Li and colleagues [203] studied the effects of glutamine-enriched TPN on hepatic steatosis. They randomized adult rats to receive chow, 25% dextrose-base TPN, or 25% dextrose-base TPN with 2% glutamine. Panlobular vacuolization of the hepatocytes was noted on histology in the TPN group, whereas the chow group and the rats fed TPN + glutamine showed normal liver morphology. Hepatic lipid content was significantly elevated in the TPN (without glutamine) group, as was the portal insulin/glucagon molar ratio. In contrast, portal glucagon was significantly elevated, whereas the insulin/glucagon ratio and hepatic lipid content did not increase above control levels in the glutamine-supplemented rats. The results suggest that addition of L-glutamine to standard TPN prevents the development of hepatic steatosis, possibly by stimulating glucagon secretion and thus lowering the portal insulin/glucagon ratio and increasing hepatic lipid export. However, in this study, glucagon did not increase gut mucosal thickness, intestinal weight, or protein content in the group receiving 2% parenteral glutamine. Helton and colleagues also demonstrated the beneficial effects of glutamine-enriched enteral elemental diets in attenuating the gain in liver weight and fat content that develops after massive small bowel resection [201].

Glutamine Nutrition and Tumor Growth

Because tumors are avid glutamine consumers, several investigators have examined the effects of glutamine-supplemented diets on indices of malignant cell proliferation in vivo and in vitro. In a number of malignant cell types, it has been shown that maximal rates of proliferation occur when glutamine concentrations are maintained at 0.5 mM or above. In 1955, Eagle [10] demonstrated that proliferation of cultured HeLa cells is greatest when glutamine concentrations are greater than 1 mM. Thus, the requirement of most growing malignant cells in vitro appears to reflect a need for a continuous supply of glutamine in the absence of the normal in vivo (approximately 0.6 mM in blood) supply, rather than supraphysiologic concentrations. In vivo studies using tumor-bearing rats showed that administration of glutamine-supplemented TPN did not affect tumor weight, tumor DNA content, or tumor glutaminase activity [176]. Furthermore, DNA flow cytometric analysis did not demonstrate any difference in percentage of aneuploid tumor cells within the G1, S, or G2/M cell cycles. However, the ratio of aneuploid to diploid cells within the tumor mass increased by 20% in animals receiving glutamine. TPN + glutamine had no effect on tumor glutathione (GSH) levels. No increase in hepatic GSH levels were observed, but gut mucosal GSH levels were 20% greater in the TPN + glutamine group. Similar observations in tumor-bearing animals were made when oral glutamine-supplemented diets were used [177]. A recent study by Bartlett and associates [204] demonstrated the trophic effects of a glutamine-supplemented enteral diet on the small bowel in tumor-bearing rats and showed that they did not stimulate tumor growth. Rats were implanted with mammary adenocarcinoma (MAC)-33 mammary carcinoma cells and randomly assigned to receive standard enteral diets supplemented with either 3% glutamine or 3% glycine (control). Small bowel mucosa in the glutamine-fed group showed an increased mucosal DNA content. There was no significant difference in tumor weight or protein and DNA content and no increase in the incidence of metastases between the groups.

Glutamine Nutrition and Lymphocytes

Newsholme [205] suggests that glutamine may be essential for lymphocyte proliferation in response to an antigenic challenge both as a precursor for nucleotide biosynthesis and as a major energy source. Cell culture studies demonstrate that failure to supplement the culture media with glutamine impairs the ability of lymphocytes to respond to mitogenic stimulation [206]. In terminally differentiated macrophages, glutamine may be required for the synthesis of mRNA for producing secretory proteins (such as TNF or IL-1) during immune challenge or for the synthesis of phospholipid to support cell membrane activity during pinocytosis or phagocytosis. To examine the relationship between glutamine depletion and lymphocyte and macrophage function, Parry-Billings and colleagues [207] studied burn patients. Lymphocyte function was impaired in vitro at the low blood glutamine levels characteristic of those seen in vivo in severely burned patients. The obvious implication of these studies is that the immunodeficiency associated with critical illness may, in part, be a metabolic phenomenon amenable to therapy by nutritional support. Testing this hypothesis would involve studying the impact of glutamine-enriched diets on immune function. The decrease in clinical infections noted in bone marrow transplantation patients receiving glutamine-enriched TPN suggests a salutary effect of glutamine on the immune system [208].

Glutamine Nutrition and the Lungs

Because glutamine is required for endothelial function and because of the important role the lungs play in glutamine metabolism, Austgen and colleagues examined the effects of a glutamine infusion on lung weights after a bolus of endotoxin. Compared to endotoxin-treated animals who received a control amino acid infusion, the glutamine-infused group had a decrease in pulmonary edema after endotoxin ($p < 0.08$) [Austgen et al., unpublished data]. Hinshaw and Burger [209] demonstrated that glutamine supplementation significantly increased ATP levels and viability of endothelial cells 5 hours after hydrogen peroxide injury. These observations suggest that mitochondrial substrates that bypass glucose-dependent pathways of ATP synthesis may be useful therapeutic agents for maintenance of ATP levels in oxidant-injured cells.

Human Clinical Trials

Studies in human volunteers [19,210] and in hospitalized patients have failed to demonstrate any toxicity associated with glutamine-supplemented parenteral nutrition. Concern exists about infusing glutamine because of its biochemical relationship to ammonia, but elevated circulating levels of ammonia have not been reported to date. Glutamate, which is generated during the metabolism of glutamine, is intimately related to the neurotransmitter γ-aminobutyric acid (GABA), but no neurologic side effects were reported in these patients. Mebane [211] reported that two patients who ingested supplemental glutamine (2–4 g/d) developed an increase in energy level. Such observations may be coincidental because infusion of much larger doses (20–40 g/d) have not caused neurologic symptoms.

Glutamine in solution undergoes hydrolysis in a relatively short period of time, but this process can be slowed considerably by adjusting the pH and temperature of the solution. Breakdown is negligible when the glutamine is added to the TPN mixture at the time the pharmacist prepares the final solution. In the United States, the majority of studies evaluating the use of glutamine-supplemented diets have used free glutamine. In Europe, however, glutamine dipeptides have commonly been evaluated [212–214]. The most common dipeptides used are L-alanylglutamine and L-glycylglutamine. These dipeptides, although more expensive than free glutamine, are stable in solution and are much more soluble than free glutamine (approximately 400 g/L vs. approximately 30 g/L). These dipeptides are rapidly hydrolyzed after infusion, have a short half-life, and, in general, are as effective as free glutamine. Moreover, they are safe and without side effects.

The best study to date evaluating the effects of glutamine-enriched TPN is a randomized, double-blind controlled trial [208,215]. The investigators studied 45 adults receiving allogenic bone marrow transplants for hematologic malignancies. Patients received a standard, glutamine-free TPN solution or an experimental isonitrogenous, isocaloric solution supplemented with L-glutamine (0.57 g/kg body weight per day). Patients received the diets for approximately 1 month after bone marrow transplants. Patients receiving glutamine-supplemented parenteral nutrition after bone marrow transplants had improved nitrogen balance, a diminished incidence of clinical infections, less fluid accumulation, and a shortened hospital stay (Table 12-4). It should be noted that positive effects of glutamine-enriched TPN may be accentuated in critically ill patients whose systems are compromised to a point where normal biochemical changes that are necessary to respond to insult are no longer possible.

Summary

Although beneficial effects of glutamine have not always been observed [203], a variety of studies from different laboratories suggest that, under certain circumstances, glutamine supplementation of the diet may be beneficial to patients. Further studies are required to determine which individuals are the best candidates for such therapy. If and when conclusive data demonstrate that glutamine nutrition will "make a difference," the enteral route of delivery should always be used unless it is contraindicated. Under certain circumstances, provision of glutamine via the parenteral route may not be as effective as enteral administration (Table 12-5) [216,217].

Table 12-4. Results of a Randomized Trial of Glutamine-Enriched TPN (GLN-TPN) versus Standard TPN (STD-TPN) After Bone Marrow Transplantation

Group	No. of Patients Studied	Nitrogen Balance (g/d)	No. of Patients With Clinical Infections	No. of Patients Without Positive Cultures	Increase in ECW (L)[c]	Hospital Stay (days)
STD-TPN	21	-4.2 ± 1.2	9 (43%)	1 (5%)	3.2 ± 0.9	36 ± 2
GLN-TPN	25	-1.4 ± 0.5[a]	3 (12%)[b]	10 (42%)[b]	0.4 ± 0.9[b]	29 ± 1[b]

Data analysis by unpaired t-test or Fisher Exact test. ECW = extracellular water.

[a] $p < 0.01$.

[b] $p < 0.05$ vs. STD-TPN.

[c] n = 10 patients per group.

Source: Modified from MR Scheltinga, et al. Glutamine-enriched intravenous feedings attenuate extracellular fluid expansion after standard stress. *Ann Surg* 214:385, 1991; and TR Ziegler, et al. Glutamine-supplemented parenteral nutrition improves nitrogen retention and reduces hospital mortality versus standard parenteral nutrition following bone marrow transplantation: A randomized, double-blind trial. *Ann Intern Med* 116:821, 1992.

Table 12-5. Incidence of Bacterial Translocation in Animals Receiving Methotrexate and Randomized to Identical Glutamine-Supplemented Elemental Diets Administered Orally (PO) or Intravenously (IV)

Diet	Incidence of Positive MLN	Incidence of Positive Liver	Incidence of Positive Spleen	Mortality
IV-GLN	10/10	8/10	8/10	10/10 (100%)
PO-GLN	10/10	6/10	4/10*	1/10 (10%)*

Enteral administration was associated with a significant decrease in the incidence of positive cultures in the spleen and a marked improvement in survival. The most commonly translocating bacteria were *E. coli* and *Proteus* sp. MLN = mesenteric lymph node; GLN = glutamine.

*$p < 0.05$ vs. IV.

Source: Modified from JC Alverdy. Effects of glutamine-supplemented diets on immunology of the gut. *JPEN* 14:109S, 1990.

References

1. Souba WW. Interorgan ammonia metabolism in health and disease: A surgeon's view. *JPEN* 11:569S, 1987.
2. Hanson PJ, Parson SDS. Metabolism and transport of glutamine and glucose in vascularly perfused rats small intestine. *Biochem J* 166:509, 1977.
3. Souba WW, et al. Current research review: The role of glutamine in maintaining a healthy gut and supporting the metabolic response to injury and infection. *J Surg Res* 48:383, 1990.
4. Windmueller HG. Glutamine utilization by the small intestine. *Adv Enzymol* 53:202, 1982.
5. Windmueller HG, Spaeth AE. Intestinal metabolism of glutamine and glutamate from the lumen as compared to glutamine from blood. *Arch Biophys Biochem* 171:662, 1975.
6. Windmueller HG, Spaeth AE. Uptake and metabolism of plasma glutamine by the small intestine. *J Biol Chem* 249:5070, 1974.
7. Windmueller HG, Spaeth AE. Respiratory fuels and nitrogen metabolism in vivo in small intestine of fed rats. *J Biol Chem* 255:107, 1980.
8. Welbourne TC, Childress D, Givens G. Renal regulation of interorgan glutamine flow in metabolic acidosis. *Am J Physiol* 251:R858, 1986.
9. Plumley DA, et al. The role of the lungs in maintaining amino acid homeostasis. *JPEN* 14:569, 1990.
10. Eagle H. Nutritional needs of mammalian cells in tissue culture. *Science* 122:501, 1955.
11. Krebs HA. Glutamine Metabolism in the Animal Body. In J Mora, R Palacios (eds), *Glutamine: Metabolism, Enzymology, and Regulation.* New York: Academic, 1980. P 319.
12. Turinsky J, Long C. Free amino acids in muscle: Effect of muscle fiber population and denervation. *Am J Physiol* 258:E485, 1990.
13. Askanazi J, et al. Muscle and plasma amino acids following injury. *Ann Surg* 192:78, 1980.
14. Roth E, et al. Metabolic disorders in severe abdominal sepsis: Glutamine deficiency in skeletal muscle. *Clin Nutr* 1:25, 1982.
15. Vinnars E, Bergstrom J, Furst P. Influence of the postoperative state on the intracellular free amino acids in human muscle tissue. *Ann Surg* 182:665, 1975.
16. Hammarqvist F, et al. Addition of glutamine to total parenteral nutrition after elective abdominal surgery spares free glutamine in muscle, counteracts the fall in muscle protein synthesism and improves nitrogen balance. *Ann Surg* 209:455, 1989.
17. Lacey J, Wilmore DW. Is glutamine a conditionally essential amino acid? *Nutr Rev* 48:297, 1990.
18. Stehle P, et al. Effect of parenteral glutamine peptide supplements on muscle glutamine loss and nitrogen balance after major surgery. *Lancet* 1:231, 1989.
19. Ziegler TR, et al. Safety and metabolic effects of L-glutamine administration in humans. *JPEN* 14:137S, 1990.
20. Kominz DR, et al. The amino acid composition of actin, myosin, tropomyosin, and the meromyosins. *Arch Biochem Biophys* 50:48, 1951.
21. Christensen HN. Role of amino acid transport and countertransport in nutrition and metabolism. *Physiol Rev* 70:43, 1990.
22. Bode BP, et al. Characteristics and regulation of hepatic glutamine transport. *JPEN* 14:51S, 1990.
23. Shotwell MA, Kilberg MS, Oxender DL. The regulation of neutral amino acid transport in mammalian cells. *Biochim Biophys Acta* 737:267, 1983.
24. Stevens BR, et al. Intestinal brush border membrane Na^+/glucose cotransporter functions in situ as a homotetramer. *Proc Natl Acad Sci USA* 87:1456, 1990.
25. Stevens BR, Wright EM. Kinetics of the intestinal brush border proline (Imino) carrier. *J Biol Chem* 262:6546, 1987.
26. Fafournoux P, et al. Bidirectional transport of glutamine across the cell membrane in rat liver. *Biochem J* 216:401, 1983.
27. Hautamaki RD, Green B, Souba WW. Characterization of L-glutamine transport by type II alveolar cells. *Am J Physiol* 262:L459, 1992.
28. Bode BP, Kilberg MS. Amino acid dependent increase in hepatic system N activity is linked to cell swelling. *J Biol Chem* 257:345, 1991.
29. Pacitti AJ, Austgen TR, Souba WW. Mechanisms of increased hepatic glutamine uptake in the endotoxin-treated rat. *J Surg Res* 53:298, 1992.
30. Ahmed A, Taylor PM, Rennie MJ. Characteristics of glutamine transport in rat sarcolemmal vesicles from rat skeletal muscle. *Am J Physiol* 259:E284, 1990.
31. Kilberg MS, Handlogten ME, Christensen HS. Characteristics of system ASC for transport of neutral amino acids in the isolated rat hepatocyte. *J Biol Chem* 256:3304, 1981.
32. Kilberg MS, Handlogten ME, Christensen HN. Characteristics of an amino acid transport system in rat liver for glutamine, asparagine, histidine, and closely related analogs. *J Biol Chem* 255:4011, 1980.
33. Souba WW, Copeland EM. Cytokine modulation of sodium-dependent glutamine transport across the brush border membrane of monolayers of human intestinal Caco-2 cells. *Ann Surg* 215:536, 1992.
34. Souba WW, Pan M, Stevens BR. Characterization of L-glutamine transport by the brush border of Caco-2 monolayers. *Biochem Biophys Res Comm* 188:746, 1992.
35. Stevens BR, Kaunitz J, Wright EM. Intestinal transport of amino acids and sugars: Advances using membrane vesicles. *Ann Rev Physiol* 417:471, 1984.
36. Stevens BR, et al. Organic and inorganic solute transport in renal and intestinal membrane vesicles preserved in liquid nitrogen. *Membr Biochem* 4:271, 1982.
37. Said HM, et al. Transport characteristics of glutamine in human intestinal brush-border membrane vesicles. *Am J Physiol* 256:G240, 1989.
38. Salloum RM, et al. Dietary modulation of small intestinal glutamine transport in intestinal brush border membrane vesicles of rats. *J Surg Res* 48:635, 1990.
39. Schroder MT, Schafer G, Schauder P. Characterization of glutamine transport into resting and concanavalin A-stimulated peripheral human lymphocytes. *J Cell Physiol* 145:155, 1990.
40. Dudrick PS, Bland KI, Souba WW. Effects of tumor necrosis factor on System ASC-mediated glutamine transport by human fibroblasts. *J Surg Res* 52:347, 1992.
41. Herskowitz K, et al. Characterization of L-glutamine transport by pulmonary artery endothelial cells. *Am J Physiol* 260:L241, 1991.
42. Sastrasinh S, Sastrasinh M. Glutamine transport in submitochondrial particles. *Am J Physiol* 257:F1050, 1989.
43. Nissim I, et al. Relative role of glutaminase, glutamate dehydrogenase, and AMP-dehydrogenase pathways in

hepatic ureagenesis: Studies with ^{15}N. *Arch Biochem Biophys* 292:393, 1992.

44. Adams RLP, Knowler JT, Leader DP. *The Biochemistry of the Nucleic Acids,* 10th ed. New York: Chapman & Hall, 1986. P 120.
45. Medina MA, et al. Relevance of glutamine metabolism to tumor cell growth. *Mol Cell Biochem* 113:1, 1992.
46. Reitzer LJ, Wice BM, Kennell D. Evidence that glutamine, not sugar, is the major energy source for cultured HeLa cells. *J Biol Chem* 254:2669, 1979.
47. Wu P, Ray NG, Shuler ML. A single-cell model for CHO cells. *Ann NY Acad Sci* 665:152, 1992.
48. Newsholme P, Newsholme EA. Rates of utilization of glucose, glutamine and oleate and formation of end-products by mouse peritoneal macrophages in culture. *Biochem J* 261:211, 1989.
49. Ardawi MSM, Newsholme EA. Glutamine metabolism in lymphocytes of the rat. *Biochem J* 212:835, 1983.
50. Brand K. Glutamine and glucose metabolism during thymocyte proliferation. *Biochem J* 228:353, 1985.
51. Gonzalez-Mateis F, et al. Inhibition of glycolysis by amino acids in ascites tumor cells. *J Biol Chem* 268:7809, 1993.
52. Guppy M, Greiner E, Brand K. The role of the Crabtree effect and an endogenous fuel in the energy metabolism of resting and proliferating thymocytes. *Eur J Biochem* 212:95, 1993.
53. Sumbilla CM, et al. Comparison of the oxidation of glutamine, glucose, ketone bodies and fatty acids by human diploid fibroblasts. *Biochim Biophys Acta* 675:301, 1981.
54. Zielke HR, et al. Lactate: A major product of glutamine metabolism by human diploid fibroblasts. *J Cell Physiol* 104:433, 1980.
55. Lazo PA. Amino acid and glucose utilization by different metabolic pathways in Ascites-tumour cells. *Eur J Biochem* 117:19, 1981.
56. Mares-Perlman JA, Shrago E. Energy substrate utilization in freshly isolated Morris hepatoma 7777 Cells. *Cancer Res* 48:602, 1988.
57. Spolarics Z, et al. Glutamine and fatty acid oxidation are the main sources of energy for Kupffer and endothelial cells. *Am J Physiol* 261:G185, 1991.
58. Zielke HR, et al. Reciprocal regulation of glucose and glutamine utilization by cultured human diploid fibroblasts. *J Cell Physiol* 95:41, 1978.
59. Krutzfeldt A, et al. Metabolism of exogenous substrates by coronary endothelial cells in culture. *J Mol Cell Cardiol* 22:1393, 1990.
60. Barbehenn EK, et al. An examination of the efficiency of glucose and glutamine as energy sources for cultured chick pigment epithelial cells. *J Cell Physiol* 118:262, 1984.
61. He Y, Chu S-HW, Walker WA. Nucleotide supplements alter proliferation and differentiation of cultured human (Caco-2) and rat (IEC-6) intestinal epithelial cells. *J Nutr* 123:1017, 1993.
62. Souba WW, Smith RJ, Wilmore DW. Glutamine metabolism by the intestinal tract. *JPEN* 9:608, 1985.
63. Ewart HS, Brosnan JT. Rapid activation of hepatic glutaminase in rats fed on a single high-protein meal. *Biochem J* 293:339, 1993.
64. Ardawi MSM, Koja SM. Effect of hyperthyroidism on glucose, glutamine and ketone-body metabolism in the gut of the rat. *Int J Biochem* 25:619, 1993.
65. Haussinger D, Lamers WH, Moorman AF. Hepatocyte heterogeneity in the metabolism of amino acids and ammonia. *Enzyme* 46:72, 1992.
66. Kaiser S, Curthoys NP. Effect of pH and bicarbonate on phosphoenolpyruvate carboxykinase and glutaminase mRNA levels in cultured renal epithelial cells. *J Biol Chem* 266:9397, 1991.
67. Leighton B, et al. Maximum activities of some key enzymes of glycolysis, glutaminolysis, Kreb cycle, and fatty acid utilization in bovine pulmonary endothelial cells. *FEBS Lett* 225:93, 1987.
68. Michalik M, Nelson J, Erinska M. Glutamate production in Islets of Langerhans: Properties of phosphate-activated glutaminase. *Metabolism* 41:1319, 1992.
69. Perera SY, Chen TC, Curthoys NP. Biosynthesis and processing of renal mitochondrial glutaminase in cultured proximal tubular epithelial cells and in isolated mitochondria. *J Biol Chem* 265:17764, 1990.
70. Rosa LF, Curi Y, Curi R. Effect of insulin, glucocordicoids and thyroid hormones on the activities of key enzymes of glycolysis, glutaminolysis, the pentose-phosphate pathway and the Krebs cycle in rat macrophages. *J Endocrinol* 135:213, 1992.
71. Sarantos P, Ockert K, Souba WW. Endotoxin stimulates lymphocyte glutaminase expression. *Arch Surg* 128:920, 1993.
72. Thekkumkara TJ, Patel MS. Ochatoxin-A decreases the activity of phosphoenolpyruvate carboxykinase and its mRNA content in primary cultures of rat kidney proximal convoluted tubule cells. *Biochem Biophys Res Commun* 162:916, 1989.
73. Hogstad S, et al. Glutaminase in neurons and astrocytes cultured from brain: Kinetic properties and effects of phosphate, glutamate, and ammonia. *Neurochem Res* 13:383, 1988.
74. Swierczynski J, Bereznowski Z, Makarewicz W. Phosphate-dependent glutaminase of rat skeletal muscle. *Biochim Biophys Acta* 1157:55, 1993.
75. Donnelly M, Scheffler IE. Energy metabolism in respiration-deficient and wild-type Chinese hamster fibroblasts in culture. *J Cell Physiol* 89:39, 1976.
76. Lanks KW, Li P-W. End products of glucose and glutamine metabolism by cultured cell lines. *J Cell Physiol* 135:151, 1988.
77. Zielke HR, et al. Growth of human diploid fibroblasts in the absence of glucose utilization. *Proc Natl Acad Sci USA* 73:4110, 1976.
78. Zielke HR, Zielke CL, Ozand PT. Glutamine: A major energy source for cultured mammalian cells. *Fed Proc* 43:121, 1984.
79. Knox WE, Horowitz ML, Friedell GH. The proportionality of glutaminase content to growth rates of rat hepatomas. *Cancer Res* 29:669, 1969.
80. Linder-Horowitz M, Knox WE, Morris HO. Glutaminase activities and growth rates of rat hepatomas. *Cancer Res* 29:1195, 1969.
81. Newsholme EA, Crabtree B, Ardawi MSM. The role of glycolysis and glutamine utilization in rapidly dividing cells. *Biosci Rep* 5:393, 1985.
82. Szondy Z, Newsholme EA. The effect of various concentrations of nucleobases, nucleosides or glutamine on the incorporation of [^{3}H]thymidine into DNA in the rat mesenteric lymph node lymphocytes stimulated by phytohaemagglutinin. *Biochem J* 270:437, 1990.
83. Bilir BM, et al. Novel control of the position-dependent expression of genes in hepatocytes. *J Biol Chem* 268:19776, 1993.

84. Meister A. Glutamine Synthetase of Mammals. In PD Boyer (ed), *The Enzymes,* vol 10. New York: Academic, 1974. P 699.
85. Adde SK, Lotspeich WD. Relation between glutamine utilization and production in metabolic acidosis. *Am J Physiol* 215:269, 1968.
86. Lockwood AH, et al. The dynamics of ammonia metabolism in man. *J Clin Invest* 63:449, 1979.
87. Ruderman N. Muscle amino acid metabolism and gluconeogenesis. *Annu Rev Med* 26:245, 1975.
88. Welbourne TC. Role of the lung in glutamine homeostasis. *Contrib Nephrol* 63:178, 1988.
89. Arola L, et al. Glutamine synthetase activity in the organs of fed and 24-hour fasted rats. *Horm Metab Res* 13:199, 1981.
90. Lund PA. Radiochemical assay for glutamine synthetase, and activity of the enzyme in rat tissues. *Biochem J* 118:35, 1970.
91. Ardawi MSM. Glutamine-synthesizing activity in lungs of fed, starved, acidotic, diabetic, injured, and septic rats. *Biochem J* 270:829, 1990.
92. Curthoys NP, Lowry OH. The distribution of glutaminase isoenzymes in the carious structures of the nephron in normal, acidotic and alkalotic rat kidney. *J Biol Chem* 248:162, 1973.
93. Feng B, Hilt DC, Max SR. Transcriptional regulation of glutamine synthetase gene expression by dexamethasone in L6 muscle cells. *J Biol Chem* 265:18702, 1990.
94. Kumar S, et al. The hormonal regulation of gene expression of glial markers: Glutamine synthetase and glycerol phosphate dehydrogenase in primary cultures of rat brain and in C6 cell line. *J Neurosci Res* 16:251, 1986.
95. Lemieux G, et al. Glutamine synthetase and glutamyl transferase in the kidney of man, dog and rat. *Am J Physiol* 231:1068, 1976.
96. Muhlbacher F, et al. Effects of glucocorticoids on skeletal muscle glutamine metabolism in skeletal muscle. *Am J Physiol* 247:E75, 1984.
97. Prusiner S, Milner L. A rapid radioactive assay for glutamine synthetase, glutaminase, asparagine synthetase, and asparaginase. *Ann Biochem* 37:429, 1979.
98. Rowe WB. Glutamine Synthetase From Muscle. In A Meister (ed), *Methods in Enzymology.* New York: Academic, 1985. P 113.
99. Seiler N, Reid J, Knodgen B. A sensitive method for the assay of glutamine synthetase. *Neurochem Res* 15:301, 1990.
100. Windmueller HG. Phosphate dependant glutaminase in the small intestine. *Arch Biochem Biophys* 182:506, 1977.
101. Banner C, et al. Isolation of a cDNA for rat brain glutaminase. *Mol Brain Res* 3:247, 1988.
102. Kuo CF, Darnell JE. Mouse glutamine synthetase is encoded by a single gene that can be expressed in a localized fashion. *J Mol Biol* 208:45, 1989.
103. Kapadia CR, et al. Alterations in glutamine metabolism in response to operative stress and food deprivation. *Surg Forum* 33:19, 1982.
104. Max SR, et al. Dexamethasone regulates glutamine synthetase expression in rat skeletal muscles. *Am J Physiol* 255:E397, 1988.
105. Smith RJ, et al. Regulation of glutamine synthetase and glutaminase activities in cultured skeletal muscle cells. *J Cell Physiol* 120:197, 1984.
106. Souba WW, et al. Effects of glucocorticoids on lung glutamine and alanine metabolism. *Surgery* 108:213, 1990.
107. Sarantos P, Howard D, Souba WW. Dexamethasone regulates glutamine synthetase expression in rat lung. *Metabolism* 42:795, 1993.
108. Souba WW, Wilmore DW. Postoperative alterations of arteriovenous exchange of amino acids across the gastrointestinal tract. *Surgery* 94:342, 1983.
109. Miller BM, et al. Interorgan relationships of alanine and glutamine during fasting in the conscious dog. *J Surg Res* 35:310, 1983.
110. Souba WW, Smith RJ, Wilmore DW. Effects of glucocorticoids on glutamine metabolism in visceral organs. *Metabolism* 34:450, 1985.
111. Fox AD, et al. Dexamethasone administration induces increased glutaminase-specific activity in the jejunum and colon. *J Surg Res* 44:391, 1988.
112. Sarantos P, Abouhamze A, Souba WW. Glucocorticoids regulate intestinal glutaminase expression. *Surgery* 112: 278, 1992.
113. Dudrick PS, et al. Dexamethasone stimulates glutaminase expression in mesenteric lymph nodes. *Am J Surg* 165:34, 1993.
114. Souba WW, Wilmore DW. Gut-liver interaction during accelerated gluconeogenesis. *Arch Surg* 120:66, 1985.
115. Gebhardt R, Kleeman E. Hormonal regulation of amino acid transport system N in primary cultures of rat hepatocytes. *Eur J Biochem* 166:339, 1987.
116. Geer RJ, et al. Glucagon: An important stimulator of gut and hepatic glutamine metabolism. *Surg Forum* 38:27, 1987.
117. Sartorius OW, Calhoun D, Pitts RF. Studies on the interrelationship of the renal cortex and renal ammonia excretion by the rat. *Endocrinology* 52:256, 1953.
118. Welbourne T, et al. Triamcinolone activation of renal ammonia production. *Proc Soc Exp Biol Med* 153:539, 1976.
119. Welbourne TC. Interorgan glutamine flow in metabolic acidosis. *Am J Physiol* 253:F1069, 1987.
120. Austgen TR, Plumley DA, Souba WW. Simple method of determining pulmonary blood flow in the anesthetized rat. *J Invest Surg* 4:81, 1991.
121. Austgen TR, et al. Adaptive regulation in skeletal muscle glutamine metabolism in endotoxin-treated rats. *J Trauma* 32:600, 1992.
122. Ardawi MSM, Majzoub MF. Glutamine metabolism in skeletal muscle of septic rats. *Metabolism* 40:155, 1991.
123. Austgen TA, et al. Glutamine metabolism by the endotoxin-injured lung. *J Trauma* 31:1068, 1991.
124. Plumley DA, et al. Accelerated lung amino acid release in hyperdynamic septic surgical patients. *Arch Surg* 125:57, 1990.
125. Herskowitz K, et al. The effects of endotoxin on glutamine transport by pulmonary artery endothelial cells. *J Surg Res* 50:356, 1991.
126. Souba WW, et al. Cytokine modulation of glutamine transport by pulmonary artery endothelial cells. *Surgery* 110:295, 1991.
127. Austgen TR, et al. The effects of endotoxin on splanchnic metabolism of glutamine and related substrates in vivo. *J Trauma* 31:742, 1991.
128. Dudrick PS, et al. The early response of the brush border glutamine transporter to endotoxemia. *J Surg Res* 52: 372, 1992.
129. Souba WW, et al. The effects of sepsis and endotoxemia on gut glutamine metabolism. *Ann Surg* 211:543, 1990.

130. Von Allmen D, et al. Increased intestinal protein synthesis during sepsis. *Surg Forum* 41:68, 1990.
131. Salloum RM, Copeland EM, Souba WW. Brush border transport of glutamine and other substrates during sepsis and endotoxemia. *Ann Surg* 213:401, 1991.
132. Peitsch JB, et al. Burn injury alters intestinal glutamine transport. *J Surg Res* 46:296, 1989.
133. Austgen TR, et al. Cytokine regulation of intestinal glutamine utilization. *Am J Surg* 163:174, 1991.
134. Sarantos P, Ockert K, Souba WW. Effects of endotoxin on glutaminase expression in mesenteric lymph nodes. *Arch Surg* 128:920, 1993.
135. Brand K, et al. Metabolism of glutamine in lymphocytes. *Metabolism* 38:29S, 1989.
136. Brand K, et al. Metabolic alterations associated with proliferation of mitogen-activated lymphocytes and of lymphoblastoid cell lines: Evaluation of glucose and glutamine metabolism. *Immunobiology* 173:23, 1986.
137. Austgen TR, et al. Endotoxin and renal glutamine metabolism. *Arch Surg* 126:23, 1991.
138. Inoue Y, Pacitti AJ, Souba WW. Endotoxin stimulates Na^+-dependent amino acid transport in rat liver. *J Surg Res* 54:393, 1993.
139. Zamir O, et al. Tumour necrosis factor (TNF) and interleukin-1 (IL-1) induced muscle proelysis through different mechanisms. *Mediat Inflammation* 1:247, 1992.
140. Watkins K, Dudrick PS, Souba WW. Interleukin-6 and dexamethasone work coordinately to augment hepatic amino acid transport. *J Trauma* 36:523, 1994.
141. Ganada OP, Ruderman N. Muscle nitrogen metabolism in chronic hepatic insufficiency. *Metabolism* 25:427, 1976.
142. Jepson MM, et al. Relationship between glutamine concentration and protein synthesis in rat skeletal muscle. *Am J Physiol* 18:E166, 1988.
143. Rennie MJ, et al. Characteristics of a glutamine carrier in skeletal muscle have important consequences for nitrogen loss in injury, infection, and chronic disease. *Lancet* 1:1008, 1986.
144. Rennie MJ, et al. Skeletal muscle glutamine transport, intra-muscular glutamine concentration, and muscle protein turnover. *Metabolism* 38:47, 1989.
145. Newsholme EA, Parry-Billings M. Properties of glutamine release from muscle and its importance for the immune system. *JPEN* 14:63S, 1990.
146. Furst P, et al. Amino Acid Metabolism in Cancer. In R Kluthe, GW Lohr (eds), *Nutrition and Metabolism in Cancer.* Stuttgart: Thieme, 1981. P 75.
147. Kovacevic Z, Morris HP. The role of glutamine in the oxidative metabolism of malignant cells. *Cancer Res* 32:326, 1972.
148. Kovacevic Z. The pathway of glutamate oxidation in isolated mitochondria from mammalian cells. *Biochem J* 125:757, 1971.
149. Wu C, Bauer JM. A study of free amino acids and of glutamine synthesis in tumor-bearing rats. *Cancer Res* 20:848, 1960.
150. Yamamoto H, et al. Relative uptake of plasma amino acids by fetal and tumor tissues. *Metabolism* 23:1017, 1974.
151. Quesada AR, et al. Contribution by host tissues to circulating glutamine in mice inoculated with Ehrlich ascites tumor cells. *Cancer Res* 48:1551, 1988.
152. Sauer LA, Stayma JW III, Dauchy RT. Amino acid, glucose, and lactic acid utilization in vivo by rat tumors. *Cancer Res* 46:3469, 1986.
153. Chen MK, et al. Tumor glutamine use exceeds intestinal glutamine use in cachectic tumor-bearing rats. *Surg Forum* 41:12, 1990.
154. Chen MK, et al. Tumor regulation of hepatic glutamine metabolism. *JPEN* 15:159, 1991.
155. Fischer JE, Chance WT. Total parenteral nutrition, glutamine, and tumor growth. *JPEN* 14:86S, 1990.
156. Pacitti AJ, et al. Mechanisms of accelerated hepatic glutamine efflux in the tumor-bearing rat. *Surg Oncol* 1:173, 1992.
157. Salloum RM, et al. Selective stimulation of brush border glutamine transport in the tumor-bearing rat. *J Surg Res* 50:391, 1992.
158. Salloum RM, et al. Selective inhibition of intestinal glutaminase activity in the tumor-bearing rat. *Surg Forum* 50:115, 1991.
159. Souba WW, et al. Tumor modulation of intestinal glutaminase activity. *FASEB J* 4:A1042, 1990.
160. Souba WW, et al. Interorgan glutamine metabolism in the tumor-bearing rat. *J Surg Res* 44:720, 1988.
161. Chen MK, et al. Influence of progressive tumor growth on glutamine metabolism in skeletal muscle and kidney. *Ann Surg* 217:555, 1993.
162. Chance WT, et al. Hypothalamic concentration and release of neuropeptide Y into microdialysates is reduced in anorectic tumor-bearing rats. *Life Sci.*
163. Stovroff MC, Norton JA. Cachectin levels in the serum of tumor-bearing rats. *Arch Surg* 124:94, 1989.
164. Warren RS, Jeevanandam M, Brennan MF. Comparison of hepatic protein synthesis in vivo versus in vitro in the tumor-bearing rat. *J Surg Res* 42:43, 1987.
165. Warren RS, Jeevanandam M, Brennan MF. Protein synthesis in the tumor-influenced hepatocyte. *Surgery* 98:275, 1985.
166. Dudrick PS, et al. Na^+-dependent glutamine transport in the liver of tumour-bearing rats. *Surg Oncol* 2:205, 1993.
167. Norton JA, et al. Parabiotic transfer of cancer cachexia/anorexia in male rats. *Cancer Res* 45:5547, 1985.
168. Illig KA, Maronian N, Peacock JL. Cancer cachexia is transmissible in plasma. *J Surg Res* 52:353, 1992.
169. Argiles JM, et al. The role of cytokine in muscle wasting: Its relation to cancer cachexia. *Med Res Rev* 12:637, 1992.
170. Stovroff MC, Fraker DL, Norton JA. Cachectin activity in the serum of cachectic, tumor-bearing rats. *Arch Surg* 124:94, 1989.
171. Pacitti AJ, Inoue Y, Souba WW. Tumor necrosis factor stimulates Na^+-dependent amino acid transport in plasma membrane vesicles from rat liver. *J Clin Invest* 91:474, 1993.
172. Ardawi MSM. Skeletal muscle glutamine production in thermally injured rats. *Clin Sci* 74:165, 1988.
173. Kapadia CR, et al. Maintenance of skeletal muscle intracellular glutamine during standard surgical trauma. *JPEN* 9:583, 1985.
174. MacLennan PA, Brown RA, Rennie MJ. A positive relationship between protein synthetic rate and intracellular glutamine concentration in perfused rat skeletal muscle. *FEBS Lett* 215:187, 1987.
175. Millward DJ, Jepson MM, Omer A. Muscle glutamine concentration and protein turnover in vivo in malnutrition and in endotoxemia. *Metabolism* 38:6, 1989.
176. Austgen TR, et al. The effects of glutamine-enriched total parenteral nutrition on tumor growth and host tissues. *Ann Surg* 215:107, 1992.

177. Klimberg VS, et al. Glutamine-enriched diets support muscle glutamine metabolism without stimulating tumor growth. *J Surg Res* 48:319, 1990.

178. Baskerville A, Hambleton P, Benbough JE. Pathologic features of glutaminase toxicity. *Br J Exp Pathol* 61:132, 1980.

179. Okabe S, et al. Inhibitory effect of L-glutamine on gastric irritation and back diffusion of gastric acid in response to aspirin in the rat. *Dig Dis Sci* 20:626, 1975.

180. Shive W, et al. Glutamine in treatment of peptic ulcer. *Texas State J Med* 36:840, 1957.

181. Hwang TL, et al. Preservation of small bowel mucosa using glutamine-enriched parenteral nutrition. *Surg Forum* 38:56, 1987.

182. Klimberg VS, et al. Glutamine-enriched total parenteral nutrition supports gut metabolism. *Surg Forum* 40:175, 1989.

183. Salloum RM, Herskowitz K, Souba WW. Intravenous glutamine stimulates brush border gut glutamine transport. *Surg Forum* 41:195, 1990.

184. Barber AE, et al. Glutamine or fiber supplementation of a defined formula diet: Impact on bacterial translocation, tissue composition, and response to endotoxin. *JPEN* 14:335, 1990.

185. Grant J. Use of L-glutamine in total parenteral nutrition. *J Surg Res* 44:506, 1988.

186. Salloum RM, et al. Glutamine is superior to glutamate in supporting gut metabolism, stimulating intestinal glutaminase activity and preventing bacterial translocation. *Surg Forum* 40:6, 1989.

187. Jacobs DO, et al. Combined effects of glutamine and epidermal growth factor (EGF) on GI mucosal cellularity. *Surgery* 104:358, 1988.

188. Burke D, et al. Glutamine supplemented TPN improves gut immune function. *Arch Surg* 124:1396, 1989.

189. Alverdy JC, et al. The effect of glutamine-enriched TPN on gut immune cellularity. *J Surg Res* 52:34, 1992.

190. Cardona MA, et al. Bacterial translocation through intact ileal mucosa in vitro: An active metabolic process [Abstract]. Presented at Surgical Infection Society, Fort Lauderdale, Florida, April 8–10, 1991.

191. Fox AD, et al. Effect of a glutamine supplemented enteral diet on methotrexate-induced enterocolitis. *JPEN* 12:325, 1988.

192. Jacobs DO, et al. Disparate effects of 5-fluorouracil on the ileum and colon of enterally fed rats with protection by dietary glutamine. *Surg Forum* 38:45, 1987.

193. O'Dwyer ST, et al. 5-Fluorouracil toxicity on small intestinal mucosa but not white blood cells is decreased by glutamine [Abstract]. *Clin Res* 35:369A, 1987.

194. Souba WW, et al. Oral glutamine reduces bacterial translocation following abdominal radiation. *J Surg Res* 48:1, 1990.

195. Klimberg VS, et al. Oral glutamine accelerates healing of the small intestine and improves outcome after whole abdominal radiation. *Arch Surg* 125:1040, 1990.

196. Klimberg VS, et al. Prophylactic glutamine protects the intestinal mucosa from radiation injury. *Cancer* 66:62, 1990.

197. Nath SK, et al. [15N]- and [14C]glutamine fluxes across rabbit ileum in experimental diarrhea. *Am J Physiol* 262:G312, 1992.

198. Frankel W, et al. Glutamine enhancement of structure and function in transplanted small intestine in the rat. *JPEN* 17:47, 1993.

199. Yoshida S, et al. Effect of total parenteral nutrition, systemic sepsis, and glutamine on gut mucosa in rats. *Am J Physiol* 26:E368, 1992.

200. Helton S, et al. Effects of glutamine-enriched parenteral nutrition on the exocrine pancreas. *JPEN* 14:344, 1990.

201. Helton S, et al. Enteral glutamine prevents pancreatic atrophy and hepatic steatosis following small bowel resection. *J Surg Res* 48:297, 1990.

202. Opara EC, Burch W, Akwari OE. Characterization of glutamine-regulated pancreatic islet hormone release. *Surg Forum* 41:16, 1990.

203. Li S, et al. Addition of L-glutamine to total parenteral nutrition (TPN) and its effects on portal insulin and glucagon and the development of hepatic steatosis in rats. *J Surg Res* 48:421, 1990.

204. Bartlett D, Kalish BA, Torosian M. Effects of oral glutamine on tumor and host growth. *Ann Surg Oncol* 2:71, 1995.

205. Newsholme EA, et al. A role for muscle in the immune system and its importance in surgery, trauma, sepsis, and burns. *Nutrition* 4:261, 1988.

206. Taudou G, Wiart J, Panijel J. Influence of amino acid deficiency and tRNA aminoacylation on DNA synthesis and DNA polymerase activity during the secondary immune response in vitro. *Mol Immunol* 20:255, 1983.

207. Parry-Billings M, et al. Does glutamine contribute to immunosuppression after major burns? *Lancet* 336:523, 1990.

208. Ziegler TR, et al. Glutamine-supplemented parenteral nutrition improves nitrogen retention and reduces hospital mortality versus standard parenteral nutrition following bone marrow transplantation: A randomized, double-blind trial. *Ann Intern Med* 116:821, 1992.

209. Hinshaw DB, Burger JM. Protective effect of glutamine on endothelial cell ATP in oxidant injury. *J Surg Res* 49:222, 1990.

210. Lowe DL, et al. Glutamine-enriched total parenteral nutrition is safe in normal humans. *Surg Forum* 40:9, 1989.

211. Mebane AH. L-glutamine and mania. *Am J Psychiatry* 141:1302, 1984.

212. Adibi SA. Intravenous use of glutamine in peptide form: Clinical applications of old and new observations. *Metabolism* 38:89S, 1989.

213. Furst P, Albers S, Stehle P. Glutamine-containing dipeptides in parenteral nutrition. *JPEN* 14:118S, 1989.

214. Lochs H, Hubl W. Metabolic basis for selecting glutamine-containing substrates for parenteral nutrition. *JPEN* 14:114S, 1990.

215. Scheltinga MR, et al. Glutamine-enriched intravenous feedings attenuate extracellular fluid expansion after standard stress. *Ann Surg* 214:385, 1991.

216. Alverdy JC. Effects of glutamine-supplemented diets on immunology of the gut. *JPEN* 14:109S, 1990.

217. Scott TE, Moellman JR. Intravenous glutamine fails to improve gut morphology after radiation therapy. *JPEN* 16:440, 1992.

Selected Readings

Newsholme EA, et al. A role for muscle in the immune system and its importance in surgery, trauma, sepsis, and burns. *Nutrition* 4:261, 1988.

An excellent review discussing the role of skeletal muscle as the major glutamine producer and its role in supporting other tissues that require glutamine in large amounts, especially during critical illness.

Souba WW, et al. Current research review: The role of glutamine in maintaining a healthy gut and supporting the metabolic response to injury and infection. *J Surg Res* 48:383, 1990.

The authors review the studies that have demonstrated the benefits of glutamine-enriched nutrition in supporting intestinal metabolism and function. Attention is focused on both the gut mucosa as well as the gut immune system.

Windmueller HG. Glutamine utilization by the small intestine. *Adv Enzymol* 53:202, 1982.

An outstanding early review by the "father" of glutamine metabolism that summarizes an elegant series of experiments describing the important role of the small intestine in glutamine metabolism.

Ziegler TR, et al. Glutamine-supplemented parenteral nutrition improves nitrogen retention and reduces hospital mortality versus standard parenteral nutrition following bone marrow transplantation: A randomized, double-blind trial. *Ann Intern Med* 116:821, 1992.

The best controlled, blinded, randomized, prospective clinical trial to date that demonstrates the benefits of glutamine-enriched TPN in patients treated with bone marrow transplantation. Glutamine supplementation diminished the incidence of infections and reduced hospital stay. The savings associated with such therapy is substantial.

Zielke HR, et al. Growth of human diploid fibroblasts in the absence of glucose utilization. *Proc Natl Acad Sci USA* 73:4110, 1976.

A classic paper that indicates that cultured cells can proliferate in the absence of glucose if glutamine is added to the medium. The work pioneered the way to additional investigations that have indicated that glutamine is the principal fuel used by many dividing cells.

13

Intestinal Fuels: Implications for Improvement of Intestinal Growth and Function

John L. Rombeau
John I. Lew

Significant recent advances have occurred in understanding the molecular and metabolic events contributing to intestinal cell growth and function. Intrinsic to these events is the recognition that nutrients are important mediators of enterotrophism. Moreover, specific nutrients such as glutamine and butyrate are preferentially oxidized by the enterocyte and colonocyte respectively. This chapter reviews the processes of proliferation and differentiation in the intestinal epithelium with emphasis on the effects of starvation, stress, and nutrient-induced reparation. A more detailed discussion is provided for glutamine and butyrate.

Normal Intestinal Epithelium

Cellular Proliferation and Differentiation

Intestinal epithelial cells have one of the fastest turnover rates in the human body. Turnover of the intestinal epithelium involves the proliferation, migration, differentiation, maturation, and eventual exfoliation of its component cells. Intestinal epithelial cell replacement depends on the continual division of proliferating stem cells deep within mucosal crypts. Stem cells of the small intestine and colon are undifferentiated cells capable of proliferation, self-maintenance, production of differentiated, functionally competent cells, and tissue regeneration after injury [1,2]. Newly synthesized cells migrate and differentiate from the lower half of crypts to the mucosal surface, where they mature and eventually extrude into the lumen. Under normal conditions, proliferation is balanced by exfoliation so that epithelial cell populations are preserved at a steady state [3].

Proliferation is a process that involves a consecutive pattern of cyclic changes in gene expression that eventually lead to cell division [2]. These cyclic changes may be associated with either slight or dramatic alterations in the cellular concentration of proliferative gene products that are represented by transitional points within the cell cycle. The initiation and termination of the S (DNA synthesis) and M (mitosis) phases delineate four transitional points or end points commonly used to characterize proliferative cells (Figure 13-1). Thus, certain gene products or proteins required for DNA synthesis and mitosis serve as indices of cell proliferation. For example, increased and decreased concentrations of the precursor nucleic acid enzyme, thymidylate synthetase, may define the DNA synthesis phase of the cell cycle and function as an applicable marker for proliferative cells.

In addition to proliferation, intestinal epithelial cells are capable of differentiation. Differentiation is the qualitative change in cellular phenotype resulting from new or noncyclic gene product synthesis that eventually renders cells functionally competent [1,2]. As cells differentiate from one functional state to another, the expression of specific genes within these cells is increased while the expression of other genes is decreased. Such changes in noncyclic gene expression may be detected by modifications in cell morphology or the presence of novel protein [2]. In certain cases, some of these products of gene expression may serve as markers of cell differentiation.

Because differentiation is also a qualitative change, cells are considered differentiated only in comparison to other cells that may have the ability to further undergo this process. Moreover, in contrast to differentiation, maturation can be considered as a quantitative change in cellular phenotype or novel protein expression related to functional competence [1,2]. Degree of cell maturation, therefore, can be measured on a quantitative scale, such as weight of specific or novel protein per cell. Consequently, in the course of time, a differentiated cell eventually matures to become a fully functional competent cell of its tissue domain [2].

As cells differentiate from one functional state to another, changes in gene expression are primarily regulated by either activation or repression of gene transcription [2]. Although post-tran-

Figure 13-1. Cell cycle including transitional points for measurement of proliferation.

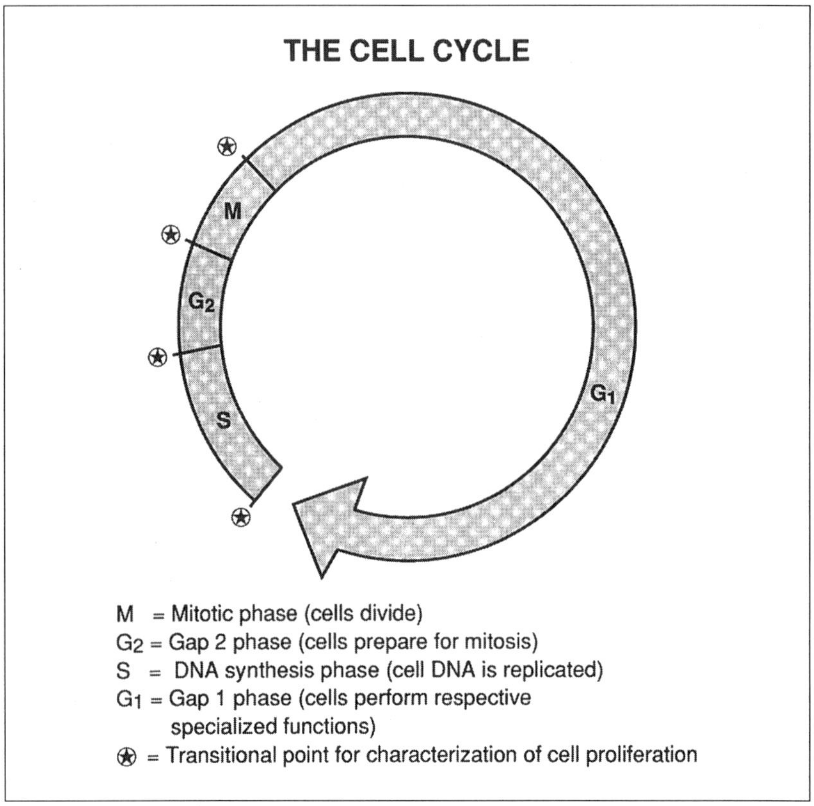

scriptional and post-translational regulation play important processing roles for final protein expression, gene transcription is the main mechanism responsible for significant changes of cellular phenotype and function in differentiation (Figure 13-2) [4,5]. Transcription is activated when multiple nuclear proteins or transcription factors bind specific DNA sequences, called *DNA regulatory elements,* that lie on the same DNA strand as the structural gene that encodes mRNA [6]. These transcriptional factors are encoded by other genes on different DNA strands as well as by genes on the same transcribed DNA strand. Thus, the interaction between transcription factors and DNA regulatory elements play a key role in the regulation of gene transcription in intestinal cell differentiation [6].

In summary, cell proliferation and differentiation are processes that are mutually inclusive [2]. Many cells in the adult human display well-developed structures that classify them as differentiated relative to other less structured cells. Furthermore, these same cells may also have the capability to proliferate. Bone marrow and mesenchymal cells clearly demonstrate both qualities [2,7]. Therefore, proliferation, differentiation, and maturation are cellular processes that coexist and occur as stem cells develop into fully functional competent cells. These events may be regarded as a transition from an utmost degree of proliferation

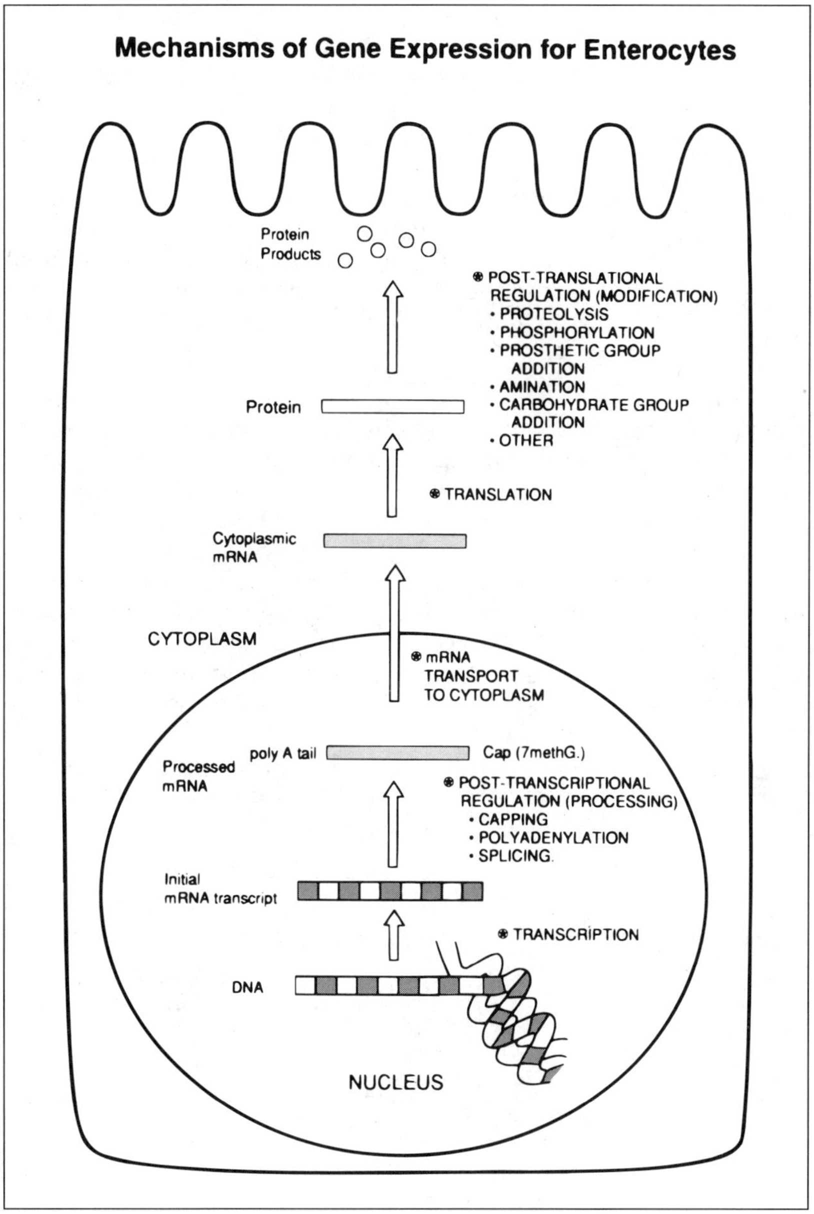

Figure 13-2. Proposed mechanisms of gene expression for enterocytes.

and no differentiation/maturation to the opposite degree of utmost differentiation/maturation and no proliferation (Figure 13-3). Within the transitional state, the coexistence of proliferation and differentiation allows cells the flexibility to increase or decrease one or both processes [2].

Small Intestine

The epithelium of the small intestine consists of a lower proliferative zone found in crypts and an upper nonproliferative zone located on villi. Stem cells anchored slightly above the crypt base give rise to four types of small intestinal cells: absorptive columnar cells (enterocytes), goblet cells, enteroendocrine cells, and Paneth cells [2,8]. Most of the precursors arising from the crypt cells are immature enterocytes, whereas more than 95% of villus cells consist of mature absorptive enterocytes [9].

Absorption is greatly enhanced by the villi that extend into the small intestinal lumen. Furthermore, the enterocytes that cover these projections possess well-developed brush borders composed of microvilli, which increase the lumenal absorptive surface many-fold. These cells are bound together by tight junctions that maintain an impermeable barrier between the lumenal contents and intestinal submucosa [10].

Enterocyte precursors migrate in a linear fashion from crypts to villus tips, where they ultimately exfoliate into the lumen. In humans, the time for differentiating enterocytes to reach the lumen and mature is 5 to 6 days in most of the small bowel and 3 days in the ileum [11]. Similar to enterocytes, immature goblet cells migrate linearly from crypts onto villi, where they mature to become mucus-secreting goblet cells. Enteroendocrine cells also migrate toward the villus tip, taking about 4 days to reach the surface. As these cells differentiate, they acquire an increasing number of cytoplasmic granules and lose the ability to divide. Finally, Paneth cells do not divide and reside only in crypt bases, where they are eventually engulfed by macrophages. These cells produce lysosomes and have a longer life span—several weeks—than that of the other intestinal cell types [2,8,11].

In human small intestine, sucrase-isomaltase is an enterocyte specific, brush-border enzyme that has insignificant activity in crypt cells and maximal activity in lower and middle villus enterocytes. Accordingly, levels of sucrase-isomaltase mRNA are low in crypt cells, dramatically increased in crypt-villus junctional enterocytes, maximal in lower and middle villus enterocytes, and decreased in villus tip enterocytes [5]. Such evidence suggests that sucrase-isomaltase gene expression is regulated primarily by the level of mRNA concentration at the several transitional points up the crypt-villus axis. Increased mRNA levels, therefore, may be the principal mechanism for gene expression changes in enterocyte differentiation. Furthermore, the dramatic mRNA expression in enterocytes at the crypt-villus junction coincides with the coexistent transitional cellular process of proliferation to nonproliferation. Finally, the decreased levels of sucrase-isomaltase mRNA in villus tip enterocytes, caused possibly by decreased transcription or increased mRNA degradation, may characterize a senescent state prior to lumenal exfoliation of these cells [5].

Large Intestine

The large intestine (colon) has no villi, and its epithelium shares similar patterns of proliferation and differentiation with the small intestine. The absorptive colonic epithelium is planar and consists of straight tubular crypts that extend into the lamina propria. Stem cells in lower crypt bases differentiate into three types: absorptive columnar cells (colonocytes), mucus-secreting goblet cells, and hormone-producing enteroendocrine cells. In humans, the time for these cells to reach the lumenal surface, where they are extruded, is about 3 to 8 days [3,11]. Although lined with enteroendocrine cells, colonic crypts consist primar-

Figure 13-3. Characteristics of enterocyte proliferation, differentiation/maturation.

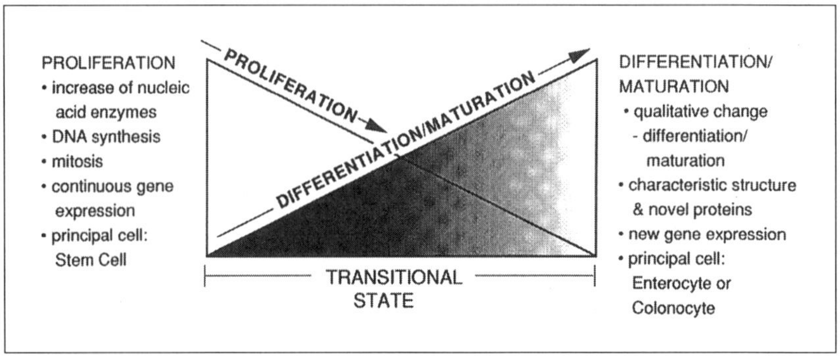

ily of goblet cells. The lumenal surface, however, comprises mainly colonocytes, which have fewer microvilli than enterocytes of the small intestine [12].

Although they appear as small columnar cells in the ascending colon, stem cells (vacuolated cells) of the descending colon and rectum contain secretory vesicles. Before reaching the lumenal surface, these vacuolated cells lose their vesicles and differentiate into absorptive colonocytes with microvilli [13]. Differentiating colonocyte precursors migrate upward toward the crypt orifice and exit into a narrow, surrounding cuff of surface epithelium. These hexagonal-shaped cuffs, from a lumenal view, demonstrate the intricate pattern of cell migration in the large intestine and may represent the colonic counterpart to small intestinal villi [14].

Intestinal Mucosal Growth and Function

The most important stimulus for intestinal mucosal growth and function is the presence of food or nutrients in the gut lumen. Nutrient-lumenal contact is responsible for a number of physiologic responses that maintain intestinal cell mass. The routes of nutrient delivery, dietary constituents, and intestinal fuels influence these gut regulatory mechanisms. Mucosal atrophy and hypofunction, for example, occur in patients during prolonged periods of parenteral feeding. The small intestine and colon are metabolically active organs that require specific nutrients to continually function properly. When not maintained adequately, these organs are susceptible to injury that may impair digestive, absorptive, and barrier function [3,15].

As mentioned, cell replacement in the intestinal epithelium or mucosa is dependent on continual stem cell proliferation located deep within intestinal crypts. Intestinal mucosal growth is determined by the rates of intestinal cell proliferation and exfoliation (loss). Normal gut mucosa is maintained at a steady state when the rate of cell proliferation is balanced by the rate of cell exfoliation [3]. For mucosal growth or hyperplasia to occur, the rate of cell proliferation must be greater than the rate of cell exfoliation. This physiologic state may result from one of three conditions: (1) increased cell proliferation rate and constant cell exfoliation rate; (2) increased cell proliferation rate and decreased cell exfoliation rate; and (3) constant cell proliferation rate and decreased cell exfoliation rate (Table 13-1). In contrast, for mucosal atrophy or hypoplasia to occur, the rate of cell exfoliation must be greater than the rate of cell proliferation. This state may also result from one of three conditions: (1) decreased cell proliferation rate and constant cell exfoliation rate; (2) decreased cell proliferation rate and increased cell exfoliation rate; and (3) constant cell proliferation rate and increased exfoliation rate (see Table 13-1). Thus, the rate of intestinal cell turnover determines mucosal growth, and any changes in these processes result in different physiologic states [3].

Several factors regulate the growth of intestinal mucosa. The small intestine and colon are not only influenced by the effects of nongastrointestinal hormones (for example, glucocorticoids, growth hormone, insulin, thyroxine), but also by many other factors regulated by ingested nutrients. The physical presence of nutrients in the intestinal lumen (lumenal nutrition) directly affects mucosal growth by providing local nutrition and increasing surface cell exfoliation [3]. Furthermore, specific dietary constituents may directly stimulate mucosal growth independent of their nutritional value. Such compounds (for example, dietary fiber) may also be converted into trophic factors of the intestine by the action of digestive enzymes or bacteria within the gut lumen [3,16].

Lumenal nutrition indirectly affects mucosal growth by regulating release of gastrointestinal peptides (for example, gastrin, enteroglucagon), stimulating intestinal neural circuits, enhancing

Table 13-1. Characterization of Changes in Rate of Intestinal Mucosal Proliferation and Exfoliation

	Rate of Proliferation	Rate of Exfoliation
Normal mucosa (steady state)	same	same
Mucosal growth (hyperplasia)	↑	no change, *or*
	↑	↓, *or*
	no change	↓
Mucosal atrophy (hypoplasia)	↓	no change, *or*
	↓	↑, *or*
	no change	↑

↑ = increases, ↓ = decreases

intestinal blood flow, and increasing gut motility and secretion. These mechanisms are interrelated because blood flow, motility, and secretion are regulated by nerves and peptides, and nerves and blood flow may release and deliver peptides to the intestinal mucosa [3,17,18]. Accordingly, there is evidence to suggest that gastrointestinal hormones and nerve stimulation directly affect mucosal growth [19,20].

Although its primary function is the digestion and absorption of nutrients into blood and lymph circulation, the normal intestinal mucosa also serves as a protective physical barrier against the absorption of intralumenal bacteria and their toxins. The epithelial cell membranes prevent transcellular migration of such antigens, and the tight junctions between these cells hinder particle movement through paracellular channels. Furthermore, mucus cell secretions prevent the adherence and invasion of enteric bacteria and toxins.

The intestinal barrier is characterized by several immunologic components. The mucosa and submucosa are replete with lymphocytes, macrophages, neutrophils, and Peyer patches, which are lymphoid aggregates of the terminal ileum. Found abundantly in bile and intestinal secretions, IgA binds and mediates the recognition of such antigens as bacteria and their toxins. Furthermore, hepatic Kupffer cells are in a key position to collect and detoxify antigens that penetrate beyond the intestinal wall and regional lymphatic tissue. The intact epithelium and its immunologic constituents are the major components of intestinal barrier function, although cell-mediated immunity may play a supportive role to the mucosa [15].

Effects of Nutrient Deprivation on Intestinal Mucosal Growth and Function

When deprived of lumenal nutrients, the intestinal mucosa undergoes profound changes in morphology and function. Starvation, malnutrition, critical illness, and total parenteral nutrition (TPN) are states of nutritional deprivation that impair the digestive, absorptive, and barrier function of the gut mucosa. Such conditions are associated with reduced intestinal cell proliferation, diminished rate of cell turnover, and mucosal hypoplasia. Several animal studies reveal that nutrient deficits compromise the intestinal mucosa. However, the findings from these animal models may not accurately delineate these processes in humans. Thus, the consequences of nutritionally stressed states on human intestinal mucosal growth and function remain to be studied.

Starvation

During periods of starvation, mucosal atrophy occurs due to decreased rates of intestinal cell proliferation and increased rates of cell exfoliation. In adult rats, weight loss of the small intestine (53%) after starvation is greater than the rest of the whole body (32%) [21]. Starvation reduces intestinal villus height and crypt cell depth and progressively diminishes levels of DNA, RNA, and protein content [21–23]. The decreases in villus height and mucosal thickness are caused by diminished intestinal crypt cell production. Studies with [^{3}H]thymidine incorporation reveal decreased rates of crypt cell proliferation throughout the intestines of starved rats [23,24]. Furthermore, the rate of enterocyte migration and exfoliation from villus tips also decreases [24]. When adult rats are starved for several days and then refed, enterocyte proliferation and renewal occurs after 7 days [23,25].

Starvation also causes decreased enzyme function in rat small intestine. Alterations in enzyme function are evaluated mainly by enzyme activity per unit mucosal length. Consequently, the activity of certain enzymes can be measured under conditions of starvation and, in some cases, may not indicate any significant changes [26]. Although brush-border disaccharidase activity per unit mucosal length is usually decreased in starved rats, lactase activity may be increased, while maltase and sucrase activity may remain unchanged [27–29]. Nevertheless, the overall decrease of disaccharidase activity corresponds well to the degree of villus atrophy. Furthermore, the intestinal enzyme activity in starved rats returns to normal levels after several days of refeeding [29,30]. In some instances, certain disaccharidases reach maximal activity at 12 hours after carbohydrate ingestion [31].

The previously mentioned animal studies suggest that starvation also causes significant changes in mucosal permeability. Indeed, such evidence supports the hypothesis that starvation compromises the intestinal mucosa leading to increased permeability and subsequent detrimental sequelae. However, acute starvation for 4 to 5 days in humans does not produce significant changes in mucosal permeability [32].

Malnutrition

In developed countries such as the United States, malnutrition associated with chronic illness, chronic hospitalization, or postsurgical recovery is far more common than prolonged starvation [26]. During malnutrition, gastric acid secretion decreases, thereby providing a milieu favorable for bacterial overgrowth in the proximal small intestine. Furthermore, cell-mediated immunity and secretion of IgA may be reduced. These factors predispose the small bowel to enteric bacteria, which may lead to mucosal injury, diarrhea, and increased nutrient losses [26]. However, the evidence to support the notion that malnutrition alone compromises the intestinal mucosal barrier to pathogens and increases the possibility of host infection in humans has not been conclusive.

In infant rabbits (at 7 days postpartum), malnutrition by litter expansion alters intestinal growth and function compared to *ad libitum* fed controls [33]. In young rabbits, malnutrition decreases jejunal and ileal mucosal mass as indicated by: (1) lowered mucosal weight, DNA, and protein content; (2) decreased enterocyte proliferation and differentiation; (3) delayed cell maturation as measured by mucosal enzyme activity; and (4) increased glucose-stimulated sodium transport. Refeeding of these malnourished rabbits at 28 days leads to rapid and complete recovery as shown by: (1) restored jejunal and ileal mass within 4 days; (2) increased enterocyte renewal and differentiation by 7 days; (3) complete return of normal mucosal enzyme activity by 14 days; and (4) depressed glucose-sodium transport to control levels within 7 days [33]. In malnourished infant rats, a similar effect occurs as shown by recovery of disaccharidase activity and intestinal weight after 14 and 21 days of refeeding, respectively [28].

Although malnutrition etiologically is divided into two groups, namely marasmus and kwashiorkor, both forms often appear together in hospitalized patients [26]. Marasmus is a condition of chronic undernourishment primarily caused by caloric and protein deficiency. In contrast, kwashiorkor is a condition of severe protein undernourishment with adequate caloric intake.

Mucosal structure virtually remains normal in marasmus, but some patients can manifest mild changes [34]. These alterations in the small intestine include shortened villus height with lengthened crypt depth, increased lymphocytes and plasma cells, reduced mucosal thickness, decreased crypt mitotic indices, and depressed rate of cell differentiation [34]. Ultrastructural findings reveal irregular microvilli that are sparse, short, and branched. In addition to thickening of the basement membrane, autophagosomes that contain swollen mitochondria are found widespread in enterocytes [34]. During nutritional repletion, microvilli return to regular morphology while autophagosomes become scarce. Although its thickness and mitotic indices approach normality, mucosal structure overall still remains aberrant. The amount of time for the entire mucosa to normalize in malnourished patients receiving therapeutic diets is not known [34].

Functional abnormalities associated with marasmus in the small intestine are rare. Mild forms of steatorrhea can occur and may result from mucosal barrier injury. Additionally, decreased levels of alkaline phosphatase, peptidase, and disaccharidases are found in some patients with marasmus [26,35].

In patients with kwashiorkor, mucosal injury of the small intestine is more severe [34]. Whereas most patients have flat villi, some reveal moderately severe patchy lesions. In kwashiorkor, mucosal thickness and mitotic indices are relatively normal in the small bowel while intestinal crypt cell proliferation and migration are noticeably impaired [34]. The presence of large lipid deposits in enterocytes is an outstanding feature of some patients and may possibly reflect reduced apolipoprotein synthesis associated with severe protein malnutrition. In extreme cases, severe enterocyte destruction may result from the formation of flat villus lesions. With protein repletion, the epithelial abnormalities of the small intestine in kwashiorkor patients quickly improve, although not fully to normal [34].

In contrast to marasmus, malabsorption is a common characteristic of kwashiorkor. Steatorrhea caused by mucosal injury involves the decreased uptake of fatty acids by small bowel mucosa. Such mucosal lesions may depress chylomicron transport into villus lacteals [26,34]. Furthermore, brush-border dipeptidase activity is decreased in kwashiorkor due to damaged microvilli and changes in protein synthesis caused by amino acid deficiency. These enzyme defects may increase fecal nitrogen losses in patients with this condition [34]. The lack of disaccharidases and glucose transport proteins may also worsen existing conditions of carbohydrate malabsorption caused by mucosal injury. Finally, diminished absorption of fat-soluble and water-soluble vitamins often occurs. These functions fortunately are regained with the initiation of a therapeutic nutritional regimen [26,34].

Critical Illness

The intestinal tract is one of several main target organs that are compromised in the critically ill patient. Stresses such as cardiogenic shock, hypovolemia, sepsis, and thermal injury can produce necrotic lesions in the intestinal mucosa. These conditions, with low mesenteric blood flow, disrupt the integrity of the intestinal barrier [36]. In addition to these stresses, nutritional deprivation and altered intestinal flora caused by broad-spectrum antibiotics further impair intestinal absorption. Stress-induced lesions of the intestinal mucosa begin at the apices of the villi and progress downward to separate the epithelium from the lamina propria. If such lesions continue, destruction of the lamina propria, ulceration, and transmural necrosis of the intestinal barrier may occur. Such disruption of mucosal integrity allows for invasion by intralumenal constituents such as bacteria and endotoxin into the portal circulation [36]. Thus, the eroded mucosa becomes an ineffective barrier.

Hypoxia, associated with low blood flow, is an important cause of intestinal mucosa lesions during stress [37]. Exfoliation of intestinal epithelial cells, decreased mucus production, and increased mucosal permeability to intralumenal particles occurs with hemorrhagic shock. Furthermore, in such states of shock, lysosomal rupture renders the intestinal mucosa more susceptible to digestion by released enzymes. The lumenal presence of pancreatic enzymes such as elastase and trypsin also play an important role in the pathogenesis of barrier dysfunction in intestinal ischemia. Accordingly, preservation of blood flow and perfusion of the intestinal lumen with nutrients and oxygen may protect the mucosa from damage in the ischemic gut [36].

Although intestinal ischemia is a major cause of mucosal barrier lesions, past studies suggest reperfusion of such ischemic tissue promotes oxygen-free (superoxide) radical formation, which causes further barrier damage and eventual organ destruction. Generated by xanthine oxidase, superoxide radicals are eliminated by endogenous oxygen radical scavengers such as superoxide dismutase, catalase, and glutathione [36,38]. Glutathione, a tripeptide and major antioxidant, consists of glutamate derived from glutamine, cysteine, and glycine. Recent studies suggest prophylactic administration of glutamine after intestinal shock and ischemia-reperfusion preserves glutathione stores, which may enhance antioxidant protection [39,40].

Bacterial Translocation

Bacterial translocation is defined as the process by which bacteria migrate across the intestinal mucosal barrier to invade the liver, spleen, and mesenteric lymph nodes. Any combination of these conditions, often found in critically ill patients, will promote bacterial translocation. These conditions are physical disruption of mucosal barrier (i.e., hemorrhagic shock, sepsis), microflora imbalance resulting in bacterial overgrowth of enteric bacilli (i.e., broad-spectrum antibiotic therapy), and impaired host immune system (i.e., immunosuppressive drugs, protein deficiency) [15,41].

Intestinal barrier failure and bacterial translocation is not an "all or none" phenomenon [38]. Disintegration of any one component of the intestinal barrier facilitates translocation of bacteria to the mesenteric lymph nodes, liver, and spleen. However, in the healthy host, translocated bacteria do not multiply and spread systematically. [*Editor's Note:* This may be the key to understanding the translocation phenomenon. A little translocation is, as stated elsewhere, energy-requiring and may be a good thing as part of immune surveillance.] Microorganisms are localized in the aforementioned organs and eventually eliminated by tissue macrophages. In conditions of severe or complete intestinal barrier failure, translocating bacteria invade mesenteric lymph nodes, systemic organs, and the circulatory system. The majority of animal models with this condition usually survive. However, those animals with thermal injury or protein deficiency receiving nonlethal doses of endotoxin frequently die from the translocation of bacteria [38].

While a physical mucosal barrier and host immune system are important for effective barrier function, an intact epithelial barrier will preclude bacterial translocation despite impaired cell-mediated immunity. Thus, the intestinal mucosal barrier may play a primary role in preventing bacterial translocation, and host immune defenses may serve a secondary role in intestinal barrier function [38].

Endotoxemia

Bacterial endotoxins may also cross an impaired intestinal barrier. Normally, endotoxins enter the portal system in small amounts and are detoxified rapidly by hepatic Kupffer cells. Intestinal ischemia markedly potentiates the systemic effects of endotoxemia. If the superior mesenteric artery is temporarily occluded in rabbits, fatal endotoxemia can occur. Interestingly, when the intestinal microflora of these animals is removed, fatal endotoxemia does not occur when the same artery is occluded [42]. In mice, endotoxin enhances bacterial translocation from the intestinal lumen to the mesenteric lymph nodes in a dose-dependent fashion. Lethal doses of bacterial toxins disrupt intercellular tight junctions, increasing permeability to bacteria and maintaining or amplifying endotoxemia [43].

Endotoxemia occurs in critically ill patients with low blood flow (i.e., cardiogenic or hypovolemic shock). A large percentage of trauma patients in shock have endotoxemia without evidence of visceral perforations. Of those with systolic blood pressures less than 80 mm Hg at hospital admission, 56% of patients have endotoxemia. Furthermore, of those with systolic blood pressures greater than 80 mm Hg at admission, endotoxemia occurs in 9% of these patients [44]. Thus, severe hypotension leads to marked increases in endotoxemia. [*Editor's Note:* A note of caution: These studies were carried out with radiolabel; however, when the radiolabel was counted, there was no exclusion of the label as being recirculated to other molecules.]

Systemic Inflammatory Response Syndrome

Systemic inflammatory response syndrome (SIRS), previously referred to as the multiple organ failure syndrome, is defined as the sequential failure of lungs, liver, and kidney following multiple trauma, severe burns, hemorrhagic shock, and infection, especially in immunocompromised patients. This syndrome is a significant cause of morbidity and mortality in critically ill patients. Initially, SIRS was thought to be exclusively due to sepsis [38,45]; however, recent evidence suggests it can occur in the absence of infection [46,47]. Enteric bacteremia is found in some critically ill patients dying of SIRS, and no septic focus can be found either clinically or by autopsy in such individuals. Consequently, increasing attention has been directed to the investigation of gut-derived bacteria as translocating pathogens responsible for initiating sepsis and perpetuating SIRS.

In the gut origin hypothesis of SIRS, translocated enteric bacteria and endotoxins travel to organs and tissues causing sepsis, macrophage cytokine secretion, neutrophil protease stimulation, oxidant production, proinflammatory endothelial cell promotion, and complement and coagulation system activation. It has been hypothesized that these processes are self-sustaining and responsible for initiating SIRS [45,48].

Despite this interesting hypothesis, there is no definitive evidence in humans to support the gut origin sepsis as a cause of SIRS. In fact, evidence for this hypothesis rests primarily on laboratory experiments with animal models. In the opinion of one of the authors (JLR), gut-induced SIRS occurs only in a very small percentage of malnourished, critically ill patients who are severely septic and immunosuppressed with significantly compromised gut barrier function. [*Editor's Note:* I agree!] While studies have demonstrated that increased bacterial translocation plays a major role in determining survival in animal models of critical illness, strong clinical evidence for this idea is lacking. Although increased gut barrier permeability to hydrophilic particles has been seen in both animal models and critically ill patients, the clinical significance of this finding is still unclear.

Total Parenteral Nutrition

Because many hospitalized patients are unable to eat voluntarily, total parenteral nutrition (TPN) is administered to avoid complications of starvation and malnutrition. Although used in patients with intestinal dysfunction throughout the world, there is some concern that TPN may actually be detrimental to the gut. As mentioned, the most important stimulus for mucosal growth is the physical presence of nutrients in the intestinal lumen. Because TPN does not directly stimulate the intestinal lumen and lacks intestinal fuels (glutamine and butyrate), this alimentation method deprives the gut of essential nutrients, thereby promoting mucosal atrophy, malabsorption, and other detrimental sequelae. While studies with parenterally fed animals are the bases for these findings, human studies show disparate results. Such differences bring into question whether such findings obtained from animals are relevant to hospitalized patients.

Marked mucosal atrophy and impaired intestinal enzyme activity occurs in rat small intestine after prolonged TPN administration [49–51]. Intestinal weight, mucosal weight, mucosal DNA, and protein decrease by 22%, 28%, 25%, and 35%, respectively, in rats fed TPN for one week. Furthermore, disaccharidase levels fall, with a 46% decrease in maltase and sucrase specific activity, and no change in lactase activity [49]. The most significant decreases in mucosal weight, villus height, DNA, and protein content appear in the ileum and subsequently in the jejunum only after three days of TPN [51].

In human studies with TPN, mucosal structure and brush-border enzyme function undergo separate degrees of change in the small intestine [52,53]. Although mucosal thickness decreases and permeability increases in normal human subjects fed TPN for two weeks, microvillus height and mucosal DNA, RNA, and protein content remain unchanged [53]. After 21 days of TPN, biopsies of proximal and nondiseased small bowel from patients with inflammatory bowel disease reveal slight decreases in microvillus height and significantly lower enzyme activity (sucrase, maltase, lactase, glucoamylase, acid aminopeptidase, dipeptidyl peptidase) [52]. Most of these detectable structural and functional changes are reversed by enteral feeding [52,53].

The process of bacterial translocation has been postulated to occur in hospitalized patients with TPN-induced mucosal atrophy and accounts for some episodes of sepsis encountered in these patients. In one study, rats administered TPN demonstrated increased levels of bacterial translocation presumably due to increased cecal bacterial count and impaired intestinal immunity [54]. In another study, however, TPN-induced gut atrophy in rats did not lead directly to bacterial translocation [55]. Although 10 days of TPN caused mucosal hypoplasia, bacterial overgrowth, and a ten-fold increase in permeability to lactulose, such developments did not increase the rate of bacterial translocation when compared to pair-fed controls. Thus, mucosal atrophy, bacterial translocation, and increased macromolecular permeability may be independent processes. Indeed, gut origin sepsis in humans during TPN administration may be caused by increased gut permeability to macromolecules such as endotoxin, and bacterial translocation is more likely the result rather than the cause of such septic states [55].

Enteral Nutrition

Because many critically ill patients are unable to eat voluntarily, nutrients must be administered either enterally or parenterally. Enteral feeding or enteral nutrition (EN) may be more beneficial than TPN, which has contributed significantly to the management of hospitalized patients. As mentioned, prolonged TPN administration in patients leads to mucosal atrophy, increased barrier permeability, and decreased intestinal enzyme activity. Similar to lumenal nutrients, enteral nutrients directly stimulate and nourish the intestinal lumen, and indirectly induce trophic factors to promote mucosal growth and function. Several animal and human studies demonstrate that even when deficient in intestinal fuels, EN effectively reverses TPN-induced morphologic and functional changes in the gut. Other studies indicate that route of enteral delivery also influences the mucosal response to lumenal nutrients and that early EN reduces septic complications in critically ill patients.

When fed TPN intravenously, rats develop marked intestinal atrophy compared to rats fed either TPN orally or standard rat chow [56]. Total intestinal weight, mucosal weight, and villus height significantly differ among the three groups of rats, with these study variables best maintained in the standard rat chow group. The mucosal weight, DNA, and protein contents of the proximal intestine in rats fed chemically defined diets intragastrically are significantly higher than in rats fed TPN [57]. Although chemically defined diets maintain mucosal structure in the proximal bowel, this effect diminishes rapidly in the distal small intestine and colon, where mucosal atrophy occurs similar to that after TPN administration. Furthermore, EN is more effective than TPN in stimulating gut adaptive hyperplasia after surgical resection [58–60]. Additionally, enteral nutrients may directly nourish the intestine and stimulate the release of trophic gut peptides that are important for intestinal growth and adaptation.

In humans, EN reverses mucosal atrophy associated with TPN administration. When normal volunteers are given either standard diets (Osmolyte, Ross, Columbus, OH) or glutamine and arginine diets (Alitrac, Ross, Columbus, OH) via tube after two weeks of TPN, jejunal mucosal thickness returns to near-normal levels [53]. However, in this study, EN increased rather than reduced intestinal permeability induced by TPN. Additionally, glutamine and arginine supplementation provided no additional enterotrophic benefit in normal human subjects after prolonged TPN when compared to enteral nutrition alone. Clearly, studies in hospitalized patients are needed to determine the clinical significance of these findings.

The route of enteral delivery also influences intestinal mucosal growth. When compared to jejunal delivery, orally ingested diets better maintain the proximal gut mucosa of rats fed identical liquid diets [61]. Additionally, mucosal weight, DNA, and protein content in orally fed rats display a normal decreasing proximal to distal gut gradient, while jejunally fed rats display marked mucosal growth at sites adjacent to intrajejunal infusion and significant distal mucosal atrophy. Furthermore, regular solid nutrients maintain intestinal mucosal integrity better than enteral elemental formulas [57,60,62]. In rats fed several formula diets intragastrically, mucosal weight, DNA, and protein content decreased significantly compared to rats fed regular chow diets [62]. These studies indicate that intestinal mucosal growth and function are determined by several factors, which include presence of intraluminal nutrients, route of enteral delivery, and composition of enteral nutrients.

The intestinal tract in critically ill patients has traditionally been considered to be inactive as a consequence of primary disease, infection, injury, or side effects of certain medications. Paralytic ileus usually occurs at some point in the course of treating these patients. Different components of the intestinal tract are not equally susceptible to paralytic ileus. The small intestine is somewhat resistant to ileus development, and impaired absorption and dysmotility usually resolve within the first 24 hours following insult. The colon and stomach, however, may take more than three days to regain normal motility after injury [63]. Consequently, early postoperative EN, which bypasses the stomach and delivers nutrients directly into the small bowel, is often used in critically ill patients [64,65]. Paralytic ileus also promotes enteric bacterial overgrowth. Thus, in addition to rapid repair or prevention of intestinal mucosal injury, control of microfloral overgrowth and the provision of medication to up-regulate the host immune system against translocating bacteria and endotoxins may be efficacious in the treatment of critically ill patients. Accumulating evidence suggests early administration of EN preserves intestinal barrier function by maintaining mucosal mass, preventing disruption of normal microflora balance, and modulating host immune defenses [66].

In a well-controlled comparative study, EN and TPN altered immunologic and metabolic responses to endotoxemic injury in normal human volunteers [67]. These subjects received either isocaloric, isonitrogenous EN or TPN for seven days and were then given intravenous injections of *Escherichia coli* endotoxin. TPN significantly worsened systemic manifestations of endotoxemia when compared to EN. Parenterally fed subjects demonstrated increased arterial and hepatic vein cachectin production consistent with activated reticuloendothelial cell response. Furthermore, TPN subjects showed greater adverse effects of endotoxemic injury as indicated by increased peripheral lactate production and increased peripheral amino acid release. This study suggests that either TPN or the lack of enteral nutrients impairs intestinal barrier function and increases hepatic and splanchnic host exposure to bacteria and endotoxin. These events may amplify cytokine response by increasing splanchnic and reticuloendothelial cell activation to subsequent injury. Cytokines produced and secreted by hepatic Kupffer cells and splanchnic lymphocytes also enhance production of counterregulatory hormones that may transiently down-regulate cytokine production, increase output of hepatic-produced acute phase proteins, and reduce gluconeogenesis [66]. Thus, antecedent route of nutritional support may influence immunologic and metabolic responses in critically ill patients to subsequent insults.

Several controlled clinical trials demonstrate that EN improves clinical outcome and decreases sepsis in critically ill postoperative trauma patients. After a three-week period, critically ill patients receiving more enteral protein (0.61 g/kg/day) and less intravenous protein (0.47 g/kg/day) have lower rates of sepsis by varied metabolic criteria than patients receiving no enteral protein and all intravenous protein (1.82 g/kg/day) [68]. Indeed, larger amounts of protein given intravenously to the patients with no enteral protein do not compensate for increased rates of sepsis. Furthermore, patients that receive EN within 12 hours after surgery are less prone to develop infection (17%) compared to patients who receive TPN (37%) [69]. The incidence of major septic morbidity is 3% in patients fed EN compared to 20% in patients given TPN. Finally, patients that receive enteral feeding within 24 hours of injury develop fewer pneumonias, intraabdominal abscesses, and line sepsis than parenterally fed patients [70]. Among the most severely injured subpopulation, enterally fed patients have significantly fewer septic complications than parenterally fed patients. These clinical trials illustrate that EN is well tolerated in severely injured patients and that early enteral feeding reduces septic complications in critically ill patients.

Intestinal Fuels

The absorptive surface area of the small intestine and colon contains the most metabolically active cell population in the human body. The enterocytes and colonocytes that cover this lumenal surface have tremendous energy requirements that make the metabolic needs of the intestine immense. Fortunately, the intestinal tract has the remarkable ability to obtain nutrients from both its lumen and vascular blood supply [15,71]. Specific nutrients known as *intestinal fuels* are metabolic substrates that have trophic and functional effects on the gut mucosa. Glutamine is the preferred intestinal fuel of the small intestine, whereas short-chain fatty acids (SCFAs) are favored fuels of the colon. Of the SCFAs, butyrate is the preferred metabolic fuel of the colon. The small intestine is capable of utilizing lumenal and systemic glutamine to feed its mucosa, while the colon primarily obtains SCFAs by means of indigenous bacterial fermentation of dietary fiber or undigested starch from its lumen [72,73].

Most commercially available EN and TPN formulations for hospitalized patients do not provide these essential intestinal fuels. In fact, glutamine is absent in all currently available formulations of TPN in the United States. Furthermore, SCFAs are not administered enterally to patients with colon dysfunction, and concomitant antibiotic therapy suppresses colonic microflora that normally produce SCFAs from dietary fiber and undigested starch. Thus, at a time when the intestinal tract might conceivably benefit from physiologically appropriate feeding, the prescribed nutritional therapy paradoxically starves the gut and leads to mucosal atrophy [15]. Current studies suggest that provision of EN or TPN supplemented with glutamine or SCFAs may be more efficacious in hospitalized patients with intestinal dysfunction than provision of such nutritional formulations without these intestinal fuels.

Glutamine

Glutamine is a nonessential amino acid that plays a major role in the metabolism, structure, and function of the small intestine. A detailed discussion of glutamine is included elsewhere in this text (see Chapter 12). The principal intestinal fuel for enterocytes, glutamine may be especially important in critically ill patients when the intestinal barrier becomes vulnerable [74,75]. The mucosa of the small intestine obtains glutamine from both its lumen and blood supply. In fact, enterocytes are optimally fed by glutamine when this intestinal fuel is obtained simultaneously through both the apical and basolateral cell membranes. In studies of glutamine kinetics in the rat jejunum, CO_2 contribution from lumenal input is 39% while supply from blood glutamine is 38.8% (Figure 13-4) [72].

In the small intestine, enterocytes possess very active glutaminases that hydrolyze glutamine to glutamate and ammonia. Additionally, enterocytes use glutamine from the vascular supply, and the majority of its nitrogen end products appear in ammonia, alanine, and citrulline. Such nitrogen end products are released into the portal circulation after enteral glutamine administration and are metabolized by the liver before reaching the systemic circulation. Thus, glutamine is metabolized when it enters enterocytes either across the lumenal brush border or through the basolateral membrane from the systemic circulation [74,75].

In critically ill patients, increased protein catabolism provides amino acids for other systemic organs. Skeletal muscle is the primary organ of glutamine synthesis and storage. Accordingly, the concentration of this amino acid is 30 times higher in skeletal muscle than in the systemic blood supply [75]. Glutamine release from skeletal muscle markedly increases during critical illness, and circulating concentrations of this amino acid are decreased because of its increased uptake by other tissues [15,75]. Indeed, the rationale for use of glutamine in the parenteral diets of critically ill patients is based in part on the premise that such supplements may maintain the intracellular glutamine pool and conserve muscle protein [76]. In patients with multisystem trauma, increased and selective uptake of glutamine occurs in the intestinal tract [77]. In stressed conditions, glutamine depletion surpasses that of all other amino acids and endures during recovery after all other amino acids have returned to normal levels [78].

There is controversy concerning which forms of glutamine are too unstable and poorly soluble for addition to previously formulated solutions [76]. Some investigators assert that glutamine dipeptides are more stable and soluble for parenteral supplementation than free glutamine preparations. In hospitalized patients, glutamine dipeptide-supplemented TPN preserves mucosal structure and permeability of the small intestine in contrast to standard TPN formulations [79].

There is some concern that glutamate, a byproduct of free glutamine decomposition at higher temperatures and pH, may have neurotoxic effects in humans [76]. When free glutamine is added to high concentrations of amino acid preparations, its solubility may decrease and its rate of decomposition may increase [76]. Serious consequences

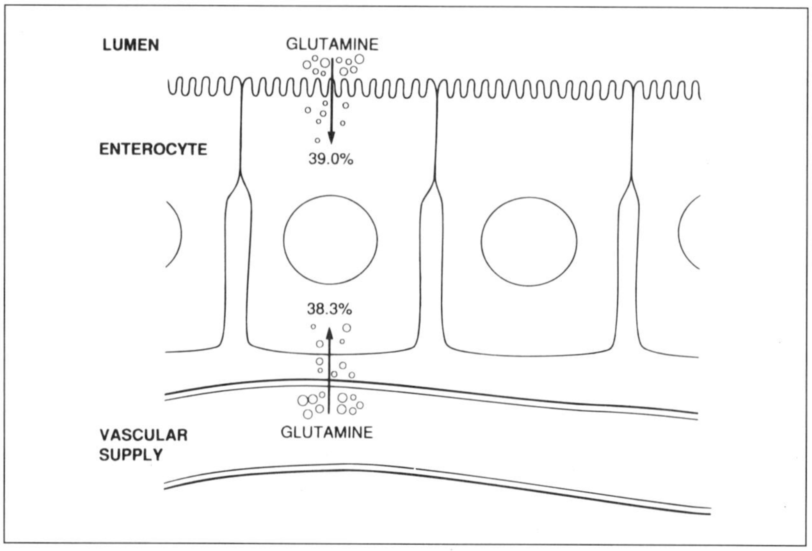

Figure 13-4. Percentage contribution of enterocyte utilization of glutamine-lumen vs. vascular supply.

purportedly arise if very high amounts of free glutamine are used with resultant formation of glutamate. Furthermore, parenteral diets supplemented with free glutamine are contraindicated in patients with hepatic or renal dysfunction because ammonia is coincidentally an end product of glutamine.

In normal human volunteers, however, infusions of parenteral nutrients with increasing doses of free glutamine are well tolerated with no toxic effects [80,81]. Plasma glutamine increases significantly with glutamine infusion but stabilizes at concentrations 25% above control values. The toxic metabolites of glutamine, ammonia, and glutamine do not increase significantly with parenteral administration of free glutamine. Additionally, nitrogen balance, hormonal concentrations, mental status, and cognitive performance remain unchanged [80]. Clearly, with these differing viewpoints, several aspects of glutamine utilization and efficacy remain to be studied before final judgment can be made.

Included in some current EN formulations, in most instances glutamine is administered in insufficient amounts to support intestinal mucosal growth. Furthermore, current TPN formulas do not contain glutamine, which may explain in part why mucosal atrophy occurs in patients receiving prolonged parenteral feeding. Additional causes for such mucosal atrophy may be the result of decreased nutrient contact or insufficient production of enterotrophic GI hormones. Elevated plasma glutamine levels above control values cause trophic effects on rat intestinal mucosa [82]. Additionally, TPN with glutamine diminishes gut atrophy and stimulates small bowel disaccharidase activity [83]. Similar results occur when glutamine is administered enterally [84,85]. Finally, both enteral and parenteral glutamine infusions significantly increase mucosal mass of intestinal grafts in rats receiving heterotopic and orthotopic small bowel isografts compared to nonglutamine controls [86–88]. However, the question remains as to whether enteral glutamine provides benefits in humans similar to those seen in these animal studies. Ironically, there are commercially available enteral diets with increased glutamine contents despite no controlled data in humans to justify the prescription of these formulations.

Current TPN formulas without glutamine promote bacterial translocation in rats. Bacterial translocation is reduced in rats orally fed glutamine, while it does not occur in those animals fed regular chow diets [54]. Furthermore, EN and TPN glutamine-enriched formulas increase intestinal glutaminase activity and glutamine uptake. Accordingly, glutamine-supplemented TPN maintains immune cellularity better than standard formulations [89,90]. Glutamine-supplemented TPN maintains IgA at normal physiologic levels, which in turn prevents bacterial adherence to enterocytes. Thus, glutamine supplementation decreases bacterial translocation and preserves intestinal immune function during TPN.

Several studies suggest glutamine-enhanced EN and TPN benefit animals with intestinal mucosal injury due to chemotherapy. Glutamine-enriched EN preserves intestinal mass and improves survival of rats with methotrexate-induced enterocolitis [91]. Similar results were found in rats on glutamine-enriched TPN after receiving 5-fluorouracil (5-FU). Increased villous height and mucosal DNA content were found in these rats. When the supplemented TPN was given before 5-FU administration, there was further increased mucosal cellularity and significantly lower mortality compared to controls [92].

As mentioned, glutathione (GSH) is a major antioxidant consisting of glutamate derived from glutamine. Although this tripeptide protects normal tissue from oxidant injury, GSH also enhances tumor tissue resistance to chemotherapy and radiation. Oral glutamine supplementation may restore depleted GSH to normal levels in cancer patients, thereby providing the intestinal tract and other organs a form of acquired resistance to oxygen-free radicals generated by chemotherapy and radiation therapy. Thus, enteral glutamine supplementation may enhance the selectivity of antitumor drugs by protecting normal tissue and sensitizing tumor cells to chemotherapy-related injury [78].

In a double-blind, randomized, controlled clinical trial, patients given glutamine-supplemented TPN after bone marrow transplantation demonstrated improved nitrogen balance, reduced infection, lower rates of microfloral overgrowth, and shortened hospital stay compared to patients receiving standard TPN [93]. Although nutrient intake was similar in both groups, nitrogen balance improved in glutamine-supplemented TPN patients compared to controls (-1.4 ± 0.5 g/day versus -4.2 ± 1.2 g/day; $p = 0.002$). Furthermore, a smaller number of patients (13%) developed clinical infections in contrast to controls (43%). Finally, patients receiving glutamine had significantly lower incidences of microfloral colonization and shortened hospitalizations (29 ± 1 days versus 36 ± 2 days; $p = 0.017$) [93]. [*Editor's Note:* It may be that the beneficial effects of glutamine-supplemented TPN may be discernible, if at all, only in very sick patients. Two studies in perioperative patients [94,95] reveal statistically, but not likely biologically, significant differences.]

In a subsequent study using a similar protocol, patients given glutamine-supplemented TPN after bone marrow transplantation showed decreased total body water and shortened hospital stay compared to patients receiving TPN [96]. However, incidence of bacterial overgrowth, clinical infections, and mortality did not differ significantly between the two groups. Additionally, in hospitalized patients receiving standard TPN, substitution with glutamine-supplemented TPN did not cause any untoward effects and appeared to be safe [96].

While enteral diets supplemented with glutamine alone maintain intestinal mucosal integrity, the addition of epidermal growth factor (EGF) has a synergistic effect on mucosal growth in rat small intestine [97]. Indeed, there is evidence to suggest that the mitogenic effects of EGF, which include DNA, RNA, and protein synthesis, are in fact glutamine-dependent [98]. Additionally, glucocorticoid hormones may increase intestinal glutamine utilization by increasing glutaminase expression, thereby providing more energy for enterocytes in stress-related states [99]. Thus, growth factors and hormones may act as trophic factors in conjunction with glutamine to maintain the integrity of the intestinal mucosa.

Short-Chain Fatty Acids

Short-chain fatty acids (SCFAs) are fermentation end products of enzymatic breakdown of dietary fiber, undigested starch, or nonabsorbed simple carbohydrates by indigenous colonic microflora. In general, SCFAs are products of pyruvate metabolism that are essential for the metabolic welfare of colonocytes. The physiologic effects of SCFAs, which include energy production, increased colonocyte proliferation, blood flow enhancement, autonomic nervous system stimulation, and increased gastrointestinal hormone production, regulate the growth and maintenance of the colonic milieu. Acetate, propionate, and n-butyrate account for approximately 85% of all SCFAs produced in the human colon [16,100]. Of the SCFAs, butyrate is preferentially oxidized by normal colonocytes [73,101]. When compared to the other common fuels, butyrate is again the principal metabolic fuel for colonocytes with acetoacetate, L-glutamine, and d-glucose following in sequential order of importance [73,102].

Absorption

SCFA absorption in the colon is regarded principally as a passive, transcellular process. While SCFA absorption is mainly by non-ionic diffusion, recent studies also suggest the presence of a carrier-mediated SCFA anion exchange mechanism with bicarbonate [103,104]. The amount and rate of SCFAs absorbed across colonocyte membranes vary in different segments of the colon. Although cell membrane lipid fluidity and content may partially explain the differences of SCFA absorption in cecal, proximal, and distal colonic mucosa, the exact mechanism for this process is not known [103]. Findings obtained from different animal models vary widely and may not accurately describe SCFA transport in humans. Undoubtedly, more studies are needed to elucidate the mechanisms of SCFA absorption in humans.

SCFA transport across colonocyte membranes is a rapid process. Perfusion studies demonstrate that SCFA absorption rates in colon increase linearly with higher concentrations of SCFAs [105,106]. This evidence suggests that SCFA transport in the colon is a nonsaturable, passive process [103]. Although non-ionized lipid soluble acids are theoretically more able to permeate cell membranes in acidic environments, lowered pH values from 7.2 to 5.5 in human colon and from 7.4 to 5.4 in rat cecum have no significant effect on SCFA absorption rates [107,108]. This contradiction to theory is ascribed to a constant pH microclimate of about 6.5 that exists at the lumenal surface of the colon in humans and rats [109,110]. The pH of this microclimate is near neutral and not affected by changes in lumenal bulk pH. Therefore, lumenal contents that lower pH do not increase non-ionized SCFA concentration at the colonic mucosal surface. Several in vivo and in vitro studies reveal that approximately 50% of the three major SCFAs in the cecum and proximal colon are absorbed in the ionized form. However, in the distal colon, SCFAs are primarily absorbed according to lipid solubility (n-butyrate > propionate > acetate). This evidence indicates that most SCFAs are absorbed in the non-ionized form [103,111,112].

The main route of non-ionized SCFA absorption is by passive transport across colonocyte membranes [103,113]. For non-ionized diffusion to occur, SCFA anions need to be protonated. Protons are obtained at the apical colonocyte membrane by Na^+-H^+ exchange or by K^+-H^+ ATPase found in apical colonocyte membranes of the distal colon (Figures 13-5, 13-6) [103]. In guinea pig cecum and proximal colon, inhibition of Na^+-H^+ exchange decreases SCFA flux from mucosa to serosa by 35% and approximately 40%, respectively [114]. In guinea pig distal colon, inhibition of K^+-H^+ ATPase decreases SCFA flux from mucosa to serosa by approximately 70% [114]. Furthermore, non-ionized SCFAs increase the proton load within colonocytes when they enter these cells and dissociate. The mechanism of proton homeostasis in

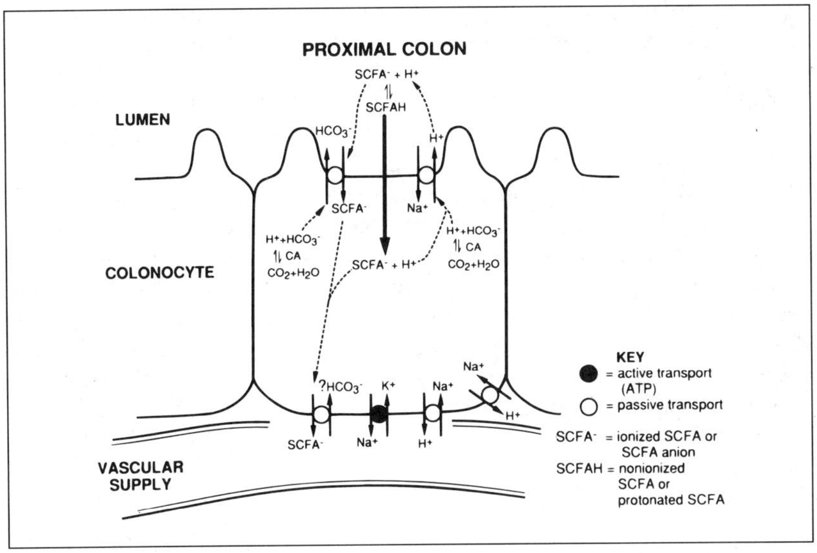

Figure 13-5. Proposed mechanisms for absorption and transport of SCFA in the proximal colon.

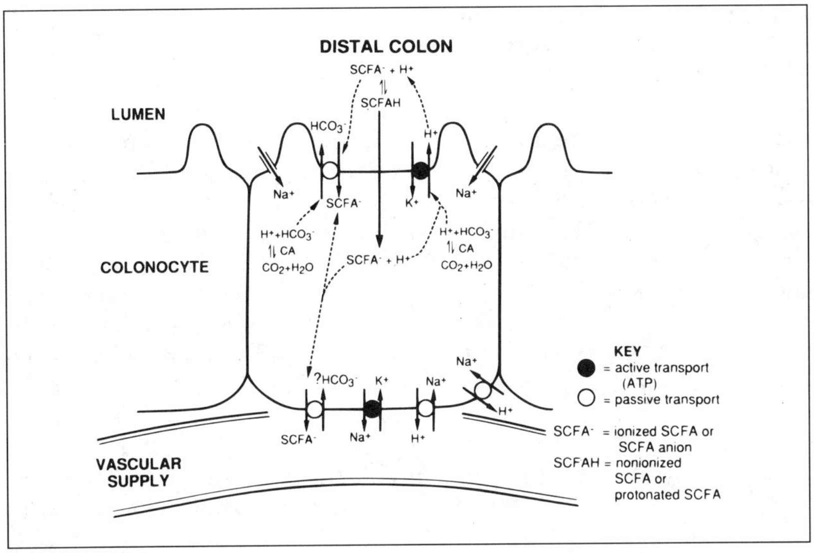

Figure 13-6. Proposed mechanisms for absorption and transport of SCFA in the distal colon.

colonocytes is unknown, but there is evidence to suggest that Na^+-H^+ exchange in the basolateral membrane of these cells regulates intracellular pH [115].

Although previous studies suggest ionized SCFA absorption occurs by means of paracellular transport, voltage clamp experiments indicate that this pathway does not play a major role in the colon. In the proximal colon of guinea pigs, SCFA absorption occurs primarily by SCFA anion diffusion as indicated by a lumen negative transepithelial potential difference [112]. Furthermore, in vitro clamping experiments with equine colon reveal that transepithelial potential differences have no effect on unidirectional SCFA fluxes [116]. These findings suggest that ionized SCFAs are primarily absorbed by transcellular transport and that a barrier to ionized SCFA diffusion across the paracellular pathway exists [103].

Ionized SCFAs are absorbed either by anion exchange or by co-transport with cations on colonocyte membranes. A possible anion exchange mechanism may involve the absorption of ionized SCFA and the secretion of bicarbonate (HCO_3^-) (see Figures 13-5, 13-6). Several studies indicate that HCO_3^- accumulates in the colonic lumen proportionately to ionized SCFA absorption [105,107,117]. In perfused rat colon, HCO_3^- secretion almost doubles in the presence of butyrate [71]. An outward HCO_3^- gradient enhances butyrate uptake by apical and basolateral membrane vesicles of rat colonocytes. These processes appear saturable and thereby suggest the presence of a butyrate-HCO_3^- exchange mechanism [118,119].

Additionally, carbonic anhydrase may be essential in supplying protons for non-ionic SCFA absorption as well as HCO_3^- for ionized SCFA-HCO_3^- exchange (see Figures 13-5, 13-6). Carbonic anhydrase activity is increased in the colon, but the significance of apical membrane-bound carbonic anhydrase compared to cytosolic carbonic anhydrase is not known [120,121].

Several colonic perfusion studies reveal a relationship between SCFA and Na^+ absorption. In human colon, Na^+ absorption is several times higher than SCFA absorption, whereas in rat colon, Na^+ absorption is twice as high as SCFA absorption [105,117,122]. The proposed mechanism between SCFA and Na^+ transport involves the recycling of protons. The dissociation of non-ionized SCFAs after transport into colonocytes may promote Na^+-H^+ exchange and thereby stimulate Na^+ absorption [123]. However, several other animal studies do not support this proposed model. In the proximal colon of the pony, SCFAs do not stimulate net Na^+ absorption [116]. In marsupials, no relationship between SCFAs and Na^+ absorption exists [124]. Finally, the presence of propionate in pig distal colon significantly reduces Na^+ absorption [125]. Clearly, further studies are needed to elucidate the relationship between SCFAs and Na^+ absorption.

In rat and guinea pig distal colon, there is a close interaction between SCFA and K^+ absorption. This relationship is attributed to K^+-H^+ ATPase activity in the apical membrane of distal colonocytes. As mentioned, the protonation of ionized SCFAs for passive absorption is dependent on K^+-H^+ ATPase activity. There is no evidence to suggest that SCFAs directly affect the activity of this ATPase pump [126].

Under voltage clamp conditions, butyrate stimulates Na-Cl absorption in the rat distal colon, possibly by coupling of Na^+-H^+ and Cl^--butyrate exchanges [123]. Several other studies, however, do not support the presence of Cl^--butyrate exchange. In rat distal colon, studies with apical membrane vesicles confirm the presence of Na^+-H^+ and butyrate-HCO_3^- exchanges, but not the presence of Cl^--butyrate exchange [118]. In the human rectum in vivo, SCFAs stimulate Na^+ absorption without Cl^- [127]. Finally, HCO_3^- accumulation in perfused rat colon is the result of increased SCFA concentration and not of Cl^- [117]. More studies are needed to clarify the relationship, if any, between SCFAs and Cl^- absorption.

Metabolism

SCFAs play an essential metabolic role in the maintenance and welfare of colonocytes, as noted by the provision of approximately 70% of the energy supply for the colonic mucosa (Figure 13-7). Of the three principal SCFAs, butyrate is the preferred respiratory fuel of normal colonocytes [73,101,128]. Several studies with labeled n-butyrate indicate that ketogenesis in colonic mucosa occurs by the HMG-CoA pathway [129,130]. In colonocytes, SCFA oxidation affects several functions such as ATP generation, lipogenesis, and Na^+ and K^+ absorption [131]. Therefore, diminished SCFA oxidation can cause severe physiologic consequences for colonocytes and thereby disrupt the colonic mucosal barrier and, presumably, its immune function. Indeed, SCFA starvation of colonocytes is hypothesized to be either a cause of or precursor to ulcerative colitis [101,131].

Although highly utilized in rat colonocytes, about 80% of glucose is converted to lactate, with

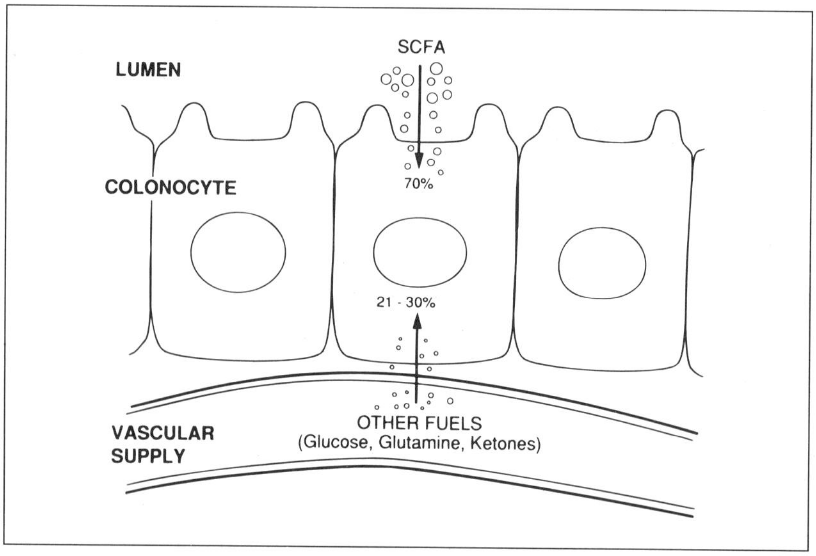

Figure 13-7. Percentage contribution and source of colonocyte energy utilization from lumen and vascular supply.

only 28% to 45% of this substrate oxidized to CO_2 [73,102]. In the presence of n-butyrate, glucose oxidation drops to 1% to 2% despite a total increase in oxygen consumption. Labeling studies with different substrates reveal that n-butyrate spares glucose and glutamine oxidation. Accordingly, glucose or glutamine does not decrease the entry of butyrate carbons in the Krebs cycle. Furthermore, total oxygen consumption by n-butyrate comprises 70% of total colonocyte oxidation [73,131]. These findings clearly indicate that n-butyrate is the principal respiratory fuel for colonocytes with acetoacetate, glutamine, and glucose following in sequential order of importance [73,102]. In humans, colonocyte preference for respiratory fuels is similar to that found in rats. In proximal or distal colonic mucosa, butyrate suppresses glucose oxidation by about 50% [101]. However, regional differences demonstrate that n-butyrate oxidation predominates in the distal colon, whereas glucose and glutamine oxidation are more pronounced in the proximal colon [73,131].

Less is known about the colonic metabolism of propionate and acetate. Butyrate and propionate are primarily metabolized by colonic mucosa or liver, whereas acetate passes predominantly into the peripheral circulation where it, in part, nourishes the colon via the basolateral membrane [132]. Furthermore, SCFA metabolism differs among species. In rabbits, acetate is primarily metabolized in the distal colon [133]. In rats, approximately 85% of the absorbed butyrate and propionate is metabolized by the liver, while only 75% of acetate is metabolized. Because the liver is extremely efficient in clearing butyrate and propionate, systemic levels of these SCFAs are practically undetectable [134].

Normal colonocytes depend on fatty acid oxidation (β-oxidation) for energy production, and SCFA availability strongly affects this oxidation process [131]. When starved of SCFAs, colonocytes oxidize butyrate at a significantly diminished rate with decreased ketogenesis [135]. The main SCFAs, which include butyrate, propionate, and acetate, are activated into their respective CoA derivatives by SCFA CoA synthetases. These activated SCFA substrates in the order of butyrate > propionate > acetate individually or collectively influence production of ATP and acetyl CoA essential for colonocyte metabolism [73]. Preferred activation of butyrate over propionate and acetate indicates that acetyl-CoA for colonocyte lipogenesis is obtained primarily from butyrate [131].

Because SCFAs are not synthesized endogenously, the colonic mucosa can only obtain these respiratory fuels from bacterial fermentation. Therefore, in states of SCFA deprivation such as decreased ingestion of dietary carbohydrate or reduction in the colonic microflora, diminished β-oxidation severely impairs colonocyte function. These pathogenic states lead to decreased ATP production, diminished absorption, reduced lipid synthesis, and impaired detoxification mechanisms in the colonic mucosa. These conditions, in turn, lead to colonocyte barrier breakdown, immune dysfunction, and other detrimental sequelae [131].

Physiologic Effects

One effect of SCFA production, absorption, and metabolism is the provision of energy for colonic mucosal growth. Although energy production depends largely on the quality and quantity of dietary carbohydrate, the exact amount from colonic fermentation in humans is not known. If undigested dietary carbohydrate is the principal substrate for colonic fermentation, and 70% of the potential energy is available for absorption as SCFAs, the theoretical yield in patients ingesting a balanced diet is about 5% of total energy requirements with a range (based on 20 to 60 g substrate fermented) of 3% to 9% in people consuming Western diets. A higher percentage is likely to be found in populations where staples are primarily starch-based. Inasmuch as the energy produced is primarily directed to the colonic epithelium, comprising a very small percentage of the total body weight, SCFAs theoretically provide most of the energy for the colon [136].

In addition to supplying the major caloric source for the colon, SCFAs have additional important effects on the colonic mucosa. Because colonocyte metabolic activity consumes most of the nutritional requirements of the large intestine, SCFAs are an important stimulus for mucosal growth and function in the colon. Several mechanisms by which SCFAs may mediate these enterotrophic effects include the following: (1) increased colonocyte proliferation; (2) enhanced production of enterotrophic gastrointestinal hormones; (3) stimulation of the autonomic nervous system; and (4) increased mesenteric blood flow.

Increased Colonocyte Proliferation. Lumenal nutrients such as soluble dietary fiber are substrate precursors of SCFAs that increase colonocyte proliferation. Studies with [^{3}H] thymidine show increased crypt cell turnover and accelerated cell migration in animals on fiber-supplemented diets [137]. Certain soluble fibers such as guar gum, pectin, and wheat bran alter the rate of cell proliferation in the specific segments of the colon [138]. In rats fed separate guar gum and pectin-supplemented diets, colonocyte proliferation increases more than in those fed cellulose and fiber-free diets. In the distal colon, the various dietary fiber constituents equally promote colonocyte proliferation [138,139].

Other studies show that fiber ingestion is important in the maintenance and growth of the colonic mucosa. Low-fiber diets produce atrophy, as noted, by mucosal hypoplasia and a decreased rate of colonocyte proliferation [140]. Dietary components such as cellulose may be important in sustaining colonic mucosal integrity, but it is generally believed that the trophic effects in the colon are mediated by the SCFA fermentation products from dietary fiber and undigested starch [141–143].

Much evidence suggests that SCFAs function primarily by an indirect systemic effect. Increased proliferation not only occurs in colonocytes exposed to lumenal SCFAs, but also in adjacent unexposed colonocytes and ileal enterocytes [141,144]. Furthermore, colonic SCFA perfusion promotes mucosal growth in isolated, nonperfused, and denervated loops of jejunum. However, a direct effect cannot be dismissed because some evidence suggests butyrate stimulates colonocyte proliferation in short-term organ cultures of human colonic mucosa independent of neural and systemic factors [145].

Of the main SCFAs, lumenal butyrate plays a major role in colonocyte proliferation and consequent mucosal growth in the colon. SCFAs have a dose-dependent stimulatory effect on crypt cell production rate in the order of effectiveness: n-butyrate > propionate > acetate [73,141]. When delivery of fermentable nutrients to the colonic lumen is diminished, butyrate production decreases and mucosal atrophy occurs [146,147]. Accordingly, infusion of butyrate into the colonic lumen promotes mucosal growth as shown by increased mucosal mass, DNA content, and mitotic indices [141,148]. In rats, intralumenal perfusion of butyrate concentrations of 20 mM, 40 mM, and 150 mM into cecectomized rat colon increase segmental DNA by 100%, 100%, and 50%, respectively. Infusion of 20 mM butyrate stimulates colonic mucosal growth similarly to physiologic concentrations of butyrate, propionate, and acetate combined. However, butyrate concentrations 7.5 times the normal colonic concentration (20 mM) do not significantly increase colonocyte proliferation and mucosal growth [144].

In vitro butyrate studies reveal disparate results when compared to in vivo studies. Some in vitro experiments show that butyrate stimulates colonocyte proliferation in 25 and 60 mM concentrations, while other studies show that butyrate concentrations of 2 to 8 mM have no effect or decrease colonocyte proliferation [145,149,150]. If these in vitro studies receive further confirmation, the possibility that butyrate acts via an intermediary found only in intact colonic mucosa appears likely. These effects of butyrate in vitro merit further investigation.

At the molecular level, the mechanisms by which butyrate promotes colonocyte proliferation are not well understood. Several studies with colon cancer cell lines demonstrate that butyrate paradoxically decreases colonocyte proliferation [151–154]. Obviously, normal and neoplastic colonocytes have different molecular and metabolic profiles that may partially explain this paradoxical effect. Because most information about the molecular effects of butyrate comes from studies with colon cancer cell lines, these findings may not accurately delineate the molecular effects of butyrate in normal colonocytes.

Butyrate has three main effects on cellular DNA. First, histone deacetylase is inhibited, which causes histone hyperacetylation. This abnormal state may alter chromatin structure, thereby down-regulating cyclic gene expression associated with cell proliferation [155–157]. Second, butyrate prevents phosphorylation of histones H1 and H2A. Phosphorylated histone H1 is usually found in proliferating cells [158]. Finally, butyrate hypermethylates cellular DNA, a process that may inactivate cyclic gene expression and arrest cell proliferation [156]. These down-regulating effects of butyrate are nonspecific and may explain the potential protective effects of dietary fiber against colon cancer.

Other studies with cancer colon cell lines indicate that butyrate stimulates expression of new gene products associated with cell differentiation in a specific manner [159]. In human colon cancer cell line HT29, butyrate induces an increase in alkaline phosphatase activity characteristic of more differentiated cells compared to untreated control cells [160]. Thus, the molecular effects of butyrate may include inhibition of cellular proliferation and stimulation of cellular differentiation. In addition to neoplastic colonocytes, these effects of butyrate may occur in colonocytes of the other pathogenic states such as ulcerative colitis.

Recent work from our laboratory confirms the hypothesized molecular effects of butyrate in colonocytes from patients with ulcerative colitis. Butyrate increased nonspecific protein synthesis and decreased DNA synthesis in ulcerative colitis-diseased colonocytes when compared to normal, Crohn's, and diverticulitis colonocytes in vitro [unpublished results]. We speculate that butyrate suppresses cyclic gene expression (i.e., DNA synthesis) and enhances new gene expression associated with differentiation in ulcerative colitis-diseased colonocytes. The higher levels of nonspecific protein synthesis from our study are possibly due to increased novel protein synthesis from heightened new gene expression that characterize differentiated cells. Clearly, more extensive colonocyte studies with butyrate are needed.

Enhanced Production of Enterotrophic Gastrointestinal Hormones. An important mechanism by which SCFAs regulate intestinal mucosal growth may involve stimulation of gastrointestinal hormone production. Gastrin, enteroglucagon, and polypeptide Y (PYY) have been implicated as the main hormones trophic for intestinal cell proliferation and mucosal growth.

Gastrin is trophic to several segments of the intestinal tract. This hormone stimulates intestinal cell proliferation and increases levels of DNA, RNA, and protein content in duodenal, ileal, and proximal colonic mucosa [3]. In rats, removal of the antrum and its gastrin-producing G cells decreases colonic DNA content [161]. Furthermore, exogenous pentagastrin administered to normal human colonic epithelial cells in vitro causes a five-fold increase in cell number compared to a three-fold increase in cells treated with saline [162].

In starved rats, plasma gastrin levels increase slowly after refeeding and correlate only with crypt cell production rate in the duodenum. However, plasma enteroglucagon levels increase rapidly to above-normal levels and correlate well with crypt cell production rates in the small bowel and colon. These findings suggest that enteroglucagon may be important in overall control of enterocyte and colonocyte replacement [163]. In the same starved rat model, fermentable fiber (i.e., SCFAs) stimulates colonocyte proliferation markedly in the distal colon [164]. Mechanical bulk in the form of kaolin, however, does not stimulate proliferation. This increased cell turnover with fermentable fiber strongly correlates with increased plasma enteroglucagon levels throughout the intestinal tract and elevated PYY levels found only in the colon. There is no significant correlation with plasma gastrin levels [164].

Although they are found throughout the intestinal tract, most enteroglucagon-producing cells are present in the terminal ileum and proximal colon. These cells are, therefore, in an optimal position to monitor digesta for SCFAs or unabsorbed nutrients. This milieu provides a potential feedback mechanism to regulate SCFA production. There is a strong correlation between increased plasma enteroglucagon levels and intestinal cell proliferation in a variety of experimental models [163,165].

In rats and humans, PYY is primarily produced in the small intestine and colon, and its receptors are localized in the small bowel [164,166,167]. In rats with normally innervated ceca, SCFAs have a systemic jejunotrophic effect that is associated with significantly elevated tissue concentrations of gastrin in the jejunum [168]. In rats with denervated ceca, SCFAs do not induce a jejunotrophic effect or elevate tissue gastrin levels. Jejunal PYY levels do not increase significantly with cecal SCFA infusions in either innervated or denervated rats.

Stimulation of the Autonomic Nervous System. There is evidence to suggest that the autonomic nervous system has a role in mediating the enterotrophic effects of SCFAs. In fasted anesthetized rats, SCFAs perfused at a rapid rate into the colon increased the mitotic and labeling indices of colonocytes [169]. This trophic stimulation is abolished by preceding surgical vagotomy or chemical sympathectomy with guanethidine sulfate [148,169]. Furthermore, SCFA infusions significantly increase crypt cell production rate in both normally innervated and extrinsically denervated jejunal segments [170]. These findings indicate that SCFAs can systemically stimulate jejunal enterocyte proliferation and, thus, do not require efferent autonomic nerve connections [170].

SCFA administration for 10 days into normally innervated rat cecum out of intestinal continuity produces trophic changes in jejunum [168]. When extrinsic denervation of rat ceca is performed, the jejunotrophic effects of cecally infused SCFAs are abolished. This study suggests that afferent innervation (i.e., from cecum to the central nervous system) is essential for the jejunotrophic effects of cecal SCFAs, whereas the previous study suggests transection of efferent innervation does not alter the trophic effects of SCFAs.

In a study to determine which component of the autonomic nervous system (i.e., parasympathetic or sympathetic) is responsible for cecal SCFA-mediated jejunotrophism, rats were given cecal infusions of either SCFAs or saline for 10 days after surgical vagotomy, chemical sympathectomy with guanethidine, or sham operation [171]. In such rats, both parasympathetic and sympathetic systems are important in mediating trophic effects of cecal SCFAs on jejunal structure. However, only disrupted parasympathetic connections fully abolish the effects on jejunal function (i.e., glucose absorption, disaccharidase activity) [171]. When considered together, these findings suggest that autonomic receptors play a key role in SCFA-induced regulation of enterocyte proliferation.

Increased Mesenteric Blood Flow. The trophic effects of SCFAs on the colonic mucosa are probably mediated in part by increased mesenteric blood flow [172,173]. Intralumenal SCFA infusion at postprandial concentrations increases colonic blood flow by 24% in dogs, which suggests that SCFAs directly dilate colonic vasculature [172]. Of the three main SCFAs, acetate produces a greater increase of blood flow than n-butyrate and propionate [132,172]. SCFAs individually and in combination produce a significant and concentration-dependent dilatation of resistant arteries in resected human colon in vitro [18]. This vasodilatory effect suggests that SCFAs may improve colonic microcirculation in vivo, thereby providing an explanation for their trophic effect on colonic mucosa. Such results might explain how modest doses of SCFAs have trophic effects on intestinal mucosa even after parenteral administration [18,174,175].

The aforementioned studies suggest that the trophic effects of SCFAs may be due in part to increased blood flow to the intestinal mucosa; the magnitude of these effects in either normal or stressed states remains to be studied. Furthermore, studies are needed to determine if the vascular dilatation is caused directly by SCFAs or indirectly by either production of enterotrophic gastrointestinal hormones or stimulation of the autonomic nervous system.

Summary. The mechanisms of action for the enterotrophic effects of SCFAs are complex and probably multifactorial. The direct addition of energy to the colonic mucosa is only a modest factor whereas the increase of blood flow may contribute more to enterotrophism. Locally mediated mechanisms do not singularly account for the trophic effects of SCFAs in the colon because mucosal trophism occurs both locally and distally from the site of SCFA infusion. Furthermore, SCFAs stimulate mucosal growth in the small bowel as well as in the colon when colonic infusions are given to rats. Enterotrophic gastrointestinal hormones and the autonomic nervous system may be additional mediators of both the local and systemic trophic effects of SCFAs.

Clinical Implications

Several clinical studies demonstrate that SCFAs play a major role in the maintenance and welfare of the colonic mucosa. Much evidence suggests varied SCFA metabolism throughout the large intestine, and certain inflammatory conditions of the distal colon appear to respond to SCFA therapy. Potential clinical indications for the utilization of SCFAs include patients with diversion colitis, pouchitis following total proctocolectomy with an ileal anal pouch, or distal ulcerative colitis. The rationale for use of SCFAs is based on the premise that colonocyte energy deficiency may contribute to the pathogenesis of these inflammatory diseases and that energy generation by SCFA production may ameliorate these conditions. Because SCFAs given orally are quickly absorbed in the small intestine and do not reach the colon, these substrates are presently administered by rectal irrigation [176].

Diversion Colitis. In a clinical study, five patients with diversion colitis were treated with SCFA irrigations (butyrate 40 mmol/L, propionate 30 mmol/L, and acetate 60 mmol/L) twice daily for 6 weeks [177]. Endoscopic appearance of colonic mucosa of patients receiving SCFA improved after 2 weeks and progressively improved after 4 to 6 weeks when compared to saline controls. Histologic degree of colonic inflammation decreased dramatically [177]. In a double blind and prospective study of 13 patients with diversion colitis, however, no marked improvement was seen after 2 weeks of SCFA administration [178]. When seven patients received SCFA enemas (butyrate 40 mmol/L, propionate 30 mmol/L, and acetate 60 mmol/L) and six patients received isotonic saline, endoscopic and histologic indices revealed no significant changes [178]. The reason for these negative results may be due to the short period of study and the inclusion of milder forms of diversion colitis, which may reveal modest improvement compared to severe forms of this disease [176,179].

Pouchitis. Pouchitis is found in patients with mucosal inflammation of the ileal reservoir ("pouch") after restorative proctocolectomy. In patients with pouchitis, SCFA concentration and production are reduced significantly when compared to patients without pouchitis [180,181]. When pouchitis patients were given SCFA enemas (butyrate 40 mmol/L, propionate 30 mmol/L, and acetate 60 mmol/L) for 4 weeks, no significant effects were found [182]. In another study, butyrate suppositories (40 mmol) given twice daily for 3 weeks ameliorated clinical conditions in only three of nine patients with pouchitis [183]. Clearly, the effects of SCFA on pouchitis remain to be studied in larger clinical trials.

Distal Ulcerative Colitis. In one clinical study, 12 patients with severe distal ulcerative colitis received SCFA rectal irrigations (butyrate 40 mmol/L, propionate 30 mmol/L, and acetate 80 mmol/L) for 6 weeks. Of the 10 patients who completed the study, 9 had significant improvement in mean disease activity index score and in mucosal histology score [184]. In another study, butyrate enemas (100 mmol/L), given twice daily for 2 weeks to 10 patients with distal ulcerative colitis, returned colonocyte proliferation to normal values and expanded proliferative zones within the mucosa. Stool frequency and rectal bleeding regressed in patients receiving butyrate enemas. Furthermore, endoscopic appearance of colonic mucosa improved considerably and histologic findings of inflammation decreased significantly. All these parameters did not change in those patients who received a placebo [185]. While these initial clinical trials are encouraging, more extended human studies with SCFA are needed.

Conclusion

The importance of the intestine as the preferred route of nutrient administration for the hospitalized patient continues to be confirmed. Recent studies demonstrate that the most important determinant of gut growth and function is the provision of nutrients into the intestinal lumen. Lumenal nutrients mediate their effects directly by physical contact and indirectly by the increased production of enterotrophic gastrointestinal hormones. Intestinal epithelial proliferation and differentiation are both enhanced by the provision of enteral nutrients. Conversely, the absence or diminution of enteral nutrients during starvation, malnutrition, critical illness, and TPN-induced bowel rest is associated with intestinal atrophy and hypofunction.

In selected conditions of intestinal dysfunction, it is hypothesized that it may be preferable to feed into the intestine those fuels that are preferentially utilized by its component epithelium. Examples of these fuels include glutamine for the small bowel and short-chain fatty acids for the colon. Clinical trials are ongoing to confirm the validity of this hypothesis in patients with critical illness, short-bowel syndrome, pouchitis, diversion colitis, and ulcerative colitis. The provision of specialized nutrients into the gut to enhance its growth and function provides exciting new therapeutic possibilities for the patient with intestinal dysfunction.

References

1. Lajtha LG. Stem cell concepts. *Differentiation* 14:23, 1979.
2. Potten CS, Loeffler M. Stem cells: Attributes, cycles, spirals, pitfalls and uncertainties. Lessons for and from the Crypt. *Development* 110:1001, 1990.
3. Johnson LR. Regulation of Gastrointestinal Growth. In LR Johnson (ed), *Physiology of the Gastrointestinal Tract,* 2nd ed. New York: Raven, 1987.
4. Maniatis T, Goodbourn S, Fischer JA. Regulation of inducible and tissue-specific gene expression. *Science* 236: 1237, 1987.
5. Traber PG, et al. Sucrase-isomaltase gene expression along crypt-villus axis of human small intestine is regulated at level of mRNA abundance. *Am J Physiol* 262: G123, 1992.
6. Traber PG, Wu GD, Wang W. Novel DNA-binding proteins regulate intestine-specific transcription of the sucrase-isomaltase gene. *Mol Cell Biol* 12:3614, 1992.
7. Evans GS, Potten CS. Stem cells and the elixir of life. *Bioessays* 13:135, 1991.
8. Gordon JI. Intestinal epithelial differentiation: New insights from chimeric and transgenic mice. *J Cell Biol* 108:1187, 1989.
9. Cheng H, Leblond CP. Origin, differentiation and renewal of the four main epithelial cell types in the mouse small intestine: I. Columnar cell. *Am J Anat* 141:461, 1974.
10. Madara JL, Trier JS. Functional Morphology of the Mucosa of the Samll Intestine. In LR Johnson (ed), *Physiology of the Gastrointestinal Tract,* 2nd ed. New York: Raven, 1987.
11. Lipkin M. Proliferation and Differentiation of Normal and Diseased Gastrointestinal Cells. In LR Johnson (ed), *Physiology of the Gastrointestinal Tract,* 2nd ed. New York: Raven, 1987.
12. Shamsuddin AM, Phelps PC, Trump BF. Human large intestinal epithelium: Light microscopy, biochemistry, and ultrastructure. *Hum Pathol* 13:790, 1982.
13. Chang WWL, Leblond CP. Renewal of the epithelium in the descending colon of the mouse: I. Presence of three cell populations: vacuolated-columnar, mucous and argentaffin. *Am J Anat* 131:73, 1971.
14. Schmidt GH, Wilkinson MM, Ponder BAJ. Cell migration pathway in the intestinal epithelium: An in situ marker system using mouse aggregation chimeras. *Cell* 40:425, 1985.
15. Wilmore DW, et al. The gut: A central organ after surgical stress. *Surgery* 104:917, 1988.
16. Cummings JH, Branch WJ. Fermentation and the Production of Short Chain Fatty Acids in the Human Large Intestine. In GV Vahouny, D Kritchevsky (eds), *Basic and Medical Aspects of Dietary Fiber.* New York: Plenum, 1986.
17. Furness JB, et al. Correlated functional and structural analysis of enteric neural circuits. *Arch Histol Cytol* 52(S):161, 1989.
18. Mortensen FV, et al. Short chain fatty acids dilate isolated human colonic resistance arteries. *Gut* 31:1391, 1990.
19. Johnson LR. New aspects of the trophic action of gastrointestinal hormones. *Gastroenterology* 72:788, 1977.
20. Kiba T, et al. Ventromedial hypothalamic lesions increase gastrointestinal DNA synthesis through vagus nerve in rats. *Gastroenterology* 104:475, 1993.
21. Steiner M, et al. Effect of starvation on the tissue composition of the small intestine in the rat. *Am J Physiol* 215:75, 1968.
22. Brown HO, Levine ML, Lipkin M. Inhibition of intestinal epithelial cell renewal and migration induced by starvation. *Am J Physiol* 205:868, 1963.

23. Altmann GG. Influence of starvation and refeeding on mucosal size and epithelial renewal in the rat small intestine. *Am J Anat* 133:391, 1972.
24. Clarke RM. The time-course changes in mucosal architecture and epithelial cell production and cell shedding in the small intestine of the rat fed after fasting. *J Anat* 120:321, 1975.
25. Aldewachi HS, et al. The effect of starvation and refeeding on cell population kinetics in the rat small bowel mucosa. *J Anat* 119:105, 1975.
26. Jackson WD, Grand RJ. The human intestinal response to enteral nutrients: A review. *J Am Coll Nutr* 10:500, 1991.
27. Raul F, et al. Modifications of brush border enzyme activities during starvation in the jejunum and ileum of adult rats. *Enzyme* 28:328, 1982.
28. Rossi TM, et al. Effect of nutritional rehabilitation on the development of brush border disaccharidases of postnatally malnourished weaning rats. *Pediatr Res* 20:793, 1986.
29. Yamada K, et al. Different effect of starvation on activity of sucrase and lactase in rat jejunoileum. *Am J Physiol* 244:G449, 1983.
30. Solimano G, Burgess EA, Levin B. Protein-calorie malnutrition: Effect of deficient diets on enzyme levels of jejunal mucosa of rats. *Br J Nutr* 21:55, 1967.
31. Gorostiza E, et al. Influence of starvation and sucrase regulation by dietary sucrose in the rat. *Am J Clin Nutr* 40:1017, 1984.
32. Elia M, et al. Effect of total starvation and very low calorie diets on intestinal permeability in man. *Clin Sci* 73:205, 1987.
33. Butzner JD, Gall DG. Impact of refeeding on intestinal development and function in infant rabbits subjected to protein-energy malnutrition. *Pediatr Res* 27:245, 1990.
34. Brunser O. Effects of malnutrition on intestinal structure and function in children. *Clin Gastroenterology* 6:341, 1977.
35. James WPT. Effects of protein-calories malnutrition on intestinal absorption. *Ann NY Acad Sci* 176:244, 1971.
36. Saadia R, et al. Gut barrier function and the surgeon. *Br J Surg* 77:487, 1990.
37. Jones WG, et al. Splanchnic vasoconstriction and bacterial translocation after thermal injury. *Am J Physiol* 261:H1190, 1991.
38. Deitch EA. Bacterial translocation of the gut flora. *J Trauma* 30:S184, 1990.
39. Hong RW, et al. Glutamine preserves liver glutathione after lethal hepatic injury. *Ann Surg* 215:114, 1992.
40. Robinson MK, et al. Glutathione deficiency increases organ dysfunction after hemorrhagic shock. *Surgery* 112:140, 1992.
41. Berg RD. Translocation of Indigenous Bacteria from the Intestinal Tract Lumen. In DJ Hentges (ed), *Intestinal Microflora in Health and Disease.* New York: Academic, 1983.
42. Hammer-Hodges D, et al. Role of intraintestinal gram-negative bacterial flora in response to major injury. *Surg Gynecol Obstet* 138:599, 1974.
43. Deitch EA, Berg R, Specian R. Endotoxin promotes the translocation of bacteria from the gut. *Arch Surg* 122:185, 1987.
44. Rush BF, et al. Endotoxemia and bacteremia during hemorrhagic shock: The link between trauma and sepsis? *Ann Surg* 207:549, 1988.
45. Deitch EA. Multiple organ failure: Pathophysiology and potential future therapy. *Ann Surg* 216:117, 1992.
46. Goris RJA, et al. Multiple-organ failure and sepsis without bacteria: An experimental model. *Arch Surg* 121:897, 1986.
47. Border JR. Multiple systems organ failure. *Ann Surg* 216:111, 1992.
48. Zhi-Yong S, Yuan-Lin D, Xiao-Hong W. Bacterial translocation and multiple system organ failure in bowel ischemia and reperfusion. *J Trauma* 32:148, 1992.
49. Levine GM, et al. Role of oral intake in maintenance of gut mass and disaccharide activity. *Gastroenterology* 67:975, 1974.
50. Johnson LR, et al. Structural and hormonal alterations in the gastrointestinal tract of parenterally fed rats. *Gastroenterology* 68:1177, 1975.
51. Hughes CA, Dowling RH. Speed of onset of adaptive mucosal hypoplasia and hypofunction in the intestine of parenterally fed rats. *Clin Sci* 59:317, 1980.
52. Guedon C, et al. Decreased brush border hydrolase activities without gross morphologic changes in human intestinal mucosa after prolonged total parenteral nutrition of adults. *Gastroenterology* 90:373, 1986.
53. Buchman AL, et al. Parenteral nutrition leads to a decrease in intestinal mucosal thickness and an increase in intestinal permeability in man. *Gastroenterology* 104: A612, 1993.
54. Alverdy JC, Aoys E, Moss GS. Total parenteral nutrition promotes bacterial translocation from the gut. *Surgery* 104:185, 1988.
55. Illig KA, et al. Total parenteral nutrition-induced changes in gut mucosal function: Atrophy alone is not the issue. *Surgery* 112:631, 1992.
56. Thompson JS, et al. The effect of the route of nutrient delivery on gut structure and diamine oxidase levels. *JPEN* 11:28, 1987.
57. Morin CL, Ling V, Bourassa D. Small intestinal and colonic changes induced by a chemically defined diet. *Dig Dis Sci* 25:12, 1980.
58. Feldman EJ, et al. Effects of oral versus intravenous nutrition on intestinal adaptation after small bowel resection in the dog. *Gastroenterology* 70:712, 1976.
59. Ryan GP, et al. Effects of various diets on colonic growth in rats. *Gastroenterology* 77:658, 1979.
60. Ecknauer R, Sicar B, Johnson LR. Effect of dietary bulk on small intestinal morphology and cell renewal in the rat. *Gastroenterology* 81:781, 1981.
61. Young EA, et al. Gastrointestinal response to oral versus gastric feeding of defined formula diets. *Am J Clin Nutr* 35:715, 1982.
62. Young EA, et al. Comparative study of nutritional adaptation to defined formula diets in rats. *Am J Clin Nutr* 33:2106, 1980.
63. Rolandelli RH, Rombeau JL. Enteral nutrition in critically ill patients. *Perspect Crit Care* 2:1016, 1989.
64. Ryan JA. Jejunal Feeding. In JE Fischer (ed), *Surgical Nutrition,* 1st ed. Boston: Little, Brown, 1983.
65. Muggia-Sullam M, et al. Postoperative enteral versus parenteral nutritional support in gastrointestinal surgery. *Am J Surg* 149:106, 1985.
66. Lowry SF. The route of feeding influences injury responses. *J Trauma* 30:S10, 1990.
67. Fong Y, et al. Total parenteral nutrition and bowel rest modify the metabolic response to endotoxin in humans. *Ann Surg* 210:449, 1989.

68. Border JR, et al. The gut origin septic states in blunt multiple trauma (ISS = 40) in the ICU. *Ann Surg* 206: 427, 1987.

69. Moore FA, et al. TEN versus TPN following major abdominal trauma: Reduced septic morbidity. *J Trauma* 29:916, 1989.

70. Kudsk KA, et al. Enteral versus parenteral feeding: Effects on septic morbidity after blunt and penetrating abdominal trauma. *Ann Surg* 215:503, 1992.

71. Roediger WEW, et al. Anion control of sodium absorption in the colon. *Q J Exp Physiol* 71:195, 1986.

72. Windmueller HG, Spaeth AE. Respiratory fuels and nitrogen metabolism in vivo in small intestine of fed rats. *J Biol Chem* 255:107, 1980.

73. Roediger WEW. Utilization of nutrients by isolated epithelial cells of the rat colon. *Gastroenterology* 83:424, 1982.

74. Windmueller HG. Glutamine utilization by the small intestine. *Adv Enzymol* 53:201, 1982.

75. Souba WW, et al. Glutamine nutrition: Theoretical considerations and therapeutic impact. *JPEN* 14:237S, 1990.

76. Furst P, Albers S, Stehle P. Glutamine-containing dipeptides in parenteral nutrition. *JPEN* 14:118S, 1990.

77. McAnena OJ, et al. Selective uptake of glutamine in the gastrointestinal tract: Confirmation in a human study. *Br J Surg* 78:480, 1991.

78. Herskowitz K, Souba WW. Intestinal glutamine metabolism during critical illness: A surgical perspective. *Nutrition* 6:199, 1990.

79. van der Hulst RRWJ, van Kreel BK, von Meyenfeldt MF. Glutamine and the preservation of gut integrity. *Lancet* 341:1363, 1993.

80. Lowe DK, et al. Safety of glutamine-enriched parenteral nutrient solutions in humans. *Am J Clin Nutr* 52:1101, 1990.

81. Ziegler TR, et al. Safety and metabolic effects of L-glutamine administration in humans. *JPEN* 14:137S, 1990.

82. O'Dwyer ST, et al. Maintenance of small bowel mucosa with glutamine-enriched parenteral nutrition. *JPEN* 13:579, 1989.

83. Grant J, Snyder PJ. Use of L-glutamine in total parenteral nutrition. *J Surg Res* 44:506, 1988.

84. Jacobs DO, et al. Disparate effects of 5-fluorouracil on the ileum and colon of enterally fed rats with protection by dietary glutamine. *Surg Forum* 38:45, 1987.

85. Smith RJ, et al. The Gastrointestinal Response to Injury, Starvation and Enteral Nutrition. In *Report of the Eighth Ross Conference on Medical Research.* Columbus, OH: Ross Laboratories, 1988.

86. Schroeder P, et al. Glutamine prevents mucosal injury after small bowel transplantation. *Transplant Proc* 24: 1104, 1992.

87. Frankel WL, et al. Glutamine enhancement of structure and function in the transplanted small intestine in the rat. *JPEN* 17:47, 1993.

88. Zhang W, et al. Improvement of structure and function in orthotopic small bowel transplantation in the rat by glutamine. *Transplantation* 56:512, 1993.

89. Burke D, et al. Glutamine supplemented TPN improves gut immune function. *Arch Surg* 124:1396, 1989.

90. Alverdy IC, et al. The effect of glutamine-enriched TPN on gut immune cellularity. *J Surg Res* 52:34, 1992.

91. Fox AD, et al. Effect of a glutamine-supplemented enteral diet on methotrexate-induced enterocolitis. *JPEN* 12:325, 1988.

92. O'Dwyer ST, et al. 5-fluorouracil toxicity on small intestinal mucosa but not white blood cells is decreased by glutamine. *Clin Res* 35:369A, 1987.

93. Ziegler TR, et al. Clinical and metabolic efficacy of glutamine-supplemented parenteral nutrition after bone marrow transplantation. *Ann Intern Med* 116:821, 1992.

94. Hammarqvist F, et al. Addition of glutamine to total parenteral nutrition after elective abdominal surgery spares free glutamine in muscle, counteracts the fall in muscle protein synthesis, and improves nitrogen balance. *Ann Surg* 209:455, 1989.

95. Stehle P, et al. Effect of parenteral glutamine peptide supplements on muscle glutamine loss and nitrogen balance after major surgery. *Lancet* 1:231, 1989.

96. Schloerb PR, Amare M. Total parenteral nutrition with glutamine in bone marrow transplantation and other clinical applications (a randomized, double-blind study). *JPEN* 17:407, 1993.

97. Jacobs DO, et al. Combined effects of glutamine and epidermal growth factor (EGF) on GI mucosal cellularity. *Surgery* 104:358, 1988.

98. Ko TC, et al. Glutamine is essential for epidermal growth factor-stimulated intestinal cell proliferation. *Surgery* 114:147, 1993.

99. Sarantos P, Abouhamze A, Souba WW. Glucocorticoids regulate intestinal glutaminase expression. *Surgery* 112:278, 1992.

100. Cummings JH. Colonic absorption: The importance of short chain fatty acids in man. *Scand J Gastroenterol* 19:90, 1984.

101. Roediger WEW. Role of anaerobic bacteria in the metabolic welfare of the colonic mucosa in man. *Gut* 21:793, 1980.

102. Ardawi MSM, Newsholme EA. Fuel utilization on colonocytes of the rat. *Biochem J* 231:713, 1985.

103. Engelhardt WV, Luciano L, Reale E. Transport of SCFA across the large intestinal epithelium of guinea pig. *Acta Vet Scand (Suppl)* 86:103, 1989.

104. Engelhardt WV, Rechkemmer G. Segmental differences of short-chain fatty acid transport across guinea pig large intestine. *Exp Physiol* 77:491, 1992.

105. Ruppin H, et al. Absorption of short-chain fatty acids by the colon. *Gastroenterology* 78:1500, 1980.

106. Rechkemmer G, Engelhardt WV. Concentration and pH dependence of short-chain fatty acid absorption in the proximal and distal colon of guinea pig (Cavia porcellus). *Comp Biochem Physiol* 91A:659, 1988.

107. McNeil NI, Cummings JH, James WPT. Short-chain fatty acid absorption by the human large intestine. *Gut* 19:819, 1978.

108. Fleming SE, Choi SY, Fitch MD. Absorption of short chain fatty acids from the rat cecum in vivo. *J Nutr* 121:1787, 1991.

109. Rechkemmer G, et al. pH microclimate at the luminal surface of the intestinal mucosa of guinea pig and rat. *Pflugers Arch* 407:33, 1986.

110. McNeil NI, Ling KLE, Wager J. Mucosal surface pH of the large intestine of the rat and of normal and inflamed large intestine in man. *Gut* 28:707, 1987.

111. Luciano L, et al. Structure of zonulae occludentes and the permeability of the epithelium to short-chain fatty acids in the proximal and the distal colon of guinea pig. *J Membr Biol* 82:145, 1984.

112. Ronnau K, Guth D, Engelhardt WV. Absorption of dissociated and undissociated short-chain fatty acids across the

colonic epithelium of guinea pig. *Q J Exp Physiol* 74:511, 1989.

113. Soergel KH, et al. Colonic fermentation and absorption of SCFA in man. *Acta Vet Scand* 86:107, 1989.

114. Engelhardt WV, et al. Effect of amiloride and oubain on short-chain fatty acid transport in guinea pig large intestine. *J Physiol* 460:455, 1993.

115. Bugaut M. Occurrence, absorption and metabolism of short chain fatty acids in the digestive tract of mammals. *Comp Biochem Physiol* 86B:439, 1987.

116. Argenzio RA, et al. Interrelationship of Na, HCO_3 and volatile fatty acid transport by equine large intestine. *Am J Physiol* 233:E469, 1977.

117. Umesaki Y, et al. Effect of organic acid absorption on bicarbonate transport in rat colon. *Pflugers Arch* 379:43, 1979.

118. Mascolo N, Rajendran VM, Binder HJ. Mechanism of short chain fatty acid uptake by apical membrane vesicles of rat distal colon. *Gastroenterology* 101:331, 1991.

119. Reynolds D, Rajendran VM, Binder HJ. Butyrate transport in rat distal colon basolateral membrane vesicles: Evidence for bicarbonate/butyrate exchange. *Gastroenterology* 100:A838, 1991.

120. Lonnerholm G. Carbonic anhydrase in the intestinal tract of the guinea pig. *Acta Physiol Scand* 99:53, 1977.

121. Charney AN, et al. Functional role of carbonic anhydrase in intestinal electrolyte transport. *Am J Physiol* 251: G682, 1986.

122. Roediger WEW, Moore A. Effect of short-chain fatty acid on sodium absorption in isolated human colon perfused through the vascular bed. *Dig Dis Sci* 26:100, 1981.

123. Binder HJ, Mehta P. Short chain fatty acids stimulate active sodium and chloride absorption in vitro in the rat distal colon. *Gastroenterology* 96:989, 1989.

124. Rubsamen K, et al. Regional differences in electrolyte, short-chain fatty acid and water absorption in the hindgut of two species of arboreal marsupials. *Pflugers Arch* 399:68, 1983.

125. Holtug K, Rasmussen HS, Mortensen PB. An in vitro study of short-chain fatty concentrations, production and absorption in pig (Sus Scrofa) colon. *Comp Biochem Physiol* 103A:189, 1992.

126. Stingelin Y, Wolffram S, Scharrer E. Evidence for Potassium/Acetate Cotransport in Rat Distal Colon. In F Alvarado, CH van Os (eds), *Ion Gradient-Coupled Transport.* Amsterdam: Elsevier, 1986.

127. McNeil NI, Cummings JH, James WPT. Rectal absorption of short-chain fatty acids in the absence of chloride. *Gut* 20:400, 1979.

128. Roediger WEW. Metabolic basis of starvation diarrhea: Implications for treatment. *Lancet* 1:1082, 1986.

129. Henning SJ, Hird FJR. Concentrations and metabolism of volatile fatty acids in the fermentative organs of two species of kangaroo and the guinea pig. *Br J Nutr* 24:145, 1970.

130. Henning SJ, Hird FJR. Ketogenesis from butyrate and acetate by the caecum and the colon of rabbits. *Biochem J* 130:785, 1972.

131. Roediger WEW. The Place of SCFAs in Colonocyte Metabolism in Health and Ulcerative Colitis: The Impaired Colonocyte Barrier. In JH Cummings, T Sakata, JL Rombeau (eds), *Physiologic and Clinical Aspects of Short-Chain Fatty Acids.* Cambridge: Cambridge University, 1993.

132. Cummings JH, et al. Short chain fatty acids in human large intestine, portal, hepatic and venous blood. *Gut* 28:1221, 1987.

133. Marty JF, Vernay MY, Abravanel GM. Acetate absorption and metabolism in the rabbit hind-gut. *Gut* 26:562, 1985.

134. Remesy C, Demigne C, Chartier F. Origin and utilization of volatile fatty acids in the rat. *Reprod Nutr Dev* 20:1339, 1980.

135. Firmansyah A, Penn D, Lebenthal E. Metabolism of glucose, glutamine, n-butyrate, β-hydroxybutyrate in isolated rat colonocyte following acute fasting and chronic malnutrition. *Gastroenterology* 97:622, 1989.

136. Cummings JH, Gibson GR, MacFarlane GT. Quantitative estimates of fermentation in the hindgut of man. *Acta Vet Scand* 86:76, 1989.

137. Vahouny GV, Cassidy MM. Dietary Fiber and Intestinal Adaptation. In GV Vahouny, D Kritchevsky (eds), *Basic and Medical Aspects of Dietary Fiber.* New York: Plenum, 1986.

138. Jacobs LR. Dietary Fiber and the Intestinal Mucosa. In JH Cummings (ed), *The Role of Dietary Fiber in Enteral Nutrition.* Abbott Park: Abbott International, 1989.

139. Jacobs LR, Lupton JR. Relationship between colonic luminal pH, cell proliferation and colon carcinogenesis in 1,2-dimethyl-hydrazine treated rats fed high fiber diets. *Cancer Res* 46:1727, 1986.

140. Bristol JB, Williams CN. Large bowel growth. *Scand J Gastroenterol* 19(S93):25, 1984.

141. Sakata T. Stimulatory effect of short chain fatty acids on epithelial cell proliferation in the rat intestine: A possible explanation for trophic effects of fermentable fibre, gut microbes and luminal trophic factors. *Br J Nutr* 58:95, 1987.

142. Cameron IL, et al. Quantitative contribution of factors regulating rat colonic crypt epithelium: Role of parenteral and enteral feeding, caloric intake, dietary cellulose level and the colon carcinogen DMH. *Cell Tissue Kinet* 23:227, 1990.

143. Cummings JH. Production and Metabolism of Short-Chain Fatty Acids in Humans. In *Short-Chain Fatty Acids: Metabolism and Clinical Importance. Report of Tenth Ross Conference on Medical Research.* Columbus, OH: Ross Laboratories, 1991.

144. Kripke SA, et al. Stimulation of intestinal mucosal growth with intracolonic infusion of short chain fatty acids. *JPEN* 13:109, 1989.

145. Scheppach WM. Short-Chain Fatty Acids Are a Trophic Factor for the Human Colonic Mucosa In Vitro. In *Short-Chain Fatty Acids: Metabolism and Clinical Importance. Report of Tenth Ross Conference on Medical Research.* Columbus, OH: Ross Laboratories, 1991.

146. Goodlad RA, Wright NA. Effects of addition of kaolin or cellulose to an elemental diet on intestinal cell proliferation in the rat. *Br J Nutr* 50:91, 1983.

147. Sakata T. Depression of intestinal epithelial cell production rate by hindgut bypass in rats. *Scand J Gastroenterol* 23:1200, 1988.

148. Sakata T, Yajima T. Influence of short chain fatty acids on the epithelial cell division of digestive tract. *Q J Exp Physiol* 69:639, 1984.

149. Friedman E, Lightdale C, Winawer S. Effects of psyllium fiber and short-chain organic acids derived from fiber breakdown on colonic epithelial cells from high risk patients. *Cancer Lett* 43:121, 1988.

150. Young GP, Gibson PR. Contrasting Effects of Butyrate on Proliferation and Differentiation of Normal and Neoplastic Cells. In *Short-Chain Fatty Acids: Metabolism and Clinical Importance. Report of Tenth Ross Conference on Medical Research.* Columbus, OH: Ross Laboratories, 1991.

151. Tsao D, et al. Differential effects of sodium butyrate, dimethyl sulfoxide, and retinoic acid on membrane-associated antigen, enzymes and glycoproteins of human rectal adenocarcinoma cells. *Cancer Res* 42:1052, 1982.

152. Whitehead RH, Young GP, Bhathal PS. Effects of short chain fatty acids on a new human colon carcinoma cell line (LIM1215). *Gut* 27:1457, 1986.

153. Colony PC. The Identification of Cell Types in the Normal Adult Colon. In LH Augenlicht (ed), *Cell and Molecular Biology of Colon Cancer.* Boca Raton: CRC, 1989.

154. Barnard JA, Warwick G. Sodium butyrate rapidly induces "enterocytic-like" differentiation and growth inhibition of HT-29 cells. *Gastroenterology* 102:A199, 1992.

155. Kruh J. Effects of sodium butyrate, a new pharmacological agent, on cells in culture. *Mol Cell Biochem* 42:65, 1982.

156. deHaan JB, Gevers W, Parker MI. Effects of sodium butyrate on the synthesis and methylation of DNA in normal cells and their transformed counterparts. *Cancer Res* 46:713, 1986.

157. Toscani A, Soprano DR, Soprano KJ. Molecular analysis of sodium butyrate-induced growth arrest. *Oncol Res* 3: 223, 1988.

158. D'Anna JA, Tobey RA, Gurley LR. Concentration-dependent effects of sodium butyrate in Chinese hamster cells: Cell-cycle progression, inner histone acetylation, histone H1 dephosphorylation and induction of an H1-like protein. *Biochemistry* 19:2656, 1980.

159. Foss FM, et al. Alteration of the expression of pp60c-src and p561ck associated with butyrate-induced differentiation of human colon carcinoma cells. *Oncol Res* 5:13, 1989.

160. Gamet L, Daviaud D, Denis-Pouxviel C. Effects of short-chain fatty acids on growth and differentiation of the human colon-cancer cell line HT29. *Int J Cancer* 52:286, 1992.

161. Dembinski AB, Johnson LR. Growth of pancreas and gastrointestinal mucosa in antrectoma and gastrin treated rats. *Endocrinology* 105:769, 1979.

162. Sirinek KR, Levine BA, Moyer MP. Pentagastrin stimulates in vitro growth of normal and malignant human colon epithelial cells. *Am J Surg* 149:35, 1985.

163. Goodlad RA, et al. Cell proliferation plasma enteroglucagon and plasma gastrin levels in starved and refed rats. *Virchows Arch Cell Pathol* 43:55, 1983.

164. Goodlad RA, et al. Effects of an elemental diet, inert bulk, and different types of dietary fiber on the response of the intestinal epithelium to refeeding in the rat and relationship to plasma gastrin, enteroglucagon, and PYY concentrations. *Gut* 28:171, 1987.

165. Sagor G, et al. Evidence for a humoral mechanism after small intestinal resection. *Gastroenterology* 84:902, 1983.

166. Calam J, et al. Regional differences in concentrations of regulatory peptides in human colon mucosal biopsy. *Dig Dis Sci* 34:1193, 1989.

167. Hill FLC, et al. Peptide YY, a new gut hormone (a mini-review). *Steroids* 56:77, 1991.

168. Frankel W, et al. Stimulation of the autonomic nervous system mediates short-chain fatty acid induced jejunotrophism. *Surg Forum* 43:24, 1992.

169. Sakata T, Engelhardt WV. Stimulatory effect of short-chain fatty acids on the epithelial cell proliferation in the rat large intestine. *Comp Biochem Physiol* 74A:459, 1983.

170. Sakata T. Stimulatory effect of short-chain fatty acids on epithelial cell proliferation of isolated and denervated jejunal segment of the rat. *Scand J Gastroenterol* 24:886, 1989.

171. Reilly K, et al. The parasympathetic (PSNS) and sympathetic (SNS) nervous systems mediate the systemic effects of short-chain fatty acids (SCFA) on jejunal structure and function. *Surg Forum* 44:20, 1993.

172. Kvietys PR, Granger ND. Effect of volatile fatty acids on blood flow and oxygen uptake by the dog colon. *Gastroenterology* 80:962, 1981.

173. Demigne C, Remesy C. Stimulation of absorption of volatile fatty acids and minerals in the cecum of rats adapted to a very high fiber diet. *J Nutr* 115:53, 1985.

174. Koruda MJ, et al. Parenteral nutrition supplemented with short-chain fatty acids: Effect on the small bowel mucosa in normal rats. *Am J Clin Nutr* 51:685, 1990.

175. Karlstad MD, et al. Parenteral nutrition with short- and long-chain triglycerides: Triacetin reduces atrophy of small and large bowel mucosa and improves protein metabolism in burned rats. *Am J Clin Nutr* 55:1005, 1992.

176. Scheppach WM, Bartram P, Richter F. Management of Diversion Colitis and Other Conditions. In JH Cummings, T Sakata, JL Rombeau (eds), *Physiologic and Clinical Aspects of Short-Chain Fatty Acids.* Cambridge: Cambridge University, 1993.

177. Harig JM, et al. Treatment of diversion colitis with short chain fatty acid irrigation. *N Engl J Med* 320:23, 1989.

178. Guillenot F, et al. Treatment of diversion colitis by short-chain fatty acids. *Dis Colon Rectum* 34:861, 1991.

179. Roediger WEW. Oxidative and synthetic functions of n-butyrate in colonocytes [Letter]. *Dis Colon Rectum* 35:511, 1992.

180. Wischmeyer PE, et al. Fecal short chain fatty acids in patients with pouchitis after ileal pouch anal anastomosis. *Gastroenterology* 100:A848, 1991.

181. Clausen MR, Tvede M, Mortensen PB. Short-chain fatty acids in pouch contents from patients with or without pouchitis after ileal pouch-anal anastomosis. *Gastroenterology* 103:1144, 1992.

182. DeSilva HJ, et al. Short-chain fatty acid irrigation in severe pouchitis. *N Engl J Med* 321:1416, 1989.

183. Wischmeyer PE, et al. Treatment of pouchitis after ileal-anal anastomosis with glutamine and butyric acid. *Gastroenterology* 102:A617, 1992.

184. Breuer RI, et al. Rectal irrigation with short-chain fatty acids for distal ulcerative colitis. *Dig Dis Sci* 36:185, 1991.

185. Scheppach WM, et al. Effect of butyrate enemas on the colonic mucosa in distal ulcerative colitis. *Gastroenterology* 103:51, 1992.

Selected Readings

Breuer RI, et al. Rectal irrigation with short-chain fatty acids for distal ulcerative colitis. *Dig Dis Sci* 36:185, 1991.

A clinical trial of short-chain fatty acid (SCFA) rectal irrigations in 12 patients with severe distal ulcerative colitis. Of the 10 patients who completed the study, 9 showed decreased disease activity and improved mucosal histology scores after 6 weeks of SCFA treatment.

Potten CS, Loeffler M. Stem cells: Attributes, cycles, spirals, pitfalls and uncertainties. Lessons for and from the Crypt. *Development* 110:1001, 1990.

A thought-provoking overview of cell proliferation and differentiation remarkably illustrated for the epithelial crypts of the small intestine. This review allows the reader to grasp the basic concepts of cell proliferation and differentiation that are essential to understanding the effects of intestinal fuels at the molecular level.

Scheppach WM, et al. Effect of butyrate enemas on the colonic mucosa in distal ulcerative colitis. *Gastroenterology* 103: 51, 1992.

A single-blind trial of butyrate enemas and placebo in 10 patients with refractory distal ulcerative colitis. Butyrate enemas decreased stool frequency and reduced degree of inflammation in patients of this study.

Ziegler TR, et al. Clinical and metabolic efficacy of glutamine-supplemented parenteral nutrition after bone marrow transplantation. *Ann Intern Med* 116:821, 1992.

A double-blind, randomized, controlled trial of glutamine-supplemented and standard parenteral nutrition in 45 patients receiving bone marrow transplants (BMT) for hematologic malignancies. Glutamine-supplemented parenteral nutrition improved nitrogen balance, decreased incidence of clinical infection, lowered rates of microbial colonization, and shortened overall hospital stay in patients after BMT compared to those receiving standard parenteral nutrition.

14

Arginine

Adrian Barbul

It is generally accepted that adequate nutritional support is an essential component in the successful treatment of the critically ill patient. Nutritional intervention affects how the hospitalized patient responds to infection, injury, and neoplasia. In the past two decades, the concept of nutrition support for the hospitalized patient has evolved considerably. The aim of most therapeutic nutritional regimens is to maintain positive nitrogen balance to preserve or restore lean body tissue. More recent interest has focused on the use of various nutrients, solely or as part of a complete nutritional regimen, to modulate the immune system and positively enhance patient outcome. Among these dietary factors, the amino acid arginine has been found to possess a number of extremely useful and unique effects on immune function, post-traumatic nitrogen metabolism, and wound healing. All of these effects, coupled with relative safety, make the use of arginine attractive for the care of traumatized or seriously ill patients.

Biochemistry and Physiology of Arginine

Arginine, a dibasic amino acid, is considered to be a dietary, conditionally dispensable amino acid [1]. Arginine is synthesized endogenously in the kidney from gut-derived citrulline. The small intestine converts dietary amino acids, including glutamine, to citrulline. Supplemental dietary glutamine leads to enhanced intestinal citrulline synthesis with increased renal arginine production. The quantities of arginine produced normally are sufficient to maintain muscle and connective tissue mass but may be less than that required for optimal protein biosynthesis and, therefore, optimal growth. In times of immaturity and severe stress, such as sepsis, trauma, and nitrogen overload, endogenous synthesis of arginine is insufficient to meet the heightened demands that increased protein turnover requires. Therefore, in such situations, arginine becomes an indispensable amino acid for optimal growth and maintenance of positive nitrogen balance (Figure 14-1) [2–4].

Arginine is a normal constituent of numerous body proteins and is associated with a variety of essential reactions of intermediary metabolism. The intestinal absorption of arginine involves a transport system shared with lysine, ornithine, and cysteine. This system is energy and sodium dependent and has substrate specificity. Arginine, ornithine, and lysine also share a common uptake and transport system in the brain, leukocytes, erythrocytes, and fibroblasts [5].

Arginine serves as a vehicle for the transport, storage, and excretion of nitrogen. The transamination between arginine and glycine results in guanidinoacetic acid, which is further methylated to form the high-energy phosphagen creatine phosphate. The reversible release of fumaric acid by dismutation of arginosuccinic acid further links arginine metabolism with cellular energetics via the tricarboxylic acid cycle. Arginine and its metabolite ornithine are also utilized for polyamine biosynthesis, an important requirement for cellular division (see Figure 14-1).

The urea cycle represents the major metabolic pathway for ammonia detoxification, and arginine plays a key regulatory role within this cycle (see Figure 14-1) [6]. Any condition that increases the demand for ammonia detoxification is likely to increase arginine requirements. Approximately twice as much ornithine and four times as much citrulline are needed to achieve the same degree of protection against hyperammonemia as that provided by arginine.

Recently, L-arginine has been shown to be the unique substrate for the production of the biologic effector molecule, nitric oxide (NO). This important pathway has been shown to be present in many tissues and cells, including endothelium, brain, inflammatory cells (lymphocytes, macrophages, neutrophils, mast cells), platelets, and he-

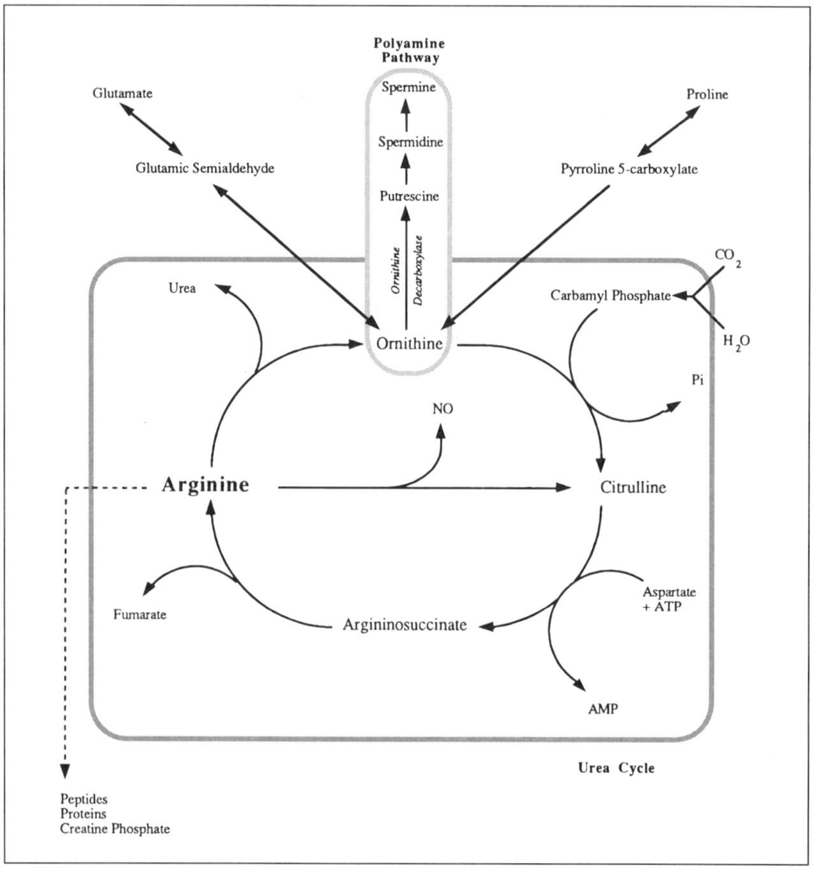

Figure 14-1. Schematic representation of the major metabolic cycles of arginine.

patocytes [7]. NO, which is pharmacologically and chemically identical to endothelial-derived relaxing factor (EDRF), is a recently identified biologic effector molecule. In addition to its role in vasodilatation, NO is a putative neurotransmitter and cytotoxic effector molecule. NO is formed by oxidation of one of two identical terminal guanidine groups of L-arginine by the enzyme NO synthase (provisionally EC 1.14.13.39), a dioxygenase of which there are at least two identified isoforms. The enzyme has been found in almost all tissue types examined and occurs in all animal species from mammals, reptiles, and birds to the horseshoe crab [8–11]. The latter animal has survived unchanged during 500 million years of evolution, indicating that the generation of NO is one of the oldest phylogenetically preserved regulatory systems. Both isoforms of NO synthase have been identified as flavoproteins [12–14], each containing flavine adenine dinucleotide and flavine adenine mononucleotide, and both inhibited by diphenyleneiodonium, a flavoprotein inhibitor [15].

NO synthase type I is cytosolic, expressed constitutively, and activated by Ca^{2+}/calmodulin [16]. Following stimulation by various agonists, the generation of NO by this isoform is quantitatively smaller in both amount and duration than that of NO synthase type II [8]. NO synthase I has been identified in the brain [16–18], lung [19], retina [20], adrenal glands [21], platelets [22], endocardial cells, vascular endothelial cells [23,24], skeletal muscle, spleen, and skin [25].

NO synthase type II has been cloned [26,27] and identified as two 125-135,000 KDa monomer proteins, which form a 250,000 KDa dimer [14,28]. The enzyme is inducible by endotoxins, exotoxins, and/or cytokines and is found in macrophages [29–31], Kupffer cells [32], parenchymal liver cells [33,34], neutrophils [35], fibroblasts [36], chondrocytes [37], and smooth muscle cells [38]. Mouse macrophage NO synthase II shares 51% homology with the rat cerebellar NO synthase I [27]. Like NO synthase I, macrophage NO synthase II contains binding sites for both flavine adenine dinucleotide and NADPH [26,27]. It is soluble and has an absolute requirement for tetrahydrobiopterin and possibly for Mg^{2+} and reduced thiols such as dithiothreitol or glutathione [39]. The induction of this isoform is inhibited by glucocorticoids [40–42] transforming growth factor-β 1,2 and 3 [43], IL-4, and IL-10 [44]. These compounds have no inhibitory activity on the formation of NO once the enzyme is expressed.

There are still many questions regarding the physiology of NO synthesis and its alterations in different pathologic states. There is no evidence yet that exogenous arginine, even in large doses, modulates the rate of synthesis of NO (for one possible exception, see the next section). Conversely, plasma and tissue levels of arginine are usually high enough to meet the demands of the NO synthase enzyme in healthy individuals. The two exceptions noted thus far involve the local wound environment, where arginine levels are very low [45], and the atherosclerotic vessel, where again, low arginine concentrations may be responsible for the lack of endogenous vasodilatation [46]. A great deal of current research is focusing on modulating NO synthase activity, whether endogenous or induced by different disease states.

Arginine and Hormone Secretagogue Activity

Increased plasma levels of arginine lead to enhanced secretion of several hormones, including insulin, glucagon, growth hormone, prolactin, and adrenal catecholamines (Table 14-1) [5]. While arginine is not the only amino acid that stimulates the release of these hormones, it is certainly the most potent.

The strong endocrine secretagogue action of arginine occurs via a largely unexplained mechanism that appears to be linked to cholinergic activity. This fact and the recent demonstration of NO synthase immunoreactivity and functional activity in several secretory organs support evidence that NO is involved in arginine-induced hormone secretion. For example, both L-arginine and L-ornithine are potent insulotrophic agents [47]. The depolarizing activity of these two cationic amino acids has been proposed as being responsible for their ability to stimulate insulin release [48]; however, this explanation is insufficient to account for all of the insulin release. In vivo, pancreatic NO is produced in response to D-glucose and L-arginine or tolbutamide, a hypoglycemic drug [49,50]. As opposed to this constitutive NO synthesis, large

Table 14-1. Endocrine Secretagogue Effects of Arginine

Pituitary gland
Growth hormone
Prolactin
Pancreas
Insulin
Glucagon
Somatostatin
Pancreatic polypeptide
Adrenal gland
Catecholamines
Aldosterone
Brain
Vasopressin

NO production is induced by interleukin-1β [51], probably in intrapancreatic macrophages and endothelial cells. This mechanism has been implicated in the pathologic damage found in autoimmune insulitis characteristic of type I diabetes mellitus. Inhibition of constitutive NO production by N-monomethyl-arginine (a competitive inhibitor of arginine for NO synthase) reduces insulin secretion in response to L-arginine [52]. Inhibition of inducible NO synthesis by N-monomethyl-arginine is effective in reducing the onset of streptozotocin-diabetes [53].

NO synthase immunoreactivity and functionality have been also located in the adrenal gland [21]. NO modulates adrenal medullary vasodilatation that may increase the release of adrenal hormones due to increased perfusion. In addition, L-arginine [53] as well as other agents that increase intracellular cGMP levels, such as NO, stimulate catecholamine release from the adrenal gland [54,55]. Endogenously formed NO facilitates the release of adrenaline in the rabbit [56].

Because L-arginine causes the release of many other hormones by cholinergic actions, it is reasonable to speculate that NO may be involved in the secretion of other hormones such as pituitary growth hormone and prolactin. The lack of NO synthase immunoreactivity in the anterior pituitary is given as evidence against this possibility. However, a form of the enzyme that does not react with NO synthase type I may be present there.

If increased NO synthesis is the mechanism by which arginine leads to enhanced hormone secretion, this would be one of the first known instances whereby exogenous arginine can directly regulate levels of NO synthesis, whether by the constitutive or the inducible NO synthase systems.

Arginine and Post-Traumatic Nitrogen Metabolism

Based on the concept that post-trauma nutritional requirements approximate those of the growing

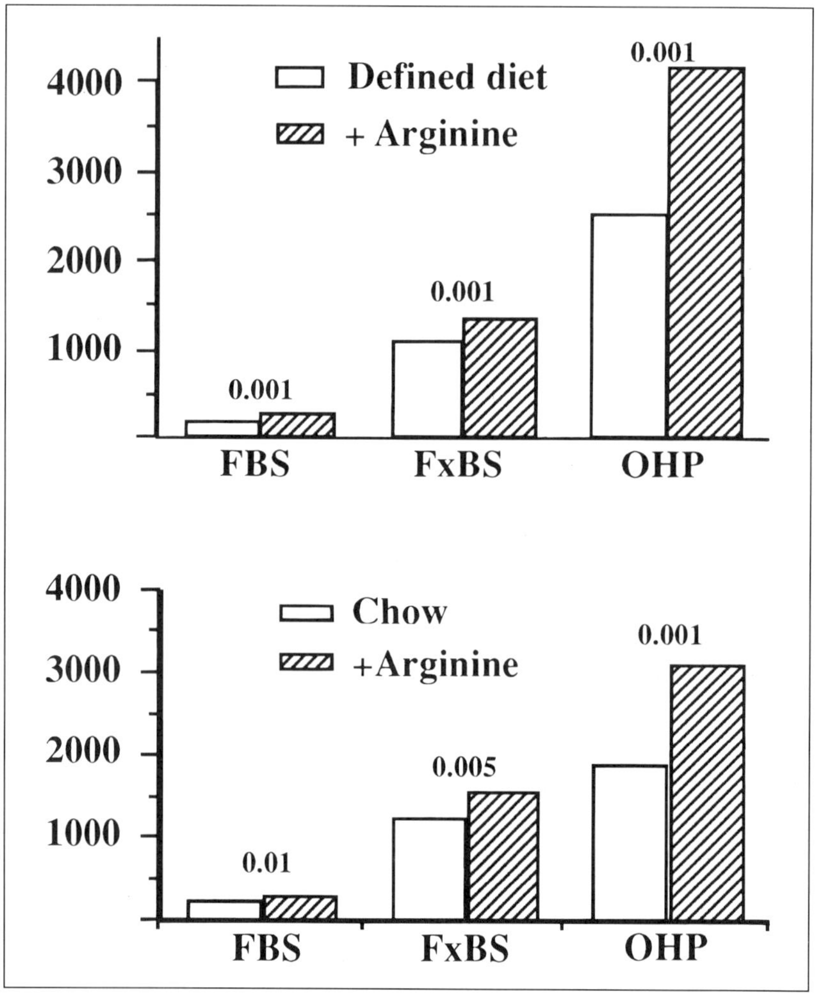

Figure 14-2. Effect of arginine on wound healing in rats. *Top:* Effect of arginine deficiency (defined diet) on wound healing. *Bottom:* Effect of 1% arginine supplementation on wound healing. FBS-fresh wound breaking strength (g); FxBS = formaldehyde-fixed wound breaking strength (g); OHP-hydroxyproline (μg/100 mg of polyvinyl alcohol sponge inserted).

rather than the adult organism, Seifter has shown that arginine is required for the survival and weight gain of mildly injured rats [4]. Animals subjected to either partial starvation or bilateral closed femoral fractures have improved nitrogen retention when given amino acid mixtures containing a larger proportion of arginine [57,58].

Healthy elderly human volunteers demonstrate increased nitrogen retention following supplementation with 30 g of arginine aspartate (17 g of free arginine) for two weeks [59]. Clinically, arginine given alone or in conjunction with complete nutritional support has been shown to reduce nitrogen loss in postoperative patients. Thus, elective surgical patients given 30 g/day of arginine hydrochloride intravenously for the first three days post-cholecystectomy had a 60% reduction in urinary nitrogen excretion [60]. Following major abdominal surgery for gastrointestinal malignancies, patients receiving immediate enteral feedings supplemented with 25 g of arginine had a mean positive nitrogen balance when compared to glycine-supplemented controls [61].

Supplemental ornithine also increases nitrogen retention following surgery in man [62,63]. As ornithine cannot replace arginine for nutritional requirements [64], this similar mode of action on nitrogen balance suggests a common pharmacologic mechanism of action. The amounts of arginine and ornithine required to achieve the above effects are in excess of those achieved by normal nutritional means and represent a pharmacologic dose.

Arginine and Wound Healing

Successful wound healing is the cornerstone of recovery following surgical procedures. Nearly half of all postoperative morbidity involves wound complications [65]. One of the most common problems encountered among critically ill patients is a delay in the efficiency of wound healing. In particular, the elderly are more prone to certain wound healing complications, including abdominal wound dehiscence and bowel anastomosis breakdown. Both animal and human experimental evidence demonstrate that arginine can positively modulate the wound healing process, mainly by enhancing wound collagen deposition.

The role of arginine in wound healing was first demonstrated in studies of animals placed on arginine-deficient diets. When such animals are subjected to the minor trauma of a dorsal skin incision and closure, they have increased postoperative weight loss and increased mortality when compared to rats fed a similar defined diet containing arginine. Furthermore, the arginine deficiency results in decreased wound breaking strength and wound collagen accumulation (Figure 14-2) [4]. Subsequently, it was noted that chow-fed rats (thus not arginine-deficient) given a 1% arginine HCl supplementation also have enhanced wound breaking strength and collagen synthesis when compared to chow-fed controls (see Figure 14-2) [4]. A similar enhancement of both of these wound healing parameters was observed in parenterally fed rats given an amino acid mixture containing high doses (7.5 g/L) of arginine in rats [66]. Mature or old rats fed a diet supplemented with a combination of both arginine and glycine also have an enhanced rate of wound collagen deposition when compared to controls [67]. The effect of arginine on wound healing in rats is dependent on the presence of an intact hypothalamo-pituitary axis because hypophysectomized rats, whether or not treated with growth hormone, do not demonstrate any beneficial effects on wound healing when given arginine supplementation [68].

Two studies have been carried out in healthy human volunteers examining the effect of arginine supplementation on collagen accumulation. Young healthy human volunteers (25 to 35 years old) were found to have significantly increased wound collagen deposition following oral supplementation with either 30 g of arginine aspartate (17 g of free arginine) or 30 g of arginine HCl (24.8 g of free arginine) daily for 14 days (Figure 14-3) [69].

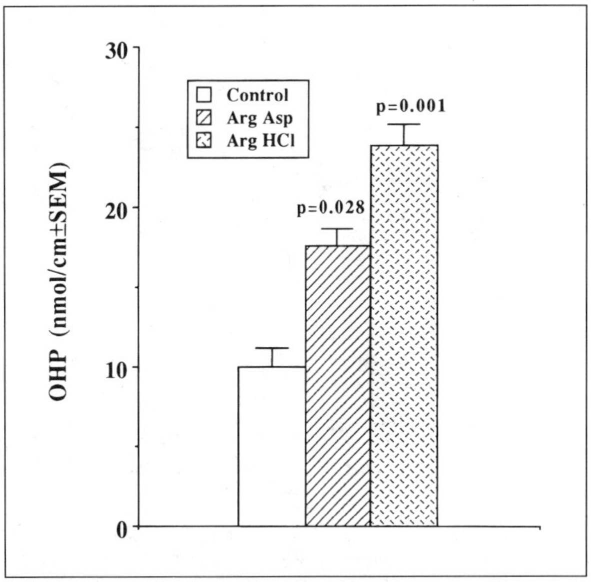

Figure 14-3. Effect of two weeks of arginine supplementation on hydroxyproline (OHP) accumulation in subcutaneously implanted polytetrafluoroethylene catheters in young human volunteers. Each group of 12 volunteers received a placebo syrup (control), 30 grams of arginine aspartate (Arg Asp), or 30 grams of arginine HCl (Arg HCl) for two weeks. (From A Barbul et al. Arginine enhances wound healing in humans. *Surgery* 108:331, 1990.)

In a subsequent study of healthy aged humans (67 to 82 years old), daily supplements of 30 g of arginine aspartate for 14 days resulted in significantly enhanced collagen and total protein deposition at the wound site when compared to placebo controls. There was no enhanced DNA present in the wounds of the arginine-supplemented subjects, suggesting that the effect of arginine is not mediated by an inflammatory mode of action (Figure 14-4) [59]. In this study, arginine supplementation had no effect on the rate of epithelialization of a superficial skin defect, further suggesting that the main effect of arginine on wound healing is to enhance wound collagen deposition.

Gains in breaking strength during the first weeks of healing are directly related to new collagen synthesis. An early progressive gain in tensile strength is an important factor in determining the competence of surgical incisions. Previous studies suggest that an increased deposition of collagen early in the wound healing process correlates with an increase in wound strength. Thus, arginine supplementation may result in an improvement in wound strength as a consequence of enhanced collagen deposition.

The T-cell-dependent immune system has been shown to play an important role in the regulation of wound healing. T-lymphocytes are necessary for the progression and orderly outcome of the normal wound healing process. Activated T-lymphocytes are capable of recruiting, expanding,

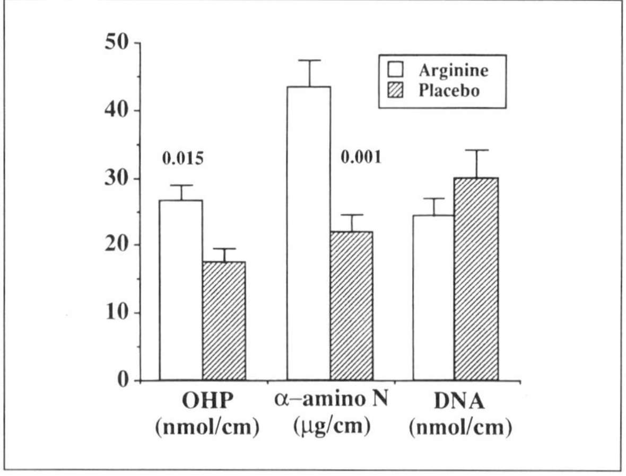

Figure 14-4. Effect of arginine on wound healing parameters in healthy elderly human volunteers. The hydroxyproline (OHP), total alpha-amino nitrogen (α-amino N), and DNA accumulation in subcutaneously implanted polytetrafluoroethylene catheters was measured at the end of two weeks. Controls (n = 15) received a placebo syrup, while the arginine group (n = 30) received 30 grams of arginine aspartate in double-blind fashion. (From SJ Kirk et al. Arginine stimulates wound healing and immune function in aged humans. *Surgery* 114: 155, 1993.)

and activating the fibroblasts that are primarily responsible for this repair process [70]. Perhaps the effect of arginine in enhancing T-cell function (*v.i.*) may also underlie its beneficial effect on wound collagen accumulation and/or maturation.

Arginine and Immune Function

Depressed immune responsiveness is a prominent feature of critical surgical illness, significant trauma, or burn injury. It has become apparent that less catastrophic traumatic insults, including elective moderate surgical operative procedures, also induce significant alterations in immune competence. Changes in the functional ability of the immune system have also been observed with the aging process. In particular, alterations in the T-cell population have been observed, with a decrease in overall numbers and a shift in the proportions of subpopulation toward a predominance of the Ts/c subset. These alterations in immune function are reflected in a decreased proliferative capacity in older animals and humans in response to a challenge with mitogenic and allogeneic target cells. There is evidence to suggest that the addition of post-traumatic immune suppression to the coexisting decrease in immunity contributes to morbidity and mortality in the elderly patient. In animals, thymic involution is one of the hallmarks of stress, injury, and aging. Because the thymus plays a critical role in T-cell-mediated immune responses, thymic involution likely represents a deleterious aspect of the general reaction to stress and injury.

Arginine given in large doses has numerous beneficial effects on the immune system, particularly on the thymus-dependent and T-cell-dependent immune reactions (Table 14-2). Additionally, arginine plays a key role in the metabolic intracellular activity of lymphocytes. In vitro, there is an absolute requirement for arginine in the normal growth of lymphocytes [71,72]. As in vivo, this requirement for arginine can be substituted by citrulline but not by ornithine. If the cultures are carried in arginine-free media, the mitogenic response of lymphocytes to PHA and Con A is reduced by 60% to 80%, while RNA and protein synthesis is diminished by approximately 25% [73,74]. Arginine is also required for the effective induction of cytotoxic T cell function in vitro [75]. All of these parameters of lymphocyte function are restored at a media concentration of 0.04 mM arginine; further increases in arginine concentration do not result in further enhancement of response.

Adult human plasma arginine concentration

Table 14-2. Immune Effects of Arginine

Action	Animals	Humans
↑ Mitogenic response of lymphocytes		
Health	yes	yes
Injury/stress	yes	yes
↑ Allograft rejection	yes	not done
↑ Number of T cells, mitogenic reactivity and DTH responses in immunocompromised host	yes[a]	yes[b]
↑ Anti-tumor cytotoxicity in vitro	yes	yes
↑ Anti-tumor responses in vivo	yes	not done
↑ Response to sepsis	yes	not done

[a]Athymic nude animals
[b]HIV-infected

ranges from 0.04 to 0.1 mM. Some of the in vitro arginine requirement for optimal lymphocyte proliferation relates to the induction of NO synthesis following mitogenic stimulation. This is supported by the fact that NO donors, such as S-nitrosoacetyl penicillamine or sodium nitroprusside, can totally replace the need for exogenous arginine for optimal lymphocyte DNA synthesis [72].

In animals, arginine supplementation leads to an increase in thymic weight and minimizes the thymic involution that normally occurs with injury [76]. Subsequently it was demonstrated that the gain in thymic weight is due to a significant increase in the number of lymphocytes present in the thymic glands. This increase in the number of thymic gland lymphocytes is accompanied by a significant enhancement of the lymphocyte blastogenic response to mitogens [77,78].

In healthy humans, arginine supplementation (15 to 30 g/day) stimulates peripheral blood mononuclear cell responses to the mitogens Con A, PHA, and PWM, and to allogeneic target cells [59,69,79]. An increase in the activity of these parameters is thought to correlate with enhanced T-cell function in vivo. This enhanced mitogenic response of peripheral blood mononuclear cells is noted both in healthy young and elderly human subjects supplemented with arginine. In aged humans and rodents, arginine restores plasma levels of thymulin, a thymic hormone, to values found in younger subjects [80], an effect that may underlie in part the enhanced T-cell function noted with arginine supplementation.

In injured animals, arginine is capable of abrogating the deleterious effects of trauma on T-cell responses as well as restoring thymic-mediated function earlier than in controls [58,66,76,77]. Following 30% total body surface area third-degree burn, guinea pigs supplemented with 1% to 2% arginine have enhanced immune responses, as assessed by increased delayed hypersensitivity responses to dinitrofluorobenzene or diminished abscess formation following *Staphylococcus aureus* inoculation [81]. In rats subjected to a lethal peritonitis model, survival rates were greatly increased by arginine administered either intragastrically or intravenously [82].

A reversal of the alteration in T-cell function associated with trauma or surgery has been demonstrated in patients fed enteral diets rich in arginine [61]. Patients undergoing major abdominal operations for gastrointestinal malignancies had increased in vitro immune responses that correlated with decreased wound infections and decreased length of hospital stay when supplemented with arginine [83]. In addition, moderately stressed ICU patients given an enteral diet containing large amounts of arginine demonstrated preservation or enhancement of T-lymphocyte blastogenesis [84]. In children with severe burn injuries, maintenance of normal plasma levels of arginine correlates with parameters of enhanced host immune and nutritional status [85]. Subsequently, the administration of an enteral diet supplemented with arginine was shown to result in reduced rates of wound infections and shortened hospital stay in a small group of young burn patients [86]. In a preliminary study, patients infected with HIV showed a significant enhancement of the mitogenic responses to Con A and PHA following a two-week dietary arginine supplementation (Table 14-3) [87].

The exact mechanism whereby arginine stimulates T-cell function is unknown (Figure 14-5). As mentioned above, thymic hormone secretion is enhanced by arginine. In athymic nude mice, arginine increases the number of T cells and enhances their response to mitogens in vitro, which

Table 14-3. Effect of Arginine Supplementation on Peripheral Blood Mononuclear Cell Responses to Mitogens in Different Patient Populations

	Concanavalin A		Phytohaemagglutinin	
Subjects	Pre-arginine	Post-arginine	Pre-arginine	Post-arginine
Healthy	58	217[a]	84	307[a]
Postoperative	45	88[a]	94	145[a]
Intensive care unit	—	+172%[b]	—	+68%[b]
HIV-infected	5	15[a]	28	75[a]

[a]Stimulation index
[b]Percentage change from baseline

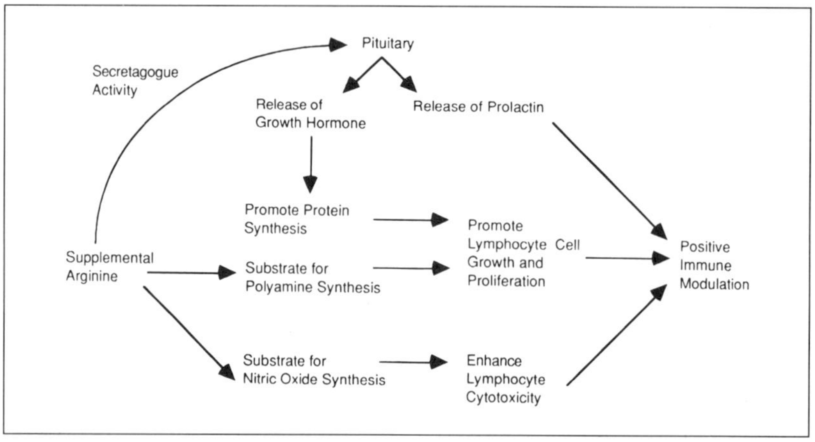

Figure 14-5. Postulated mechanisms of action for the immunomodulating effects of arginine.

results in the acquisition of delayed hypersensitivity responses in vivo [88]. This suggests that arginine can enhance T-cell maturation and differentiation at extrathymic sites independent of functioning thymus.

Ornithine also exhibits strong thymotrophic activity [89]. Because both arginine and ornithine are precursors for polyamine synthesis, which is required for heightened cellular proliferation, one could propose this as a possible mechanism of action. However, experimental data suggest that the thymotrophic effect of arginine and ornithine are not mediated directly via polyamine synthesis. Seifter has suggested that the thymic effects may be related to the pituitary secretagogue activity of the two basic amino acids [4]. Further supporting this hypothesis is the requirement for an intact hypothalamo-pituitary axis for arginine to exert its immune stimulatory function [90].

The arginine-induced release of prolactin and growth hormone is possibly most important in terms of its immunologic effects. Recent evidence indicates that prolactin has a direct effect on both cellular and humoral immunity. Lymphocytes have been shown to both produce and respond to prolactin, and part of the in vivo immune effect of arginine may be due to its ability to elevate serum prolactin levels [91]. Receptors for growth hormone are found on both monocytes and lymphocytes [92]. Growth hormone has been shown to potentiate the activity of lymphocytes, natural killer cells, and cytotoxic T-lymphocytes in vitro and to enhance lectin-induced T-cell proliferation and IL-2 synthesis in vivo [93,94]. All of the above actions of growth hormone can be replicated by arginine administration, strongly supporting the hypothesis that enhanced pituitary hormone secretion may underlie, at least in part, the mechanism of action of arginine on the immune system.

Arginine and Sepsis

Both enteral and parenteral administration of arginine were found to increase survival of mice and rats subjected to cecal ligation and puncture [95,96], but not in a guinea pig model of established peritonitis [97]. In addition, arginine improves histone and acute-phase protein synthesis during gram-negative sepsis in the rat [98]. Thus, the enhanced survival may be related to both an improved immune response as well as support of acute-phase responses.

Of concern, however, is that the intestinal absorption of arginine is significantly decreased during experimental sepsis and after resuscitation from experimental hemorrhagic shock [99,100]. Furthermore, the utilization of arginine may be decreased and its biosynthesis may be impaired during sepsis, as suggested by the significantly decreased plasma arginine levels in septic patients [101]. This implies that for optimal therapeutic effect of arginine during sepsis, the parenteral route may need to be employed, although further studies are required to clarify this recommendation.

Clinical Recommendations

As noted above, arginine possesses numerous pharmacologic actions that can have great potential benefit in clinical practice. Although the animal experimental data are compelling, continued clinical studies are necessary to better define the role of arginine in the care of patients. There is always the danger that because arginine is relatively safe, well tolerated, and with mild or no untoward effects being noted following administration of large doses, there may be indiscriminate application of arginine in a variety of conditions where it may be ineffectual at best or harmful at worst. The need to define its role and use for wound healing, states of diminished immune function, or as part of anticancer therapy is critical. Even issues such as minimal effective dosage in human clinical practice have not been fully defined. This plea for careful studies is not meant to hinder the application of arginine in the clinic, but it is meant as a call for judicious and scientific usage. Such application should result in arginine playing an important role in the nutritional and pharmacologic management of patients.

References

1. Rose WC. The nutritive significance of the amino acids and certain related compounds. *Science* 86:298, 1937.
2. Rose WC. Amino acid requirements of man. *Fed Proc* 8:546, 1949.
3. Nakagawa I, et al. Amino acid requirements of children: Minimal needs of tryptophan, arginine, histidine based on nitrogen balance method. *J Nutr* 80:305, 1963.
4. Seifter E, et al. Arginine: An essential amino acid for injured rats. *Surgery* 84:224, 1978.
5. Barbul A. Arginine: Biochemistry, physiology and therapeutic implications. *JPEN* 10:227, 1986.
6. Fahey JL. Toxicity and blood ammonia rise resulting from intravenous amino acid administration in man: The protective effect of L-arginine. *J Clin Invest* 36:1647, 1957.
7. Moncada S, Higgs EA (eds). *Nitric Oxide From Arginine: A Bioregulatory System.* New York: Elsevier, 1990.
8. Moncada S, Palmer RM, Higgs EA. Nitric oxide: Physiology, pathophysiology, and pharmacology. *Pharmacol Rev* 43:109, 1991.
9. Miller V, Vanhoutte P. Endothelium-dependant relaxation in isolated blood vessels of lower vertebrates. *Blood Vessels* 23:411, 1986.
10. Sung YJ, et al. L-arginine-dependent production of a reactive nitrogen intermediate by macrophages of a uricotelic species. *J Leukocyte Biol* 50:49, 1991.
11. Radomski MM, Martin JF, Moncada S. Synthesis of nitric oxide by the haemocytes of the American horseshoe crab (Limulus polyphemus). *Philos Trans R Soc Lond [Biol]* 334:129, 1991.
12. Mayer B, et al. Brain nitric oxide synthase is a biopterin- and flavin-containing multi-functional oxido-reductase. *FEBS Lett* 288:187, 1991.
13. Stuehr D, et al. Purification and characterization of the cytokine-induced macrophage nitric oxide synthase: An FAD- and FMN- containing flavoprotein. *Proc Natl Acad Sci USA* 88:7773, 1991.
14. Hevel JM, White KA, Marletta MA. Purification of the inducible murine macrophage nitric oxide synthase. *J Biol Chem* 266:22789, 1991.
15. Stuehr DJ, et al. Inhibition of macrophage and endothelial cell nitric oxide synthase by diphenyleneiodonium and its analogs. *FASEB J* 5:98, 1991.
16. Bredt DS, Snyder SH. Isolation of nitric oxide synthetase, a calmodulin-requiring enzyme. *Proc Natl Acad Sci USA* 87:682, 1990.
17. Knowles RG, et al. Formation of nitric oxide from L-arginine in the central nervous system: A transduction mechanism for stimulation of the soluble guanylate cyclase. *Proc Natl Acad Sci USA* 86:5159, 1989.
18. Förstermann U, et al. Enzymes synthesizing guanylate cyclase-activating factors in endothelial cell, neuroblastoma cells, and rat brain. *J Cardiovasc Pharmacol* 17:S57, 1991.
19. Mayer B, Böhme E. Ca^{2+}-dependent formation of an L-arginine-derived activator of soluble guanylate cyclase in bovine lung. *FEBS Lett* 256:211, 1989.
20. Venturini CM, et al. Synthesis of nitric oxide in the bovine retina. *Biochem Biophys Res Comm* 180:920, 1991.
21. Palacios M, et al. Nitric oxide from L-arginine stimulates the soluble guanylate cyclase in adrenal glands. *Biochem Biophys Res Comm* 165:802, 1989.
22. Radomski MW, Palmer RM, Moncada S. An L-arginine/nitric oxide pathway present in human platelets regulates aggregation. *Proc Natl Acad Sci USA* 87:5193, 1990.
23. Palmer RM, Moncada S. A novel citrulline-forming enzyme implicated in the formation of nitric oxide by vascular endothelial cells. *Biochem Biophys Res Comm* 159:348, 1989.
24. Mülsch A, Bassenge E, Busse R. Nitric oxide synthesis in endothelial cytosol: Evidence for a calcium-dependent and a calcium-independent mechanism. *Naunyn Schmiedebergs Arch Pharmacol* 340:767, 1989.
25. Salter M, Knowles RG, Moncada S. Widespread tissue distribution, species distribution and changes in activity of Ca^{2+}-dependant and Ca^{2+}-independant nitric oxide synthases. *FEBS Lett* 291:145, 1991.
26. Lyons CR, Orloff GJ, Cunningham JM. Molecular cloning and functional expression of an inducible nitric oxide synthase from a murine macrophage cell line. *Proc Natl Acad Sci USA* 267:6370, 1992.
27. Xie Q, et al. Cloning and characterization of inducible nitric oxide synthase from mouse macrophages. *Science* 256:225, 1992.
28. Yui Y, et al. Purification of nitric oxide synthase from rat macrophages. *J Biol Chem* 266:12544, 1991.

29. Stuehr DJ, Marletta MA. Induction of nitrite/nitrate synthesis in murine macrophages by BCG infection, lymphokines, or interferon-γ. *J Immunol* 140:518, 1987.

30. Hibbs JB, Taintor RR, Vavrin Z. Macrophage cytotoxicity: Role for L-arginine deaminase and imino nitrogen oxidation to nitrite. *Science* 235:473, 1987.

31. Marletta MA, et al. Macrophage oxidation of L-arginine to nitrite and nitrate: Nitric oxide is an intermediate. *Biochemistry* 27:8706, 1988.

32. Billiar TR, et al. An L-arginine-dependent mechanism mediates Kupffer-cell inhibition of hepatocyte protein synthesis in vitro. *J Exp Med* 169:1467, 1989.

33. Curran RD, et al. Hepatocytes produce nitrogen oxides from L-arginine in response to inflammatory products of Kupffer cells. *J Exp Med* 170:1769, 1989.

34. Knowles RG, et al. Differential induction of brain, lung and liver nitric oxide synthase by endotoxin in the rat. *Biochem J* 270:833, 1990.

35. McCall TB, et al. Synthesis of nitric oxide from L-arginine by neutrophils: Release and interaction with superoxide anion. *Biochem J* 261:293, 1989.

36. Werner FG, et al. Tetrahydrobiopterin-dependent formation of nitrite and nitrate in murine fibroblasts. *J Exp Med* 172:1599, 1990.

37. Stadler J, et al. Articular chondrocytes synthesize nitric oxide in response to cytokines and lipopolysaccharide. *J Immunol* 147:3915, 1991.

38. Busse R, Mülsch A. Induction of nitric oxide synthase by cytokines in vascular smooth muscle cells. *FEBS Lett* 275:87, 1990.

39. Stuehr DJ, Kwon NS, Nathan CF. FAD and GSH participate in macrophage synthesis of nitric oxide. *Biochem Biophys Res Comm* 168:558, 1990.

40. DiRosa M, et al. Glucocorticoids inhibit the induction of nitric oxide synthase in macrophages. *Biochem Biophys Res Comm* 172:1246, 1990.

41. Radomski MW, Palmer RM, Moncada S. Glucocorticoids inhibit the expression of an inducible, but not the constitutive, nitric oxide synthase in vascular endothelial cells. *Proc Natl Acad Sci USA* 87:10043, 1990.

42. Knowles RG, et al. Anti-inflammatory glucocorticoids inhibit the induction by endotoxin of nitric oxide synthase in the lung and aorta of the rat. *Biochem Biophys Res Comm* 172:1042, 1990.

43. Förstermann U, et al. Induced RAW 264.7 macrophages express soluble and particulate nitric oxide synthase: Inhibition by transforming growth factor-β. *Eur J Pharmacol* 225:161, 1992.

44. Nathan C. Nitric oxide as a secretory product of mammalian cells. *FASEB J* 6:3051, 1992.

45. Albina JE, et al. Arginine metabolism in wounds. *Am J Physiol* 254:E459, 1988.

46. Drexler H, et al. Correction of endothelial dysfunction in coronary microcirculation of hypercholesterolemic patients by L-arginine. *Lancet* 338:1546, 1991.

47. Floyd JCJ, et al. Stimulation of insulin secretion by amino acids. *J Clin Invest* 45:1487, 1966.

48. Sener A, et al. Stimulus-secretion coupling of arginine-induced insulin release: Comparison with histidine-induced insuline release. *Endocrinology* 127:107, 1989.

49. Laychock SG, Modica ME, Cavanaugh CT. L-arginine stimulates cyclic guanosine 3′,5′-monophosphate formation in rat islets of Langerhans and RINm5F insulinoma cells: Evidence for L-arginine:nitric oxide synthase. *Endocrinology* 129:3043, 1991.

50. Schmidt HHHW, et al. Insulin secretion from pancreatic B cells caused by L-arginine-derived nitrogen oxides. *Science* 255:721, 1992.

51. Welsh N, et al. Interleukin 1β-induced nitric oxide production in isolated rat pancreatic islets requires gene transcription and may lead to inhibition of the Krebs cycle enzyme aconitase. *Endocrinology* 129:3167, 1991.

52. Lukic ML, et al. Inhibition of nitric oxide generation affects the induction of diabetes by streptozocin in mice. *Biochem Biophys Res Comm* 178:913, 1991.

53. Imms FJ, London DR, Neame RLB. The secretion of catecholamines from the adrenal gland following arginine infusion in the rat. *J Physiol (Lond)* 200:55, 1969.

54. Dohi T, Morita K, Tsujimoto A. Effect of sodium azide on catecholamine release from isolated adrenal gland and on guanilate cyclase. *Eur J Pharmacol* 94:331, 1983.

55. O'Sullivan AJ, Burgoyne RD. Cyclic GMP regulates nicotine-induced secretion from cultured bovine adrenal chromaffin cells: Effects of 8-bromo-cyclic GMP, atrial natriuretic peptide, and nitroprusside (nitric oxide). *J Neurochem* 54:1805, 1990.

56. Halbrügge T, et al. Role of nitric oxide formation in the regulation of haemodynamics and the release of noradrenaline and adrenaline. *Naunyn Schmeidebergs Arch Pharmacol* 344:720, 1991.

57. Steffe CH, et al. Studies in amino acid utilization: V. The determination of minimum dietary essential amino acid requirements in protein depleted adult male albino rats. *J Nutr* 40:483, 1950.

58. Barbul A, et al. Metabolic and immune effects of arginine in post-injury hyperalimentation. *J Trauma* 21:970, 1981.

59. Kirk SJ, et al. Arginine stimulates wound healing and immune function in aged humans. *Surgery* 114:155, 1994.

60. Elsair J, et al. Effect of arginine chlorhydrate on nitrogen balance during the three days following routine surgery in man. *Biomedicine* 29:312, 1978.

61. Daly J, et al. Immune and metabolic effects of arginine in the surgical patient. *Ann Surg* 208:512, 1988.

62. Leander U, et al. Nitrogen sparing effect of ornicetil in the immediate postoperative state: Clinical biochemistry and nitrogen balance. *Clin Nutr* 4:43, 1985.

63. Wernerman J, et al. Ornithine-alpha-ketoglutarate improves skeletal muscle protein synthesis as assessed by ribosome analysis and nitrogen use after surgery. *Ann Surg* 206:674, 1987.

64. Levenson SM, et al. Citrulline replaces arginine as a dietary essential in rats; ornithine does not. *Fed Proc* 726:2421, 1980.

65. Bucknall T. Factors Affecting Wound Healing. In T Bucknall, H Ellis (eds), *Wound Healing for Surgeons.* London: Bailliere Tindall, 1984. P 42.

66. Barbul A, et al. Intravenous hyperalimentation with high arginine levels improves wound healing and immune function. *J Surg Res* 38:328, 1985.

67. Chyun J, Griminger P. Improvement of nitrogen retention by arginine and glycine supplementation and its relation to collagen synthesis. *J Nutr* 114:1697, 1984.

68. Barbul A, et al. Wound healing and thymotropic effects of arginine: A pituitary mechanism of action. *Am J Clin Nutr* 37:786, 1983.

69. Barbul A, et al. Arginine enhances wound healing in humans. *Surgery* 108:331, 1990.

70. Regan MC, Barbul A. Regulation of Wound Healing by the T Cell-Dependent Immune System. In H Janssen, R Rooman, JIS Robertson (eds), *Wound Healing.* Petersfield, UK: Wrightson Biomedical, 1991. P 21.

71. Eagle H. Amino acid metabolism in mammalian cell cultures. *Science* 130:432, 1959.

72. Efron D, et al. Nitric oxide generation from L-arginine is required for optimal peripheral blood lymphocyte DNA synthesis. *Surgery* 110:327, 1991.

73. Chisari FV, et al. Production of two distinct and independent hepatic immunoregulatory molecules by the perfused rat liver. *Hepatology* 5:735, 1985.

74. Her-Lin S, et al. The mechanism of inhibitory effects of liver extract on lymphocyte proliferation: II. Inhibition of DNA, RNA, and protein synthesis and their relationship to the effects of metabolic inhibitors. *Clin Exp Immunol* 72:228, 1988.

75. Moriguchi A, et al. Functional changes in human lymphocytes and monocytes after in vitro incubation with arginine. *Nutr Res* 7:719, 1987.

76. Barbul A, et al. Arginine: A thymotropic and wound healing promoting agent. *Surg Forum* 28:101, 1977.

77. Barbul A, et al. Immunostimulatory effects of arginine in normal and injured rats. *J Surg Res* 29:228, 1980.

78. Barbul A, et al. Thymic and immune stimulatory actions of arginine. *JPEN* 4:446, 1980.

79. Barbul A, et al. Arginine stimulates lymphocyte immune responses in healthy humans. *Surgery* 90:244, 1981.

80. Fabris N, Mocchegiani E. Arginine-containing compounds and thymic endocrine activity. *Thymus* 19:S21, 1992.

81. Saito H, et al. Metabolic and immune effects of dietary arginine supplementation after burn. *Arch Surg* 122:784, 1987.

82. Madden HP, et al. Stimulation of T cell immunity enhances survival in peritonitis. *J Surg Res* 44:658, 1988.

83. Daly JM, et al. Enteral nutrition with arginine, RNA, and omega-3 fatty acids in patients after operation: Immunologic, metabolic, and clinical outcome. *Surgery* 112:56, 1992.

84. Cerra FB, et al. Effect of enteral nutrient on in vitro tests of immune function in ICU patients: A preliminary report. *Nutrition* 6:84, 1990.

85. Alexander JW, et al. Beneficial effects of aggressive protein feeding in severely burned children. *Ann Surg* 192:505, 1980.

86. Alexander JW, Gottschlich M. Nutritional immunomodulation in burn patients. *Crit Care Med* 18:S149, 1990.

87. Barbul A. Arginine and immune function. *Nutrition* 6:S51, 1990.

88. Kirk SJ, et al. Arginine enhances T cell responses in athymic nude mice. *JPEN* 16:429, 1992.

89. Barbul A, et al. Thymotropic actions of arginine, ornithine and growth hormone [Abstract]. *Fed Proc* 37:264, 1978.

90. Barbul A, et al. Supplemental arginine, wound healing and thymus: Arginine-pituitary interaction. *Surg Forum* 29:93, 1978.

91. Kirk SJ, et al. Inhibition of prolactin secretion reduces the T cell immunostimulatory effects of arginine. *Surg Forum* 42:3, 1991.

92. Kiess W, Butenandt O. Specific growth hormone receptors on human peripheral mononuclear cells: Re-expression, identification, and characterization. *J Clin Endocrinol Metab* 60:740, 1985.

93. Davila DR, et al. Role of growth hormone in regulating T-dependant immune events in aged, nude, and transgenic rodents. *J Neurosci Res* 18:108, 1987.

94. Snow EC, Feldbush TL, Oakes JA. The effects of growth hormone and insulin upon MLC responses and the generation of cytotoxic lymphocytes. *J Immunol* 126:161, 1981.

95. Madden HP, et al. Stimulation of T cell immunity by arginine enhances survival in peritonitis. *J Surg Res* 44:658, 1988.

96. Gianotti L, et al. Arginine-supplemented diets improve survival in gut-derived sepsis and peritonitis by modulating bacterial clearance. *Ann Surg* 217:644, 1993.

97. Gonce SJ, et al. Arginine supplementation and its effect on established peritonitis in guinea pigs. *JPEN* 14:237, 1990.

98. Léon P, et al. Arginine supplementation improves histone and acute-phase protein synthesis during gram-negative sepsis in the rat. *JPEN* 15:503, 1991.

99. Gardiner KR, Barbul A. Intestinal amino acid absorption during sepsis. *JPEN* 17:277, 1993.

100. Sodeyama M, et al. The effect of hemorrhagic shock on intestinal amino acid absorption in vivo. *Circ Shock* 38:153, 1992.

101. Freund HR, et al. Plasma amino acids as predictors of the severity and outcome of sepsis. *Ann Surg* 190:571, 1979.

Selected Readings

Barbul A. Arginine: Biochemistry, physiology and therapeutic implications. *JPEN* 10:227, 1986.

A complete and still up-to-date review of the use of supplemental arginine in a variety of experimental and clinical settings.

Daly J, et al. Immune and metabolic effects of arginine in the surgical patient. *Ann Surg* 208:512, 1988.

First study to demonstrate the benefit of supplemental enteral arginine in postoperative surgical patients. Thirty patients undergoing total cystectomy and immediate postoperative enteral feeding were randomized to receive either supplemental arginine (25 g/day) or glycine (43 g/day). The arginine-supplemented group achieved positive nitrogen balance, had increased CD4+ counts, and demonstrated enhanced peripheral lymphocyte mitogenesis.

Efron D, et al. Nitric oxide generation from L-arginine is required for optimal peripheral blood lymphocyte DNA synthesis. *Surgery* 110:327, 1991.

This study offers a possible mechanism for the need of arginine for optimal lymphocyte function and suggests a pathway by which arginine may improve immune function. Nitric oxide synthesis in a variety of immune-mediated reactions is a new and exciting topic.

Gardiner KR, Barbul A. Intestinal amino acid absorption during sepsis. *JPEN* 17:277, 1993.

A review of the intestinal absorption of amino acids, including arginine, during sepsis. The decrease in absorption has implications for the administration of amino acids during clinical sepsis.

Kirk SJ, et al. Arginine stimulates wound healing and immune function in aged humans. *Surgery* 114:155, 1993.

A randomized double-blind study that demonstrates that supplemental arginine stimulates wound collagen accumulation and peripheral blood lymphocyte mitogenesis.

15

Nutrition in Wound Healing

Thomas K. Hunt
Harriet Williams Hopf

Surgeons have noted for centuries that surgery and sepsis produce malnutrition and that once it exists, recovery—that is, healing—is seriously prolonged. The first insight into healing was nutritional: Lind's 1753 discovery that citrus fruit juices cure scurvy. Yet, disagreements still exist on the role of nutrition in prevention of serious complications. Surgery and trauma induce a catabolic state that may lead rapidly to protein-calorie malnutrition, as well as vitamin and mineral deficiencies. Up to 50% of hospitalized patients may have significant preexisting protein or protein-calorie malnutrition, which is associated with increased morbidity and mortality and which is exacerbated by the catabolic effects of injury. Both protein-calorie malnutrition and cofactor deficiency impair host defenses against infection and wound repair. The mechanisms by which malnutrition impairs vital cell functions are well delineated in some instances, as with vitamin C deficiency. Although malnutrition impairs healing, excess repletion does not appear to enhance healing or other outcomes and may, in fact, be detrimental [1–7].

This chapter will review: (1) normal wound healing; (2) the effects of protein-calorie malnutrition on wound repair; (3) the role of vitamins and minerals in normal wound repair and the effects of specific deficits; and (4) evidence that nutritional repletion improves wound healing and other outcomes.

Mechanisms of Wound Repair

The healing process results from disruption of the normal extracellular environment by interruption of local blood perfusion, which in turn elicits coagulation and inflammatory cell recruitment. Eventually, inflammatory cells and their products elicit angiogenesis and a new extracellular matrix of collagen and proteoglycans [8]. This process normally ceases when the extracellular environment is restored. Mechanisms of repair and resistance to infection are complex and depend first on circulatory factors and then on nutrition. Healing proceeds through a series of mechanisms that are often redundant (Figure 15-1).

Coagulation and Homeostasis

Disruption of tissue and cells leads to complement release, which attracts polymorphonuclear leukocytes to the site of injury. The main purpose of these cells is to defend against infection. The coagulation cascade in response to endothelial cell injury and platelet degranulation leads to release of further chemoattractants and other factors [9]. Thrombin (itself a mitogen and angiogenic stimulus) causes platelets to release platelet-derived growth factor (PDGF), platelet factor IV, transforming growth factor beta (TGF-β), and insulin-like growth factor 1 (IGF-1). All stimulate fibroblast replication. Fibrin deposition is followed by fibrinolysis and release of chemoattractive peptides, particularly fibrinopeptide E, which attract monocytes, and fibrinopeptide B, which is angiogenic. Residual fibrin activates monocytes to release cytokines. Macrophages also release most of the growth factors found in platelets. Plasmin digests fibrin and basement membranes of vessels. This and other proteolytic events contribute to angiogenesis.

Coagulation, while it is necessary to prevent exsanguination and initiates the cascade that leads to healing, also presents a problem. When bleeding of cut vessels is ended by thrombosis, the local microvasculature becomes occluded. Thus the delivery of nutrients, including most notably oxygen, is impaired or lost. Bruising or crushing trauma, in particular, injures the vascular supply and produces large volumes of ischemic tissue that is, as a result, at high risk of poor healing.

Inflammation

After an early predominance of granulocytes, by 48 hours after injury macrophages dominate the cellular response. Granulocytes are more im-

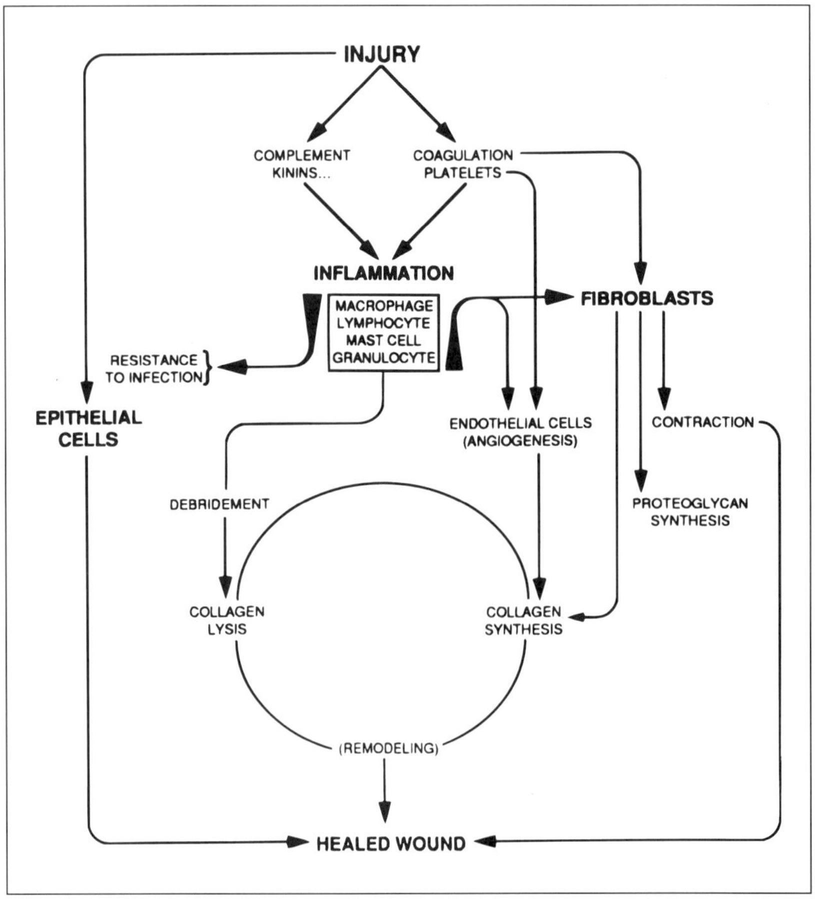

Figure 15-1. Wound healing represents a complex interaction of cellular processes that is initiated by injury. Cellular signals are imperative for the control of inflammation, angiogenesis, and collagen production. (From DD Zabel, TK Hunt. Skin, peritoneum and colonic healing processes. *Perspect Colon Rectal Surg* 6:191, 1993. Reprinted with permission.)

portant to antibacterial defense than to repair. Repair, however, is severely impeded by the absence of macrophages. Stimulated macrophages stimulate replication and movement of both fibroblasts and vascular endothelial cells. When macrophagic inflammation is prevented by large doses of anti-inflammatory steroids or by malnutrition, repair is inhibited.

Macrophages, with some help from lymphocytes, release a number of "growth factors" when stimulated by injured tissue, fibrin, foreign bodies, and especially by the low oxygen and high lactate concentrations found in wounds [10]. The exact details are unknown, but TGF-β, IL-1, IL-6, IL-8, TNF-α, IGF-1, and LDGF (a gene family of FGF-like molecules) have been traced to macrophages. With the addition of these substances, and probably others like them, the local environment begins to encourage cell growth as well as to attract inflammatory cells, new fibroblasts, and endothelial cells into the conditioned area. Many of the growth factors are also chemoattractants. Some of them, TNF-α and IL-1, for example, also serve as messengers to the liver and other distant tissues to produce the so-called acute-phase response. [*Editor's Note:* As time goes on, more cytokines are being implicated in the acute-phase response. At present, IL-6 seems particularly important, at least for acute-phase protein synthesis.]

Granulocytes and macrophages are activated or "primed" on entering the wound space. Among the many consequences of this is the oxidative burst, which is the rapid conversion of molecular (dissolved) oxygen to superoxide. This conversion is the starting point for the production of a series of oxygen radicals, which are central to oxidative bacterial killing. The overall reaction is:

$$\text{glucose} + O_2 \rightarrow O_2^- + \text{lactate} + H^+$$

This is a central event in healing and performs two important functions: (1) superoxide is essential to intraleukocytic killing of bacteria; (2) lactate stimulates collagen synthesis and angiogenesis (see below). One side effect is that the oxidative burst increases oxygen consumption, thus decreasing oxygen available in the wound, which may limit new matrix formation and ultimately bacterial killing capacity.

Macrophages and granulocytes also release proteolysins, including several collagenases. Ordinarily, these serve useful functions: debridement of denatured tissue, remodeling of the new scar tissue so that it can acquire strength without undue mass, and assistance of angiogenesis. On the other hand, if proteolysis becomes excessive, as it does in chronic wounds and during sepsis, an enormous amount of lysis will eventually require an equally large amount of rebuilding with huge nutritional consequences.

Fibroplasia

After a few days, under the intense stimulation of the wound environment, fibroblasts migrate in, multiply, and begin to synthesize and deposit collagen and proteoglycans. Fibroblasts originate locally, and replication rates are proportional to oxygen availability.

Neovascularization

Wound healing is critically dependent on angiogenesis to replace the damaged vascular supply. New vessels start as blind-ended endothelial cell buds from venules and accompany the macrophages and fibroblasts. The original capillaries seem to coalesce, and some vessels become as large as 3 to 5 mm in diameter in the final scar. Clearly, new vessels, like collagen, also "turn over."

Neovascularization occurs along the steep oxygen gradient that characterizes wounds. The major angiogenic stimulus in wounds is derived from macrophages, which produce a chemoattractant, angiogenic polypeptide, when placed in a hyperlactated or hypoxic environment.

The Wound Module

By the end of the third or fourth day, full-thickness wounds have a characteristic cellular architecture. Macrophages surround the wound space. Beneath is a layer of immature fibroblasts. Under these is a layer of replicating fibroblasts, which lie just on the injury side of the most distal functioning vessel and accompany the proliferating endothelial buds. Mature fibroblasts and the earliest visible traces of scar collagen lie just behind. This module advances into the wound space, drawn by products of activated macrophages, and supports its new vessels with new collagen matrix (Figure 15-2).

Dead spaces heal until filled. This happens for several reasons: (1) immature vessels leak fibrin, which releases angiogenic peptides and activates macrophages to produce growth and chemoattractant factors; and (2) growth of vessels follows the oxygen and lactate gradients (above). The high lactate, 10 to 15 mmol, also stimulates macrophages to produce endothelial chemoattractant factor(s). Fibrin, lactate, and/or hypoxia elicit TNF-α, TGF-1, IL-8, and IL-1 from macrophages, which in turn make more lactate in response to EGF, IGF-1, and possibly other factors. Healing continues until the new vessels unite with others, establish mature circulatory loops, stop leaking fibrin, and decrease the lactate gradient. As circu-

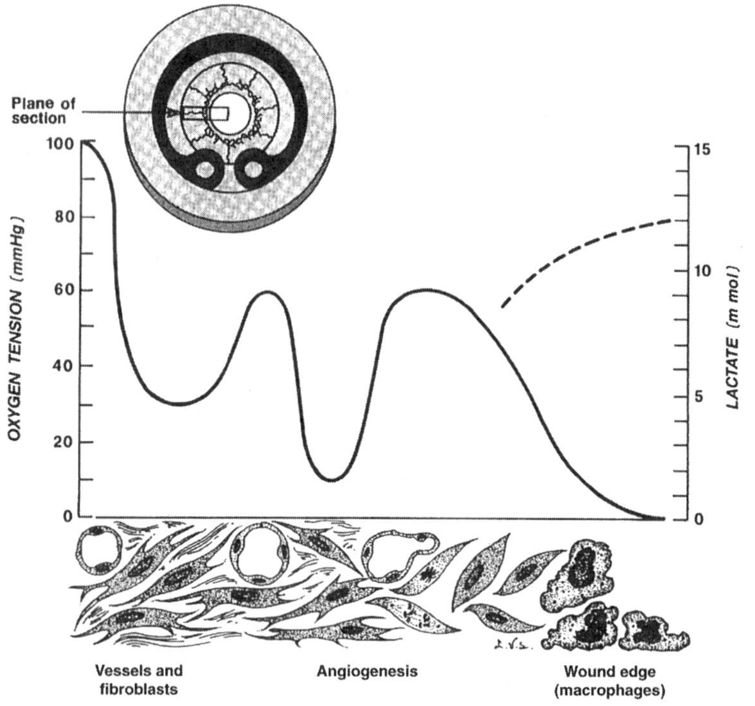

Figure 15-2. The wound module. Cross section of the wound module in a rabbit ear chamber (diagram of chamber is in left upper corner of diagram). Note that PO_2, depicted graphically above the cross section, is highest next to the vessels, with a gradient down to near zero at the wound edge. Note also the lactate gradient, high in the dead space and lower (but still above plasma) toward the vasculature. (From IA Silver. The physiology of wound healing, in TK Hunt, JE Dunphy [eds], *Fundamentals of Wound Management.* New York: Appleton-Century-Crofts, 1980, p. 30. Reprinted with permission.)

lations unite, the oxygen and lactate gradients are obliterated. If foreign bodies, antigen-antibody complexes, infection, and/or other processes continue to elicit inflammation, the gradients will not disappear and healing will continue, perhaps to excessive scarring.

Collagen Synthesis

Collagen is the mechanical mainstay of repair in humans (Table 15-1). Collagen polymers, or fibers, are composed of long, thin monomers in the form of triple helices, approximately 289 × 1.4 nm in

Table 15-1. Types of Vertebrate Collagen

Type	Locus of Human Gene (Chromosome)	Composition	Distribution	Function
I	17 7	$[\alpha 1(I)]_2\alpha 2(I)$	Skin, tendon, bones, cornea; the most prevalent collagen	Formation of striated fibers of varying diameter
II	12	$[\alpha 1(II)]_3$	Hyaline cartilages, vitreous humor, intervertebral disc	Formation of striated fibrils of generally smaller diameter than type I fibers
III	2	$[\alpha 1(III)]_3$	Fetal skin, cardiovascular system	Formation of small fibrous elements, similar to type II, but may also form cofibers with type I collagen molecules
IV	13	$[\alpha 1(IV)]_2\alpha 2(IV)$	Basement membranes	Formation of meshlike scaffold
V–XIII	2,6,12,21	Minor collagens	Essentially all tissues	Largely unknown, form coaggregates with major collagens

dimension, that "glue" the sides of the wound together (Figure 15-3).

Assembly of the collagen monomer begins with synthesis of three alpha chains that are long sequences of trimers with the basic structures of glycine-X-R in which X is often proline, hydroxyproline, lysine, or hydroxylysine. The gene, however, does not code for hydroxylysine or hydroxyproline. Some of its prolines and lysines are hydroxylated as each growing alpha chain comes off the polyribosome and is inserted into the endoplasmic reticulum. These clinically significant reactions are catalyzed by prolyl and lysyl hydroxylase and require molecular oxygen, ferrous iron, ascorbic acid, and α-ketoglutarate [11]. If a minimal number of prolines are not hydroxylated, the alpha chains cannot form the thermostable triple helix that characterizes the collagen monomer and therefore cannot be exported from the cell. The defective collagen is hydrolyzed and the amino acids recycled. Current information, noting the importance of the characteristic hypoxia found in wounds, suggests that a considerable amount of collagen is turned over in this manner. Without hydroxylysines, a later step in which the monomers cross-bind and provide strength to the final fiber cannot occur. The amount of oxygen that is available for these hydroxylations controls the rate at which collagen is deposited into the extracellular space and the rate at which wounds can support new vessels and gain strength.

The major stimulus for collagen formation is closely related to the low oxidation-reduction potential in the healing area. This low potential is due largely to the high concentration of lactate, which is contributed by leukocytes and macrophages during aerobic glycolysis. Lactate stimulates the formation of collagen-synthesizing enzymes and collagen synthesis in aerobic fibroblast cultures. The mechanism is complex and depends on the rate at which nicotinamide can be removed from NAD^+ (*not* NADH) to form adenosine diphosphoribose (ADPR). Various forms of ADPR normally suppress collagen gene expression and post-translational hydroxylations. However, when lactate accumulates, the NAD^+ pool shrinks, the inhibitory ADPR is removed, collagen mRNA production rises, and synthesis ensues. Thereafter, the critical hydroxylations (similarly controlled by ADPR) that control export and depend on oxygen occur (Figure 15-4). In this reducing environment, ascorbate (vitamin C) exists as dihydroascorbate, its reduced form. Ascorbate is an essential cofactor (oxygen radical) for hydroxylation.

This at first appears paradoxical. The mechanism for collagen synthesis and deposition relies on a low NAD^+, i.e., a low oxyredox potential. However, collagen deposition is critically dependent on PO_2 in the cell. The paradox is resolved by the fact that the low NAD^+ is a direct consequence of the lactate released (aerobically) by leukocytes. When PaO_2 is elevated, wound PO_2 rises slightly, but little effect on lactate is seen in the wound space. A larger effect on PO_2 is seen in the zone of collagen synthesis, and consumption rises there when PO_2 rises. For this reason, elevating PaO_2 can raise collagen deposition without materially changing the oxyredox state.

Collagen synthesis requires structural amino acids, glucose to meet the energy needs of protein synthesis, iron and ascorbate (to transfer oxygen

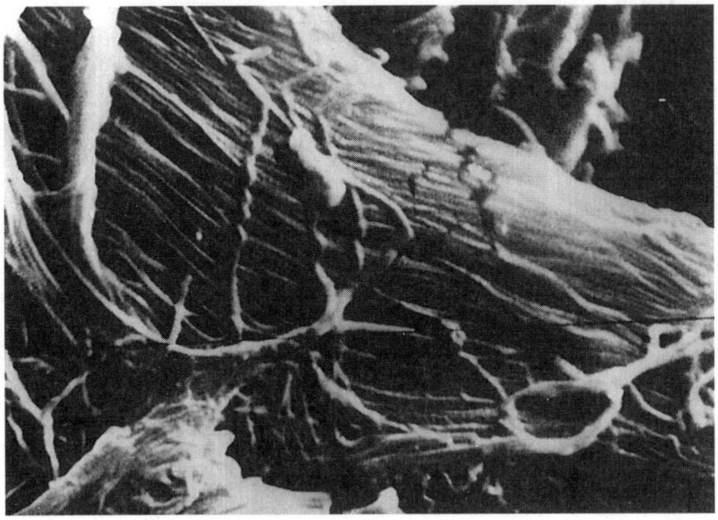

Figure 15-3. Scanning electron micrograph of the cut edge of a normal collagen fiber showing that it is made up of bundles of cross-banded fibrils (13,000X). (From JC Forrester, et al. Scanning electron microscopy of healing wounds. *Nature* 221:373, 1969. Reproduced by permission from Nature, © 1969, Macmillan Magazines Limited.)

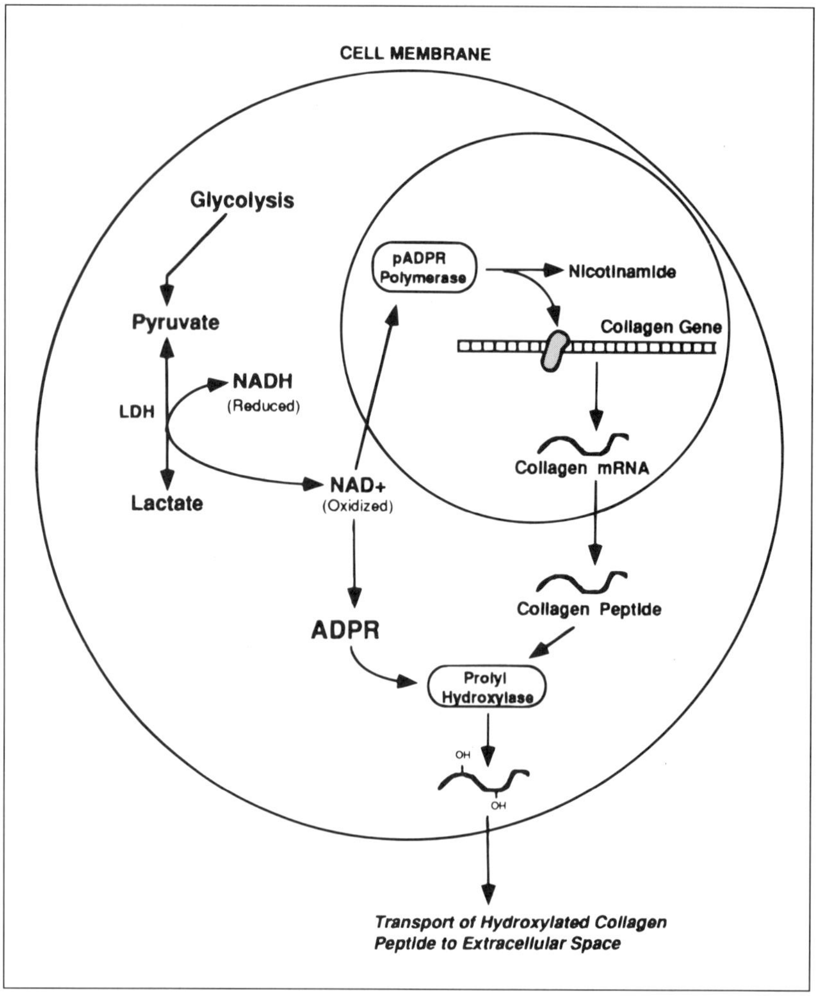

Figure 15-4. Schematic diagram of metabolic control of collagen synthesis. Elevated wound lactate reduces NAD^+ by lactate dehydrogenase (LDH). Thus, the synthesis of nuclear poly-ADPR (pADPR) and cytoplasmic ADPR is substantially decreased. This in turn releases the repression of collagen genes and inhibition of prolyl hydroxylase. As a result, both collagen transcription and prolyl hydroxylase are activated causing an enhanced production of extracellular hydroxylated collagen, provided that vitamin C and oxygen are present as substrate for prolyl hydroxylase. Some evidence implicates a negative action of certain growth factors and poly-ADPR production. (From DD Zabel, TK Hunt. Skin, peritoneum and colonic healing processes. *Perspect Colon Rectal Surg* 6:191, 1993. Reprinted with permission.)

for proline and lysine hydroxylation), oxygen, sulfated amino acids, arginine, lysine, vitamin A, and probably other vitamins, if only for energy metabolism. The remarkable point about this mechanism is the number of factors that are required for synthesis but that do not appear in the final product.

Growth factors, particularly IGF-1 and TGF-β, also stimulate collagen synthesis and deposition. Mechanisms are unknown except that some evidence unites this observation with the ADPR system, namely that IGF-1 inhibits ADPR synthetase.

Collagen Lysis

Collagen turns over rapidly in wounds because of two types of enzymes: (1) collagenases, which are normally released by inflammatory cells and fibroblasts in catabolic situations such as starvation, stress, and inflammation; and (2) lysosomal enzymes, which leak from leukocytes. The plasmin/plasminogen system may also contribute.

Collagen synthesis consumes energy and nutrients and depends heavily on vascular resources. Collagen lysis, on the other hand, uses little, if any, energy in the wound and does not depend on blood supply. Wound edge fusion depends on net collagen synthesis and deposition. If lysis predominates, healing may stop or even regress. The balance between collagen synthesis and lysis is delicate enough to be tipped in either direction and is particularly sensitive to circulatory status and nutrition.

Epithelization

Epithelial cell growth and migration are led largely by growth substances released by epithelial stem cells. As epithelium advances, the underlying connective tissue contracts and mitotic and synthetic activity in the deeper tissue decreases. Epithelization is easily hindered, especially in zinc, oxygen, and vitamin A deficiencies.

Wound surfaces exposed to ambient conditions usually dry out and form eschars. Because eschar cannot support overlying cells, epithelium must advance underneath by enzymatically cleaving the boundary between eschar and live tissue. This is a slow process. On the other hand, epithelia migrate quickly over moist, viable surfaces. For this reason, new dressing techniques have been designed to retain moisture and the extracellular milieu that fosters repair. They are truly improvements over the old wet-to-dry gauze and probably minimize nutritional requirements by conserving protein, decreasing leukocyte turnover, and minimizing water evaporation and calorie loss. [*Editor's Note:* These are biologically well-founded concepts. It is surprising that except in "wound healing centers" there is little knowledge and use of these dressings.]

Resistance to Infection

Many years of surgical experience have demonstrated that the incidence of wound infection is inversely proportional to tissue vascularity. Wounds of the tongue, although frequent, are rarely infected. Infection of face or neck wounds is far less frequent than infection in the extremities. Muscle is rarely infected and then only when ischemic. Subcutaneous tissues, which have the most vulnerable blood supply, are most commonly the site of infection.

Resistance to infection is one of the most important contributions of healing. The first break in the host defense occurs when cutaneous (or mucosal) immune mechanisms are broached. Clearly, rapid repair is the ultimate defense mechanism. Early closure of large open wounds is an important strategy and goal.

In one way or another most of the known immune functions contribute to host defenses. However, one of the distinctive properties of healing is its dependence on nonspecific immunity. One aspect of nonspecific immunity, oxidative bacterial killing, is put at great disadvantage in wounds and becomes, therefore, a conspicuous vulnerability.

Leukocytes migrate into wounds where complement factors facilitate bacterial phagocytosis. Leukocyte granules fuse with the developing phagosome and release into it so-called nonoxidative killing substances such as defensins, cationic protein, myeloperoxidase, and lactoferrin, which are bactericidal. All this occurs in anaerobic as well as aerobic environments. The nonoxidative system is remarkably efficient. Organisms that are sensitive to it are rarely causes of wound infections, becoming more frequent only in leukopenic conditions.

On the other hand, phagocytosis also activates the so-called oxidative killing system. This begins with a burst of oxygen consumption, often more than 50 times the baseline level. This is due to assembly ("activation") of the NADPH-linked oxygenase of leukocytes [12]. As noted above, the reactants are glucose and molecular oxygen. The products, superoxide, lactate, and hydrogen ion, are secreted into phagocytic vacuoles. Note that this constitutes aerobic glycolysis. Any superoxide that is not immediately fixed onto bacterial membranes is dismutated to hydrogen peroxide. This and halide and myeloperoxidase (from the granule fusion) form hypohalites, such as hypochlorite, that are also bactericidal. Any excess peroxide is then reconverted to molecular oxygen that, presumably, is recycled (Figure 15-5). Clearly, this is a fast-moving set of reactions that maintains a pool of bactericidal oxygen radicals, provided that oxygen is present in adequate amounts.

The size of the radical pool is determined by the rate at which oxygen is converted to superoxide. The Km with respect to oxygen for the NADPH-linked oxygenase is about 60 mmHg. In plain terms, this means that the rate of superoxide production for bactericidal purposes occurs at only half-maximal speed at 60 mmHg and is maximal only when intracellular PO_2 is about 600 mmHg. Therefore, bacterial killing capacity for bacteria not susceptible to nonoxidative enzymes is limited by PO_2 in the range from 0 to about 600 mmHg. In clinical terms, this means that no one breathing air at only one atmosphere can kill bacteria at maximal rate. Certainly, in the oxygen-starved environment of wounds, bacterial killing is seriously impaired [13]. This appears to be the Achilles heel of wounds. [*Editor's Note:* This does not translate into a role for hyperbaric oxygen in wounds. The data simply are not there.]

Wound perfusion is as important as arterial PO_2 in determining wound PO_2. Thus, most wounds are hypoxic even in the presence of supranormal PaO_2 because of vascular disruption and vasoconstriction (caused by such factors as hypovolemia, hypothermia, and pain—all common to surgical or traumatic wounds). Attention to support of perfusion is as important as supporting PaO_2. On the other hand, there is clear evidence that in tissues where increasing perfusion can be accomplished only by angiogenesis (radiated or ischemic tissue, for example), administration of oxygen at > 1 atm may be of significant benefit [62,63,64].

We know that the lack of superoxide production presents a serious clinical problem because children who inherit a deficiency of the NADPH-linked oxygenase (chronic granulomatous disease) die of infections early in life unless constantly protected by antibiotics. Even with antibiotics, they are plagued with infections by organisms that commonly infect wounds, including *Staphylococ-*

Figure 15-5. A schematic diagram of the phagocytic vacuole of a polymorphonuclear leukocyte. Dissolved oxygen is converted to superoxide by the membrane-bound NADPH-linked oxygenase. Superoxide radicals are converted to hydrogen peroxide by superoxide dismutase. Peroxide is further converted to hypochlorite by myelo-peroxidase. Catalase can reconvert hydrogen peroxide to dissolved oxygen. (From DD Zabel, TK Hunt. Skin, peritoneum and colonic healing processes. *Perspect Colon Rectal Surg* 6:191, 1993. Reprinted with permission.)

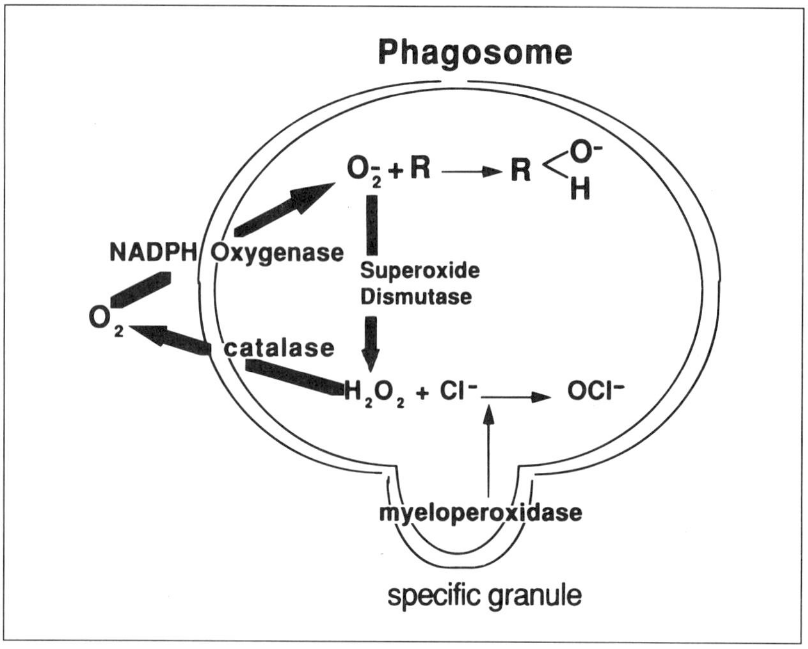

cus aureus, group A *Streptococcus, Escherichia coli, Pseudomonas aeruginosa, Candida,* and some *Proteus* species. In short, a lack of substrate oxygen is equivalent to a lack of the NADPH-linked oxidase, the local equivalent of chronic granulomatous disease.

Killing capacity is also limited somewhat by pH. If extracellular pH is low, the pH of the phagosome is similarly low, and the back pressure of mass action limits superoxide production [14]. The pH optimum is rather broad, and pH is probably not as important to bacterial killing as oxygen until severe acidosis is reached.

Data are emerging that hypoxia is a stimulus for TNF and IL-1 secretion by leukocytes in culture. Cytokines are clearly made in wounds, and almost certainly these perform a useful normal function in stimulating acute-phase protein synthesis in the liver after injury. However, cytokines also have well-known deleterious functions when excessively stimulated. Extensive hypoxic tissue after multiple injuries theoretically could lead to excessive levels of cytokines. This may be one of the insults necessary to produce full syndrome of "sepsis" and multiple organ failure. It could be the only one necessary in elderly or already-ill patients. There are only two known and useful therapeutic responses to the presence of extensive hypoxic tissue: (1) reperfuse and reoxygenate, or (2) debride the ischemic tissue. These are not, of course, mutually exclusive.

Massive open wounds as are encountered in burns depress immune functions in several ways. Leukocyte turnover becomes massive and prolonged, and nutritional demands increase. Contamination is prolonged, and a greater number and type of organisms are present than in clean, primarily closed wounds. The specific immune system plays a greater role in such an environment. Injury-related defects of this system are disclosed by the fact that extensively burned patients become infected by organisms that do not flourish in simple wounds and are not killed by either oxidative or nonoxidative, nonspecific functions of granulocytes. In burns or severely traumatized patients saprophytic and fungal infections became more troublesome.

Nutritional Factors in Wound Repair

Protein-Calorie Malnutrition

Malnutrition, whether chronic or acute, impairs wound healing and host defenses. Vitamin and mineral deficits seldom occur in surgical patients in the absence of protein-calorie malnutrition. Malnutrition may preexist, and may be induced or exacerbated by the catabolic state that results from injury and sepsis. Injury leads to a number of acute consequences that cause nutritional deficits in proportion to the degree of injury and infection. These include: (1) increased metabolic rate and calorie loss resulting from fever (IL-1, TNF-α); increased cell, collagen, and bone turnover; pain and other sources of increased catecholamine levels; and increased cardiac output; (2) increased water loss resulting from evaporative loss, fever, sweating, and diarrhea; and (3) increased bone loss from immobilization. Both calorie and protein needs are proportional to the extent of injury and infection. Patients recovering from uncomplicated cardiac surgery need little protein and only minimal calories, whereas patients who have had simple colostomies for peritonitis resulting from diverticulitis may need supplements for both. Correction of deficits preoperatively and maintenance of adequate nutrition (enterally or parenterally) postoperatively may prevent complications or reduce their severity. Adequate and timely assessment of nutritional status is therefore critical [15].

Normal Metabolism

Energy requirements in humans are met by the metabolism of carbohydrates, proteins, and fats. Carbohydrates and proteins provide about 4 kcal/g, while fats provide about 9 kcal/g [16].

Carbohydrates are stored mainly in the liver and muscle as glycogen. These stores are sufficient to supply basal calorie requirements for less than one day. Even during starvation, however, glycogen stores remain largely intact because most tissues preferentially use fat and protein. Brain, red blood cells, and leukocyte functions are glycogen dependent [17]. In hypoxic areas, such as the leading edge of a wound, anaerobic metabolism requires glucose as a substrate, produces lactate, and increases the caloric demand to recycle the lactate to glucose. In wounds, leukocytes and macrophages make lactate aerobically, which is recycled to glucose in the liver. Lactate is also produced anaerobically in hypoxic wounds, and this lactate must also be converted to glucose by the liver. This inefficient cycle consumes calories and becomes more prominent as injury increases.

Body protein makes up a large potential energy source that can be converted to glucose in the liver through gluconeogenesis. All proteins in the body, however, serve a function. Therefore, metabolism of protein to glucose leads to a negative nitrogen balance, with the loss of muscle, plasma proteins, and enzymes.

Excess protein in the diet is converted to fat for storage. Under normal circumstances, the majority of calories are supplied by fat metabolism. After several days of starvation, the brain begins to use ketones (derived from fat) as an alternate energy source. After trauma or surgery, the stress response leads to a decreased ability to use fat energy sources [17].

Prevalence of Malnutrition

A significant proportion of elective surgery patients have long-standing malnutrition resulting from chronically reduced intake. Warnold and Lundholm [18] in Sweden found evidence of malnutrition in 12% of 215 noncancer patients preoperatively. About 50% of both medical and surgical patients at an urban Boston hospital showed evidence of malnutrition [19]. [*Editor's Note:* The patient population of this oft-quoted study is skewed, as it is composed of a large population of urban indigent, with all that implies. It is therefore not representative of most hospitals, at least in the United States.] Muller and associates [20] found severe malnutrition in 12% of German patients scheduled for major gastrointestinal surgery. In a New Zealand hospital, 43% of inpatients awaiting surgery had evidence of impaired nutrition, although malnutrition was evident in only 5% of patients scheduled for routine elective surgery [17]. In a study of 129 orthopedic patients in Houston, 42% showed evidence of malnutrition. These included 29% of patients presenting for total hip arthroplasty and 57% of multiple trauma patients five days post-injury [21]. [*Editor's Note:* One must be careful about statistics for malnutrition, which is obviously dependent on the definitions and parameters utilized. In at least elective surgery, mild or moderate malnutrition does not seem to increase the risk to an extent beyond the complication rate of our efforts to replenish these patients [22]. However, more precise and less expensive methods of restoration may make it possible to consider for therapy even mild malnutrition, if one can agree on definition.]

Effects of Malnutrition on Outcome

Surgery, trauma, and infection result in a catabolic state with a negative nitrogen balance [23]. Glucagon, glucocorticoid, and catecholamine levels are elevated, while insulin levels are depressed. Growth hormone is also elevated, while IGF-1 and thyroxin are decreased. In the presence of this ongoing stress response, the administration of glucose does not prevent protein catabolism as it does in pure starvation. Net fat oxidation persists despite high serum glucose, largely because of inappropriately low insulin levels. The degree of catabolism is proportional to the severity of injury. Long bone fractures induce a 20% to 30% increase in basal energy expenditure, multiple trauma and sepsis a 50% to 80% increase, and extensive thermal injury up to a 100% to 150% increase [21]. [*Editor's Note:* These are the standard figures given in the literature and are oft-quoted. My personal bias is that the numbers are high: with trauma and sepsis—30%; with long bone fractures uncomplicated by sepsis—15% to 20%; with burns—these figures are variable, in my opinion.] In patients who are unable to take in adequate protein and calories to meet the increased demand, the negative nitrogen balance will increase and be prolonged. Even maximal enteral or parenteral nutritional support cannot restore an anabolic state until physiologic stresses and the resultant high levels of stress hormones resolve.

Protein-calorie malnutrition, with its resultant loss of essential proteins, leads to inadequate wound healing and impaired host defenses. Tensile strength is decreased in subcutaneous, fascial, and anastomotic wounds, with anastomotic wounds generally the most sensitive. Sulfur-containing amino acids such as methionine and cysteine seem particularly important to restore normal healing. Although branched-chain amino acids improve nitrogen balance after trauma, they do not appear to improve wound healing. Glutamine, which has been shown to be a precursor for nucleotide biosynthesis in fibroblasts and appears essential for lymphocyte proliferation, does not improve healing in wounded animals [24].

Numerous immune defects result from malnutrition. Protein depletion appears to affect cellular immunity more than it does humoral immunity. Malnourished patients show decreased T cell numbers, decreased response to mitogen stimulation, and loss of delayed hypersensitivity reactions. Phagocytic cell function, antibody production, and complement levels may also be impaired [25], however, and these are the key elements in host defense of the wound.

Nutritional Factors in Wound Healing

Arginine

Arginine is an amino acid that appears to play a unique role in wound healing. Arginine appears to have both purely nutritional functions (protein synthesis) as well as pharmacologic functions. It decreases urinary nitrogen excretion, enhances collagen synthesis, increases total lymphocyte count, and enhances T cell function [26].

Arginine-deficient rats show impaired wound strength and collagen deposition, while arginine supplementation improves these variables even in normally nourished rats [27]. Similarly, oral arginine supplementation increased collagen deposition in subcutaneous implants in nonoperated, healthy volunteers [28,29]. The mitogenic response of lymphocytes was also increased in these normal subjects. Similar effects have been shown in elderly volunteers and surgical patients. Supplemental arginine did not, however, alter the rate of epithelization of a split thickness donor site. The mechanisms by which arginine achieves these beneficial effects are not known but are likely multifactorial.

Arginine stimulates pituitary growth hormone (GH) secretion [30]. Growth hormone plays a major role in wound repair, at least in part by stimulating the release of IGF-1 and increasing collagen gene expression (see below), and this may be one mechanism for the increased collagen deposition induced by supplemental arginine. This is supported by two observations: (1) an intact hypothalamic-pituitary axis is required for supplemental arginine to exert its beneficial effect on healing, and (2) IGF-1 levels were significantly increased in elderly human volunteers after two weeks of dietary arginine supplementation.

Arginine may also serve as an indirect precursor for proline biosynthesis, through increased production of ornithine. Proline is a major component of collagen. Arginine is metabolized to ornithine in the urea cycle, and ornithine can be converted to proline. Supporting this hypothesis, arginine levels are low within the wound, and this corresponds to high levels of arginase and ornithine. The current evidence, however, indicates that the rate of conversion of ornithine to proline within the wound is low, so this is likely a minor mechanism.

Wound healing is impaired in rats in which function of all T cells is blocked by a monoclonal antibody (OX-19). Arginine is thymotropic and increases the mitogenic responses of T cells and macrophages. The importance of this observation to the salutary effect of arginine on wound healing has yet to be examined.

Finally, arginine is involved in the production of nitric oxide (a potent, locally acting, vasodilator), which may also be a potent stimulus to collagen gene expression.

The many beneficial effects, with few apparent deleterious effects, may lead to routine supplementation with arginine in the perioperative period regardless of nutritional status in the future. In patients with malnutrition or other compromise (especially immune), it may prove particularly useful [28].

Growth Hormone and IGF-1

A number of studies have shown a role for growth hormone in the restoration of healing parameters in malnourished animals. Wound tensile strength 6 days after laparotomy was 2 times greater in malnourished rats given 3 days of preoperative and 5 days of postoperative growth hormone than in malnourished controls, and 18% greater than in normally nourished controls. All animals were fed normal diets postoperatively, and the differences disappeared by 14 days. In another study, growth hormone administration postoperatively returned wound tensile strength to normal in malnourished rats given corticosteroids for 3 weeks preoperatively. In more severely injured rats, however, growth hormone administration had no beneficial effects on wound healing.

When administered in prolonged starvation, growth hormone exacerbates ketoacid production and increases urinary nitrogen losses. Therefore, growth hormone should be given only in combination with nutritional repletion and adequate caloric intake. In pediatric burn patients, growth hormone administration in combination with enteral nutrition resulted in improved wound healing and increased IGF-1 levels compared to a placebo.

Growth hormone appears to exert its favorable effects in part by stimulating IGF-1 synthesis. IGF-1 mediates the anabolic effects of growth hormone by inhibiting protein degradation and also by promoting protein synthesis and glycogen deposition. However, IGF-1 is much more potent than growth hormone in inhibiting protein degradation, and the converse is true for the stimulation of protein synthesis. IGF-1 combined with IGF binding protein 3 (IGFBP-3), the principal IGF binding protein that transports IGF-1 in the plasma, is a more powerful stimulant of healing than IGF-1 alone when applied directly to wounds. Growth hormone may have further beneficial effects by increasing IGF-1 concentrations in specific tissues, including liver and skeletal muscle [31].

IGF-1 has many actions in wound healing. These include priming neutrophils for the respiratory burst, increasing the number of macrophages in wounds [32], and stimulation of fibroblast proliferation and collagen synthesis by increasing gene transcription.

IGF-1 plasma levels are decreased in malnutrition, trauma, burn injury, and critical illness. After injury, plasma IGF-1 decreases despite an increase in plasma growth hormone. In more severe injury/stress states, growth hormone production decreases. Decreased plasma growth hormone in these circumstances is associated with increased mortality.

Tissue repair proceeds more slowly in IGF-1 deficient rats. Administration of IGF-1 alone also has been shown to reverse the healing defect induced by starvation or corticosteroid treatment. In corticosteroid-treated rats, IGF-1 concentration is decreased in wound fluid obtained from subcutaneously implanted wound chambers, and this is associated with decreased collagen deposition in the chambers. Infusion of IGF-1 for 14 days into wound chambers in these corticosteroid-treated rats returned collagen deposition to normal [33].

Vitamin C

Adequate vitamin C (ascorbic acid) is essential for normal healing; however, in uninjured subjects, wound healing is impaired only after about six months of dietary vitamin C deficiency (scurvy). Inadequate vitamin C in the diet leads to increased capillary permeability and fragility, with frequent rupture and hemorrhage. In healing wounds angiogenesis may be decreased or absent. These abnormalities reflect inadequate production of basement membrane collagen. Tensile strength of the wound is diminished because of inadequate collagen deposition, as well as synthesis of abnormal collagen [34]. Wound infections are more frequent.

Vitamin C performs multiple functions, both direct and indirect, in wound repair. It increases procollagen production by fibroblasts. It increases lipid peroxidation, leading to the formation of reactive aldehydes. In vitro, malondialdehyde, one of these lipid peroxidation products, induces a two- to three-fold increase in procollagen mRNA and collagen secretion in fibroblasts. Inhibition of lipid peroxidation by the addition of vitamin E inhibits collagen gene expression. Vitamin C is "amphoteric." In leukocytes, vitamin C can act as a radical, a radical generator, or a radical scavenger in oxidative stress. Thus it probably protects cell membranes from radical damage, while at the same time acting as a radical or radical generator for the purpose of intraphagosomal oxidative bacterial killing and intranuclear induction of collagen synthesis.

Vitamin C is concentrated in leukocytes and promotes bactericidal function. The intracellular concentration is decreased in vitamin C deficiency. Hyperglycemia also decreases transport of vitamin C into leukocytes, apparently because glucose and vitamin C compete for the same (insulin-independent) transport mechanism. No matter the cause, intracellular ascorbate deficiency appears to decrease bacterial killing by neutrophils. Ascorbic acid is a cofactor for superoxide dismutase, which catalyzes the conversion of superoxide to hydrogen peroxide [35]. Within neutrophil phagosomes, this reaction is central to the cycle, described above, that generates bactericidal oxygen and nitroso-radicals. Ascorbate may participate in other reactions in this cycle as well. Neutrophils (and macrophages) produce a large quantity of these radicals in response to phagocytosis of bacteria. Although neutrophils also produce bactericidal lysosomal enzymes, these are relatively ineffective against some organisms, including *Staphylococcus aureus, Escherichia coli, Klebsiella, Candida,* and anaerobes. Thus, vitamin C deficiency may also impair resistance to infection in wounded tissue. In corticosteroid-treated neutrophils, vitamin C improves bacterial killing by restoring bactericidal radical production.

Vitamin C also participates as a cofactor in the hydroxylation of proline and lysine during the post-translational modification of collagen. As discussed above, this step is critical in allowing collagen to be exported from the cell, as well as in the formation of the cross-linked triple-helical structure that confers strength to connective tissue. In this reaction, vitamin C is one of the radical formers that support the reaction of proline or lysine with oxygen. In physiology, it seems one of the most important [36].

Wound remodeling is a continuous process in which collagen deposition and lysis are in equilibrium. With vitamin C deficiency, collagen lysis proceeds normally, despite the decreased collagen deposition. Thus mature, well-healed wounds have been reported to break down in patients with scurvy.

Peterkovsky [36] has elucidated another mechanism by which ascorbate deficiency may impair wound repair. Vitamin C deficiency appears to induce two IGF-binding proteins (not IGFBP-3) that prevent IGF-1 from reaching fibroblasts. This decreases collagen mRNA transcription, collagen synthesis, and lactate formation. The addition of IGF-1 to vitamin C-deficient fibroblast cultures returns collagen synthesis to normal.

IGF-1 also performs several other functions, as described in detail above, which may also contribute to the improved wound healing seen in IGF-1 treated, vitamin C-deficient cells. It primes neutrophils to the respiratory burst and increases the number of macrophages in wounds. These functions may also be impaired by the decrease in available IGF-1 in ascorbate deficient states.

Ascorbate-deficient guinea pigs also lose weight, and the degree of weight loss correlates with the degree of inhibition of collagen synthesis. In these animals, proteoglycan, DNA, and procollagen mRNA synthesis, which do not require ascorbate, are also decreased. Fasting alone induces a decrease in available IGF-1 equivalent to that produced by ascorbate deficiency. These observations may help explain clinical findings of impaired collagen deposition (wound healing) after only a brief (one to three days) period of starvation combined with catabolism, and of restored collagen deposition after only a brief duration of nutritional repletion (seven days), and before other markers of malnutrition, including total lymphocyte count, albumin, and lean body mass, begin to return toward normal.

Normal, uninjured humans require about 20 to 30 mg vitamin C daily to prevent the development of scurvy; however, daily vitamin C requirements are increased in the burned or trauma patient. After trauma, plasma and white cell levels of ascorbic acid fall immediately and in proportion to the severity of injury. This appears to be a result of increased vitamin C metabolism and accumulation of vitamin C at the site of injury, although the predominant mechanism is unknown. In most reactions, ascorbate is consumed. It has rapid turnover in trauma and sepsis. Urinary excretion, however, does not increase. Supplementation with vitamin C (100 to 2000 mg per day, depending on the severity of injury) prevents development of the changes seen with ascorbic acid deficiency [34].

B Vitamins

Several B vitamins contribute to normal healing. Vitamin B_1 (thiamine) is a cofactor for lysyl oxidase, the enzyme that catalyzes the formation of lysine-lysine bonds, which, along with proline-proline bonds, increase the strength of collagen. Thiamine deficiency decreases collagen deposition, particularly of type III collagen [37].

Vitamin B_5 (pantothenic acid) appears to play a role in cell replication. Deficiency of the vitamin impairs wound strength. Histologically, wound sections show a decreased density of fibroblasts [37].

Open skin wounds heal abnormally in rats fed diets deficient in pyridoxine (vitamin B_6) and riboflavin (vitamin B_2) for five weeks before injury. The healing tissue shows increased vascularity and cellularity with decreased collagen matrix deposition. Biotin-deficient rats show similar changes but to a very mild degree [34].

Healing of bone may also be impaired by nutritional deficiencies. For example, fracture healing is abnormal in rats fed a diet deficient in pyridoxine for 21 days prior to injury. Deficiency of this vitamin decreases periosteal glucose-6-phosphate dehydrogenase activity. Pyridoxine deficiency also appears to create an imbalance between osteoblastic and osteoclastic activity. Callus size and new bone production are significantly decreased. Some regions of the fracture site may appear osteoporotic [38].

Megaloblastic anemia resulting from folate or vitamin B_{12} (cyanocobalamin) deficiency may occur in surgical patients. Anemia, however, unless it is severe (hematocrit less than about 17%), does not affect wound repair [39]. Anemia that severe would be corrected perioperatively for other reasons. On the other hand, wound oxygenation may be impaired in these patients in the absence of severe anemia because megaloblastic red cells increase blood viscosity, which decreases tissue perfusion.

Rats deficient in vitamins B_5, B_6, and folate produce fewer antibody-forming cells, and thus less antibody, in response to an antigenic stimulus. B vitamin deficiency may also impair bacterial killing, especially in chronic wounds, in which opportunistic and fungal infections are prominent [34]. The mechanism is unknown.

Traumatic injury and sepsis lead to a decrease in total body levels of the B vitamins, particularly B_1, B_2, and nicotinamide. Therefore, it is recommended that severely injured patients receive five to ten times the usual daily requirement for the B vitamins.

Vitamin A

Although the mechanisms are poorly understood, vitamin A clearly plays a significant role in wound healing. Known processes in which vitamin A is required include epithelial growth, synthesis of glycoproteins and proteoglycans, labilizing lysosomal membranes, cellular immunity, reproduction, and vision [34]. Particularly important to wounds is that the inflammatory response is dependent on the presence of adequate vitamin A. Vitamin A opposes the anti-inflammatory effect of steroids, and, when administered topically or systemically, can correct wound healing impairment in patients on chronic steroids [34,35,37]. Vitamin A has also been shown to improve healing after radiation therapy and in diabetics, presumably by a similar mechanism [40,41].

The systemic administration of vitamin A in patients who require steroids for treatment of inflammatory disease could potentially cause exacerbation of disease. It appears, however, that this is not the case, or at least happens only rarely. For example, vitamin A does not reverse the weight loss in corticosteroid-treated rats. Nonetheless, caution should be used in administering large doses of vitamin A to such patients.

In vitamin A-deficient animals, epithelization, collagen synthesis, wound contraction, prolylhydroxylase activity, and collagen cross-linking are all impaired. In humans, isolated vitamin A deficiency is uncommon. It is associated with epithelial metaplasia, increased infection, delayed wound healing, and diminished stress tolerance [34].

Vitamin A may become depleted during prolonged stress or infection as a result of increased urinary excretion. Large doses of corticosteroids also rapidly deplete liver stores of vitamin A. Daily supplementation with 25,000 international units (IU) of vitamin A (five times the recommended daily dose) should be adequate to avoid impaired wound healing, even in severely injured or ill patients [34,37].

Large doses of vitamin A do not appear to improve healing beyond normal. In fact, prolonged large doses of vitamin A (over 50,000 IU per day) can be toxic. Toxicity includes excessive inflammatory response, visual disturbances, coma, pseudotumor cerebri, and loss of collagen in soft tissues, especially cartilage [34,37].

Vitamin E

Vitamin E stabilizes membranes, partly by protecting them against oxidative damage. There are few studies of its role in wound healing. They indicate that large doses of vitamin E given at the time of injury retard fibrosis and healing. Vitamin E also possesses anti-inflammatory properties similar to steroids. Ehrlich and Hunt [42,43] demonstrated that administration of vitamin A in the first few days after wounding reverses the wound healing impairment induced by vitamin E, similar to the effect of vitamin A in reversing the effects of corticosteroids on healing.

The anti-inflammatory properties of vitamin E, which are similar to those of steroids, may stem in part from stabilization of macrophage membranes [34,35,37]. Vitamin E is clearly one of the molecules that regulates the oxidant state of wounds and shares this effect with vitamin C. It also has antioxidant properties, which may decrease the usual increase in collagen gene expression induced by lipid peroxidation products. On the other hand, vitamin E could potentially decrease damage to the wound induced by excessive radical release by inflammatory cells [37]. After the healing process is established, provision of increased vitamin E might reduce excess scar formation seen in chronic wounds.

Vitamin K

Vitamin K is required for the post-translational carboxylation of glutamate in Factors II, VII, IX, and X. Vitamin K deficiency leads to deficient coagulation, which may impair wound healing, as wound hematomas predispose to infection and poor tissue repair [34,37].

Recent evidence indicates that vitamin K may also be required for bone repair. Osteocalcin is a vitamin K-dependent, calcium-binding protein synthesized by osteoblasts. Osteocalcin is chemotactic for osteoclast precursors and monocytes, and thus appears to be involved in bone remodeling. Some studies have demonstrated impaired histologic fracture healing in dicumarol-treated rats. Einhorn and associates [44] found no difference in mechanical or histologic measurements in rats fed a vitamin K-deficient diet. The effects of chronic vitamin K deficiency (dietary or warfarin-induced) have not been evaluated.

Macrominerals

Magnesium is essential for wound repair, as it is a cofactor for a large number of enzymes involved in protein synthesis. Magnesium deficiency, which is usually related to alcoholism or malabsorption, induces depression, muscular weakness, dizziness, potential seizures, and metabolic acidosis [34].

Trace Minerals

Copper, manganese, and zinc are also essential cofactors for many synthetic enzymes. Copper, for example, is required for the function of lysyl oxidase, clearly an important enzyme for wound repair [34,37]. Manganese is a cofactor for superoxide dismutase, which is involved in the cycle of bactericidal-free radical production by neutrophils. Thus, bacterial killing may be impaired by a deficiency of manganese [34].

Zinc is a cofactor for RNA and DNA polymerase. Inadequate serum zinc ($< 100\ \mu g/100$ mL) is associated with poor wound healing and impaired immune function. Repletion to normal levels returns the healing to normal. Some studies have shown that excess zinc may improve wound healing beyond normal, but others have shown no effect. Serum and total body zinc levels may decrease rapidly after trauma [34,35,37]. Long-term steroid therapy decreases serum zinc levels. Patients on steroids with impaired wound healing should receive both supplemental vitamin A and zinc to restore healing [37]. Topical zinc is well absorbed by granulation tissue.

Inadequate iron (Fe^{2+}) can impair collagen synthesis and wound healing because iron is required for the hydroxylation of proline and lysine. However, this effect has been noted only in immature animals. Iron is also part of the oxidant state. Iron deficiency is quite common and may result from prolonged or severe blood loss, infection, or inadequate dietary intake. Iron deficiency is easily detected and treated. Treatment should be aggressive [34,35].

Iron deficiency may also cause anemia. As with vitamin B_{12} deficiency, anemia must be quite severe before wound healing is impaired by decreased oxygen delivery to the wound.

Molybdenum, cobalt, chromium, selenium, vanadium, and tin are all essential, although at very low levels. The role of these elements in wound healing is largely unknown. Selenium, acting with vitamin E, stabilizes membranes. Excessive replacement of selenium may therefore impair wound healing [34].

Correction and Prevention of Nutritional Deficits

Evaluation of Nutritional Status

Before nutritional deficits can be corrected, they must be recognized. Particularly, the severity of the deficit must be estimated. The identification of predictive markers that are easily and inexpensively measured in a clinical setting is crucial. Hill and associates [17] measured total body water, total body protein, and total body fat using tritiated water dilution and in vivo neutron activation analysis. Their results have uncovered inaccuracies in several commonly used markers for malnutrition. Total body water increases (as extracellular fluid accumulates) at about the same rate that total body protein decreases. Thus, measurements of weight loss may be misleading in acute malnutrition. Anthropometric measurements (e.g., triceps skin fold) underestimate total body fat by about 19%. Changes in total body water with ongoing nutritional depletion also render anthropometric measurements inadequate [46].

While total body analysis provides accurate and precise information, these measurements require tritiated water dilution and in vivo neutron activation, which are not widely available. Other assessments that have been used as predictive markers include weight loss and weight as percentage of ideal body weight; anthropometric measurements; creatinine/height index; serum proteins including albumin and transferrin; total iron-binding capacity; total lymphocyte count; tests of anergy-delayed hypersensitivity; and urinary nitrogen measurements for estimates of nitrogen balance. Of these, serum albumin and total lymphocyte count appear to be the most useful as wound prognosticators [17,18,21]. [*Editor's Note:* Albumin is well established as a prognostic indicator of outcome with respect to nutritional status, as are transferrin, functional status [17], and anergy to injected antigens [25]. Lymphocyte count, in my opinion, is not.] One limitation is that serum albumin and total lymphocyte count are also markers for sepsis or infection; however, unrecognized infection will impair wound healing even in the absence of malnutrition [47], and, in any case, infection will likely induce a catabolic state.

Among 23 patients undergoing a Syme amputation, all of whom met Wagner's criteria, the wound healed in 6 out of 7 with normal albumin and total lymphocyte count and 1 out of 1 with low total lymphocyte count. However, the wound healed in only 1 out of 4 with a low-serum albumin, and 2 out of 11 with both a low total lymphocyte count and a low-serum albumin [48].

Although more than 10% weight loss is frequently cited as increasing the risk of postoperative complications [18], Windsor and Hill [49] found that weight loss of greater than 10% was predictive of increased complications only if it was associated with clear physical impairment such as fatigue, weakness, shortness of breath, mood changes, unhealed or infected wounds, and/or albumin less than 3.2 g/dl. In patients with more than 10% weight loss without physical impairment, total body protein and fat were no different than that of controls, but these were significantly diminished in patients with physical impairment.

Nitrogen balance may also be an inappropriate marker for adequacy of nutritional replacement. In a study comparing two TPN formulations in rats, Barbul and associates [50] found that rats in the group with more negative nitrogen balance in fact showed improvement in wound healing and immune function variables. In fact, changes in hydroxyproline content/tensile strength may occur before changes in other nutritional parameters. Return of normal intestinal anastomotic healing may, however, lag behind that of subcutaneous tissue.

Efficacy of Perioperative Nutritional Support

Clearly, perioperative malnutrition impairs wound healing and resistance to infection. Nutritional repletion may lead to improvements in these outcomes. Interventions to improve the nutritional status of surgical patients are indicated only if they clearly improve outcome in these patients. Animal studies are generally encouraging. In malnourished dogs, decreased serum IgG and complement, total lymphocyte count, and neutrophil chemotaxis all correct with nutritional repletion [51]. Early postoperative TPN in previously normally nourished rats leads to weight gain, improved wound tensile strength, and increased anastomotic bursting pressure [52]. There is no evidence that nutritional support in excess of calculated requirements is beneficial, however, and some evidence that it may be detrimental.

Nutritional support, whether enteral or parenteral, however, is not without risk. Aspiration and diarrhea are common with feeding tubes, and central line placement may be complicated by pneumothorax, hemothorax, subclavian vein thrombosis, and catheter sepsis [17]. The decision to implement perioperative nutritional supplementation or repletion, therefore, requires the surgeon to weigh the benefits (improved healing and resistance to infection, among others) against the risks. Careful outcome studies of different methods of nutritional repletion are required to allow for informed decisions. There is strong and growing evidence that nutritional repletion reduces surgical complications, at least in certain populations. The formulation and route of administration also appear to be important. The data, however, are somewhat conflicting, and further studies are clearly needed.

In 167 malnourished patients scheduled for surgery for gastrointestinal cancer, 10 days of preoperative total parenteral nutrition (TPN) with glucose and protein resulted in a 2-kg weight gain, improvement in serum protein levels and measures of immunocompetence, and a reduction in wound complications and mortality when compared with patients who received a regular hospital diet for 10 days [20]. [*Editor's Note:* This "trial" was in reality a retrospective review.] The severity, but not the incidence, of infectious complications was decreased. Patients who received 50% of their nonprotein calories as lipid had a significantly higher mortality than either of the other groups, and this arm of the study was discontinued early on. The reasons for this increase in mortality associated with fat administration are unclear, but the results are supported by several other studies.

In a cooperative Veterans Administration (VA) study [22], patients received either 7 to 15 days of preoperative TPN, and at least 3 days of postoperative TPN, or no TPN until at least 3 days after surgery. Patients who received TPN had an increased risk of infections (including pneumonia, catheter sepsis, UTI, and wound infections). In patients with mild malnutrition, there was no decrease in noninfectious complications. In patients with moderate malnutrition, there was a decrease in noninfectious complications (generally wound complications), but this was offset by the increase in infectious complications. In severely malnourished patients, the significant decrease in wound complications was much greater than the slight increase in infectious complications.

TPN administered for at least 7 days preoperatively in 50 severely malnourished surgical patients decreased the incidence of complications by

59%, of sepsis by 60%, and of death by 81% compared to 95 controls [53]. In another randomized study of 70 patients with gastric carcinoma, those who received 7 to 10 days of preoperative TPN had a significantly lower rate of wound infection [54]. Conversely, in 26 patients with gastric carcinoma with a weight loss of more than 10 pounds, there was no difference in complication rate between those who received 48 hours of preoperative and 10 days of postoperative TPN and those who received no TPN [55]. [*Editor's Note:* As a coauthor of this study, I am convinced that if we had an adequate number of patients, say 300, with the same statistical trend, it would have been significant. As it was, in this small prospective trial, we showed a trend. This is a type II statistical error.] More than 2 days of preoperative repletion may be required to show an effect. On the other hand, prolonged delay of surgery may not be feasible or advisable in some patients.

Wound healing has fairly specific requirements. The turnover of sulfated amino acids—in particular, lysine, proline, and arginine—is high. Most nutritional replacements are not specifically designed to meet these needs. It is to be expected that the best replacement is the most specific, and further research should be done in this regard. Moreover, wound repair suffers early. Goodson and associates [37] showed that even a 1- to 2-day period of starvation in concert with systemic illness was enough to decrease hydroxyproline (collagen) deposition in subcutaneously placed, expanded polytetrafluoroethylene (ePTFE) implants significantly in the immediate postoperative period. Haydock and Hill [15,56], using the same technique, evaluated wound healing in 36 normally nourished, 21 mildly malnourished, and 9 moderately malnourished surgical patients. They found that even in mildly malnourished patients, or patients in whom inadequate dietary intake was of short duration, collagen deposition was about half of normal.

On the other hand, wound healing seems to be more rapidly restored than other processes affected by malnutrition. Haydock and Hill [15] also found that collagen deposition was increased in 47 malnourished patients after one week of TPN, despite no change in serum proteins or other markers of malnutrition.

Even the short period of postoperative starvation may have a negative effect on wound repair. Collagen deposition was greater in 32 normally nourished general surgery patients who received immediate postoperative total enteral nutrition (TEN) than in control patients, who received only 5% dextrose solutions intravenously until clinically able to tolerate oral intake [57].

In a study of immediate (12 to 18 hours postinjury) TEN in major abdominal trauma patients, Moore and associates [58] found a 69% decrease in septic complications. In a follow-up study comparing TEN with TPN, there were 117% more infectious complications and 600% more major septic complications (abdominal abscess, pneumonia) in the TPN than in the TEN group [59]. Infection rates in the TEN groups were similar in the two studies. Many studies corroborate these findings of the superiority of TEN over TPN. The mechanism is likely improved gut integrity with use, and resultant decrease in bacterial translocation. [*Editor's Note:* It is unfortunate that the superior results of TEN are automatically linked to increased gut integrity, without any evidence. There are many other beneficial results of gut feeding that may beneficially influence the outcome, including, for example, improved hepatic protein synthesis.]

Nutrition affects both healing and immunity to infection. Unfortunately, the relationships are vague. Sound surgical judgment depends on nutritional assessment. When possible, most surgeons postpone major elective operations until patients are nutritionally ready, although what "ready" means is far from clear. Readiness does not require weight gain. It appears mainly to mean that pools of rapidly turning-over substances are restored. A few days' repletion even of chronic losses seems to restore wound healing. The corollary is that acute starvation, even for a few days, is surgically important. The patients at risk seem to be those who have not eaten *recently*.

Guidelines for Nutritional Therapy

The data on the efficacy of perioperative nutritional support are somewhat conflicting. Parenteral nutrition is indicated only when risks of that support are less than the risk inherent in the patient's nutritional state. When feasible, enteral nutrition is preferable to parenteral because it maintains gut integrity and may decrease bacterial translocation [60]. In patients with severe malnutrition who are scheduled for major surgery, delay of surgery for TPN/TEN is probably indicated when appropriate. The length of delay is again controversial, but probably should be at least 7 to 10 days. [*Editor's Note:* I believe this period to be between 5 and 7 days.] With mild or moderate malnutrition, delay for TPN/TEN is probably contraindicated. However, postoperative nutritional support should be considered, particularly if the patient may remain without oral intake for a prolonged period.

In patients whose surgery is delayed for other

reasons, TPN/TEN should be instituted if severe malnutrition exists. If mild to moderate malnutrition is present and the patient is expected to be without oral intake or to receive limited calories for 5 to 7 days, TPN/TEN should be initiated early. Three liters of 5% dextrose supplies only 600 calories, so patients undergoing multiple tests for which they remain without oral intake for much of the day may in effect be starved [15,17,61].

Nutritional support should be started early in trauma patients who are expected not to take adequate oral nutrition for 3 to 4 days. These patients are stressed and, thus, will progress to significant protein depletion more rapidly than other patients [15].

Appropriate formulations of TPN and TEN, including caloric content, ratio and type of protein, fat, and carbohydrate, and other considerations are covered extensively elsewhere in this text. To ensure optimal wound healing, however, particular attention should be paid to replacing vitamin C, zinc, vitamin A, B vitamins, sulfated proteins (especially arginine), and possibly vitamin E. Pharmacologic use of arginine, growth hormone, and IGF-1 may also be useful, although the data are still preliminary.

Conclusions

Many surgical patients are at high risk of developing protein-calorie malnutrition, potentially in association with one or more vitamin or mineral deficiencies. Because of the dependence of injury repair on many proteins, enzymes, and cofactors, as well as intact host defenses (particularly nonspecific neutrophil and macrophage modulated), such nutritional deficits increase the incidence of wound infection and impaired wound healing.

While it is clear that appropriate nutritional support will benefit the malnourished patient, it is not yet clear that it is the best way to prevent the development of malnutrition or to replete mild to moderate malnutrition in the surgical setting. Further investigation into the optimal replacement of nutritional factors perioperatively is needed. Development of techniques that rapidly, accurately, and inexpensively assess nutritional status is crucial for providing guidelines for therapy.

The poor wound healing found in scurvy was part of the subject of one of the first controlled studies in the history of medicine when Lind did his experiment on scorbutic sailors aboard the HMS *Salisbury.* Since then, many investigators have contributed to knowledge on the importance of nutrition to wound healing. Despite this long history, specifics remain vague. Wound healing recruits so many body processes that the complexity of nutritional problems remains beyond full understanding. If wound healing is or is expected to be a problem, the general approach is to repair the deficits recognizing that there may be some excessive replacement in order to repair unknown specific defects. It is rarely useful to measure any one substance (for example, vitamin A, arginine, etc.). It is generally best to design a good nutritional repletion and let the body and the wound take care of the specific details.

References

1. Adzick NS, Lorenz HP. Cells, matrix, growth factors, and the surgeon. *Ann Surg* 220:10, 1994.
2. Barbul A. Postoperative Wound Infection. In JL Cameron (ed), *Current Surgical Therapy,* 4th ed. St Louis: Mosby, 1992. P 960.
3. Cohen IK, Diegelmann RF. Wound Healing. In KT Oldham et al (eds), *Surgery: Scientific Principles and Practice.* Philadelphia: Lippincott, 1993. P 86.
4. Edington HD. Wound Healing. In DL Steed, RC Simmons (eds), *Basic Science Review for Surgeons.* Philadelphia: Saunders, 1992. P 41.
5. Goodson WH, et al. The influence of a brief preoperative illness on postoperative healing. *Ann Surg* 205:250, 1987.
6. Hunt TK, Muller RV, Goodson WH III. Wound Healing. In LW Way (ed), *Current Surgical Diagnosis and Treatment.* Norwalk, CT: Appleton & Lange, 1994. P 80.
7. Jennings RW, Hunt TK. Overview of Postnatal Healing. In MT Longaker, NS Adzick (eds), *Fetal Wound Healing.* New York: Elsevier, 1992. P 25.
8. Dvonch VM, et al. Changes in growth factor levels in human wound fluid. *Surgery* 112:18, 1992.
9. Folkman J, Klagsburn M. Angiogenic factors. *Science* 235:442, 1987.
10. Zabel DD, Hunt TK. Peritoneum and colonic healing processes. *Perspect Colon Rectal Surg* 6:191, 1993.
11. Duncan BW, et al. Regulation of Prolyl Hydroxylase Activity in Fetal and Adult Fibroblasts. In MT Longaker, NS Adzick (eds), *Fetal Wound Healing.* New York: Elsevier, 1992. P 303.
12. Sbarra AJ, Strauss R. The Respiratory Burst and the NADPH Oxidase of Phagocytic Leukocytes. In R Lutter, D Roos, B Bolscher (eds), *The Respiratory Burst and Its Significance.* New York: Plenum, 1988.
13. Edwards S, Hallett M, Campbell A. Oxygen-radical production during inflammation may be limited by oxygen concentration. *Biochem J* 217:851, 1984.
14. Rotstein OD, et al. The deleterious effect of reduced pH and hypoxia on neutrophil migration in vitro. *J Surg Res* 45:298, 1988.
15. Haydock DA, Hill GL. Improved wound healing response in surgical patients receiving intravenous nutrition. *Br J Surg* 74:320, 1987.
16. Schwartz SI. *Principles of Surgery.* New York: McGraw-Hill, 1994.
17. Streat SJ, Hill GL. Nutritional support in the management of critically ill patients in surgical intensive care. *World J Surg* 11:194, 1987.
18. Warnold I, Lundholm K. Clinical significance of preoperative nutritional status in 215 noncancer patients. *Ann Surg* 199:299, 1984.

19. Bistrian BR, Blackburn GL, Hallowell E. Protein status of general surgical patients. *JAMA* 230:858, 1974.
20. Muller JM, et al. Indications and effects of preoperative parenteral nutrition. *World J Surg* 10:53, 1986.
21. Jensen JE, et al. Nutrition in orthopaedic surgery. *J Bone Joint Surg* 64A:1263, 1982.
22. Buzby GP, et al (Veterans Affairs Total Parenteral Nutrition Cooperative Study Group). Perioperative total parenteral nutrition in surgical patients. *N Engl J Med* 325:525, 1991.
23. Rhoads JE. Memoir of a surgical nutritionist. *JAMA* 272:963, 1994.
24. McCauley R, et al. Effects of glutamine infusion on colonic anastomotic strength in the rat. *JPEN* 15:437, 1991.
25. Christou N. Perioperative nutritional support: Immunologic defects. *JPEN* 14:186S, 1990.
26. Kirk SJ, Barbul A. Role of arginine in trauma, sepsis, and immunity. *JPEN* 14:226S, 1990.
27. Seifter E, et al. Arginine: An essential amino acid for injured rats. *Surgery* 84:224, 1978.
28. Barbul A, et al. Arginine enhances wound healing and lymphocyte immune response in humans. *Surgery* 108: 331, 1990.
29. Barbul A, et al. Arginine stimulates lymphocyte immune response in healthy human beings. *Surgery* 90:244, 1981.
30. Barbul A, et al. Wound healing and thymotropic effects of arginine: A pituitary mechanism of action. *Am J Clin Nutr* 37:786, 1983.
31. Guyda HJ. Concepts of IGF Physiology. In EM Spencer (ed), *Modern Concepts of Insulin-Like Growth Factors.* New York: Elsevier, 1991. P 99.
32. Mueller RV, et al. The effect of insulin-like growth factor I on wound healing variables and macrophages in rats. *Arch Surg* 129:262, 1994.
33. Suh DY, Hunt TK, Spencer EM. Insulin-like growth factor-I reverses the impairment of wound healing induced by corticosteroids in rats. *Endocrinology* 131:2399, 1992.
34. Levenson SM, Seifter E, Van Winkle W. Nutrition. In TK Hunt, JE Dunphy (eds), *Fundamentals of Wound Management in Surgery.* New York: Appleton-Century-Crofts, 1979.
35. Orgill D, Demling RH. Current concepts and approaches to wound healing. *Crit Care Med* 16:899, 1988.
36. Peterkofsky B. Ascorbate requirement for hydroxylation and secretion of procollagen: Relationship to inhibition of collagen synthesis in scurvy. *Am J Clin Nutr* 54:1134S, 1991.
37. Goodson WH III, Hunt TK. Wound Healing and Nutrition. In KN Jeejeebhoy et al (eds), *Nutrition and Metabolism in Patient Care.* Philadelphia: Saunders, 1988. P 635.
38. Dodds RA, et al. Abnormalities in fracture healing induced by vitamin B6-deficiency in rats. *Bone* 7:489, 1986.
39. Jonsson K, et al. Tissue oxygenation, anemia, and perfusion in relation to wound healing in surgical patients. *Ann Surg* 214:605, 1991.
40. Seifter E, et al. Impaired wound healing in streptozotocin in diabetes: Prevention by supplemental vitamin A. *Ann Surg* 194:42, 1981.
41. Winsey K, et al. Effect of supplemental vitamin A on colon anastomotic healing in rats given preoperative irradiation. *Am J Surg* 153:153, 1987.
42. Ehrlich HP, Hunt TK. Effects of cortisone and vitamin A on wound healing. *Ann Surg* 167:324, 1968.
43. Hunt TK. Vitamin A and wound healing. *J Am Acad Dermatol* 15:817, 1986.
44. Einhorn TA, et al. The contributions of dietary protein and mineral to the healing of experimental fractures: A biomechanical study. *J Bone Joint Surg* 68A:1389, 1986.
45. Heppenstall RB. Fracture and Cartilage Repair. In JE Dunphy, et al (eds), *Fundamentals of Wound Management in Surgery: Selected Tissues.* New Jersey: Chirurgecom, 1977. P 1.
46. Caldwell MD. Nutritional Support in the Surgical Patient. In JL Cameron (ed), *Current Surgical Therapy,* 4th ed. St Louis: Mosby, 1992. P 946.
47. Pettigrew RA, Hill GL. Indicators of surgical risk and clinical judgement. *Br J Surg* 73:47, 1988.
48. Dickhaut SC, DeLee JC, Page CP. Nutritional status: Importance in predicting wound healing after amputation. *J Bone Joint Surg* 66A:71, 1984.
49. Windsor JA, Hill GL. Weight loss with physiologic impairment. *Ann Surg* 207:209, 1988.
50. Barbul A, et al. Intravenous hyperalimentation with high arginine levels improves wound healing and immune function. *J Surg Res* 38:328, 1985.
51. Dionigi R, et al. The effects of total parenteral nutrition on immunodepression caused by malnutrition. *Ann Surg* 185:467, 1977.
52. Delany HM, et al. Effect of early postoperative nutritional support on skin wound and colon anastomosis healing. *JPEN* 14:357, 1990.
53. Mullen JL, et al. Reduction of operative morbidity and mortality by combined preoperative and postoperative nutritional support. *Ann Surg* 192:604, 1980.
54. Williams RH, et al. A randomized controlled trial of preoperative intravenous nutrition in patients with stomach cancer. *Br J Surg* 6:667, 1976.
55. Holter AR, Rosen HM, Fischer JE. The effects of hyperalimentation on major surgery in patients with malignant disease. *Acta Chir Scand* 466:86, 1976.
56. Haydock DA, Hill GL. Impaired wound healing in surgical patients with varying degrees of malnutrition. *JPEN* 10:550, 1986.
57. Schroeder D, et al. Effects of immediate postoperative enteral nutrition on body composition, muscle function, and wound healing. *JPEN* 15:376, 1991.
58. Moore EE, Jones TN. Benefits of immediate jejunostomy feeding after major abdominal trauma: A prospective, randomized study. *J Trauma* 26:874, 1986.
59. Moore FA, et al. TEN versus TPN following major abdominal trauma-reduced septic morbidity. *J Trauma* 29:916, 1989.
60. Saito H, et al. A new model for studying nutrition in peritonitis. *Ann Surg* 209:334, 1989.
61. Smith TK. Prevention of complications in orthopedic surgery secondary to nutritional depletion. *Clin Orthop* 222:91, 1987.
62. Hammarlund C, Sundberg T. Hyperbaric oxygen reduced size of chronic leg ulcers: A randomized double-blind study. *Plast Reconstr Surg* 93(4):829–834, 1994.
63. Uhl E, et al. Hyperbaric oxygen improves wound healing in normal and ischemic skin tissue. *Plast Reconstr Surg* 93(4):835–841, 1994.
64. Brakora MJ, Sheffield PJ. Hyperbaric oxygen therapy for diabetic wounds. *Clin Podiatr Med Surg* 12(1):105–117, 1995.

Selected Readings

Barbul A, et al. Arginine enhances wound healing and lymphocyte immune responses in humans. *Surgery* 108:331, 1990.

This paper investigates the effects of a specific nutritional supplement, arginine, on wound repair and resistance to infection. It also reviews the many possible mechanisms through which arginine has its effects. The investigators used ePTFE implants, a relatively new technique, to evaluate collagen deposition/adequacy of healing in human subjects.

Goodson WH, et al. The influence of a brief preoperative illness on postoperative healing. *Ann Surg* 205:250, 1987.

The authors used ePTFE implants to demonstrate the extremely rapid impairment of wound repair caused by decreased protein-calorie intake during stress.

Haydock DA, Hill GL. Improved wound healing response in surgical patients receiving intravenous nutrition. *Br J Surg* 74:320, 1987.

The authors used ePTFE implants to evaluate the effect of TPN specifically on wound healing outcomes. The rapid response of wound healing components to nutritional repletion is clear in this paper.

Levenson SM, Seifter E, Van Winkle W. Nutrition. In TK Hunt, JE Dunphy (eds), *Fundamentals of Wound Management in Surgery*. New York: Appleton-Century-Crofts, 1979. P 286.

An excellent, albeit somewhat dated, review of the many nutritional factors that affect wound repair.

Peterkofsky B. Ascorbate requirement for hydroxylation and secretion of procollagen: relationship to inhibition of collagen synthesis in scurvy. *Am J Clin Nutr* 54:1134S, 1991.

Scurvy was the first identified condition that allowed a specific nutritional correction. This study examines mechanisms of wound healing impairment in vitamin C deficiency.

16

Nitric Oxide

Timothy R. Billiar
Richard L. Simmons

Nitric oxide (·N = O), long known as a toxic atmospheric gas, is now known to be the smallest biologic product of mammalian cells, exhibiting a diverse range of biologic functions. Mitchell first suggested that mammals produce oxides of nitrogen in 1916 [1]. In recent history, three separate lines of unrelated research led to the confirmation of nitrogen oxide formation in eukaryotic cells and the delineation of the L-arginine-·N = O pathway. First, in studies on endogenous nitrate synthesis as a source for carcinogen formation, Tannenbaum and co-workers in the late 1970s and early 1980s showed that mammals produce nitrate (NO_3^-) and that this production was enhanced by endotoxin treatment [2–5]. Subsequently in 1985, Stuehr and Marletta [6] provided conclusive evidence for nitrogen oxide synthesis in a specific cell when they showed induced NO_3^- synthesis in murine macrophages treated with lipopolysaccharide (LPS) and interferon-gamma (IFNγ).

In a second line of research on mechanisms of macrophage antitumor cytotoxicity, Hibbs et al. [7] reported that L-arginine was the substrate for murine macrophage nitrite-nitrate (NO_2^- + NO_3^-) synthesis and that N^G-substituted L-arginine analogues served as effective competitive inhibitors of this newly discovered pathway. Hibbs et al. [7] further showed that the conversion of L-arginine to nitrogen oxides is required for macrophage-induced cytotoxicity of certain tumor cell lines. In a third area of investigation, Palmer et al. [8], followed by Ignarro et al. [9], were the first to show in 1987 that ·N = O was produced by a mammalian cell when they revealed that ·N = O accounted for the endothelium-derived relaxing activity discovered by Furchgott and Zawadzki in 1980 [10]. Palmer and colleagues [11] were then the first to show that L-arginine was the substrate for ·N=O synthesis in endothelial cells. That ·N=O was the biologically active intermediate of this pathway in activated macrophages was then shown by Marletta et al. [12], Hibbs et al. [13], and Stuehr et al. [14]. By 1988, the pathway was identified in neuronal tissue [15], and the wide distribution and potential importance of ·N=O formation in mammalian physiology and pathophysiology was evident.

It is now known that ·N=O is the product of the five-electron oxidation of one of the chemically equivalent guanidino nitrogens of L-arginine by the enzyme nitric oxide synthase (NOS) [16]. NADPH provides the electrons and the oxygen for the ·N=O, and citrulline is derived from molecular oxygen (Figure 16-1) [17]. To date, three distinct isoforms of this enzyme have been isolated, purified, and the cDNAs cloned. Humans represent the only species from which cDNA clones have been isolated for all three isoforms (Table 16-1) [18–21]. As of early 1994, it is unknown whether other isoforms exist. Two of the enzymes are constantly present and are termed constitutive NOS (cNOS). These include the endothelial cNOS, which produces the endothelial-derived relaxing factor, and the neuronal cNOS, which releases ·N=O to act as a neurotransmitter. A third isoform is probably not expressed at all in resting cells, but instead must be induced by cytokines, microbes, or microbial constituents such as LPS. All three isoforms are homodimers and all contain consensus binding sites for calmodulin, flavin, and NADPH. All are also known to contain tetrahydrobiopterin (BH_4) and a heme group. Despite these similarities, these three isoforms are products of distinct genes situated on separate chromosomes, exhibiting unique tissue distribution (see Table 16-1). Gene structures have been determined for the endothelial [22] and inducible [23] isoforms, and both contain 26 exons, suggesting a common ancestor gene. However, all isoforms share only approximately 50% amino acid homology. These evolved characteristics give each isoform distinct and important differences in regulation and location, which enable each type to perform unique functions. The most important difference between the isoforms besides the constitutive or inducible expression is the regulation by calcium and calmodulin. Whereas the cNOSs are active only when calmodulin binds to the enzyme in the presence of calcium [24], inducible NOS (iNOS) is maintained in a constantly active state by a permanently bound calmodulin [25]. This important difference means that cNOS activity is tightly regulated by agonists that increase intracellular calcium, whereas iNOS activity is limited only by substrate and cofactor availability.

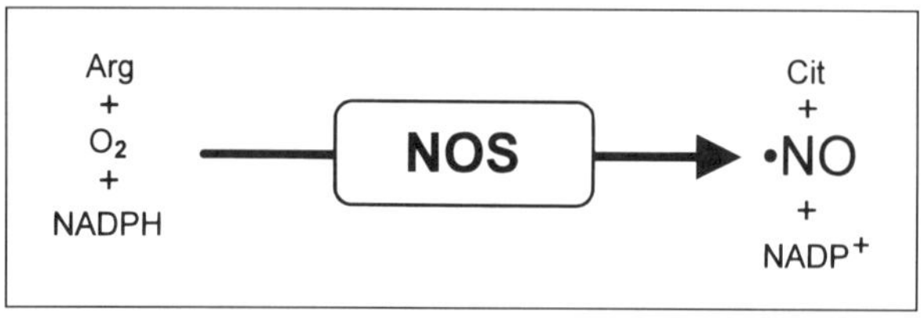

Figure 16-1. Biosynthesis of nitric oxide (·N=O) from L-arginine. Nitric oxide synthase (NOS) acts on L-arginine, deriving electrons from NADPH and oxygen from molecular O_2 to form ·N=O, citrulline (Cit), and $NADP^+$.

Distribution and Expression of Nitric Oxide Synthase (NOS)

Endothelial cNOS is known to be mostly membrane-bound and is found generally in endothelial cells. Recent data indicate that endothelial cNOS may also be in neurons [26]. The neuronal cNOS has been identified in the cytosol of central and autonomic peripheral neurons [27] and the juxtaglomerular cells of the kidney, while mRNA for neuronal cNOS has been found in skeletal muscle in humans [28]. Nitric oxide derived from the neuronal cNOS isoform in the autonomic nervous system acts as a nonadrenergic, noncholinergic neurotransmitter; ·N=O from endothelial cNOS acts to relax smooth muscle, as well as prevent platelet and neutrophil adhesion to the endothelium. Thus, endothelial ·N=O constitutes endothelial-derived relaxing factor (EDRF). The regulation of the expression of the neuronal cNOS

Table 16-1. Human Nitric Oxide Synthase (NOS) Isoforms: Tissue and Chromosomal Localization

Human NOS Isoform	Localization	Chromosome
Endothelial cNOS	Endothelium	7
Neuronal cNOS	Central and peripheral neurons	12
Inducible NOS	Multiple cell types	17

has not been characterized. The endothelial cNOS expression is up-regulated by sheer stress and down-regulated by tumor necrosis factor (TNF). Consensus sequences in the TATA-less promoter of the human endothelial cNOS for cytokines and sheer stress suggest that these changes may involve transcriptional regulation [22].

Since the initial reports of iNOS expression in murine macrophages and macrophage cell lines, it has become apparent that the capacity to express this enzyme in mammals is widespread. iNOS expression has been demonstrated in such diverse cell types as macrophages, hepatocytes, smooth muscle cells, pancreatic islets, chondrocytes, cardiac myocytes, fibroblasts, endothelial cells, and astrocytes [30]. The potential for iNOS expression extends far beyond the classic immune system and includes tissues found at essentially every site within the body. Vascular smooth muscle, cardiac myocytes, fibroblasts, and hepatocytes represent large tissue masses with the potential to produce massive amounts of $\cdot N=O$ upon induction [31–34]. The conditions under which a specific tissue is induced to express iNOS and the degree and duration of expression may vary considerably from tissue to tissue. For example, we have shown an induction of iNOS lasting several days in vivo in hepatocytes during the chronic hepatic inflammation induced by *Corynebacterium parvum* (*C. parvum*) injection [35], but a minor degree of iNOS expression lasting only a few hours after LPS injection in rats [36]. Endotoxemia results in acute expression in a number of other tissues, including the lung, heart, kidney, and brain. In contrast to endotoxemia, it is also likely that more localized inflammatory processes such as immune-mediated arthritis or type I diabetes will involve iNOS expression only at the specific site of inflammation induced by local mediators.

Common to all cells that express iNOS is the requirement for certain cytokines and/or LPS in order to induce expression of the enzyme. Following exposure to the stimulating agent, $\cdot N=O$ synthesis is delayed by several hours while enzyme (and perhaps cofactors) are synthesized. Thereafter, $\cdot N=O$ synthesis is sustained for several hours or longer. Another common theme in iNOS expression is the strong synergy observed between the inducing agents. For murine macrophages, the marked synergy between LPS and IFNγ has been shown to occur at the transcriptional level [29]. We have described synergy between IL-1, TNF, IFNγ, and LPS when added together to cultured hepatocytes [37]. iNOS mRNA levels reveal synergy between any double and most triple combination of these cytokines in rat hepatocytes, while single cytokines, but not LPS alone, stimulate minor increases in mRNA levels [38]. In some cells, single agents, including LPS in murine macrophages [6] or IL-1 in vascular smooth muscle or chondrocytes, are relatively effective alone [32,39,40]. Induction in some cell types is exquisitely sensitive to the concentration of the inducing agent. For example, IL-1 at concentrations of 5 to 50 μ/ml is relatively ineffective, but concentrations of 100 μ/ml or greater are very effective in a number of cells, including chondrocytes, smooth muscle cells, and hepatocytes [unpublished observation]. In addition, cells such as hepatocytes can be primed for iNOS expression in response to single cytokines that are ineffective by themselves. For example, hepatocytes isolated from turpentine-treated rats [41] exhibit extreme sensitivity to LPS for iNOS expression. These differences between tissues underscore the variability between cell types in the potency of stimulating agents or combinations of agents. Studies on transcriptional activation of murine macrophage iNOS have revealed a number of cytokine-responsive elements in the promoter region of this gene [42,43]. In fact, separate regions appear to control the induction of iNOS transcription in murine macrophages by LPS and IFNγ. Our characterization of the human iNOS promoter also reveals a number of potential regulatory regions responsive to cytokines [23].

Several inhibitors of iNOS induction have been reported. In all cells tested, dexamethasone at least partially prevents iNOS expression. We have shown in hepatocytes a reduction in iNOS mRNA levels by 40% to 70% when added with any cytokine or cytokine-LPS combination [38]. This finding is especially interesting because another hepatocyte response seen in inflammation, the acute-phase response, is enhanced by steroids [44]. Other inhibitors of iNOS enzyme induction in macrophages include IL-4, IL-8, IL-10, TGFβ-1, -2, -3, and macrophage deactivating factor [45]. Other cells may or may not be sensitive to these cytokines.

Cytokines most likely regulate the induction of mRNA expression either by transcriptional, post-transcriptional, or translational mechanisms. A number of other factors will, of course, regulate enzyme function. For example, many L-arginine analogues act as competitors of the natural substrate. Furthermore, flavoproteins and heme binders can substantially inhibit cNOS and iNOS activity [16]. Calmodulin inhibitors have so far only been reported to inhibit cNOS activity. The absence of enzyme cofactors such as tetrahydrobiopterin results in a loss of enzyme function. These cofactors will be discussed below.

Striking differences in iNOS expression occur between species. The best examples of these differences can be seen in macrophages and hepatocytes. As already mentioned, the iNOS pathway was first elucidated in murine macrophages [7]. Three groups independently isolated full-length cDNA clones for iNOS from the murine macrophage cell line RAW 264.7 [46–48]. Expression of iNOS by human monocytes has been observed only after prolonged exposure to GM-CSF + TNF, IFNγ + TNF, or LPS in culture [49,50]. The quantity of ·N=O produced by human monocytes-macrophages is considerably less than that seen in the murine counterpart. We have been unable to detect significant levels of NO_2^- or NO_3^- release [unpublished observation] by IL-1-, TNF-, IFNγ-, and LPS-treated human Kupffer cells. Quite the opposite is observed in human hepatocytes, which exhibit the same robust ·N=O synthesis to the very same signals seen in rat hepatocytes [33]. We have now isolated a full-length cDNA for iNOS from human hepatocytes [20]. Human hepatocyte iNOS shares 80% amino acid homology with the murine macrophage iNOS and emanates from a single gene. More recently, iNOS cDNA cloned from human chondrocytes [51] and a human adenocarcinoma cell line DLD-1 [52] exhibits high homology with our hepatocyte cDNA. An iNOS cDNA isolated from rat liver exhibited high homology to murine macrophage iNOS [53]. Presuming that sequence differences between the isolated human and rodent iNOS cDNA clones are due to species differences, the cDNA obtained from human hepatocytes may represent the sole human iNOS. This is also supported by the high homology between the different isolated human iNOS cDNA. In addition, we have cloned the human iNOS gene and found a single 37 kb locus on chromosome 17 [23], lending further support to the single iNOS gene theory. It is not clear what evolutionary pressures preserved iNOS expression in hepatocytes and reduced iNOS in macrophages in humans. Some hints may come from studies on the role of ·N=O in preventing the hepatic stages of malaria [54–56] and the potential of ·N=O as a toxic agent [57–59] or carcinogen [60–62]. The benefit derived from the antimalarial or other antiparasitic actions of ·N=O in the liver may have preserved ·N=O expression in hepatocytes, while a low threshold for macrophage iNOS expression may have had adverse consequences (for example, host cell injury). In addition, we have published data [63] showing that compared to macrophages [64], hepatocytes are equipped to efficiently resist metabolic inhibition by endogenous ·N=O and thus avoid the cytotoxic effects of ·N=O.

Molecular Actions of Nitric Oxide

Nitric oxide has many proposed and established functions. These functions, in turn, are dictated by the site and NOS isoform responsible for the functions of ·N=O. Table 16-2 lists these physiologic functions. It will become clear from the discussion below that other actions, some of which are pathologic, can be attributed to ·N=O. All of the actions of ·N=O, either physiologic or pathologic, are likely to be mediated at least in part through the mechanisms described below.

The production of ·N=O in various cell types results in several biochemical reactions that are responsible for its biologic effects within the cell. Nitric oxide is a short-lived molecule in oxygenated aqueous environments. It is also highly diffusible and rapidly crosses cell membranes, and it is now clear that ·N=O can form adducts with other molecules that may then serve as carrier molecules. Molina et al. [65] presented data that glyceraldehyde-3-phosphate dehydrogenase may serve as an intracellular shuttling molecule for ·N=O in platelets. Adducts between ·N=O and albumin [66] or glutathione [67] may act as extracellular carriers that release ·N=O to cause vasodilation or bronchodilation remote from the site of synthesis. Once at the target cell, the action of ·N=O on enzymes can be divided into activation or inactivation. The small amount of ·N=O released by cNOS isoforms is adequate to activate soluble guanylate cyclase and participate in ·N=O signaling pathways. Thus, activation of soluble guanylate cyclase by ·N=O leads to the synthesis of cGMP, which leads to relaxation [68] of vascular smooth muscle cells [69], inhibition of platelet adherence [70], aggregation [71], inhibition of neutrophil chemotaxis [72], and signal transduction in the central and peripheral nervous systems [19,27].

The larger amounts of ·N=O generated by iNOS also activate guanylate cyclase [16,73,74], but in many cell types the high output of ·N=O also exceeds the necessary concentration threshold to activate or inhibit certain other enzymes. For example, cyclooxygenase is also activated by ·N=O, adding a second heme-containing enzyme to the list of ·N=O-responsive enzyme targets [75]. It is possible that this effect is cell-type specific because we have presented evidence in rabbit chondrocytes [40] and rat Kupffer cells [76] that ·N=O impairs prostaglandin synthesis. However, most ·N=O-sensitive enzymes are inactivated by ·N=O, and the list of potential enzyme targets for ·N=O inhibition is growing. Nitric oxide appears to inactivate glyceraldehyde-3-phosphate dehydrogenase [74,77] by a process recently referred

Table 16-2. Proposed Physiologic Functions of Nitric Oxide (·N=O)

	Site	Function
Endothelial cNOS	Endothelium[a]	Vascular relaxation Inhibit platelet function Suppress vascular smooth muscle cell proliferation Inhibit PMN adherence (?)
	Neurons	Neurotransmitter
	Pancreatic islets[b]	Promotes insulin secretion
Neuronal cNOS	Central nervous system[a]	Neurotransmitter Regulates neurotransmitter release
	Autonomic nerve system[a]	Neurotransmitter
	Skeletal muscle[a]	?
	Kidney (juxtaglomerular complex)	?
	GI tract[b]	Sphincter relaxation Ion transport
Inducible NOS	Macrophage	Antimicrobial effector Antitumor effector
	Hepatocyte[a]	Antimicrobial effector Cytoprotection
	Vascular smooth muscle[a]	Vascular relaxation
	Vascular endothelial cells	Vascular relaxation
	Cardiac myocytes[a]	Antimicrobial effector (?) Cytoprotection (?)
	Bronchial epithelium	Bronchial relaxation (?) Antimicrobial effector (?)
	Renal mesangial cells	Antithrombotic Cytoprotective (?)
	Chondrocytes[a]	?
	Pancreatic islets[a]	?
	Megakaryocytes	?
	Astrocytes	?
	Fibroblasts	?

? = Function not well established.
[a] = isoform confirmed in humans.
[b] = isoform type not definite.

to as active site nitrosylation [78]. Although the consequences of the ·N=O-induced inhibition of glyceraldehyde-3-phosphate dehydrogenase is not well established, the process of protein nitrosylation may represent more generalized mechanisms for cellular regulation by ·N=O. Studies using murine tumor cell lines have shown that ·N=O inhibits three iron-containing mitochondrial enzymes—aconitase of the Krebs cycle, as well as NADPH-ubiquinone oxidoreductase and succinate-ubiquinone oxidoreductase of the electron transport chain [14,63] Nitric oxide has also been demonstrated to inhibit DNA synthesis via inhibition of ribonucleotide reductase [59,79]. Other enzymes inhibited by ·N=O include cytochrome P450 [80] and NADPH oxidase [81]. We have shown that ·N=O from either exogenous or endogenous sources profoundly suppresses total protein synthesis in hepatocytes [33,82], which is not mediated via cGMP synthesis or mitochondrial inhibition [63,72]. This, along with the capacity of ·N=O to impair enzyme function, may account for the inhibition of T-cell proliferation as well as the antimicrobial and tumoricidal activity seen by inducing ·N=O in various cell types [83].

Induced Nitric Oxide as an Antimicrobial Effector

The antimicrobial capacity of ·N=O was known long before it was recognized to be a major effector molecule in antimicrobial host defense [84,85]. The first study showing ·N=O as an antimicrobial molecule in macrophages was by Granger et al. [86], who demonstrated that L-arginine was essential for macrophage inhibition of *Cryptococcus neoformans* growth. In the ensuing years, this pathway has been confirmed, mostly in vitro, as a nonspecific defense mechanism for a variety of pathogens, including extracellular schistosomula of *Schistosoma mansoni* [87], extracellular forms of *Trypanosoma brucei* [88], and *T. cruzi* [49], intracellular *Toxoplasma gondii* [89], intracellular forms of *Mycobacterium* [90], intracellular amastigotes of *Leishmania major* [91], intrahepatic forms of murine malaria *Plasmodium yoelii* and *P. berghei* [54–56], and the human parasite *P. falciparum* [unpublished observation]. The mechanisms by which ·N = O inhibits microbial growth are not known, but most likely include the capacity of larger amounts of ·N = O to inhibit the function of many of the key metabolic enzymes (discussed above) as well as DNA synthesis (ribonucleotide reductase). Additional mechanisms could include the formation of more toxic radicals when ·N = O combines with O_2^- radicals [92,93]. For example, the combination of ·N = O and O_2^- can lead to peroxynitrite formation, which can degrade to hydroxyl radical. Recent data indicate that ·N = O can directly interfere with gene transcription in bacteria, demonstrating yet another target within microbes for ·N = O [94]. Investigators have shown that ·N = O prevents the replication of DNA viruses within cells [95,96]. This, along with a recent report implicating ·N = O in neutrophil killing of *Staphylococcal aureus* organisms using cytoplasts from these cells [97], suggests that the role of ·N = O as an antimicrobial effector molecule may be much greater than originally anticipated.

Induced Nitric Oxide as an Immune Regulator

Based on the hypothesis that ·N = O derived from macrophages could have other cellular targets and potentially regulate aspects of the immune response, studies were undertaken to determine if ·N = O was responsible for the cytostasis seen in rat splenocyte mixed lymphocyte reactions. Hoffman of our laboratories found that a robust response could be induced in such cocultures following the addition of NMA to inhibit ·N = O synthesis [98]. These observations indicated that the allogeneic immune response initiated in splenocyte mixed lymphocyte reactions included ·N = O induction most likely in the macrophages and that this ·N = O was antiproliferative to lymphocytes. This observation was confirmed by others using hemoglobin to scavenge ·N = O [99,100] or anti-IFNγ monoclonal antibodies in ConA-stimulated macrophage-splenocyte cocultures [101] to promote lymphocyte proliferation. In addition, it was found that allosensitized rat sponge matrix allograft infiltrating cells produce spontaneously higher amounts of ·N = O than infiltrating cells of syngeneic grafts [102], confirming ·N = O induction during in vivo allograft responses.

Additional observations have been made supporting ·N = O induction in vascularized allograft rejection. In experimental studies, increased plasma NO_2^- + NO_3^- levels were found in recipients of heterotopic heart, orthotopic liver, and orthotopic small bowel allografts; in contrast, animals receiving syngeneic grafts showed no increase [103]. Furthermore, our laboratory showed that electron paramagnetic resonance spectroscopy analysis of rejecting heart allograft resulted in the formation of nitrosylation heme and nonheme proteins [104]. Detection of nitrosylferrohemoglobin signals by electron paramagnetic resonance spectroscopy accompanied with increased ·N = O production was also found in animals during rejection and graft-versus-host disease following small bowel transplantation [105], demonstrating that the ·N = O was produced at the graft site.

Although it is likely that macrophages represent the primary source of ·N = O involved in immune regulation, it is possible that lymphocytes also produce ·N = O [106]. Nitric oxide exerts its immunoregulatory effects not only by impairing lymphocyte function; it also affects rodent macrophage metabolic and secretory activity, and even macrophage viability [107,108]. Drapier and Hibbs [64] showed that macrophages induced to express iNOS undergo the same metabolic inhibition as tumor cells exposed to ·N = O. We have shown that rat Kupffer cells secrete more PGE_2 and IL-6 in response to IFNγ and LPS if ·N = O synthesis is inhibited [76]. Our data suggest that the PGE_2 effect may be due to a direct effect of ·N = O in cyclooxygenase activity. Recent data indicate that macrophage ·N = O may account for the sporadic apoptosis seen in LPS-stimulated murine macrophage cultures [109].

Induced Nitric Oxide in Septic and Inflammatory Responses

iNOS expression is potentially a part of any inflammatory response, either local or systemic. There is now good in vivo evidence for iNOS expression in a number of inflammatory responses. For example, LPS infusion enhances ·N = O synthesis, detected by increased circulating nitrogen oxide levels and urinary NO_3^- excretion [4,5,110]. Endotoxin injection into rodents results in high-level iNOS expression in lung, liver, kidney, heart, vascular smooth muscle, and brain [N. Hutchinson, personal communication]. Peak iNOS mRNA expression appears to occur 6 hours, and iNOS enzymatic activity 12 hours, after LPS bolus, and both return to baseline levels by 24 hours. Peak circulating levels of NO_3^- are seen at 12 hours. Studies by Kilbourn and associates [111–113] have supported the hypothesis that iNOS expression is responsible for the vascular collapse and shock in sepsis. NOS inhibitors effectively reversed the hypotension following LPS injection in rats and TNF infusion in dogs.

It is likely that ·N = O has the same effects in humans. We have demonstrated significant increases in circulating NO_3^- levels in septic humans [114]. IL-2 therapy in cancer patients is known to result in sustained hypotension. We and others have presented evidence for increased ·N = O formation in humans following IL-2 immunotherapy [115,116]. Finally, NOS inhibitors have been used to successfully reverse hypotension in two septic patients [117]. This reversal of hypotension by NOS inhibition might seem advantageous, but there may be detrimental side effects. A number of studies, including our own, suggest that iNOS inhibition using nonspecific NOS inhibitors in endotoxemia may be detrimental. If ·N = O inhibitors are administered to animals given LPS, increases in liver and intestinal damage have been observed [118,119]. Using an exaggerated model of LPS-induced injury involving first the injection of *C. parvum* followed by LPS, we have shown that ·N = O exerts a protective function by preventing microthrombosis and oxygen radical-mediated damage [120]. Our data would suggest that prostacyclin and ·N = O function together to maintain vascular-sinusoidal integrity in hepatic inflammation [121]. Conversely, ·N = O donors have been shown to reduce acute endotoxin-induced damage to the gut [122]. To realize the beneficial effects of iNOS inhibition on vascular tone, it may be necessary to develop specific iNOS inhibitors and to establish safe doses and routes of administration. In addition, pharmacologic ·N = O doses may well have to be given simultaneously. It is likely that iNOS inhibitors will simply serve to replace other less effective or less specific vasoconstrictors. Whether iNOS induction contributes to other adverse or protective aspects of sepsis is unknown. [*Editor's Note:* This discussion is typical of the quandary of inhibiting many functions of a widely distributed intermediary that likely functions at a paracrine or autocrine level.]

While sepsis represents acute systemic inflammatory response, the role of ·N = O in chronic localized inflammatory response appears to be quite different. We have shown that chondrocytes from rabbits produce large amounts of ·N = O in response to IL-1 [40]. Synovial fluid from patients with osteoarthritis exhibits elevated NO_3^- levels [unpublished observation]. It is likely that ·N = O participates in the inflammatory reaction and subsequent joint destruction in some types of immune-mediated arthritis [123]. Inhibition of ·N = O synthesis also prevents the kidney damage and joint destruction in spontaneous autoimmune disease in MRL-1pr/1pr mice, which resembles systemic lupus erythematosis in humans [124]. A second example of potentially great importance takes place in juvenile diabetes. Experimental data suggest that IL-1-induced ·N = O synthesis in pancreatic islets may interfere with insulin secretion or even damage islets [125,126]. There is also evidence for chronic expression of iNOS in the smooth muscle in atherosclerotic aortic aneurysms in humans, a disease in which there is progressive dilation and destruction of the aortic wall often leading to rupture [Simon Watkins, personal communication]. A role for ·N = O in neurodegenerative disorders has also been postulated [127]. Taken together, unlike the situation in acute expression of iNOS in sepsis or during infection where ·N = O serves a protective role, prolonged localized expression as part of pathologic inflammatory responses appears to have adverse consequences. Clearly, understanding the roles of ·N = O in localized chronic inflammation is of paramount importance to developing therapeutic strategies to combat any adverse consequences of ·N = O in these diseases.

Regulation of Nitric Oxide Synthase (NOS) Activity

The single most important distinguishing feature of cNOS versus iNOS regulation is the role of calcium/calmodulin (Figure 16-2). cNOS is activated when calmodulin binds to the cNOS in the presence of calcium, resulting in the transfer of electrons from NADPH to the active site heme group [128], presumably through prosthetic flavin groups within the enzyme. In striking contrast, the murine iNOS has a tightly bound calmodulin that keeps the enzyme tonically activated [25]. Thus, iNOS activity is regulated by substrate and cofactors, while cNOS activity is tightly controlled by calmodulin binding and dissociation. We have shown that expressed human iNOS exhibits some calcium dependency [20]. It is possible that human iNOS binds calmodulin with less avidity and is more easily down-regulated by this mechanism. Phosphorylation also plays a role in the regulation of endothelial cNOS activity. Phosphorylation of endothelial cNOS is associated with displacement of the enzyme from the plasma membrane and loss of enzyme activity [12]. The other NOS isoforms also contain potential phosphorylation sites. Whether these are, in fact, phosphorylated and play a role in the regulation of enzyme activity is not known.

A number of cofactors are required for ·N = O synthesis [129–133]. Of these, tetrahydrobiop-

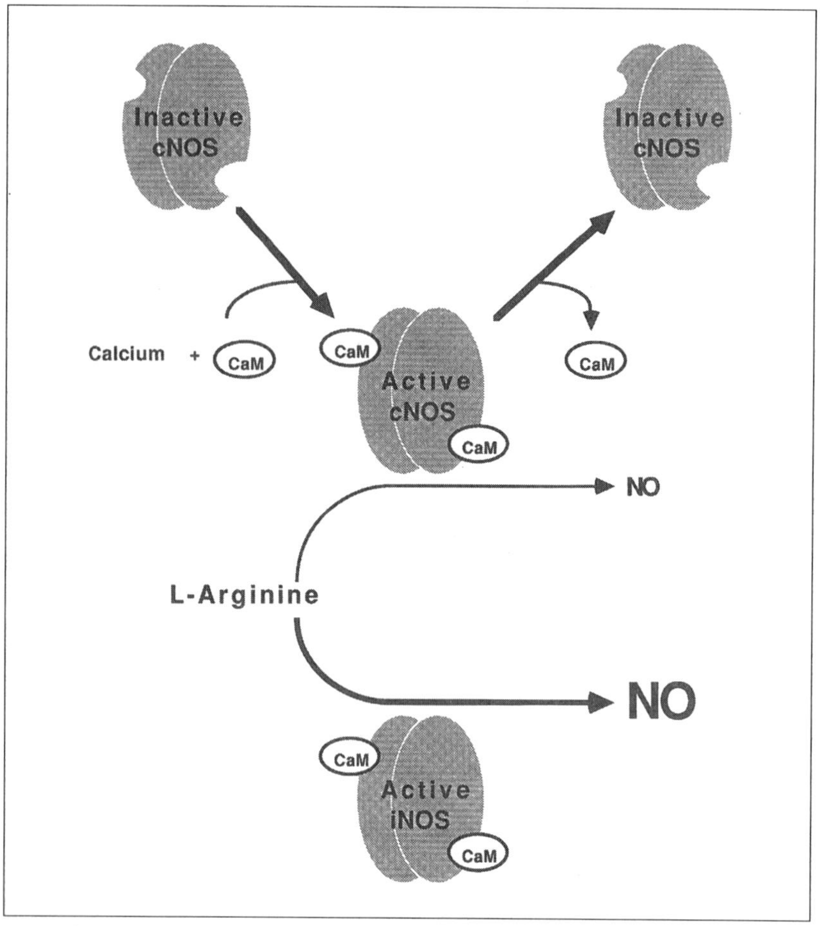

Figure 16-2. Key feature of nitric oxide synthase (NOS) regulation. The constitutive NOS (cNOS) enzymes are activated to produce ·N=O from L-arginine when, under physiologic conditions, Ca^{++} levels increase inside the cells. Ca^{++} then binds to calmodulin (CaM), which increases the affinity of the calmodulin for the cNOS enzyme. Calmodulin binding initiates ·N=O synthesis, which is believed to continue until calmodulin is no longer bound. In important contrast, calmodulin is incorporated in the inducible nitric oxide synthase (iNOS) enzyme during synthesis of the enzyme. Thus, iNOS is always in the activated state, resulting in sustained ·N=O synthesis.

terin (BH_4) appears to be rate-limiting [134]. BH_4 most likely plays a structural role in enzyme activity by maintaining the active dimeric configuration of the enzyme [135]. BH_4 levels are dependent both on de novo synthesis of BH_4 from GTP and recycling and salvage of the oxidized forms, quinone dihydrobiopterin and dihydrobiopterin, respectively. Macrophages, smooth muscle cells, and fibroblasts must co-express the rate-limiting enzyme for BH_4 synthesis, GTP-cyclohydrolase, to support iNOS activity. We have found in hepatocytes that the addition of exogenous BH_4 or the BH_4 substrate sepiapterin increases ·N=O formation [unpublished observation]. It is possible that under some conditions, iNOS activity is limited by BH_4 availability. Multiple sites for BH_4 synthesis regulation exist, and manipulations of the BH_4 pathways may provide a means to either increase or decrease ·N=O formation. For example, it has been shown that hepatocytes more effectively inhibit the pre-erythrocytic development of *Plasmodium* spp. in the presence of added BH_4 [136]. In vivo studies are needed to determine whether exogenous BH_4 sources will arrest plasmodium development at the hepatic stage in intact organisms. A recent publication suggests that NADPH synthesis may also be co-induced with iNOS [137]. The importance of NADPH availability on cNOS or iNOS activity remains to be determined.

It is likely that ·N=O may regulate its own synthesis. The first published time course of ·N=O synthesis indicated a plateau in ·N=O synthesis by 40 to 60 hours [138]. It was unknown if this was due to a feedback inhibition. Using rat hepatocytes, we have shown that maximum ·N=O production occurs 24 hours after cytokine stimulation, which is then followed by a steep decrease in ·N=O production [unpublished observation]. iNOS mRNA levels peaked in hepatocytes at 4 to 8 hours after stimulation and declined by 24 hours [38]. Added red blood cells rapidly scavenged ·N=O [139] and resulted in an increase of total NO_3^- release into the supernatant and prolonged iNOS mRNA expression. We have also found that chronic inhibition of iNOS in vivo increases iNOS levels in the liver [unpublished observation]. These data suggest that ·N=O may regulate total iNOS activity both at the mRNA level and at the level of enzyme activity. Indeed, Assreuy and co-workers [140] found that the iNOS activity can be increased by the addition of hemoglobin or decreased by ·N=O-releasing substances such as S-nitroso-acetyl-penicillamine. Rogers and Ignarro [141] gave the first evidence of a negative feedback effect of ·N=O on cNOS from cerebellum using a similar approach. Addition of exogenous ·N=O, superoxide dismutase, and electron paramagnetic resonance spectroscopy inhibited cNOS activity [141]. Delineating the mechanism of this regulation may provide additional approaches for iNOS regulation and suggests that rapid removal of ·N=O, as seen in the presence of hemoglobin, will increase total ·N=O formed.

Arginine Bioavailability and Nitric Oxide Synthase (NOS) Activity

As arginine is the only physiologic nitrogen donor for the NOS-catalyzed reaction, regulation of the availability of this essential substrate can determine cellular rates of ·N=O synthesis. Studies using ^{15}N-labeled arginine in human volunteers have indicated that less than 2% of consumed arginine is converted to ·N=O and that up to three times more orally administered arginine is converted to ·N=O than arginine given via the intravenous route. Hibbs and co-workers [115] found that about 0.1% of intravenous ^{15}N-arginine was excreted in the urine as $^{15}N_3^-$, the final product of ·N=O formation. This amount increased sevenfold in the patients given IL-2 as part of cancer immunotherapy. Ureagenesis remained constant with approximately 20% of administered arginine converted to urea. Thus, only small amounts of exogenous L-arginine are converted to ·N=O, compared to urea formation. Other sources of L-arginine are known to exist, such as endogenously produced L-arginine (discussed below). Once L-arginine enters a cell expressing iNOS, it can be utilized by several pathways. The presence of these other pathways depends on the cell type and the phenotypic status of the cell (that is, stimulated versus resting). The best-studied cell is the murine macrophage. Studies using radiotracers in unstimulated cells have shown that up to 96% of exogenous L-arginine is acted on by arginase, and the remainder goes to polyamine synthesis or protein synthesis [142]. By contrast, in stimulated cells, as much as 30% goes to ·N=O formation, with the majority of the reduction encountered in urea formation. The ultimate routes of L-arginine metabolism are likely to be very different in each organ and dependent on the presence of urea cycle enzymes that either remove or produce arginine.

Three potential sources of arginine for ·N=O synthesis exist, including L-arginine uptake via specific transmembrane transporter, endogenous biosynthesis, and free L-arginine generated by proteolysis. Recent advances have been made in understanding the relationships between L-arginine uptake, L-arginine synthesis, and induced ·N=O synthesis. Several groups have shown that arginine transport increases in macrophages stimulated to express iNOS [9,143,144]. The increased arginine transport may be due in part to the expression of an inducible transporter. In stimulated murine macrophages, recent identification of the expression of a novel arginine transporter, termed the murine cationic amino acid transporter-2B (MCAT-2B), provides evidence for the presence of an induced transporter in these cells [145]. This transporter is distinct from MCAT-1, which is expressed constitutively. Arginine transport also is stimulated by endotoxin in pulmonary artery endothelial cells [146] and is increased in liver during sepsis [147,148], suggesting that this may be a widespread adaptive response when ·N=O synthesis is induced. The basis for the increased transport in these tissues has not been established.

In tissues remote from a constant supply of arginine or where transmembrane transport of arginine may be limiting, it is likely that endogenous sources of arginine will provide substrate for ·N=O synthesis. Enzymatic biosynthesis of arginine outside of the liver is a result of the actions of argininosuccinate synthetase, which incorporates a nitrogen from aspartate into citrulline by forming argininosuccinate and argininosuccinate lyase, which converts the argininosuccinate to arginine while releasing fumerate. Low-level expression of this enzyme may be responsible for the recycling of citrulline back to arginine reported in bovine endothelial cells [149,150]. Increased conversion of citrulline to arginine has also been reported in LPS-stimulated macrophages [151]. We have shown that the expression of argininosuccinate synthetase mRNA and activity is dramatically up-regulated in murine macrophages and rat vascular smooth muscle cells stimulated to express iNOS. The expression of argininosuccinate synthetase and iNOS was similar in both cell types, suggesting that these enzymes may be co-regulated [152,153]. The functional importance of this observation was shown in experiments where exogenous citrulline enhanced macrophage ·N=O synthesis and exogenous citrulline replaced arginine for ·N=O synthesis in smooth muscle cells [unpublished observation]. It is important to point out that although the low-level expression of ar-

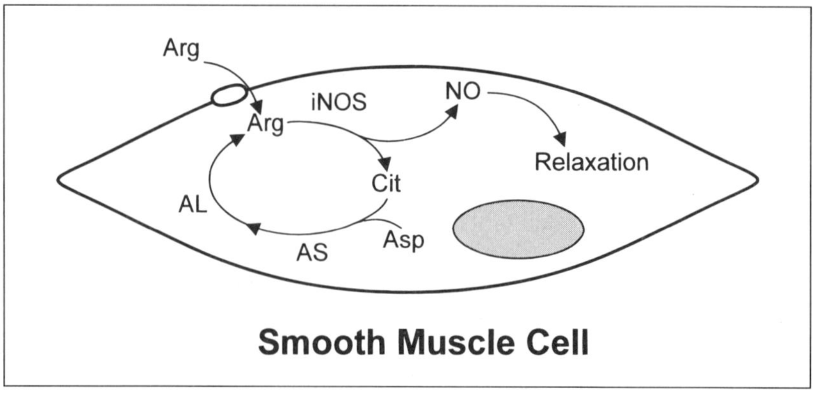

Figure 16-3. Proposed sources of L-arginine for nitric oxide (·N = O) synthesis in vascular smooth muscle. Following exposure to cytokines, inducible nitric oxide synthase (iNOS) and argininosuccinate synthetase (AS) are expressed in vascular smooth muscle cells. Arginine (Arg) taken up by the cells via specific amino acid transporters is acted upon by nitric oxide synthase (NOS), forming ·N = O and citrulline (Cit). The citrulline is then converted back to arginine by the actions of argininosuccinate synthetase and argininosuccinate lyase (AL), deriving a nitrogen from aspartate (ASP). This arginine is then available to form more ·N = O and citrulline. ·N = O causes relaxation of the smooth muscles and reduces vascular tone.

gininosuccinate lyase was not altered in these cells, the kinetics of the lyase are much more rapid than the synthetase and not likely to be limiting. The coupling of arginine and ·N = O synthesis has led us to term this pathway the *·N = O-citrulline cycle* [152,153]. We propose that increases in arginine uptake and endogenous arginine synthesis collaborate to maximize cellular capacity for ·N = O synthesis (Figure 16-3). Widespread induced expression of the arginine biosynthetic pathway may contribute to nitrogen wasting through transamination of amino acids to produce arginine. Arginine not converted to ·N = O could then be shuttled to the liver and converted to urea and citrulline. It is important to point out that even in states of maximal iNOS expression, less than 1% of total urinary nitrogen excretion occurs in the form of nitrate or nitrite [unpublished observation], indicating that the conversion of arginine to ·N = O accounts for only a fraction of nitrogen wasting. Ureagenesis represents by far the greatest source of nitrogen loss.

Compared to other cell types that express iNOS, hepatocytes are unique because they constitutively contain a complete urea cycle. Thus, hepatocytes contain high levels of arginase, which removes arginine, as well as high levels of the arginine biosynthetic enzymes. Using an isolated perfused liver system, we have studied the roles of exogenous versus endogenous sources of arginine for the synthesis of ·N = O. iNOS expression was induced by in vivo treatment with killed *C. parvum,* which results in a sustained expression of iNOS in virtually every hepatocyte with only low-level induction in the nonparenchymal cells [35]. Nitric oxide synthesis could not be detected in livers from normal rats. Livers from *C. parvum*-treated rats exhibited high-level ·N = O synthesis in the absence of exogenous arginine. This expression was doubled if excess exogenous arginine was provided. Increasing endogenous arginine synthesis via the urea cycle by providing exogenous ornithine and glutamine, which dramatically enhance urea synthesis, had no effect on ·N = O synthesis. Inclusion of physiologic levels of arginine in the perfusate increased ·N = O synthesis but not ureagenesis. Our findings indicate that ·N = O synthesis in the liver in chronic inflammation is dependent mostly on exogenous arginine, that an endogenous source of arginine separate from the urea cycle exists for ·N = O synthesis, and that arginine generated via the urea cycle is not available to iNOS [unpublished observation]. Another recent report using perfused livers from LPS-treated rats indicates that arginine derived from the urea cycle will support iNOS activity [154]. It is important to note that nonparenchymal cells are likely to represent a major source of ·N = O in this case. In addition, the LPS and *C. parvum* models are each quite unique and may account for the differences observed between the two studies.

Summary

Nitric oxide plays an important role in essentially every function vital to life and propagation of the species. Endothelial cNOS regulates the moment-to-moment changes in vascular tone throughout the body. Neuronal cNOS participates in neurotransmission in the CNS, and in the periphery it mediates critical features of GI motility and sexual function. The wide distribution of the cytokine-induced NOS has opened our eyes to the possibility that almost every cell can exhibit important antimicrobial activity via ·N = O and locally regulate the immune response. Abnormal expression of these NOS pathways is likely to play roles in many diseases.

Thus, understanding the complex regulation and functions of ·N = O synthesis is of critical importance. The key role of L-arginine and other guanidino compounds to the synthesis and regulation of ·N=O production merges the science of nutrition with numerous fields of investigation focusing on ·N=O research.

References

1. Mitchell HH, Shonle HA, Grindley HS. The origin of nitrate in the urine. *J Biol Chem* 24:461, 1916.
2. Tannenbaum SR, et al. Nitrite and nitrate are formed by endogenous synthesis in the human intestine. *Science* 200:1487, 1978.
3. Green LC, et al. Nitrate biosynthesis in man. *Proc Natl Acad Sci USA* 78:7764, 1981.
4. Green LC, Tannenbaum SR, Goldman P. Nitrate synthesis in the germfree and conventional rat. *Science* 212:56, 1981.
5. Wagner DA, Young VR, Tannenbaum SR. Mammalian nitrate biosynthesis: Incorporation of $^{15}NH_3$ into nitrate is enhanced by endotoxin treatment. *Proc Natl Acad Sci USA* 80:4518, 1983.
6. Stuehr DJ, Marletta MA. Mammalian nitrate biosynthesis: Mouse macrophages produce nitrite and nitrate in response to Escherichia coli lipopolysaccharide. *Proc Natl Acad Sci USA* 82:7738, 1985.
7. Hibbs JB Jr, Taintor RR, Vavrin Z. Macrophage cytotoxicity: Role for L-arginine deiminase and imino nitrogen oxidation to nitrite. *Science* 235:473, 1987.
8. Palmer RMJ, Ferrige AG, Moncada S. Nitric oxide release accounts for the biological activity of endothelium-derived relaxing factor. *Nature* 327:524, 1987.
9. Ignarro LJ, et al. Endothelium-derived relaxing factor produced and released from artery and vein is nitric oxide. *Proc Natl Acad Sci USA* 84:9265, 1987.
10. Furchgott RF, Zawadzki JV. The obligatory role of endothelial cells in the relaxation of arterial smooth muscle by acetylcholine. *Nature* 228:373, 1980.
11. Palmer RMJ, Ashton DS, Moncada S. Vascular endothelial cells synthesize nitric oxide from L-arginine. *Nature* 333:664, 1988.
12. Marletta MA, et al. Macrophage oxidation of L-arginine to nitrite and nitrate: Nitric oxide is an intermediate. *Biochemistry* 27:8706, 1988.
13. Hibbs JB Jr, et al. Nitric oxide: A cytotoxic activated macrophage effector molecule. *Biochem Biophys Res Commun* 157:87, 1988.
14. Stuehr DJ, et al. Activated murine macrophages secrete a metabolite of arginine with the bioactivity of endothelium-derived relaxing factor and the chemical reactivity of nitric oxide. *J Exp Med* 169:1011, 1989.
15. Garthwaite J, Charles SL, Chess-Williams R. Endothelium-derived relaxing factor release on activation of NMDA receptors suggests role as messenger in the brain. *Nature* 336:385, 1988.
16. Stuehr DJ, Griffith OW. Mammalian nitric oxide synthases. *Adv Enzymol Relat Areas Mol Biol* 65:287, 1992.
17. Feldman PL, Griffith OW, Stuehr DJ. The surprising life of nitric oxide. *Chem Engin News* 71(51):26, 1993.
18. Marsden PA, et al. Molecular cloning and characterizations of human endothelial nitric oxide synthase. *FEBS Lett* 307:287, 1992.
19. Bredt DS, et al. Cloned and expressed nitric oxide synthase structurally resembles cytochrome P-450 reductase. *Nature* 351:714, 1991.
20. Geller DA, et al. Molecular cloning and expression of inducible nitric oxide synthase from human hepatocytes. *Proc Natl Acad Sci USA* 90:3491, 1993.
21. Janssens SP, et al. Cloning and expression of cDNA encoding human endothelium-derived relaxing factor/nitric oxide synthase. *J Biol Chem* 267:14519, 1992.
22. Marsden PA, et al. Structure and chromosomal localization of the human constitutive endothelial nitric oxide synthase gene. *J Biol Chem* 268:17478, 1992.
23. Chartrain NA, et al. Molecular cloning, structure, and chromosomal localization of the human inducible nitric oxide synthase gene. *J Biol Chem* 269:6765, 1994.
24. Bredt DS, Snyder SH. Isolation of nitric oxide synthetase, a calmodulin-requiring enzyme. *Proc Natl Acad Sci USA* 87:682, 1990.
25. Cho HJ, et al. Calmodulin is a subunit of nitric oxide synthase from macrophages. *J Exp Med* 176:599, 1992.
26. O'Dell TJ, et al. Endothelial NOS and the blockade of LTP by NOS inhibitor in mice lacking neuronal NOS. *Science* 265:542, 1994.
27. Bredt DS, et al. Nitric oxide synthase protein and mRNA are discretely localized in neuronal populations of the mammalian CNS together with NADPH diaphorase. *Neuron* 7:615, 1991.
28. Nakane M, et al. Cloned human brain nitric oxide synthase is highly expressed in skeletal muscle. *FEBS Lett* 316:175, 1993.
29. Lorsbach RB, et al. Expression of the nitric oxide synthase gene in mouse macrophages activated for tumor cell killing. *J Biol Chem* 268:1908, 1993.
30. Nussler AK, Billiar TR. Inflammation, immunoregulation, and inducible nitric oxide synthase. *J Leukoc Biol* 54:171, 1993.
31. Werner-Felmayer G, et al. Tetrahydrobiopterin-dependent formation of nitrite and nitrate in murine fibroblasts. *J Exp Med* 172:1599, 1990.
32. Busse R, Mülsch A. Induction of nitric oxide synthase by cytokines in vascular smooth muscle cells. *FEBS Lett* 275:87, 1990.
33. Curran RD, et al. Hepatocytes produce nitrogen oxides from L-arginine in response to inflammatory products of Kupffer cells. *J Exp Med* 170:1769, 1989.
34. Schulz R, Nava E, Moncada S. Induction and potential biological relevance of a Ca^{2+}-independent nitric oxide synthase in the myocardium. *Br J Pharmacol* 105:575, 1992.
35. Billiar TR, et al. Inducible cytosolic enzyme activity for the production of nitrogen oxides from L-arginine in hepatocytes. *Biochem Biophys Res Commun* 168:1034, 1990.
36. Billiar TR, et al. Modulation of nitrogen oxide synthesis in vivo: N^G-monomethyl-L-arginine inhibits endotoxin-induced nitrite/nitrate biosynthesis while promoting hepatic damage. *J Leukoc Biol* 48:565, 1990.
37. Curran RD, et al. Multiple cytokines are required to induce hepatocyte nitric oxide production and inhibit total protein synthesis. *Ann Surg* 212:462, 1990.
38. Geller DA, et al. Cytokines, endotoxin, and glucocorticoids regulate the expression of inducible nitric oxide synthase in hepatocytes. *Proc Natl Acad Sci USA* 90:522, 1993.
39. Beasley D, Schwartz JH, Brenner BM. Interleukin 1 induces prolonged L-arginine-dependent cyclic guanosine monophosphate and nitrite production in rat vascular smooth muscle cells. *J Clin Invest* 87:602, 1991.
40. Stadler J, et al. Articular chondrocytes synthesize nitric

oxide in response to cytokines and lipopolysaccharide. *J Immunol* 147:3915, 1991.

41. Freeswick PD, et al. Remote tissue injury primes hepatocytes for nitric oxide synthesis. *J Surg Res* 57:205, 1994.
42. Xie Q-W, Whisnan R, Nathan C. Promoter of the mouse gene encoding calcium-independent nitric oxide synthase confers inducibility by interferon γ and bacterial lipopolysaccharide. *J Exp Med* 177:1779, 1993.
43. Lowenstein CJ, et al. Macrophage nitric oxide synthase gene: Two upstream regions mediate induction by interferon γ and lipopolysaccharide. *Proc Natl Acad Sci USA* 90:9730, 1993.
44. Heinrich PC, Castell JV, Andus T. Interleukin-6 and the acute phase response. *Biochem J* 265:621, 1990.
45. Morris SM Jr, Billiar TR. New insights into the regulation of inducible nitric oxide synthesis. *Am J Physiol* 266:E829, 1994.
46. Xie QW, et al. Cloning and characterization of inducible nitric oxide synthase from mouse macrophages. *Science* 256:225, 1992.
47. Lowenstein CJ, et al. Cloned and expressed macrophage nitric oxide synthase contrasts with the brain enzyme. *Proc Natl Acad Sci USA* 89:6711, 1992.
48. Lyons CR, Orloffs GJ, Cunningham JM. Molecular cloning and functional expression of an inducible nitric oxide synthase from a murine macrophage cell line. *J Biol Chem* 267:6370, 1992.
49. Muñoz-Fernandez MA, Fernandez MA, Fresno M. Activation of human macrophages for the killing of intracellular Trypanosoma cruzi by TNF-α and IFN-g through a nitric oxide-dependent mechanism. *Immunol Lett* 33:35, 1992.
50. Hunt NCA, Goldin RD. Nitric oxide production by monocytes in alcoholic liver disease. *J Hepatol* 14:146, 1992.
51. Charles IG, et al. Cloning, characterization, and expression of a cDNA encoding an inducible nitric oxide synthase from the human chondrocyte. *Proc Natl Acad Sci USA* 90:11419, 1993.
52. Sherman PA, et al. Purification and cDNA sequence of an inducible nitric oxide synthase from a human tumor cell line. *Biochemistry* 32:11600, 1993.
53. Wood ER, et al. Hepatocytes and macrophages express an identical cytokine inducible nitric oxide synthase gene. *Biochem Biophys Res Commun* 191:767, 1993.
54. Mellouk S, et al. IFN-γ inhibits development of Plasmodium berghei exoerythrocytic stages in hepatocytes by an L-arginine-dependent effector mechanism. *J Immunol* 146:3971, 1991.
55. Nussler A, et al. L-arginine-dependent destruction of intrahepatic malaria parasites in response to tumor necrosis factor and/or interleukin 6 stimulation. *Eur J Immunol* 21:227, 1991.
56. Nussler AK, et al. In vivo induction of the nitric oxide pathway in hepatocytes after injection with irradiated malaria sporozoites, malaria blood parasites or adjuvants. *Eur J Immunol* 23:882, 1993.
57. Li L, et al. Role of nitric oxide in lysis of tumor cells by cytokine-activated endothelial cells. *Cancer Res* 51:2531, 1991.
58. Drapier J-C, Weitzerbin J, Hibbs JB Jr. Interferon-γ and tumor necrosis factor induce the L-arginine-dependent cytotoxic effector mechanism in murine macrophages. *Eur J Immunol* 18:1587, 1988.
59. Kwon NS, Stuehr DJ, Nathan CF. Inhibition of tumor cell ribonucleotide reductase by macrophage-derived nitric oxide. *J Exp Med* 174:761, 1991.
60. Miwa M, et al. Nitrosation of amines by stimulated macrophages. *Carcinogenesis* 8:955, 1987.
61. Iyengar R, Stuehr DJ, Marletta MA. Macrophage synthesis of nitrite, nitrate, and N-nitrosamines: Precursors and role of the respiratory burst. *Proc Natl Acad Sci USA* 84:6369, 1987.
62. Kosaka H, et al. Nitrosation by stimulated macrophages: Inhibitors, enhancers and substrates. *Carcinogenesis* 10:563, 1989.
63. Stadler J, et al. Effect of exogenous and endogenous nitric oxide on mitochondrial respiration of rat hepatocytes. *Am J Physiol* 260:C910, 1991.
64. Drapier J-C, Hibbs JB Jr. Differentiation of murine macrophages to express nonspecific cytotoxicity for tumor cells results in L-arginine-dependent inhibition of mitochondrial iron-sulfur enzymes in the macrophage effector cells. *J Immunol* 140:2829, 1988.
65. McDonald B, et al. Glyceraldehyde-3-phosphate dehydrogenase is required for the transport of nitric oxide in platelets. *Proc Natl Acad Sci USA* 90:11122, 1993.
66. Keaney JF Jr, et al. NO forms an adduct with serum albumin that has endothelium-derived relaxing factor-like properties. *J Clin Invest* 91:1582, 1993.
67. Gaston B, et al. Endogenous nitrogen oxides and bronchodilator S-nitrosothiols in human airways. *Proc Natl Acad Sci USA* 90:10957, 1993.
68. Waldman SA, Murad R. Cyclic GMP synthesis and function. *Pharmacol Rev* 394:163, 1987.
69. Ignarro LJ, et al. Endothelium-derived relaxing factor produced and released from artery and vein is nitric oxide. *Proc Natl Acad Sci USA* 84:9265, 1987.
70. Radomski MW, Palmer RMJ, Moncada S. Endogenous nitric oxide inhibits human platelet adhesion to vascular endothelium. *Lancet* 2:1057, 1987.
71. Mellion BT, et al. Evidence for the inhibitory role of guanosine 3′:5′-monophosphate in ADP induced human platelet aggregation in the presence of nitric oxide and related vasodilators. *Blood* 57:946, 1981.
72. Kaplan SS, et al. Inhibition of neutrophil chemotaxis with N^G-monomethyl-L-arginine: A role for cyclic GMP. *Blood* 74:1885, 1989.
73. Billiar TR, et al. Association between synthesis and release of cGMP and nitric oxide biosynthesis by hepatocytes. *Am J Physiol* 262:C1077, 1992.
74. Molina y Vedia L, et al. Nitric oxide-induced S-nitrosylation of glyceraldehyde-3-phosphate dehydrogenase inhibits its enzymatic activity and increases endogenous ADP-ribosylation. *J Biol Chem* 267:24929, 1992.
75. Salvemini D, et al. Nitric oxide activates cyclooxygenase enzymes. *Proc Natl Acad Sci USA* 90:7240, 1993.
76. Stadler J, et al. Endogenous nitric oxide inhibits the synthesis of cyclooxygenase products and interleukin-6 by rat Kupffer cells. *J Leukoc Biol* 53:165, 1993.
77. Dimmeler S, Lottspeich F, Brune B. Nitric oxide causes ADP-ribosylation and inhibition of glyceraldehyde-3-phosphate dehydrogenase. *J Biol Chem* 267:1, 1992.
78. McDonald LJ, Moss J. Stimulation by nitric oxide of an NAD linkage to glyceraldehyde-3-phosphate dehydrogenase. *Proc Natl Acad Sci USA* 90:6238, 1993.
79. Lepoivre M, et al. Alteration of ribonucleotide reductase activity following induction of the nitrite-generating pathway in adenocarcinoma cells. *J Biol Chem* 265:14143, 1990.
80. Khatsenko OG, et al. Nitric oxide is a mediator of the decrease in cytochrome P450-dependent metabolism caused by immunostimulants. *Proc Natl Acad Sci USA* 90:11147, 1993.

81. Clancy RM, Leszczynska-Piziak J, Abramson SB. Nitric oxide, an endothelial cell relaxation factor, inhibits neutrophil superoxide anion production via a direct action on the NADPH oxidase. *J Clin Invest* 90:1116, 1992.

82. Billiar TR, et al. An L-arginine-dependent mechanism mediates Kupffer cell inhibition of hepatocyte protein synthesis in vitro. *J Exp Med* 169:1467, 1989.

83. Nathan CF, Hibbs JB Jr. Role of nitric oxide synthesis in macrophage antimicrobial activity. *Curr Opin Immunol* 3:65, 1991.

84. Reddy D, Lancaster JR Jr, Cornforth DP. Nitrite inhibition of Clostridium botulinum: Electron spin resonance detection of iron-nitric oxide complexes. *Science* 221:769, 1983.

85. Woods LFJ, Wood JM, Gibbs PA. The involvement of nitric oxide in the inhibition of the phosphoro-clastic system in Clostridium sporogenes by sodium nitrite. *J Gen Microbiol* 125:399, 1981.

86. Granger DL, et al. Specific amino acid (L-arginine) requirement for the microbiostatic activity of murine macrophages. *J Clin Invest* 81:1129, 1988.

87. James SL, Glaven J. Macrophage cytotoxicity against schistosomula of Schistosoma mansoni involves arginine-dependent production of reactive nitrogen intermediates. *J Immunol* 143:4208, 1989.

88. Vincendeau P, et al. Nitric oxide-mediated cytostatic activity on Trypanosoma brucei gambiense and Trypanosoma brucei brucei. *Exp Parasitol* 75:353, 1992.

89. Adams LB, et al. Microbiostatic effect of murine-activated macrophages for Toxoplasma gondii: Role for synthesis of inorganic nitrogen oxides from L-arginine. *J Immunol* 144:2725, 1990.

90. Adams LB, et al. L-arginine-dependent macrophage effector functions inhibit metabolic activity of Mycobacterium leprae. *J Immunol* 147:1642, 1991.

91. Green SJ, et al. Activated macrophages destroy intracellular Leishmania major amastigotes by an L-arginine-dependent killing mechanism. *J Immunol* 144:278, 1990.

92. Beckman JS, et al. Apparent hydroxyl radical production by peroxynitrite: Implications for endothelial injury from nitric oxide and superoxide. *Proc Natl Acad Sci USA* 87:1620, 1990.

93. Nathan CF, et al. Identification of interferon-gamma as the lymphokine that activates human macrophage oxidative metabolism and antimicrobial activity. *J Exp Med* 158:670, 1983.

94. Nunoshiba T, et al. Activation by nitric oxide of an oxidative-stress response that defends Escherichia coli against activated macrophages. *Proc Natl Acad Sci USA* 90:9993, 1993.

95. Croen KD. Evidence for an antiviral effect of nitric oxide: Inhibition of herpes simplex virus type 1 replication. *J Clin Invest* 91:2446, 1993.

96. Karupiah G, Xie Q-w, Buller RML, et al. Inhibition of viral replication by interferon-γ-induced nitric oxide synthase. *Science* 261:1445, 1993.

97. Malawista SE, Montgomery RR, Van Blaricom G. Evidence for reactive nitrogen intermediates in killing of staphylococci by human neutrophil cytoplasts. *J Clin Invest* 90:631, 1992.

98. Hoffman RA, et al. Alloantigen-induced activation of rat splenocytes is regulated by the oxidative metabolism of L-arginine. *J Immunol* 145:2220, 1990.

99. Albina JE, Henry WL Jr. Suppression of lymphocyte proliferation through the nitric oxide synthesizing pathway. *J Surg Res* 50:403, 1991.

100. Mills CD. Molecular basis of "suppressor" macrophages: Arginine metabolism via the nitric oxide synthetase pathway. *J Immunol* 146:2719, 1991.

101. Albina JE, Abate JA, Henry WL Jr. Nitric oxide production is required for mouse resident peritoneal macrophages to suppress mitogen-stimulated T cell proliferation: Role of IFN-γ in the induction of the nitric oxide-synthesizing pathway. *J Immunol* 147:144, 1991.

102. Langrehr JM, et al. Nitric oxide synthesis in the in vivo allograft response: A possible regulatory mechanism. *Surgery* 110:335, 1991.

103. Langrehr JM, et al. Nitric oxide production in host-versus-graft and graft-versus-host reactions in the rat. *J Clin Invest* 90:679, 1992.

104. Lancaster JR Jr, et al. EPR detection of heme and nonheme iron-containing protein nitrosylation by nitric oxide during rejection of rat heart allograft. *J Biol Chem* 267:10994, 1992.

105. Langrehr JM, et al. Detection of nitric oxide by EPR spectroscopy during rejection and graft-versus-host disease following small-bowel transplantation in the rat. *Surgery* 112:395, 1992.

106. Kirk SJ, Regan MC, Barbul A. Cloned murine T lymphocytes synthesize a molecule with the biological characteristics of nitric oxide. *Biochem Biophys Res Commun* 173:660, 1990.

107. Albina JE, et al. Regulation of macrophage physiology by L-arginine: Role of the oxidative L-arginine deiminase pathway. *J Immunol* 143:3641, 1989.

108. Albina JE, et al. Regulation of macrophage functions by L-arginine. *J Exp Med* 169:1021, 1989.

109. Albina JE, et al. Nitric oxide-mediated apoptosis in murine peritoneal macrophages. *J Immunol* 150:5080, 1993.

110. Granger DL, Hibbs JB Jr, Broadnax LM. Urinary nitrate excretion in relation to murine macrophage activation: Influence of dietary L-arginine and oral N^G-monomethyl-L-arginine. *J Immunol* 146:1294, 1991.

111. Kilbourn RG, et al. Reversal of endotoxin-mediated shock by N^G-methyl-L-arginine, an inhibitor of nitric oxide synthesis. *Biochem Biophys Res Commun* 172:1132, 1991.

112. Kilbourn RG, et al. N^G-methyl-L-arginine inhibits tumor necrosis factor-induced hypotension: Implications for the involvement of nitric oxide. *Proc Natl Acad Sci USA* 87:3629, 1990.

113. Klabunde RE, Ritger RC. N^G-monomethyl-L-arginine (NMA) restores arterial blood pressure but reduces cardiac output in a canine model of endotoxic shock. *Biochem Biophys Res Commun* 178:1135, 1991.

114. Ochoa JB, et al. Nitrogen oxide levels in patients after trauma and sepsis. *Ann Surg* 214:621, 1991.

115. Hibbs JB Jr, et al. Evidence for cytokine-inducible nitric oxide synthesis from L-arginine in patients receiving interleukin-2 therapy. *J Clin Invest* 89:867, 1992.

116. Ochoa JB, et al. Increased circulating nitrogen oxides after human tumor immunotherapy: Correlation with toxic hemodynamic changes. *J Natl Cancer Inst* 84:864, 1992.

117. Petros A, Bennett D, Vallance P. Effect of nitric oxide synthase inhibitors on hypotension in patients with septic shock. *Lancet* 338:1557, 1991.

118. Seekamp A, et al. Requirements for neutrophil products and L-arginine in ischemia-reperfusion injury. *Am J Pathol* 142:1217, 1993.

119. Hutcheson AR, Whittle BJR, Boughton-Smith NK. Role of nitric oxide in maintaining vascular integrity in endotoxin-induced acute intestinal damage in the rat. *Br J Pharmacol* 101:815, 1990.

120. Harbrecht BG, et al. Inhibition of nitric oxide synthesis during endotoxemia promotes intrahepatic thrombosis and an oxygen radical-mediated hepatic injury. *J Leukoc Biol* 52:390, 1992.

121. Harbrecht BG, et al. Nitric oxide and prostacyclin interact to prevent hepatic damage during murine endotoxemia. *Am J Physiol* 266:G1004, 1994.

122. Boughton-Smith NK, et al. Protective effect of S-nitroso-N-acetyl-penicillamine in endotoxin-induced acute intestinal damage in the rat. *Eur J Pharmacol* 191:485, 1990.

123. McCartney-Francis N, et al. Suppression of arthritis by an inhibitor of nitric oxide synthase. *J Exp Med* 178:749, 1993.

124. Weinberg JB, et al. The role of nitric oxide in the pathogenesis of spontaneous murine autoimmune disease: Increased nitric oxide production and nitric oxide synthase expression in MRL-1pr/1pr mice, and reduction of spontaneous nephritis and arthritis by orally administered N^G-monomethyl-L-arginine. *J Exp Med* 179:651, 1994.

125. Corbett JA, et al. Interleukin-1-β-induced formation of EPR-detectable iron-nitrosyl complexes in Islets of Langerhans: Role of nitric oxide in interleukin-1-β-induced inhibition of insulin secretion. *J Biol Chem* 266:21351, 1991.

126. Corbett JA, et al. Nitric oxide and cGMP formation induced by interleukin-1β in Islets of Langerhans: Evidence for an effector role of nitric oxide in islet dysfunction. *Biochem J* 287:229, 1992.

127. Koprowski H, et al. In vivo expression of inducible nitric oxide synthase in experimentally induced neurological diseases. *Proc Natl Acad Sci USA* 90:3024, 1993.

128. Abu-Soud HM, Stuehr DJ. Nitric oxide synthases reveal a role for calmodulin in controlling electron transfer. *Proc Natl Acad Sci USA* 90:10769, 1993.

129. Nathan C. Nitric oxide as a secretory product of mammalian cells. *FASEB J* 6:3051, 1992.

130. Stuehr DJ, Kwon NS, Nathan CF. FAD and GSH participate in macrophage synthesis of nitric oxide. *Biochem Biophys Res Commun* 168:558, 1990.

131. Stuehr DJ, et al. Purification and characterization of the cytokine-induced macrophage nitric oxide synthase: An FAD- and FMN-containing flavoprotein. *Proc Natl Acad Sci USA* 88:7773, 1991.

132. Kwon NS, Nathan CF, Stuehr DJ. Reduced biopterin as a cofactor in the generation of nitrogen oxides by murine macrophages. *J Biol Chem* 264:20496, 1989.

133. Mayer B, John M, Heinzel B. Brain nitric oxide synthase is a biopterin- and flavin-containing multi-functional oxido-reductase. *FEBS Lett* 288:187, 1991.

134. Gross SS, Levi R. Tetrahydrobiopterin synthesis: An absolute requirement for cytokine-induced nitric oxide generation by vascular smooth muscle. *J Biol Chem* 267:25722, 1992.

135. Baek KJ, et al. Macrophage nitric oxide synthase subunits: Purification, characterization, and role of prosthetic groups and substrate in regulating their association into a dimeric enzyme. *J Biol Chem* 268: 21120, 1993.

136. Mellouk S, et al. Nitric oxide-mediated antiplasmodial activity in human and murine hepatocytes induced by gamma interferon and the parasite itself: Enhancement by exogenous tetrahydrobiopterin. *Infect Immun* 62:4043, 1994.

137. Corraliza IM, et al. Parallel induction of nitric oxide and glucose-6-phosphate dehydrogenase in activated bone marrow derived macrophages. *Biochem Biophys Res Commun* 196:342, 1993.

138. Stuehr DJ, Marletta MA. Induction of nitrite/nitrate synthesis in murine macrophages by BCG infection, lymphokines or interferon-gamma. *J Immunol* 139:518, 1987.

139. Stadler J, et al. Nonheme iron-nitrosyl complex formation in rat hepatocytes: Detection by electron paramagnetic resonance spectroscopy. *Arch Biochem Biophys* 302:4, 1993.

140. Assreuy J, et al. Feedback inhibition of nitric oxide synthase activity by nitric oxide. *Br J Pharmacol* 108:833, 1993.

141. Rogers NE, Ignarro LJ. Constitutive nitric oxide synthase from cerebellum is reversibly inhibited by nitric oxide formed from L-arginine. *Biochem Biophys Res Commun* 189:242, 1992.

142. Granger DL, et al. Metabolic fate of L-arginine in relation to microbiostatic capability of murine macrophages. *J Clin Invest* 85:264, 1990.

143. Bogle RG, et al. L-arginine transport is increased in macrophages generating nitric oxide. *Biochem J* 284:15, 1992.

144. Sato H, Fujiwara M, Bannai S. Effect of lipopolysaccharide on transport and metabolism of arginine in mouse peritoneal macrophages. *J Leukoc Biol* 52:161, 1992.

145. Closs EI, et al. Characterization of the third member of the MCAT family of cationic amino acid transporters: Identification of a domain that determines the transport properties of the MCAT proteins. *J Biol Chem* 268:20796, 1993.

146. Lind DS, Copeland EM III, Souba WW. Endotoxin stimulates arginine transport in pulmonary artery endothelial cells. *Surgery* 114:199, 1993.

147. Sax HC, et al. Amino acid uptake in isolated, perfused liver: Effect of trauma and sepsis. *J Surg Res* 45:50, 1988.

148. Inoue Y, et al. Arginine transport in human liver: Characterization and effects of nitric oxide synthase inhibitors. *Ann Surg* 218:350, 1993.

149. Mitchell JA, et al. Cultured endothelial cells maintain their L-arginine level despite the continuous release of EDRF. *Eur J Pharmacol* 182:573, 1990.

150. Hecker M, et al. The metabolism of L-arginine and its significance for the biosynthesis of endothelium-derived relaxing factor: Cultured endothelial cells recycle L-citrulline to L-arginine. *Proc Natl Acad Sci USA* 87:8612, 1990.

151. Wu G, Brosnan JT. Macrophages can convert citrulline into arginine. *Biochem J* 281:45, 1992.

152. Nussler AK, et al. Coinduction of nitric oxide synthase and arginino-succinate synthetase in a murine macrophage cell line: Implications for regulation of nitric oxide production. *J Biol Chem* 269:1257, 1994.

153. Morris SM Jr, et al. Co-induction of NO Synthase and Arginino-succinate Synthase Gene Expression: Implications for Regulation of NO synthesis. In *Proceedings of the Third International Meeting on the Biology of Nitric Oxide,* in press.

154. Wettstein M, Wolfgang G, Haussinger D. Endotoxin-induced nitric oxide synthesis in the perfused rat liver: Effects of L-arginine and ammonium chloride. *Hepatology* 19:641, 1994.

Selected Readings

Geller DA, et al. Cytokines, endotoxin, and glucocorticoids regulate the expression of inducible nitric oxide synthase in hepatocytes. *Proc Natl Acad Sci USA* 90:522, 1993.

This article provides conclusive evidence that humans express an inducible nitric oxide synthase and describes the gene that encodes for this enzyme.

Granger DL, et al. Metabolic fate of L-arginine in relation to microbiostatic capability of murine macrophages. *J Clin Invest* 85:264, 1990.

This article describes the fate of L-arginine once it enters a cell such as a macrophage.

Granger DL, Hibbs JB Jr, Broadnax LM. Urinary nitrate excretion in relation to murine macrophage activation: Influence of dietary L-arginine and oral N^G-monomethyl-L-arginine. *J Immunol* 146:1294, 1991.

This article describes urinary excretion of nitrogen oxides and the influence of dietary arginine on this excretion in mice.

Morris SM Jr, Billiar TR. New insights into the regulation of inducible nitric oxide synthesis. *Am J Physiol* 266:E829, 1994.

This recent review delves more deeply into the molecular mechanisms of inducible nitric oxide synthase regulation.

Ochoa JB, et al. Nitrogen oxide levels in patients after trauma and sepsis. *Ann Surg* 214:621, 1991.

This article describes nitrogen oxide, arginine, and citrulline levels in septic human adults.

17

Translocation as It Applies to Metabolism

J. Wesley Alexander
Roberto Gennari

The intestinal tract is one of the most complex organs in the body, being composed of dozens of different types of cells that produce hundreds of hormones, mediators, and cytokines that have thousands of biologic effects. In addition, the metabolic capacity of the intestine is comparable to that of the liver, and the absorptive area of the intestine, only one cell layer in thickness, covers approximately 2 million square centimeters in man: about 100 times the skin surface area. This acts as a barrier to an enormous number of intestinal microbes, numbering more than 1000 times the total number of people inhabiting the earth. Moreover the lymphoid mass of the intestine approximates that of the spleen and produces a large amount of circulating antibody; 90% of antibodies in the blood have specificity for intestinal microorganisms.

Metabolically, enterocytes are extremely active with a repletion rate of approximately three to five days in man, and 17 billion intestinal cells are replaced daily. Medical scientists have been concerned primarily with the absorptive, digestive, and excretory functions of the gut, and the barrier function of the gut has been largely ignored until the past few decades. This lack of interest is, perhaps, because of the incredibly efficient ability of the epithelial cells to prevent the passage of microbes through them despite a highly developed function to absorb digested and partially digested foods and even intact proteins and particles. There is more recent evidence, however, that failure of

Supported in part by USPHS Grant AI-12936.

gut barrier function may contribute to poor outcome, including death, in critically ill patients.

This review summarizes the highlights of both human and animal studies on the barrier function of the gut to place in perspective the potential importance of the process in human disease and modern therapy.

Historical Background

Fraenkel, in 1891, was the first to suggest that viable bacteria could pass through an intact intestinal wall [1]. This process was first called Durchwanderungs, or "wandering through," and was felt to be a cause of peritonitis.

In 1895, Flexner [2] provided pathologic evidence from two patients with pneumococcal peritonitis that the microorganisms had penetrated through the nonperforated intestinal wall to invade deeper structures and finally appear in the peritoneal cavity. He demonstrated that these organisms invaded the glandular layer reaching near, but not quite to, the muscularis mucosa. They could also be found in the lymphatic spaces in the subserosal coat. Shortly after the turn of the century, Hornemann [3] provided evidence that intestinal disease increased the likelihood that bacteria could migrate through to the peritoneum. Further, in 1923 Mandl [4] showed that peritonitis could occur from bacteria translocating from the normal intestine to the peritoneal cavity.

The concept of bacterial translocation was even more clearly defined in a series of experiments published by Arnold and his colleagues from 1928 to 1930 [5–7]. His experiments used dogs with thoracic duct cannulation under local anesthesia and subcutaneous placement of the duodenum to make injection of bacteria into it relatively easy. When bacteria were introduced into the duodenum, they generally could not be found in the thoracic duct lymph or blood. However, because previous experiments showed that alkalinization of the duodenum was accompanied by peripheral leukocytosis, it was reasoned that alkalinization might have an influence on microbial permeability of the gut wall. When these investigators injected bacteria mixed with an alkaline solution and egg white into the duodenum, high numbers of bacteria (500 to 1000/ml) could be recovered from thoracic duct lymph beginning as early as 5 minutes after the infusion. Appropriate controls using injection of bacteria mixed with an alkaline solution and no egg white or bacteria and egg white in a neutral solution failed to cause translocation. Translocation in these experiments was associated with an elevation of body temperature and blood leukocytosis. In some experiments, leukopenia was seen when there were high levels of bacteria in the blood during the initial 30 minutes after inoculation. These experiments showed beyond a doubt that translocation could occur across the normal mucosa of an experimental animal under certain conditions, especially with alkalinization of the duodenal contents in the presence of protein. Further experiments showed that elevation of the external environmental temperature of the animal could cause enough stress to alter the typical flora in the post-pyloric region, shifting it to a fecal type. These studies appeared to be the first to demonstrate translocation from the gut to the lymphatic system.

In 1931, Fisher [8] demonstrated that translocation of yeast could occur through the intestinal mucosa of normal dogs. Using an experimental model similar to Arnold's, one cake of yeast was suspended in 25 ml of saline and injected into the duodenum of fasting anesthetized animals. Other animals received the yeast by oral administration. Fisher was able to demonstrate translocation of the yeast to the liver and lymph in 20% to 40% of the animals within one hour, and viable colonies of yeast could be cultured from the portal vein. In another experiment, direct injection of less than 1 million yeast into the portal vein failed to be associated with dissemination to lungs, spleen, and kidney. These experiments were the first to demonstrate translocation of fungi across the intact intestinal mucosa and the first to demonstrate translocation from the gut to distant organs.

An incredibly incisive experiment done by Flory, the discoverer of penicillin, was reported in 1933 [9]. He showed that inert carbon particles (graphite) were prevented from contacting intestinal mucosal cells by the mucous layer. However, when *B. aertrycke,* a pathogenic organism, was injected into bowel loops of guinea pigs and then examined histologically, the organism could be seen to penetrate directly into the epithelial cells with no evidence of damage to the epithelial cells by light microscopy. Less frequently, bacteria were felt to penetrate between cells or through minute ulcerations. His observations showed that the bacteria could pass into the lamina propria from the basal end of the epithelial cells. This was, perhaps, the first evidence showing how bacteria penetrate directly through enterocytes.

In 1949, Schweinburg and Heimburg [10] produced chemical peritonitis in rabbits and dogs by repeated injections of monilate or gum-tragacanth, which resulted in the appearance of *E. coli* in the peritoneal exudate. This was interpreted to represent the passage of bacteria through the intact bowel wall.

Although during the 1940s several other investigators demonstrated transmural migration of organisms from the intestine in uremia, there seemed to be little attention paid to the early, clear demonstrations of translocation in experimental models until the concept was resurrected by Fine and his colleagues in the 1950s [11,12]. These investigators provided evidence that irreversible shock following hemorrhage was a result of invasion of the body by intestinal flora and endotoxin instead of the consequence of tissue hypoxia itself. In their studies, which used a standard model of hemorrhagic shock in dogs, the administration of antibiotics improved survival from 14% to 88%. The best results were with oral aureomycin or oral neomycin given as a large priming dose prior to the experiment. Interestingly, other experiments showed that aureomycin given in the portal vein was more effective than aureomycin given intravenously. They recommended that all patients in shock who were not responsive to transfusions receive antibiotic therapy. Schweinburg and Fine [13] provided further evidence that the animals subjected to several different types of shock developed toxic substances in their plasma that could be reduced by the administration of oral antibiotics before the induction of shock. They reasoned that endotoxemia derived from the gut organisms was the major source of the toxic factors in the plasma of animals subjected to shock. However, the concept that loss of gut barrier function played a role in disease was hotly debated at the time and soon lost popularity. More refined studies on bacterial translocation by Berg and Garlington in the late 1970s [14] and subsequently by Deitch, Berg, and their colleagues [15–17] in the early 1980s suggested that translocation might, indeed, be an important pathophysiologic event that leads to sepsis and infections of remote sites. The importance of the translocation event in causing sepsis and infections has been further substantiated by studies primarily in the laboratories of Rush, Wells, and ourselves [18–20].

How Does Translocation Occur?

There are at least two ways by which translocation can occur through the intact epithelial barrier of the intestine. The first is by direct penetration through the enterocytes, and the second is by uptake via M cells, which are specialized phagocytic cells found in the intestinal epithelium. It has been proposed that bacteria and other microbes can enter through the intracellular junctions, but this mechanism in fact has not been observed when using electron microscopy. Bacteria can also cross the epithelial surface through ulcerations that characteristically occur at the tips of the villi at the site where epithelial cells become detached and are extruded into the intestinal lumen, the zone of intrusion. Such ulcerations occur with high frequency in animals subjected to hemorrhagic shock, ionizing radiation, or cytotoxic agents. While we consider this to be direct invasion rather than translocation in the classic sense, the end results are the same: penetration of microbes into the lamina propria with subsequent transport to distant sites. Unfortunately, it is impossible to separate clearly the effects of the two processes in either experimental or clinical situations.

Translocation of Inert Particles

Many studies have examined the uptake of a wide variety of substances from the intestine, and some of these may have relevance to translocation of intact microbes. It is known that intact protein can be absorbed across the intestinal mucosa of newborn mammals to a much greater degree than in adults. The luminal protein is taken up by pinocytosis and transverses the cells in membrane-lined vesicles. This pathway "closes" within a few days after birth, but transport of intact proteins occurs to a much lesser degree throughout adult life. Warsaw and his colleagues [21] studied the transport of intact bovine serum albumin across the intestine of rats and found that approximately 2% was transferred in the macromolecular form to the blood and lymph in normal animals. Carter et al. [22] studied the transport of horseradish peroxidase across the intestinal epithelium after burn injury using electron microscopy. Within 6 hours after injury, this substance was found in the portal and systemic bloods, peaking at 18 hours post-injury. The uptake was found to be transcellular through normally appearing enterocytes. However, Owen [23] showed that the transport of horseradish peroxidase across the gut epithelium of normal mice was primarily by M cells via intact vesicles.

Numerous studies have shown that inert particles can be absorbed directly through the intact intestine (Table 17-1). Sanders and Ashworth [24] used polystyrene latex particles and showed that within one hour of installation of a latex emulsion into the stomach, latex particles were demonstrable within the jejunal epithelial cells. These were always enclosed in vesicles. Within two hours, the latex particles could be demonstrated in the hepatic sinusoids.

Sass et al. [25] used closed loops of jejunum of Wistar rats to study the "absorption" of latex particles of different sizes. Within 10 minutes of the time of application of the latex beads, they

Table 17-1. Inert Particles Shown to Translocate Across the Intact Mucosal Barrier

Cellulose particles
Starch granules (corn and potato)
Polystyrene latex particles
Polyvinyl chloride particles
Iron particles
Carbon particles

were found concentrated on the surface of the M cells, particularly of Peyer's patches, and the beads could be found deep within the Peyer's patch in follicles shortly thereafter. The attachment and ingestion were related to the size of the bead, with larger particles penetrating less frequently. Using confocal microscopy, Porta et al. [26] studied the uptake of latex beads coated with secretory IgA instilled into mouse intestinal loops. Bead absorption and uptake were greater at the edge compared with the apex of the follicular domes, consistent with the known distribution of the M cells in the Peyer's patches. Interestingly, adsorption and uptake were not concordant. Coating the beads with bovine serum albumin resulted in a 4-fold reduction in adsorption and a 20-fold reduction in the uptake.

Some of the most interesting studies on the translocation of inert particles were done by Volkheimer and his colleagues [27–30]. This investigator used ingestion of large amounts of potato starch granules to study passage of large particles through the intact intestinal barrier in both experimental animals and man. Within minutes after ingestion, starch granules could be found in the blood in relatively high concentrations. There was a fall in the blood concentration at about 30 minutes with a secondary rise, reaching a peak at about 1½ to 2 hours. Microscopic examination of the intestines of rats showed passage of the starch particles through the intact mucosa, seemingly between enterocytes, particularly at the zone of extrusion. Subsequently, particles were found within the lymphatics, and later they could be found in the mesenteric veins. "Persorption" (as he called this process) of cornstarch appeared to be as good or better than potato starch, and the effect was dose-dependent, more granules being found in the blood with higher ingested doses than with lower doses. The administration of caffeine or Prostigmin simultaneously with the starch granules resulted in an increase in the rate of translocation, whereas atropine administered concurrently resulted in a decrease in translocation. Translocation of iron particles ranging up to 52 microns in diameter could also be demonstrated after oral ingestion. Polyvinyl chloride particles were tested for their ability to translocate in dogs. The pattern of mucosal penetration was similar to potato starch, and the granules could be found in the blood within one minute after oral ingestion, consistent with the earlier findings of Arnold [5] using live bacteria in dogs. More particles could

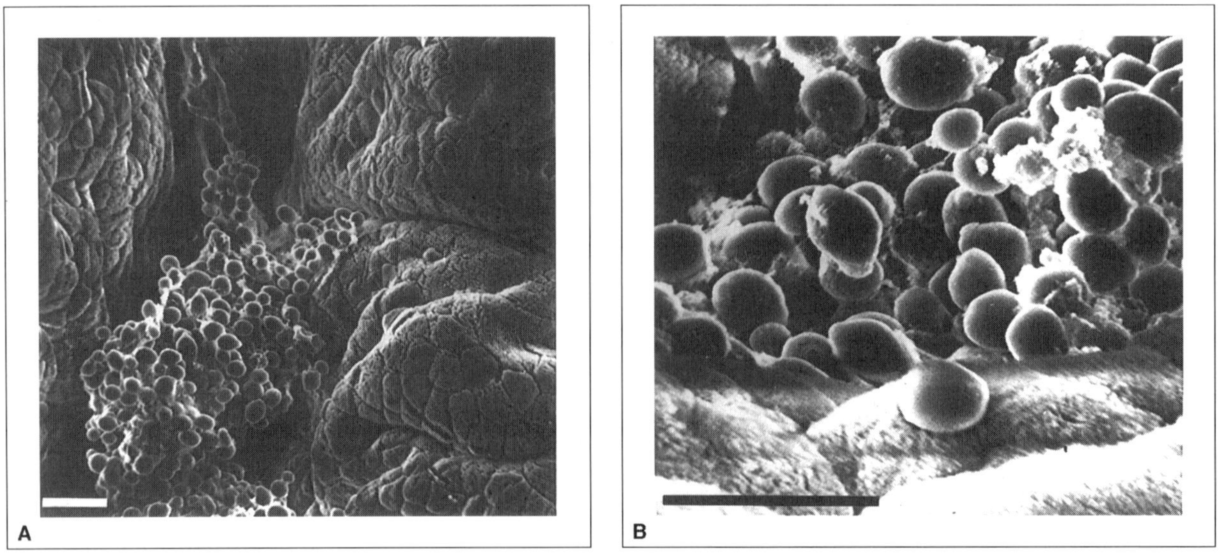

Figure 17-1. (**A**) Scanning electron microscopy of the mucosal surface of guinea pig Thiry-Vella loops instilled with *C. albicans.* Immediately after instillation clumps of *Candida* are seen over the surface of the villi. There is already attachment of the *Candida* to the epithelium, but the major part of the microorganisms are entrapped by the mucous. (**B**) Same image at a higher magnification. Scale bar = 10μm. (From JW Alexander, et al. The process of microbial translocation. *Ann Surg* 212:496, 1990. Used with permission.)

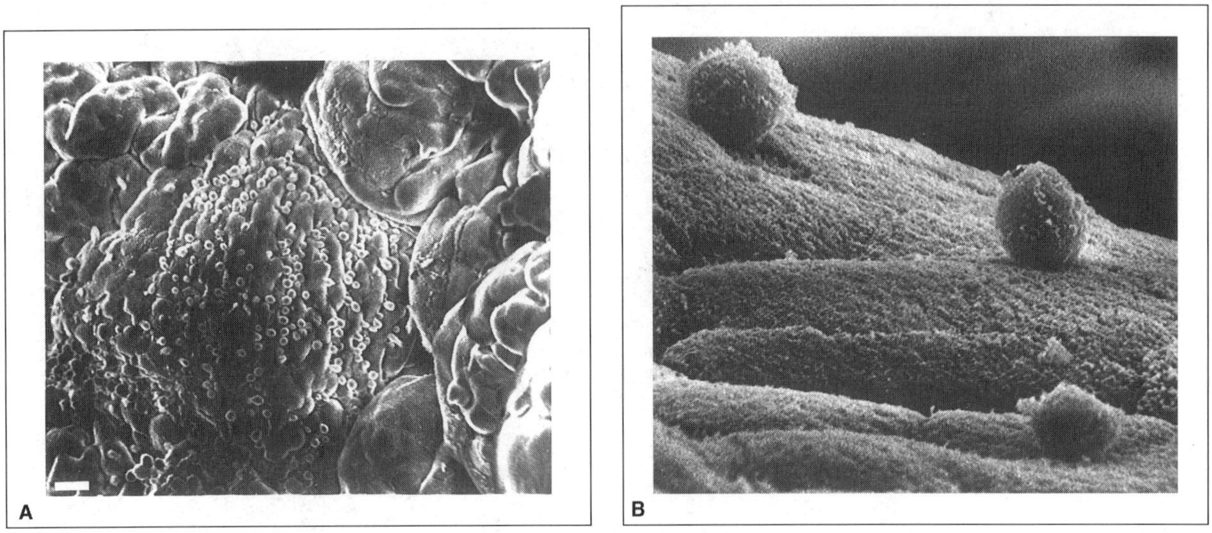

Figure 17-2. **(A)** Within a short period of time, the *Candida* became attached to the microvilli of individual epithelial cells. A characteristic of the sections examined was the diffuse attachment to one of the villi but not to the others. Scale bar = 10 μm. (From JW Alexander, et al. The process of microbial translocation. *Ann Surg* 212:496, 1990. Used with permission.) **(B)** Higher magnification tangential view showing attachment of two *Candida*.

be found in the portal blood than in arterial blood taken simultaneously. It should be noted that injury was not produced in any of these experimental animals.

Microbial Translocation

Not surprisingly, all types of microbes tested (i.e., viruses, aerobic and anaerobic bacteria, and fungi) have been found to translocate. The process whereby translocation across the intact epithelial cells occurs has been studied morphologically to the greatest extent using *Candida albicans*. Alexander et al. [31] placed suspensions of *Candida albicans* into Thiry-Vella loops in rats and guinea pigs shortly before infliction of a 30% total body surface area burn. The Thiry-Vella loops were harvested at various times up to 24 hours during the postburn period and examined by both scanning and transmission electron microscopy, as well as light microscopy using toluidine blue stains of semithin sections. *Candida* were easily recognized by their characteristic morphologic appearance (in EM studies) and intense uptake of the toluidine blue (in the light microscopy studies). Immediately after installation, clumps of *Candida* were seen scattered over the surfaces of the villi (Figure 17-1). Within a short period of time, these clumps dissociated, and individual *Candida* became attached to the microvilli of individual epithelial cells (Figure 17-2). This intimate attachment was associated with distortion (Figure 17-3) and disruption (Figure 17-4) of the outer membranes of the microvilli with subsequent penetration of the *Candida* as if by dissolution into the

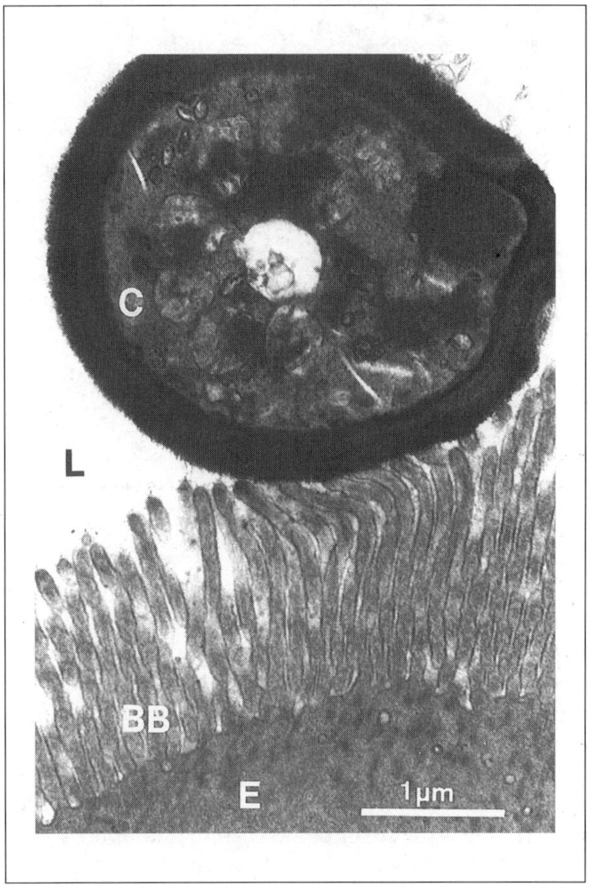

Figure 17-3. Transmission electron microscopy of the attachment of the *Candida* to the microvillus layer. The attachment is causing distortion of the outer portion of the microvillus layer, with disorientation of their linear alignment, suggesting enzymatic alterations. BB = brush border; C = *C. albicans;* E = enterocyte; L = lumen. (From JW Alexander, et al. The process of microbial translocation. *Ann Surg* 212:496, 1990. Used with permission.)

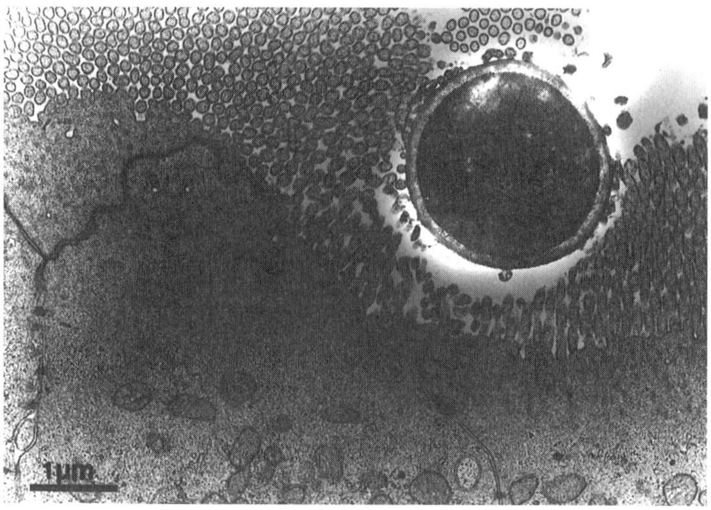

Figure 17-4. The intimate attachment of the *Candida* to the microvilli causes disruption of the membranes of microvilli, with further penetration. (From JW Alexander, et al. The process of microbial translocation. *Ann Surg* 212:496, 1990. Used with permission.)

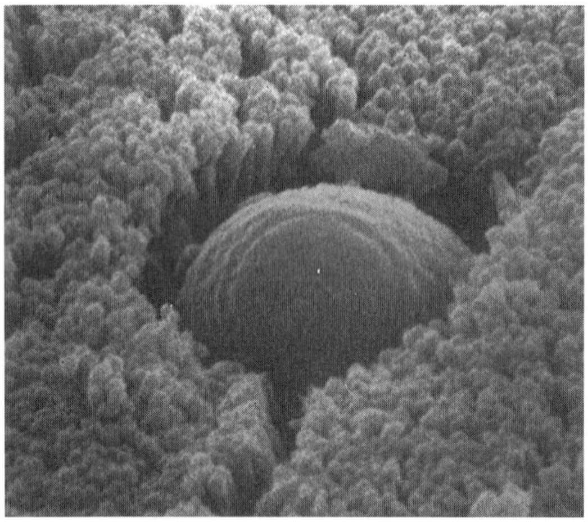

Figure 17-5. Scanning electron microscopy of the penetration of the *Candida* as if by dissolution into the microvillus layer.

microvillus layer (Figure 17-5). Passage across the outer cell membrane occurred very rapidly with rapid sealing of the defect (Figure 17-6). Entrance of the *Candidal* body into the cytoplasm occurred without a defined membrane around the *Candida,* suggesting that the process was not classical phagocytosis (Figure 17-7). As the organisms passed from the apical to the basal portion of the cell, the enterocytes appeared morphologically intact, and there was no evidence of degranulation of lysosomal bodies or other organelles into a space around the *Candida,* which was in direct contact with the cytoplasm (Figure 17-8). When the *Candida* reached the basal portion of the cell, the basal membrane of the cell opened, allowing extrusion of the *Candida* into the lamina propria along with some of the cytoplasm of the cell (Figure 17-9). Whether this caused death of the cell could not be determined in the studies done so far. Once within the lamina propria, the individual *Candidal* bodies either remained free or were phagocytized by macrophages. Both free and phagocytized *Candida* were seen within the central lacteals and venules, and they were carried to the regional lymph nodes and distal parts of the body (Figure 17-10). Wells, in very elegant studies using bacteria, showed that these organisms passed directly through the cytoplasm of the enterocytes and in a manner similar to the *Candida* [19]. In her studies, as well as our own, there was never the observation that *Candida* or bacteria passed between cells.

In the 1960s, Wolochow and Hildebrand [32] performed some very interesting studies trying to explain the mechanism of entry of bacteria from the lumen of the intestine to the blood and other body fluids. In one of their first experiments, they observed that an *E. coli* phage appeared in the blood within minutes after oral administration in rats. The primary path after translocation of the *E. coli* phage was via the intestinal lymph rather than the intestinal blood. From that observation they suggested that the passage of bacteria through the intestinal wall might be significant in the pathogenesis of certain infections. In another study [33], they examined some factors such as size, concentration, and types of bacteria that were able to influence the passage of microorganisms from the intestine to the blood via the regional lymphatic system. In a rat model, microorganisms differing widely in size were instilled into the duo-

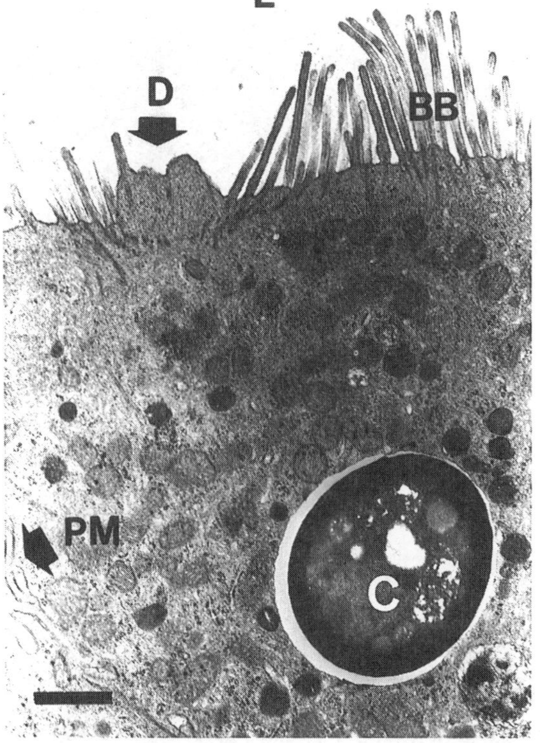

Figure 17-6. This transmission electron micrograph shows the passage across the outer cell membrane by the *Candida*. There is gross distortion of the plasma membrane and brush border at the presumed site of entry in the enterocyte, which could represent loss of continuity of the actin filament network within the brush border. BB = brush border; C = *Candida;* D = distortion of the brush border and of the plasma membrane (PM); L = intestinal lumen. Scale bar = 1 μm. (From JW Alexander, et al. The process of microbial translocation. *Ann Surg* 212:496, 1990. Used with permission.)

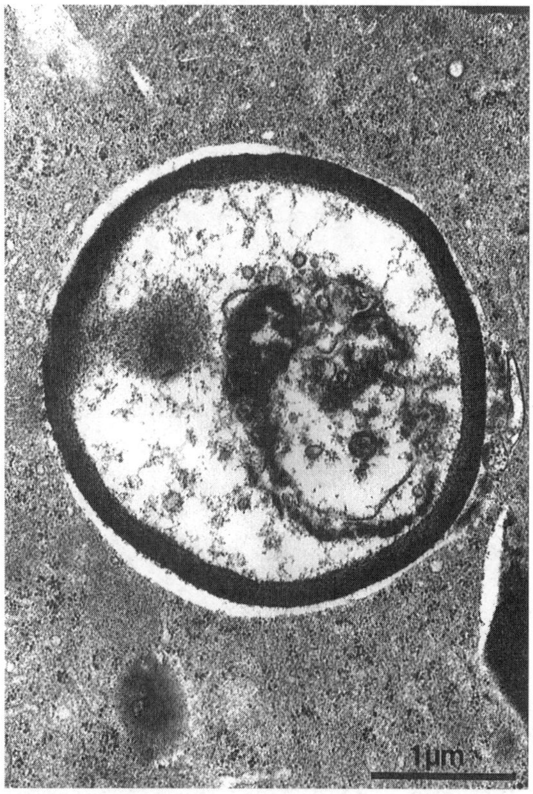

Figure 17-7. The *Candida* is not surrounded by a defined membrane, suggesting that internalization occurred by process other than classic phagocytosis. (From JW Alexander, et al. The process of microbial translocation. *Ann Surg* 212:496, 1990. Used with permission.)

denum in varying quantities and concentrations. After cannulation of the cisterna chyli, they collected the intestinal lymph for one hour after the gavage of bacteria into the intestinal tract. The frequency of recovery tended to vary directly with the concentration of the instilled suspension. Studies also suggested that particular combinations of microorganisms could act synergistically with regard to the passage through the intestinal wall. Moreover, they observed that the passage of bacteria into the blood depended not only on the size of the organisms alone but also on the different biologic properties of the bacteria.

M cells are specialized phagocytes that have a portion of the cell pass between the enterocytes to the surface of the epithelium. Viewed by scanning electron microscopy, these can be differentiated because of randomly projecting villi that are somewhat larger and less numerous than the microvilli of enterocytes (Figure 17-11). The area at the luminal surface is also generally smaller than that of the enterocytes. The M cells are more highly concentrated in the area of Peyer's patches, especially at the periphery of the domes, and are in close association with lymphocytes. In guinea pigs at least, there are approximately 50 enterocytes per M cell. Being phagocytic cells, M cells ingest particulate matter by formation of a phagocytic vacuole and may partially digest or kill some of the ingested microbes (Figure 17-12). In normal circumstances, M cells are felt to be a site for immunologic sampling of intestinal contents, ingesting the majority of particulate matter that passes across the epithelial barrier and transferring these to immunocompetent cells. Processing of antigenic material is felt to occur primarily by M cells, and the majority of inert particles are felt to pass through M cells rather than the enterocytes, despite the overwhelming preponderance of enterocytes relative to M cells [26].

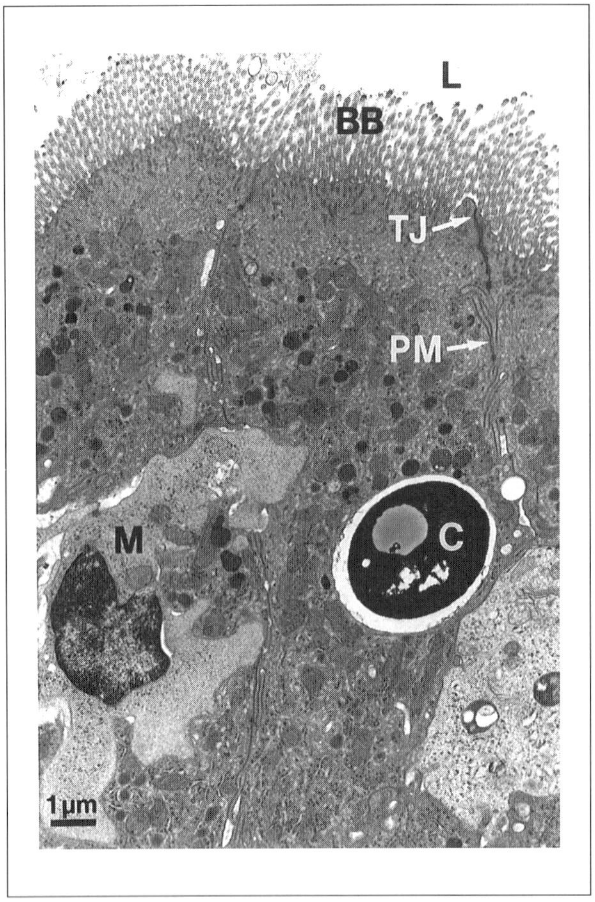

Figure 17-8. This transmission electron micrograph shows the *Candida* as it passes from the apical to the basal portion of the cell in direct contact with the cytoplasm. The enterocyte appears morphologically intact and is bordered on both sides by intraepithelial macrophages migrating through the mucosa via the intracellular junctions. BB = brush border; C = *Candida;* L = intestinal lumen; M = macrophages; PM = plasma membrane; TJ = tight junction. (From JW Alexander, et al. The process of microbial translocation. *Ann Surg* 212:496, 1990. Used with permission.)

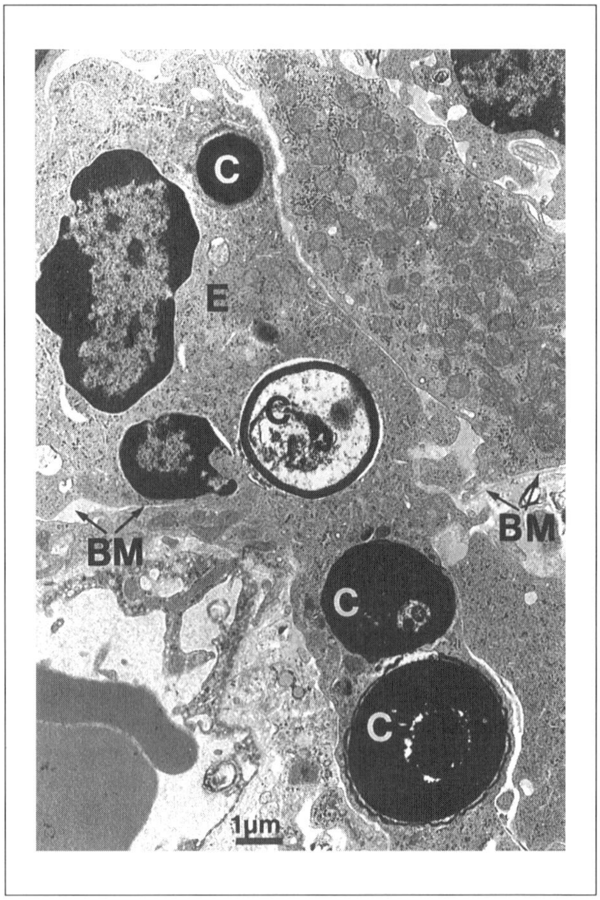

Figure 17-9. The *Candida* appears to be extruded through the basal layer of the enterocyte into the lamina propria, along with some of the cytoplasm and organelles of the cell. BM = basal membrane; C = *Candida;* E = enterocyte. (From JW Alexander, et al. The process of microbial translocation. *Ann Surg* 212:496, 1990. Used with permission.)

It thus appears that translocation of microbes by M cells is a normal event that is necessary for antigen processing to support the immunologic functions of the intestine. Translocation of microbes through the enterocytes, however, occurs at a very low level in normal individuals, but this active transport can be up-regulated by a variety of insults, most of which have reduced blood flow in the microcirculation as a common event. Finally, microbes can gain entrance through the intestinal barrier by invading ulcerations, as has been shown by Deitch et al. and many others [34,35]. Unfortunately, this "invasion" is difficult to distinguish from physiologic "sampling" or transepithelial "translocation" except at the microscopic level. All three processes may have similar physiologic consequences and may be additive.

Quantitation of Translocation Events

Measurement of translocation in experimental animals is, superficially, a straightforward event: kill the animal, culture the tissues, and count the viable organisms in those tissues. The vast majority of studies on translocation have used this simple technique. However, it provides an incomplete picture because counting the live bacteria in the tissues reflects both host and nonhost factors and does not differentiate abnormalities of barrier function from abnormalities of host defense. The number of viable bacteria culturable from the tissues associated with translocation from the intestine is determined by three factors: (1) the numbers and types of bacteria in the intestine, (2) the intrinsic barrier function of the intestine, (3) and the ability of the host to kill translocated bacteria. Estimation of translocation by measurement of viable counts alone is a quick and easy

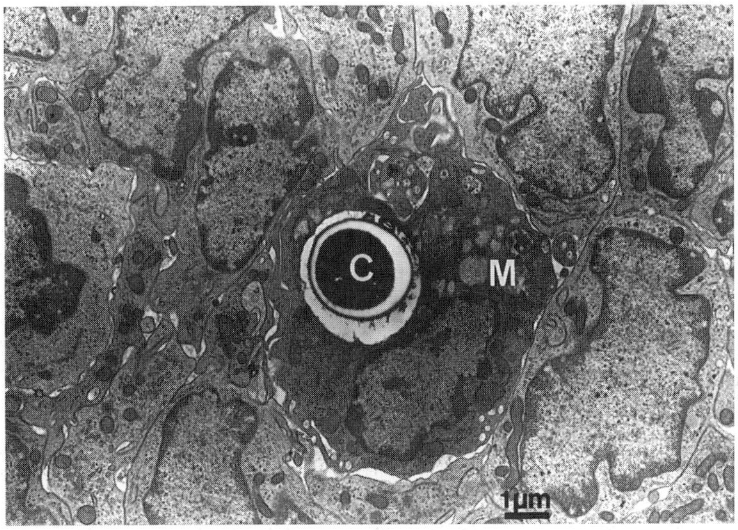

Figure 17-10. Transmission electron microscopy shows a *Candida* within a macrophage in the periocortical area of a mesenteric lymph node. C = *Candida;* M = macrophage. (From JW Alexander, et al. The process of microbial translocation. *Ann Surg* 212:496, 1990. Used with permission.)

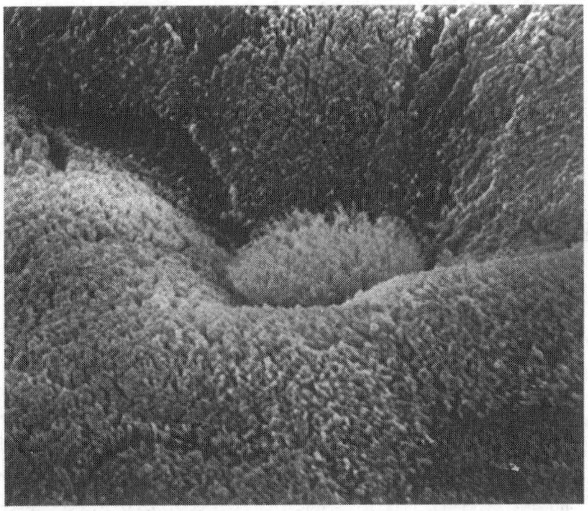

Figure 17-11. Scanning electron micrograph of an M cell in a guinea pig Thiry-Vella loop that can be differentiated because of randomly projecting villi that are somewhat larger and less numerous than the microvilli of the enterocyte.

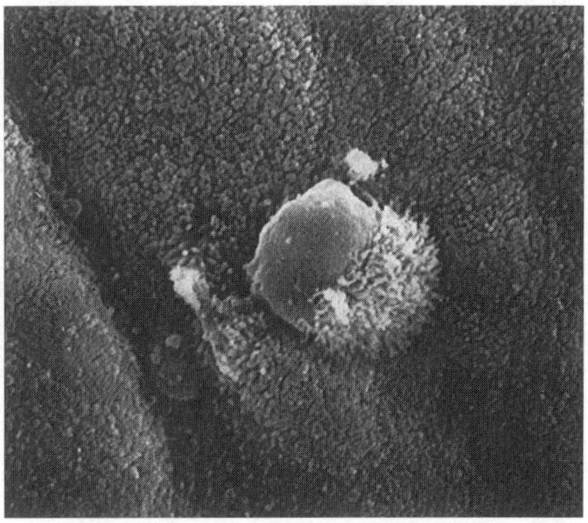

Figure 17-12. A *Candida* is being ingested by an M cell. Translocation of microorganisms by M cells is a normal event that is necessary for antigen processing to support the immunologic functions of the intestine.

way, but it does not differentiate between alterations of the intrinsic barrier function and host defense variables. Using ^{14}C glucose to radioisotopically label bacteria, we have determined that the label associated with approximately 10,000 bacteria can be found in the tissues for every single residual viable bacteria that can be cultured. However, using ^{111}Indium oxine (^{111}In), which labels existing macromolecules in intact bacteria, there is the label from approximately 100 bacteria for every viable bacteria in the tissues. Estimating from this label, the normal host kills approximately 99% of *E. coli,* consistent with what might be expected with in vitro culture of bacteria with phagocytic cells. Comparing this with the studies using ^{14}C, it would appear that for every intact bacteria that translocates, the products from an additional 100 bacteria pass through the epithelial barrier. Therefore, translocation of toxins such as endotoxin and a variety of exotoxins may play a very important role in the pathophysiologic events that occur as a consequence of translocation. In most of our experiments, we have preferred to use a gavage of a large number of radioisotopically labeled bacteria so that the numbers of organisms in the intestinal lumen is held relatively constant,

Table 17-2. Molecules that Translocate Intact Across the Mucosal Barrier

Lactulose
Mannose
Proteins (e.g., albumin)
Horseradish peroxidase
Polythylene glycol
Clostridum botulinum toxin
Endotoxin

Table 17-3. Factors that Increase Microbial Translocation as Measured by Bacterial Culture of Tissues

Changes in the luminal microbes
Antibiotic therapy (resistant organism overgrowth)
Elemental diet
Total parenteral nutrition
Damage to the epithelium
Irradiation
Cytotoxic agents
Irritants (e.g., ricinoleic acid)
CMV infection
Mucosal disease
Bowel manipulation
Bowel obstruction
Oxygen free radicals
Diminished blood flow or O_2 delivery
Hemorrhagic shock
Burn injury
Zymosan
Endotoxin
Mesenteric occlusion
Hypoxia
Fever
Immunosuppression
Prednisone (high dose)
Blood transfusion

preferring this to measuring random translocation from the indigenous flora, which may vary considerably in numbers and type. Abnormalities of the barrier function of the intestine and host defense are then easily distinguishable using radioactive counts reaching tissues to determine the integrity of the barrier function and calculation of the percentage of bacteria that survive in the tissue after translocation as a reflection of the host defense (i.e., the ability to kill translocated bacteria).

Simple measurement of the amount of radioactivity in various tissues following the ingestion of radiolabeled bacteria is increasingly difficult with the passage of time because of redistribution of the label; it depends, to a great extent, on the label used (e.g., ^{14}C redistributes very rapidly whereas ^{111}In redistributes very slowly). Translocation is sometimes estimated by surrogate markers such as lactulose or polyethylene glycol (Table 17-2). However, there is no clear evidence that these relatively small permeability markers accurately reflect the barrier function of the intestine to bacteria or their products.

Things That Increase Translocation

A large number of studies have now been reported describing manipulations that increase microbial translocation as measured primarily by culturing of microbes from the mesenteric lymph nodes and other tissues. A partial listing of these is shown in Table 17-3. Basically, these can be divided into four categories: (1) an increase in the luminal microbes, (2) damage of the epithelium, (3) diminished blood flow or oxygen delivery, and (4) immunosuppression. There is no evidence that antibiotic therapy changes the intrinsic barrier function of the intestine, and overgrowth of resistant organisms appears to be the primary reason for increased translocation associated with antibiotic therapy. The bowel flora are also altered with the administration of elemental diets or with intravenous hyperalimentation, usually with an increase of gram negative aerobic organisms. Abnormalities of the intestinal epithelium that allow a decrease in the barrier function have not yet been demonstrated with either antibiotic therapy or intravenous hyperalimentation. However, lack of specific nutrients may well be associated with alterations of host defense.

It is certainly not surprising that damage of the epithelium would increase translocation. Radiation and cytotoxic agents may cause ulcerations, as may many types of mucosal disease including viral infections. The increase in translocation by bowel manipulation, or with bowel obstruction, also seems to be associated with mucosal damage, although alterations in blood flow may be an additional feature.

Diminished intestinal blood flow is a common factor underlying many conditions that lead to translocation. These include hemorrhagic shock [18], burn injury [15], administration of a complement activating agent such as zymosan [36], or endotoxin and simple vascular occlusion [37]. Diminished blood flow results in a number of biologic changes including altered pH and decreased tissue oxygen concentrations and an increase in metabolic products, none of which have been shown to be the dominant feature in inducing translocation. Gianotti et al. [38] have shown that there is an association between the blood flow to the individual villi and translocation of *Candida* within those villi. Moreover, Gennari et al. [39]

have shown that hyperoxia in burned animals will decrease translocation. In another study he showed that treatment with heparan sulphate, an acid polysaccharide with antithrombogenic properties, was able to improve the outcome during gut-derived sepsis, probably by improving intestinal microcirculation [40]. Together, all these studies suggest a role for oxygen in regulating the transepithelial transport of intact microbes. While diminished blood flow may be associated with ulcerations of the intestinal tract, the primary mechanism of epithelial transport appears to be through the transcellular route. Once the bacteria crosses the epithelial barrier, the ability of the animal to kill the bacteria markedly influences subsequent events. Both blood transfusion and the administration of immunosuppressive agents such as prednisone will decrease the ability of the host to clear bacteria and increase the mortality related to translocation, therefore becoming models of gut origin sepsis. Burn injury has a dual effect, both diminishing barrier function and impairing host defense. As might be expected, combinations of these manipulations such as blood transfusion or steroids and burn injury have additive effects [41].

Reduction of Translocation

Extensive investigations have shown that translocation can be reduced in experimental animals using a variety of experimental models where reduction of intestinal blood flow is a prominent feature. In these models, prevention of abnormal blood flows will usually prevent translocation. Because bacterial translocation normally occurs at an almost undetectably low rate, studies to prevent translocation have all been done using pathologic or abnormal conditions. In those models where intestinal ischemia is a prominent feature, it is not surprising that prevention of mesenteric blood flow disturbances will reduce translocation. Also, because integrity of the mucosal barrier is a central feature for preventing translocation, it is logical that nutrients might also have an effect. The summary of experiments done on the subject is shown in Table 17-4. In general, arginine [42], glutamine [43], ω-3 fatty acids [44], and the insoluble fibers [45], especially lignin, will reduce translocation and improve survival. [*Editor's Note:* A contrary view concerning glutamine has been presented by another laboratory, but to my knowledge it is not yet published in manuscript form.] However, only glutamine and, to a lesser extent, the ω-3 fatty acids improve barrier function. Recently Gennari and his colleagues [46] showed that different combinations of immunoenhancing nutrients added to base diets may have additive effects in preventing bacterial translocation. They observed that diets supplemented with different combinations and percentages of arginine, glutamine, and fish oil were able to improve survival in a septic model that included immunosuppression with blood transfusions. In fact, feeding with arginine + glutamine, fish oil + arginine, or fish oil + glutamine positively affected survival during gut-derived sepsis, both improving gut barrier function and enhancing host defense. In agreement with our studies, other authors showed a protective effect of nutrients such as glutamine on the intestinal barrier function and morphologic structure. Burke et al. [47] showed that glutamine-supplemented total parenteral nutrition (TPN) protected against bacterial translocation

Table 17-4. Effects of Nutrients on Translocation

	Effect on Barrier Function	Effect on Bacterial Killing	Effect on Survival
Arginine	—	↑	↑
Glutamine	↑	↑	↑
RNA	—	—	—
ω-3 fatty acids	↑	↑	↑
ω-6 fatty acids	—	—	—
Glycine	—	—	—
Medium-chain fatty acids	—	—	—
Dietary fibers (insoluble)	NS	NS	↑
Arginine + glutamine	↑	↑	↑
Fish oil + arginine	↑	↑	↑
Fish oil + glutamine	↑	↑	↑
Riboflavin (vitamin B_2)	↑	—	↑

NS = Not studied

from the gut compared to standard formula, with an effect thought to be mediated by the secretory IgA immune system. Fox et al. [48] observed in an experimental model of a high mortality methotrexate-induced enterocolitis that a glutamine-supplemented diet resulted in a significantly longer survival time and decreased mortality. This was associated with decreased weight loss, improved nitrogen retention, increased mucosal weight, increased protein and DNA contents of the jejunal and colonic mucosa, and decreased bacterial translocation. Souba et al. [49] demonstrated that glutamine helped to maintain the gut mucosal barrier, decreasing the incidence of mesenteric lymph node (MLN)-positive culture after abdominal radiation. This study was confirmed by Klimberg et al. [50], who showed an intact gut epithelium by scanning electron microscopy in all animals receiving prophylactic glutamine compared to control animals. The effects of several important nutrients such as vitamins C and A on the translocation process have not yet been studied.

Numerous drugs affect translocation, and many of them improve survival in models of gut-origin sepsis caused by translocation. A summary of these is shown in Table 17-5. The effects can be multiple and sometimes quite complex. As an example, the prostaglandins of the E series, in general, improve barrier function, and low doses may improve bacterial killing [51]. However, high doses of some of these, especially $^{16\text{-}16}$dimethyl PGE_2, impair bacterial killing, counteracting the beneficial effect of improved barrier function. In general, the growth factors such as EGF, FGF [52], and GM-CSF [53] improve barrier function and improve survival. In addition, GM-CSF improves host defense with an additional beneficial effect on survival. Moreover, in a recent study we showed that IFN-γ treatment was able to affect both barrier function and bacterial killing in a dose-related manner [54].

Consequences of Translocation

Healthy individuals can withstand relatively large inocula of bacteria and/or endotoxin given intravenously. The response is dose related, as might be expected, and individuals often recover spontaneously. Natural experiments of the infu-

Table 17-5. Effect of Drugs on Bacterial Translocation

	Effect on Barrier Function	Effect on Bacterial Killing	Effect on Survival
Verapamil	—	±	↓
Enalapril	↑	—	↑
Indomethacin	—	↑	↑
Misoprostol	↑	↑↓	↑
Enisoprost	↑	↑↓	↑
16,16 dimethyl PGE	↑	↓	—
GM-CSF	↑	↑	↑
bFGF	↑	—	↑
Epidermal growth factor (EGF)	NS	NS	↑
Bombesin	NS	NS	↑
IGF_1	NS	NS	↑
Pentagastrin	NS	NS	—
Sucralfate	↑	—	↑
Erythromycin	—	—	—
Tetracycline	—	—	—
Neomycin	—	—	—
Anti-IL-6	↑	↑	↑
Allopurinol	NS	NS	↑
Prednisone (high dose)	↓	↓	↓
Dehydroepiandrosterone (DHEA)	—	↑	↑
IFN-γ	↑	↑	↑
Heparan sulfate	↑	↑	↑

NS = Not studied

sion of large numbers of bacteria in man have occurred, especially with infusion of contaminated blood and/or intravenous solutions. Doses exceeding several billions of bacteria or more have not always resulted in fatalities, but subjects have developed typical sepsis syndromes consisting of fever, leukopenia followed by leukocytosis, and septic shock. In both experimental animals and man, infusion of endotoxin causes a well-defined sequence of cytokine release, especially IL-1, IL-6, and tumor necrosis factor (TNF).

Infusion of bacteria into the portal vein of animals causes similar responses but may be tolerated even better than infusion intravenously because of better clearance mechanisms. Infusion of endotoxin intravenously in experimental animals does not result in a hypermetabolic response, although infusion into the portal vein does, suggesting that the liver plays a significant role in the hypermetabolism associated with translocation [55].

Gianotti et al. [56] used guinea pigs to demonstrate a clear relationship between the magnitude of bacterial translocation from the intestinal tract and the hypermetabolic response. Burn injury was induced in guinea pigs and they were then divided into two groups, one fed enterally and the other maintained only on an equal volume of lactated Ringers given by gastrostomy. Forty-eight hours later, radioactive labeled bacteria were infused into the gastrostomy. Resting energy expenditure (REE) was measured afterwards, and the animals were sacrificed for measurement of the magnitude of translocation into the portal vein and the measurement of catabolic hormones. The degree of translocation into the portal vein was directly proportional to blood cortisol levels, urinary catecholamine excretion, and the elevation in REE. These experiments were consistent with prior experiments by Mochizuki et al. [57], which showed a correlation between decreased mucosal mass in the intestine and the hypermetabolic response following burn injury. Studies in human burn patients have supported these initial studies. Chirarelli et al. [58] performed a prospective, randomized study in which one half of the patients were fed with aggressive early enteral feeding and one half had delayed enteral feeding. The patients with early enteral feeding had reduced levels of plasma glucagon, a lower incidence of bacteremia, and a shortened hospital stay. Thus, there is clear evidence that aggressive enteral feeding following burn injury may reduce the incidence of bacterial translocation, thus reducing the magnitude of the hypermetabolic response, the incidence of bacteremia, and the need for prolonged hospitalization.

Fukushima et al. [59] provided evidence that the magnitude of bacterial translocation from the intestine predicted length of survival and mortality in experimental animals. Previously transfused mice were burned and gavaged with radioactive labeled *E. coli.* Four hours after burn injury blood was drawn by retro-orbital puncture and the amount of radioactivity measured, reflecting the degree of translocation from the intestinal tract. Animals were then followed for survival. There was an inverse correlation between the amount of translocation and length of survival in the animals that died. There was also a statistically higher amount of translocation in animals that died than those that survived.

Similar findings were found by Gianotti and his colleagues [51] in a subsequent experiment using a similar experimental model. When misoprostol or eniosoprost was used to reduce translocation, there was an associated improvement in survival that was related to the amount of reduction in translocation. These experiments showed that the magnitude of translocation influences survival and that therapeutic intervention to reduce translocation will improve survival. Unfortunately, there is no good way to quantitate translocation in man, and there are few good methods to estimate the degree of multiple organ failure in experimental animals in the setting of translocation studies. Nevertheless, Fukushima and his colleagues [60] have shown that the degree of translocation from the intestine has a direct correlation with the sequestration of neutrophils in the liver as measured by myeloperoxidase content.

We and others have recently shown that the intestinal tract is an important source of IL-1, TNF, and IL-6 as well as PGE_2 [61,62]. Some of these cytokines and ecosanoids are produced by macrophages within the lamina propria that seem to be in a constantly activated state. However, large amounts of cytokines are produced by the enterocytes themselves, and these increase in response to injury, especially TNF and IL-6. It is of particular interest that anti-IL-6 antibodies improve survival following burn injury in animals that have been gavaged with bacteria [63]. It is well known that the cytokines can prime neutrophils, and Poggetti and his colleagues [64] have recently shown that neutrophils can be primed by the gut in injured animals.

Finally, bacterial translocation may serve as a source of organisms for distant infections. Howerton and Kolmen [65] were among the first to show that *Pseudomonas aeruginosa* translocated from the intestine via lymph and blood to the wound in thermally injured rats. *Pseudomonas aeruginosa* appeared in high concentrations in the lymph cisterna chyli within 1 hour of the time of burn injury, then fell progressively to undetectable levels by 6 hours. Bacterial counts rose in the blood to reach a peak three hours postburn but were not detectable by 7 hours postburn. *Pseudomonas* was present in the mesenteric lymph nodes 12 hours after burn and appeared in the burn wound by 84 hours. Secondary spread to other organs and subsequent death occurred as a consequence of growth of the translocated *Pseudomonas* in the burn wound. We have also shown that organisms translocated directly from the gastrointestinal tract to the wounds of burn animals [66].

Some of the outcome effects of bacterial translocation appear to be mediated by macrophages. Nieuwenhuijzen et al. [36] chemically depleted macrophages before inducing translocation with zymosan in rats and found that the animals depleted of macrophage had a significantly higher survival rate than the control animals, which were not depleted, thus suggesting a strong role for macrophages in the development of multiple organ failure.

There is also a gray zone between translocation and invasion by pathogenic organisms. Ordinarily, translocation is thought to involve the transport of nonpathogenic organisms. However, most organisms can become pathogenic under certain circumstances. *Listeria monocytogenes* is a systemic, intracellular pathogen that causes disease in mice. Pine et al. [67] showed that the 50% lethal doses of *Listeria monocytogenes* for mice were comparable whether given by the intragastric or intraperitoneal route. However, death occurred earlier by intragastric feeding.

Translocation in Man

There are several pathologic conditions where the passage of microorganisms from the intestine to different organs or body fluids occur, demonstrating that translocation has occurred in man (Table 17-6). Perhaps the most convincing evidence that translocation can occur in a healthy human is the single experiment done by Krause et al. [68]. This 38-year-old surgeon, in an attempt to convince his colleagues that *Candida albicans* in the gut was of no consequence, ingested a beaker of a suspension of this organism. Within a few hours he became symptomatic with fever and chills and had positive blood cultures for *Candida* as well as candiduria. He recovered from the event, but this was a clear demonstration that simply increasing numbers of an organism within the lumen of the gut could be associated with clinical sepsis from that organism. Further evidence that bacterial translocation occurs in man was provided by Tancrede and Andremont [69]. Prospective fecal and blood cultures were obtained from 55 patients with leukemia. Thirteen of 16 patients (81%) who had bacteremia caused by *Pseudomonas aeruginosa* were intestinal carriers of the same strain, compared to only 2 of 39 patients (5%) with bacteremia caused by enteral bacteria who were carriers of *P. aeruginosa.* Rush and his colleagues [70] also showed that patients who were seriously injured with hemorrhagic shock had positive blood cultures within three hours after their injury. Ten of 18 patients with admission blood pressures of less than 80 mm Hg had positive blood cultures compared to 3 of 32 patients with admission blood pressures of greater than 80 mm Hg. Only 2 of 18 patients with hypotension (less than 80 mm systolic) survived, compared to 28 of 32 patients without severe hypotension. These findings are consistent with the series of experiments by Deitch and his colleagues [34,71] on the translocation of bacteria in hemorrhagic shock. Further studies by Brathwaite et al. [72] showed that trauma patients had evidence of a galactosidase enzyme from *E. coli* in the MLN at the time of operation for trauma even though the MLN were negative for bacterial growth.

Table 17-6. Diseases Associated with Translocation

Pneumatosis intestinalis
Nonocclusive intestinal gangrene
Necrotizing enterocolitis
Irradiation
Cytotoxic drugs
Cytokine release syndrome
Crohn's disease
Ulcerative colitis
Hemorrhagic shock and severe trauma
Burn injury
Leukemia and neutropenia
Colon cancer

Marshall and his colleagues [73] performed a prospective study in 41 patients in the surgical ICU. Specimens of gastric and upper small bowel contents were obtained for quantitative culture, and the severity of organ dysfunction was quantitated by numeric score. Infectious complications developed in 33 patients and involved at least one organism concomitantly cultured from the upper GI tract in all but 3. Gut colonization correlated with the development of invasive infection within one week of intestinal culture for *Pseudomonas aeruginosa* (90% vs. 13% in noncolonized patients, $p < 0.001$) and *Staphylococcus epidermidis* (80% vs. 6%, $p < 0.001$). Pneumonia, wound infection, urinary tract infections, tertiary peritonitis, and bacteremia were all associated with GI colonization. Organ dysfunction was most marked in patients colonized with *Candida, Pseudomonas,* or *S. epidermidis*. The authors concluded that the upper GI tract was an important reservoir for organisms causing infections in the ICU. In another study, Levy et al. [74] also showed that contamination of enteral feedings was associated with positive blood cultures by organisms having the same plasmid profile as the organisms contaminating the feedings. Ambrose and associates [75] harvested and cultured samples from the ileal serosa and MLN of patients with and without Crohn's disease before noncontaminated surgical procedures and antibiotic administration. Pathogenic enteric bacteria were isolated from the MLN in 33% of Crohn's patients compared to 5% in controls and from the serosa in 27% versus 15% respectively.

Recently, Vincent and his colleagues [76] showed that patients with colorectal cancer (CRC) have an increased amount of translocation compared to noncancer patients. In a very elegant study, they compared 20 patients who had surgery for CRC to 20 patients who had surgery for noncolorectal digestive disease. Pericolonic lymph nodes, portal blood, and liver were harvested at laparotomy before antibiotics were given, and cultures performed with identification of species. They observed that translocation was present in 43% of patients who had abdominal surgery and was more frequent in the CRC group than in controls. Moreover, a greater variety of bacterial species was identified in the CRC group (15 species vs. 2 in non-CRC patients). The increased amount of bacterial translocation in patients with CRC was mainly due to the presence of bacteria in the involved pericolonic lymph nodes. In neither group were bacteria isolated from the portal blood.

Several authors have argued that translocation may not be an important event in man. Moore et al. [77] studied trauma patients who had a laparotomy for abdominal trauma. Catheters were placed in the umbilical vein to sample portal blood. Serial sampling showed no evidence of endotoxin or high levels of cytokines, such as IL-6, following the injury, and there was no relationship between levels of cytokines or endotoxin and the development of multiple organ failure. Cultures were also negative. The problem with this study is that patients had aggressive enteral feeding and prophylactic antibiotics as a part of their routine treatment protocol, which also involved aggressive resuscitation. Therefore, the investigators did many things that would reduce bacterial translocation.

Another argument against translocation occurring as an important event in man is the failure of selective decontamination to alter outcome in ICU patients [78]. However, selective decontamination could fail because of overgrowth by the remaining indigenous gastrointestinal flora followed by bacterial translocation and systemic infection [79] or because of the translocation of toxic bacterial products. It may well be that translocation of microbial products in the intestinal lumina continues to occur even though few viable bacteria can be detected in the blood. Also, anaerobic bacteria translocate to the same extent as aerobic bacteria and could trigger many of the adverse events associated with translocation. [*Editor's Note:* The authors have raised cogent arguments against accepting the data from selective decontamination in ICU patients as an argument against the decontamination hypothesis of causality in multiple organ failure. However, the decontamination studies that fail to change outcome are so numerous—23 at last count—that one is almost obliged to accept the notion of nonrelationship.]

A final argument against translocation by Munster et al. [80] is that there seems to be no direct relationship between the level of measurable endotoxin in the blood and the occurrence of multiple organ failure in burn patients. However, measurement of endotoxin in the blood is notoriously difficult and may not reflect true endotoxin concentrations or effects. Translocation of bacterial products, especially endotoxin, may result in the stimulation of large amounts of cytokines from the intestine. This may not necessarily be dose related, and it has been shown that there is a great variability from individual to individual. The intestine is a prime producer of IL-1, TNF, and IL-6, and these all rise following injury. Studies have not yet been conducted to determine associations between the magnitude of translocation and the magnitude of rise of the cytokines, but it is possible that the septic syndrome and multiple organ failure may be the result of gut responses to translocation rather than systemic responses of translocation.

Summary

The gut is a complex organ system that is highly efficient in preventing the entrance of viable bacteria and their products into the body. However, a number of insults may increase microbial translocation, which can trigger adverse effects including the development of sepsis, distant infection, and the inflammatory response syndromes. That translocation occurs in man is indisputable. However, the lack of effective tools to quantitate the magnitude of translocation has raised questions about the biologic importance of this event in humans. Therapeutic interventions are now available that decrease the incidence and severity of translocation. Some of these, such as early enteral feeding and the administration of glutamine, have proven to have beneficial effects in man, although it is unclear as to how much these are related to improvement of gut barrier function. Biologic agents such as prostaglandin E-1 analogues, anti-IL-6 antibody, and growth factors (EGF, FGF, and GM-CSF) also improve gut barrier function. Therapeutic trials with some of these agents in combination with dietary supplements seem warranted in critically ill patients.

References

1. Fraenkel A. Ueber peritoneale infektion. *Weiner Klin Wochenschr* 4:241,265,285, 1891.
2. Flexner S. Peritonitis caused by invasion of the micrococcus lanceolatus from the intestine. *Johns Hopkins Hosp Bull* 6:64, 1895.
3. Hornemann F. Beitraz zur frage ueber die Bakteriendurchlassigkleit der schleimhaut des magendarmkanals. *Zschr Hyg* 64:39, 1911.
4. Mandl F. Beitrag zur frage ler kryptogenetischen peritonitis. *Deut Zschr Chir* 182:289, 1923.
5. Arnold L. The passage of living bacteria through the wall of the intestine and the influence of diet and climate upon intestinal auto-disinfection. *Am J Hyg* 8:605, 1928.
6. Arnold L, Brody L. Passage of bacteria through the intestinal mucosa. *Proc Soc Exp Biol Med* 24:832, 1928.
7. Arnold L. Alterations in the endogenous enteric bacterial flora and microbic permeability of the intestinal wall in relation to the nutritional and meteorological changes. *J Hyg* 29:82, 1930.
8. Fisher V. Intestinal absorption of viable yeast. *Proc Soc Exp Biol Med* 28:948, 1931.
9. Flory HW. Observations on the functions of mucus and the early stages of bacterial invasion the intestinal mucosa. *J Pathol Bacteriol* 37:283, 1933.
10. Schweinburg FB, Heimburg F. Effect of chemical irritation of the peritoneum on transmural migration of intestinal organisms. *Proc Soc Exp Biol Med* 71:146, 1949.
11. Fine J, et al. The bacterial factor in traumatic shock. *Ann NY Acad Sci* 55:429, 1952.
12. Schweinburg FB, Frank HA, Fine J. Bacterial factor in experimental hemorrhagic shock: Evidence for development of a bacterial factor which accounts for irreversibility to transfusion and for the loss of the normal capacity to destroy bacteria. *Am J Physiol* 179:532, 1954.
13. Schweinburg FB, Fine J. Evidence for a lethal endotoxemia as the fundamental feature of irreversibility in three types of traumatic shock. *J Exp Med* 112:793, 1960.
14. Berg RD, Garlington AW. Translocation of certain indigenous bacteria from the gastrointestinal tract to MLN and other organs in a gnotobiotic mouse model. *Infect Immun* 23:403, 1979.
15. Deitch EA, Winterton J, Berg DD. Promotion by burn stress of the translocation of bacteria from the gastrointestinal tracts of mice. *Arch Surg* 119:166, 1984.
16. Berg RD. Promotion of the translocation of enteric bacteria from the gastrointestinal tracts of mice by oral treatment with penicillin, clindamycin or metronidazole. *Infect Immun* 33:854, 1981.
17. Deitch EA, Berg RD. Bacterial translocation from the gut: A mechanism of infection. *J Burn Care Rehab* 8:475, 1987.
18. Rush BP Jr, et al. Does the bacteremia observed in hemorrhagic shock have clinical significance? A study in germ free animals. *Ann Surg* 210:324, 1989.
19. Wells CL, Maddaus MA, Simmons RL. Proposed mechanism for the translocation of intestinal bacteria. *Rev Infect Dis* 10:958, 1988.
20. Fukushima R, et al. The degree of bacterial translocation is a determinant factor for mortality after burn injury and is improved by prostaglandin analogs. *Ann Surg* 216:438, 1992.
21. Warsaw AL, Walker WA, Eiselbacher KJ. Protein uptake by the intestine: Evidence for absorption of intact macromolecules. *Gastroenterology* 66:987, 1974.
22. Carter EA, Gonnella A, Tompkins RG. Increased transcellular permeability of rat small intestine after thermal injury. *Burns* 18:117, 1992.
23. Owen RL. Sequential uptake of horseradish peroxidase by lymphoid follicle epithelium of Peyer's patches in the normal unobstructed mouse intestine: An ultrastructural study. *Gastroenterology* 72:440, 1977.
24. Sanders E, Ashworth CT. A study of particulate intestinal absorption and hepatocellular uptake. *Exp Cell Res* 22:137, 1961.
25. Sass W, Dreyer HP, Seifert J. Rapid insorption of small particles in the gut. *Am J Gastroenterol* 85:255, 1990.
26. Porta C, et al. Confocal analysis of fluorescent bead uptake by mouse Peyer's patch follicle-associated M cells. *Exp Physiol* 77:929, 1992.
27. Volkheimer G, et al. Persorption of particles. *Digestion* 1:78, 1968.
28. Volkheimer G, et al. The effect of drugs on the rate of persorption. *Pharmacology* 1:8, 1968.
29. Volkheimer G, et al. Persorption of metallic iron particles. *Gut* 10:32, 1969.
30. Volkheimer G. Hematogenous dissemination of ingested polyvinyl chloride particles. *Ann NY Acad Sci* 246:164, 1975.
31. Alexander JW, et al. The process of bacterial translocation. *Ann Surg* 212:496, 1990.
32. Hildebrand GJ, Wolochow H. Translocation of bacteriophage across the intestinal wall of rats. *Proc Soc Exp Biol Med* 109:183, 1962.
33. Wolochow H, Hildebrand GJ, Lamanna C. Translocation of microorganisms across the intestinal wall of the rat effect of microbial size and concentration. *J Infect Dis* 116:523, 1966.
34. Deitch EA, et al. Hemorrhagic shock induced bacterial translocation is reduced by xanthine oxidase inhibition or inactivation. *Surgery* 104:191, 1988.
35. Alexander JW. Nutrition and translocation. *JPEN* 14: 1705, 1990.
36. Nieuwenhuijzen GAP, et al. Macrophage elimination increases bacterial translocation and gut-origin septicemia but attenuates symptoms and mortality rate in a model of systemic inflammation. *Ann Surg* 218:791, 1993.
37. Papa M, et al. The effect of ischemia of the dog's colon on transluminal irrigation of bacteria and endotoxin. *J Surg Res* 35:264, 1983.
38. Gianotti L, et al. Translocation of *Candida albicans* is related to the blood flow of individual villi. *Circ Shock* 40:250, 1993.

39. Gennari R, Alexander JW. Effect of hyperoxia on bacterial translocation and mortality during gut derived sepsis. *Arch Surg* (in press).

40. Gennari R, et al. Heparan sulfate increases survival during gut-derived sepsis by decreasing bacterial translocation and enhancing host defense. *Shock* 2:246, 1994.

41. Gianotti L, et al. Impact of blood transfusion and burn injury on microbial translocation and bacterial survival. *Transfusion* 32:312, 1992.

42. Gianotti L, et al. Arginine-supplemented diets improve survival in gut-derived sepsis and peritonitis by modulating bacterial clearance: The role of nitric oxide. *Ann Surg* 217:644, 1993.

43. Gianotti L, et al. Oral glutamine decreases bacterial translocation and improves survival in experimental gut-origin sepsis. *JPEN* 14:69–74, 1995.

44. Gianotti L, Alexander JW, Pyles T. Dietary fatty acids modulate host bactericidal response of microbial translocation and outcome following blood transfusion burn injury. Submitted for publication.

45. Nelson JL, et al. Influences of dietary fiber on microbial growth *in vitro* and bacterial translocation following burn injury in mice. *Nutrition* 10:32, 1994.

46. Gennari R, Alexander JW, Pyles T. Effect of different combinations of dietary additives on bacterial translocation and survival in gut-derived sepsis. *JPEN* 19(4):319–325, 1995.

47. Burke DJ, et al. Glutamine-supplemented total parenteral nutrition improves gut immune function. *Arch Surg* 124:1369, 1989.

48. Fox AD, et al. Effect of glutamine-supplemented enteral diet on methotrexate-induced enterocolitis. *JPEN* 12:325, 1988.

49. Souba WW, et al. Oral glutamine reduces bacterial translocation following abdominal radiation. *J Surg Res* 48:1, 1990.

50. Klimberg VS, et al. Prophylactic glutamine protects the intestinal mucosa from radiation injury. *Cancer* 66:62, 1990.

51. Gianotti L, et al. Prostaglandin E1 analogues, misoprostol and enisoprost, decrease microbial translocation in thermally injured mice. *Circ Shock* 40:243, 1993.

52. Gianotti L, et al. Reduction of bacterial translocation with oral fibroblast growth factor and sucralfate. *Am J Surg* 163:195, 1993.

53. Gennari R, et al. Granulocyte-macrophage colony stimulating factor improves survival in two models of gut-derived sepsis by improving gut barrier function and modulating bacterial clearance. *Ann Surg* 220:68, 1994.

54. Gennari R, Alexander JW, Pyles T. IFN-γ decreases translocation and improves survival following transfusion and thermal injury. *J Surg Res* 56:530, 1994.

55. Arita H, et al. Induction of hypermetabolism in guinea pigs by endotoxin infused through the tail vein. *Arch Surg* 123:1420, 1988.

56. Gianotti L, et al. The post-injury hypermetabolic response is correlated with the magnitude of translocation: Prevention by early enteral nutrition. *Nutrition* 10:225, 1994.

57. Mochizuki H, et al. Mechanisms of prevention of postburn hypermetabolism and catabolism by early enteral feeding. *Ann Surg* 200:297, 1984.

58. Chiarelli AP. Very early enteral nutrition supplementation in burned patients. *Am J Clin Nutr* 51:1035, 1990.

59. Fukushima R, Gianotti L, Alexander JW. The degree of bacterial translocation is a determinant factor for mortality after burn injury and is improved by prostaglandin analogs. *Ann Surg* 216:438, 1992.

60. Fukushima R, et al. Bacterial translocation related mortality may be associated with neutrophil mediated organ damage. *Shock* 3(5):323–328, 1995.

61. Ogle CK, et al. The production of TNF, IL-1, IL-6 and PGE_2 by isolated enterocytes and gut macrophages: Effect of LPS and thermal injury. *J Burn Care Rehab* 15:470, 1994.

62. Mainous HR, et al. The gut as a cytokine producing organ in systemic inflammation. *Shock* 1:537, 1994.

63. Gennari R, et al. Effect of anti-IL-6 antibacterial translocation. *Arch Surg* 129:1191, 1994.

64. Poggetti RS, et al. Liver injury is a reversible neutrophil-mediated event following gut-ischemia. *Arch Surg* 127: 175, 1992.

65. Howerton EE, Kolmen SN. The intestinal tract is a port of entry of Pseudomonas in burned rats. *J Trauma* 12:335, 1972.

66. Gianotti L, et al. Relationship between extent of burn injury and magnitude of microbial translocation from the intestine. *J Burn Care Rehab* 14:336, 1993.

67. Pine L, Malcom GB, Plikaytis BD. Listeria monocytes intragastric and intraperitoneal approximate 50% lethal doses for mice are comparable, but death occurs earlier by intragastric feeding. *Infect Immun* 58:2940, 1990.

68. Krause W, Matheis H, Wulf K. Fungaemia and funguria after oral administration of *Candida albicans. Lancet* 1:598, 1969.

69. Tancrede LH, Andremont AO. Bacterial translocation and gram-negative bacteremia in patients with hematological malignancies. *J Infect Dis* 152:99, 1985.

70. Rush BF, et al. Endotoxemia and bacteremia during hemorrhagic shock. *Ann Surg* 207:549, 1988.

71. Deitch EA, Bridges W, Berg RD. Hemorrhagic shock-induced bacterial translocation: The role of neutrophils and hydroxyl radicals. *J Trauma* 8:942, 1990.

72. Brathwaite CEM, et al. Bacterial translocation occurs in humans after traumatic injury: Evidence using immunofluorescence. *J Trauma* 34:586, 1993.

73. Marshall JL, Christou NV, Meakins JL. The gastrointestinal tract: The "undrained abscess" of multiple organ failure. *Ann Surg* 218:111, 1993.

74. Levy J, et al. Contaminated enteral nutrition solutions as a cause of nosocomial infections. *JPEN* 13:228, 1989.

75. Ambrose NS, et al. Incidence of pathogenic bacteria from mesenteric lymph nodes and ileal serosa during Crohn's disease. *Br J Surg* 71:623, 1984.

76. Vincent P, et al. Bacterial translocation in patients with colo-rectal cancer. *J Infect Dis* 158:1395, 1988.

77. Moore FA, et al. Gut bacterial translocation via the portal vein: A clinical perspective with major torso trauma. *J Trauma* 31:629, 1991.

78. Cerra FB, et al. Selective decontamination reduces nosocomial infections and length of stay but not mortality or organ failure in surgical intensive care unit patients. *Arch Surg* 127:163, 1992.

79. Jackson RJ, Smith SD, Rowe MI. Selective bowel decontamination results in gram-positive translocation. *J Surg Res* 48:444, 1990.

80. Munster AW, et al. Translocation: Incidental phenomenon or true pathology? *Ann Surg* 218:321, 1993.

Selected Readings

Alexander JW, et al. The process of microbial translocation. *Ann Surg* 212:496, 1990.

In this study the authors used translocation probes (viable *C. albicans* and *E. coli* and partially purified endotoxin) to observe and document the anatomic process of translocation by light and electron microscopy.

Arnold L. Alterations in the endogenous enteric bacterial flora and microbic permeability of the intestinal wall in relation to the nutritional and meteorological changes. *J Hyg* 29:82, 1931.

This is one of the first studies to show the passage of bacteria across an intact mucosal wall to the lymphatics and the importance of the environment in the phenomenon of microbial translocation. This experiment showed that translocation could occur across the normal mucosa of an animal under certain conditions, especially with alkalinization of the duodenal contents.

Krause W, Matheis H, Wulf K. Fungaemia and funguria after oral administration of Candida albicans. *Lancet* 1:598, 1969.

Within a few hours after ingesting a beaker of a suspension of live *Candida,* this 38-year-old surgeon became symptomatic with chills and fever and had positive blood cultures for *Candida* as well as candiduria—the first indisputable evidence for translocation of a fungus in man.

Marshall JL, Christou NV, Meakins JL. The gastrointestinal tract: the "undrained abscess" of multiple organ failure. *Ann Surg* 218:111, 1993.

The study showed a strong positive association between proximal gastrointestinal colonization and the development of nosocomial infection and multiple organ failure in a population of critically ill surgical patients.

Volkheimer G, et al. The effect of drugs on the rate of persorption. *Pharmacology* 1:8, 1968.

The authors showed in 34 healthy human subjects that, within minutes after ingestion, potato starch granules could be found in the blood in relatively high concentrations. The concentration of particles in the blood was related both to the amount ingested and concomitant medications.

18

Omega-3 and Other Polyunsaturated Fatty Acids: Modulation of the Inflammatory Response

Michael D. Peck

Omega-3 (ω-3) polyunsaturated fatty acids (PUFA) belong to a biochemically unique family of essential fatty acids that are necessary for growth, reproduction, and the maintenance of health. Although ω-3 PUFA occur naturally in the oils of certain vegetables and fish, the usual dietary intake of most humans includes very little ω-3 PUFA. In the last 20 years, there has been increased interest in the medical uses of ω-3 PUFA for both preventative and treatment purposes.

Fish oils have been reported to be antiatherogenic and antihypertensive and to lower serum lipid levels [1]. Dyerberg and associates [2] observed that Greenland Eskimos had lower serum cholesterol levels than their Danish peers, despite a diet relatively high in fat and cholesterol. They proposed the hypothesis that the high content of ω-3 PUFA in the Eskimo diet was responsible for the reduced blood lipids and low incidence of myocardial infarction [3]. Although it is now controversial whether fish oils are more efficacious at reducing serum cholesterol than ω-6 PUFA, it is agreed that they are effective in the treatment of hypertriglyceridemia [1]. Some clinical trials have suggested that supplemental fish oil may reduce mortality from coronary artery disease in patients surviving myocardial infarction and may reduce the rate of restenosis after coronary artery angioplasty [1].

Fish oil supplements have been shown to slow the progression of autoimmune disease. Diets enriched with fish oil prolong survival in autoimmune-prone mice; they may do so by reduced production of pro-inflammatory prostaglandins and leukotrienes [4,5]. The results from clinical studies, however, have been mixed. Although some investigators have reported that supplementing fish oil improves symptoms associated with rheumatoid arthritis [6], others have shown that there is no apparent beneficial effect in patients with psoriasis [7] or systemic lupus nephritis [8].

Interest has grown in preventing neoplastic tumors by diets rich in fish oils because studies have shown that mice or rats fed diets high in fish oil consistently show inhibition of mammary tumorigenesis [9] and prostate tumorigenesis [10]. Furthermore, epidemiologic studies have suggested that populations consuming higher amounts of fish oil tend to have lower rates of breast, colon, and prostate cancer [11].

Omega-3 PUFA have a role in the treatment of stressed surgical patients. Excessive activation of the arachidonic acid pathway occurs in these patients, which can be inhibited by ω-3 PUFA. For example, Alexander and associates [12] found that fish oil given enterally to guinea pigs following burn injury results in improvement in a number of metabolic and immune parameters. These observations were followed by a number of animal studies investigating the effects of ω-3 PUFA on immune function in traumatized, burned, or septic models, culminating in the development of commercially available enteral feeding products supplemented with ω-3 PUFA. Clinical trials have been conducted with these products, and the preliminary results from one of these trials suggest an improvement in infection rate and length of stay in patients fed diets supplemented with ω-3 PUFA [13].

The results from these clinical studies and animal experiments, however, are not all consistent with the hypothesis that ω-3 PUFA are uniformly beneficial to stressed surgical patients. This chapter will review the basic biochemical mechanism by which ω-3 and other PUFA exert their effect on cellular function, focusing on the cell membrane. It further will suggest that the effects of polyunsaturated fatty acids are quite diverse, including not only modulation of arachidonic acid metabolites, but also of changes in the physical characteristics of the cell membrane and of the production of lipid peroxides. Such an understanding of the multiple effects of PUFA will help guide our use of them in treating stressed surgical patients.

Lipid Biochemistry

The structure of lipids determines their functional characteristics. Fatty acids are alkyl chains terminating in carboxyl groups and are primarily classified on the basis of chain length and degree of unsaturation (Table 18-1). In a saturated fatty acid, such as stearic acid, the alkyl chain has no double bonds. Monounsaturated fatty acids, such as oleic acid, have only one double bond, and PUFA, such as linoleic acid, have two or more double bonds. Some investigators further classify the polyunsaturated fatty acids into highly unsaturated fatty acids if there are four or more double bonds present.*

PUFA are classified by the position of the first double bond. Four classes of unsaturated fatty acids are recognized, the parent molecules being palmitoleic acid (16:1 ω-7), oleic acid (18:1 ω-9), linoleic acid (18:2 ω-6), and α-linolenic acid (18:3 ω-3) (Figure 18-1). Each class is made up of a family of fatty acids that can be synthesized from the parent fatty acids, but a fatty acid of one class cannot be converted biologically to another class. For example, although oleic acid (18:1 ω-9) can be elongated and desaturated to eicosatrienoic acid (20:3 ω-9), it cannot be converted to arachidonic acid (20:4 ω-6).

Very few ω-3 fatty acids are naturally present in most oils and fats. Perilla and linseed oils are high in α-linolenic acid (58% and 54%, respectively); those oils that are commonly used for human consumption, such as canola and soybean oils (10% and 7%, respectively), are lower in α-linoleic acid. Medical foods are constructed with soybean, corn, sunflower, safflower, or canola oils, most of which are high in ω-6 fatty acids (Table 18-2) [14].

In contrast to vegetable oils, some fish oils contain up to 35% ω-3 fatty acids (see Table 18-2). These oils are isolated from fish that live on vegetation growing in cold water. The phytoplankter *Monochrysis lutheri,* for example, which is

*The nomenclature of fatty acids is based on chain length and unsaturation. Fatty acid structure is abbreviated as the length, followed by the number of double bonds, and finally by the position of the first double bond. The position of the first double bond can be identified in two ways: in the delta system (Δ), the carbon atoms are numbered from the carboxyl end; in the omega system (ω or n), the carbons are numbered from the methyl end. For example, 20:4 ω-6 refers to arachidonic acid, which is a 20-carbon acid with 4 double bonds, the first of which starts 6 carbons from the methyl end. Naturally occurring fatty acyl double bonds are in the *cis* position. *Trans*-unsaturation may occur during hydrogenation or processing by intestinal bacteria in ruminants.

Table 18-1. Names and Classes of Fatty Acids

Abbreviation	Common name	Chemical name*	Melting Point (°C)
2:0	acetic	ethanoic	16.7
4:0	butyric	butanoic	−7.9
6:0	caproic	hexanoic	−3.4
8:0	caprylic	octanoic	16.7
10:0	capric	decanoic	31.6
12:0	lauric	dodecanoic	44.2
14:0	myristic	tetradecanoic	53.6
16:0	palmitic	hexadecanoic	63.1
16:1 ω-7	palmitoleic	hexadecanoic	0
18:0	stearic	octadecanoic	69.6
18:1 ω-9	oleic	*cis*-octadecenoic	13.2
18:1 ω-9	elaidic	*trans*-octadecenoic	44.0
18:2 ω-6	linoleic	*cis,cis*-octadecadienoic	5.0
18:2 ω-6	linoelaidic	*trans, trans*-octadecadienoic	28.5
18:3 ω-3	α-linolenic	9, 12, 15-octadecatrienoic	−11.0
18:3 ω-6	γ-linolenic	6, 9, 12-octadecatrienoic	
20:3 ω-9		11, 14, 17-eicosatrienoic	
20:3 ω-6	γ-homolinolenic	8, 11, 14-eicosatrienoic	
20:4 ω-6	arachidonic	eicosatetraenoic	−49.5
20:5 ω-3	EPA	eicosapentaenoic	−54.1
22:1 ω-9	erucic	docosenoic	34.7
22:6 ω-3	DHA	docosahexaenoic	−44.3

*Unless otherwise indicated, all double bonds are *cis*.

Source: Adapted from GD Fasman (ed). *CRC Handbook of Biochemistry and Molecular Biology, Lipids, Carbohydrates, and Steroids* (3rd ed). Boca Raton: CRC Press, 1975–1977.

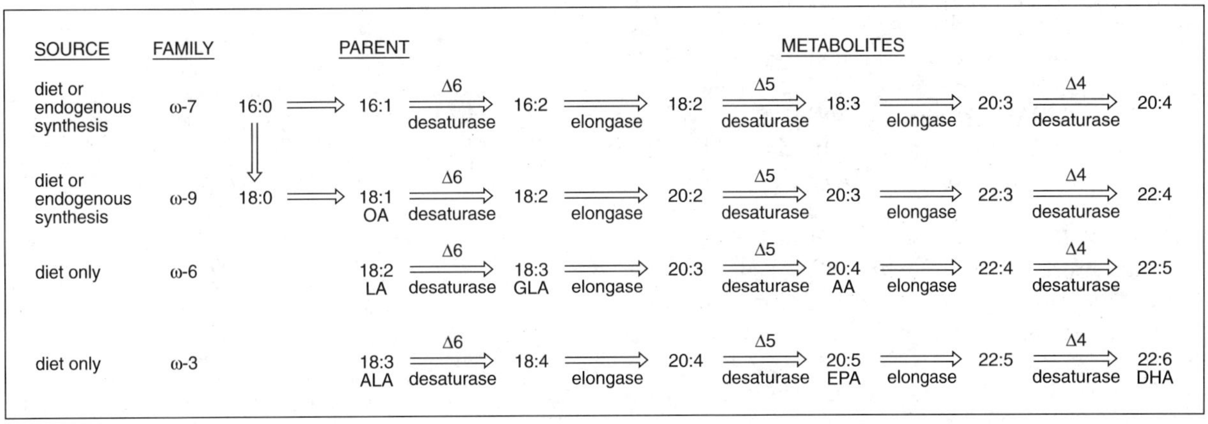

Figure 18-1. The four families of polyunsaturated fatty acids and their metabolism. Both palmitic (16:0) and stearic (18:0) acids are present in the diet and can be synthesized endogenously. Linoleic (18:2 ω-6) and linolenic (18:3 ω-3) acids can only be obtained from the diet. All four families of unsaturated fatty acids compete for the same desaturase and elongase enzymes. AA = arachidonic acid; ALA = alpha-linolenic acid; DHA = docosahexaenoic acid; EPA = eicosapentaenoic acid; GLA = gamma-linolenic acid; LA = linoleic acid; OA = oleic acid. (Based on data from R Montgomery, TW Conway, AA Spector (eds). Biochemistry: A Case-Oriented Approach. St Louis: Mosby, 1990; and MI Gurr. *Role of Fats in Food and Nutrition*. London: Elsevier, 1992.)

Table 18-2. Fatty Acid Composition of Fats and Oils (% Composition)

	SFA	MFA	PFA	OA	LA	ALA	EPA	DHA	MP(°C)	Iodine Value
Coconut oil	82	5	1	5	1				25	10
Palm kernel oil	81	11	2	11	2				24	37
Beef tallow	54	39	2	36	2				42	50
Palm oil	49	37	37	9	2				35	54
Olive oil	13	79	7	79	7				−6	81
Peanut oil	17	46	32	45	32				3	93
Cottonseed oil	22	18	60	18	60				−1	106
Sesame oil	14	40	42	40	42				−6	107
Canola oil	6	61	30	61	21	9				115
Corn oil	12	31	56	31	56				−20	123
Sunflower oil	10	20	66	20	66				−17	126
Soybean oil	14	24	54	24	47	7			−16	130
Herring oil	19	60	16				7	4		140
Safflower oil	7	17	76	17	76					145
Cod liver oil	37	41	22	17	2	2	9	9		165
Menhaden oil	34	33	30				13	8		170
Linseed oil	8	20	72	20	18	54			−24	179
Perilla oil	8	18	73	18	15	58				195
MaxEPA oil	44	29	27	15	1	3	14	9		

Source: Based on S Watanabe et al. Effect of dietary α-linolenate/linoleate balance on lipopolysaccharide-induced tumor necrosis factor production in mouse macrophages. *Life Sci* 48:2013, 1991; ME Shils, VR Young. Average Values for Triglycerides, Fatty Acids, and Cholesterol in Selected Foods and Oils. In ME Shils, V Young (eds), *Modern Nutrition in Health and Disease*. Philadelphia: Lea & Febiger, 1988. P 1547; KM Chee, et al. Fatty acid content of marine oil capsules. *Lipids* 25:523, 1990; PL Altman, DS Dittmer (eds). *Biology Data Book*. Bethesda: Federation of American Societies of Experimental Biology, 1972.

found in the North Atlantic Ocean, has 22% eicosapentaenoic acid (EPA) and 11% docosahexaenoic acid (DHA) (w/w) [15]. Fatty fish, such as mackerel, herring, tuna, sardines, salmon, and menhaden, store high amounts of ω-3 fatty acids as triglycerides in their flesh.

Some PUFA, including ω-3 PUFA, are essential to the diet. These essential lipids include fat-soluble vitamins (vitamins A, D, and E), and PUFA of the linoleic acid and α-linolenic acid groups (ω-6 and ω-3 PUFA). Omega-6 and ω-3 PUFA are destined more for structural lipids of membranes rather than for storage fats. In addition, they have unique roles as substrates for eicosanoid synthesis.

Essential fatty acids are metabolized differently. The fate of dietary α-linolenic acid is different from that of its 18-carbon ω-6 counterpart, linoleic acid, or from that of the highly unsaturated ω-3 fatty acids, EPA and DHA. When only low levels of α-linolenic acid are fed, elongation and desaturation proceed all the way to EPA and DHA. For the most part, however, α-linolenic acid is much more rapidly oxidized than dietary linoleic acid [16], bringing into question its efficacy as a modulator of eicosanoid synthesis.*

*__α-Linolenic Acid versus Fish Oil.__ There are concerns that α-linolenic acid and very long-chain polyunsaturated ω-3 fatty acids (EPA and DHA) are not biologically equivalent [17]. The first concern is that α-linolenic acid is β-oxidized to a greater extent than other essential fatty acids. For example, in humans dietarily deficient in all ω-3 fatty acids, the increase in long-chain ω-3 fatty acids after α-linolenic acid supplementation is not larger [18]. Hepatic mitochondria oxidize α-linolenic acid at twice the rate of linoleic acid [19]. There is also a suggestion that a dietary deficiency of α-linolenic acid has no pathologic significance if longer-chain ω-3 fatty acids are present in the diet. Nonetheless, if α-linolenic acid is the only ω-3 fatty acid in the diet (such as in vegans eating no animal products), long-chain ω-3 fatty acids in serum lipids are present, although low, and there are no obvious pathologic consequences [20]. Alpha-linolenic acid, in comparison to fish oil, does not reduce plasma triglycerides [20,21]. There is a discrepancy between α-linolenic acid and fish oil, described in the brief report by Dyerberg and associates [22], which noted that a volunteer given 15 ml linseed oil thrice daily for eight days increased total ω-3 fatty acid in plasma lipid fractions only four-fold, compared to over seven-fold after taking an equal amount of cod liver oil, which contains one sixth the ω-3 fatty acid content of linseed oil.
Not only are α-linolenic acid and longer-chain ω-3 fatty acids

There are ample data to confirm that dietary PUFA are incorporated into tissue lipids [20,29–35]. For example, Mori and associates found that daily supplementation of MaxEPA capsules (2.67 g EPA/day and 1.72 g DHA/day) for three weeks decreases arachidonic acid and increases EPA and DHA in platelet phospholipids from healthy males [30].

Of particular interest to the discussion of the immune system is that dietary lipids alter phospholipid profiles of leukocytes, such as lymphocytes [31], macrophages [32], and polymorphonuclear cells [33,36]. For example, Cleland and associates [33] found that membrane phospholipid fatty acid profiles reflect dietary lipid intake (olive, sunflower, linseed, or fish oils). They examined both induced peritoneal neutrophils and resting splenic mononuclear cells from rats for four weeks on diets that contained 10% (w/w) lipid, and found no differences in fatty acid profiles. Although the length of time for maximal fatty acid incorporation into lymphocytes is four to six weeks [31], significant incorporation of ω-3 fatty acids occurs as early as two weeks of feeding [32]. Clinical studies with an enteral formula containing ω-3 PUFA have confirmed that modification for plasma PUFA is altered within seven days [37].

Thus it is clear that PUFA, present in the fats and oils of natural foods, are distributed ubiquitously throughout the cell membranes of the body. As we will see, the unique structural characteristics of PUFA and their key location in biomembranes enable them to influence the structure and function of cells.

Cell Membranes

The lipid bilayer forms the structural framework for all biomembranes [38]. It serves to define outside and inside compartments, and it regulates the nature of communication between outside and inside the cell (such as the passage of ions or molecules, or the conformational changes in membrane components). Enzymes that catalyze transmembrane or intramembrane reactions may be attached to membranes. Most fundamental biochemical processes involve membranes at some point; examples include protein biosynthesis and secretion, bioenergetic reactions, and hormonal responses. The diversity of function of biomembranes is primarily due to different proteins present in the membrane. There are structural similarities for prokaryotic and eukaryotic (both animal and plant) cell membranes and for all organelle membranes.

Our present concepts of the structure of biomembranes are based on the fluid-mosaic model suggested by Singer and Nicholson [39]. This model (Figure 18-2) suggests a fluid-like phospholipid bilayer with freely diffusing globular proteins that are embedded to various degrees. Although the traditional model suggests a rather homogeneous interior, recent evidence would suggest that membrane proteins do not diffuse freely, possibly directly affecting their function [38]. The lateral domains of membranes are heterogeneous and differentiated, and some regions may not be structured in the traditional phospholipid bilayer.

The major components of biomembranes are proteins and lipids. Protein content ranges from 20% in myelin to 75% in mitochondria (Table 18-3). There are several classes of lipids present in membranes. One class is the glycerophospholipids, which are glycerophosphates with fatty acids esterified to two hydroxyl groups. These molecules are amphoteric, with a polar phosphate-containing head group and a nonpolar fatty acid tail. The phosphate at the *sn*-3 position is linked to choline, ethanolamine, inositol, serine, or glycerol. Although phospholipids are technically any lipids that contain phosphoric groups (such as plasmalo-

---

metabolized differently, but they appear to have different effects on cellular function. For example, Ehringer and associates [23] found that DHA causes a much greater enhancement than α-linolenic acid of the rates of fusion and permeability of phosphatidylcholine bilayers. Neither fatty acid has any effect on the fluidity of these artificial bilayers. These results suggest a role for DHA in increasing the susceptibility of target cells, such as tumor cells, to damage by increasing membrane permeability, and also that cellular functions requiring movement, such as phagocytosis, may also be modulated by longer-chain ω-3 fatty acids.

Alpha-linolenic acid and longer-chain ω-3 fatty acids have different strengths of effect on production of trienoic prostanoids and pentaenoic leukotrienes. For example, Hwang and associates [24] found in rats that longer-chain ω-3 fatty acids fed fish oil are more effective than α-linolenic acid in suppressing arachidonic acid levels and cyclooxygenase-derived products in platelets and lung homogenates. Several investigators have observed that dietary fish oil is several times more effective than α-linolenic acid in increasing 5-hydroxyeicosapentaenoic acid (5-HEPE) and pentaenoic leukotrienes such as LTB_5 and LTE_5 [24–26].

Because of these differential effects on membrane biophysical characteristics and eicosanoid production, α-linolenic acid and fish oil have differential effects on the immune system. For example, Kelley and associates [27] observed that T-cell blastogenesis is increased only by linseed oil, but not by fish oil in rabbits fed 23 en% of the diet as fat. In contrast, Wu and associates [28] found that α-linolenic acid fed to monkeys induces no changes in lymphocyte subsets, whereas fish oil decreases the number of T cells and increases the number of B cells. Although preliminary, these results are intriguing enough to suggest that more complex studies be done in animal models of infection to compare the relative efficacy of α-linolenic acid and longer-chain ω-3 fatty acids.

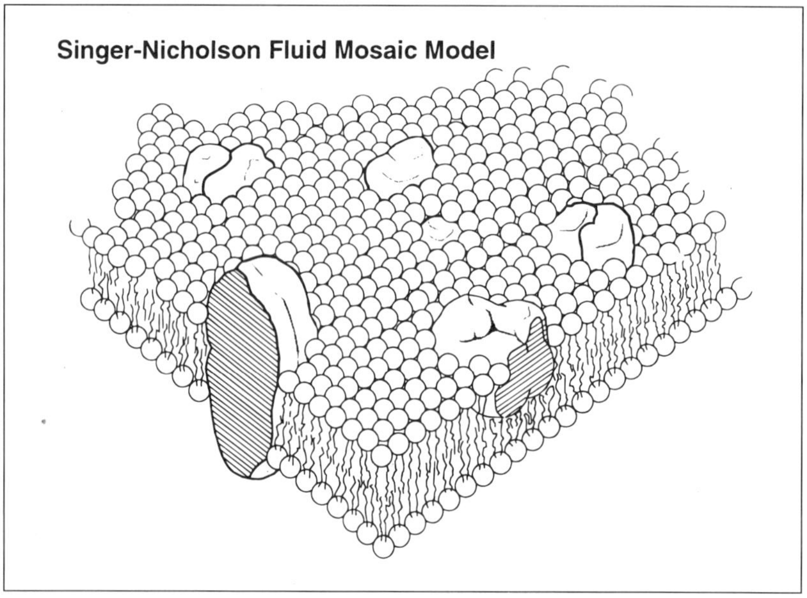

Figure 18-2. The Singer-Nicholson fluid mosaic model. The matrix of the membrane is formed by the phospholipid bilayer. Proteins are scattered throughout the bilayer of the plasma membrane in the pattern of a mosaic. Various types of proteins are associated with the lipid bilayer, including surface and transmembrane proteins. Proteins are not fixed in position and have lateral mobility and rotational freedom. Flip-flop, however, does not occur, so that the surface of a protein exposed to extracellular fluid does not flip over and become exposed to the cytoplasm. (Based on SJ Singer, GL Nicholson. The fluid mosaic model of the structure of cell membranes. *Science* 175:720, 1972.)

Table 18-3. Composition of Cell Membranes

	Composition by weight		
Membrane	Protein (%)	Lipid (%)	Carbohydrate (%)
Myelin	20	75	5
Erythrocyte	49	43	8
Hepatocyte plasma membrane	54	39	7
Outer mitochondrial membrane	50	46	4
Inner mitochondrial membrane	75	23	2

Source: R Montgomery, TW Conway, AA Spector (eds). Biochemistry: A Case-Oriented Approach. St Louis: Mosby, 1990.

gens, cardiolipins, or sphingolipids), the term is used to describe 1,2-diacylphosphoglycerides, which are the predominant lipids in eukaryotic and prokaryotic membranes. (In animal cells, phosphatidylcholine predominates; in bacteria, phosphatidylethanolamine predominates.) The acyl chains at the *sn*-1 and the *sn*-2 positions are usually even-numbered fatty acids ranging from 14 to 24 carbons. The most common acyl chains are 16, 18, and 20 carbons in length. The *sn*-1 position is occupied by saturated fatty acids, and the *sn*-2 position by unsaturated fatty acids, most commonly 18:1, 18:2, 18:3, and 20:4 (all *cis*).

The biophysical properties and chemical behaviors of the lipids in the bilayer support the functional properties of the membrane. There is a nonrandom distribution of over 100 species of lipids in biomembranes; the reasons for this heterogeneity and the mechanism responsible for it are not known. Nonetheless, studies have shown that cell viability can be maintained within a wide range of lipid composition [40].

The diverse properties of biomembranes are related to the phase of lipids in lipid-water mixtures [38]. Mixtures of lipids in water can exist in four different phases [41,42]. The bulk of lipids in biological membranes exists in the lamellar liquid crystalline phase, in which there is a high degree of order of the polar head groups and disorder of the acyl chains (Figure 18-3). At lower temperatures, under experimental conditions, this mixture can exist as the lamellar gel phase, in which there is tighter packing and more order of the acyl chains. In the hexagonal I phase (H_I), lipids exist as cylinders packed in a hexagonal pattern with the polar head groups outside. In the hexagonal II phase (H_{II}), the polar head groups are inside. Hexagonal structures exist in small domains in biomembranes, such as hepatic microsomes, mitochondrial inner membranes, and retinal rod outer

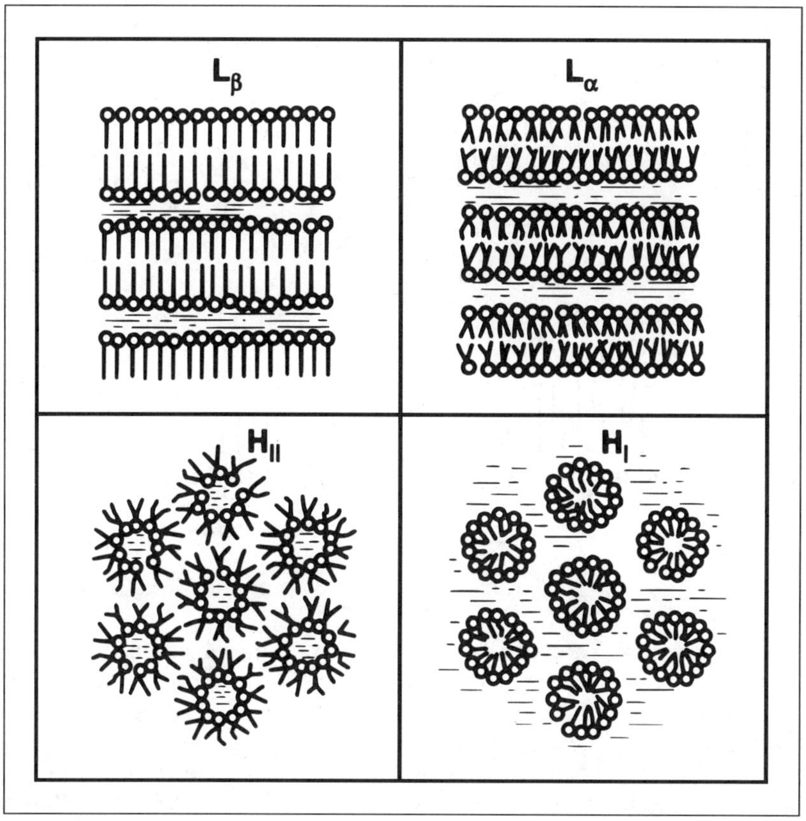

Figure 18-3. Schematic representations of lipid-water phases. L_β: lamellar gel phase, which is formed at low temperatures and in which the fatty acyl chains are packed more tightly together and are more highly ordered; L_α: lamellar liquid crystalline phase, which represents the bulk of lipids in biologic membranes and in which there is considerable disorder of the acyl chains; H_{II}: Hexagonal II phase, in which the lipids are in the form of cylinders with the polar groups facing the inside where there is a column of water; H_I: Hexagonal I phase, in which the lipids are in the form of cylinders with the polar groups on the outside in contact with water. (Diagram based on RB Gennis. *Biomembranes: Molecular Structure and Function.* New York: Springer, 1989, adapted from GG Shipley. Recent X-ray Diffraction Studies of Biological Membrane Components. In D Chapman, DFH Wallach (eds), *Biological Membranes.* New York: Academic, 1973.)

segments, and may be especially critical to membrane fusion [43–45]. In fact, membrane lipids are polymorphic and can exist in different phases. For example, phosphatidylethalomine prefers the H_{II} hexagonal phase [41,46].

The transition of lipids from gel to liquid crystalline phases (conceptually similar to the transition of ice to liquid water) is characterized by the melting temperature, which is the midpoint of this transition. Iodine values represent the number of double bonds present in natural lipids and vary directly with the melting temperature (see Table 18-1). Several factors determine the melting temperature. Although interactions among polar head groups can influence the melting temperature, the interaction among acyl chains is the most important determinant. The longer the acyl chain length, the higher is the melting temperature, because of increased Van der Waals forces. The presence of double bonds lowers the melting temperature because of increased disorder among the acyl chains; *cis*-double bonds lower the melting temperature much more than *trans*-double bonds. The double bond forces a 37° bend in the chain. The maximal effect on melting temperature occurs when the double bond is in the middle of the acyl chain (for example, oleic acid, in which the double bond is at the ω-9 position in an 18-carbon chain). In addition, the differences among the effects of increasing unsaturation (oleic, linoleic, and arachidonic acids) on membrane fluidity are relatively small compared to the changes noted between saturated (palmitic) and monounsaturated (oleic) fatty acids, suggesting that the first double bond plays the most important role [47]. Moreover, there appears to be increasing disorder of the membrane with increasing depth of the first double bond from the phospholipid head group, suggesting that the position of the fatty acyl double bonds is more important than the quantity [48].

The different phases of phospholipids may create microscopic lipid heterogeneities with distinct composition and physical properties within the membrane. There may be regions of different fluidity, as both gel and liquid crystalline phases exist in different domains (Figure 18-4). These different domains could be responsible for sequestration of enzymes or could be areas for phase transitions that would allow increased flip-flop of proteins, increased permeability, or increased adhesion of lipid vesicles. For example, fusion between membrane organelles may involve a transition of lamellar liquid crystalline to H_{II} phases [49].

In summary, fatty acids from the diet are incorporated into the phospholipids of cell mem-

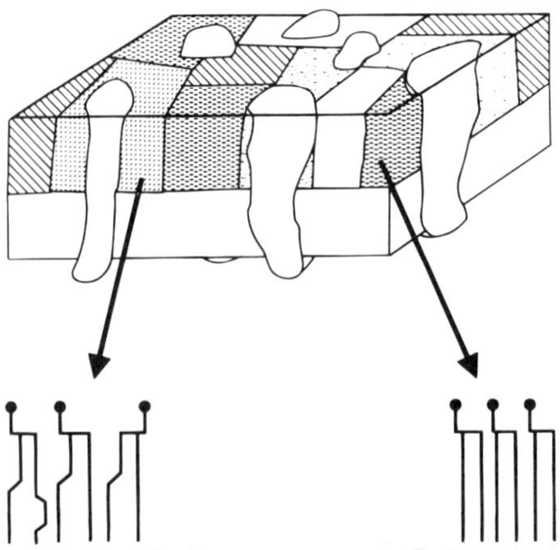

Figure 18-4. The structurally distinct domains of plasma membranes. In this highly schematized diagram of a plasma membrane, Klausner and associates have illustrated the diversity of lipid domains within membranes. These domains may represent lamellar gel, liquid crystalline, or hexagonal phases. Indeed, some may represent areas of increased or decreased fluidity of liquid crystalline phases. For instance, cis-unsaturated fatty acids may partition into a more disordered region than saturated or trans-unsaturated fatty acids; the function of the protein embedded in this domain may be altered by this difference in fluidity. (Based on RD Klausner, et al. Lipid domains in membranes. *J Biol Chem* 255:1286, 1980.)

branes. There they form a dynamic structural framework for all intra- or transmembrane processes. The physical properties of the fatty acyl tails of the membrane phospholipids modulate these processes. The next section will review the manner by which membrane fluidity influences the function of cell membranes.

Membrane Fluidity

Membrane fluidity is a biophysical concept used to describe the resistance to movement of various types of molecules within membranes; it is strongly related to lipid packing or order. Biomembranes generally are in liquid crystalline phases, in which fluidity is maintained to support life functions because, in general, membranes in gel states do not support biochemical reactions. For example, trout biomembranes will adjust their fatty acid content by increasing unsaturation to maintain membrane fluidity when they are exposed to cold waters [50].

Membrane fluidity can be altered by dietary lipids and disease. Increasing the amount of polyunsaturated fat in the diet increases the membrane P-S ratio (ratio of polyunsaturated to saturated fatty acids) and membrane fluidity [48,51,52]. Clinical studies have shown that membrane fluidity changes in injured patients, with both severe injury and sepsis resulting in decreased fluidity of peripheral blood cells [53,54], although major burn injury increases fluidity of human peripheral blood lymphocytes [55].

As noted above, changes in membrane fluidity alter the function of cells. For example, evidence shows that increases in membrane fluidity increase the mobility of intramembranous proteins. In addition, Fernandes [51] has noted that dietary fish oil increases lymphocyte IL-2 receptor expression, which may be caused by an increase in membrane fluidity. Interestingly, there may be an optimal range of fluidity within which cellular function is optimized. Schroit and Gallily [56] have noted that macrophage phagocytic activity is not linearly related to the cholesterol-phospholipid ratio (which is a major function determining membrane fluidity), but has an optimal value at a ratio of 0.425, and gradually decreases at both reduced and elevated ratios. Phagocytic activity is, however, linearly related to the unsaturation index and the saturated-unsaturated fatty acid ratios of the membrane, suggesting that cholesterol itself may have a regulatory role [56].

Patching (the cross-linking of plasma membrane proteins into large clusters following ligand-binding) and capping (coalescence of these clusters into one cap) of surface molecules are early events in cellular activation and may be modulated by membrane fluidity. Patching occurs when multivalent antibodies bind to surface molecules. It is an energy-independent event, the result of the lateral movement of intramembranous glycoproteins in the phospholipid bilayer until they combine with free binding sites on the multivalent antibodies. Capping is an energy-dependent process, related closely to the cytoskeleton, and is linked to the transfer of information into the cell. Klausner and associates [57] found that murine lymphocytes incubated with *cis*-unsaturated fatty acids have increased membrane fluidity and inhibited capping by antimouse gamma globulin. Although others have also shown that free fatty acids inhibit patching and capping [58,59], we have shown that mice fed diets with 40 en% safflower or fish oil have lymphocytes in which capping with anti-CD44 monoclonal antibodies is increased, compared to those from animals fed diets from coconut or olive oil [60]. In addition, murine lymphocytes incubated with oleic acid show an increase in expression of CD44 antigens and also an increase in CD44 receptor capping [61]. It is not yet known how these changes in receptor capping relate to modulation of cell function, but they are thought to alter early events in cell activation.

Experimental models in which receptor capping is altered, for example, have shown that lymphocyte blastogenesis is changed. We have shown that murine lymphocyte membrane fluidity decreases with both safflower and fish oil diets, and that lymphocyte blastogenesis in response to mitogens is inhibited in parallel to the change in fluidity [62]. These results are similar to those of Hoover and associates [63], who found that murine lymphocytes incubated with linoleic acid show an increased expression of surface antigen but decreased mitogenesis [63]. They note that their results were similar with α-linolenic acid, suggesting that these effects are not mediated by prostaglandins, but related more to the physical characteristics of PUFA.

Macrophage function may also be altered by lipids via changes in membrane fluidity. Phagocytosis by macrophages is a special form of endocytosis in which large particles such as microorganisms and cell debris are ingested via large endocytic vesicles called phagosomes. After particles bind to the surface of the phagocyte, activated receptors transmit signals to the cell interior to initiate the response. Pseudopods are subsequently extended and engulf the particle and fuse at their tips. Incubation with *cis*-unsaturated fatty acids increases phagocytosis by macrophages [56,64–68]. For example, Calder and associates [68] found that murine thioglycollate-elicited peritoneal macrophages, incubated with albumin-complexed unsaturated fatty acids (linoleic acid, α-linolenic acid, arachidonic acid, EPA, and DHA) have decreased adhesion to plastic plates and increased phagocytosis of zymosan particles. The rate of phagocytosis correlates with the P-S ratio ($r = 0.747$). The correlation between phagocytosis and membrane phospholipid PUFA content is also very high ($r = 0.928$). The effects that DHA and EPA have on phagocytosis, however, are not as marked as predicted based on the degree of unsaturation. Specifically, although linoleic acid increases phagocytosis to 145% of control, EPA increases it only to 126% and DHA to 135% [68].

Thus, dietary PUFA can insert into cell membranes and modulate cell function, such as phagocytosis or proliferation, by altering fluidity. The next section will review a completely different mechanism by which PUFA insert into membranes and alter cellular function. This mechanism is secondary to the generation of lipid peroxides and often leads to significant cellular damage.

Lipid Peroxides

Free radicals are molecules with unpaired electrons in the outer orbit [69–72]. As such, they are highly reactive and play integral roles as intermediates in normal biochemical reactions. They are produced either by radiation effects or through reduction-oxidation reactions with transition metals or enzymes. Tissue injury increases the production of free radicals, which in turn contribute to the pathophysiology of injury or disease.

Lipid peroxides are formed from autoxidation (from exposure of unsaturated fatty acids to molecular oxygen) or from peroxidation from attack by other free radicals. The consequences of lipid peroxidation include decreased membrane fluidity (although the effect may vary with the model [72]), oxidation of thiol groups and, in addition, enzymes in the membranes, and liberation of breakdown products (such as malondialdehyde), which produce damage elsewhere. In fact, measurements of malondialdehyde or conjugated dienes, are used as evidence of lipid peroxidation processes.

Plasma membranes are critical sites for free radical reactions (Figure 18-5) [71]. The plasma membrane, as the first site of contact with the cell's environment, encounters extracellular free radicals before other cell components. The perhydroxyl radical (the protonated form of the superoxide radical), partitions into lipids in the membrane, at which time unsaturated fatty acid and transmembrane proteins with oxidizable amino acids are attacked. Subsequent reactions may proceed to the interior of the cell.

One of the consequences of attack by lipid peroxides is modulation of eicosanoid synthesis. Farrukh and associates [73] found that lipid peroxides increase cyclooxygenase and lipoxygenase products of arachidonic acid. On the other hand, Mosconi and associates [74] found that platelet thromboxane production is decreased in rats gavaged with fish oil and restored to normal by the antioxidant vitamin E.

Cellular defenses against free radical damage include chain-breaking scavengers, which act by scavenging the chain-carrying oxygen radicals; many are lipid-soluble [75]. Although β-carotene and retinoic acid play minor roles, vitamin E (espe-

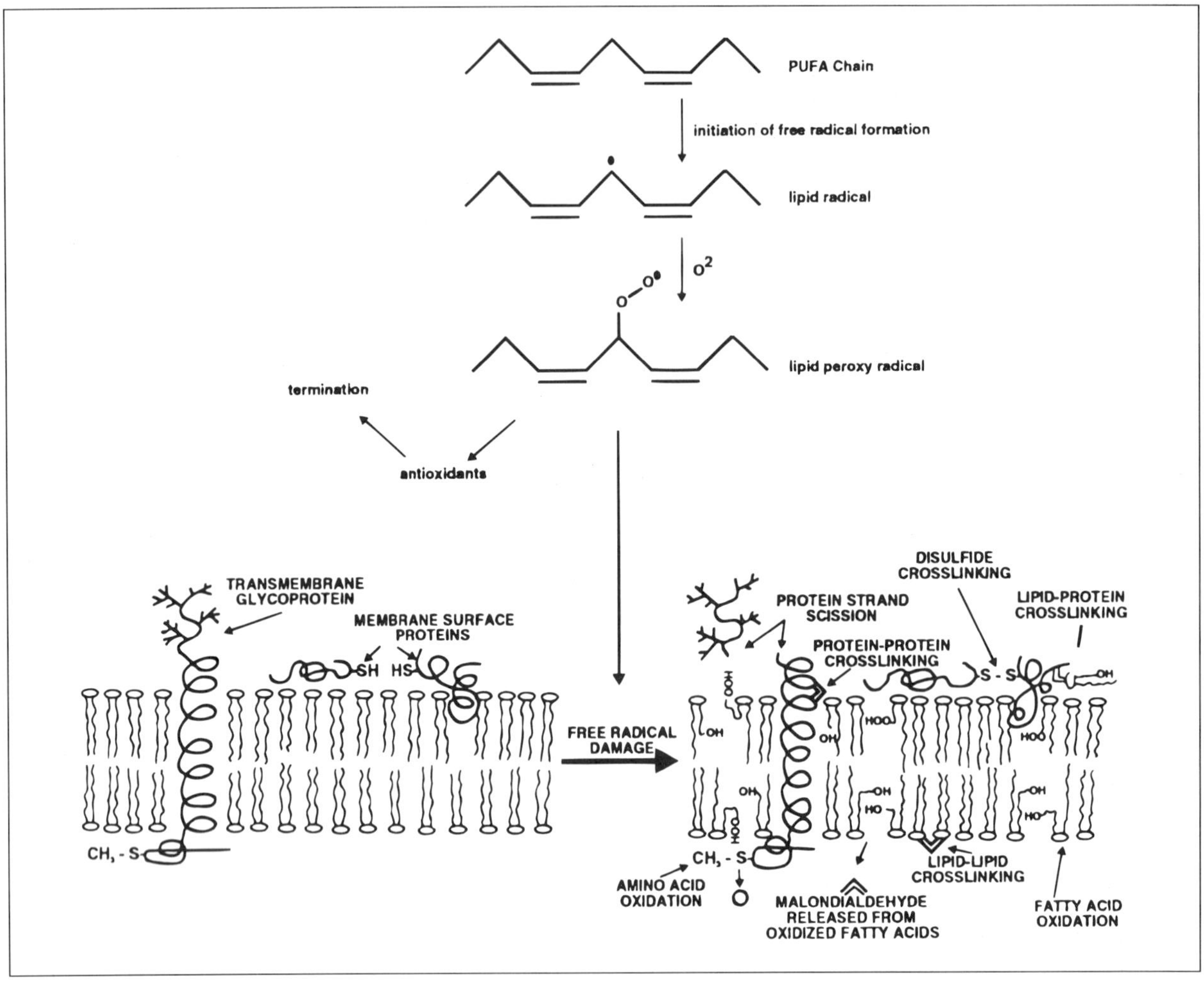

Figure 18-5. Free radical damage to membranes. Lipid peroxides are initiated by oxygen free radicals, forming lipid free radicals. Following initiation there is rapidly accelerating propagation through chain reactions in which lipid radicals collide with each other and generate more lipid radicals. Often these react with oxygen to form lipid peroxy radicals. If antioxidants (such as vitamin E) do not convert the lipid radicals into inactive molecules, these radicals can catalyze a number of damaging reactions in cell membranes, including amino acid oxidation, protein-protein cross-linking and protein strand scission. Malondialdehyde is released from some of these reactions and can mediate other damaging consequences. (Based on BA Freeman, JD Crapo. Free radicals and tissue injury. *Lab Invest* 47:412, 1982.)

cially α-tocopherol) is the major lipid peroxide scavenger. Lymphocyte function is dependent on the intake of antioxidant vitamins, such as β-carotene, selenium, and vitamins A and E [76].

Intake of dietary PUFA leads to consumption of free-radical scavengers, especially vitamin E. Dietary fish oil alters the fatty acid composition of tissues decreasing arachidonic acid and raising EPA and DHA, and it decreases tissue stores of vitamin E [77–83]. Fish oil diets are also associated with increased plasma hepatic malondialdehyde and conjugated dienes, and there appears to be an inverse correlation of tissue vitamin E and circulating malondialdehyde levels [77–84]. However, neither linseed nor canola oils (sources of α-linolenic acid) produce the same degree of lipid peroxidation as fish oil [81,83], although both are sources of ω-3 PUFA. The difference appears to be related to chain length and number of unsaturated double bonds (3 in α-linolenic acid versus 5 in EPA and 6 in DHA). While in some cases, supplemental vitamin E in the diet protects against lipid peroxidation [80], it is not uniformly protective [77,78,81,84].

The high degree of lipid peroxide production by dietary fish oil has effects on cell function and also on cell survival. Lymphocyte proliferation, for example, is suppressed by PUFA in vitro; because lymphocytes in culture are unable to elongate and desaturate 18-carbon fatty acids to arachidonic acid, this phenomenon is probably due to lipid peroxidation [85]. In healthy males fed defined diets with 40 en% fish oil, the suppression of peripheral blood mononuclear cell proliferation in response to mitogens is reversed by vitamin E, and there is a direct correlation between plasma α-tocopherol levels and blastogenesis [86]. More directly, PUFA have a pronounced cytotoxic effect in culture. Gram-positive cocci are sensitive to arachidonic acid in culture and can be protected by catalase and iron chelators [87]. Cytotoxicity of lymphocytes incubated with fatty acids is increased by decreasing fatty acyl chain length and by increasing unsaturation [88]. Finally, Begin [89,90] has shown that PUFA have cytotoxic effects on both normal and transformed cells and can stimulate growth when fatty acid concentration is low (less than 20 μM) but are cytotoxic when levels are high (greater than 100 μM). The cytotoxicity of the fatty acids is associated with their ability to induce lipid peroxidation and can be blocked by vitamin E, although, paradoxically, EPA and DHA did not always increase levels of malondialdehyde [90].

As mentioned above, free radical production is increased in disease or by injury. Shock states, in which there is inadequate tissue perfusion due to hemorrhage or inflammation, are associated with free radical production [91]. Allopurinol improves outcome in canine hemorrhagic shock [92–95]. Scavenging of oxygen free radicals by superoxide dismutase also decreases the production of lipid peroxides in the plasma of endotoxin-shocked dogs [96]. Alpha-tocopherol is protective against mortality from endotoxin in mice, restoring liver ATP stores by reducing the lipid peroxide load [97,98]. Because free radical scavengers improve survival in these studies, we assume that their production contributes significantly to the pathophysiology of shock.

Oxygen free radical scavengers protect against lung, liver, and kidney damage in the experimental models of multiple organ failure syndrome (MOFS) [69]. MOFS is characterized by the failure of two or more organ systems, commonly kidneys, liver, heart, or lungs, following a variety of inciting events, such as trauma, sepsis, or hemorrhagic shock. Not all experimental evidence, however, supports the hypothesis that free radicals are positive agents in MOFS. Van Bebber and associates [99] have found that although superoxide dismutase and catalase prevent plasma malondialdehyde appearance in zymosan-treated rats (an experimental model of MOFS), the clinical condition and mortality is not changed. If free radicals play a significant role in MOFS, they may do so indirectly, such as by damaging intestinal mucosa and allowing bacterial translocation from the gut lumen to occur [100]. Alternatively, free radicals may have their greatest effect by modulating mediators, such as endothelium-derived relaxing factor (nitric oxide), which exacerbates the vasodilation of septic shock [101,102].

Injuries are also associated with increased appearance of lipid peroxidation products. Demling and LaLonde [103] have shown an increase in plasma malondialdehyde and conjugated dienes following burn injury in sheep. The increase in plasma peroxidation products is associated with increased oxygen consumption, lung inflammation, and liver dysfunction and is attenuated by allopurinol [104]. (The beneficial effects of allopurinol are limited to the lung; liver function is not improved.) Similarly, Horton and White [105] have found lazaroids (inhibitors of lipid peroxidation) improve the cardiac dysfunction associated with burn injury.

Although lipid peroxidation may play a significant role in the pathophysiology of disease and injury, the role of dietary PUFA in increasing the body's burden of lipid peroxides is unknown. Polyunsaturated fatty acid, especially highly unsaturated fatty acids such as EPA and DHA, can undergo rapid autoxidation. At room temperature with exposure to atmosphere oxygen, fish oils will lose a significant portion of their EPA and DHA to autoxidation [106]. (Preservatives such as BHA or BHT are needed ex vivo because vitamin E is ineffective at preventing autoxidation of highly polyunsaturated fatty acids outside the body.)

Although rancid fish oil is absolutely unpalatable to man, enteral products that include fish oil may be delivered to patients without the extent of lipid peroxidation being obvious. Nonetheless, there is little direct evidence that dietary lipid peroxides produce organ dysfunction, and Kinsella [106] has concluded that the intake of dietary ω-3 PUFA should not exert any deleterious effects via peroxidation as long as adequate vitamin E is consumed. Formulas for estimating the amount of vitamin E supplementation in man required for PUFA intake are available [107].

Eicosanoids

The discussion thus far has shown that dietary PUFA exert their effects on cellular function both by altering membrane fluidity and by challenging membrane antioxidant defense systems. This section will review the relationship of essential PUFA to the production of eicosanoids, a diverse group of lipid mediators.

Eicosanoids are products formed from 20-carbon PUFA. They share a 5-carbon ring structure and differ at sites of oxygenation. Most mammalian cells, except erythrocytes, can metabolize arachidonic acid, but different cells generate different profiles of arachidonic acid end products [108–110]. Only a few cell lines, however, including leukocytes, hepatocytes, and gastric and adrenal cells, have specific prostaglandin receptors [111]. Only minimal concentrations (10^{-9} g/g) are needed for physiologic effects in target cells. The very small concentrations necessary, coupled with very short half-lives, suggest that eicosanoids have autocrine or paracrine effects on nearby cells rather than on distant organ systems [110,112].

Eicosanoid release is stimulated by a variety of substances. Collagen, thrombin, bradykinin, antigen-antibody complexes, oxygen free radicals, growth factors, and cytokines are all capable of stimulating release of esterified arachidonic acid and further enzymatic modification to eicosanoid products [108]. The two major pathways of arachidonic acid metabolism begin with the enzymes cyclooxygenase, leading to prostanoids (prostaglandins and thromboxanes), and lipoxygenase, which produces leukotrienes, hydroxyeicosatetraenoic acids, and lipoxins (Figure 18-6). (A third pathway, through cytochrome P_{450}, forms epoxides, which are converted to hydroxy-fatty acids.)

The metabolism of arachidonic acid to eicosanoid end products starts with the peroxidation of arachidonic acid and the formation of free-radical intermediates. The main source of arachidonic acid is membrane phospholipids. Esterified arachidonic acid is released by the action of phospholipase A_2, a membrane-bound enzyme activated by calcium that releases arachidonic acid primarily from phosphatidylcholine, and by phospholipase C, which is specific for phosphatidylinositol (see Figure 18-6) [109].

Arachidonic acid pathways are regulated both by dietary and pharmacologic means. Omega-3 fatty acids directly suppress the activity of cyclooxygenase, inhibiting formation of dienoic prostanoids (such as TXA_2 and PGE_2). In addition, dietary ω-3 PUFA provide substrates for eicosanoid production that result in less biologically potent end products, such as prostaglandin E_3 and LTB_5 [113–117]. There are also pharmacologic inhibitors specific for cyclooxygenase (such as aspirin, ibuprofen, and indomethacin) and for lipoxygenase (although none have been approved for clinical use) [118].

Eicosanoids primarily regulate cellular activity by altering intracellular levels of cAMP and cGMP. For example, PGE_2 suppresses lymphocyte blastogenesis by increasing cAMP levels. Other eicosanoids, such as leukotrienes, increase cGMP levels, which have opposing effects to increases in cAMP levels; the cAMP-cGMP ratio, rather than

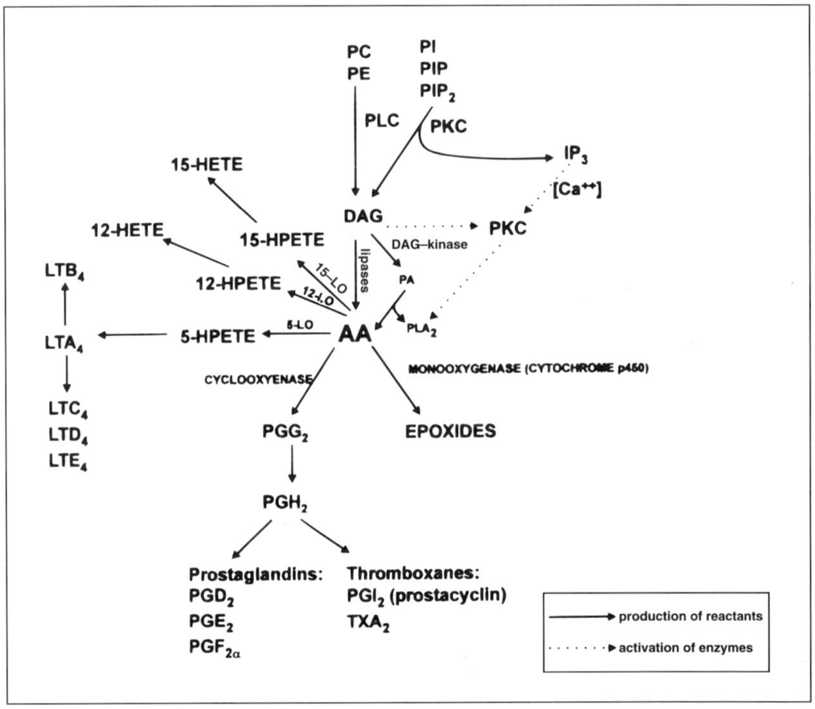

Figure 18-6. Proposed reactions that lead to the formation of eicosanoids from membrane phospholipids. Hydrolysis of PC or PE by PLC produces DAG, which is acted on by lipases to liberate arachidonic acid. In addition, DAG-kinase phosphorylates DAG to form PA, a substrate for PLA_2, also producing arachidonic acid. PKC hydrolyzes PI, PIP, and PIP_2 to generate DAG and IP_3. IP_3 increases cytosolic calcium, which in turn stimulates PKC. DAG also stimulates PKC, which increases arachidonic acid production by PLA_2. These lines of metabolism converge to liberate arachidonic acid, which in turn is the substrate for oxygenase systems (see text). AA = arachidonic acid; DAG = diacylglycerol; HETE = hydroxyeicosatetraenoic acid; HPETE = hydroperoxyeicosatetraenoic acid; IP_3 = inositol trisphosphate; LTA_4 = leukotriene A_4; LTB_4 = leukotriene B_4; LTC_4 = leukotriene C_4; LTD_4 = leukotriene D_4; LTE_4 = leukotriene E_4; PA = phosphatidic acid; PC = phosphatidyl choline; PE = phosphatidyl ethanolamine; PI = phosphatidyl inositol; PIP = phosphatidylinositol phosphate; PIP_2 = phosphatidylinositol bisphosphate; PKC = protein kinase C; PLA_2 = phospholipase A_2; PLC = phospholipase C. (Based on L Levine. Introduction. *Prog Allergy* 44:1, 1988.)

the absolute amount of either cyclic nucleotide, ultimately determines the magnitude and direction of the cellular response [109].

Prostaglandins are formed from the activity of cyclooxygenase on arachidonic acid and perform major regulatory functions in the immune response. Lymphocytes and macrophages both have receptors for and can secrete prostaglandins [119]. The role of prostaglandins in modulation of immune processes is complex, depending on the concentration of prostaglandin, the length of prostaglandin-target cell interaction, and the state of differentiation of the target cell [110].

PGE_2 in particular plays important roles in modulating immune function. Its proinflammatory effects include fever, erythema, increased vascular permeability, vasodilation, and enhancement of the pain and edema caused by bradykinin and histamine [111]. PGE_2 also modulates leukocyte function, probably by increasing intracellular cAMP levels.

Both T and B lymphocyte function are sensitive to regulation by PGE_2. PGE_2 generally suppresses T-cell function, such as mitogen-induced blastogenesis, clonal expansion, antigenic stimulation, E-rosette formation, lymphokine production, generation of cytotoxic cells, and lymphocyte migration, and can do so at physiologically relevant concentrations [109–111,120–123]. One subset of T cells, suppressor T cells, may be stimulated by prostaglandins, but the contribution of this effect overall will still be one of suppression of T-cell function [121]. The effects of PGE_2 on B-cell function and antibody production in comparison is dose dependent. At low doses, PGE_2 tends to enhance antibody production [109,110,121,124] while suppressing B-cell proliferation [109,111,122]. These effects of PGE_2 on both T and B cells can be blocked by cyclooxygenase inhibitors.

PGE_2 suppresses cytokine release [109,111,122,123,125], including IL-1 and tumor necrosis factor (TNF). Indeed, one of the primary roles of PGE_2 is to down-regulate the release of cytokines such as TNF, which has been implicated in the pathogenesis of septic shock [121,125,126]. [*Editor's Note:* While the cytokines, including TNF, apparently play some role in shock-like states, one cannot ascribe all the symptomatology to one or even a few cytokines. Our own data concerning TNF, for example, suggests that at least some of the effects of TNF on sepsis are indirect, possibly mediated by steroids.] Prostaglandins also suppress phagocyte function, such as chemotaxis, chemokinesis, aggregation, spreading, and oxidative metabolism of leukocytes [111,122].

With injured patients PGE_2 production is increased and blockade of cyclooxygenase is often associated with improvement of immune function. For instance, burn injury is associated with increased levels of plasma PGE_2, although plasma levels do not correlate well with the degree of immunosuppression in these patients [120,127]. The immunosuppression seen in these patients, however, is restored by addition of indomethacin or monoclonal anti-PGE_2 antibodies [120,127]. Indeed, it is true that cyclooxygenase inhibitors such as indomethacin or ibuprofen restore cytokine production in lymphocyte blastogenesis to normal levels in both animal models [118,128–130] and in human studies [131–133]. Faist and associates [131,132] have found that postoperative administration of indomethacin, with or without thymopentin, also restores helper T-cell subsets, IL-2 receptor expression, and normal delayed-type hypersensitivity responses and is associated with a decrease in early opportunistic infections.

The beneficial effects of cyclooxygenase blockade can be significant. Pretreatment of ibuprofen in dogs challenged with infusion of *E. coli* restores mean arterial blood pressure and is associated with decreased plasma prostanoid levels, although TNF and IL-6 are unchanged [130]. Revhaug and associates [133] found that pretreatment with ibuprofen prior to challenge with endotoxin in healthy human males results in suppression of the usual symptoms and signs of endotoxemia, namely the flu-like symptoms, fever, tachycardia, caloric expenditure, and elevation of stress hormones.

Leukotrienes are another class of arachidonic acid metabolites that are produced by 5-lipoxygenase activity. Leukotrienes play important roles in allergic and immune reactions and are produced by all leukocytes except lymphocytes [111,122]. LTC_4, LTD_4, and LTE_4 are the slow-reacting substances released in response to IgE and are responsible for the smooth muscle restriction of anaphylactic reactions; they may play an important but yet undefined role in the pathogenesis of shock [134]. The major 5-lipoxygenase product involved in modulation of the immune system, however, is LTB_4.

LTB_4 is a major mediator of leukocyte activity [135]. It stimulates aggregation, lysosomal release, and chemotaxis of polymorphonuclear cells. Most leukocytes do not synthesize 5-lipoxygenase products on a constitutive basis; the main source of LTB_4 is polymorphonuclear cells [135]. The significance of 5-lipoxygenase products in the immunosuppression associated with injury or infection is not well described. However, Schonfeld and associates [136] have shown that polymorphonuclear cells isolated from trauma patients show a decreased capacity to generate LTB_4 in the first week after injuries.

The role of 5-lipoxygenase products on lymphocyte function is not clear, for not as much work has been done in this area as has been done in the relationship of PGE_2 and lymphocytes. Lymphocytes do not synthesize lipoxygenase products, but lymphocyte function does seem to be suppressed by LTB_4 [135]. Lipoxygenase inhibitors, on the other hand, have also been shown to suppress blastogenesis and natural killer cell function [135,137].

To understand the role of eicosanoids in immune function requires above all an appreciation for the complexity of the eicosanoid system. Although PGE_2 and LTB_4 are clearly the most potent regulators of leukocyte function, other eicosanoids may have some role, however minor, to play. The actions of eicosanoids are dose dependent and may counteract each other. For example, PGE_2 and LTB_4 have opposite effects on phagocyte functions, yet both are metabolites of the same precursor, linoleic acid. The importance of eicosanoids in the immune response is highlighted by studies of cyclooxygenase inhibition, which generally improves immune function and survival from sepsis.

Thus, in summary, dietary PUFA, distributed throughout the cell membranes of the body, modulate the inflammatory response by increasing membrane fluidity, producing lipid peroxides, and modulating eicosanoid synthesis by the availability of substrates. The next section will review the effect of PUFA on several effector arms of the immune system.

Lipids and Immune Function

Cytokines

Many studies indicate that PUFA depress cytokine production. For example, Santoli and Zurier [138] found that lymphocytes cultured with arachidonic acid and EPA have suppressed IL-2 synthesis. Similarly, Billiar and associates [139] found that both fish oil and safflower oil fed to rats suppress Kupffer cell production of IL-1 and TNF. The suppression of IL-2 production may be correlated with an increase in malondialdehyde because arachidonic acid both suppresses IL-2 production and increases malondialdehyde in a transformed lymphocyte cell line [140]. In contrast, Ertel and associates [141] have shown that fish oil restores IL-1 and IL-2 release in hemorrhagic-shocked mice.

The effect of lipids on cytokine production may be species-specific. Although fish oil allows for increased TNF production by endotoxin-stimulated resident peritoneal macrophages due to suppression of PGE_2 synthesis [142,143], fish oil supplements in healthy men and women suppress peripheral blood mononuclear cell production of not only TNF, but also of IL-1, IL-2, and IL-6 [144,145]. Interestingly, this suppression of cytokine production by fish oil supplements in humans persists up to 10 weeks after the supplements have been discontinued [144].

Although in many cases indomethacin reverses the effects of fatty acids on cytokine production [142,146], variations in prostaglandin production are not the only factors responsible for the modulation of cytokine production by fatty acids. For example, Karmiol and associates [146] found that IL-6 production by human lung fibroblasts cultured with oleic, linoleic, or linolenic acids is stimulated by linoleic acid the greatest, followed by linolenic, and then by oleic acids. Although indomethacin suppressed IL-6 production by all fatty acids, the pattern remained the same, suggesting that suppression of cyclooxygenase products such as PGE_2 is not the only factor responsible for IL-6 production in the cells. Santoli and Zurier [138] found that the ability of fatty acids to suppress IL-2 production in cultured lymphocytes is independent of prostaglandin synthesis. Similarly, Hardardottir and Kinsella [142] found that although indomethacin increases and exogenous PGE_2 decreases TNF production from peritoneal macrophages, those mice fed sardine oil still produce more TNF than mice fed safflower oil. This again suggests that the modulation of TNF by lipids is multifactorial [142].

Phagocytes

Phagocytosis is one of a number of nonspecific antimicrobial systems that constitute innate immunity. The cells responsible for engulfment and digestion of microorganisms are polymorphonuclear neutrophils and mononuclear phagocytes (monocytes and macrophages). Polymorphonuclear cells and monocytes circulate in the bloodstream; on the other hand, macrophages are fixed in tissues throughout the body. Phagocytes are attracted to sites of inflammation or bacterial invasion, following a gradient of chemical stimuli (chemotaxis). The phagocytes adhere to the microbe and engulf it with pseudopods extended around the particle. Cytoplasmic granules fuse with the phagocytosed microbe and discharge their contents, killing the organism. Killing mechanisms are both oxygen dependent, in which superoxide anion, hydrogen peroxide, singlet molecular oxygen and hydroxyl radicals are generated, and oxygen independent, including enzymes and lactoferrin. The degranulation of phagocytes during the killing of microbes can be measured by chemiluminescense or by assays of superoxide generation and oxidative burst.

Accumulation of phagocytes at sites of acute inflammation is generally not affected by lipids [147–149], although ω-3 fatty acids increase the influx of polymorphonuclear cells in response to zymosan [150] and increase the number of polymorphonuclear cells and mononuclear phagocytes in chronic inflammation [147]. Phagocytosis, on the other hand, is suppressed by saturated fats [151,152]. Interestingly, the type of PUFA to which phagocytes are exposed, however, whether ω-6 or ω-3 PUFA, has no effect on phagocytosis [115,149].

The effect of dietary lipids on bactericidal killing by phagocytes is not clear. Although Hawley and Gordon [152] found that human polymorphonuclear cells incubated with palmitic acid have decreased bactericidal capacity compared to those incubated with oleic acid, Blonk and associates [153] have shown that healthy human males supplemented with EPA-DHA capsules for 12 weeks have polymorphonuclear cells that kill *S. aureus* normally ex vivo.

There are distinct changes in the oxygen-dependent intracellular killing mechanisms with lipids. Unsaturated fatty acids in culture media suppress the degranulation and respiratory burst of phagocytes [154–156]. On the other hand, PUFA increase hydrogen peroxide production and superoxide release [148,149,157]. Indomethacin has no effect on chemiluminescense of peritoneal macrophages incubated with either arachidonic acid or EPA [156], suggesting that the changes associated with these PUFA are not related to alterations in eicosanoid synthesis. In fact, Costa Rosa and associates [148] have found that mononuclear intracellular concentrations of the enzymes hexokinase, glutathione peroxidase, and citrate synthetase are modified by dietary PUFA, suggesting modulation within the cell at the level of protein transcription and synthesis. However, phagocytes from injured patients may not respond to dietary lipid manipulation, suggested by Gadd and Hansbrough [158], who have shown that the polymorphonuclear cell oxidative burst, suppressed by burn injury, is not ameliorated by the addition of fish oil to the diet of mice.

Lymphocytes

Cell-mediated immunity, effected by T lymphocytes, begins with proliferation of lymphocyte populations following appropriate ligand binding to cell surface receptors. Lymphocyte proliferation (or blastogenesis) can be induced experimentally by mitogens, such as plant lectins, or in culture with allogeneic lymphocytes in the mixed lymphocyte response. The ability of lymphocytes to respond to stimuli such as mitogens has been used as a measurement of lymphocyte responsiveness and activation. Lipids, introduced exogenously both through the diet and as free fatty acids bound to carriers in cell culture media, affect lymphocyte proliferation.

Diets high in fat suppress blastogenesis [151,159,160]. In fact, growing rats fed diets with 15% (w/w) fat, compared to 3% in controls, develop thymic involution after three months [161]. The suppressive effects of high-fat diets appear consistent in all studies when T cells are used as the responding population, but are inconsistent when B cells are studied [151,159]. The degree of unsaturation of the dietary fatty acids is a less potent regulator of lymphocyte proliferation than high amounts of dietary fat, as safflower and corn oil have the same effect as lard and coconut oil when diets with 20 en% are fed to mice [151]. Splenic lymphocytes from septic animals do not, however, share this sensitivity to high-fat diets (162).

When high amounts of dietary fat are not the major determinant of the responsiveness of lymphocytes, the degree of unsaturation and specifically the family of PUFA can be a powerful modulator of blastogenesis. Diets that are high in ω-6 fatty acids, such as safflower or corn oils, lead to increased PGE_2 production and suppression of lymphocyte blastogenesis [159,163,164]. In contrast, diets enriched with ω-3 fatty acids enhance lymphocyte proliferation [27,51,165] and are associated with a decrease in PGE_2 production [51]. Oddly enough, fish oil, however, does not enhance lymphocyte blastogenesis in burned mice [158,166].

Delayed-type hypersensitivity reactions result from interaction of T lymphocytes with antigens, peaking at two to three days. Antigen is encountered and initially processed by macrophages, which are activated to release cytokines such as IL-1 and TNF. The macrophages present the processed antigen to T lymphocytes, which then produce other cytokines such as IL-2 and interferon. Macrophages and lymphocytes accumulate and often fuse to form multinucleated giant cells and granulomas. Delayed-type hypersensitivity reactions are probably important for host defense against intracellular pathogens, such as *Mycobacteria, Listeria,* and *Salmonella* species, and viruses. Although some studies have shown that the type or amount of dietary fat does not affect delayed-type hypersensitivity responses in experimental animals [27,151,167], the majority of studies have shown that the delayed-type hypersensitivity response can be significantly suppressed by lipids.

Dietary PUFA suppress the delayed-type hypersensitivity response, whether they are from the ω-6 [168,169] or ω-3 family [147,165]. Even so, some studies have noted that fish oil diets increase the delayed-type hypersensitivity response in septic or burned guinea pigs [12,162]. Because the other studies were done in animals that were not stressed, these findings suggest that infection or injury may permit the eicosanoid-modulating properties of fish oil to improve the delayed-type hypersensitivity response.

B lymphocytes produce antibodies, which are glycoproteins that bind to antigens and are the primary component of humoral immunity. Blastogenesis of B cells can be increased by feeding rats diets with soybean oil [161]. Production of antibodies by B cells, however, may not be affected by dietary lipids [147,166,170]. The results from studies that have shown that dietary lipids change antibody production are not consistent enough to formulate any general conclusion. For example, corn oil diets (which would increase PGE_2 production) suppress antibody production [169], but it is also depressed by essential fatty acid deficient diets (170) and by fish oil diets [51] (both of which would decrease PGE_2 production). Adding to the confusion are observations that antibody production can be increased by corn oil (ω-6 PUFA) [151] and linseed oil (ω-3 PUFA) [27]. Although it is tempting to pass these discrepancies off as being due to differences in animal models or in assays used to measure antibody production, the fact is that the mechanisms by which dietary lipids modulate B-cell populations and antibody production are unknown.

Cytotoxicity

Another major effector arm of the immune system is the lysis or killing of one cell type by another, involving macrophages, natural killer cells, and cytotoxic T lymphocytes. These cells are involved in protecting the body against viral and intracellular bacteria and surveying the body against tumors. They are also the cells involved in mediating the rejection of allograft tissues after transplantation and in the chronic self-destruction of autoimmune diseases. These killing mechanisms often involve the presentation of antigen to the lymphocytes by macrophages acting as antigen-presenting cells. The antigen-presenting capacity of macrophages and also the tumoricidal properties can be up-regulated by interferon-γ (IFN-γ).

Diets high in fat suppress cytolysis [171]. Although essential fatty acid deficiency suppresses cytotoxicity, so do diets with PUFA [171]. In some studies, unsaturated fatty acids in culture inhibit cytolysis [172], whereas in others they enhance cytolysis [58,173]. The effect is due to more than changes in membrane fluidity alone, as elaidic acid (with a melting point of 53°F) has a higher cytotoxic index than 15:0 (with a melting point of 52°F) [58]. Because lymphocytes in culture do not have the enzymes necessary to elongate and desaturate 18-carbon fatty acids from the medium into eicosanoid by-products, it is also unlikely that this effect is due to changes in eicosanoid metabolism.

Omega-3 fatty acids have mixed effects on cytotoxicity. Meydani and associates [174] found that young mice respond to fish oil diets by suppressing natural killer cell activity (although this effect is not seen in old mice), and Yamashita and associates [175] found EPA emulsions also suppress natural killer cell activity. DHA suppresses macrophage tumoricidal activity, although bacterial phagocytosis and intracellular killing are not affected [176]. The suppression by ω-3 PUFA of macrophage killing of mastocytoma cells in mice can be overcome by higher concentrations of IFN-γ, suggesting that ω-3 PUFA create an imbalance in cytokine production [177]. In contrast, Fernandes and associates [51] have found that fish oil diets restore natural killer cell activity in mice prone to autoimmune disease. Similarly, Schlager and associates [178] have shown that incubation with α-linolenic acid enhances cytotoxicity of murine macrophages against fibrosarcoma cells.

Antigen presentation by accessory cells such as macrophages may also be modulated by lipids. Omega-3 highly polyunsaturated fatty acids depress antigen-presenting cell function in normal mice [179], an effect that may be due to suppression of IFN release [151]. The opposite effect, however, is seen in hemorrhagic-shocked mice, in which fish oil restores antigen-presenting cell function [141].

Lipids may exert their effects on tumor surveillance by altering the susceptibility of tumor cells to attach and of lysis by cytotoxic host cells. Although some investigators have not confirmed that alterations in target cell membrane phospholipid fatty acid profiles are associated with changes in susceptibility to cytolysis [180], others have found that unsaturated fatty acids introduced to the cells in the culture media are associated with increased lysis [181,182]. The increases in susceptibility to lysis appear to parallel the increase in unsaturation of the fatty acids and also the increase in fluidity of the membrane [182].

Lipids and Specific Disease States

Given the diverse and potent effects of lipids on the immune system, it is logical to postulate that outcome in disease states in which the immune system is a primary component will be modulated by PUFA. This, in fact, has been true in a number of models of hypermetabolism, transplantation, cancer, and sepsis; these findings will be reviewed in this section.

Metabolism

Although metabolism is independent of the immune system, it is governed by many of the same control mechanisms, such as cytokines. In addition, diseases or injuries that are associated with immunosuppression also tend to increase the metabolic response. Thus this section begins with a discussion of the effects of PUFA, especially ω-3 PUFA, on metabolism.

Awad and associates [183] found that rats fed on beef tallow, safflower oil, or fish oil maintain body weight and composition regardless of the type of lipid in the diet. In addition, there are no differences in lipolysis or lipogenesis. Dietary lipids, however, may alter the uptake of ω-3 PUFA. Pan and Storlien [184] found that rats fed saturated fat in combination with ω-3 PUFA had greater uptake of ω-3 PUFA and less weight gain, compared to those fed either olive oil or safflower oil with the same amount of ω-3 PUFA.

Dietary fish oil dampens the hypermetabolic response to burn injury. Both burned rats and burned guinea pigs exhibit less of an increase in resting metabolic expenditure following burn injury, and there is better preservation of protein synthesis and lean body mass [12,185].

Prefeeding of fish oil may prevent deposition of lipids in the liver during sepsis. Lanza-Jacoby and associates [186] found that rats fed with fish oil diets prior to injection with *E. coli* had decreased hepatic lipid deposition compared to animals fed corn oil. The rats fed fish oil diets also have decreased triglyceride, phospholipid, and cholesterol synthesis in the liver, as well as decreased levels of glycerol-3-phosphate acyltransferase. The hypertriglyceridemia of sepsis, however, is not affected by fish oil feedings.

Although the down-modulation of metabolic processes by fish oil may be due to diminished PGE_2 production, there are also direct effects on mitochondrial enzymes. Malis and associates [187] found that mitochondria of renal cortical cells from rats fed fish oil diets (compared to beef tallow-fed controls) have reductions in respiratory control, uncoupled respiration, and site I (NADH coenzyme Q reductase) activity of the electron transport chain. Bhathena and associates [188] have also found that fish oil supplements given to healthy men suppress the release of the stress hormones insulin, glucagon, and growth hormone.

Transplantation

Mertin and associates [189,190] found that subcutaneous injection with PUFA prolongs the survival of skin allografts in mice. Thrice weekly injections of linoleic acid, α-linolenic acid, or arachidonic acid in mice increased the median survival time of skin allografts. Interestingly, the increase in median survival times of allografts was directly correlated with the degree of unsaturation of the fatty acids used, suggesting that this effect was related more to the physical properties of PUFA, such as increasing membrane fluidity or peroxidation, than to the differential production of eicosanoid metabolites [189]. These investigators also found that primary and subsequent memory cytotoxic allograft responses decreased in animals treated with linoleic acid. The immunosuppressant effects of linoleic acid, however, disappear in splenectomized mice, suggesting that this effect is not a direct one on lymphocytes themselves, but rather mediated through other effector cells in the immune system [191].

Others have found, in contrast to the Mertin studies, that ω-3 PUFA are immunosuppressive. For example, Kelley and associates [192] found that cyclosporine given in fish oil vehicle compared to olive oil increases the survival of rat heart transplants; delayed-type hypersensitivity is also suppressed. The results of a nonblinded, noncontrolled trial of fish oil supplements in renal transplant patients have also shown a decrease in the rate of deterioration of renal allograft function [193]. These observations indicate that ω-3 PUFA, through an unspecified immunosuppressive effect, prolong allograft survival, just as do ω-6 PUFA. Because both families of PUFA have the same effect on allograft survival, the effect is more likely due to the shared physical properties of PUFA on cell membranes than the production of divergent eicosanoid metabolites with different biologic potency.

Cancer

Both the amount and type of dietary lipid affect neoplastic disease in laboratory animals. Diets that are high in fat lead to increases in the incidence and number of dimethylhydrazine-induced colon carcinomas in rats [163], decreased tumor latency and lymphocyte cytotoxicity in mice with melanoma [171], and increased incidence and growth rate of mammary carcinoma in rats

[194,195]. These experimental data parallel epidemiologic studies that suggest that high fat diets increase the risk of neoplastic disease in humans [11].

PUFA also tend to generally facilitate tumor growth. For example, both King and Kollmorgen [194,195] found that diets with 20% (w/w) corn oil increase the incidence and growth rate of mammary carcinoma in rats. And yet some investigators have found that dietary lipids have no effect on tumor yield [148]. Nonetheless, others have found that both corn and safflower oil diets lead to increased tumor incidence and volume in rats with liver tumors [163] or in mice with melanoma [171]. There is concern that as PUFA intake in the American diet has increased to replaced saturated fat to reduce the risk of atherosclerotic disease, the incidence of neoplastic disease has risen [11].

Not all PUFA facilitate tumor growth. Supplementation with fish oil on a daily basis decreases the weight and volume of mammary tumors in rats [195]. Supplementation with fish oils in this model is associated with decreased PGE_2 in tumor microsomes and with increased ω-3 PUFA in tumor cell phosphatidylcholine. In parallel to the studies with fish oil, Mertin and Hunt [190] showed that essential fatty acid deficient diets lead to decreased incidence of methylcholanthrene tumors in mice, adding weight to the hypothesis that depression of PGE_2 production is associated with improved tumor surveillance. It is known from specimens of human hepatocellular carcinoma that membrane α-linolenic acid and DHA are lower and that thromboxane and prostacyclin are higher than in reference specimens [196]. An interesting observation is that permeability of tumor cells is increased after incubation with DHA [197], suggesting another mechanism for the suppressive effects of fish oil on tumor growth. On the whole, fish oil may benefit the tumor-bearing host both by decreasing prostanoid production and by destabilizing effects on tumor cell membranes. [*Editor's Note:* There is preliminary evidence from a study in Scotland that ω-3 PUFA do increase metastasis in some human tumors.]

Outcome from Infection

Cyclooxygenase products play a role in the morbidity and mortality that accompanies gram-negative bacterial infections. Essential fatty acid deficient rats, which produce prostaglandins in smaller quantities, are more resistant to endotoxin shock than controls [198], and ibuprofen protects against mortality after cecal ligation and puncture (a model of bacterial peritonitis) in mice that have been subjected to hemorrhagic shock [129].

As expected, diets rich in PUFA also modulate the response to bacterial infection, although the experimental results are not all consistent with each other. On the one hand, several investigators have found that fish oil, given either enterally or parenterally, improves survival from endotoxin or bacterial shock [199–202]. On the other hand, some investigators have found that the type and amount of dietary lipid have no effect on survival from bacterial infection [203], and in one study we reported that fish oil paradoxically increases mortality from *Pseudomonas* infection in burned mice [166]. In another study, we found that diets based either on ω-6 PUFA-rich vegetable oils or on fish oils have no difference in their effect on survival from bacterial peritonitis in guinea pigs fed enterally for two weeks during the infection [162]. Interestingly, the best survival rates were achieved with a diet composed of a mixture of vegetable and fish oils, with a resultant ω-6 to ω-3 ratio of approximately 2 to 1. Although the pure fish oil diets were associated with a decrease in splenocyte PGE_2 production and an increase in delayed-type hypersensitivity responses, these changes in prostanoid production and immune function appear to be insufficient by themselves to improve survival.

Conclusions

PUFA, from their location on phospholipid tails within cell membranes, are positioned to regulate the immune response in at least three ways: (1) by increasing membrane fluidity, (2) by introducing free-radical lipid peroxides, and (3) by providing precursors for eicosanoid metabolism. As clinicians, we must judge whether the inclusion of PUFA into the diet of stressed surgical patients is safe and efficacious.

The first issue is that of safety. The most serious concern is the relationship between dietary PUFA and lipid peroxide production. Several tentative connections can be made. First, it is clear that diets high in PUFA, especially fish oil, can lead to increases in tissue lipid peroxides and consumption of the natural scavenger, vitamin E. Second, free radicals, including lipid peroxide, produce cellular and tissue damage. Third, what is not clear is if the additional burden of lipid peroxide associated with PUFA diets exacerbates ongoing tissue destruction in disease or injury. In light of these relationships, we can conclude that dietary PUFA definitely raise lipid peroxide breakdown products associated with injury or infection but are not necessarily the cause of defects in cellular function. Future studies of PUFA supplementation in injury or infection should include documentation of lipid peroxidation products.

The next issue is that of efficacy. Evaluation of the prevention or control of surgical infections is challenging, all the more so because these patients represent a complex collection of independent variables that are not present in simple laboratory models. Is it reasonable to prescribe fish oil, for example, to surgical patients based on the response of guinea pigs to purified endotoxin? In my experience, as the animal models become more complex, the results become more difficult to interpret.

For this reason, we should have very clear end points established for our therapy before we begin manipulation of dietary PUFA. For example, the use of ω-3 PUFA in stressed patients has been rationalized based on the suppression of PGE_2 synthesis. However, the regulation of the immune response by eicosanoids is complex with a multitude of products released and designed to act in a coordinated manner at the autocrine or paracrine level. While we are able to quantitate the degree to which dietary PUFA alter tissue lipid profiles and changes in isolated cell function, what is needed are quantitative measurements of physiologic function that can be correlated with tissue levels of fatty acids.

Indeed, the absolute levels of ω-3 and ω-6 PUFA achieved in tissues may not be as important as their ratio to each other [35]. As Boudreau and associates [204] have observed, "assessment of the minimum or desirable amounts of n-3 fatty acids to suppress 20:4n-6 metabolism would be difficult without knowing the ratios of n-3 to n-6 fatty acids in the diets." In evaluating the appropriate ω-3 to ω-6 ratio for stressed patients, it may be useful conceptually to observe the diet of the hominid prior to the era of supermarket diets. Estimates of the fatty acid intake of our late Paleolithic ancestors suggest that ω-3 PUFA were about 3% of total fat intake from wild game, compared to 0.4% in today's commercially available meat [205]. Thus, although ω-3 PUFA played a more prominent role in the diet of our ancestors, it certainly was not the predominant lipid in the diet. Therefore, we should be cautious about arbitrarily increasing the ω-3 PUFA content, such as by giving large amounts of fish oil. In the end, as indicated above, it is the ratio rather than the absolute amounts of ω-3 and ω-6 PUFA that determine efficacy.

Finally, the issue of membrane fluidity should be addressed when PUFA intake is increased. The relationship of membrane fluidity to outcome in surgical patients has not yet been thoroughly addressed. Nevertheless, there are sufficient data to justify measurements of membrane fluidity during manipulation of dietary lipids and to perform correlations with cellular function and outcome. It is likely that there is an optimal range of membrane fluidity, above or below which cellular function is impaired.

In conclusion, ω-3 and other PUFA have the potential to be used to modulate the immune response in surgical patients. Their exact efficacy, and therefore their role, has yet to be defined. In addition, like pharmacologic agents to which immunomodulating nutrients are often compared, safe doses need to be established and toxicities avoided. As long as we can use them wisely, PUFA are another weapon in the surgeon's armament against infection. [*Editor's Note*: The author has cogently stated the case for consideration of ω-3 PUFA and other agents as immunomodulators and is appropriately cautious. Previous experience has shown that immunomodulation at an unfortunate or inopportune time (for example, during spreading rampant infection) may lead to mortality. An example may be the increased mortality with fish oil in burned mice with *Pseudomonas aeruginosa* [166].]

References

1. Harris WS. Effects of Dietary Fatty Acids on Cholesterol, Triglyceride and Lipoprotein Distribution. In GJ Nelson (ed), *Health Effects of Dietary Fatty Acids.* Champaign, IL: American Oil Chemists' Society, 1991. P 69.
2. Dyerberg J. Observations of Populations in Greenland and Denmark. In SM Barlow, ME Stansby (eds), *Nutritional Evaluation of Long Chain Fatty Acids in Fish Oil.* London: Academic, 1982.
3. Dyerberg J, Bang HO, Stofferson E. Eicosapentaenoic acid and prevention of thrombosis and atherosclerosis? *Lancet* 2:117, 1978.
4. Prickett JD, Robinson DR, Steinberg AD. Effects of dietary enrichment with eicosapentaenoic acid upon autoimmune nephritis in female NZB X NZW/F_1 mice. *Arthritis Rheum* 26:133, 1983.
5. Kelley VE, et al. A fish oil diet rich in eicosapentaenoic acid reduces cyclooxygenase metabolites, and suppresses lupus in MRL-1PR mice. *J Immunol* 134:1914, 1985.
6. Kremer JM, et al. Fish oil fatty acid supplementation in active rheumatoid arthritis. *Ann Intern Med* 106:497, 1987.
7. Soyland E, et al. Effect of dietary supplementation with very long chain ω-3 fatty acids in patients with psoriasis. *N Engl J Med* 328:1812, 1993.
8. Clark WF, et al. Fish oil in lupus nephritis: Clinical findings and methodological implications. *Kidney Int* 44:75, 1993.
9. Welch CW. Relationship between dietary fat and experimental mammary tumorigenesis: A review and critique. *Cancer Res* 52:2040s, 1992.
10. Rose DP, Connolly JM. Dietary fat, fatty acids and prostate cancer. *Lipids* 27:798, 1992.
11. Henderson MM. Correlations Between Fatty Acid Intake and Cancer Incidence. In GJ Nelson (ed), *Health Effects*

of Dietary Fatty Acids. Champaign, IL: American Oil Chemists' Society, 1991. P 136.

12. Alexander JW, et al. The importance of lipid type in the diet after burn injury. *Ann Surg* 204:1, 1986.
13. Daly JM, et al. Enteral nutrition with supplemental arginine, RNA, and omega-3 fatty acids in patients after operation: Immunologic, metabolic, and clinical outcome. *Surgery* 112:56, 1992.
14. Gottschlich M. Selection of optimal lipids. *Nutr Clin Pract* 7:155, 1992.
15. Ackman RG. Fatty Acid Composition of Fish Oil. In SM Barlow, ME Stansby (eds), *Nutritional Evaluation of Long-Chain Fatty Acids in Fish Oil.* New York: Academic, 1982. P 12.
16. Sprecher H. Metabolism of Dietary Fatty Acids. In GJ Nelson (ed), *Health Effects of Dietary Fatty Acids.* Champaign, IL: American Oil Chemists' Society, 1991.
17. Nettleton JA. ω-3 fatty acids: Comparision of plant and seafood sources in human nutrition. *J Am Diet Assoc* 91:331, 1991.
18. Cunnane SC, Chen ZY, Yang J. α-Linolenic acid in humans: Direct functional role or dietary precursor? *Nutrition* 7:437, 1991.
19. Clouet P, Niot I, Bezard J. Pathway of α-linolenic acid through the mitochondrial outer membrane in the rat liver and influence on the rate of oxidation. *Biochem J* 263:867, 1989.
20. Sanders TA, Roshanai F. The influence of different types of ω3 polyunsaturated fatty acids on blood lipids and platelet function in healthy volunteers. *Clin Sci* 64:91, 1983.
21. Kelley DS, Nelson GJ, Love JE. Dietary α-linolenic acid alters tissue fatty acid composition, but not blood lipds, lipoproteins or coagulation status in humans. *Lipids* 28:533, 1993.
22. Dyerberg J, Bang HO, Aagaard O. α-Linolenic acid and eicosapentaenoic acid. *Lancet* 1:199, 1980.
23. Ehringer W, et al. A comparison of the effects of linolenic (18:3Ω3) and docosahexaenoic (22:6Ω3) acids on phospholipid bilayers. *Chem Phys Lipids* 54:79, 1990.
24. Hwang DH, Boudreau M, Chanmugam P. Dietary linolenic acid and longer-chain ω-3 fatty acids: Comparison of effects on arachidonic acid metabolism in rats. *Lipids* 118:427, 1988.
25. Brouard C, Pascaud M. Effects of moderate dietary supplementations with ω-3 fatty acids on macrophage and lymphocyte phospholipids and macrophage eicosanoid synthesis in the rat. *Biochim Biophys Acta* 1047:19, 1990.
26. Whelan J, Broughton KS, Kinsella JE. The comparative effects of dietary α-linolenic acid and fish oil on 4- and 5-series leukotriene formation in vivo. *Lipids* 26:119, 1991.
27. Kelley DS, et al. Effects of type of dietary fat on indices of immune status of rabbits. *J Nutr* 118:1376, 1988.
28. Wu D, Meydani SN, Hayek M. Immunological effects of (ω-3) polyunsaturated fatty acids (PUFA) in non-human primates. *FASEB J* 7:A73, 1993.
29. Cunnane SC, Manku MS, Horrobin DF. Essential fatty acids in the liver and adipose tissue of genetically obese mice: Effect of supplemental linoleic and γ-linolenic acids. *Br J Nutr* 53:441, 1984.
30. Mori TA, et al. New findings in the fatty acid composition of individual platelet phospholipids in man after dietary fish oil supplementation. *Lipids* 22:744, 1987.
31. Tiwari RK, Clandinin MT, Cinader B. Effect of high polyunsaturated fat diets on the composition of B cell and T cell membrane lipids. *Nutr Res* 7:489, 1987.
32. Chapkin RS, Carmichael SL. Effects of dietary ω-3 and ω-6 polyunsaturated fatty acids on macrophage phospholipid classes and subclasses. *Lipids* 25:827, 1990.
33. Cleland LG, et al. Comparison of cell membrane phospholipid fatty acids in five rat strains fed four test diets. *Lipids* 25:559, 1990.
34. Diboune M, et al. Composition of phospholipid fatty acids in red blood cell membranes of patients in intensive care units: Effects of different intakes of soybean oil, medium-chain triglycerides, and black-currant seed oil. *JPEN* 16:136, 1992.
35. Lands WEM, Morris A, Libelt B. The Function of Essential Fatty Acids. In GJ Nelson (ed), *Health Effects of Dietary Fatty Acids.* Champaign, IL: American Oil Chemists' Society, 1991.
36. Sprecher H. Metabolism of Dietary Fatty Acids. In GJ Nelson (ed), *Health Effects of Dietary Fatty Acids.* Champaign, IL: American Oil Chemists' Society, 1991.
37. Cerra FB, et al. Improvement in immune function in ICU patients by enteral nutrition supplemented with arginine, RNA, and menhaden oil is independent of nitrogen balance. *Nutrition* 7:193, 1991.
38. Gennis RB. *Biomembranes: Molecular Structure and Function.* New York: Springer, 1989.
39. Singer SJ, Nicholson GL. The fluid mosaic model of the structure of cell membranes. *Science* 175:720, 1972.
40. Sparrow CP, Ganorg BR, Raetz CR. Escherichia coli membrane vesicles with elevated phosphatidic acid levels. *Biochim Biophys Acta* 796:373, 1984.
41. Shipley GG. Recent X-Ray Diffraction Studies of Biological Membrane Components. In D Chapman, DFH Wallach (eds), *Biological Membranes.* New York: Academic, 1973.
42. Cullis PR, de Kruijff B. Structural Properties of Lipids and Their Functional Roles in Biological Membranes. In RC Aloia (ed), *Membrane Fluidity in Biology.* New York: Academic, 1983.
43. Seddon JM. Structure of the inverted hexagonal (H_{II}) phase and non-lamellar phase transitions of lipids. *Biochim Biophys Acta* 1031:1, 1990.
44. Cullis PR, de Kruijff B. Lipid polymorphism and the functional roles of lipids in biological membranes. *Biochim Biophys Acta* 559:399, 1979.
45. Gruner SM. Intrinsic curvature hypothesis for biomembrane lipid composition: A role for non-bilayer lipids. *PNAS USA* 82:3665, 1985.
46. Cullen J, Phillips MC, Shipley GG. The effects of temperature on the composition and physical properties of the lipids of Pseudomonas fluorescens. *Biochem J* 125:733, 1971.
47. Stubbs CD, et al. Effect of double bonds on the dynamic properties of the hydrocarbon region of lecithin bilayers. *Biochemistry* 20:4257, 1981.
48. Léger CL, et al. Evidence for a structurally specific role of essential polyunsaturated fatty acids depending on their peculiar double-bond distribution in biomembranes. *Biochemistry* 29:7269, 1990.
49. Quinn PJ. Dynamics and receptor function of membranes. *Biochem Soc Trans* 18:133, 1990.
50. Hazel JR, Williams EE. The role of alterations in membrane lipid composition in enabling physiological adaptation of organisms to their physical environment. *Prog Lipid Res* 29:167, 1990.
51. Fernandes G. Effect of Dietary Fish Oil Supplement on Autoimmune Disease: Changes in Lymphoid Cell Subsets, Oncogene mRNA Expression and Neuroendocrine

Hormones. In RK Chandra (ed), *Health Effects of Fish and Fish Oil*. St John's: ARTS Biomedical, 1989.

52. Berlin E, Bhathena SJ, Judd JT. Dietary fat and hormonal effects on erythrocyte membrane fluidity and lipid composition in adult women. *Metabolism* 38:790, 1989.
53. Todd JC, Mollitt DL. Erythrocyte membrane alterations induced by sepsis. *J Trauma* 31:1040, 1991.
54. Franceschi D, et al. Trauma alters the lymphocyte's plasma membrane fluidity. *J Trauma* 28:1029, 1989.
55. Tolentino MV, et al. Peripheral lymphocyte membrane fluidity after thermal injury. *J Burn Care Rehabil* 12:498, 1991.
56. Schroit AJ, Gallily R. Macrophage fatty acid composition and phagocytosis: Effect of unsaturation on cellular phagocytic activity. *Immunology* 36:199, 1979.
57. Klausner RD, et al. Lipid domains in membranes. *J Biol Chem* 255:1286, 1980.
58. Mandel G, Clark W. Functional properties of EL-4 tumor cells with lipid-altered membranes. *J Immunol* 120:1637, 1978.
59. Hoover RL, Lynch RD, Karnovsky MJ. Decrease in adhesion of cells cultured in polyunsaturated fatty acids. *Cell* 12:295, 1977.
60. Peck MD, et al. Diets high in polyunsaturated oils decrease lymphocyte membrane anistropy and B-cell mitogenesis. *Nutrition* 11:755, 1995.
61. Peck MD, et al. Fatty acid unsaturation increases expression and capping of murine lymphocyte CD44 and CD45. *Nutrition*. In press.
62. Peck MD, Li Z, Pressman BC. Lymphocyte membrane anistropy is affected by dietary lipids and is correlated with the lymphocyte blastogenic response to LPS. *Surg Forum* 43:19, 1992.
63. Hoover RL, et al. Effects of linoleic acid on capping, lectin mediated mitogenesis, surface antigen expression, and fluorescent polarization in lymphocytes and BHK cells. *J Cell Physiol* 103:399, 1980.
64. Schroit AJ, Rottem S, Gallily R. Motion of spin-labeled fatty acids in murine macrophages: Relation to cellular phagocytic activity. *Biochim Biophys Acta* 426:499, 1976.
65. Lokesh BR, Wrann M. Incorporation of palmitic acid or oleic acid into macrophage membrane lipids exerts differential effects on the function of normal mouse peritoneal macrophages. *Biochim Biophys Acta* 792:141, 1984.
66. Mahoney EM, et al. Response of endocytosis to altered fatty acyl composition of macrophage phospholipids. *Proc Natl Acad Sci USA* 74:4895, 1977.
67. Mahoney EM, et al. Influence of fatty acyl substitution on the composition and function of macrophage membranes. *J Biol Chem* 255:4910, 1980.
68. Calder PC, et al. Uptake and incorporation of saturated and unsaturated fatty acids into macrophage lipids and their effect upon macrophage adhesion and phagocytosis. *J Biol Chem* 269:807, 1990.
69. Gerdin B, Haglund U. Possible Involvement of Oxygen-Free Radicals in Shock and Shock-Related States. In EA Neugebauer, JW Holaday (eds), *Handbook of Mediators in Septic Shock*. Boca Raton: CRC, 1993. P 457.
70. Pryor WA. Free radical biology: Xenobiotics, cancer, and aging. *Ann NY Acad Sci* 393:1, 1982.
71. Freeman BA, Crapo JD. Free radicals and tissue injury. *Lab Invest* 47:412, 1982.
72. Slater TF, et al. Symposium on nutritional aspects of free radicals. *Proc Nutr Soc* 46:1, 1987.
73. Farrukh IS, et al. The role of cyclooxygenase and lipoxygenase mediators in oxidant-induced lung injury. *Am Rev Respir Dis* 137:1343, 1988.
74. Mosconi C, et al. Vitamin E influences the effects of fish oil on fatty acids and eicosanoid production in plasma and circulating cells in the rat. *Biochem Pharmacol* 37:3415, 1988.
75. Niki E. Lipid antioxidants: How they may act in biological systems. *Br J Cancer* 55:153, 1987.
76. Bendich A. Antioxidant Vitamins and Immune Responses. In RK Chandra (ed), *Nutrition and Immunology*. New York: Alan R. Liss, 1988.
77. Hu ML, et al. Effect of dietary lipids and vitamin E on in vitro lipid peroxidation in rat liver and kidney homogenates. *J Nutr* 119:1574, 1989.
78. Leibovitz BE, Hu ML, Tappel AL. Lipid peroxidation in rat tissue slices: Effect of dietary vitamin E, corn oil-lard and menhaden oil. *Lipids* 25:125, 1990.
79. Meydani SN, et al. Effect of long-term fish oil supplementation on vitamin E status and lipid peroxidation in women. *J Nutr* 121:484, 1991.
80. Haglund O, et al. The effects of fish oil on triglycerides, cholesterol, fibrinogen and malondialdehyde in humans supplemented with vitamin E. *J Nutr* 121:165, 1991.
81. Kaasgaard SG, Holmer G, Hoy CE. Effects of dietary linseed oil and marine oil on lipid peroxidation in monkey liver in vivo and in vitro. *Lipids* 27:740, 1992.
82. D'Aquino M, et al. Effect of fish oil and coconut oil on antioxidant defence system and lipid peroxidation in rat liver. *Free Radic Res Commun* 12–13;147, 1991.
83. Lenz PH, Watkins T, Bierenbaum M. Effect of dietary menhaden, canola and partially hydrogenated soy oil supplemented with vitamin E upon plasma lipids and platelet aggregation. *Thromb Res* 61:213, 1991.
84. Brown JE, Wahle KWJ. Effect of fish-oil and vitamin E supplementation on lipid peroxidation and whole-blood aggregation in man. *Clin Chim Acta* 193:147, 1990.
85. Chow SC, Sisfontes L, Björkhem I, et al. Suppression of growth in a leukemic T cell line by ω-3 and ω-6 polyunsaturated fatty acids. *Lipids* 24:700, 1989.
86. Kramer TR, et al. Increased vitamin E intake restores fish-oil-induced suppressed blastogenesis of mitogen-stimulated T lymphocytes. *Am J Clin Nutr* 54:896, 1991.
87. Knapp HR, Melly MA. Bactericidal effects of polyunsaturated fatty acids. *J Infect Dis* 154:84, 1986.
88. Kageyama K, et al. Cytotoxic activity of unsaturated fatty acids to lymphocytes. *Can J Biochem* 58:504, 1980.
89. Begin ME. Effects of polyunsaturated fatty acids and of their oxidation products on cell survival. *Chem Phys Lipids* 45:269, 1987.
90. Begin ME, Ellis G, Horrobin DF. Polyunsaturated fatty acid-induced cytotoxicity against tumor cells and its relationship to lipid peroxidation. *J Natl Cancer Inst* 80:188, 1988.
91. LaLonde C, et al. Relationship between liver oxidant stress and antioxidant activity after zymosan peritonitis in the rat. *Crit Care Med* 21:894, 1993.
92. Crowell JW, Jones CE, Smith EE. Effect of allopurinol on hemorrhagic shock. *Am J Physiol* 216:744, 1969.
93. Baker CH. Protection against irreversible hemorrhagic shock by allopurinol. *Proc Soc Exp Biol Med* 141:694, 1972.
94. Lazarus HM, Owens ML, Hopfenbeck A. Allopurinol protection of hepatic nuclear function during hemorrhagic shock. *Surg Forum* 25:10, 1974.
95. Cunningham SK, Keaveny TV. Effect of a xanthine oxi-

dase inhibitor on adenine nucleotide degradation in hemorrhagic shock. *Eur Surg Res* 10:305, 1978.

96. Morgan RA, Manning PB, Coran AG. New findings in the fatty acid composition of individual platelet phospholipids in man after dietary fish oil supplementation. *Lipids* 25:319, 1987.
97. Sugino K, et al. The role of lipid peroxidation in endotoxin-induced hepatic damage and the protective effect of antioxidants. *Surgery* 101:746, 1989.
98. Sugino K, et al. Changes in the levels of endogenous antioxidants in the liver of mice with experimental endotoxemia and the protective effects of the antioxidants. *Surgery* 105:200, 1989.
99. van Bebber IP, et al. Superoxide dismutase and catalase in an experimental model of multiple organ failure. *JPEN* 11:521, 1992.
100. Haglund U. Systemic mediators released from the gut in critical illness. *Crit Care Med* 21:S15, 1993.
101. Rubanyi GM, Vanhoutte PM. Superoxide anions and hyperoxia inactivate endothelium-derived relaxing factor. *Am J Physiol* 250:H822, 1986.
102. Gryglewski RJ, Palmer AMJ, Moncada S. Superoxide anion is involved in the breakdown of endothelium-derived vascular relaxing factor. *Nature* 320:454, 1986.
103. Demling RH, LaLonde C. Systemic lipid peroxidation and inflammation induced by thermal injury persists into the post-resuscitation period. *J Trauma* 30:69, 1990.
104. Demling RH, LaLonde C. Early postburn lipid peroxidation: Effect of ibuprofen and allopurinol. *Surgery* 107:85, 1990.
105. Horton JW, White DJ. U-74, 500A inhibition of burn-induced cardiac dysfunction. *J Surg Res* 52:251, 1992.
106. Kinsella JE. Dietary ω-3 Polyunsaturated Fatty Acids of Fish Oils, Autoxidation Ex Vivo and Peroxidation In Vivo: Implications. In M Friedman (ed), *Nutritional and Toxicological Consequences of Food Processing.* New York: Plenum, 1991.
107. Muggli R. Dietary Fish Oils Increase the Requirement of Vitamin E in Humans. In SK Chandra (ed), *Health Effects of Fish and Fish Oil.* St. Johns: ARTS Press, 1989.
108. Levine L. Introduction. *Prog Allergy* 44:1, 1988.
109. Janniger CK, Racis SP. The arachidonic acid cascade: An immunologically based review. *J Med* 18:69, 1987.
110. Goodwin JS, Ceuppens J. Regulation of the immune response by prostaglandins. *J Clin Immunol* 3:295, 1983.
111. Parker CW. Leukotrienes and prostaglandins in the immune system. *Adv Prostaglandin Thromboxane Leukotriene Res* 16:113, 1986.
112. Samuelsson B, Paoletti R (eds). *Leukotrienes and Other Lipoxygenase Products.* New York: Raven, 1982.
113. Lee TH, et al. Characterization and biologic properties of 5,12,-dihydroxy derivatives of eicosapentaenoic acid, including leukotriene B_5 and the double lipoxygenase product. *J Biol Chem* 259:2383, 1984.
114. Terano T, Salmon JA, Moncada S. Biosynthesis and biological activity of leukotriene B_5. *Prostaglandins* 27:217, 1984.
115. Lokesh BR, Kinsella JE. Modulation of prostaglandin synthesis in mouse peritoneal macrophages by enrichment of lipids with either eicosapentaenoic or docosahexaenoic acids in vitro. *Immunobiology* 175:406, 1987.
116. Lands WEM. Differences in ω-3 and ω-6 eicosanoid precursors. *Adv Prostaglandin Thromboxane Leukotriene Res* 19:602, 1989.
117. Needleman P, et al. Triene prostaglandins: Prostacyclin and thromboxane biosynthesis and unique properties. *Proc Natl Acad Sci USA* 76:944, 1979.
118. Rockwell WB, Ehrlich HP. Ibuprofen in acute-care therapy. *Ann Surg* 211:78, 1990.
119. Robertson RP. Characterization of prostaglandin and leukotriene receptors: An overview. *Prostaglandins* 31:395, 1986.
120. Ninnemann JL, Stockland AE. Participation of prostaglandin E in immunosuppression following thermal injury. *J Trauma* 24:201, 1984.
121. Plescia OJ, Racis S. Prostaglandins as physiological immunoregulators. *Prog Allergy* 44:153, 1988.
122. Parker CW. Lipid mediators produced through the lipoxygenase pathway. *Ann Rev Immunol* 5:65, 1987.
123. Kunkel SL. The importance of arachidonate metabolism by immune and nonimmune cells. *Lab Invest* 58:119, 1988.
124. Staite ND, Panayi GS. Prostaglandin regulation of B-lymphocyte function. *Immunol Today* 5:175, 1984.
125. Waymack JP, et al. Effect of prostaglandin E in multiple experimental models. *J Surg Res* 49:328, 1990.
126. Waymack JP, Yurt RW. Effect of prostaglandin E on immune function in multiple animal models. *Arch Surg* 123:1429, 1988.
127. Grbic JT, et al. The role of prostaglandin E_2 in immune suppression following injury. *Ann Surg* 214:253, 1991.
128. Freeman BA, Crapo JD. Free radicals and tissue injury. *Lab Invest* 47:412, 1982.
129. Ertel W, et al. Ibuprofen restores cellular immunity and decreases susceptibility to sepsis following hemorrhage. *J Surg Res* 53:55, 1992.
130. Coran AG, et al. Ibuprofen intervention in canine septic shock: Reduction of pathophysiology without decreased cytokines. *J Surg Res* 53:272, 1992.
131. Faist E, et al. Immunoprotective effects of cyclooxygenase inhibition in patients with major surgical trauma. *J Trauma* 30:8, 1990.
132. Faist E, et al. Immunomodulatory therapy with thymopentin and indomethacin. *Ann Surg* 214:264, 1991.
133. Revhaug A, et al. Inhibition of cyclooxygenase attenuates in the metabolic response to endotoxin in humans. *Arch Surg* 123:162, 1988.
134. Keppler D, Hagmann W, Denzlinger C (eds). Leukotrienes as Mediators in Endotoxin Shock and Tissue Trauma. In *First Vienna Shock Forum, Part A: Pathophysiological Role of Mediators and Mediator Inhibitors in Shock.* New York: Alan R. Liss, 1987.
135. Davies P. Lipoxygenase products in immunity. *Immunol Invest* 16:623, 1987–1988.
136. Schonfeld W, et al. Leukotriene generation in patients with multiple injuries. *J Trauma* 33:799, 1992.
137. Kelly JP. Effect of inhibitors of arachidonic acid metabolism on mitogenesis in human lymphocytes: Possible role of thromboxanes and products of the lipoxygenase pathway. *J Immunol* 122:1563, 1979.
138. Santoli D, Zurier RB. Prostaglandin E precursor fatty acids inhibit human IL-2 production by a prostaglandin E-independent mechanism. *J Immunol* 143:1303, 1989.
139. Billiar TR, et al. Fatty acid intake and Kupffer cell function: Fish oil alters eicosanoid and monokine production to endotoxin stimulation. *Surgery* 104:343, 1988.
140. Venkatraman JT, Fernandes G. Differential effects of fatty acids on proliferative response and IL-2 production by EL-4 cells. *FASEB J* 7:A56, 1993.

141. Ertel W, et al. Modulation of macrophage membrane phospholipids by ω-3 polyunsaturated fatty acids increases interleukin-1 release and prevents suppression of cellular immunity following hemorrhagic shock. *Arch Surg* 128:15, 1993.

142. Hardardottir I, Kinsella JE. Tumor necrosis factor production by murine resident peritoneal macrophages is enhanced by dietary ω-3 polyunsaturated fatty acids. *Biochim Biophys Acta* 1095:187, 1991.

143. Watanabe S, et al. Effect of dietary α-linolenate/linoleate balance on lipopolysaccharide-induced tumor necrosis factor production in mouse macrophages. *Life Sci* 48:2013, 1991.

144. Endres S, et al. The effect of dietary supplementation with ω-3 polyunsaturated fatty acids on the synthesis of interleukin-1 and tumor necrosis factor by mononuclear cells. *N Engl J Med* 320:265, 1989.

145. Meydani SN. Oral (ω-3) fatty acid supplementation suppresses cytokine production and lymphocyte proliferation: Comparison between young and older women. *J Nutr* 121:484, 1991.

146. Karmiol S, Curry R, Phan SH. Fatty acid modification of human lung fibroblasts (HLFS) results in differential IL-6 production due to IL-1β stimulation. *FASEB J* 7:A429, 1993.

147. Yoshino S, Ellis EF. Effect of a fish-oil-supplemented diet on inflammation and immunological processes in rats. *Int Arch Allergy Appl Immunol* 84:233, 1987.

148. Costa Rosa LF, et al. Effects of various dietary fatty acids on enzyme activities of carbohydrate and glutamine metabolism and the metabolic response of lymphocytes and macrophages during Walker-256 ascites cell tumour growth in rats. *Biochem Mol Biol Int* 29:33, 1993.

149. Hubbard NE, Somers SD, Erickson KL. Effect of dietary fish oil on development and selected functions of murine inflammatory macrophages. *J Leukoc Biol* 49:592, 1991.

150. Lefkowith JB, et al. Manipulation of the acute inflammatory response by dietary polyunsaturated fatty acid modulation. *J Immunol* 145:1523, 1990.

151. Morrow WJW, et al. Dietary fat and immune function. I. Antibody responses, lymphocyte and accessory cell function in (NZB X NZW) F_1 mice. *J Immunol* 135:3857, 1985.

152. Hawley HP, Gordon GB. The effects of long chain free fatty acids on human neutrophil function and structure. *Lab Invest* 34:216, 1976.

153. Blonk MC, et al. Dose-response effects of fish-oil supplementation in healthy volunteers. *Am J Clin Nutr* 52:120, 1990.

154. Naccache PH, et al. Modulation of rabbit neutrophil aggregation and degranulation by free fatty acids. *J Leukoc Biol* 36:333, 1984.

155. Wong K, Chew C. The respiratory burst of human neutrophils treated with various stimulators in vitro is dampened by exogenous unsaturated fatty acids. *J Cell Physiol* 119:89, 1984.

156. Magrum LJ, Johnston PV. Effect of culture in vitro with eicosatetraenoic (20:4(ω-6)) and eicosapentaenoic (20:5(ω-3)) acids on fatty acid composition, prostaglandin synthesis and chemiluminescense of rat peritoneal macrophages. *Biochim Biophys Acta* 836:354, 1985.

157. Badwey JA, et al. Effects of free fatty acids on release of superoxide and on change of shape by human neutrophils. *J Biol Chem* 259:7870, 1984.

158. Gadd MA, Hansbrough JF. Postburn suppression of murine lymphocyte and neutrophil functions is not reversed by prostaglandin blockade. *J Surg Res* 48:84, 1990.

159. Ossman JB, Erickson KL, Canolty NL. Effects of saturation and concentration of dietary fats on lymphocyte transformation in mice. *Nutr Rep Int* 22:279, 1980.

160. Kelly JP, Parker CW. Effects of arachidonic acid and other unsaturated fatty acids on mitogenesis in human lymphocytes. *J Immunol* 122:1556, 1979.

161. Egami MI, et al. Effect of fatty acid-rich diets on thymocyte proliferation and thymus involution during growing. *Physiol Behav* 53:531, 1993.

162. Peck MD, et al. Composition of fat in enteral diets can influence outcome in experimental peritonitis. *Ann Surg* 213:74, 1991.

163. Newberne PM. Dietary fat, immunological response, and cancer in rats. *Cancer Res* 41:3783, 1981.

164. Locniskar M, Nauss KM, Newberne PM. The effect of quality and quantity of dietary fat on the immune system. *J Nutr* 113:951, 1983.

165. Fowler KL, Chapkin RS, McMurray DN. Effects of purified dietary ω-3 ethyl esters on murine T-lymphocyte function. *FASEB J* 7:A72, 1993.

166. Peck MD, et al. The effect of dietary fatty acids on response to *Pseudomonas* infection in burned mice. *J Trauma* 30:445, 1990.

167. Trocki O, et al. Effects of fish oil on postburn metabolism and immunity. *JPEN* 11:521, 1987.

168. Bennett M, Uauy R, Grundy SM. Dietary fatty acid effects on T-cell-mediated immunity in mice infected with mycoplasma pulmonis or given carcinogens by injection. *Am J Pathol* 126:103, 1987.

169. Friend JV, et al. Effect of different dietary lipids on the immune responses of Hartley strain guinea pigs. *Int Arch Allergy Appl Immunol* 62:292, 1980.

170. DeWille JW, Fraker PJ, Romsos DR. Effects of essential fatty acid deficiency, and various levels of dietary polyunsaturated fatty acids, on humoral immunity in mice. *J Nutr* 109:1018, 1979.

171. Erickson KL. Dietary fat influences on murine melanoma growth and lymphocyte-mediated cytotoxicity. *J Natl Cancer Inst* 72:115, 1984.

172. Richieri GV, Mescher MF, Kleinfeld AM. Short term exposure to *cis* unsaturated free fatty acids inhibits degranulation of cytotoxic T lymphocytes. *J Immunol* 144:671, 1990.

173. Bialick R, et al. Modulation of cell-mediated cytotoxicity function after alteration of fatty acid composition in vitro. *J Immunol* 132:81, 1984.

174. Meydani SN, et al. Fish oil and tocopherol-induced changes in natural killer cell-mediated cytotoxicity and PGE_2 synthesis in young and old mice. *J Nutr* 118:1245, 1988.

175. Yamashita N, et al. Effect of eicosapentaenoic and docosahexaenoic acid on natural killer cell activity in human peripheral blood lymphocytes. *Clin Immunol Immunopathol* 59:335, 1991.

176. Dustin LB, et al. Docosahexaenoic acid, a constituent of rodent fetal serum and fish oil diets, inhibits acquisition of macrophage tumoricidal function. *J Immunol* 144:4888, 1990.

177. Somers SD, Chapkin RS, Erickson KL. Alteration of in vitro murine peritoneal macrophage function by dietary enrichment with eicosapentaenoic and docosahexaenoic acids in menhaden fish oil. *Cell Immunol* 123:201, 1989.

178. Schlager SL, Meltzer MS, Madden LD. Role of membrane lipids in the immunological killing of tumor cells: II. Effector cell lipids. *Lipids* 18:483, 1983.

179. Huang SC, Misfeldt ML, Fritsche KL. Dietary fat influ-

ences Ia antigen expression and immune cell populations in the murine peritoneum and spleen. *J Nutr* 122:1, 1992.

180. Gill R, Clark W. Membrane structure-function relationships in cell-mediated cytolysis. *J Immunol* 125:689, 1980.
181. Schlager SI, Ohanian SH. A role for fatty acid composition of complex cellular lipids in the susceptibility of tumor cells to humoral immune killing. *J Immunol* 123:146, 1979.
182. Yoo TJ, et al. Effect of fatty acid modifications of cultured hepatoma cells on susceptibility to complement-mediated cytolysis. *Cancer Res* 40:1084, 1980.
183. Awad AB, Fink CS, Horvath PJ. Alteration of membrane fatty acid composition and inositol phosphate metabolism in HT-29 human colon cancer cells. *Nutr Cancer* 19:181, 1993.
184. Pan DA, Storlien LH. Dietary lipid profile is a determinant of tissue phospholipid fatty acid composition and rate of weight gain in rats. *J Nutr* 123:512, 1993.
185. Teo TC, et al. Administration of structured lipid composed of MCT and fish oil reduces net protein catabolism in enterally fed burned rats. *Ann Surg* 210:100, 1989.
186. Lanza-Jacoby S, et al. Adaptation to a fish oil diet before inducing sepsis in rats prevents fatty infiltration of liver. *JPEN* 16:353, 1992.
187. Malis CD, et al. Incorporation of marine lipids into mitochondrial membranes increases susceptibility to damage by calcium and reactive oxygen species: Evidence of enhanced activation of phospholipase A_2 in mitochondria enriched with ω-3 fatty acids. *Proc Natl Acad Sci USA* 87:8845, 1990.
188. Bhathena SJ, et al. Effects of ω-3 fatty acids and vitamin E on hormones involved in carbohydrate and lipid metabolism in men. *Am J Clin Nutr* 54:684, 1991.
189. Mertin J. Effect of polyunsaturated fatty acids on skin allograft survival and primary and secondary cytotoxic response in mice. *Transplantation* 21:1, 1976.
190. Mertin J, Hunt R. Influence of polyunsaturated fatty acids on survival of skin allografts and tumor incidence in mice. *Proc Natl Acad Sci USA* 73(3):928, 1976.
191. Mertin J, et al. Importance of the spleen for the immunoinhibitory action of linoleic acid in mice. *Int Arch Allergy Appl Immunol* 53:469, 1977.
192. Kelley VE, et al. Enhancement of immunosuppression by substitution of fish oil for olive oil as a vehicle for cyclosporine. *Transplantation* 48:98, 1989.
193. Sweny P. Use of dietary fish oils in renal allograft recipients with chronic vascular rejection. *Transplant Proc* 25:2089, 1993.
194. King MM, et al. Incidence and growth of mammary tumors induced by 7,12-dimethylbenz[a]anthracene as related to the dietary content of fat and antioxidant. *J Natl Cancer Inst* 63:657, 1979.
195. Kollmorgen GM, et al. Inhibition of lymphocyte function in rats fed high-fat diets. *Cancer Res* 39:3458, 1979.
196. Hanai T, et al. Comparison of prostanoids and their precursor fatty acids in human hepatocellular carcinoma and noncancerous reference tissues. *J Surg Res* 54:57, 1993.
197. Stillwell W, Ehringer W, Jenski LJ. Docosahexaenoic acid increases permeability of lipid vesicles and tumor cells. *Lipids* 28:103, 1993.
198. Ball HA, et al. Role of thromboxane, prostaglandins and leukotrienes in endotoxic and septic shock. *Intensive Care Med* 12:116, 1986.
199. Mascioli EA, et al. Enhanced survival to endotoxin in guinea pigs fed IV fish oil emulsion. *Lipids* 23:623, 1988.
200. Mascioli EA, et al. Endotoxin challenge after menhaden oil diet: Effects on survival of guinea pigs. *Am J Clin Nutr* 49:277, 1989.
201. Barton RG, et al. Dietary omega-3 fatty acids decrease mortality and Kupffer cell prostaglandin E_2 production in a rat model of chronic sepsis. *J Trauma* 31:768, 1991.
202. Murray MJ, et al. Effects of a fish oil diet on pigs' cardiopulmonary response to bacteremia. *JPEN* 15:152, 1991.
203. Clouva-Molyvdas P, Peck MD, Alexander JW. Short-term dietary lipid manipulation does not affect survival in two models of murine sepsis. *JPEN* 16:343, 1992.
204. Boudreau MD, et al. A-linolenic acid and prostaglandin synthesis. *Nutrition* 8:211, 1992.
205. Eaton SB. Humans, lipids and evolution. *Lipids* 27:814, 1992.
206. Shils ME, Young VR. Average Values for Triglycerides, Fatty Acids, and Cholesterol in Selected Foods and Oils. In ME Shils, V Young (eds), *Modern Nutrition in Health and Disease.* Philadelphia: Lea & Febiger, 1988. P. 1547.
207. Chee KM, et al. Fatty acid content of marine oil capsules. *Lipids* 25:523, 1990.
208. Altman PL, Dittmer DS (eds). *Biology Data Book.* Bethesda: Federation of American Societies of Experimental Biology, 1972.
209. Montgomery R, Conway TW, Spector AA (eds). *Biochemistry: A Case-Oriented Approach.* St. Louis: Mosby, 1990.

Selected Readings

Gennis RB. *Biomembranes: Molecular Structure and Function.* New York: Springer, 1989.

This book provides a comprehensive and comprehensible overview of the biologic properties of cell membranes.

Gurr MI. *Role of Fats in Food and Nutrition.* London: Elsevier, 1992.

This monograph, by one of the pioneers of research into the interactions of lipids and immunity, strives to assess the many attributes of dietary fats that contribute to the nutrition of man, especially in the context of other food components.

Kinsella JE. Dietary ω-3 Polyunsaturated Fatty Acids of Fish Oils, Autoxidation Ex Vivo and Peroxidation In Vivo: Implications. In M Friedman (ed), *Nutritional and Toxicological Consequences of Food Processing.* New York: Plenum, 1991.

This thorough review was written to address concerns about the potential deleterious effects resulting from peroxidation of dietary ω-3 PUFA.

Nelson GJ. *Health Effects of Dietary Fatty Acids.* Champaign, IL: American Oil Chemists' Society, 1991.

This monograph includes distillations of oral presentations given in 1990 and is intended to be both a reference work for the active investigator and an overview for the practicing clinician.

Plescia OJ, Racis S. Prostaglandins as physiological immunoregulators. *Prog Allergy* 44:153–171, 1988.

This is one of the more recent comprehensive reviews of the immunoregulatory role of prostaglandins.

III

Patient Evaluation

19

Nutritional Assessment: The Assessment of the Nutritional and Metabolic Status of Surgical Patients

John A. Windsor
Graham L. Hill

Many surgical diseases are associated with weight loss, and protein-energy malnutrition (PEM) is not uncommon in surgical patients [1]. The PEM may be due to an absolute (when nutritional intake does not meet normal requirements) or relative (when nutritional intake meets normal requirements but the person has increased requirements) deficiency in protein and energy intake. While mild PEM associated with uncomplicated surgery in a well-nourished patient is an accepted part of surgical illness and does not require intervention, the same cannot be said for moderate to severe PEM, which is often unrecognized and therefore untreated. There are a number of reasons why nutritional assessment has not become an integral part of the clinical evaluation of all surgical patients. These include a recognition that PEM is only one of many potential risk factors in a surgical patient, a genuine concern about the relevance and reliability of current methods of nutritional assessment, and the paucity of evidence indicating the efficacy of nutritional therapy in improving the outcome of malnourished patients.

What then is the justification for the nutritional assessment of surgical patients? Put simply, it is that PEM adversely affects patient outcome. It was over 50 years ago that Hiram Studley demonstrated a relationship between preoperative weight loss and postoperative morbidity and mortality in patients undergoing gastric resection for peptic ulcer disease [2]. Many factors in modern surgery now make this relationship less apparent, and these include minimally invasive approaches, prophylactic antibiotics, rational intravenous fluid therapy, better anesthesia and postoperative analgesia, improved suture materials, and expert physiotherapy. Nevertheless, a number of recent prospective studies have shown that severely malnourished patients are still at an increased risk of developing complications after major surgery [3,4]. The accurate identification of such patients justifies nutritional assessment, as long as cost-effective nutritional therapy can be prescribed.

Objectives of Nutritional Assessment

The objectives of nutritional assessment were quite straightforward up to a decade ago, for example, "the determination of the caloric requirements and the weight status of the patient" [5]. Today, we must think more carefully about what is required of nutritional assessment in the surgical context. Any technique of nutritional assessment must be based first on a concept of nutritional status that is appropriate to surgical patients. Second, it must be able to diagnose malnutrition on the basis of a clinically relevant defect, that is, when protein-energy malnutrition is already or soon will be of sufficient intensity to impact adversely on the course of the patient's illness. This technique of nutritional assessment must be able to select individual patients who warrant nutritional and/or metabolic intervention, and the technique ought to be able to provide a means of monitoring changes in nutritional status in response to any such treatment. Although sophisticated methods for assessment are being developed (for example, methods for estimating the components of energy and protein and methods to measure body composition), the widespread applicability of any technique of nutritional assessment requires it to be simple enough to be incorporated into the routine clinical evaluation of patients.

Traditional Approaches to Nutritional Assessment

The chapter on nutritional assessment in the first edition of this text concluded that "current nutritional assessment tools fall short of critical expectations" because they lack "a clearly defined defect to treat, and an end-point to strive for" [6]. Confidence in traditional nutritional assessment techniques has eroded in recent years. In retrospect, it was rather naive to attempt to adapt descriptive tools developed for the survey of starving populations into prognostic clinical tools to assess individual patients [7]. Many of the traditional markers of PEM have such a large variance and a poor sensitivity-specificity profile in the sick surgical patient [8] that their usefulness is limited to serial measurements of groups of patients or populations.

The use of body weight indices as markers of nutritional status has come under scrutiny. The errors in determining weight loss from a single measurement of body weight are greater if predicted rather than recalled well weight is used. Even so, random error in the determination of weight loss based on recalled weight is up to 7.2 kg [9]. The poor sensitivity (67%) and predictive power (75%) means that one third of patients with at least 10 kg of weight loss would be missed, and one quarter of patients without this degree of weight loss would be considered to have lost at least 10 kg of body weight [9]. Nevertheless, when weight loss is correctly interpreted in its clinical context and not overinterpreted, it remains a vital global marker of nutritional status.

Anthropometric methods of nutritional assessment (for example, skinfold thickness and arm muscle circumference) have been used in two ways: (1) to compare measured values with those of a reference population, and (2) to compare serial data from the same patient. The main pitfall of the first method is its dependence on age-, sex-, and race-matched reference values. Even when these have been available, studies of preoperative patients have failed to demonstrate any increased incidence of postoperative complications in patients with PEM diagnosed by anthropometric techniques [10]. The large variance between serial measurements for an individual patient is another pitfall. Hall et al. [11] found that the coefficient of variation was 22.6% for triceps skinfold thickness (TSF) and 4.7% for arm circumference (AC). Therefore, to confirm a true change in arm muscle circumference, which is derived from TSF and AC, a change of around 3 cm is required. The traditional anthropometric methods of measuring PEM are not appropriate for assessing adult hospital patients because they, unlike children, are not growing. In addition, a number of nonnutritional factors affect the anthropometric status of individuals [12,13], for example, the size of muscles and skeleton is partly dependent on exercise, bedridden patients undergo some disuse atrophy of muscle independent of PEM, and, more importantly in critically ill surgical patients, expansion of interstitial fluid may mask any reduction of skinfold thickness [14,15].

The use of plasma proteins as markers of PEM requires a disregard for the evidence that their concentration is more likely to be affected by factors other than nutritional status (for example, sepsis chronic liver disease and inflammatory bowel disease) [13,16]. Plasma protein levels are best considered as an index of the severity of illness rather than nutritional status [17], and any prognostic nutritional indices that rely on them tend to select septic rather than malnourished patients [18]. In following ward patients receiving nutritional support, plasma protein levels broadly reflect nitrogen balance [19], but it is far from clear that this applies in critically ill septic or traumatized surgical patients. Furthermore, the derivation of these indices from a number of different nutritional markers defies statistical logic because the limitations and errors of each marker are compounded rather than lessened. Bayes probability analysis demonstrates that single or multiple associations of nutritional markers do not improve their ability to predict postoperative outcome [17,20].

Many clinicians rely on the weekly assessment of nitrogen balance to assess nutritional status. Unfortunately, in clinical practice the performance of nitrogen balance is full of difficulties unless a very strict protocol is used [21]. More often than not, this is impossible or impractical in a busy surgical service.

There is little doubt that most currently used techniques of nutritional assessment flounder in the face of the stated objectives. A fresh approach to nutritional assessment is required [22], one that takes into account the importance of surgical illness in producing PEM and that is based on concepts that are relevant to the surgical patient.

Metabolic Stress and Surgical Patients

Surgical patients are rarely victims of pure starvation. While semi-starvation is often present, the presence or absence of metabolic stress is of far greater significance to the patient in terms of the development of PEM and clinical outcome. While patients who are chronically starved adapt by reducing the extent of body protein loss, patients who are metabolically stressed (for example, due to sepsis, trauma, major surgery, burns, or malignancy) lose this response. The metabolic basis for this loss of adaptive response involves not only the well-characterized neuroendocrine "stress response" but various cytokines, reactive oxygen species, and lipid mediators that act as the link between sepsis and trauma and the metabolic and immunologic responses observed. There are data implicating tumor necrosis factor in this protein breakdown [23]. It is clear that this cytokine, as well as the interleukins 1 and 6, are associated with redistribution of body protein and massive lipolysis [24]. Cytokines, particularly TNF, may prime neutrophils to generate increased amounts of superoxide radicals and many of their effects may be mediated through intracellular radical generation [25].

Consequences of Metabolic Stress in Surgical Patients

One of the important consequences of metabolic stress in surgical patients is the acceleration of protein and fat loss, over and above what would occur due to starvation alone. Another consequence is the expansion of the extracellular fluid volume that accompanies the protein depletion, especially in the presence of metabolic stress [15]. This may mask subtle changes in body weight and certainly makes its interpretation more difficult. The rate of change in body weight that occurs in serious sepsis (after resuscitation), uncomplicated surgery, and major injury compared with the rate of loss of body weight that occurs with total starvation are shown in Figure 19-1 [26].

A third consequence of the metabolic stress in surgical patients is the reduced ability to retain administered protein because of continuing net protein catabolism. The net changes in total body protein that occur in patients given nutritional support are determined by the relative effects of two competing processes: protein depletion and metabolic stress. In a recent study of surgical patients receiving a two-week course of total parenteral nutrition [27], it was found that those patients with 20% to 30% depletion in body protein stores had a marked tendency to gain body protein. When similar patients had a raised metabolic expenditure, this tendency to gain protein was still present, but it was less (Figure 19-2). Patients with mild protein depletion and a raised metabolic expenditure had continuing net losses of protein despite aggressive nutrition support.

Because of the impact of metabolic stress on nutritional status, any approach to nutritional assessment must incorporate a relevant marker of it. Much research effort is directed at exploring new ways (for example, growth factors, using nutrients as pharmacologic agents, and the use of anticytokines) in which the continuing catabolism of surgical illness might be consistently reversed.

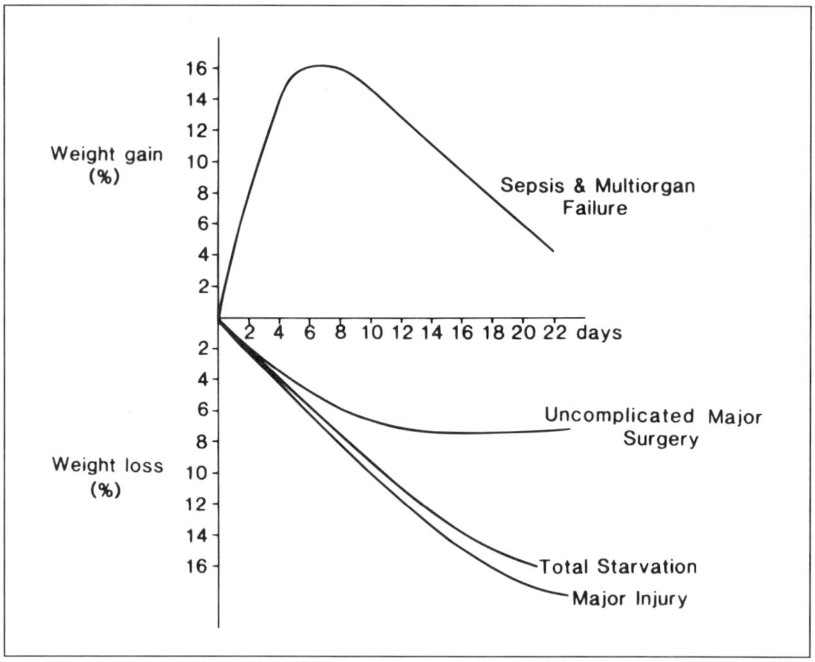

Figure 19-1. Changes in body weight that occur in serious sepsis (after resuscitation), uncomplicated surgery, and major injury compared to the rate of loss of body weight that occurs with total starvation. (From GL Hill, AH Beddoe. Dimensions of the human body and its compartments. In JM Kinney et al. [eds], *Nutrition and Metabolism in Patient Care.* Philadelphia: Saunders, 1988. Reproduced by permission.)

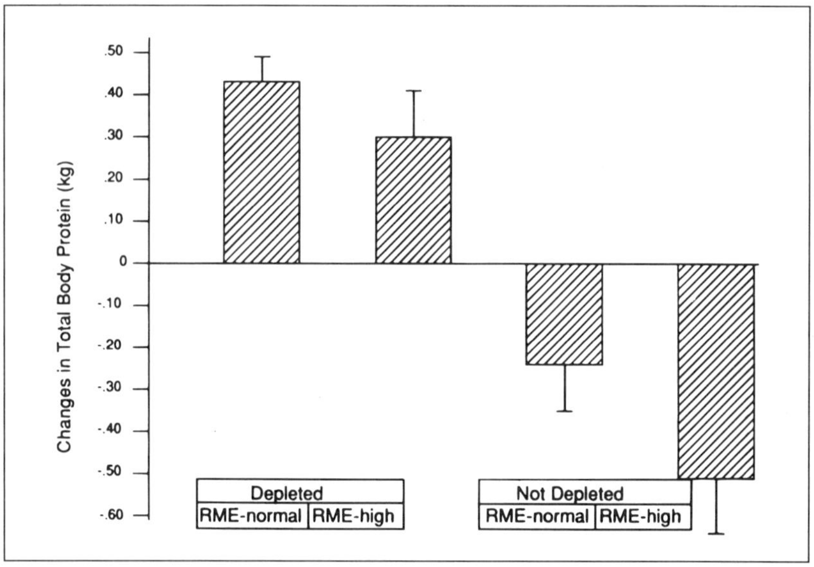

Figure 19-2. Surgical patients who are depleted of body stores of protein have a marked tendency to gain protein within total parenteral nutrition. When metabolic expenditure is raised in similar patients, this tendency to gain protein is still present, but it is less. RME = resting metabolic expenditure. (From GL Hill et al. Protein status and metabolic expenditure determine the reponse to intravenous nutrition: A basis for a new classification of surgical malnutrition. *Br J Surg* 78:109, 1991. Reproduced by permission of Blackwell Scientific Publications.)

A New Approach to Nutritional Assessment: Assessment of Physiologic Function

Patients with significant PEM do not face increased surgical risks because they have lost a certain amount of body weight, fat, or protein. Malnourished patients develop complications and die because of the impairment and eventual failure of vital physiologic and protein-dependent functions (Figure 19-3). The most important component of the lost weight is body protein. Its loss is responsible for the impairment of a wide range of physiologic functions. It is suggested that this dysfunction underlies the increased surgical risk found in patients with significant PEM [3].

The importance of impaired function has been recognized in a relatively recent definition of malnutrition as "[t]he state induced by alterations in dietary intake resulting in changes in subcellular, cellular and/or organ function which exposes the individual to increased risks of morbidity and mortality and which can be reversed by adequate nutritional support" [28]. There are, however, two obvious deficiencies with this definition. The first is that it does not acknowledge the importance

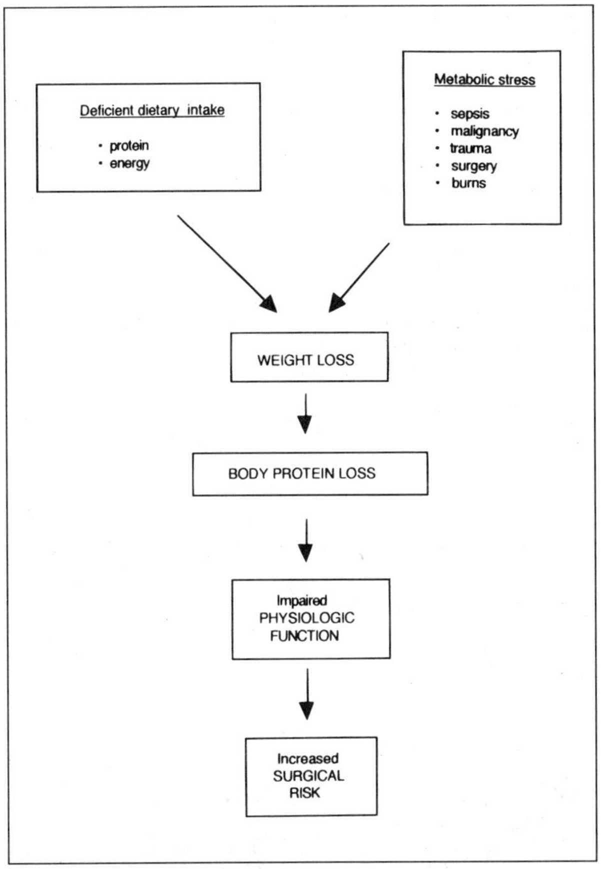

Figure 19-3. The relationship of deficient dietary intake, metabolic stress, nutritional status, physiologic function, and surgical risk. (From JA Windsor. Underweight patients and the risks of surgery. *World J Surg* 17:165, 1993. Reproduced by permission.)

of metabolic stress. Second, there are as yet no markers of cellular or subcellular function that can be put to use in the routine clinical assessment of nutritional status.

The purpose of this chapter is not to review all the physiologic alterations that can accompany PEM, but to emphasize a number of physiologic functions that are affected by protein depletion and that have particular relevance to the surgical patient. These are summarized in Table 19-1.

To explore this concept of impaired physiologic function further, it is clear that an impairment would be more likely to occur during the development of PEM if the relevant organ system was already affected by disease. For instance, respiratory function can be severely limited by underlying obstructive airways disease (immune function by steroid therapy), cardiac function limited by atherosclerosis, and exercise tolerance limited by cardiorespiratory disease, peripheral vascular disease, or arthritis. These factors reduce the "reserve capacity" of a particular physiologic function, making it more likely that the loss of body protein will cause a significant impairment of that function [3]. In this way, the assessment of nutritional status by physiologic function is the assessment of both the influence of PEM and that of comorbid disease. The assessment of function does not help to isolate PEM as an independent risk factor, but it does make the assessment more relevant by placing the evaluation of PEM within the individual patient's clinical context.

In summary, the impact of the loss of body protein on vital physiologic functions provides an appropriate starting point for defining PEM in surgical patients. This approach has the potential for fulfilling the objectives for nutritional assessment in providing a clinically relevant defect to diagnose and treat. Early studies have confirmed that it is possible to monitor the response to treatment on the basis of measurements of physiologic functions [39,40].

Modern Approaches to Nutritional Assessment

In the surgical context, and from the previous discussion, it is clear that nutritional assessment must evaluate the following aspects: protein and energy balance, body composition, relevant physiologic function, and the degree of metabolic stress. These aspects can be evaluated both in the clinic and in the laboratory.

Clinical Nutritional Assessment

The reliability of clinical judgment in evaluating the nutritional status of surgical patients should be more widely recognized [41]. It was in 1987 that Detsky et al. [42] published evidence to suggest that clinical examination was the best way to identify patients at risk for nutrition-associated complications. They compared seven techniques of nutritional assessment (including plasma proteins, anthropometry, creatinine-height index, delayed cutaneous hypersensitivity, and prognostic nutritional index) in terms of the ability to predict one nutrition-associated complication (infection) by dividing a sample of 59 surgical patients into high- and low-risk groups. The results showed that a subjective global assessment (SGA), consisting of a dietary and medical history with a functional assessment and a physical examination, offered the best combination of sensitivity and specificity in predicting outcome. Studies conducted in Auckland Hospital also found that a thorough clinical evaluation was as effective in identifying a subset of patients at high risk of nutrition-associated postoperative complications as anthropometric measurements, plasma protein

Table 19-1. Physiologic Functions of Relevance to Surgical Patients; Examples of Measurements Used in the Assessment of Nutritional Status

Surgically Relevant Physiologic Functions	Clinical Relevance	Example of Measurements	References
Psychological	Motivation Fatigue Coping	Self-Questionnaire —Profile of Mood Score [POMS] —Symptom Check List [SCL]	17, 29
Respiratory Muscle	Ventilation Oxygenation Expectoration	Respiratory Function Tests —peak expiratory flow rate —vital capacity —forced expiratory volume (1 sec) —respiratory muscle strength —maximum voluntary ventilation	30, 31, 32
Skeletal Muscle	Mobilization	Voluntary Tests —hand grip strength —hand grip endurance	33, 34
		Involuntary Strength —ulnar stimulation of adductor pollicis (force & force/frequency ratio)	35, 36
		Involuntary Endurance —fade of force —relaxation rate	
Wound Healing	Tissue repair	Hydroxyproline accumulation	37
Immune Function	Resistance to infection	Lymphocyte count Lymphocyte function	38
		Cytokines	24
Liver Function	Protein synthesis	Plasma proteins Acute-phase proteins	16, 19

concentrations, grip strength, and the most commonly used prognostic indices (Philadelphia, Boston, and Leeds) [10]. Based on this work, we developed the following method of clinical nutritional assessment. It is not as advanced as the definitive approach, but it does take nutritional assessment in a new direction by abandoning inappropriate traditional techniques and deliberately incorporating an assessment of metabolic stress and relevant physiologic functions [22].

Assessment of Protein and Energy Balance

In practice the clinician may obtain an overview of protein and energy balance by assessing the frequency and size of the patient's meals and comparing the results obtained with an estimate of rate of loss of body weight. Table 19-2 shows the relationship between meal size and the loss of body weight over time [43]. It can be seen that if meal size has been only 50% of normal over a period of three months, the patient will have a weight loss of 15%. If energy intake is 20% of normal over a period of six months, then the patient will suffer from near lethal loss of body weight (45%). [*Editor's Note:* We know from the hunger strikes of IRA prisoners, in whom protein and energy deprivation was near total, death from (pulmonary) infection took place in 60 to 70 days.]

Over shorter time periods, changes in body weight reflect either overhydration or the combined effects of starvation and major metabolic stress. With major injury or serious sepsis, negative protein and energy balance is the rule, but simple bedside assessment of the magnitude of this imbalance is not precise. A more comprehensive assessment of protein and energy intake can be performed by a dietitian. A 24-hour recall with a food frequency cross-check is the technique used most frequently, although an analysis of a food record diary of a calorie count is also used. Once the diet information is collected, the data are processed by a computer using food composition tables, and the amount and adequacy of the total protein and energy intake are assessed by comparison with recommended daily allowances. For clinical purposes, protein and energy output in surgical patients is calculated at the bedside; 1.5 g of protein/kg/day and 40 kcal/kg/body weight are reasonable approximations of protein and energy requirements. When the output calculated in this way is related to dietary assessment of intake,

Table 19-2. Relationship between meal size and loss of body weight (expressed as a percentage of original body weight) over time

Meal Size (% of normal)	Weight Loss (% over time)		
	3 months	6 months	9 months
20	30	45	—
30	25	35	40
50	15	25	30
70	10	15	20
80	8	12	15

Source: Data derived from A Keys, et al. *The Biology of Human Starvation.* Minneapolis: University of Minnesota Press, 1950.

then an approximation of protein and energy deficit is obtained.

Assessment of Body Composition

In the assessment and subsequent evaluation of patients with nutritional and metabolic disorders, measurements of body weight should always be made.

Weight loss can be determined easily if a patient's weight before and after the occurrence of the loss has been measured. Usually, however, patients have already lost weight when they are first seen, and the size of the weight loss then needs to be evaluated by comparing the measured weight with some other estimate of well weight. The accuracy of the result depends on the accuracy with which well weight can be measured. There is a lot of research on the measurement of well weight (ideal weight), and it is now clear that it is more reliable to estimate weight loss by using the patient's recalled well weight than by using published tables of ideal weight [9]. Even then, estimating weight loss can be quite misleading in individual subjects, and it is important therefore to relate the estimate of weight loss to the physical examination of the patient.

General Appearance. The severely malnourished patient is readily recognized by the loss of body contours that result from the loss of muscle tissue and subcutaneous fat. The face is thin and the cheekbones are prominent; the patient looks haggard and emaciated. The wasting of soft tissues is particularly marked in the region of the buttocks, which are thin and flat. The shoulder girdle is square and prominent. Patients with major injury and serious sepsis may be profoundly protein depleted with severe erosions of muscle mass, and yet not have this classic appearance due to a relative preservation of body fat mass and an overlying layer of extracellular water.

Body Fat Stores. Gross loss of body fat can be observed not only from the patient's appearance by also by palpating a number of skinfolds between the finger and thumb. When the dermis can be felt between the finger and thumb on pinching the triceps and biceps skinfolds, considerable losses of body fat have occurred. We call this a positive finger-thumb test. Body composition studies have shown that the body mass is composed of less than 10% body fat when this physical sign is present [44].

Body Protein Stores. In a similar manner, protein stores may be assessed by inspection and palpation of a number of muscle groups. The temporalis muscles, deltoids, suprascapular and infrascapular muscles, the bellies of biceps and triceps, and the interossei of the hands should all be looked at and palpated. The long muscles in particular are considered to be profoundly protein depleted when the tendons are prominent to palpation. Body composition studies have shown that when the tendons are prominent to palpation and the bony prominences of the scapula are obvious, patients have lost more than 30% of their total body protein stores [44]. We call this a positive tendon-bone test.

Hypoalbuminemia and Excess Body Water. Although albumin is affected by a host of factors unrelated to nutrition, when a patient with PEM has low levels of plasma albumin, it usually indicates an expanded extracellular fluid space [44] that occasionally may be large enough to be clinically detectable as pitting edema.

Assessment of Physiologic Function

Functional impairment secondary to loss of body protein is the most important part of the assessment of nutritional status. Weight loss without evidence of physiologic abnormality is probably of no consequence [3]. The loss of function to note is that which is clinically quite obvious and which has occurred over the same time period as the loss of body weight. The patient should be questioned about unhealed scratches or sores, easy tiredness, or substantial changes in exercise tolerance. Function is observed while performing the physical examination and by watching the patient's activity around the ward. Grip strength can be assessed by asking the patient to squeeze strongly the surgeon's index and middle fingers for at least 10 seconds. Impairment is judged in the light of patient's age, sex, and body habitus. Respiratory muscle function is assessed by asking the patient to blow hard holding a strip of paper 10 cm from the lips. Severe impairment is present when the paper does not move appreciably, when there is shortness of breath at rest and normal conversation is not possible, and when there is virtually no chest expansion.

Assessment of Metabolic Stress

Although methodology does exist for the precise calculation of metabolic expenditure, its assessment is primarily based on the estimated metabolic demand for a given clinical setting. Metabolic stress can usually be revealed during the course of a history and physical examination. It is present if the patient has had major trauma or major surgery in the previous week or there is evidence of serious sepsis (fever > 33°C, pulse > 100 per min, respiratory rate > 30 per min, white blood count < 3 or > 12×10^9 per liter, positive blood culture, active inflammatory bowel disease, defined focus of infection).

Applying the Clinical Nutritional Assessment to Risk Assessment

This approach to clinical nutritional assessment was investigated in a prospective study of preoperative patients awaiting major gastrointestinal surgery. Objective measurements were also made of both nutritional status and a range of relevant physiologic functions [3]. On the basis of this clinical assessment, patients were assigned to one of three categories: (1) patients with normal nutritional status and no impairment of physiologic function, (2) patients with evidence of PEM but no impairment of physiologic function, and (3) patients who had both PEM and impairment of physiologic function. These patient categories were well matched for other perioperative risk factors, including the magnitude of surgery, operating surgeon, perioperative sepsis, and malignancy. Objective measurements of body stores of proteins and liver, skeletal muscle, respiratory, and psychological function confirmed the validity of the clinical classification. Patients with both PEM and impaired physiologic function had more major and septic complications, a higher incidence of pneumonia, and longer hospital stays than patients in the other two categories. The results of this study confirm that weight loss is a basic indicator of surgical risk in modern surgical practice, providing it is associated with clinically obvious impairment of physiologic function.

From an economic standpoint, the proportion of patients identified as having significant PEM is important. Not only is nutritional intervention costly, but data from the Veteran Affairs trial suggest that less than 5% of surgical candidates, or only those who are most severely malnourished, stand to benefit from preoperative feeding [4]. In our own study described above, the data suggest that a lot more than 5% of our patients were at increased risk of postoperative complications. If a more rigorous definition of significant PEM is applied to our patients, for instance requiring at least three physiologic functions to be impaired rather than two, then just over 10% of our patients would have been selected as having significant PEM [unpublished data]. An analysis of the postoperative clinical course of this subgroup of patients revealed that a significantly higher proportion of them sustained complications.

Applying Clinical Nutritional Assessment to Patient Selection for Preoperative Nutritional Support

Although sophisticated decision trees have been suggested for selecting patients for preoperative nutrition, in clinical practice the process can be more straightforward (Figure 19-4). There are three factors that must be considered when a patient is being assessed for preoperative nutritional support: (1) the nutritional state with its associated functional impairment, (2) the magnitude of the projected operative procedure, particularly in terms of the known postoperative risks, and (3) the anticipated response to the nutritional therapy.

Laboratory Nutritional Assessment

A number of the more important laboratory nutritional assessment techniques have been selected as examples of what is now possible. And while most of the techniques for the measurement of body composition, physiologic function, and metabolic stress are likely to remain research tools, some will become part of routine clinical practice, at least in centers responsible for the care of patients with complex nutritional and metabolic problems.

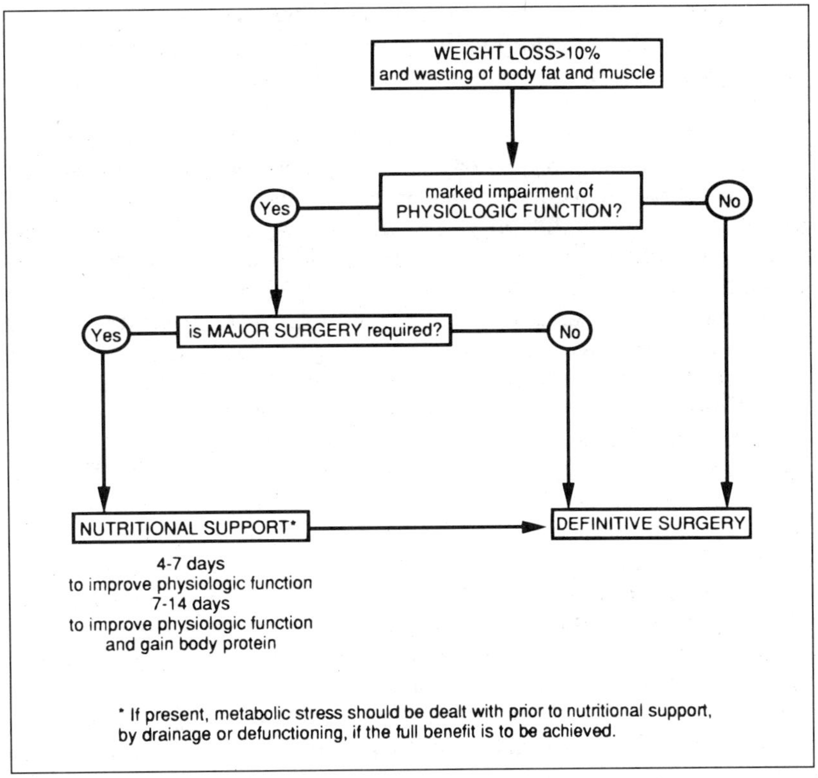

Figure 19-4. Simplified decision tree for selecting surgical patients for preoperative nutritional therapy. (From GI Hill. Malnutrition and surgical risk: Guidelines for nutritional therapy. *Ann J Royal Coll Surg Engl* 69:264, 1987. Reproduced by permission.)

Measuring Body Composition

Atomic Level

At the atomic level, the body can be described in terms of approximately 50 elements, 9 of which (O, C, H, N, Ca, P, K, Na, Ci) account for greater than 98% of body weight. Although these can be measured, the clinical usefulness of such measurement has not been demonstrated. The in vivo neutron activation analysis measurement of changes in total body carbon may yet prove useful in assessing changes in body energy stores [45]. Nuclear magnetic resonance imaging techniques allow the measurement of a number of nuclei (for example, ^{1}H, ^{13}C, ^{23}Na, ^{31}P, ^{39}K) that have yielded a large body of information on metabolic changes in various organs and tissues. Take, for example, phosphorous, which comprises approximately 1% of lean body weight but plays a crucial role in many metabolic processes [46]. Many phosphate compounds (for example, adenosine triphosphate, inorganic phosphate, phosphocreatine) are relevant to cellular energetics and can be detected in vivo by phosphorous magnetic resonance spectroscopy (MRS). Thus, phosphorous MRS may represent a powerful new tool for evaluating energetics in the cells of living subjects under different nutritional conditions. Skeletal muscle protein catabolism is ultimately responsible for the many metabolic derangements associated with metabolic stress and starvation. One important index of energy state that can be measured in vivo is the phosphorylation potential (ratio of ATP to ADP × Pi). This ratio modulates a number of metabolic processes such as whether tissue amino acids will be synthesized into tissue protein or broken down to glucose, the extent of the plasma membrane gradients of the essential electrolytes, the intracellular pH, and the distribution of water between various cellular compartments. As such it is critically related to a number of essential properties of living cells and is a critical parameter of cellular function that might be used to monitor nutritional and metabolic interventions. Phosphorous MRS scans of the liver are also possible. These scans will likely prove useful in the study of hepatocellular energetics associated with increased oxidative stress and sepsis and in monitoring the liver's response to specific therapies [47].

Molecular Level

The measurement of body composition at the molecular level has been of considerable clinical value. A five-compartment model comprising water, protein, fat, glycogen, and mineral, measured by in vivo neutron activation analysis, tritium dilution, and dual energy x-ray absorptiometry (DEXA) has proved to be very useful in a number of clinical settings [44,48].

Neutron Activation Analysis, DEXA and Dilution Techniques. Prompt gamma in vivo neutron activation analysis (IVNAA) is presently the only technique available that allows the multi-elemental composition of the human body to be measured [49]. By this means total body calcium, sodium, chloride, phosphorus, and nitrogen can be determined safely and efficiently. The technique involves the subject passing through a collimated neutron field produced by plutonium-beryllium neutron sources. Capture of neutrons by atoms of the target elements creates unstable isotopes that revert to their stable baseline condition by emission of one or more gamma rays of characteristic energy, which are detected by sodium-iodide detectors. The energy emitted identifies the particular elements, and the level of activity shows its abundance. The most abundant nuclear reaction observed when the human body is irradiated is the capture of thermal neutrons by hydrogen. The use of hydrogen as an internal standard permits partial body irradiation to be used to determine whole body abundances of other elements relative to hydrogen. In critically ill patients, with vastly expanded extracellular fluid volumes, there are difficulties with an excessive hydrogen background and varying ratios of total body hydrogen to total body nitrogen [48]. Phantom and cadaver studies have demonstrated that the IVNAA facility is able to measure total body nitrogen with a precision of 4%. Total body lipid (90% of which is the "nonessential" lipids in the triglyceride form) has usually been calculated as the difference between body weight and the combined measurements of total body protein, minerals, and glycogen. The problem with this approach is that there is no direct way of measuring total body glycogen, which has to be estimated from skeletal size [49]. Dual energy x-ray absorptiometry can also be used to estimate total body fat. The techniques of measuring total body water by tritium dilution and extracellular water by bromide dilution have several problems in relation to sick surgical patients. Not only are there expanded water spaces, often involving collections of free fluid within body cavities that have unpredictable mixing with the circulation, but there are also potential losses of tritium or bromide during the period of equilibration. Despite these problems, the measurement precision is less than 2% [50].

Molecular Biology and Nutritional Assessment. Molecular biology is transforming many aspects of surgical practice, and nutritional assessment is no exception. In primarily dealing with the regulation of gene and protein synthesis, there is a great deal of study encompassing the synthesis and degradation of all structural proteins, functional enzymes, and peptide hormones. Many nutrients act at the molecular level and are known to be important substrates and cofactors for protein synthesis. A range of molecular biologic techniques (for example, chromatin structure analysis, RNA-DNA sequencing, and recombinant DNA technology) are becoming an integral part of nutrition research, and it is highly likely that a number will become important diagnostic tools in nutritional assessment [51]. The advantage of this approach is that the assays tend to require very small tissue amounts and are more direct and specific.

Cellular Level

At the cellular level, the body can be described as being composed of four main compartments: (1) the body cell mass (BCM), (2) extracellular fluid, (3) extracellular solids, and (4) fat [52]. The BCM represents the total cellular mass and is the living, metabolically active component of the body [53]. The measurement of BCM has traditionally been based on the measurement of total body potassium. By assuming an average ratio for the intracellular K to intracellular N of 3 mmol K/g N and by assuming that one quarter of wet cell weight is protein, Moore pointed out that the BCM could be derived from the total exchangeable potassium [53]. Thus, the quantification of BCM is dependent on the assumptions that it has an average K-N ratio of 3 in all states of sickness and health, and that protein comprises 25% of cell mass even in sick surgical patients [54].

Although the concept of BCM has proven fundamental to our understanding of metabolic changes in critically ill patients, the assumptions that allow total body protein to be used to quantify it cannot always be made without resorting to complicated tables or nomograms. In the cellular model, the extracellular mass is the component of the fat-free mass that exists outside the cell and is composed of both fluids and solids. As has been discussed, extracellular fluid volume in sick patients invariably expands [53]. Traditionally, extracellular water has been measured by radiosulfate or bromide dilution [55,56], but there are great difficulties interpreting isotope dilution studies in ill surgical patients. The measurement of total body chlorine by in vivo neutron activation analysis may prove to be a useful means of estimating changes in extracellular water [57].

Isotope Dilution Techniques. Body compositional changes have classically been quantified by isotope dilution techniques. For example, if a fixed known amount of ^{22}Na is administered intravenously, total exchangeable sodium (Na_e) can be determined from the specific activity of the isotope. Total exchangeable potassium (K_e) can be derived from this measurement if the total body water (TBW) is known according to $K_e = TBW \times R - Na_e$, where R is the ratio of the sum of sodium and potassium in a sample of whole blood divided by its water content. The validity of determining exchangeable potassium by using this method has been demonstrated in normal humans and animals [58]. Once these quantities are derived, other measurements of body composition such as the BCM, lean body mass, extracellular mass, and body fat can be calculated by using standard equations.

The ratio of Na_e to K_e is a sensitive measure of nutritional status [59] and is a dynamic expression of the extracellular mass expressed as a function of the body cell mass. The ratio increases significantly under various conditions including sepsis, malnutrition, and after major abdominal surgery [59,60].

There are inherent difficulties in using total body potassium as an index of cellular depletion and repletion. It is generally accepted that changes in total body potassium reflect changes in the body's somatic protein stores and its BCM because these variables are normally closely correlated. Furthermore, total body potassium is linearly related to both the intracellular water volume and to total body nitrogen. However, this mathematical relationship may not be present in sick surgical patients who are, for example, significantly depleted of potassium. And in these patients, the characteristic relationship between BCM and total body water may no longer exist. The ability to determine BCM accurately will vary as the potassium content of the cell changes because of changes in intracellular water. These techniques may also be inaccurate if the composition of the cell changes because of alterations in nitrogen content that occur independently of changes in intracellular potassium and water. In other words, a decrease in total body potassium is usually interpreted as a change in lean body mass of normal composition. In fact, changes of intracellular potassium concentration may occur independently of changes in lean body mass [61].

Whole Body Level

There are other ways of measuring body composition at the whole body level [52]. Computed tomographic body scanning has been used to measure volume of subcutaneous and adipose tissue [62]. Magnetic resonance imaging has also been advanced as a tool for the measurement of body fat [63].

Dual Energy X-ray Absorptiometry. Dual energy x-ray absorptiometry (DXA) is being developed to measure not only fat and minerals but also the total lean tissues of the body. Photons of defined energy are directed at the subject, and there is a loss of energy as some photons are absorbed. The amount of attenuation depends on the nature of the tissue through which the photo beam passes. These changes can be used to quantify the mineral, fat, lean-tissue compartments of the body, as well as the tissue content of different regions of the body [64], and the appendicular muscle mass [65]. At 5 mrad the radiation dose is small, which means that serial measurements are possible to track changes in body composition over time. This technology is becoming increasingly available in many hospitals, and it may open up a new era in the measurement of body composition in surgical patients.

Bioelectrical Impedance Analysis (BIA). The impedance techniques have become increasingly popular as noninvasive and relatively inexpensive methods of estimating the fat-free mass, total body water, and its compartments. Single-frequency BIA appears to be most sensitive to changes in body water, but because of the expansion of extracellular water that accompanies illness, the prediction of lean body mass may be unreliable in patients, particularly the regression equations used that are derived from healthy populations [66]. Multiple-frequency bioelectrical impedance analysis is still largely an experimental technology, but it holds promise. The advantage over single-frequency BIA is that it allows differential current flow through the intra- and extracellular spaces to be assessed, and this should improve the accuracy with which the hydration status and fluid distribution can be determined [67,68]. We recently conducted a clinical trial comparing multifrequency BIA with other methods of measurement of fluid spaces in critically ill surgical patients and were disappointed to find the large errors present when measurements of total body water and extracellular water are compared with those obtained from tritium and bromide dilution.

Measuring Physiologic Function

Skeletal Muscle Function

The function of skeletal muscle is important in surgical convalescence because early mobilization reduces the incidence of postoperative venous thrombosis and pneumonia. Measurements of skeletal muscle function, both voluntary and involuntary, have been used as markers of nutritional status [33–36,69].

The measurement of voluntary hand grip strength has been shown to be an excellent marker of total body protein, as directly measured by in vivo neutron activation analysis, and an even better indicator of the extent of body protein loss [34]. As a predictor of postoperative complications, grip strength is often superior to biochemical and anthropometric markers of nutritional status [10,33,69]. Serial measurements of grip strength have been shown to have a role in monitoring a patient's response to nutritional therapy [39,40]. Although voluntary tests have been criticized because of the influence of psychological factors, motivation and cooperation are important in a patient's recovery from major surgery.

Involuntary tests of skeletal muscle function have also been found to be reliable measures of nutritional status [36]. Some groups are now using maximal relaxation rate as a primary marker of nutritional status, and it is possible that a user-friendly clinical device will be widely available in the near future. The force-frequency characteristics and endurance properties of the adductor pollicis muscle in humans and the gastrocnemius muscle in rats have been extensively studied [35]. Hypocalorically fed and fasted humans and untreated patients with anorexia were shown to have a decreased force of contraction at higher stimulation frequencies, with maintenance of force at lower ones. In addition, the muscle relaxation rate was significantly slower and there was a significant increase in muscle fatiguability in fasting subjects and in the untreated anorexic. Refeeding fasted, morbidly obese subjects and the anorexic patients resulted in a correction of the muscle function abnormalities within two to four weeks and before a measurable restoration of normal body composition and, in particular, muscle bulk. This latter feature has promoted research to elucidate the basis for the impaired muscle function. Preliminary work has suggested that the reduced force reflects the reduced availability of energy during contraction, the reduced relaxation rate reflects the reduced availability of ATP for the energy-dependent uptake of calcium into the endoplasmic reticulum, and the increase in muscle fatiguability reflects an accumulation of calcium and possible Z band degeneration [36].

The alteration of skeletal muscle function and composition in malnourished patients appears to be due to a limitation of energy production. In such patients given nutritional support, the early restitution of body potassium without a parallel rise in body nitrogen suggests that cell ion uptake occurs earlier than protein synthesis [70]. The fall in intracellular potassium that occurs in PEM and that is thought to reflect changes in body cell mass may be explained on the basis of altered membrane pump activity. Transmembrane potential difference falls with starvation and can persist despite restoration of positive nitrogen balance, which again implicates changes in cellular energetics in the genesis of impaired skeletal muscle function. One or more defects in cellular membrane function in patients with surgical illness may provide a common marker of PEM and metabolic stress at the cellular level.

Defects in muscle fiber types and a reduction in key enzymes of glucose oxidation and intracellular substrates have been found in patients with PEM. It has been shown that both type I (high oxidation and low glycolytic capacity) and type II (low oxidation and high glycolytic capacity) fibers are smaller in patients with PEM, and there is also a smaller proportional number of type II fibers [71]. These changes result in a significant reduction of fructose biphosphatase, phosphofructokinase, and hexokinase activities. It is likely that these alterations contribute to the syndrome of impaired glucose tolerance, muscle weakness, and fatigue that is characteristic of PEM [71].

Respiratory Function

The ability to maintain tissue oxygen levels and to expectorate effectively are important to the patient undergoing major surgery. Pneumonia continues to be one of the most important causes of postoperative morbidity and mortality, and its incidence has not changed appreciably over the past 30 years [72].

A striking loss of the periodic deep breaths that provide reinflation of atelectatic areas has been noted in chronically starved subjects [73], which when combined with a reduction in tidal volume [74] may well increase the susceptibility to pulmonary infections. In addition, it has been suggested that protein-depleted patients are more susceptible to pulmonary complications because of an ineffective cough secondary to expiratory muscle weakness [30]. Because of the known effects of PEM on skeletal muscle function, it is not surprising to find that protein depletion is associated with an impairment of respiratory muscle function. In particular, PEM is associated with a reduction in respiratory muscle strength, maximum voluntary ventilation [30], and diaphragmatic muscle mass [75]. There are other well-documented changes in respiratory function after surgery and anesthesia [31], and these affect lung volume, mechanics, gas exchange, and patterns of ventilation [76].

The impact of PEM on respiratory function and the risk of postoperative respiratory complications has been studied in a prospective series of

80 patients undergoing major elective gastrointestinal surgery [77]. The patients were divided into two groups on the basis of the extent of body protein loss, which was measured directly by in vivo neutron activation analysis. There was no significant difference between the two groups for the recognized risk factors for postoperative atelectasis and pneumonia, including age, height, sex, surgical diagnosis, the presence of chronic lung disease, smoking, proportion of upper abdominal incisions, the degree of obesity, the duration of anesthesia, and the use of prophylactic antibiotics and physiotherapy. However, there was a significant difference between these two groups of patients for respiratory muscle strength, vital capacity, and peak expiratory flow rate. A significantly higher proportion of protein-depleted patients with atelectasis went on to develop pneumonia and, as a result, spent longer in the hospital. Using logistic regression analysis, the loss of body protein was shown to be an important and independent risk factor for postoperative pneumonia.

Wound Healing

From a survival point of view, the functions of tissue repair and wound healing would be expected to have a high priority in the face of developing PEM. However, it has not been easy to show a close association between wound healing and PEM in adult surgical subjects. Although the incidence of wound dehiscence and anastomotic leakage is more dependent on technical factors than on the rate of collagen synthesis and cross-linkage, PEM is still considered to be a risk factor in the development of these complications. Using a technique in which the accumulation of hydroxyproline is measured in subcutaneous polytetrafluoroethylene implants, it has been possible to demonstrate an improvement in the wound healing response in patients who were given intravenous nutrition [37]. More recently, it has been shown that the maintenance of a normal preoperative food intake is more important in preventing an impairment in the wound healing response than the degree of PEM [78].

Immune Function

An acquired immune incompetence is thought to be responsible for the increased incidence and virulence of infections that are observed in surgical patients with PEM [79]. Although many immunologic deficits have been demonstrated in the malnourished patient [80], the data linking these to patient outcome are sparse [81]. The very act of surgery is immunosuppressive, and the surgeon can modulate the patient's immune response in several different ways [82]. For instance, the effect of a bacterial inoculum can be reduced by the restoration of blood volume, oxygenation, and perfusion. In addition, immune competence is probably aided by competent surgery, which reduces the stress response and the need for blood transfusion [82]. Definite anatomic changes in lymphoid tissues in patients with PEM were first recognized almost 150 years ago, when the thymus was noted to be a "barometer of malnutrition, and a very sensitive one" [83]. Histologically there are fewer lymphoid cells within the thymus, a loss of corticomedullary differentiation, and the Hassall bodies become enlarged. Related to this is the depletion of lymphocytes in the spleen and in the thymus-dependent paracortical areas of the lymph node. The reduction in thymic activity observed in PEM is thought to be responsible for impaired maturation of T lymphocytes and therefore, along with decreased help provided by T lymphocytes, a reduction in the number of antibody-producing cells [84]. As a result, the response to new and recalled antigens is markedly depressed. The process of phagocytosis is also affected in PEM. The complement is an essential opsonin, and the concentrations and activity of most complement components are decreased [85]. There is also recent evidence for the reduced production of several cytokines, including interleukins-1 and -2 and γ-interferon, in patients with PEM [80]. Moreover, the ability of T lymphocytes to respond appropriately to cytokines is impaired [86].

Despite these known associations between nutritional and immune status, specific markers of immune function have not been found to be useful in routine monitoring of critically ill surgical patients. Not only are there confounding effects of surgery and sepsis, but the time frame in which improved nutrition might result in improved immune function further limits the usefulness of these tests.

Psychological Function

Although not well understood, there is no doubt that a patient's psychological function is very important in preparing for and recovering from surgery. There are a number of self-questionnaires that have been used to attempt to characterize the psychological profile of surgical patients, especially with studies of convalescence and postoperative fatigue [17,29,87,88].

Measuring Metabolic Stress

Indirect Calorimetry

Direct measurement of resting metabolic expenditure (RME) by indirect calorimetry is the best way of quantifying the intensity of metabolic stress. Indirect calorimetry measures gas exchange (oxygen consumption and carbon dioxide production) and allows the heat produced by oxidative processes to be determined. The measurements are readily performed at the bedside with the patient lying in a darkened, quiet, and thermoneutral environment. The RME varies with the size of the patient and, in particular, the metabolic body size, which is the body compartment that consumes energy. Although the measurements of total body potassium and through them estimates of the body cell mass are the gold standard for metabolic body size [89], fat-free body mass is more practical in the clinical setting. Fat-free mass (FFM) may be measured either by skinfold measurement or simply by bioelectrical impedance. In normal subjects, RME is related closely to the size of the fat-free body regardless of age or sex [90]. The RME can then be calculated by derived regression equations, such as the following obtained from a normal population in our laboratory [91]:

$$\text{RME (kcal/24 h)} = 13.6 \text{ FFM (kg)} + 550 \text{ (males and females)}$$

The mean ratio (+ standard deviation) of the measured to predicted RME for normal subjects was 1.00 ± 0.09. This means that a patient with a ratio greater than 1.18 is considered to have a significantly elevated RME and metabolic stress.

Catabolic Index

The catabolic index separates urinary urea excretion into urea excretion due to dietary protein intake and urea excretion due to increased protein catabolism [92]. The measurements required are 24-hour nitrogen intake and 24-hour urinary urea over the same period. The catabolic index (CI) is then calculated as follows:

$$\text{CI} = \text{urinary urea N (g)} - [\text{dietary N (g)} + 3]$$

The degree of metabolic stress is assigned as follows:

Metabolic Stress	*Catabolic Index*
nil	< 0
moderate	0–5
severe	>5

Scoring Systems

Metabolic stress can also be measured and monitored on the basis of a number of physiologic measurements. The most commonly used scoring system is the APACHE II score, which combines 11 physiologic variables (as the acute physiology component of the score) with points for age and chronic health [93]. [*Editor's Note:* APACHE II scores have been disappointing in many studies, particularly nutritional studies as correlating with defined nutritional risk.]

Circulating Markers of Metabolic Stress

Levels of counterregulatory hormones, acute-phase reactants, and the measurement of the circulating levels of a number of cytokines are also used to estimate the degree of metabolic stress [94]. For example, the systemic response to sepsis is mediated in part through the action of various cytokines, including interleukin-1, which is released by activated macrophages. One of the actions of interleukin-1 is to increase the hepatic synthesis of acute-phase proteins. As such, C-reactive protein is an attractive marker because in normal subjects it has a very low serum concentration that rises exponentially within four hours of the onset of infection. Although no clinician would base the likelihood of significant metabolic stress being present solely on changes in the serum CRP values, this is a good example of the type of information about a patient's metabolic status that can be derived from blood testing.

Conclusion

In this chapter we have set out a theoretical basis and a practical application for the clinical assessment of nutritional status. If this clinical assessment indicates that a patient has lost 10% or more of body weight, confirmed by physical examination of body fat and muscle, and that there is impairment of vital physiologic functions as detailed above, a period of nutritional support can be justified. The duration of nutritional support depends on whether the end point is the restoration of physiologic function, which can often be achieved within a week, or the restoration of near-normal body composition.

The straightforward clinical techniques that have been described are readily applicable to the daily care of surgical patients and can be easily understood by clinical staff. This approach to bedside clinical nutritional assessment will be refined with further studies, but it represents an important step towards a method of nutritional assessment that defines a clinically relevant "defect to treat and end-point to strive for" [6].

This chapter also describes how modern research laboratories are exploring new and sometimes complex ways of assessing nutritional status. As for the future, there is little doubt that some of the important developments in the areas of cellular energetics, membrane function, and regulation of protein synthesis will result in new tools for the accurate and relevant detection of surgical patients who require nutritional and/or metabolic intervention.

References

1. Hill GL, et al. Malnutrition in surgical patients: An unrecognized problem. *Lancet* 1:689, 1977.
2. Studley HO. Percentage of weight loss: A basic indicator of surgical risk in patients with chronic peptic ulcer. *JAMA* 106:458, 1936.
3. Windsor JA, Hill GL. Weight loss with physiologic impairment: A basic indicator of surgical risk. *Ann Surg* 207:290, 1988.
4. The Veterans Affairs Total Parenteral Nutrition Cooperative Study Group. Perioperative total parenteral nutrition in surgical patients. *N Engl J Med* 325:525, 1991.
5. MacBurney M, Wilmore DW. Rational decision-making in nutritional care. Symposium on Surgical Nutrition. JL Mullen, LO Crosby, JL Rombeau (eds). *Surg Clin North Am* 61:571, 1981.
6. Kudsk KA, Sheldon GF. Nutritional Assessment. In JE Fisher (ed), *Surgical Nutrition.* Boston: Little, Brown, 1983. P 407.
7. Windsor JA. Underweight patients and the risks of surgery. *World J Surg* 17:165, 1993.
8. Jeejeebhoy KN, Detsky AS, Baker JP. Assessment of nutritional status. *JPEN* 14:193S, 1990.
9. Morgan DB, Hill GL, Burkinshaw L. The assessment of weight loss from a single measurement of body weight: Problems and limitations. *Am J Clin Nutr* 33:2101, 1980.
10. Pettigrew RA, Hill GL. Indicators of surgical risk and clinical judgement. *Br J Surg* 73:47, 1986.
11. Hall JC, et al. Upper limb anthropometry: The value of measurement variance studies. *Am J Clin Nutr* 33:1846, 1980.
12. Jeejeebhoy KN, Meguid MM. Assessment of nutritional status in the oncologic patient. *Surg Clin North Am* 66:1077, 1986.
13. Rich AJ. The assessment of body composition in clinical conditions. *Proc Nutr Soc* 41:389, 1982.
14. Streat SJ, Beddoe AH, Hill GL. Measurement of body water in intensive care patients with fluid overload. *Metabolism* 34:688, 1985.
15. Streat SJ, Hill GL. Nutrition in the management of critically ill patients in surgical intensive care. *World J Surg* 11:194, 1987.
16. Golden MHN. Transport proteins as indices of protein status. *Am J Clin Nutr* 35:1159, 1982.
17. Indicators of surgical risk [Editorial]. *Lancet* 2:1422, 1986.
18. Rainey-MacDonald CG, et al. Validity of a two variable nutritional index for use in selecting candidates for nutritional support. *JPEN* 7:15, 1983.
19. Church JM, Hill GL. Assessing the efficacy of intravenous nutrition in general surgical patients: Dynamic nutritional assessment with plasma proteins. *JPEN* 11:135, 1987.
20. Leite JFMS, et al. Value of nutritional parameters in the prediction of postoperative complications in elective gastrointestinal surgery. *Br J Surg* 74:426, 1987.
21. Konstantinides FN, et al. Urinary urea nitrogen: Too insensitive for calculating nitrogen balance studies in surgical clinical nutrition. *JPEN* 15:189, 1991.
22. Windsor JA, Hill GL. Nutritional assessment: A pending renaissance. *Nutrition* 7:377, 1991.
23. Zamir O, et al. Evidence that TNF participates in the regulation of muscle proteolysis in sepsis. *Arch Surg* 127:170, 1992.
24. Fong Y, et al. TNF or IL-I induces cachexia with redistribution of body proteins. *Am J Physiol* 256:R659, 1989.
25. Tsujimoto M, et al. TNF promotes superoxide anion generation from neutrophils. *Biochem Biophys Res Commum* 137:1094, 1986.
26. Hill GL, Beddoe AH. Dimensions of the human body and its compartments. In JM Kinney, et al (eds), *Nutrition and Metabolism in Patient Care.* Philadelphia: Saunders, 1988. P 89.
27. Hill GL, et al. Protein status and metabolic expenditure determine the response to intravenous nutrition: A basis for a new classification of surgical malnutrition. *Br J Surg* 78:109, 1991.
28. Grant JP. Current practices of nutritional assessment: Functional assessment. In SM Levenson (ed), *Nutritional Assessment: Present Status, Future Directions and Prospects.* Columbus, Ohio: Ross Laboratories, 1981. P 137.
29. Schroeder D, Hill GL. Postoperative fatigue: a prospective physiological study of patients undergoing major abdominal surgery. *Aust N Z J Surg* 61:774, 1991.
30. Rochester DF, Esau SA. Malnutrition and the respiratory system. *Chest* 85:411, 1984.
31. Schoonover GA, Olsen GN. Pulmonary function testing in the preoperative period: A review of the literature. *J Clin Surg* 1:125, 1982.
32. Windsor JA, Hill GL. Risk factors for postoperative pneumonia: The importance of protein depletion. *Ann Surg* 208:209, 1988.
33. Hunt DR, Rowlands BJ, Johnson D. Hand grip strength: A simple prognostic indicator in surgical patients. *JPEN* 9:701, 1985.
34. Windsor JA, Hill G. Grip strength: A measure of the extent of protein loss in surgical patients. *Br J Surg* 75:880, 1988.
35. Greig PD, Jeejeebhoy KN. Muscle function testing in the hospitalized patient: Implications for starvation and refeeding. *IEEE Engineering in Medicine and Biology Magazine,* June 1986. P 36.
36. Jeejeebhoy KN. Bulk or bounce: The object of nutritional support. *JPEN* 12:539, 1988.
37. Haydock DA, Hill GL. Impaired wound healing in surgical patients with varying degrees of malnutrition. *JPEN* 10:550, 1986.
38. Twomey P, Ziegler D, Rombeau JL. Utility of skin testing in nutritional assessment; a critical review. *JPEN* 6:50, 1982.
39. Christie PM, Hill GL. Effect of intravenous nutrition on nutrition and function in acute attacks of inflammatory bowel disease. *Gastroenterology* 99:730, 1990.
40. Stokes MA, Hill GL. Improvement in physiological function with enteral nutrition. *Br J Surg* 78:758, 1991.
41. Lupo L, et al. Reliability of clinical judgement in evaluation of the nutritional status of surgical patients. *Br J Surg* 80:1553, 1993.
42. Detsky AS, et al. What is subjective global assessment of nutritional state? *JPEN* 11:440, 1987.
43. Keys A, et al. *The Biology of Human Starvation.* Minneapolis: University of Minnesota Press, 1950, P 129.
44. Hill GL. Body composition research: Implications for the practice of clinical nutrition. *JPEN* 16:197, 1992.

45. Kinney JM, Moore FD. Carbon balance: A clinical approach to energy exchange. *Surgery* 40:16, 1956.

46. Jacobs DO, Scheltinga MRM. Metabolic assessment. In JL Rombeau, MD Caldwell (eds), *Clinical Nutrition: Parenteral Nutrition.* Philadelphia: Saunders, 1993. P 245.

47. Kobayashi T, *Robinson MK, Rounds JD* et al. Depression of hepatocyte energy status during systemic infection: An in vivo ^{31}P magnetic resonance spectroscopy study. *Surg Forum* 43:11, 1992.

48. Hill GL, Monk D, Plank LD. Measuring body composition in intensive care patients. In DW Wilmore, YA Carpentier (eds), *Metabolic Support of the Critically Ill Patient.* Berlin: Springer, 1993.P 89.

49. Beddoe AH, Streat SJ, Hill GL. Evaluation of an in vivo prompt gamma neutron activation facility for body composition studies in critically ill intensive care patients: Results on 41 normals. *Metabolism* 33:270, 1984.

50. Mazess RB, et al. Dual-energy X-ray absorpiometry for total body and regional bone mineral and soft tissue composition.*Am J Clin Nutr* 51:1106, 1990.

51. Fong Y, Moldawer LL, Lowry SF. Experimental and clinical applications of molecular cell biology in nutrition and metabolism. *JPEN* 16:477, 1992.

52. Wang ZM, Peirson RN Jr, Heymsfield SB. The five level model: A new approach to organizing body composition research. *Am J Clin Nutr* 56:19, 1992.

53. Moore FD, et al. The body cell mass and its supporting environment. In FD Moore (ed), *Body Composition in Health and Disease.* Philadelphia: Saunders, 1963.

54. Moore FD. Energy and maintenance of body cell mass. *JPEN* 4:228, 1980.

55. Shires GT, Williams J, Brown F. Simultaneous measurement of plasma volume, extracellular fluid volume, and red blood cell mass in man utilizing I^{131}, $S^{35}O^{4}$, and Cr^{51}. *J Lab Clin Med* 55:776, 1960.

56. Barratt TM, Walser M. Extracellular fluid in individual tissues and in whole animals: The distribution of radiosulfate and radiobromide. *J Clin Invest* 48:56, 1969.

57. Yasumura S, Cohn SH, Ellis KJ. Measurement of extracellular space by total body neutron activation. *Am J Physiol* 244:R360, 1983.

58. Shizgal HM, et al. Indirect measurement of total exchangeable potassium. *Surgery* 85:496, 1979.

59. Shizgal HM. Body composition. In JE Fischer (ed), *Surgical Nutrition.* Boston: Little, Brown, 1983. P 3.

60. Shizgal HM, Milne CA, Spanier AH. The effect of nitrogen sparing intravenously administered fluids on postoperative body composition. *Surgery* 85:496, 1979.

61. Jeejeebhoy KN, et al. Critical evaluation of the role of clinical assessment and body composition in patients with malnutrition before and after total parenteral nutrition. *Am J Clin Nutr* 35:1117, 1982.

62. Tokunaga K, et al. A novel technique for the determination of body fat by computed tomography. *Int J Obes* 7:437, 1988.

63. Fowler PA, et al. Validation of the in vivo measurement of adipose tissue by magnetic resonance imaging of lean and obese pigs. *Am J Clin Nutr* 56:7, 1992.

64. Schlemmer A, et al. Direct measurement of abdominal fat by dual photon absorptiometry. *Int J Obes* 14:603, 1990.

65. Khaled MA, et al. Electrical impedance in assessing human body composition: The BIA method. *Am J Clin Nutr* 47:789, 1988.

66. Schroeder D, Christie PM, Hill GL. Bioelectrical impedance analysis for body composition: Clinical evaluation in general surgical patients. *JPEN* 14:129, 1990.

67. Duerenberg P, Schouten FJM. Loss of total body water and extracellular water assessed by multifrequency impedance. *Eur J Clin Nutr* 46:247, 1992.

68. Segal KR, et al. Estimation of extracellular and total body water by multiple-frequency bioelectrical-impedance measurement. *Am J Clin Nutr* 54:26, 1991.

69. Klidjian AM, et al. Relation of anthropometric and dynamometric variables to serious postoperative complications. *Br Med J* 281:899, 1980.

70. Almond DJ, King RFGJ, Burkinshaw L. Potassium depletion in surgical patients: Intracellular cation deficiency is independent of loss of body protein. *Clin Nutr* 6:45, 1987.

71. Church JM, Choong SY, Hill GL. Abnormalities of muscle metabolism and histology in malnourished patients awaiting surgery: Effects of a course of intravenous nutrition. *Br J Surg* 71:563, 1984.

72. Garibaldi RA, et al. Risk factors for postoperative pneumonia. *Am J Med* 70:677, 1981.

73. Bendixen HH, Smith FM, Mead J. Pattern of ventilation in young adults. *J Appl Physiol* 19:195, 1964.

74. Rosenbaum SH, Askanazi J, Hyman AL. Respiratory patterns in profound nutritional depletion [abstract]. *Anesthesiology* 51:S366, 1979.

75. Arora NS, Rochester DF. Effect of body weight and muscularity on human diaphragm muscle mass, thickness and area. *J Appl Physiol Resp (Environ Exercise Physiol)* 52:64, 1982.

76. Bartlett RH, Gassaniga AB, Gerahty TR. Respiratory maneuvers to prevent postoperative pulmonary complications: A critical review. *JAMA* 224:1017, 1973.

77. Windsor JA, Hill GL. Risk factors for postoperative pneumonia: the importance of protein depletion. *Ann Surg* 208:209, 1988.

78. Windsor JA, Knight GS, Hill GL. Wound healing response in surgical patients; recent food intake is more important than nutritional status. *Br J Surg* 75:135, 1988.

79. MacLean LD. Host resistance in surgical patients. *J Trauma* 19:297, 1979.

80. Chandra RK. Nutrition and immunity: Lessons from the past and new insights into the future. *Am J Clin Nutr* 53:1087, 1991.

81. Dempsey DT, Mullen JL, Buzby GP. The link between nutritional status and clinical outcome: Can nutritional intervention modify it? *Am J Clin Nutr* 47:352, 1988.

82. Meakins JL. Surgeons, surgery and immunomodulation. *Arch Surg* 126:494, 1991.

83. Simon J. *A Physiological Essay on the Thymus Gland.* London: Renshaw, 1845.

84. Chandra RK. Numerical and function deficiency in T helper cells in protein energy malnutrition. *Clin Exp Immunol* 51:126, 1983.

85. Rochester DF, Arora NS, Braun NMT. Maximum contractile force of human diaphragm muscle, determined in vivo. *Trans Am Clin Climatol Assoc* 93:200, 1981.

86. Haller I, Zubler RH, Lambert PH. Plasma levels of complement components and complement hemolytic activity in protein-energy malnutrition. *Clin Exp Immunol* 34:248, 1978.

87. Christensen T, Bendix T, Kehlet H. Fatigue and cardiorespiratory function following abdominal surgery. *Br J Surg* 69:417, 1982.

88. Schroeder D, Hill GL. Predicting postoperative fatigue: Importance of preoperative factors. *World J Surg* 17:226, 1993.

89. Kinney JM, Lister J, Moore FD. Relationship of energy expenditure to total exchangeable potassium. *Ann N Y Acad Sci* 110:711, 1963.

90. Roza AM, Shizgal HM. The Harris-Benedict equation reevaluated: Resting energy requirements and the body cell mass. *Am J Clin Nutr* 40:168, 1984.

91. Hill GL. *In Disorders of Nutrition and Metabolism in Clinical Surgery: Understanding and Management.* Edinburgh: Churchill Livingstone, 1992. P 287.

92. Bistrian BR. A simple technique to estimate severity of stress. *Surg Gynecol Obstet* 148:675, 1979.

93. Knaus WA, et al. APACHE II: A severity of disease classification system. *Crit Care Med* 13:818, 1985.

94. Michie HR, Wilmore DW. Sepsis and tumor necrosis factor: Bedfellows that cannot be ignored. *Ann Surg* 212:653, 1990.

Selected Readings

Baker JP, et al. Nutritional assessment: A comparison of clinical judgement and objective measurements. *N Engl J Med* 306:969, 1982.

This was the original paper that showed that a clinical nutritional assessment was effective in identifying patients at risk of nutrition-associated postoperative complications.

Bernstein LH. Utilizing laboratory parameters to monitor effectiveness of nutritional support. *Nutrition* 10:58, 1994.

The report from a Consensus meeting to examine the continuation of the laboratory to monitor effectiveness of nutritional support. Although many laboratory measurements were discussed, one of the main recommendations of this conference was to use urinary nitrogen loss and serum prealbumin on a weekly basis in patients receiving nutritional support as measures of catabolism and return to anabolism.

Hill GL. Body composition research: Implications for the practice of clinical nutrition. *JPEN* 16:197, 1992.

In this paper the author describes the use of modern body composition technology in understanding protein-energy malnutrition in surgical patients.

Meakins JL, et al. Delayed hypersensitivity: Indication of acquired failure of host defenses in sepsis and trauma. *Ann Surg* 186:241, 1977.

This is the original paper describing the profound effect of anergy in predicting the prognosis of critically ill surgical patients.

Windsor JA, Hill GL. Weight loss with physiologic impairment: A basic indicator of surgical risk. *Ann Surg* 207:290, 1988.

This paper took the original concept of Hiram Studley that weight loss was a risk factor for postoperative complications and demonstrated that with modern surgical care this is only true when the weight loss is associated with clinically detectable impairment of relevant physiologic functions. It introduced a method of clinical nutritional assessment that incorporated both somatic and functional dimensions and validated it with objective measurements.

IV

Physiologic Response

20

Starvation: Metabolic and Physiologic Responses

Stanley M. Levenson
Obi J. Imegwu
Tsueng H. Chang

For at least 2500 years physicians have been aware of the effects of diet and nutritional status on health and on the body's response to injury and disease [1]. A large number of clinical and experimental studies during the past 80 years, including the early classic studies of Dubois [2], Benedict [3], Cuthbertson [4], and their associates, have confirmed and extended this understanding. This chapter deals with some of the metabolic and physiologic responses to food deprivation, per se, to lay the basis for later discussions in this volume of the metabolic and physiologic responses to injury and disease and how these are affected by food intake, for it is clear that the latter plays a critical modulating role in these responses. We will be concerned primarily with effects of inadequate food intake in the presence of adequate water intake. The reader is referred to the book by Wolf entitled *Thirst* [5]. Vitamin, unsaturated fatty acid, and trace mineral deficiencies, per se, will not be discussed, except to point out that the appearance of such deficiencies is slowed during uncomplicated starvation [6]. Nor will we discuss the psychological changes associated with (caused by?) starvation; this complicated subject is beyond the scope of this book, and the interested reader is referred to the references [7,8].

Food deprivation can occur as a primary event in previously healthy individuals, as in famine or

*Supported in part by NIH (NIGMS) Research Grant R01 GM 48161-02

voluntary starvation, or it may come about as a secondary result of injury or disease. Also, in recent years, purposeful fasting of obese patients has become an increasingly popular therapeutic regimen. The metabolic responses to food deprivation are quantitatively and often qualitatively different in these various circumstances, and one of our efforts will be to point out some of the major differences in the metabolic responses to starvation by otherwise healthy individuals and by seriously ill and injured patients.

Historical Survey

Never in history has there been enough food for all people. Throughout evolution, man's existence has been facilitated by his ability to survive long periods of enforced fasting. It is a sad commentary on our civilization that severe hunger is rampant throughout much of the world, even in developed countries, including the United States. Paradoxically, in some of these same countries, obesity is a major health problem. A discussion of the complex social, economic, political, and cultural causes for this situation is beyond the scope of this chapter, but the primacy of their solution is self-evident.

Descriptions of some of the overall physical, functional, and psychological effects of severe food deprivation can be found in the earliest writings, but it was not until the late nineteenth century that prospective studies of experimental animals (Voit) and of men who subjected themselves to voluntary food deprivation began (Succi in Italy, Tanner in the United States, and Merlotti in France).

Early studies established the relative rates of weight loss during starvation and demonstrated that after several days the percentage of expended calories obtained from carbohydrate was minimal (less than 5%), 10% to 15% were the result of protein metabolism, and about 85% were the result of fat metabolism. Liver and muscle glycogen fell very rapidly during the first 24 hours of starvation, but some glycogen was present even after three weeks. These early investigations showed also that urinary nonprotein nitrogen and sulfur fell during the first weeks of starvation of men (Figure 20-1) and the proportion of urea in urinary nonprotein nitrogen fell from about 85% to 55% within three weeks, while urinary ammonium increased substantially, paralleling the developing metabolic acidosis reflected by the appearance of large quantities of β-hydroxybutyric acid and acetone in the urine. It was noted that gluconeogenesis increased fairly promptly but later declined in parallel with the decreased rate of body protein loss, as evidenced by a gradual decline in urinary nitrogen. There followed a prolonged period in which urinary nitrogen plateaued at a level of about 3 g daily.

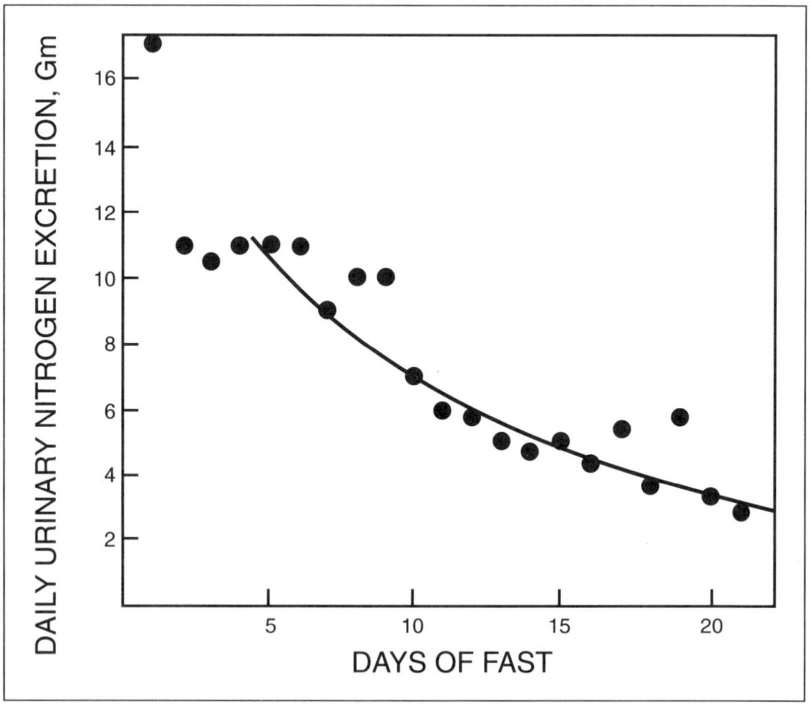

Figure 20-1. Daily urinary nitrogen excretion during one of Succi's prolonged fasts. (From E Freund, O Freund. Beitrage zum Stoffweensei im Hunger-zustande. *Weiner Klin Rundschau* 15:91, 1901.)

It was found that survival during starvation depended on the amount of fat present in the organism at the beginning of food deprivation. When the fat stores became markedly depleted, there was an increase in urinary nitrogen excretion, the so-called premortal rise. Body temperature and the normal diurnal variations in temperature were generally maintained close to normal until just a short time before death, when there was a marked decline in body temperature.

These early observations have been elucidated further during the past 80 years, owing to an increased understanding of mammalian biochemical and physiologic processes in general. Key advances were made between 1915 and 1920, when Dubois [2] began his classic studies of metabolic rates in healthy volunteers and in patients (especially those with infectious diseases). In the same period, Benedict [9] began his equally classic studies on the biochemical, physiologic, and psychological responses of young men subsisting voluntarily on a modestly reduced diet that led to a weight loss of about 10% over many months. He found that their metabolic rates gradually declined about 12% to 18% per kilogram body weight (16% to 22%/m^2 body surface), demonstrating that the fall in metabolic rate was proportionately greater than the loss of total body mass.

Benedict [3,9] also studied (a *tour de force*) the effects of total nutrient deprivation (other than water) for 31 days in a male volunteer living in a whole-body calorimeter. His caloric expenditure dropped gradually from an average of 1650 calories per day during the first week to an average of 1290 calories per day during the third week, remaining at or near the latter level for the duration of the study. A calculation of the amounts of carbohydrate, protein, and fat metabolized during the first week was made some years later from Benedict's published data by Peters and Van Slyke (Table 20-1) [10]. As mentioned, after a few days the percentage of expended calories obtained from carbohydrate was minimal (less than 5%), whereas the proportions of calories derived from protein and fat were essentially constant for the next three and one-half weeks, about 15% to 18% and 80% to 85%, respectively. Gamble et al. [11] reported similar findings in fasting children; these children, like fasting adults, showed a prompt decline in urinary nitrogen excretion during the first 10 days of fasting.

Wars have always accentuated the problems of supplying adequate nutrition to populations and have provided opportunities to study the effects of undernutrition on large numbers of people of all ages. Notable among the studies and publications describing the effects of undernutrition in Western Europe during and after World War II are those edited by McCance and Widdowson [8], Burger et al. [12], Winick [13], Lindtjorn [14], and Bittles et al. [15]. In 1944, Keys et al. [16] began their remarkable study of semistarvation in 32 men, all healthy conscientious objectors to war. The reader is urged to read their excellent book, *The Biology of Human Starvation* [16].

The 1950s saw relatively few studies of starvation, per se, but there were large numbers of studies dealing with the metabolic effects of injury and illness in which reduction of food intake plays such an important role. In 1959, there began a great resurgence of investigative interest in the effects of starvation, per se, when Bloom [17], and later Duncan [18], introduced prolonged total fasting with free access to water for weight reduction of obese people. This stimulated a great number of studies in the 1960s that have continued un-

Table 20-1. Calculation of Amounts of Carbohydrate, Protein, and Fat Metabolized by Benedict's Fasting Man

		Food Metabolized		
Days of Fast	Nitrogen Excreted (g)	Carbohydrate (g)	Protein (g)	Fat (g)
1	7.1	69	43	135
2	8.4	42	50	142
3	11.3	39	68	130
4	11.9	4	71	136
5	10.4	—	63	133
6	10.2	—	61	133
7	9.8	—	59	134

Source: JP Peters, DD Van Slyke. *Quantitative Clinical Chemistry Interpretations*, Vol. 1. Baltimore: Williams & Wilkins, 1946.

abated. Cahill [19,20], Owen [21,22], Felig [23–25], Waterlow [26], Carlson and Campbell [27], and Lowry [28], and their co-workers have been among the major contributors in this field.

Current Concepts of the Effects of Starvation

At the basis for all the responses to starvation lies a common denominator: lack of exogenous energy substrates and of essential dietary nutrients, such as certain amino acids. Man's survival is based in large measure on his ability to produce and renew regulatory peptides and proteins. This, in turn, involves a wide range of other reactions involving all metabolites. In starvation, the range of metabolic activity is altered, sometimes drastically. Some metabolic pathways that are active in the normal state are partially or completely turned off; others that normally are minimally active achieve major importance; and some pathways are newly developed and function only during prolonged starvation. The ability to respond adaptively to a variety of external stimuli becomes impaired during starvation, and at times a response will be elicited only when the stimulus poses a threat to survival. The organism faced with severe food deprivation channels its metabolic activity to one goal: survival. Regulatory neuroendocrine mechanisms control the levels of certain major metabolic fuels. This is particularly important for organs like the brain, which have constant and high-energy demands but minimal fuel depots.

Metabolic Rate: Energy Conservation

Paramount among the metabolic tasks is the need for the starving organism to regulate its energy expenditure and, therefore, energy requirement. Among the important adaptations to starvation are two that result in a lowering of caloric expenditure and a slowing of the rate of deterioration. One of these is voluntary, a reduction in physical work, while the other is involuntary, a reduction in basal metabolic rate proportionately greater than the loss of both body weight (Figure 20-2) and lean body mass [3,16,29,30]. Body temperature decreases slightly at this time, but the level of decrease is a relatively minor factor in the lowered metabolic rate. A major difference between the response to food deprivation, per se, and the response to injury or sepsis, with or without a concomitant reduction in food intake, is an increase

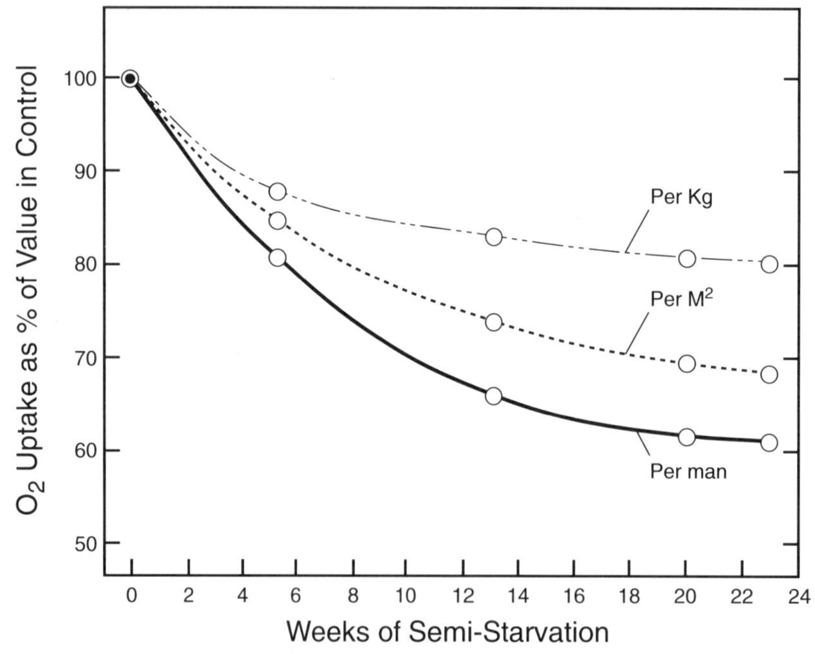

Figure 20-2. Mean basal metabolism for 32 men before and during 24 weeks of semistarvation. All values are expressed as percentage of the prestarvation (control) values for the oxygen uptake per man, per square meter of body surface, and per kilogram of body weight (Minnesota experiment). (From A Keys, et al. *The Biology of Human Starvation.* Minneapolis: University of Minnesota Press, 1950.)

in metabolic rate in the latter and a lowering in the former [31]. While basal metabolic rate increases with falling weight in nonstarved individuals, it *falls* with decreasing weight during starvation [26]. Waterlow points out that in the classic semistarvation work of Keys, an average fall in basal metabolic rate of 16% was recorded compared to an anticipated increase in basal metabolic rate of 12% based on body weight alone [26].

Much of an animal's (including humans') resting energy expenditure is devoted to maintenance of ionic and other compartments against diffusion gradients and to maintenance of a certain amount of mechanical work, for example, respiration, cardiac contractility, and peristalsis. Resting energy expenditure is also involved in peptide and protein synthesis, particularly the synthesis of hormones and enzymes, which permit the body to respond to alterations in the internal or external environments. In the body's dynamic response to starvation, per se, regulatory neuroendocrine and other metabolic mechanisms lower the metabolic rate to help safeguard survival and maintain the blood levels of certain major metabolic fuels within relatively narrow limits. Concomitant with the reduced overall metabolic rate is the possible loss of cell mass by certain metabolically active tissues, such as the liver, pancreas, and gut, but not the brain. While many tissues adapt to starvation by lowering their basal energy demands, and even supplying energy substrates for use by other tissues, the central nervous system continues to consume 20% of basal calories and is a main beneficiary of the "sparing" effect just mentioned [19,20,32,33].

Kleiber [34] has shown that the changes in metabolic rate differ for various organs in starving rats, but no such comparable comprehensive measurements are available in humans. The sparing of critical proteins at the "expense" of others results in a disproportionately large reduction in the weight of certain viscera—notably the liver, gastrointestinal tract, and pancreas—during starvation. This reduction is rapid (a matter of days) in small mammals such as rats [35]. Significant amounts of protein are lost from these viscera (Table 20-2), and the activities of certain enzymes are altered. As a result of the selective loss of liver proteins in early starvation, those enzymes related directly to fatty acid oxidation and gluconeogenesis appear to be conserved best, whereas those enzymes concerned with urea synthesis are decreased. The early starvation period results also in a loss of intestinal mucosal digestive hydrolases. At the same time, the rate of regeneration of gut mucosal epithelial cells is slowed. During starvation, exocrine pancreatic function is diminished because of decreased synthesis of pancreatic and gastrointestinal enzymes, and digestion of dietary protein, fat, and polysaccharides is inhibited. The gastrointestinal tract may become relatively intolerant of food, and the refeeding of starving patients becomes a challenge.

Cardiac work is sharply reduced (bradycardia, decreased cardiac output) as starvation progresses. The resting metabolic rate of skeletal muscle is likely to be lowered for the following reasons: (1) Maintenance of muscle mass is dependent on physical activity and on active (i.e., endergonic) reactions involving substrate uptake (glucose, amino acids) and the uptake of ions (K^+, Mg^{2+}, HPO_4^{2-}) against concentration gradients.

Table 20-2. Relative Losses of Protein from Various Organs and Tissues of Albino Rats in a Seven-Day Fast, as Percentages of Control Values

Organ or Tissue	% Loss
Liver	40
Prostate	29
Seminal vesicles	29
Gastrointestinal tract	28
Kidneys	20
Drawn blood	20
Heart	18
Muscle, skin, and skeleton	8
Brain	5
Eyes	0
Testicles	0
Adrenals	0

Source: T Addis, LJ Poo, W Lew. The quantities of protein lost by the various organs and tissues of the body during a fast. *J Biol Chem* 115:111, 1936.

Because muscle glycogen and protein synthesis are depressed in starvation, the energy required even in the basal state is lessened. (2) Because muscle tone is decreased (characteristic of starved individuals), resting energy need is decreased. (3) There is a disproportionate loss of white muscle fibers compared to red muscle fibers. Red muscle fibers have a lower activation threshold, utilize fuel more efficiently (by metabolizing glucose oxidatively), and metabolize fats more readily than white fibers. (4) There is a voluntary decrease in muscular activity of starving individuals.

With the decreased overall metabolic rate during starvation, there is a decrease in circulating T_3. However, during starvation the metabolic rate of thyroidectomized rats also falls, showing that some mechanism(s) in addition to (other than) decrease in circulating T_3 is responsible for the progressive lowering of metabolic rate during starvation. The changes in and roles of the thyroid hormones, catecholamines, and other hormones in starvation are discussed in more detail later.

General Appearance and Weight Loss

Progressive weight loss is an inevitable consequence of starvation. Haggard-faced, lean, bony, chronically starved people are recognized at a glance, even by the layman [36,130]. The skin is loose, flaccid, rough, and flaking. There are areas of overkeratinization and increased pigmentation. Plugs of hardened protein material distend the hair follicles and often project as spikes. Children are particularly (much more rapidly) affected by starvation because of their relatively greater nutrient requirement. The following graphic, horrifying description was reported from Phnom Penh, Cambodia, by a journalist:

> Waves of mothers carrying gravely ill children—swollen children [kwashiorkor], children with stick-like concentration camp bodies [marasmus], children with parchment skin hanging in flaccid folds, coughing children, weeping children, silent children too weak to respond anymore. . . . The child had been malnourished before. Now she is a skeletal horror, little more than bulging eyes and a protruding rib cage. Every few seconds she produces a wail that racks her body. In three hours she is dead. [37]

The rate of weight loss, which is proportional to the reduction in food intake, generally is greatest at the beginning of food deprivation, reflecting a disproportionate loss of water. The rate then decreases gradually, leveling off as physical activity lessens and metabolic rate falls (Table 20-3). Previously healthy nonobese adults can tolerate a weight loss of 5% to 10% with little functional disorganization. At the other extreme, save for exceptional individuals, most nonobese human beings and animals deprived of all food (but not water) do not survive weight losses greater than 40%, which occur in two to three months. Experimental studies in laboratory animals have shown, as mentioned, that early in starvation there is a rapid reduction in the weight of certain viscera, notably the liver, gastrointestinal tract, and pancreas. Autopsy studies [38] of people dead of prolonged starvation showed that the greatest organ weight losses were by the pancreas, spleen, kidney, liver, genitals, gut, and muscles, and least by the brain, eyes, and skeleton.

Body Composition

The overall changes in body composition during prolonged (24 weeks) semistarvation and later refeeding of previously healthy young men are depicted in Figure 20-3 [16]: the increase in extracellular fluid, the disproportionate loss of fat, the lesser loss of lean body mass, and the maintenance of bone mineral. The mechanisms underlying the relative increase in extracellular water, which is general in most tissues and may accumulate as gross edema in dependent areas, are not fully known:

> It is not yet clear if any local abnormality need be invoked to explain the edema, but it may be that a reduction of muscle size and intercellular colloid, and a loss of elastic fibers from a skin now too large for the structures it was designed to

Table 20-3. Weight Loss (%) During Food Deprivation of Varying Degrees as Measured Over Time

	Caloric Intake as % of Normal Balance							
Duration (mo)	90	80	70	60	50	40	30	20
3	5	8	10	12	15	20	25	30
6	8	12	15	20	25	30	35	45
12 or more	10	15	20	25	30	35	40	—

Source: A Keys, et al. *The Biology of Human Starvation,* Vol. 1. Minneapolis: University of Minnesota Press, 1950. P 129.

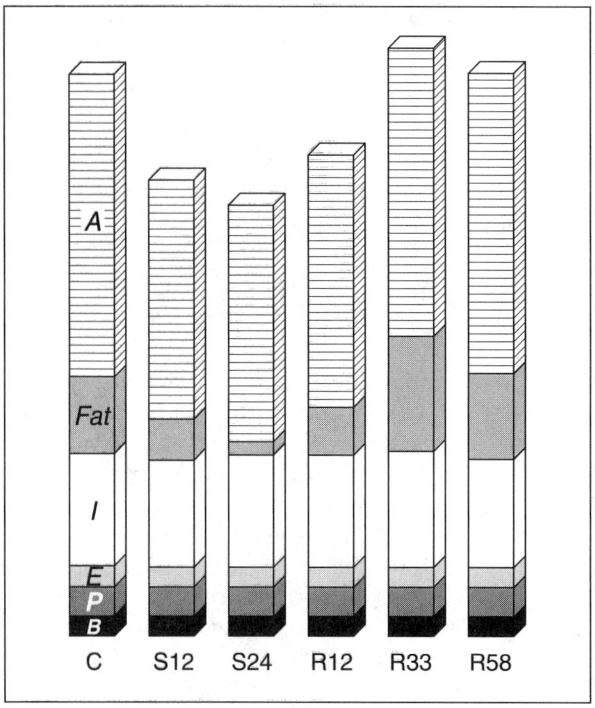

Figure 20-3. The major compartments, as weight, of the bodies of young men in a normal state of nutrition, in semistarvation, and in subsequent rehabilitation. Columns: C = control (prestarvation); S12 and S24 = 12 and 24 weeks of semistarvation; R12, R33, and R58 = 12, 33, and 58 weeks of rehabilitation. Compartments: B = bone; P = blood plasma; E = erythrocytes; I = interstitial fluid (thiocyanate space less plasma volume); A = active tissue (total body weight less the other indicated compartments). (From A Keys, et al. *The Biology of Human Starvation.* Minneapolis: University of Minnesota Press, 1950.)

> enclose, will all favor localized collection of fluid in the dependent parts. If and when there is a fall in the concentration of serum proteins, it is natural to suppose that this will also operate, and a large intake of salt must also help. Theories based on overactivity of the hormones of the suprarenal cortex, a deficiency of aneurin [vitamin B_1], and abnormalities of renal function must be regarded for the moment as not proven. [8]

Some have suggested that abnormal amounts of ferritin are released from the liver and stimulate the production of antidiuretic hormone. Other aspects of sodium and water metabolism and renal function are discussed later.

The caloric value of the tissue lost during semistarvation (and starvation) is much greater *later* than *earlier*, a reflection of the increasing utilization of body fat. During the *early* periods of semistarvation, the body loses a mixture of fat, protein, and water; the caloric equivalent of the lost tissue may be about 2000 cal/kg, which does not correspond to the composition of any tissue of the body. Fat storage tissue is about 90% fat, and 1 kg of storage fat would be expected to supply about 8100 calories. A figure very close to the aforementioned (8000 cal/kg tissue) was found by Grande [39] as the caloric equivalent of the tissue lost *late* in semistarvation (Figure 20-4).

The energy density of weight loss in semistarvation was calculated by Alpert [40] using the two-reservoir model and was found to be 4436 ± 869 kcal/kg (18.57 ± 3.60 MJ/kg). For the first 12 weeks of the semistarvation period, the coefficient of variation was 0.19, indicating that the energy density was reasonably constant. Alpert points out that the value reported by him is considerably less than the commonly accepted value. Calculation of the energy density of the change in the lean body mass showed a general decline in value, which Alpert attributed to a decrease in the rate of protein catabolism. The initial protein loss rate was 0.48 ± 0.12 kg/week while the average protein loss rate for the second 6 weeks of semistarvation was found to be 0.12 ± 0.03 kg/week. It was also shown that the response time of the lean body mass decrease was 64 ± 2 days while that of the fat store decrease was 135 ± 4 days.

The reason why fat becomes the major fuel metabolized during starvation is evident from Table 20-4. The body composition of a typical 65 kg man includes 12 kg of triglyceride, 6 kg of "mobilizable" muscle protein, and 0.8 kg of carbohydrate, which includes free serum glucose as well as liver and muscle glycogen [19,20,32,33]. The amount of stored carbohydrate is minimal, whereas the amount of potential calories in fat, especially in storage depots such as the subcutaneous tissue, is proportionately very large. Most organs appear to lose fat in proportion to their initial fat content. Exceptions are the brain and nervous tissues and possibly the kidney. As fat is lost, the

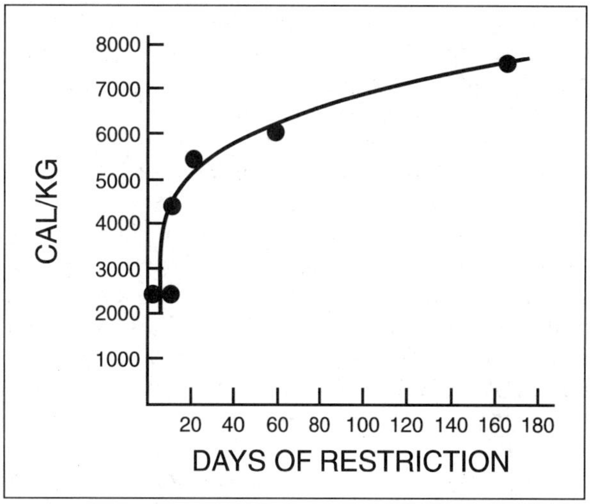

Figure 20-4. Caloric equivalent of the weight loss and duration of the restriction period. (From F Grande. Energetics and weight reduction. *Am J Clin Nutr* 21:305, 1968.)

Table 20-4. Normal Stores of Available Energy and Rates of Utilization in a Man Weighing Sixty-Five Kg

	Total Body Content (g)	Available Store			Daily Utilization* (g)	Exhaustion Time (days)
		(g)	(mj)	(kcal)		
Carbohydrate	500	150	2.5	600	All used in first 24 hr.	Less than 1
Protein	11,000	2,400	40	9,600	60	About 40
Fat	9,000	6,500	235	58,500	150	About 40

*Assuming an energy expenditure of about 6.7 mj (1600 kcal)/day.
Source: R Passmore, JS Robson. *A Companion to Medical Studies,* Vol. 3. Oxford: Blackwell, 1974.

fat cells shrink until the cytoplasm becomes merely a limiting membrane.

There is potentially a fairly large caloric source in protein, but there is relatively little "labile" protein that can be "burned" to help meet the caloric expenditure without some loss of important cellular and enzymatic functions. Protein must be conserved if organ and body functions are to continue. The metabolic events and adaptations that occur during starvation and underlie the greater utilization of fat and relative preservation of protein are discussed in the following sections.

Intermediary Metabolism

The increase in metabolic economy that accompanies starvation requires the cooperative interaction of multiple organ systems. When dietary intakes of fat, carbohydrate, and protein are inadequate, glucose homeostasis and "sparing" of certain critical proteins and lipids (for example, nervous system proteolipids, lipoproteins) are central factors. Although stored fat is an expendable fuel source, the dependency of the central nervous system, peripheral nerves, red blood cells, white blood cells, active fibroblasts, and certain phagocytes on glucose as their main or sole energy substrate makes provision of glucose (gluconeogenesis) during starvation essential. Because hepatic glycogen is limited and muscle glycogen unable to be mobilized for extracellular use, the carbon skeletons of proteins become an important source of necessary glucose.

We have mentioned that during fasting the following occur: (1) a gradual drop in urinary nitrogen (chiefly urea), which begins within a few days and plateaus in man after about two weeks until shortly before death, when it rises moderately; (2) a prompt but modest lowering of blood sugar, after which it plateaus until the end stages of the fast, when it falls sharply; (3) a gradual increase in plasma fatty acids, keto acids, and ketones leading to metabolic acidosis and ketonuria; (4) a gradual increase in urinary NH_4^+ (Figure 20-5); and (5) an increase in urinary sodium and potassium excretions. In normal men fasted for 10 days, the early loss includes a negative water balance (500 ml/day), nitrogen loss (averaging 8.5 g/day), and mineral losses (1.85 g sodium and 1.5 g potassium) [29]. As starvation continues, nitrogen losses are reduced to 2 to 4 g/day; some glucose-burning organs, for example, the brain, are by this time utilizing chiefly ketones derived from the fat stores. Urinary nitrogen losses are much greater following injury than during uncomplicated starvation. The data presented by Kinney [41,42] suggest that the proportionate amounts of protein and fat lost are not much different than their proportions in healthy, fed subjects; the disproportionate higher utilization of fat seen during starvation, per se, is not seen following injury. In addition, water and sodium conservation are immediate following injury, and although administration of carbohydrate to the starved individual has an immediate protein-sparing effect, this effect is less in the injured individual.

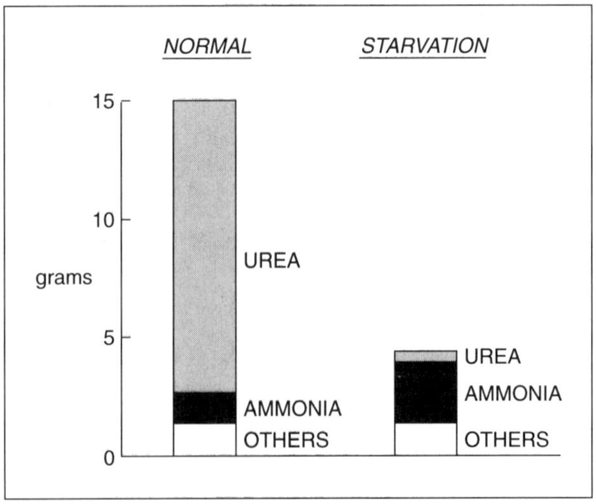

Figure 20-5. Urinary nitrogen excretion in the postabsorptive state after a standard diet of 90–100 grams of protein and after five to six weeks of starvation, showing marked reduction in total nitrogen, the relative increase in ammonia, and the relatively unchanged excretion of the sum of uric acid, creatinine, and other nonprotein-nitrogen metabolites. (From GJ Cahill Jr. Starvation in man. *N Engl J Med* 282:668, 1970. Reprinted by permission.)

Amino acid and protein turnover and cell loss involve the breakdown of a portion of the protein, amino acid, and nucleic acid pools. This breakdown results in an obligatory loss of nitrogen, largely in the form of urea, but also as free amino acids, peptides, creatine, creatinine, uric acid, and ammonia. The amount of nitrogen lost is a function of the balance of energy intake and output and the size of the protein and amino acid pools, which in turn are affected by dietary intake of all nutrients and the physiologic state. Protein intake increases the size of the amino acid pool, as do exercise and other stimuli for gluconeogenesis and glycogenolysis, such as injury or glucocorticoid administration. The amino acid pool size can be increased by states in which both protein synthesis and breakdown are speeded up, but overall breakdown exceeds synthesis, as in hyperthyroidism. The mechanism of salvage or recycling of amino acids (for example, hydrolysis of digestive enzymes and absorption and reutilization of the amino acids) conserves amino acids, but at a significant expenditure of energy. This salvage, however, makes possible many different metabolic and physiologic responses by various organs regardless of their size.

In prolonged starvation, the amino acid pool is decreased for three reasons: (1) amino acid intake is nil; (2) protein breakdown decreases gradually and reaches a near-plateau because metabolic rate and physical activity fall and fat becomes the major fuel; and (3) turnover of certain proteins may be decreased. One consequence is that the starving animal may not synthesize certain enzymes in amounts adequate to respond appropriately to environmental stimuli. For example, as starvation proceeds, the liver urea cycle enzymes decrease. As a result, the starving individual cannot respond quickly to a load of ammonia by synthesizing more urea. The body may become less or nonresponsive in a variety of other ways. For example, the liver may not respond adequately to catecholamine stimuli for glucogenesis because (a) it has decreased numbers of catecholamine receptors or decreased levels of adenylate cyclase, or both; (b) it has decreased amounts of glycogen; or (c) it has decreased amounts of enzymes and cofactors required for glycogenolysis and gluconeogenesis.

Normal adults can make metabolic adjustments to a wide variety of nutrient intakes. When caloric and protein intakes are adequate, the proportions of fat, carbohydrate, and protein may be varied within wide limits without upsetting the steady state, once a small amount of unsaturated fatty acids (about 2% to 4% of calories) and small amounts of glucose (75 to 100 g daily) are included. Once the minimal intake requirement of protein (about 0.3 to 0.5 g/kg body weight/day) for nitrogen equilibrium in healthy adults is met, "extra" amino acids absorbed as the result of a higher protein intake are deaminated, transaminated, and their nitrogen is converted to urea and excreted. Some of the carbon chain is oxidized and/or converted to carbohydrate and fat. A new steady state is again reached within three to four days. If less than adequate amounts of protein are ingested, there is a gradual depletion of body protein, with certain organs and tissues being more affected than others, as already described. The rate of protein depletion is hastened when dietary nonprotein calories are low. When the protein intake is marginal or inadequate, the protein-sparing effect of carbohydrate is somewhat greater than that of fat, because carbohydrate may be used for the synthesis of nonessential amino acids.

Body protein losses by injured patients with limited food intakes are much larger than protein losses by uninjured people with comparable levels of decreased food intake. Also, as mentioned, the disproportionately high utilization of fat seen during prolonged food deprivation, per se, is not seen following injury. Whereas administration of small amounts of glucose (50 to 100 g) to the starved but uninjured individual has an immediate protein-sparing effect, this effect is considerably less in the severely injured individual.

When dietary intakes of fat, carbohydrate, and protein are all inadequate, glucose homeostasis and "sparing" of certain critical proteins and lipids (for example, nervous system proteolipids, lipoproteins) are central factors. Stored fat is expendable. Glucose is normally the major or sole energy source for certain key tissues, including the central nervous system. The brain normally oxidizes the glucose to CO_2 and water, and glycolysis goes on in the other tissues and cells and the lactic acid is recycled into glucose by the liver and kidney (the Cori cycle). Provision of glucose (gluconeogenesis) during starvation is thus essential [43].

The trigger that induces the initial metabolic adaptations during starvation is the arterial glucose level, which begins to fall in humans within 15 hours of fasting. This fall occurs because the peripheral organs continue to utilize glucose, while endogenous glycogen stores decrease and the supply of exogenous energy substrates is abolished. As the blood glucose level falls, the stimulus for insulin secretion diminishes, and this is reflected by the falling serum insulin levels. The falling glucose and insulin levels are accompanied by rising glucagon and growth hormone levels (Figure 20-6). Boyle et al. [44] concluded from their findings of a three-day fast by four healthy men

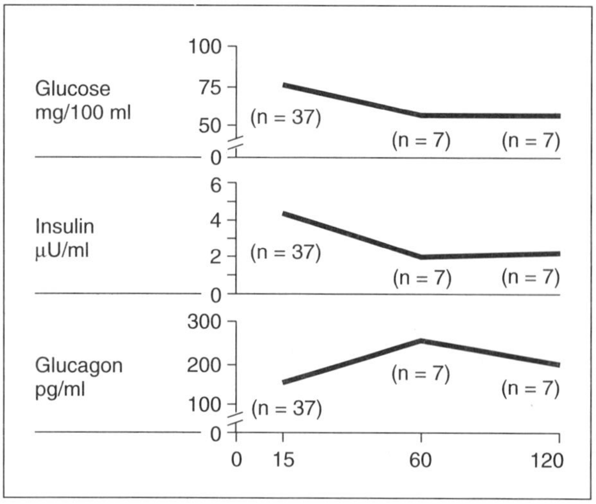

Figure 20-6. Arterial glucose, insulin, and glucagon levels after 15, 60, and 120 hours of fasting. (From FW Ahnefeld, et al. *Parenteral Nutrition.* New York: Springer, 1976.)

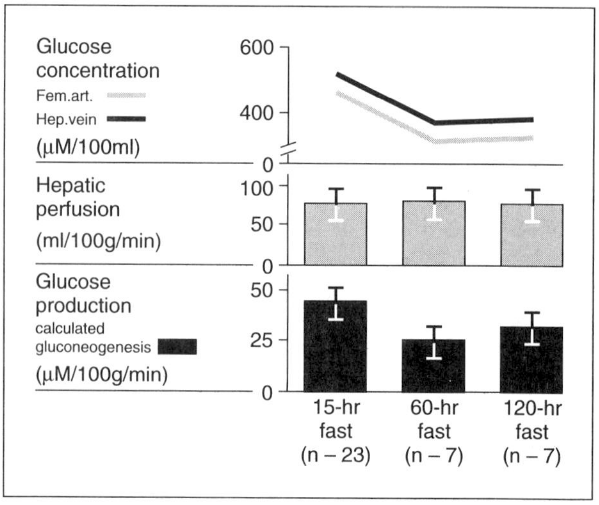

Figure 20-7. Arterial and hepatic-venous glucose concentrations, liver perfusion, and contributions of gluconeogenesis and glycogenolysis to glucose production after 15, 60, and 120 hours of fasting. (From FW Ahnefeld, et al. *Parenteral Nutrition.* New York: Springer, 1976.)

and four healthy women that the reason the plasma glucose did not fall to hypoglycemic levels was not due solely to decreased insulin secretion, but that glucagon plays a primary counterregulatory role and that while epinephrine and norepinephrine (principally epinephrine) are normally not critical for the prevention of hypoglycemia, they are if glucagon is deficient. Only limited data are available regarding the catecholamines, and the findings are conflicting. (Hormonal changes are discussed in more detail later in this chapter.)

In the first 24 hours of starvation, hepatic glycogenolysis provides most of the necessary blood sugar, but at the end of this time hepatic glycogen is nearly exhausted, and gluconeogenesis becomes the main route for the provision of glucose (Figure 20-7). The rate of gluconeogenesis then diminishes gradually, coincident with the overall decline in metabolic rate and an increase in ketone utilization by the central nervous system.

The brain does not metabolize fatty acids directly. Fatty acids generally do not cross the blood-brain barrier, but ketones and keto acids provided by the liver do. During starvation, adaptive changes occur in the transport system that result in an increase in the rate at which ketones cross the blood-brain barrier [45]. In addition, competitive inhibition for ketone transport by lactate and pyruvate is decreased because of their lower levels in starvation.

The brain begins to metabolize ketones and keto acids increasingly in starvation as glucose availability decreases [46]. Current evidence indicates that enzyme induction for this is not necessary; the brain is set to use ketones even when the individual is well fed, but under that circumstance the brain uses glucose preferentially [33]. However, starvation leads to depression of β-hydroxybutyrate dehydrogenase and β-keto acid CoA transferase, thereby increasing the levels of these two enzymes, which are important for ketone oxidation. It should be noted that certain areas of the brain metabolize glucose preferentially (solely?), while other areas of the brain may metabolize either glucose or ketones depending on their relative availability. The metabolism of ketones by the brain seems to be limited to specific regions by their permeability characteristics—areas with no blood-brain barrier show the highest rate of utilization [47]. During starvation, the brain's respiratory quotient (RQ) may be about 0.8. This indicates that either the ketones or the glucose, or both, are not completely oxidized to CO_2 and H_2O, because in that case the RQ would be significantly higher (1.0 for glucose and acetoacetic acid and 0.9 for β-hydroxybutyric acid), or that CO_2 fixation is taking place.

Some glucose is derived from the glycerol released as a result of fat mobilization, but the amount so provided is inadequate by itself to meet the starving individual's need. The additional necessary glucose is provided by gluconeogenesis. The amount of gluconeogenesis required has been estimated to be about 60 g of glucose/day early in starvation; stored or recycled glucose is of the order of 120 g/day at this time. Later, as the brain begins to metabolize certain ketones and keto acids, its glucose requirement falls substantially, about 70%, and the amount of gluconeogenesis required falls about 50%; at this time the amount of stored or recycled glucose falls to about 80 g/day [19].

During the first two to four days of starvation, roughly half of the 100 g/day of glucose oxidized by the central nervous system derives from amino acid carbon released by skeletal muscle [48]. The remaining 50 g/day of glucose utilized by the central nervous system derives from glycerol, lactate, and pyruvate, as well as splanchnic amino acids via hepatic gluconeogenesis. Although skeletal muscle glycogen does not supply glucose directly due to an absence of muscle glucose-6-phosphatase, carbon for glucose can be released from muscle by metabolization of glycogen to pyruvate and lactate [49]. Because skeletal muscle represents the largest pool of glycogen in the body (500 g vs. 100 g contained in the liver), the glucose resynthesized following muscle glycogenolysis may be substantial during the first days of starvation.

Amino Acids and Protein Turnover

Gluconeogenesis requires the presence of gluconeogenic substrates, either in the form of glucose metabolites (pyruvate and lactate), which can be recycled, or in the form of amino acids. As mentioned, skeletal muscle in a 65 kg healthy male provides roughly 6 kg of mobilizable protein representing 24,000 potential calories while liver contains about 100 g of mobilizable protein or 400 potential calories [32]. In adults, even moderate undernutrition results in reduction in body cell mass, and muscle mass is affected substantially [26]. Mobilization of liver and muscle protein, while it is necessary for gluconeogenesis in early fasting, would be detrimental to the organism if maintained at the early high rates later in starvation. Hence, rates of protein catabolism as high as 75 g daily during the second and third day of starvation are reduced to less than half this value by the second and third week of starvation (Figures 20-8 and 20-9) [20].

During early starvation when protein losses are highest (see Table 20-2), the greatest percent contributions come from organs with high rates of protein turnover. These tissues are capable of sequestering "more than their share" of amino acids during the postprandial period (in the form of protein), and tend to "export" amino acids during periods of fasting [50]. Liver protein-pool turnover rates of 90% per day in rats have been suggested, emphasizing the potential role of the liver as a source of metabolites in the acute phases of starvation [35].

A detailed account of the mechanisms of protein turnover are beyond the scope of this chapter, but it should be noted that protein turnover serves several important functions in cell homeostasis,

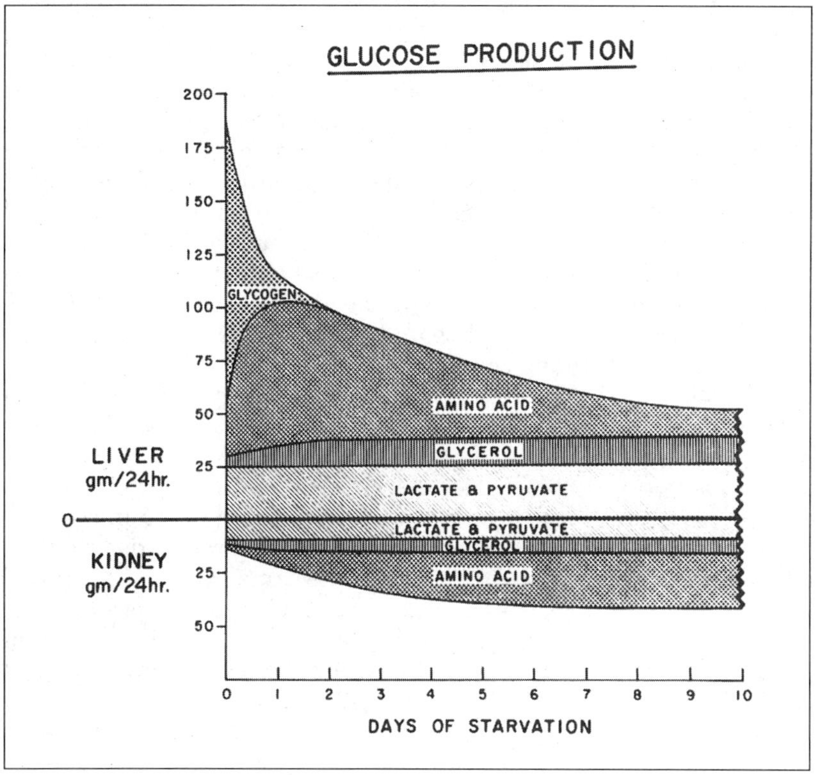

Figure 20-8. Glucose production from various precursors by liver and kidney in starving humans. Not shown is the 10–15 grams of glucose derived from ketoacids after the first week or so of starvation. (From GF Cahill Jr. Starvation: Some Biological Aspects. In JM Kinney, et al. *Nutrition and Metabolism in Patient Care.* Philadelphia: Saunders, 1988.)

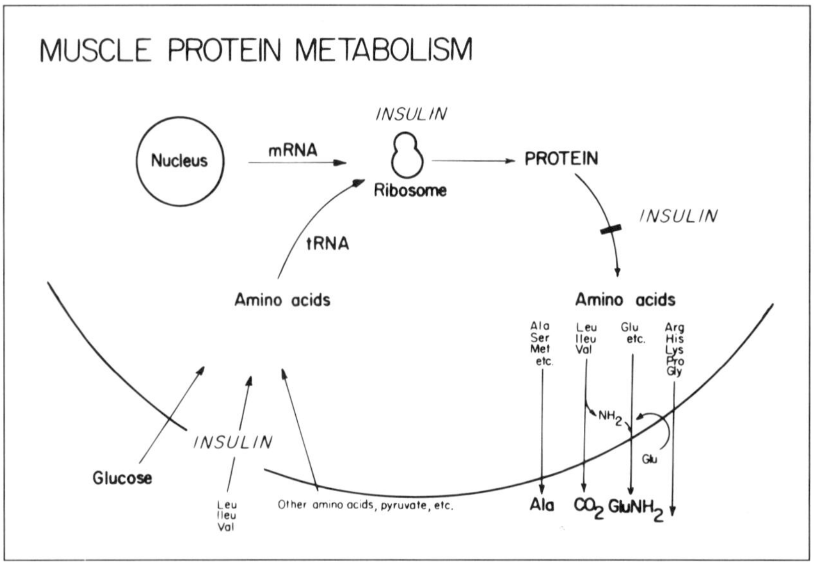

Figure 20-9. Effect of insulin in promoting glucose and amino acid uptake into muscle, activation of protein synthesis at the ribosome, and inhibition of proteolysis. Also shown is the predominant release of alanine (Ala) and glutamine ($GluNH_2$). (From GF Cahill Jr. Starvation: Some Biological Aspects. In JM Kinney et al. *Nutrition and Metabolism in Patient Care.* Philadelphia: Saunders, 1988.)

including: (1) removal of abnormal and denatured proteins, (2) post-translational processing of newly manufactured proteins, and (3) disposal of enzymes not currently useful to the cell [50]. Recent investigations into protein turnover have identified lysosomal-vacuolar pathways as the dominant mechanisms determining resident protein turnover [51], although nonlysosomal pathways have also been identified [52]. In perfused rat liver studies, hormone and substrate manipulation can initiate profound changes in the rates of lysosomal-vacuolar protein degradation. Increased glucagon, decreased insulin, and other hormone substrate changes characterizing starvation each results in increased rates of protein degradation in the perfused rat liver [53–55]. Similar findings have been demonstrated in other tissues, including skeletal muscle, heart, and adipose, although evidence suggests that in muscle changes the rates of lysosomal-vacuolar protein degradation may be limited to nonmyofibrillar protein [56–58]. Other processes underlie the increase in myofibrillar protein degradation in skeletal muscle consequent to starvation. [*Editor's Note:* One cannot assume that increased protein degradation is the result of the same mechanisms being activated in different disease states. In sepsis, for example, degradation of myofibrillar protein is most prominent and is secondary, at least in part, to the activation of the energy-dependent ubiquitin system [59]. There is no assurance that a similar mechanism is activated in starvation.]

Liver and Muscle Protein Turnover

When rats are fed diets free of protein but adequate in calories, the liver loses protein immediately, without an apparent change in the fractional rate of protein synthesis [60]. During the next three weeks, the liver continues to lose protein but more slowly, despite an increase in the fractional rate of hepatic protein synthesis. In contrast, when rats are starved, liver protein synthesis falls about 30% within two days [61], and liver protein falls rapidly. The decrease in liver protein synthesis correlates with a decrease of liver ribosomal RNA [62], but liver DNA is not altered.

Millward [63] has pointed out that the rapid loss of liver protein by the rat early in starvation is almost exactly equal to the rate of export protein synthesis that is maintained at the expense of liver cytoplasmic protein. He has stated that the liver's role in exporting protein may explain why the regulation of liver protein balance is achieved principally through regulation of protein degradation (increased in starvation) [64] rather than protein synthesis [65], because a regulatory mechanism affecting principally protein synthesis would likely affect export protein synthesis, and this would be undesirable, at least as far as acute changes are concerned.

A decrease in skeletal muscle protein of starved rats occurs much more slowly. During the feeding of protein-free diets adequate in calories, a net loss of muscle protein occurs after eight to nine days, a result principally of a reduced rate of muscle protein synthesis. Protein degradation falls also, but not to the same extent as synthesis [60]. In contrast, starvation depresses synthesis and increases degradation of muscle protein in rats [66–69]. The skeletal muscle (but not cardiac muscle) of starved rats (two to four days) shows increased levels of ribosomal subunits along with a reduced rate of protein synthesis in vitro, demonstrating a starvation-induced inhibition of peptide chain initiation [70]. A decrease in skeletal muscle protein synthesis occurs also in starving humans [71]. Wernerman and colleagues [72,73] have reported alterations in skeletal muscle ribosomes and polyribosomes in starved humans.

The changes in muscle protein synthesis during starvation may depend in part on the changes in circulating insulin. Insulin not only stimulates amino acid transport into muscle but also regulates muscle protein synthesis at the level of initiation of translation; in addition, insulin suppresses muscle protein breakdown [74]. Jenkins et al. [75] have reported that the starvation-induced increase in muscle protein degradation is nonlysosomal in origin. Supporting this conclusion is the finding that insulin and other agents known to decrease lysosomal protein degradation do not inhibit myofibrillar protein degradation [76,77].

Waterlow [26] notes that the reduction in the rate of protein turnover may have three possible adaptive advantages during protein-calorie deficiency. First, an energy saving of 70 kcal could be realized assuming that 15% of the BMR is related to the energy cost of protein synthesis. Second, if there is less protein synthesis, the demand for dietary essential amino acids would diminish, making survival possible on an intake of lower biologic value. Third, by diminishing protein catabolism, there would be a smaller amino acid flux into the free pool and, subsequently, lesser loss of amino acid carbon through oxidation [26].

Of the amino acids liberated from muscle protein during fasting, two-thirds leave directly as amino acids, especially alanine and glutamine, while others are deaminated [78,79]. Amino acid deamination and oxidation in muscle are important because the dietary essential amino acids involved (the branched-chain amino acids, particularly leucine) can be rate-limiting for tissue protein synthesis: the amount of leucine in proteins is relatively high, whereas the amount in the free amino acid pool is relatively low. The amino acids effluxing from muscle tend to be relatively low in branched-chain amino acids, and Millward [66] has pointed out that this may interfere with the ability of the liver to maintain normal export protein synthesis.

The aforementioned findings regarding protein turnover in muscle and liver are confirmatory of earlier findings by Waterlow and Stephen [80], who showed that the uptake of ^{14}C-lysine by skeletal muscle of protein-deficient animals is reduced, indicating a substantially slowed rate of protein synthesis, while liver protein synthesis is reduced only moderately. Waterlow and Stephen [81] have shown in humans and animals that this latter finding is reflected by an increase in liver amino acid activating enzymes in protein depletion and a fall with refeeding, whereas the activity of argininosuccinase (a urea cycle enzyme) falls with protein depletion and rises with refeeding. In contrast, the amino acid activating enzymes of muscle fall rapidly with protein depletion and rise with refeeding.

Dice et al. [82] found that the enhanced protein degradation in starvation is fundamentally different from normal protein catabolism; that is, correlations among molecular size, acidity, and nature of the proteins (for example, glycoproteins vs. nonglycoproteins), which are present normally, are absent in starvation (liver and muscle) and diabetes, suggesting that starvation and diabetes alter the general characteristics of intracellular protein degradation in target tissues affected by insulin. Studies in skeletal muscle, for example, demonstrate a decreased ratio of total protein to myofibrillar protein degradation [83].

Wannemacher and Dinterman [84] have reported a gradual loss during starvation of the day-night differential in the rate of protein catabolism (normally greater at night). The differential in the normally fed rat may be related to the differential food intake (principally at night) as well as the diurnal variations in secretion of various hormones.

Lowry and associates [28,85–89] have reported an extensive series of studies carried out in 10 previously healthy young men and women who starved voluntarily, generally for 10 days, and were then repleted nutritionally by intravenous alimentation. Among their findings during starvation were an increase in urinary 3-methylhistidine (3-MH) excretion, a decrease in arterial 3-MH concentration, a decrease in total body protein turnover (particularly a decrease in protein synthesis; there was a slight increase (not statistically significant) in total body protein breakdown); an increased efflux of amino acids from the forearm muscles, a decrease in plasma dietary essential amino acids, a reduction in skeletal muscle intracellular free glutamine, and an increase in isoleucine and leucine. Serum albumin was unchanged while serum bilirubin increased about 50% and serum SGOT declined about 50%. There was a slight drop in plasma K^+ and Mg^{++} concentrations and a doubling of uric acid concentration in comparison with ambulatory subjects. Muscle biopsies showed no significant changes in cellular hydration, intracellular and extracellular water distribution, and Na^+, K^+, and Cl^- concentrations; there was a significant decrease in Em, indicating a change in the ratio of intracellular to intracellular K^+ and perhaps of other ions.

In a follow-up study in rats, Fong and colleagues [90] from this same laboratory found that after three and five days of starvation, there was a significant decrease in gastrocnemius muscle mass and protein content and an associated decrease in mRNA for the three myofibrillar proteins assessed (myosin heavy chain, myosin light chain, and α-actin).

In obese men fasting for 20 days, excretion of urinary 3-methylhistidine was found to be decreased (34%), whereas the decrease in creatinine excretion and calculated loss of muscle mass was much less (15%), suggesting a decrease in skeletal muscle protein degradation [91]. No comparable reports are available of normal nonobese adults starving for long periods of time. Many investigators have ascribed the reduction in nitrogen excretion observed during long-term undernutrition to the decreased gluconeogenic demand imposed by the central nervous system through its adaptation to ketone oxidation. This view focuses on changing fuel patterns as the reason for protein sparing, but Henry et al. [92] have observed that this concept is based largely on studies of obese subjects. Supported by data obtained by Benedict [3], they argue that the fractional rates of protein catabolism in normal weight individuals does not change during starvation and that the observed protein economy is due to a reduction in metabolic rate rather than to a selective reduction in protein as a fuel.

Muscle as an Energy Store and Its Metabolic Role in Starvation

In the starved state the skeletal muscle becomes a tissue necessary for the survival of the organism because it provides biochemical intermediates essential to the maintenance of vital metabolic activities, particularly of the brain and kidneys.

Skeletal muscle normally uses glucose and fatty acids as its main energy sources. The glucose is derived directly from the circulation or indirectly from muscle glycogen. Uptake of glucose by muscle from blood is dependent in part on the blood glucose concentration, but it is most strongly dependent on serum insulin levels. This insulin effect can be blocked by other hormones, notably growth hormone. Consoli et al. [93] found that after two and one-half days of starvation, acetyl CoA entered the Krebs cycle significantly faster than in the postabsorptive state.

Once glucose enters the muscle cells, its fate depends largely on whether the muscle is resting or at work. If the latter, the glucose enters the glycolytic pathway, and, depending on the amount of work, the pyruvate either enters the Krebs cycle or is converted to lactate, which goes to the liver where it is partially converted to glucose. Muscle glycogen is utilized in normal metabolism and work by conversion of glucose-1-phosphate to glucose-6-phosphate to pyruvate in the extramitochondrial portion of the cytoplasm. The pyruvate is largely converted to acetyl coenzyme A and metabolized in the mitochondria to carbon dioxide and water. Under these conditions only a small amount of the pyruvate goes to lactate and is then transported to the liver. If the muscle is at rest, glucose in the muscle is preferentially converted to glycogen. There is a limit to the amount of muscle glycogen that can be stored, namely, about 0.75% of muscle mass. Because of the proportionately large mass of skeletal muscle, however, muscle glycogen constitutes the largest store of carbohydrate calories in the body; it is three to four times as large as the store of liver glycogen. Very early in starvation (in rats), 60% of the glucose derived from glycogen comes from the liver and 40% from the muscle [94]. However, stored liver and muscle glycogen are of little quantitative significance in the fuel economy of the starving individual because they could supply less than a day's energy during total starvation, even if totally metabolized. Fatty acids are key energy sources for muscle during starvation.

Additional Aspects of Skeletal Muscle Metabolism

Muscle fibers are classified as either fast- or slow-twitch depending on the myofibrillar ATPase they express. Fast-twitch, or white, fibers can be further classified as type IIA (fast-twitch-oxidative glycolytic) or type IIB (fast-twitch glycolytic) [48,95]. Slow-twitch, or red, fibers are better suited metabolically to limitations of glucose utilization such as occur during starvation [48]. The low insulin levels that accompany fasting diminish the use of glucose as a fuel by skeletal muscle, a metabolic condition that favors substrate oxidation in muscle fibers capable of fatty acid oxidation. In addition, evidence suggests that slow-twitch fibers consume less ATP than fast-twitch fibers per unit of isometric tension developed [96,97].

Because glucose supply is limited, and fuel economy is essential during periods of starvation, muscles depending heavily on glycolysis become a liability to the organism. Furthermore, glycolysis results in the generation of intermediates (pyruvate and lactate) that require recycling, thus imposing the additional high cost of gluconeogenesis on the organism [48]. These findings imply that selective atrophy of fast- rather than slow-twitch fibers would carry a greater benefit than proportionately equal losses of both. Indeed, several studies have demonstrated a reduction in fast-twitch over slow-twitch fibers, both in anorexia and in chronically undernourished patients [98,99]. [*Editor's Note:* Interestingly, in sepsis, proteolysis is increased preferentially in white, fast-twitch muscle (59,100–102).]

A number of aspects of muscle metabolism are relevant to the metabolic responses and adaptations to starvation:

1. Uptake of glucose and the subsequent conversion to glycogen are largely under insulin control. In starvation, glucose uptake by muscle is affected mainly by the low levels of serum insulin. There is evidence that in starvation the insulin effect on glucose uptake by muscle is increased. The glucose uptake in vivo of starved animals is independent of the elevated fatty acid or ketone levels in the blood [103]. Ruderman et al. [104] have shown in studies of the isolated perfused rat hindquarter that after a 48-hour fast, glucose oxidation decreased 75%. The decrease in lactate oxidation was in general paralleled by changes in the activity of the active form of pyruvate dehydrogenase, indicating that glucose metabolism was inhibited at the step of pyruvate oxidation.
2. Muscle cannot provide blood glucose from its own glycogen because it lacks the enzyme glucose-6-phosphatase.
3. Formation of creatine phosphate by muscle.
4. Muscle glycogenesis.
5. Gluconeogenesis from alanine via pyruvate does not occur in the muscle because muscle has very little pyruvate carboxylase, the enzyme that generates oxaloacetate, a precursor of phosphoenolpyruvate (PEP) needed for de novo hexose synthesis.

$$\text{Pyruvate} + \text{ATP} + CO_2 \xrightarrow[\text{almost absent in muscle}]{\text{pyruvate carboxylase}} \text{oxaloacetate} + \text{ADP} + \text{Pi}$$

$$\text{Oxaloacetate} + \text{GTP} \xrightarrow[\text{present in muscle}]{\text{phosphoenol pyruvate carboxykinase}} \text{PEP} + \text{GDP} + CO_2$$

Sum:

$$\text{Pyruvate} + \text{ATP} + \text{GTP} \longrightarrow \text{PEP} + \text{ADP} + \text{GDP} + \text{Pi}$$

6. Muscle provides amino acids to the liver and kidney for gluconeogenesis. (A detailed discussion of these points follows.)

Muscle Creatine Phosphate

As mentioned, skeletal muscle activity is diminished in starvation to a near basal amount of ATP-dependent muscle contraction. Under conditions of minimum ventilatory activity and decreased muscle perfusion, glycolysis in white muscle is favored. The PEP formed in glycolysis can go into various pathways. In cells that are at low energy levels and therefore have increased levels of ADP and AMP (starvation), the system is driven in the direction of making ATP. That is,

$$\text{ATP} + \text{PEP} \xrightarrow{\text{pyruvate kinase}} \text{ATP} + \text{pyruvate}$$

The energetics of the reaction strongly favor ATP formation. The formation of this ATP acts to moderate (slow down) both glycolysis and the Krebs cycle by the inhibitory allosteric effects of ATP on glycolytic enzymes and by the depletion of ADP, which is both a necessary substrate and a positive allosteric effector of some glycolytic enzymes. The relative lack of ATP is an appropriate response to starvation. High amounts of ATP could favor synthetic reactions (glycogen or fat synthesis) or could limit the amount of PEP that could phosphorylate ADP. These synthetic reactions would be inappropriate in the starving individual because they would be energy-consuming.

One factor that modulates the amounts of ATP and ADP in muscle cells is the amount of creatine present. The energetics of the reaction ATP + Creatine $\rightleftarrows$ Cr~P + ADP favor ATP synthesis. This is a very good adaptive mechanism for energy storage when high levels of ATP are present because high levels of ATP (which would be generated by high levels of respiration or glycolysis) would favor the synthetic reaction $\rightarrow$ Creatine phosphate (Cr~P) at times when the cells can afford the energy expenditure. Thus, the potential energy of glucose or fatty acid oxidation would yield a high amount of immediately available ~P. A reasonably small proportion of this ATP energy is spent to synthesize the high energy compound Cr~P, which represents a readily available store of ~P. Thus, during oxidations, ADP + Pi stimulate respiration and ATP synthesis and stimulate the reaction ATP + Cr $\rightarrow$ Cr~P + ADP.

Under the conditions of glycolysis and respiration the net synthesis of high energy bonds is limited by available inorganic phosphorus. Therefore, oxidation increases the amount of ATP and Cr~P and decreases the amounts of Pi. As the ATP is used for muscle or other work, Cr~P is converted to ATP until the Cr~P is used up. This gives rise to increased levels of ADP + Pi, which in turn stimulate glycolysis and respiration leading to ATP synthesis. Therefore, glycolysis and respiration are stimulated by ADP and inorganic P and tend to be inhibited by ATP. This is a useful adaptive phenomenon because low energy levels in the cell stimulate respiration and glycolysis, which then produce the energy (ATP) that slows glycolysis and respiration.

The presence of high concentrations of creatine permits the muscle to store five times as much readily available phosphate bond energy as would be the case if ATP and ADP were the only reservoirs of ~P energy. The creatine phosphate reservoir is a useful mechanism for the nourished active muscle. For starved, inactive muscle, it represents an unnecessary and perhaps useless or futile cycle. Certain events that occur in the starving muscle decrease the activity of the creatine kinase system and therefore have adaptive value in starvation. The muscle wasting that occurs in starvation involves the loss of the enzymatically active protein, creatine kinase, and the loss of small substrate molecules such as creatine. This means that Cr~P mechanism in starvation decreases the amount of work muscle can carry out, but it represents a way of conserving energy and muscle mass. It is clear that the decreased work in starvation has adaptive value. What may not be obvious is that the decrease in the amounts of ATP + Cr~P inhibits the ATP-dependent synthetic phases of wasteful "futile" metabolic cycles and the ATP-dependent phases of glucose assimilation, thus conserving body glucose mainly for nonmuscle uses, for example, brain and blood cell metabolism.

Muscle Glycogenesis

Although muscle is the source of metabolites that provide energy for other tissues, it cannot provide this in the form of glucose from its own glycogen because muscle lacks the enzyme glucose-6-phosphatase. Thus, although muscle can synthesize glycogen from blood glucose and can degrade glycogen to glucose-6-phosphate, the glucose-6-phosphate so formed must be used within the muscle cell.

In addition to muscle's ability to synthesize glycogen from glucose, it has a limited ability to synthesize glycogen or glucose-6-phosphate from the carbon chains of some glucogenic amino acids, especially those that can be converted to oxaloacetate by either transamination or the Krebs cycle, but at a considerable energy cost.

Cytosol Reactions

$$\text{Aspartate} + \alpha\text{-ketoglutarate} \xrightarrow{\text{glutamic acid oxaloacetate transaminase}} \text{oxaloacetate (OAA)} + \text{glutamate} \quad (1)$$

$$\text{OAA} + \text{NADH} + \text{H}^+ \xrightarrow{\text{malic dehydrogenase}} \text{malate} \quad (2)$$

Malate Shuttle (malate in cytosol ⟶ malate in mitochondria) (3)

Mitochondrial Reactions

$$\text{NAD}^+ + \text{malate} \xrightarrow{\text{malic dehydrogenase}} \text{OAA} + \text{NADH} + \text{H}^+ \quad (4)$$

$$\text{OAA} + \text{GTP} \xrightarrow{\text{phosphoenol pyruvate carboxykinase}} \text{phosphoenol pyruvate (PEP)} + \text{CO}^2 + \text{GDP} \quad (5)$$

PEP transport (mitochondrial PEP ⟶ cytosol PEP) (6)

The glutamate generated in reaction 1 is used to regenerate the α-ketoglutarate necessary for reaction 1 in the following way:

Glutamate transport (cytosol glutamate ⟶ mitochondrial glutamate)

$$\text{Mitochondrial glutamate} + \text{NAD} + \text{H}_2\text{O} \quad (7)$$

$$\xrightarrow{\text{glutamic dehydrogenase}} \alpha\text{-ketoglutarate} + \text{NH}_4^+ + \text{NADH} \quad (8)$$

As is evident from the following summation of the foregoing reactions, the flow of carbon from aspartate to PEP and to glycogen requires the OAA-malate shuttle, while the flow of aspartate N requires the glutamate-α-ketoglutarate shuttle:

$$\text{Aspartate carbon} \xrightarrow{\text{OAA-malate shuttle}} \text{PEP} + \text{CO}_2$$

$$\text{Aspartate nitrogen} \longrightarrow \text{N of other amino acids, amides, and NH}_4^+$$

The PEP produced from aspartate and some other glycogenic amino acids can be resynthesized into glycogen, but at a considerable energy cost. However, it is not only the energetics that limit muscle glycogen synthesis from amino acids, but in starvation there are mechanisms that limit the availability of amino acids for this purpose. The synthesis of muscle glycogen from glucogenic amino acids depends on a net synthesis of PEP.

The shuttle mechanisms could give rise to a net formation of PEP and, therefore, a net synthesis of glucose from aspartate as illustrated.

PEP can be formed also from some other amino acids by similar types of reactions involving the various shuttles:

Valine, Methionine, Isoleucine → succinyl CoA → succinate → OAA → PEP → glycogen

and

Glutamic acid, Glutamine, Histidine, Proline → glutamic acid → α-ketoglutarate → succinate

succinate → OAA → PEP → glycogen

However, for gluconeogenesis to proceed from these amino acids in addition to a functional malate oxaloacetate shuttle, it is necessary that mitochondria carry out the oxidation of some substrates derived from the amino acids (for example, α-ketoglutarate and succinate) at a more rapid rate than usual to provide PEP. Additionally, mitochondrial oxidation of the reduced cofactors (mainly NADH generated by substrate oxidation) by the electron transport chain would have to proceed at normal or greater-than-normal rates. Aoki et al. [105] have pointed out that in starvation, proteolysis of muscle is diminished because of the existence of large amounts of reduced nicotinamide coenzymes. Chua and associates [106] have pointed out that in the fed state both reduced blood flow of muscle and muscle hypoxia without ischemia favor proteolysis over protein synthesis. Thus the effect on proteolysis may be mediated by both the tissue O_2 levels and failure to remove metabolites, both of which lead to a reduced environment. In contrast to the fed state, muscle protein is conserved in starvation by mechanisms that inhibit proteolysis and gluconeogenesis. Cahill and colleagues [19,20,32,33] suggest that control over muscle metabolism by thyroid hormone is important in conserving muscle mass and energy in starvation because thyroid hormone creates an oxidizing environment in the cell. We have pointed out elsewhere in this chapter that circulating T_3 is low in starvation.

How else may increased reducing power lessen mitochondrial PEP synthesis and glycogen synthesis? High NADH concentration in the cytosol favors the formation of malate from OAA, the first part of the shuttle. However, in the reducing environment of the mitochondria, malate would not readily be reoxidized. Therefore, PEP synthesis would be inhibited. In the reducing environment, malate participates in coupled reactions that result in lactate and alanine formation. Increased reducing power, then, favors cytosol reactions involving the formation of lactate, malate, glycerophosphate, and alanine. Of these, only alanine and lactate leave the cell. Both may be synthesized into glycogen by the liver, or they may be oxidized by the heart. Additionally, reducing power favors the formation of amino acids from their more highly oxidized keto analogues. Thus glutamine synthesis is favored in muscle under starving conditions; as this glutamine can be exported, it influences the flow of carbon and nitrogen throughout the body.

Gluconeogenesis

Gluconeogenesis, the biosynthesis of glucose from noncarbohydrate precursors such as amino acids, pyruvate, lactate, and glycerol, is a universal pathway in animals, plants, fungi, and microorganisms and shares a large portion of the glycolytic pathway. Seven of the 10 steps in glycolysis are reversed in gluconeogenesis. However, three reactions (out of the ten in glycolysis) are essentially irreversible in vivo from the standpoint of free energy changes: (1) the conversion of glucose to glucose-6-phosphate catalyzed by hexokinase, (2) phosphorylation of fructose-6-phosphate to fructose-1,6-bisphosphate catalyzed by phosphofructokinase-1, and (3) the conversion of phosphoenolpyruvate (PEP) to pyruvate catalyzed by pyruvate kinase. Therefore, in gluconeogenesis, three bypasses exist to drive these three steps in the opposite direction. Among these, the gluconeogenic conversion of pyruvate to PEP (that is, the reverse of (3) above) is central to the gluconeogenic pathway. In contrast to glycolysis, this conversion is carried out in several steps, the initial portion of which takes place in mitochondria. Pyruvate entering the mitochondria is sequentially converted into oxaloacetate and malate; the latter is then transported into the cytosol and converted into oxaloacetate, then PEP. However, if lactate is the precursor, it is first converted to pyruvate in the cytosol, and the PEP is formed inside the mitochondria and transported out (Figures 20-10 and 20-11) [107].

It should be emphasized that gluconeogenesis is costly in terms of energy expenditure. The synthesis of one molecule of glucose requires the expenditure of six high-energy phosphate groups (four from ATP, two from GTP). We should be reminded that to conserve energy, anabolic and catabolic activities are regulated *reciprocally* by regulatory enzymes. That is, when the conditions

Figure 20-10. Alternative pathways in mitochondria in gluconeogenesis for pyruvate and lactate as precursor. (From AL Lehninger, DL Nelson, MM Cox. *Principles of Biochemistry* [2nd ed]. New York: Worth, 1993.)

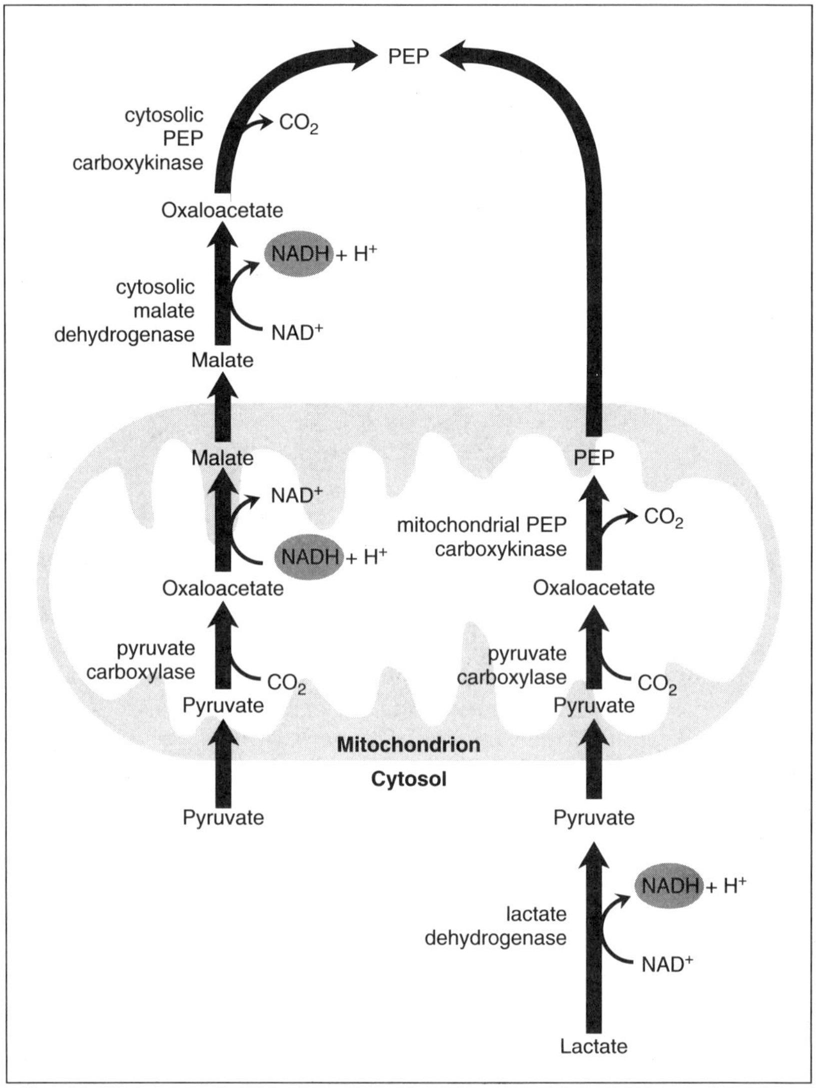

favor catabolism (of glucose), anabolic pathway (or synthesis) of glucose is inhibited, and vice versa. The regulation of gluconeogenesis also differs in different animals and from tissue to tissue in the same animal.

Synthetic and degradative pathways are controlled *reciprocally* by different regulatory enzymes. The energy-requiring biosynthetic pathways and energy-yielding breakdowns of ATP molecules are coupled.

The cycle described by Cori demonstrated that lactate produced by skeletal muscle could be converted to liver glycogen and glucose at high rates and suggested that (1) the mechanism involved a reversal by the liver of a number of steps in the glycolytic sequence, and (2) this was an important normal metabolic phenomenon by which two major organ systems (muscle and liver) interacted. At about the same time Krebs described the citric acid cycle as (1) a mechanism for the oxidation of pyruvate to carbon dioxide and water, and (2) a way of generating alanine and glutamic and aspartic acids by emanation of the appropriate keto acids. Because the latter reactions are reversible, Krebs suggested that the metabolites of this cycle, including pyruvate, could be used as a way of coupling amino acid metabolism to carbohydrate metabolism. Later, he singled out alanine as key among the amino acids whose carbon skeleton is converted to glucose.

Corroboratory data concerning the close relationship between alanine and glucose metabolism were obtained from the study of amino acid metabolism in exercising healthy male subjects in postabsorptive states. During mild exercise, alanine release increased by 25%, whereas with more intense exercise, alanine release increased by 60% to 96%. Increases in arterial alanine concentrations

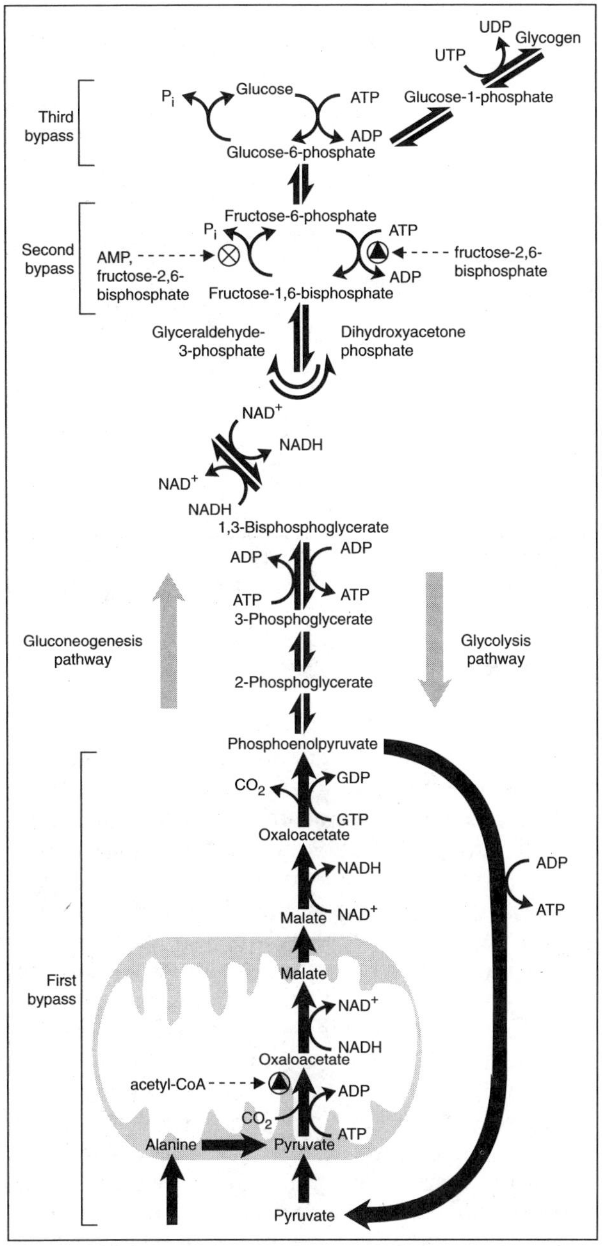

Figure 20-11. Outline of opposing pathways in glycolysis and gluconeogenesis. Note specifically the three bypasses in the gluconeogenesis. (From AL Lehninger, DL Nelson, MM Cox. *Principles of Biochemistry* [2nd ed]. New York: Worth, 1993.)

were directly proportional to the rise in arterial pyruvate and to the intensity of the work; glutamine measurements were not obtained [108].

Some quantitation of the early skeletal muscle metabolic changes in starvation was achieved by measurements of arteriovenous differences of amino acids across the deep tissues (largely skeletal muscles) of the forearm and leg [21,109]. When normal and obese subjects were fasted for a 12- to 14-hour overnight period, there was a consistently negative arteriovenous difference, indicating a net output of amino acids from the skeletal muscle. Alanine output exceeded that of all other amino acids, representing, together with glutamine, over 50% of the total amino acid release (Figure 20-12). Similar results were obtained from measurements of the amino acid output from the myocardium [110] and gut [111].

Muscle alanine is produced from several sources including the transamination of pyruvate produced in glycolysis and the alanine liberated by proteolysis. Felig [23] proposed the following metabolic scheme, called the glucose-alanine cycle (Figure 20-13). In this reaction sequence involving liver and muscle, some blood glucose (derived from the liver) is taken up by muscle and converted to pyruvate via glycolysis. The pyruvate is then transaminated using, in particular, the amino groups of branched-chain amino acids to yield alanine and a keto acid capable of metabolism by the muscle. There is a linear correlation between circulating concentrations of alanine and pyruvate in humans in the basal state; no other amino acid has this relationship to pyruvate. Following exercise or fasting there is increased muscle pyruvate production and release of alanine. The alanine is then transported to the liver, where oxidative deamination of the substrate provides the energy for gluconeogenesis.

Although the glucose-alanine cycle accounts for some aspects of carbohydrate and protein metabolism, it does not account for a net flow of amino acid carbon to carbohydrate during starvation because no carbon is lost in the glucose-alanine cycle. Several groups of authors (ourselves included) have pointed out that the carbon of alanine released by muscle must have its origin in the amino acids released by proteolysis or in the carbon chain of one of the acids of the Krebs cycle [33,112]. In the example cited below, Eli Seifter speculated on the critical importance of malate, malic enzyme, and the Krebs cycle in such a scheme [112].

$$\text{Malate} + \text{NAD}^+ \xrightarrow[\text{malic enzyme}]{\text{Mn}^{2+}} \text{Pyruvate} + \text{NADH} + \text{HCO}_3^-$$

$$\text{Pyruvate} + \text{aspartate} \longrightarrow \text{alanine} + \text{oxaloacetate}$$

$$\text{Oxaloacetate} + \text{acetyl CoA} \longrightarrow \text{citrate}$$

$$\text{Citrate via Krebs cycle} \longrightarrow \text{malate}$$

Pertinent sum:

$$\text{Malate} + \text{aspartate} \longrightarrow \text{alanine} + \text{malate} + \text{HCO}_3^-$$

The following concepts advanced by Seifter [112] derived from this scheme:

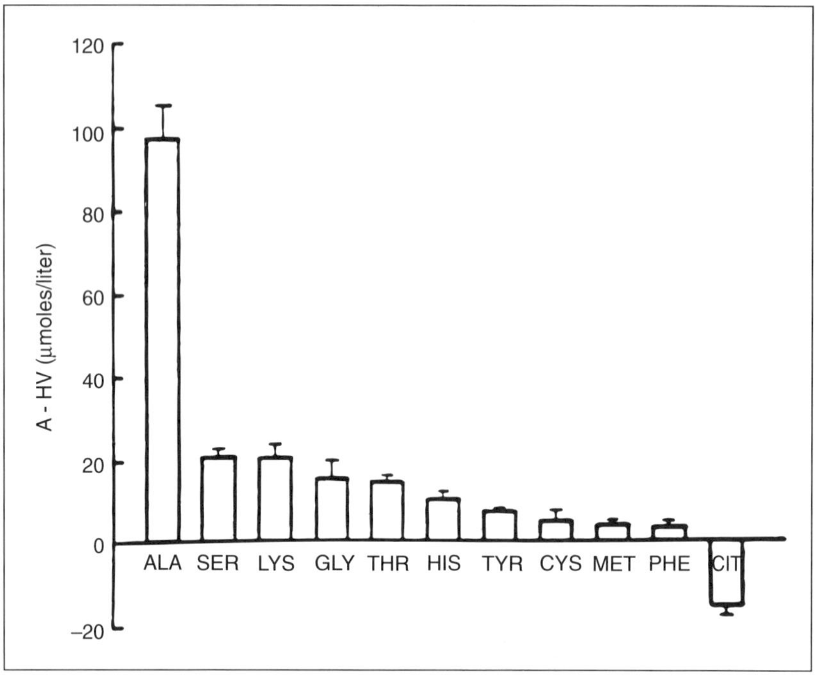

Figure 20-12. Net balance of individual amino acids across the splanchnic bed (arterio-hepatic venous differences) in 12 subjects in the resting postabsorptive state. Only those amino acids whose mean A-HV differences were significantly different from zero are shown. (From P Felig, J Wahren. Amino acid metabolism in exercising man. *J Clin Invest* 50:2703, 1971. Reproduced by permission.)

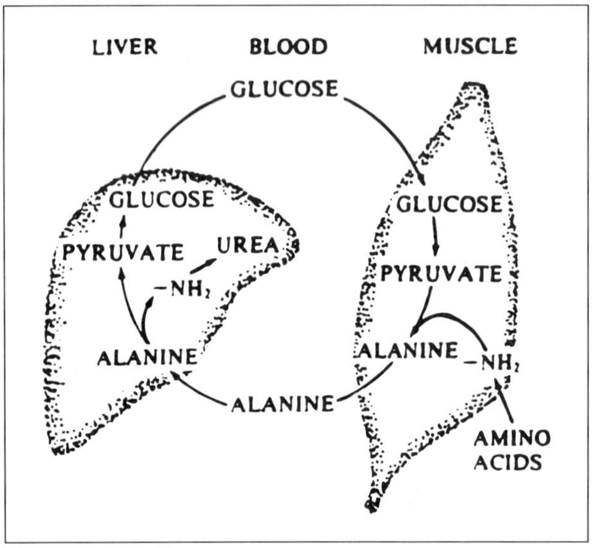

Figure 20-13. The glucose-alanine cycle. (From P Felig. The glucose-alanine cycle. *Metabolism* 22:179, 1973.)

1. The synthesis of extra alanine (other than alanine derived from 3-carbon amino acids) by muscle is possible because of the presence of malic enzyme in the muscle.
2. Because malate is both a reactant and a product (Krebs cycle), the net carbon transfer involved in alanine biosynthesis comes from the degradation of muscle amino acids (for example, aspartate, glutamate, and valine).
3. Most amino acids metabolized in the muscle according to this scheme would yield (a) some alanine, (b) carbon dioxide, (c) fatty acid derivatives in a partially oxidized state, and (d) energy.

Clarification of amino acid metabolism and transport in and out of muscle was brought by Garber et al. [79] in a series of *in vitro* experiments with rat epitrochlear muscle. The pattern of amino acid release by this muscle preparation is remarkably similar to that observed in studies of arteriovenous differences across skeletal muscle in postabsorptive humans; alanine and glutamine account for more than 60% of the total amino acid release. Despite the disproportionately high release of alanine and glutamine, the tissue levels of these amino acids were found to be virtually unchanged. The following observations support the view that alanine carbon is not derived from glucose:

1. No correlation was found between glucose uptake and alanine release.
2. Muscle alanine and glutamine release were not changed by added insulin.
3. When glycolysis was blocked by iodoacetate, alanine and glutamine release were not decreased.
4. Using amino-oxyacetate, which inhibits alanine aminotransferase, a decrease in alanine release and a reciprocal increase in glutamine formation were noted, showing that an alanine transaminase rather than alanine dehydrogenase was involved in alanine synthesis.
5. Addition of amino acids such as aspartate, leucine, and valine increased the total carbon ef-

TRANSAMINATION

$$(1a)\ AA_{(t)} + aKGA \rightleftharpoons aKA_{(t)} + GLU$$

OXIDATIVE DEAMINATION

$$AA_{(d)} \longrightarrow aKA_{(d)} + NH_3\ (1b)$$

$$aKGA + NH_3 \rightleftharpoons GLU\ (2)$$

$$(3)\ aKA_{(t\ or\ d)} \longrightarrow \longrightarrow \longrightarrow MAL + nCO_2$$

$$(4)\ MAL \longrightarrow PYR + CO_2$$

$$(5)\ PYR + GLU \rightleftharpoons ALA + aKGA$$

$$(1a \longrightarrow 5)\ \text{or}\ (1b \longrightarrow 5) \quad AA_{(t\ or\ d)} \longrightarrow ALA + (n_{(t\ or\ d)} + 1)CO_2$$

Figure 20-14. Equations for the postulated reactions involved in synthesis of alanine (ALA) in skeletal muscle. Amino acid may transaminate ($AA_{(t)}$) with alpha-ketoglutarate (α-KGA) (1a) or may be oxidatively deaminated ($AA_{(d)}$) (1b) with subsequent glutamate (GLU) formation (2). For amino acids that form pyruvate directly, Equations 3 and 4 are to be omitted. Equation 3 represents the number of steps necessary to form malate (MAL) in the citric acid cycle, with the subsequent formation of pyruvate by $NADP^+$-malate dehydrogenase (4). Identical equations of summation (for carbon atoms) result regardless of the mechanism of glutamate formation (1a versus 1b and 2). (From AJ Garber, IE Karl, DM Kipnis. Alanine and glutamine synthesis and release from skeletal muscle. *J Biol Chem* 251:836, 1976.)

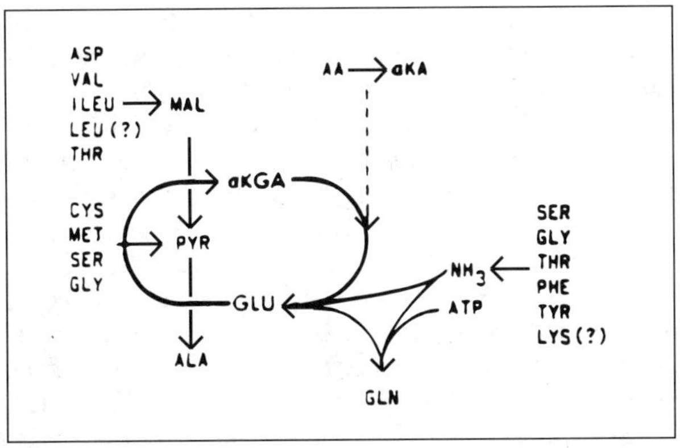

Figure 20-15. Summary of the intracellular mechanisms leading to alanine and glutamine formation. AA = amino acid; KA = ketoacid. (From AJ Garber, IE Karl, DM Kipnis. Alanine and glutamine synthesis and release from skeletal muscle. *J Biol Chem* 251:836, 1976.)

flux from muscle, as measured by pyruvate + lactate + alanine + glutamate + glutamine release, by 70%, 54%, and 40%, respectively, in the presence of iodoacetate.

6. Addition of pyruvate did not increase the rate of alanine formation above that produced by aspartate, leucine, serine, and valine. These findings demonstrate that the increased carbon efflux from muscle is derived principally from metabolic transformation of amino acids to alanine and glutamine (Figures 20-14 and 20-15). Alanine formation from pyruvate and glutamate via transamination by alanine aminotransferase represents the final common pathway. Carbon derived from glycolysis and metabolic transformation of amino acids contributes to the intracellular pyruvate pool. The rate of glycolysis is not rate-limiting for alanine formation, whereas pyruvate formation from amino acids is reflected in corresponding changes in alanine synthesis and release.

Net synthesis of alanine from cysteine, methionine, glycine, and serine can be accounted for because they all lead ultimately to formation of pyruvate and glutamate. Methionine, isoleucine, and valine can lead to net alanine formation by generating succinyl CoA, which then becomes oxidized to malate via the Krebs cycle. The malic enzyme action is now known to possess sufficient activity in skeletal muscle to divert 4-carbon intermediates to pyruvate formation as suggested by Seifter [112].

Pozefsky et al. [114] found in normal men that the plasma concentrations of most amino acids in arterial blood had fallen after a 12-hour overnight fast, but those of the branched-chain amino acids (valine, leucine, and isoleucine) and α-aminobutyrate had risen. The arterial concentration of the branched-chain amino acids rose even more at 60 hours of starvation. The glutamine-asparagine peak remained unchanged. The A-V difference (forearm) of several other amino acids (threonine, glycine, alanine, α-aminobutyrate, methionine, tyrosine, and lysine) became increasingly more negative with starvation (12 to 60 hours). The A-V difference for the branched-chain amino acids was somewhat more negative at 60 hours than at 12 hours, but not significantly so. Serine was actively taken up by muscle during the postabsorptive state, whereas it was released after the 60-hour fast. The 60-hour fast increased the rate of total amino acid (notably alanine) release from the forearm muscles by 69% over the postabsorptive levels.

Intracellular skeletal muscle amino acid concentrations were studied by Bergstrom et al. [115] in quadriceps muscle biopsies obtained from healthy subjects after an overnight fast. They found that eight dietary essential amino acids represent only 8.4% of the total pool of muscle free amino acids, whereas glutamine, glutamic acid, and alanine constitute about 79%. The intracellular concentrations of the branched-chain dietary essential amino acids (valine, leucine, and isoleucine) were greater than the plasma concentrations.

In many areas of nutrition and metabolism there is currently a good deal of interest in the branched-chain amino acids [43] and their keto analogues [116]. There are some special aspects of the metabolism of branched-chain amino acids that relate to starvation. Muscle, particularly red and heart muscle, is capable of utilizing leucine, isoleucine, and valine for energy to a greater extent than is the liver. It is this property that permits these compounds and their metabolites to act as regulators of muscle protein breakdown. Some of the intermediates of branched-chain amino acid can give rise to either muscle or liver glycogen.

Among factors that regulate muscle protein breakdown it has been found that the branched-chain amino acids, their keto derivatives, and their decarboxylated products inhibit muscle protein catabolism. For example, in muscle, valine, a branched-chain amino acid, is converted to α-ketoisovaleric acid and then oxidized to isobutyric acid. All of these compounds inhibit muscle protein breakdown. It is not known whether the subsequent metabolites of valine also share this property. It has been suggested that the partial oxidation of the branched-chain amino acids and the partial oxidation of ketoacids by muscle contributes to the reducing environment of the muscle cell and that the inhibition of proteolysis is due to this reducing environment.

Insulin, in addition to promoting muscle protein synthesis, also inhibits protein breakdown. In starvation, insulin levels are low and therefore the control (inhibition) of protein breakdown derives in greater part from the branched-chain amino acids and their metabolites. In an earlier discussion of this, Seifter and Levenson had suggested an analogous approach using aromatic and branched-chain α-hydroxy and α-keto analogues of the amino acids; supporting evidence for the effectiveness of this approach using the α-keto analogues has since been reported by Sapir and colleagues [117–120].

The branched-chain amino acids (which by themselves inhibit protein breakdown) do not augment the inhibitory action of insulin on protein breakdown. Some investigators [121] have speculated that leucine plays a special role in the inhibition of proteolysis. Because other branched-chain amino acids and some of their metabolites also are active in this regard [32], the existence of a special role for leucine has been questioned. Seifter and we suggest that the latter view is probably correct for the fasted or starved animal. For the fed animal, though, it is likely that circulating leucine is an important regulator of insulin secretion. It is not by accident that leucine, the one purely ketogenic amino acid, is a stimulus for hormonal changes that can abrogate the ketotic state.

Most studies directed toward evaluating the role of the liver and gut in amino acid exchange in normal humans have used measurements of arterial-hepatic venous differences, because the portal vein is not readily accessible for catheterization. Felig and Wahren [111] showed in normal, healthy volunteers that alanine predominates in the amino acid uptake across the splanchnic bed in the postabsorptive state. Studies of overnight fasted patients undergoing elective cholecystectomy and intraoperative portal vein sampling showed that the organs (principally the gastrointestinal tract) drained by the portal vein consistently released alanine, and that liver took up alanine, glycine, leucine, and isoleucine. The splanchnic bed (chiefly the gut) takes up glutamine and releases glutamate and alanine [111,122]. The importance of the gut in glutamine metabolism is indicated by the observation that removal of the gastrointestinal tract, pancreas, and spleen, but not the liver, which was left in situ with its blood supply ligated, causes a greater rise in plasma glutamine than does nephrectomy [123].

Shulman et al. [124] have reported observations suggesting that the plasma glucose level can itself, independently of insulin or glucagon, modify the metabolism of the two main gluconeogenic precursors. They studied dogs that were fasted and given somatostatin and constant infusions of insulin and glucagon. They found that hyperglycemia leads to an elevation in the plasma lactate concentration primarily as a consequence of decreased lactate uptake by the liver. In addition, hyperglycemia causes the plasma alanine level to rise as a result of an increase in the production rate of the amino acid and a fall in its fractional extraction by the liver. Finally, hyperglycemia not only alters the net rate of entry of the aforementioned gluconeogenic precursors into the liver, but also decreases the efficiency with which they are converted to glucose.

Importance of Oxaloacetate in Muscle and Liver Metabolism

Muscle and liver oxaloacetate (OAA) is a key metabolite in gluconeogenesis because it acts as a link between the carbon chain of some glucogenic amino acids and the carbon chain of glucose. For example, in muscle net OAA is generated from amino acids such as aspartate derived from protein:

$$\text{Aspartate} + \text{keto glutamate} \longrightarrow \text{OAA} + \text{gutamate}$$

$$\text{OAA} \longrightarrow \text{Krebs cycle} \longrightarrow CO_2 + H_2O$$
$$\text{OAA} \longrightarrow \text{Krebs cycle} \longrightarrow \text{malate}$$
$$\text{OAA} \longrightarrow \text{PEP} \longrightarrow \text{limited muscle gluconeogenesis}$$

Muscle OAA also is critical because it provides the carbon chain for gluconeogenesis in liver and because it provides substrates for heart muscle metabolism. In muscle:

$$\text{OAA} + \text{NADH} + H^+ \xrightarrow[\text{dehydrogenase}]{\text{malic (MDH)}} \text{malate} + NAD^+$$

$$\text{Malate} + NAD^+ \xrightarrow[\text{enzyme}]{\text{malic}} \text{pyruvate} + CO^2 + \text{NADH} + H^+$$

$$\text{Pyruvate} + \text{NADH} + H^+ \xrightarrow[\text{dehydrogenase}]{\text{lactic}} \text{lactate} + NAD^+$$

Sum:

$$\text{Muscle OAA} + \text{NADH} + H^+ \longrightarrow \text{muscle lactate} + CO^2 + NAD^+$$

$$\text{Muscle lactate} \longrightarrow \text{liver lactate} \longrightarrow \text{glucogen}$$
$$\text{Muscle lactate} \longrightarrow \text{uptake and utilization by heart}$$

Thus OAA serves to carry the carbon chain of amino acids (as lactate) to the liver for resynthesis into glycogen. It should be noted that lactate here also functions as part of an interorgan transport of excess reducing power generated by muscle because the starving muscle carries out less complete oxidation than does well-nourished and perfused muscle.

In addition to providing lactate to liver for gluconeogenesis and to heart for further oxidation, OAA is the key in supplying muscle *alanine* to the liver for gluconeogenesis:

$$\text{Aspartic acid} + \alpha\text{-ketoglutarate} \xrightarrow[\text{transaminase (GOT)}]{\text{glutamic oxaloacetic}} \text{OAA} + \text{glutamate}$$

$$\text{OAA} + \text{NADH} + H^+ \xrightarrow{\text{malic dehydrogenase}} \text{malate} + NAD^+$$

$$\text{Malate} + NAD^+ \xrightarrow[\text{enzyme}]{\text{malic}} \text{pyruvate} + CO_2 + \text{NADH} + H^+$$

$$\text{Pyruvate} + \text{glutamate} \xrightarrow[\text{transaminase (GPT)}]{\text{glutamic pyruvic}} \text{alanine} + \alpha\text{-ketoglutarate}$$

Sum:

$$\text{Aspartic acid} \xrightarrow[\alpha\text{-ketoglutarate, } H^+\text{, } NAD^+\text{, NADH + pyruvate}]{\text{GOT, MDH, GPT, OAA, malate,}} \text{alanine} + CO_2$$

Thus muscle OAA provides some carbon for muscle gluconeogenesis or liver gluconeogenesis, or lactate for peripheral utilization. There exists a group of glucogenic amino acids that cannot provide OAA or PEP in muscle. Therefore, they are not glucogenic in muscle, but give rise to alanine and lactate, which can be converted to glycogen in liver and several other tissues:

$$\text{Glycine, Alanine, Serine, Cysteine, Hydroxyproline, Threonine (in part)} \longrightarrow \text{pyruvate}$$
$$\text{pyruvate} \longrightarrow \text{muscle alanine}$$
$$\text{pyruvate} \longrightarrow \text{muscle lactate}$$

Role of Glutamine

Glutamine plays a major function in transporting some of the ammonia from muscle catabolism and a related function in providing a carbon skeleton that can be utilized for gluconeogenesis, although recent work of Goldberg [125] emphasizes this latter function. From the quantitative standpoint, about equal amounts of alanine and glutamine leave muscle under various metabolic states. Because the carbon of glutamine (as α-ketoglutarate) is convertible to the carbon of alanine (as pyruvate), either one can transport the carbon and nitrogen of other muscle amino acids to the liver or the kidney. In the muscle, glutamine is formed from glutamate that originates either from proteolysis or from transamination of α-ketoglutarate and can be derived by a net synthesis from fatty acid oxidation and oxidation of the carbon skeleton of some amino acids, such as aspartic acid, via the Krebs cycle. Glutamine synthesis is an energy-dependent reaction requiring a glutamyl phosphate intermediate, which reacts with ammonia to yield the amino acid. Formation of glutamine by glutamine synthetase requires ammonia, glutamate, and ATP. The required glutamate is derived from either muscle protein glutamate, methionine, valine, or isoleucine. The latter three amino acids are precursors of succinyl CoA, therefore of α-ketoglutaric acid, and can contribute to a net synthesis of glutamine.

The preceding data are highly relevant to the

glucogenic events in starvation. Alanine, the prime substrate for liver gluconeogenesis, and glutamine, the prime substrate for renal gluconeogenesis, are both derived from amino acid metabolism in muscle. Factors that regulate the rate of synthesis and release of these amino acids could directly affect the rate and importance of these two gluconeogenic pathways in different stages of starvation. Dependence on alanine as a gluconeogenic source poses problems to the body in terms of disposing of the ammonia formed in deamination. In the fed or postabsorption state, the ammonia is fed into the urea cycle in the liver and is synthesized into urea at the expense of considerable energy. In the prolonged starved state, urea is no longer the major nitrogen excretory product, but ammonium ion is; to a major extent this is because of the large amounts of ketones and ketoacids excreted at this time.

The adaptation of the kidneys to starvation becomes a major feature of the responses to food deprivation. Thus, early in starvation 90% of gluconeogenesis goes on in the liver and 10% in the kidney, but later in starvation 45% goes on in the kidney and 55% in the liver.

Kidney glutamine also contributes to the homeostasis of acid-base balance. By use of the enzyme glutaminase, glutamine becomes the immediate source of the ammonia, which accepts hydrogen ion and acts to neutralize some of the acidic products of metabolism. This reaction is quantitatively small in fed individuals, but in starvation becomes critical for survival for two reasons: (1) during starvation the body becomes depleted of sodium, potassium, and other fixed bases, and (2) the amounts of base required to neutralize the excreted keto acids (100 mEq/day) are large and require the production of a base by metabolism. The glutaminase reaction fulfills this requirement, permitting the excretion of ammonium and preserving the glutamate. The glutamate then acts as an acceptor of circulating ammonia and is converted to glutamine in the kidney, which can then give rise to urinary ammonium again. With a drop in circulating ammonia, some of the glutamate is cycled to the liver for glutamine or other syntheses and some of the glutamate is deaminated. Under similar conditions, α-ketoglutarate formed in the kidney is converted to kidney glycogen, and the ammonia handled by remaining glutamate as just described. Thus, deamination of glutamate is a major factor in the kidney's role as a glucose source during starvation. In acidosis (1) kidney glutamine arriving from the muscle is hydrolyzed by glutaminase to give NH_3, which picks up H^+ that is then excreted as NH_4^+; (2) the glutamate formed in this reaction is deaminated by glutamic dehydrogenase yielding a second molecule of ammonia, which combines with H^+ to be excreted as NH_4^+; (3) α-ketoglutaric acid in reaction 2 and under acidotic conditions tends to be used for renal gluconeogenesis. This means that the kidney can dispose of both the carbon and nitrogen of glutamine arriving from muscle (Figure 20-16).

The kidney also contains enzymes capable of carrying out a glutamate-based cycle, which converts glucogenic amino acids arriving from the circulation (muscle) into kidney glycogen and produces urinary ammonia.

$$\text{Glutamic acid} + \text{NAD}^+ \xrightarrow[\text{H}_2\text{O}]{\text{glutamic dehydrogenase (GDH)}} \text{NADH} + \text{NH}_4^+ + \alpha\text{-ketoglutaric acid NH}_4^+ \xrightarrow{\text{excretion}} \text{urinary ammonium} \quad (1)$$

$$\alpha\text{-ketoglutaric acid} + \text{incoming glycogenic amino acid (e.g., alanine)} \xrightarrow[\text{transaminase (GTP)}]{\text{glutamic pyruvic}} \text{pyruvate} + \text{glutamate} \quad (2)$$

$$\text{Pyruvate} \longrightarrow \text{glycogen} \quad (3)$$

Sum:

$$\text{Glycogenic amino acid} \xrightarrow[\text{GDH, GPT}]{\text{glutamic acid, NAD}^+,} \text{renal glycogen} + \text{urinary} + \text{NH}_4^+$$

Erythrocyte Amino Acids

Early equilibration studies of amino acids using red blood cells showed long equilibration times, and it was assumed that the plasma is the most important vehicle for amino acid transport. However, later studies indicate that large amounts of interorgan and tissue amino acid exchange occur via the blood cellular elements, probably the erythrocytes, although a role for the leukocytes has not been ruled out [126]. Although the mechanism of the erythrocyte uptake and release of amino acids is not known, we think that the erythrocyte glutamyl transport system of Meister [127] could explain the transfer of amino acid into and out of the red blood cells. Moreover, this may provide the explanation for the existence of an amino acid transport system in cells that do not carry out protein synthesis. The situation parallels another function of red blood cells, i.e., oxygen transport by cells that utilize only minimal amounts of oxygen.

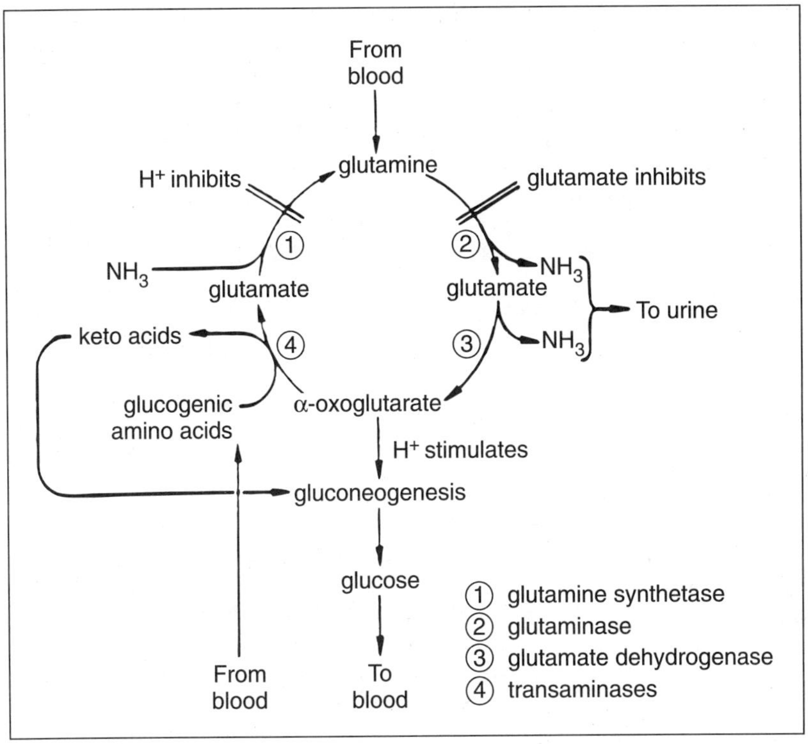

Figure 20-16. Relationship between gluconeogenesis and ammonia production in the kidney. (From P Banks, W Bartley, LM Birt. *The Biochemistry of the Tissues.* London: Wiley, 1976. Reprinted by permission.)

Erythrocyte and Leukocyte Glucose

In starvation, the brain and blood cells account for about 57% and 40%, respectively, of the glucose utilized [32]. Most brain glucose is oxidized to CO_2 and H_2O, but about 10% leaves the brain as lactate or pyruvate. Almost all the glucose used by blood cells is released as lactate. In starvation, the contribution of blood cell and brain lactate to the carbon of hepatic gluconeogenesis is as great as the carbon contribution from gluconeogenic amino acids and the glycerol from triglycerides.

Fat Metabolism

One of the important adaptive changes of starvation is the increase in the absolute and relative amounts of fat consumed for energy purposes compared to the calories derived from protein. If the rate of protein breakdown and nitrogen excretion observed in the initial phases of starvation were to continue unchanged, the organism's protein stores would soon be depleted, resulting in dysfunction and death significantly sooner than, in fact, happens. Thus, after the early phase of starvation, when gluconeogenesis is prominent, a later phase supervenes during which protein breakdown is minimized by switching over to fat as the main source of energy, thereby decreasing the need for glucose and gluconeogenesis. This is accomplished by increasing the pool of free fatty acids by lipolysis, so that muscle increases its utilization of free fatty acids to a point at which 90% of its calories may be derived from their oxidation. Additionally, the liver increases its utilization of fatty acids. The main products of hepatic oxidation of fatty acids are the ketone bodies, acetoacetic acid, and β-hydroxybutyric acid, which are then transported to tissues (muscle, brain) that would otherwise require glucose. The accelerated hepatic ketogenesis during starvation is a result of both an enhanced activity of the enzymatic system(s) involved in ketone production and an increased FFA load (enhanced activity of fatty acid synthesizing enzymes) [113,128]. Once the early phase of starvation is over, the ketones are produced by the liver in greater amounts than glucose (130 g vs. 110 g) [129]. During this phase, hepatic glucose output accounts for less than 30% of the total calories utilized by the body. As a result of these changes, in contrast to early starvation, when the body uses about 4.8 calories derived from fat for each calorie derived from protein, the body in the adapted state uses about 17 calories from fat for each calorie derived from protein. It is this change in the relative amounts of protein catabolized during starvation, a drop from about 75 g/day early in starvation to about 20 g/day later in starvation, that makes survival of two to three months and longer possible [32]. Caloric supply is the limiting factor in starvation, and examples of very obese individuals surviving starvation for a year have been described [54,122].

Fatty acids are released from adipocytes following the hydrolysis of triglycerides by lipases [54,122]. Fatty acids are present in plasma in increased amounts under conditions of low circulating insulin, a characteristic of starvation; high insulin levels inhibit the lipolytic (lipase) activity of fat cells. Fatty acids are present in the serum in combination with either albumin or lipoproteins. In the former case, the linkage is a salt one with positively charged lysyl groups of albumin. In the latter case (lipoproteins), free fatty acids are taken up by the liver and secreted as part of macrostructures containing lipoprotein, triglyceride, phospholipid, cholesterol, and fatty acids. The binding of some of these structures involves noncovalent, hydrophobic associations. In advanced starvation the synthesis of lipoproteins declines, and fatty acid transport may become dependent on the albumin-bound complex.

Entrance of free fatty acids into muscle cells appears not to be directly under special hormonal regulation; rather, the concentration of serum fatty acids is critical in determining the rate of entry of fatty acids into the muscle cell. To the extent that insulin (or lack thereof) regulates release of free fatty acids from adipose tissue, it can be considered to regulate free fatty acid uptake by the muscle indirectly. Long-chain fatty acids cannot permeate the outer mitochondrial membrane, whereas some smaller-chain fatty acids are capable of permeating the outer, but not the inner, mitochondrial membranes. Fatty acids must be primed for utilization by mitochondria. The priming process consists of reactions occurring in the outer mitochondrial membrane and in some extramitochondrial organelles, which convert a fatty acid to its acyl coenzyme A derivative:

$$\text{Fatty acid} + \text{ATP} + \text{CoA} \longrightarrow \text{fatty acid ester CoA} + \text{adenylic acid} + \text{PPi}$$

The acyl coenzyme A ester formed is now capable of crossing the outer membrane, but it is unable to permeate the inner mitochondrial membrane. This is made possible by a reaction carried out by an enzyme in the inner mitochondrial membrane:

$$\text{Acyl CoA} + \text{carnitine} \longrightarrow \text{acyl carnitine} + \text{CoA}$$

It is the acyl carnitine that is able to cross the inner membrane. The coenzyme A diffuses back to the outer aspect of the outer membrane. On the inner aspect of the inner membrane, the reverse reaction occurs:

$$\text{Acyl carnitine} + \text{CoA} \longrightarrow \text{acyl CoA} + \text{carnitine}$$

The acyl coenzyme A is now able to be oxidized inside the mitochondria, and the carnitine is free to diffuse out of the mitochondria matrix, particularly back to the inner mitochondrial membrane. These reactions can be summarized as follows:

$$\text{Fatty acid} + \text{CoA} + \text{energy} \xrightarrow{\text{(outer membrane)}} \text{fatty acid CoA ester (acyl CoA)}$$

$$\text{Acyl CoA} + \text{carnitine} \xrightarrow{\text{(inner membrane)}} \text{acyl carnitine} + \text{CoA}$$

$$\text{CoA} + \text{acyl carnitine} \xrightarrow{\text{(inside mitochondrial matrix)}} \text{acyl CoA} + \text{carnitine}$$

Sum:

$$\text{Fatty acid} + \text{CoA} + \text{energy} \xrightarrow{\text{(inside mitochondrial matrix)}} \text{acyl CoA}$$

The system is of interest from two standpoints in starving individuals:

1. The synthesis of carnitine requires methyl groups from methionine and the carbon chain of lysine. Thus it is synthesized at the expense of a nutrient that cannot be synthesized in adequate amounts (methionine) or that cannot be synthesized by the body (lysine). The biosynthesis of carnitine also involves ascorbic acid-dependent hydroxylations.
2. Carnitine levels in skeletal muscles of starved dogs and humans have been found to be higher than in samples from unstarved subjects [131]. Some investigators have considered that elevations of carnitine are essential for the adaptation to starvation, suggesting that intracellular transport of fatty acids may be limiting for fatty acid oxidation during starvation. The maintenance of high carnitine levels during starvation may be accomplished by depleting some tissues of ascorbic acid.

Grey et al. [113] have shown that the accelerated hepatic ketogenesis during starvation is a result of increased free fatty acid load and an increase in the activity of the enzyme system(s) involved in ketone body production. As the supply of fatty acids to the liver rises, there is a parallel increase in the rate of hepatic extraction of these fatty acids. Concomitantly, ketone body production in the liver increases to five to eight times the original value, and this leads to raised blood ketone levels. It has been calculated that after a 15-hour fast, 50% of the fatty acid uptake is converted to ketone bodies by the liver; this percentage increases to 80% after a 60-hour fast and to almost 100% after a 120-hour fast [132].

The increased hepatic ketogenesis is believed to result from inhibition of the citric acid cycle in the liver secondary to an accumulation of reduced coenzymes arising from increased fatty acid utilization and from substrate saturation of the citric acid cycle in the liver. Another, but quantitatively less important, source of ketone bodies is the deamination of some amino acids that are degraded via the acetyl CoA pathways. The increases in plasma ketones early in fasting reflect chiefly increased production and, to a lesser extent, some impairment of peripheral utilization, both processes being sensitive to insulin. Late in fasting, peripheral utilization of ketones is high.

Diabetes has been called "starvation in the midst of plenty." Starvation and uncontrolled diabetes both represent ketotic states, and these are compared in Figures 20-17 and 20-18. The key substance, in both the generation and utilization of ketone bodies, is acetyl CoA. In normal, fed animals, liver acetyl CoA derives from fatty acids released by adipocytes and from hepatic carbohydrate metabolism. Most of this acetyl CoA is oxidized via the Krebs cycle or resynthesized into fatty acids by the normal liver (see Figure 20-17). Only a minute amount goes to form ketones. In the liver of ketotic animals, the amount of acetyl CoA to be metabolized is greater. This is true for both the starved and diabetic state. The acetyl CoA levels rise because fatty acid synthesis becomes negligible and the amount of free fatty acids presented to the liver increases, probably owing to low plasma insulin levels or inadequate insulin activity. The activity of the Krebs cycle is only slightly decreased by ketosis, and most of the acetyl CoA goes into ketogenesis.

The liver has a mechanism for determining whether intermediates like acyl coenzyme A will go to ketone production or fatty acid synthesis. The mechanism explains why fatty acid breakdown in the liver does not usually occur at the same time as fatty acid synthesis, and how cessation of fatty acid synthesis stimulates fatty acid oxidation in the liver.

Normal State

High carbohydrate (CHO) ⟶ saturation of glycogen synthesis, then

High CHO ⟶ high levels of AcCoA

High levels of AcCoA ⟶ high levels of citrate

High levels of citrate activate AcCoA carboxylase:

$$\text{monomeric AcCoA carboxylase (inactive)} \xrightarrow{+\text{ Citrate}} \text{polymeric AcCoA carboxylase (active)}$$

$$CO_2 + \text{AcCoA} \xrightarrow[\text{AcCoA carboxylase}]{\text{polymeric}} \text{malonyl CoA}$$

$$\text{AcCoA} + 7\text{ malonyl CoA} + 14\text{ NADPH} + 14H^+ \longrightarrow \text{palmitic acid} + 7\ CO_2 + 8\text{ CoA} + 14\text{ NADP}^+ + 6H_2O$$

Fatty acid synthesis, then, is dependent (rate limited) on malonyl CoA levels, which are in turn

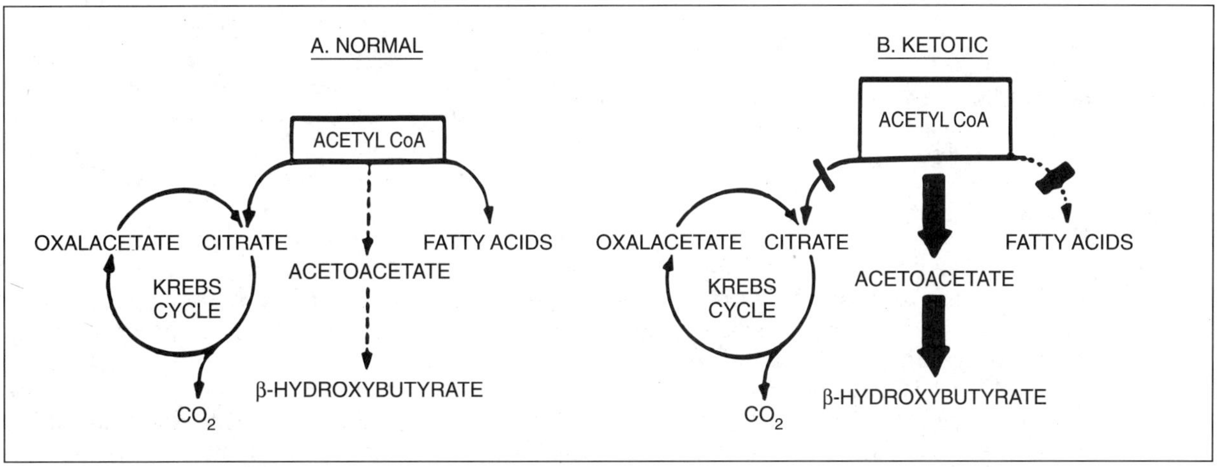

Figure 20-17. Underutilization of acetyl-CoA in genesis of ketosis. In normal liver **(A)**, acetyl-CoA is utilized primarily in Krebs cycle reactions or in fatty acid synthesis with minimal ketone formation. In ketotic states **(B)**, fatty acid synthesis becomes negligible, hepatic acetyl-CoA concentrations increase, and two-carbon flow to acetoacetate and beta-hydroxybutyrate is enhanced. Krebs cycle activity is depressed only in severe ketosis. (From JD McGarry, DW Foster. Regulation of ketogenesis and clinical aspects of the ketotic state. *Metabolism* 21:471, 1972.)

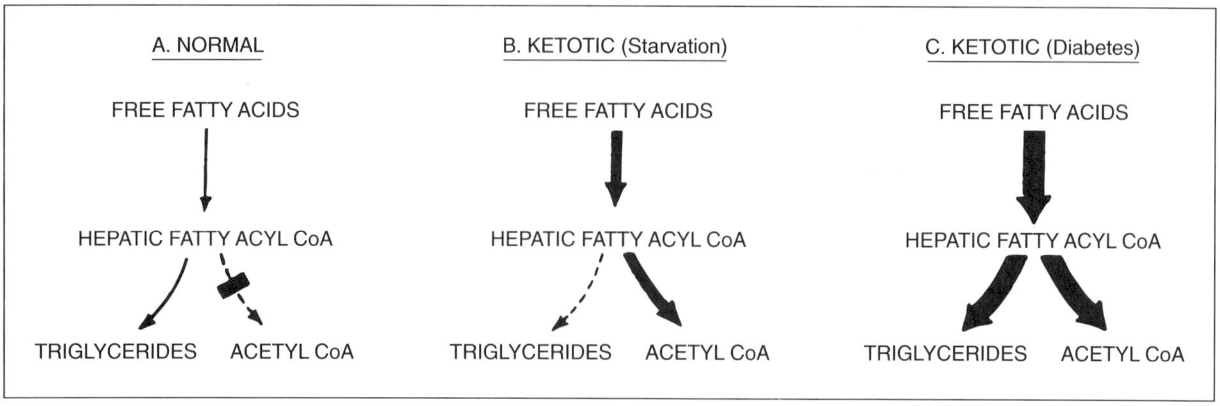

Figure 20-18. Overproduction of acetyl-CoA in the genesis of ketosis. In the normal state **(A)**, fatty acid oxidation is considered limited, probably at long-chain fatty acyl CoA-carnitine transferase reaction with hepatic fatty acids utilized primarily for triglyceride synthesis. In starvation **(B)**, entry of fatty acids into oxidative pathway is increased so that less substrate is available for triglyceride synthesis. In diabetes **(C)**, fatty acid oxidation is maximally increased and free fatty acid delivery to liver is greater than in starvation, providing substrate sufficient for both accelerated ketogenesis and enhanced triglyceride synthesis. (From JD McGarry, DW Foster. Regulation of ketogenesis and clinical aspects of the ketotic state. *Metabolism* 21:471, 1972.)

dependent on AcCoA carboxylase activity. In addition, malonyl CoA is an inhibitor of carnitine acyl transferase (CAT), and as a consequence, fatty acid CoA derivatives that are formed in fatty acid biosynthesis are prevented from being oxidized:

Palmitoyl CoA → chain elongation and triglyceride formation
Palmitoyl CoA → fatty acid oxidation

Malonyl CoA inhibits the mitochondrial transport of palmitoyl CoA by blocking the reaction

$$\text{Palmitoyl CoA} + \text{carnitine} \xrightarrow{\text{CAT}} \text{palmitoyl carnitine}$$

and therefore blocks fatty acid oxidation. As a result, fatty acid synthesis and oxidation do not occur simultaneously [133,134].

Starvation, Diabetes

In starvation, there is a decrease in malonyl CoA levels in the liver (less glucose arriving to the liver), and at the same time, high levels of free fatty acids arrive from adipocytes. The fatty acids are activated by ATP + CoA, and the acyl CoA compounds formed are able to react with carnitine to form acyl carnitine, because there is little malonyl CoA to inhibit the process. As we have already noted, carnitine, a cosubstrate for these reactions, is elevated in tissues of starved animals. These elevated carnitine levels further favor intracellular fatty acid transport and partial oxidation to ketone bodies. McGarry and Foster [133] have reported data in support of the roles of malonyl CoA and carnitine acyltransferase in the regulation of liver fatty acid oxidation and ketogenesis.

In diabetes, levels of malonyl CoA and activity of AcCoA carboxylase are modified for different reasons than they are in starvation. A relative citrate deficit (and therefore deactivation of AcCoA carboxylase) exists owing to the shunting of OAA (citrate precursor) to gluconeogenesis. The end results (ketogenesis, decreased fat synthesis), however, are similar in starvation and diabetes. Underutilization of hepatic acetyl CoA for fatty acid synthesis, therefore, underlies ketone formation in both starved and diabetic animals. Whether the increased ketogenesis leads to ketonemia depends on the level of ketogenesis and the degree of peripheral utilization of the ketones.

Diabetic ketosis differs from starvation ketosis in several important ways:

1. Peripheral utilization of ketones is low in diabetes and in early starvation, but it is high in advanced starvation. However, because of the high production of ketones in starvation, ketonemia persists.

2. Although the liver in starvation decreases its ketone production following the infusion of antiketogenic substances (lactate, pyruvate, alanine), which are converted to glucose, the diabetic liver is nonreactive and ketone formation continues high.

3. The liver of diabetics produces large amounts of triglycerides even while producing

large amounts of ketones, but this is not the case in starvation.

Influence of Fat Metabolism on Gluconeogenesis and Protein Catabolism

Lipid fuels are the most potent inhibitors of glucose utilization in the context of feeding and fasting [135–138]. Fatty acid and ketone oxidation both exert inhibitory influences on glucose utilization at the level of PDH, the rate-limiting step in glucose oxidation [107,134,139]. The PDH complex is activated by dephophosphorylation and inactivated by phosphorylation. Low circulating insulin levels are associated with net phosphorylation and hence inactivation of the PDH [137,138]. Increased fatty acid and ketone oxidation accompanied by low circulating insulin levels inhibit pyruvate oxidation and hence glucose utilization during starvation. Inhibition of PDH during starvation is an important means of maintaining glycemia; by preserving glycolytic products (pyruvate and lactate) from oxidation they can be utilized in gluconeogenesis via Cori cycle recycling [137,138]. It is likely that the block of glucose oxidation plays a regulatory role in the switch-over in energy substrate from glucose to fatty acids and ketones that occurs in starvation.

Sherwin et al. [140] have shown, after prolonged starvation in obese subjects, that plasma alanine decreases to a greater extent than any other amino acid, whereas peripheral release and splanchnic uptake of alanine are reduced to less than 50% of the levels observed in postabsorptive states. They found also that during prolonged fasting, venous alanine concentration, which had already fallen by 40% below prefast levels, fell an additional 30% in response to the ketone infusion. In parallel with this decrease of plasma alanine, urinary nitrogen excretion fell in fasted subjects given prolonged infusions of ketones. The urinary nitrogen excretion returned to basal levels after the cessation of the infusions.

In summary, it seems clear that ketones play a major regulatory role in the later phase of starvation in addition to their role as energy sources. Whereas in the early phase, the drop in insulin and increase in glucagon are key to the metabolic adaptations that occur, in the later phase, the ketone bodies play a dual role: on one hand, they represent a major energy substrate; on the other hand, they also play a major regulatory role in the metabolic adaptation, particularly in depressing gluconeogenesis as well as skeletal muscle glycolysis. The utilization of ketones by the brain during starvation has been discussed earlier in this chapter.

Whole-Body Protein Turnover

Golden and associates [141,142] found that whole-body protein synthesis and breakdown were each reduced about 40% in seriously malnourished children. These values increased above normal during the period of rapid weight gain during refeeding (70% higher for synthesis, 50% higher for degradation) and then returned to normal when the children had recovered (Figure 20-19). Millward [143] has pointed out that the average protein turnover rate of the lean tissue present in the malnourished children may not have been markedly depressed, but no measurements of lean body mass were made by Golden and his colleagues.

In the last decade, there have been a number of reports of studies of intermediary metabolism during fasting of healthy young adults using isotopically labeled tracers [27,28,86–89,144–150], which in general confirm and extend the findings already described. For example, Carlson et al. [27] have recently reported what they believe to be the first study examining simultaneous changes in carbohydrate, fat, and protein metabolism and caloric expenditure in six healthy young men 12 and 60 hours after fasting. Using labeled glucose, glycerol, palmitate, and leucine as isotopic tracers and indirect calorimetry, they found plasma glucose, hepatic glucose output, and glucose oxidation decreased significantly at 60 hours, while lipolysis, primary (intra-adipocyte) free fatty acid (FFA) reesterification, glucose disposal by nonoxidative pathways, provision of glycerol for gluconeogenesis, proteolysis, and protein and fat oxidation increased; there was a concomitant decrease in RQ. Contrary to some other studies [148] that reported an early decrease in metabolic rate, no change was observed by Carlson and colleagues. Nonoxidative leucine disposal increased, suggesting an increase in protein synthesis. As anticipated from reports by others, plasma insulin and C-peptide concentrations decreased, while plasma glucagon, epinephrine, norepinephrine, and growth hormone increased, contributing to the increased lipolysis and FFA mobilization. Plasma cortisol concentration was unchanged; others have reported an increase in plasma cortisol concentration after 72 hours fasting [44]. Carlson and colleagues [27] suggest that the increased FFA reesterification may result from the increase in plasma FFAs or possibly from increased β-adrenergic stimulation.

Earlier, Nair and associates [148], using labeled glucose and leucine and indirect calorimetry, had found in a similar but somewhat more limited study that young healthy men starved for three days showed an increase in leucine flux and oxida-

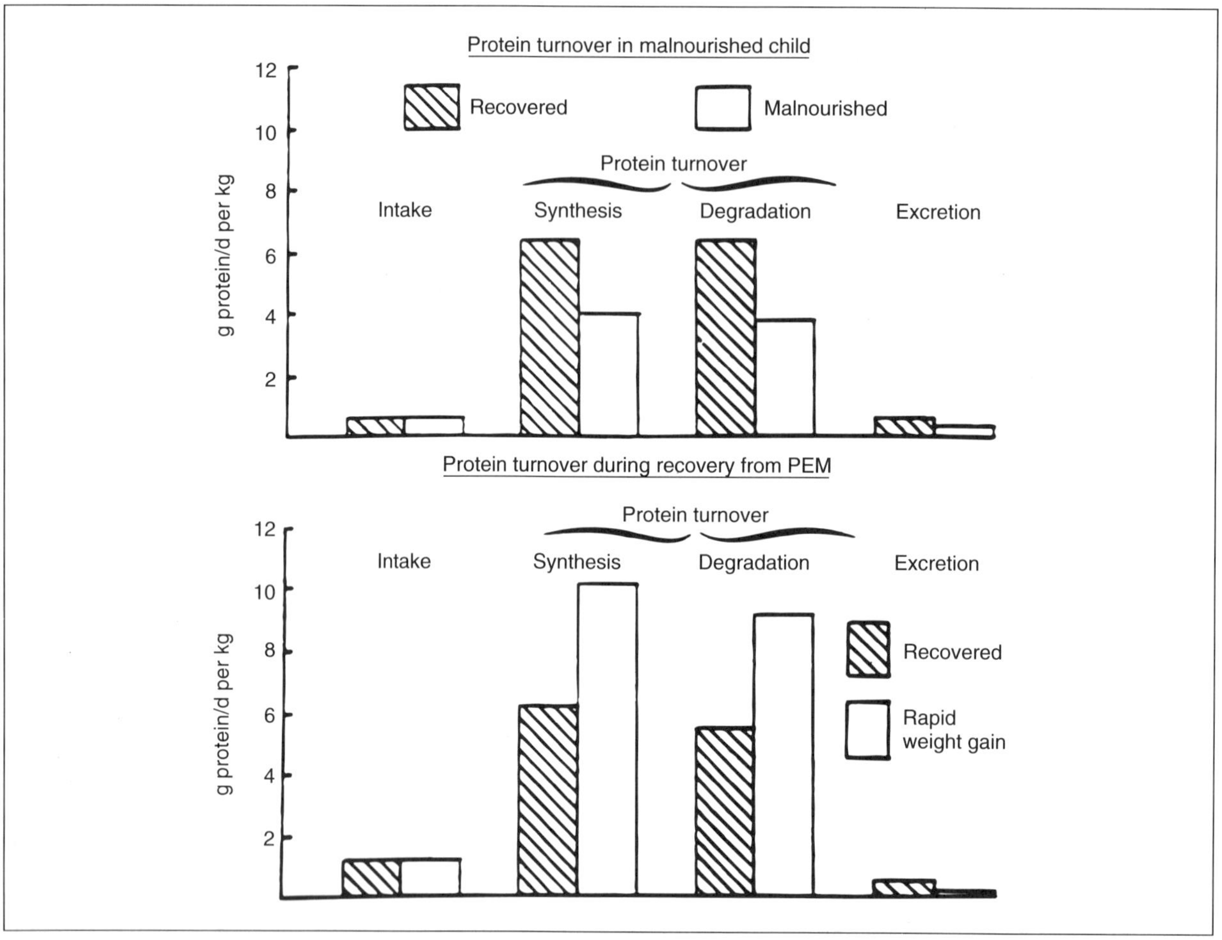

Figure 20-19. Whole-body protein turnover in malnourished, recovering, and recovered children. (From DJ Millward. Protein deficiency, starvation and protein metabolism. *Proc Nutr Soc* 38:77, 1979.)

tion, a decline in glucose production and oxidation, and an increase in fat oxidation; resting metabolic rate decreased (8%). Plasma concentrations of glutamate, serine, alanine, glycine, threonine, arginine, and tyrosine decreased while leucine and valine increased. Plasma concentrations of testosterone, insulin, and tri-iodothyronine decreased while plasma glucagon concentration increased.

Tsalikian et al. [149], using labeled leucine, also found leucine flux increased after a 30-hour fast by six healthy young adults and concluded that this reflected *increased* proteolysis. In a more extensive study, Frexes-Steed and associates [145], using labeled leucine, bicarbonate, and insulin, found in young healthy men starved for four days increased rates of leucine appearance and oxidation but no change in the rates of nonoxidative disappearance of leucine (in contrast to the findings of Carlson and colleagues after a three-day fast). Frexes-Steed and her colleagues found that elevated branched-chain (and other) amino acids were required to restore tissue sensitivity to the effects of administered insulin on protein metabolism after the four-day fast. Others have reported increases in plasma concentrations of branched-chain amino acids (leucine, valine) and decreases in a number of other amino acids [115,132].

Fryburg and colleagues [146], using labeled phenylalanine and leucine, reported in the same year that in short-term (12 and 60 hours) fasted young men and women, muscle (forearm) amino acid output accelerated due to increased proteolysis, not reduced protein synthesis. In contrast to a marked impairment in insulin-mediated glucose disposal, muscle remained sensitive to insulin's antiproteolytic action.

Using labeled glucose, Clore et al. [151] found that nocturnal modulation of hepatic glucose output (HGO) occurred in normal men during an overnight fast when glycogenolysis accounts for about 70% of hepatic glucose output and plasma concentrations of glycerol and FFA are diminished. In contrast, after a 72-hour fast, nocturnal modulation of HGO did not occur; at this time plasma FFA and glycerol concentrations were elevated, and gluconeogenesis, not glycogenolysis, predominated. They suggested that this supports a role of FFA and/or glycerol in the modulation of HGO after an overnight fast. Others have found that glycerol release provides substrate for gluconeogenesis (20% to 25% of hepatic glucose production).

Mansell and Macdonald [147], utilizing a hyperinsulinemic glucose clamp technique, found in six healthy young men subjected to a 48-hour fast that oxidative glucose disposal (consistent with relative insulin resistance) and glucose uptake by forearm muscles were decreased, but that the whole-body nonoxidative rate of glucose disposal was unchanged. The thermogenic response to infused glucose was decreased.

Wolfe and associates [150], using labeled palmitate and D-5 glycerol, had found that the rate of appearance of FFA and glycerol increased markedly after an 87-hour fast by healthy young men and that there was an increased lipolytic response to epinephrine, which they felt may have been due to an enhancement of fatty acid-triglyceride cycling. In a subsequent study, Klein and associates from this same laboratory [152] found that although β-adrenergic stimulation contributed to fat mobilization (lipolysis) in a 12-hour and 84-hour fast of healthy young men, other mechanism(s) can increase lipolysis and triglyceride-fatty acid cycling when β-adrenergic receptors are continuously blocked by propranolol infusions.

In healthy young men fasted overnight, Nurjhan and colleagues [153] found that lipolysis suppression by insulin is more sensitive than the suppression of hepatic glucose production. Jensen et al. [154], using labeled palmitate, found in young healthy subjects studied after 14 hours and 84 hours of fasting that the suppression of lipolysis by insulin during fasting was relatively less than was the stimulation of lipolysis by epinephrine. They point out that increased adipocyte sensitivity to β-adrenergic stimulation, along with decrements in insulin and increments in epinephrine plasma concentrations, may facilitate FFA mobilization during fasting.

Elia et al. [155] found that while the activity of the triglyceride-fatty acid cycle had increased considerably after a four-day fast in healthy young men, the energy expended in driving the cycle, although elevated six-fold, nevertheless accounted for only a small proportion (about 2.5%) of the total energy expenditure; total resting energy expenditure had dropped slightly (about 5%) but significantly, while the energy derived from fat oxidation had increased (about 25%); as a result, the RQ had dropped significantly from 0.80 to 0.69.

Jensen and colleagues [154], using labeled palmitate, determined palmitate flux isotopically before and during epinephrine infusion under conditions of constant plasma glucose and hormone concentrations (pancreatic clamp) in healthy young adults after 14 hours and 84 hours fast. They found that palmitate flux was greater after 84 hours of starvation, although there was little change in plasma concentrations of insulin, glucagon, growth hormone, cortisol, epinephrine, norepinephrine, and glucose. The lipolytic response to epinephrine was also greater at 84 hours. Jensen et al. concluded that lipolysis during fasting is less completely suppressed by insulin and more readily stimulated by epinephrine.

Lowell and Goodman [156] concluded from studies in fasted rats that lipid fuels may directly modulate protein metabolism in muscle during prolonged starvation and may prevent a rise in catabolic hormones. They also thought that the data indicated that free fatty acids may directly attenuate the breakdown of myofibrillar proteins in muscle during prolonged starvation and that this may be unrelated to their oxidation.

There are minimal data in humans as to changes in protein turnover of individual organs and tissues. Interpretation of changes in whole-body protein turnover during starvation poses problems similar to those we have already mentioned regarding interpretation of the changes in whole-body metabolic rate during starvation.

Albumin Synthesis and Catabolism

A consistent change during starvation is a lowering of the serum albumim level. This change reflects a decreased rate of albumin synthesis, which occurs early (one to two days) in starved rats and continues to fall, but at a slowed rate, dropping to about 20% to normal. This decrease is paralleled by a decreased ability of liver microsomes (ribosomes) from fasted rats to incorporate amino acids into protein [157].

However, James and Hay [158] observed in undernourished children that following an immediate drop in albumin synthesis there is a subsequent drop in albumin turnover as well. These changes result in albumin turnover rates 36% below baseline, but enable preservation of serum levels at only 7% below normal [159]. In humans, a decrease in serum albumin level occurs slowly during food deprivation; Keys et al. [16] found little change in serum albumin in volunteer men semistarved for as long as six months. [*Editor's Note:* One aspect of albumin metabolism missing from this equation is the percentage of albumin that is extravascular, as this in large part determines the degradative rate, and indirectly the serum albumin concentration. In many situations, serum albumin concentrations do not reflect albumin synthesis.]

The isolated perfused livers of starved rats also show lower rates of synthesis of fibrinogen, α_1 acid glycoprotein, α_2 acute-phase globulin, and haptoglobulin. Albumin catabolism of rats slows late in starvation but not proportionately to the slowing of its synthesis, as a result of which serum albumin falls.

Endocrine System

The thesis that starvation causes significant metabolic and physiologic changes, which enable the organism to better withstand food deprivation, is exemplified by the neuro-endocrinologic adaptations that occur in starvation. Hormonal adaptations occur hand in hand with other metabolic adaptations to starvation, for example, modified activities of certain enzymes. The degree to which the metabolic changes initiate and influence the hormonal modifications and the degree to which the hormonal changes initiate and influence the metabolic modifications have not been fully clarified. What is clear, however, is that the hormonal adaptations facilitate the organism's adaptation to food deprivation.

Almost all hormones are involved in the responses to food deprivation [160]. Major changes in insulin, glucagon, growth hormone, catecholamines, thyroid hormones, glucocorticoids, and antidiuretic hormone (among others) occur, and these

Table 20-5. Hormone Levels in Blood Before and During Starvation

Hormone	2 Days Before Starvation	Days of Starvation		
		3	7	14
Adrenaline (ng/ml)	0.29 ± 0.06	2.81 ± 0.26	4.05 ± 0.41	5.86 ± 0.55
Noradrenaline (ng/ml)	1.03 ± 0.10	0	0	0
ACTH (pg/ml)	48.24 ± 2.51	85.96 ± 8.94	96.31 ± 9.03	79.08 ± 6.82
β-Endorphine (pg/ml)	42.51 ± 2.36	76.03 ± 6.15	93.05 ± 9.61	87.31 ± 9.06
Cortisol (μg/dl)[a]	10.43 ± 0.54	15.10 ± 0.66	19.81 ± 0.93	18.02 ± 0.91
Cortisol (μg/dl)[b]	6.65 ± 0.62	11.29 ± 1.07	13.04 ± 1.26	15.01 ± 1.32
Aldosterone (pg/ml)	112.0 ± 4.3	146.1 ± 5.4	198.5 ± 8.1	189.9 ± 7.8
TSH (ng/ml)	4.22 ± 0.39	4.45 ± 0.43[c]	3.24 ± 0.41	3.06 ± 0.42
T_4 (μg/ml)	8.05 ± 0.72	7.53 ± 0.64[c]	6.22 ± 0.61	5.37 ± 0.59
T_3 (ng/dl)	178.0 ± 12.6	121.2 ± 10.3	93.6 ± 9.1	85.8 ± 9.0
T_3 (ng/dl)	231.1 ± 15.0	275.4 ± 16.2	386.2 ± 18.5	337.1 ± 19.4
STH (ng/ml)[a]	3.22 ± 0.26	11.88 ± 0.92	12.34 ± 1.01	10.05 ± 0.97
STH (ng/ml)[b]	2.29 ± 0.54	5.52 ± 0.63	6.01 ± 0.78	6.12 ± 0.85
Prolactin (ng/ml)	12.95 ± 0.92	6.04 ± 0.73	7.14 ± 0.81	4.87 ± 0.59
Insulin (μU/ml)[a]	18.82 ± 1.03	11.54 ± 0.94	10.03 ± 0.89	9.14 ± 0.95
Insulin (μU/ml)[b]	22.06 ± 2.09	14.32 ± 1.76	11.28 ± 1.33	10.56 ± 1.31
C-peptide (ng/ml)	2.71 ± 0.33	1.31 ± 0.25	1.35 ± 0.24	1.17 ± 0.21
Glucagon (pg/ml)	132.5 ± 9.6	188.4 ± 14.1	235.9 ± 16.3	216.7 ± 15.0
FSH (ng/ml)	1.29 ± 0.11	0.63 ± 0.07	0.65 ± 0.07	0.54 ± 0.05
LH (ng/ml)	2.18 ± 0.19	2.35 ± 0.24[c]	2.72 ± 0.26	1.63 ± 0.20
Testosterone (ng/ml)	7.47 ± 0.31	5.02 ± 0.49	4.26 ± 0.45	3.48 ± 0.56
Prostaglandin A+E (ng/ml)	3.02 ± 0.46	2.76 ± 0.38[c]	1.23 ± 0.24	1.01 ± 0.22
Prostaglandin $F_{2\alpha}$ (ng/ml)	0.78 ± 0.15	0.71 ± 0.16[c]	0.34 ± 0.10	0.26 ± 0.09
Histamine (μg/dl)	12.65 ± 0.84	8.03 ± 0.65	7.16 ± 0.61	6.78 ± 0.59
Acetylcholine (μg/dl)	1.02 ± 0.11	0.89 ± 0.10[c]	2.55 ± 0.22	3.34 ± 0.46
c-AMP (pM/ml)	15.04 ± 1.43	39.61 ± 3.24	50.56 ± 3.57	48.82 ± 3.65
c-GMP (pM/ml)	4.21 ± 0.52	6.58 ± 0.73	12.29 ± 1.15	11.87 ± 1.16
c-AMP/c-GMP ratio	3.58	6.03	4.13	4.12

[a]morning values; [b]cumulative values; [c]$p < 0.05$ compared with prestarvation level.

Source: VS Gorozhanin, VV Lobkov. Hormonal and metabolic reactions in the human body during prolonged starvation. *Kosmicheskaia Biologiia i Aviakosmicheskaia Meditsina* 24:47, 1990.

are reflected in the alterations in carbohydrate, protein, fat, water, and electrolyte metabolism.

By far the most comprehensive, but still not complete study of hormonal changes during a two-week period of starvation of 14 male volunteers (25 to 29 years of age) was reported in 1990 by Gorozhanin and Lobkov [160], whose data appear in Tables 20-5 and 20-6. The following is an English translation of their description of their findings, kindly provided by Dr. J. Rozga of the Cedars-Sinai Hospital in Los Angeles:

By day 3, there was a 10-fold increase in the blood level of adrenaline, a sharp rise in ACTH, β-endorphins and in the cumulative concentrations of cortisol and STH, aldosterone, glucagon, c-AMP, c-GMP, the c-AMP/c-GMP ratio, FFA and lactate. By day 7 and 14, there was a further statistically significant increase in the blood levels of adrenaline, the morning and cumulative concentrations of cortisol and STH, aldosterone, c-AMP, c-GMP, FFA. At the same time, the blood levels of ACTH, β-endorphin and lactate showed no significant changes. In contrast, the plasma levels of T3, prolactin, insulin (both morning and cumulative values), c-peptide, FSH, testosterone, histamine, glucose, and pH were found to be significantly lower on the 3rd day and dropped even further on the 7th and 14th day of starvation. Plasma concentrations of thyrotropic hormone, T4, PgA and E, and PgF2A were significantly lower on day 7 and 14 whereas rev-T3 was high at all time points during starvation. Plasma levels of LH were high on day 7 and low on day 14 while plasma levels of noradrenaline were below the detectable levels throughout the starvation period. Acetylcholine was increased 2.5× and 3.3× on days 7 and 14 respectively.

Urinary excretion of adrenaline gradually increased throughout the starvation period. Urinary excretions of noradrenaline and dopamine were markedly increased on day 3 but on day 4 and 14 they were at the pre-starvation levels. From day 7 on, there was a statistically significant decrease in urinary excretion of normetanephrine and of both HVA and VMA acids. Excretion of metanephrine was increased during starvation at all time points studied.

During starvation, elevated plasma and urinary concentrations of adrenaline, undetectable levels of plasma noradrenaline and increased adrenal cortex activity (ACTH and β-endorphin) reflected a strong stimulation of both adrenal-sympathetic and hypophysis-adrenal systems. Accordingly, the metanephrine:adrenaline and normetanephrine:noradrenaline ratios went rapidly down during starvation. Thus, by the end of starvation, there was a 3× decrease in metanephrine: adrenaline ratio. . . . These data suggest that o-methylation of both adrenaline and noradrenaline were markedly reduced because of an inhibitory effect of elevated ACTH and cortisol on the activity of catechol-methyl-transferase, and because hormones stimulating this enzyme (e.g., thyrotropic hormone, T3, T4, testosterone) were all decreased. A 2× decrease in urinary excretion of HVA (metabolite of dopamine, noradrenaline, and VMA) and VMA (metabolite of adrenaline and noradrenaline) together with excessive production of adrenaline, appear to suggest that elevated ACTH and cortisol inhibited mono-amine-oxidase activity as well. As a result of these interactions, the sympathetic-adrenal system during starvation was characterized not only by an excessive production of adrenaline and suppression of noradrenaline, but also by the catabolism of adrenaline, noradrenaline, dopamine and suppression of o-methylation and deamination of these compounds. This, in turn, might have led to shifting to other metabolic pathways such as chinoid oxidation, N-acetylation, demethylation, and dehydroxylation.

More detail and a description of the findings of a number of other investigators about hormonal changes during starvation follows.

Table 20-6. Urinary Excretions Before and During Starvation

Hormone	2 Days Before Starvation	Days of Starvation 3	7	14
Adrenaline (μg/24 hr)	8.81 ± 2.02	25.56 ± 4.09	31.04 ± 5.22	33.61 ± 6.12
Noradrenaline (μg/24 hr)	20.16 ± 3.51	18.34 ± 4.28*	18.87 ± 5.03*	16.58 ± 3.25*
Dopamine (μg/24 hr)	231.0 ± 20.9	348.1 ± 37.4	287.5 ± 24.4*	229.0 ± 32.6*
DOPA (μg/24 hr)	33.62 ± 4.15	38.73 ± 4.86*	26.07 ± 4.12*	39.61 ± 5.29*
Metanephrine (μg/24 hr)	123.4 ± 11.2	176.0 ± 13.1	201.6 ± 18.4	185.5 ± 16.3
Normetanephrine (μg/24 hr)	27.81 ± 5.43	23.04 ± 4.63*	14.33 ± 2.95	15.76 ± 2.42
Homovanillic acid (mg/24 hr)	2.15 ± 0.19	1.91 ± 0.17*	1.24 ± 0.16	1.19 ± 0.14
Vanilmandelic acid (mg/24 hr)	3.06 ± 0.22	2.88 ± 0.24*	1.51 ± 0.20	1.55 ± 0.22
Metanephrine-adrenaline ratio	14.02	7.03	6.48	5.52
Normetanephrine-noradrenaline ratio	1.39	1.26	0.91	0.95
Glucose (mg/dl)	89.4 ± 2.4	72.1 ± 2.6	58.6 ± 1.7	51.5 ± 1.8
Free fatty acids (mg/dl)	561.0 ± 25.5	1123 ± 38.9	1288 ± 40.1	1426 ± 41.9
pH	7.39 ± 0.02	7.27 ± 0.01	7.29 ± 0.02	7.30 ± 0.01
Lactate (mg/dl)	12.06 ± 1.11	19.51 ± 1.64	23.14 ± 1.58	21.82 ± 1.45

*$p < 0.05$ compared with prestarvation level.

Source: VS Gorozhanin, VV Lobkov. Hormonal and metabolic reactions in the human body during prolonged starvation. *Kosmicheskaia Biologiia i Aviakosmicheskaia Meditsina* 24:47, 1990.

Insulin

A key metabolic initiator of the hormonal changes is the early fall in blood sugar, which is followed by a variety of responses to maintain glucose homeostasis. Insulin secretion is decreased promptly, while glucagon, growth hormone, and possibly catecholamine secretions are increased and liver glycogenolysis is accelerated. At this early time, there is little change in circulating T_4 but a beginning decrease in circulating T_3 with an increase in rT_3 and free cortisol.

As a result of the early hormonal responses, glucose production is increased, but as starvation goes on, the rate of glucose utilization outstrips its production. Blood sugar drops somewhat further, and serum insulin continues diminished. The lowered serum insulin reduces glucose uptake by skeletal muscle and adipose tissue, promotes amino acid mobilization from muscle, and increases hepatic gluconeogenesis. The production of glucose is thereby enhanced, providing the glucose required by the brain and other glucose-using cells and tissues. Among the potential gluconeogenic precursors, only amino acids are hormonally dependent with regard to hepatic influx.

Lipolysis increases in starvation. It proceeds under the control of a number of lipases, one or more of which are under hormonal control. The functions of insulin in the inhibition, and of catecholamines, growth hormone, and glucagon in the stimulation, of lipolysis play major physiologic regulatory roles.

Insulin plays a major role in amino acid metabolism. It has long been known that insulin lowers plasma amino acid concentration and that the skeletal muscle is the main site of the insulin-mediated increased tissue amino acid uptake [161]. The in vitro sensitivity of skeletal muscle of rats to physiologic concentrations of insulin is enhanced during starvation (glucose uptake, glucose utilization, transport of α-aminoisobutyric acid) [56,162]. Splanchnic uptake of alanine and other gluconeogenic amino acids is increased by glucagon, cortisol, and growth hormone by mechanisms still undefined. Notable is the finding that insulin does not affect plasma levels of alanine in the peripheral blood or its release by muscle, but it does decrease the splanchnic uptake of alanine by 30% to 75% [111] and inhibits the incorporation of ^{14}C alanine into glucose in the perfused liver [163]. Thus, amino acid gluconeogenesis, occurring in the initial phases of food deprivation, is facilitated by the decreased plasma insulin levels.

In humans, the plasma immunoreactive insulin levels after oral and intravenous glucose administration are subnormal in prolonged starvation and in protein-calorie malnutrition ("starvation diabetes"). In the earliest phases of food deprivation, the lowered plasma insulin levels are believed to be a response to the moderate decrease in plasma glucose, and at this early time the release of insulin in response to a glucose load may be normal. In prolonged malnutrition, at least in experimental animals subjected to protein malnutrition, the diminished islet cell volume may explain the persistently low insulin levels and poor responses to glucose administration [84]; no direct damage could be observed to either A or B cells, although the B cells contained unusually pale granules, and there may be a reduction in islet size [164,165]. Evidence regarding the responsiveness of the islet B cells to glucose in starvation as assessed in vitro is unsettled [166–168].

Improved tolerance with closely spaced successive glucose loads is known as the Staub-Traugott effect. Abraira and Lawrence [169] have found that while a clear Staub-Traugott effect was shown in the fed state, this effect was conspicuously absent after long-term caloric deprivation of obese humans. Compared to the findings before fasting, insulin levels after prolonged caloric deficit were similar during the initial intravenous glucose challenge, but successive glucose loads failed to elicit incremental insulin rises, in keeping with earlier suggestions from their laboratory that distinct mechanisms mediate the insulin-initiating and potentiating actions of glucose. After starvation there was greater suppression of plasma free fatty acids and immunoreactive glucagon levels. Absence of the Staub-Traugott effect after fasting would, in their view, appear to reflect a failure of nutrient induction of improved glucose metabolism, because alterations in glucoregulatory hormones and free fatty acids do not consistently explain the presence or absence of this phenomenon in the different metabolic states so far studied by them.

A close correlation has been noted between the lowered levels of serum potassium and serum insulin in protein-calorie malnutrition. The insulin response to oral or intravenous loading of glucose is markedly improved by giving large amounts of potassium during refeeding [48,170]. When insulin was infused intravenously into obese subjects before and after a 48-hour fast and blood glucose levels were maintained by variable glucose infusion, increases in the suppression of C-peptide were observed after the 48-hour fast, but alpha cell suppression assessed by plasma glucagon levels was unchanged [171]. The author (Brodows) concluded that starvation enhances the ability of insulin to inhibit its own secretions and that this may be a physiologically important mechanism for adapting to food deprivation.

Glucagon

The role of glucagon in the early and late phases of starvation is still not fully understood. Plasma glucagon levels rise in the early phases of starvation [172]. This increase appears to be secondary to a decreased rate of glucagon clearance rather than to pancreatic hypersecretion [173]. During prolonged fasting (three to four weeks), plasma glucagon values fall to prefast levels as a consequence of reduced pancreatic secretion, despite a progressive decline in glucagon clearance.

Glucagon is a glucogenic hormone, and in the phase of maximal gluconeogenesis, it can lead to increased glucose levels by facilitating amino acid release from muscle and uptake by liver. Injected in pharmacologic doses, glucagon decreases the circulating levels of most amino acids, but its strongest effect is on alanine [25]. This decrease of the plasma amino acids occurs in parallel with an increased amino acid uptake by the splanchnic bed, especially for alanine [174,175]. Glucagon's glucogenic action is also demonstrated by the fact that it increases the negative nitrogen balance in fasted subjects [176].

In the perfused liver, glucagon increases the conversion of alanine to glucose [177]. A stimulatory effect on cellular uptake and utilization of glucogenic amino acids, particularly alanine, also has been demonstrated. Karl et al. [178], using the in vitro epitrochlaris muscle preparation, found that 10^{-6} and 10^{-8}M concentrations of glucagon had no effect on the amino acid release from the muscle. Others have shown increased amino acid output from isolated muscle in response to glucagon at a concentration of 5×10^{-6}M [179].

When hepatic glycogen stores are intact, glucagon leads to a rise in plasma glucose by activating the adenylate cyclase system, which leads to increased phosphorylase activity and glycogen degradation. In fasting obese subjects, infusion of glucagon raises plasma glucose even after long-term fasting, by which time hepatic glycogen stores are depleted, and therefore some other mechanism(s) underlies its hyperglycemic effect [180]. Glucagon favors hepatic proteolysis, and this may provide substrates for glucogenesis and glycogenolysis.

Increased serum alanine and arginine stimulate glucagon secretion. Glucagon stimulates gluconeogenesis by stimulating the conversion of pyruvate to phosphoenolpyruvate (PEP) and increases the transport of alanine into hepatic cells. This results in a lesser fall in blood glucose and, thereby, lesser inhibition of insulin secretion. Increase in serum insulin in turn diminishes the breakdown of muscle protein and synthesis of alanine and slows gluconeogenesis. Thus, glucagon and insulin play essential roles in the cyclic interrelationships between alanine and glucose. The glucocorticoids appear to play a "permissive" role. During the period of maximal gluconeogenesis in starvation, glucagon appears to inhibit insulin secretion directly.

Glucagon also leads to increased lipolysis [172]. The major influence of glucagon on hepatic FFA metabolism appears to be the diversion of circulating FFA into the pathways of oxidation (ketone body and CO_2 formation) and away from esterification products. This indicates a special role for glucagon in the metabolic switch-over to ketone bodies as starvation proceeds.

Low circulating levels of glucagon have been reported in malnourished children with severe fasting hypoglycemia [181], and in such children glucagon administration causes a prompt rise in blood sugar levels [182]. Thus, hypoglycemia, a late occurrence in protein-calorie malnutrition, may be caused in part by decreased levels of circulating glucagon.

Walter et al. [183] have reported studies in human volunteers, results of which suggest that the augmented glucagon release in man during starvation or after hypoglycemia is not significantly regulated by signals from the adrenergic nervous system.

The relationship between glucagon levels and the natriuresis that occurs at the beginning of starvation in obese subjects has been studied by Saudek et al. [184]. Both the rise in glucagon levels and the natriuresis reach their maxima on the fourth day of starvation. Both are suppressed by glucose and both start to decline by the fifth day. By the seventh day, a time when sodium balance is achieved, plasma glucagon levels have fallen to normal baseline levels. A direct action of glucagon on the kidney has been demonstrated [185].

Growth Hormone

Campbell et al. [144] have shown that severe reduction in food intake by rats decreases the release of at least five anterior pituitary hormones (GH, TSH, FSH, LH, prolactin). They suggest that this is due primarily to reduced hypothalamic stimulation rather than a reduced ability of the pituitary to secrete hormones. In five healthy women subjected to a three-week fast, half of the dexamethasome suppression tests showed decreased suppression [186].

Prior to the availability of radioimmunoassay

techniques, growth hormone (GH) secretion was thought to be diminished in malnutrition, but recent studies in starving obese subjects have shown that the circulating GH levels increased between the third and tenth day of fasting; later, between days 10 and 38, there was a steady decline in circulating GH levels to well below 50% of the starting values [21]. In normal men subjected to fasting, serum GH levels also increased (three- to fivefold) during days 3 to 5; the values returned to prefast values by the ninth day of fasting [187]. In normal women, the early increases in serum GH during the first few days were more modest (one- to threefold) [188,189]. The elevated growth hormone levels early in starvation may have a diabetogenic effect.

In prolonged protein-calorie malnutrition, Smith et al. [190] found plasma GH levels elevated (fivefold). Despite this elevation, arginine infusion led to significant rises in plasma GH; glucose infusion caused rapid and significant falls in the plasma GH levels. Plasma GH levels are elevated also in children with kwashiorkor or marasmus; marasmic children generally have lower GH levels than those suffering from kwashiorkor [191]. Marasmic children in general showed no increases in GH secretion in response to arginine [192] or to insulin hypoglycemia, and the elevated plasma GH levels in marasmus and kwashiorkor were not suppressed by intravenous or oral glucose [193,194] but did drop following the oral administration of a mixture of the dietary essential amino acids [195]. Tannenbaum and colleagues [196] found that circulating SRIF is a physiologic regulator of starvation-induced GH suppression in rats but is not involved in mediating the inhibition of insulin.

Inverse correlations between (1) plasma GH and plasma albumin levels and (2) plasma GH and plasma alanine and valine levels have been observed in children with marasmus and kwashiorkor [197]. The strong relationship between the degree of body protein depletion and plasma GH levels is demonstrated further by the finding that high-protein refeeding produces a marked drop in plasma GH levels in malnourished children [191].

Administration of human GH on alternate days, for 12 days, to fasting obese women led to increases in sodium and potassium urinary excretion, with no increase in ketoacidosis [198]. In contrast, Felig et al. [24] showed that administration of GH to obese males and females fasting for five to six weeks led to rises in serum free fatty acids, glycerol, and β-hydroxybutyrate plus acetoacetate. This was accompanied by a two- to threefold increase in plasma insulin. Urinary potassium and ketone excretion also increased significantly. There was no reduction in urinary total nonprotein nitrogen excretion. However, urinary urea excretion decreased, probably secondary to a reduction of protein catabolic processes, whereas urinary ammonia excretion increased, probably as a compensatory renal mechanism to the increased ketonemia.

GH secretion is stimulated by stress or injury. GH stimulates free fatty acid release by increasing lipolysis. Wilmore and colleagues have shown more recently that GH given to patients undergoing major elective surgery and receiving hypocaloric nutritional support lowers urinary nitrogen excretion and reduces the postoperative muscle weakness [199].

Low serum somatomedin levels have been found in children with kwashiorkor, most of whom had high serum GH levels [200]. Work with rats had already shown that serum somatomedin levels are reduced in starvation [201,202]. These findings suggest the possibility of a block in somatomedin formation in starvation. Although the somatomedins were thought initially to be dependent only on growth hormone, it now seems likely that they are regulated by insulin as well [203,204].

Plasma heat-labile inhibitors of somatomedin activity have been found in starvation, both in experimental animals and in humans [205–207]. If such inhibitors have specific effects, it raises the possibility that selective control over certain aspects of GH activity with survival benefit may exist in starvation; thus, as a compensatory mechanism, GH might influence some metabolic events, for example, lipolysis, in preference to others, for example, growth, when protein stores are being depleted.

Somatomedins and somatomedin inhibitors are produced largely by the liver, though the kidney may also produce somatomedins.

Thyroid

As noted earlier, the basal metabolic rate falls during starvation in contrast to the rise following injury, and the decrease in metabolic rate as starvation progresses is proportionately greater than the loss of weight. These observations have prompted many studies of the thyroid and thyroid hormones in both conditions.

Plasma TSH levels have been variously reported as low, normal, or high in malnourished children [208,209]. These varying results may be due to demographic factors related to nutritional and socioeconomic backgrounds or to differences in the radioimmunoassay techniques used. Diminutions of protein-bound iodine in the blood, butanol extractable iodine, and total thyroxine have been reported in infantile malnutrition. These decreases are parallel to, and may be related to, a reduction in the plasma levels of thyroxine-binding protein and pre-albumin [208]. Free plasma T_4 levels were found normal or elevated in kwashiorkor and normal or low in marasmus [210]. Thyroid involution occurs during prolonged protein-calorie malnutrition, and thyroid fibrosis has been noted in severely malnourished children [211]. In adults, prolonged protein-calorie malnutrition led to serum TSH levels that are high when compared to normal American standards but that did not change with refeeding [212].

In normal fasting adults, serum TSH levels were unchanged after a 60-hour fast [189] but significantly decreased after 10 days of fasting [187]. The secretion of TSH remains sensitive to changes in serum thyroid hormone concentrations [213,214]. Short-term (two days) starvation of rats did not alter the hypothalamic content of TRH but did decrease pituitary TSH content and serum TSH concentration [215].

In healthy adults fasted for 60 hours, mildly elevated serum levels of free T_4 were found [188], whereas at 5 and 10 days, in normal males, serum T_4 was significantly decreased as were the serum total and free T_3 concentrations [187,214,215]. In a young woman lost in the snow and deprived of food for 18 days, serum T_3 was decreased, but serum T_4 was in the normal range [216]. In obese humans, modest increases in serum free T_4 were found after 4 weeks of starvation [217]. Chopra and Smith [212] studied adult men with protein-calorie malnutrition and found that plasma bound T_4 levels were normal, but free T_4 levels were elevated, and T_3 levels were low. Although plasma albumin and thyroxine-binding pre-albumin levels were decreased, the decrease in plasma T_3 was proportionately greater. The decrease in serum T_3 (total and free) has been confirmed in short-term starvation studies, both in normal and in obese humans [187,212,218,219]. The decrease in serum T_3 levels is associated with a reciprocal rise in reverse (r) T_3 (Figure 20-20) [187,190,212, 213,220].

The high serum T_4 and low T_3 levels may reflect low peripheral conversion of T_4 to T_3 [221,222], but studies on the degradation rates of either hormone have not been carried out. The decreased hepatic T_3 generation by the starved rat is associated with decreased NPSH (nonprotein sulfhydryl groups) but not with a decrease in the absolute quantity of the enzyme 5^1-deiodinase; provision of sulfhydryl groups restored hepatic T_3 generation to normal in vitro [214,215]. There is a decrease in hepatic nuclear T_3 receptors in starved rats, and the induction of the cytosolic enzyme, malic dehydrogenase, known to be inducible by thyroid hormones, is blocked in starvation. The mechanism(s) by which T_4 is converted to the poorly calorigenic rT_3 is not known completely. The increase of serum rT_3 concentrations during starvation appears to be due to both an increase in the rate of production of rT_3 and a decrease in the rate of degradation of rT_3 [223]. It is known that administration of corticoids to hypothyroid and hyperthyroid patients leads to increased production of rT_3 [224], thus implicating raised levels of corticoids during starvation as responsible, in part, for the rise of rT_3 production.

It has been suggested that the decrease in serum T_3 during starvation spares muscle protein. Karl et al. [178], using an in vivo epitrochlaris muscle preparation, found that added thyroxine increased by 200% the amount of alanine released by the muscle, a fact that may be relevant to the early gluconeogenic events during starvation. Administration of T_3 to humans fasted for three days enhanced protein catabolism, as indicated by a doubling of urinary urea excretion [213,225], and increased fat catabolism, as demonstrated by increases in circulating free fatty acid and ketone levels [225].

Returning to the question of whether the decrease in serum T_3 may be one of the mechanisms underlying the lowered metabolic rate in starvation, it should be noted that Wimpfheimer et al. [226] have found that the decrease in resting oxygen consumption induced by starvation occurs not only in euthyroid rats but also in hyperthyroid and hypothyroid rats treated with triiodothyronine. The effectiveness of triiodothyronine in raising metabolic rate was decreased when given to hypothyroid starved rats. It is clear that some factor(s) other than the plasma levels of the thyroid hormones influenced the changes in metabolic rate following starvation in these experiments.

L-dopa, a substrate for catecholamine synthesis, given to obese patients ingesting a hypocaloric, normal protein diet, prevented the usual decline in metabolic rate, increased plasma norepinephrine to normal, and increased plasma epinephrine to levels slightly above normal. The low serum T_3 levels did not change with the administration of L-dopa, but the usual increase of plasma rT_3 was largely prevented. These data indicate that the changes in metabolic rate and T_3 can be dissociated by giving a precursor of the catecholamines. The mechanisms for the metabolic adaptation to

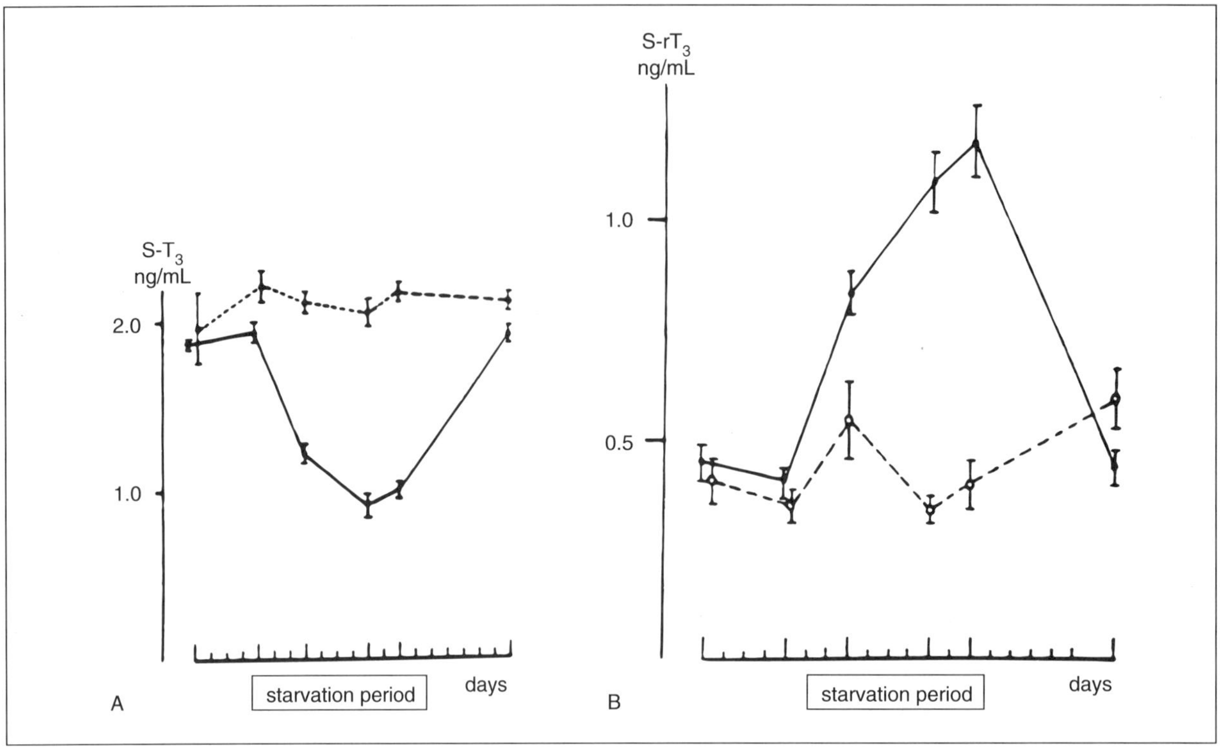

Figure 20-20. **(A)** Serum T_3 levels (mean ± SEM). **(B)** Serum rT_3 levels (mean ± SEM). ●----● = non-starved; ●——● = starved. (From J Palmblad, et al. Effects of total energy withdrawal [fasting] on the levels of growth hormone, thyrotropin, cortisol, adrenaline, noradrenaline, T_4, T_3, and r-T_3 in healthy males. *Acta Med Scand* 201:16, 1977.)

semistarvation may relate to an interplay of catecholamines and the thyroid hormones [227,228] (see under *Adrenal Medulla, Sympathetic Ganglia, Catecholamines* later in this chapter for additional discussion of the catecholamines).

Adrenal Cortex: Glucocorticoids

Data regarding histologic changes in the adrenals during starvation are conflicting. Thus, the adrenal gland has alternately been described as atrophic in infants with protein-calorie malnutrition [229] or as hyperplastic in pigs subjected to experimental protein deficiency for about one to three months [230].

Studies by Galvao-Teles et al. [231] of fasting obese humans show that rises in plasma-free cortisol and diminution of the day-night variation of these plasma levels occur. Fasting of humans of normal weight also led to increases in plasma cortisol levels; the highest levels were reached on the tenth day, the last day of the fast [187]. In a young woman lost in the snow and deprived of food for 18 days, decreased diurnal variations of serum cortisol levels were not observed [216]. In five healthy women subjected to a three-week fast, plasma cortisol level and half-life, and number and duration of cortisol secretory episodes increased [186].

There is a marked inverse correlation between plasma cortisol and albumin levels in children with protein-calorie malnutrition [197]. Thus, cortisol changed in the same direction as growth hormone in relation to serum albumin, that is, it increased as the albumin level fell.

Plasma cortisol is also elevated significantly in adults suffering from protein-calorie malnutrition; there were no significant changes in plasma ACTH [232]. Urinary free cortisol excretion was normal, but when corrections were carried out for the reduction in the creatinine clearance that occurs in starvation, free urinary cortisol excretion was elevated in protein-calorie malnutrition. Urinary 17-hydroxysteroids and 17-ketosteroids were markedly reduced.

It appears that the metabolism of cortisol is impaired in starved patients, resulting in low urinary excretion of its metabolites in the face of high circulating and high urinary excretion of free cortisol. Also, the pituitary-adrenal axis appears to be defective in its feedback control because normal response of the adrenal to ACTH persists while dexamethasone does not suppress plasma cortisol levels. In addition, normal secretion of

ACTH continues despite raised plasma cortisol levels. By contrast, lower response to ACTH, as measured by plasma cortisol levels, has been found in children with kwashiorkor [233]. Circulating cortisol-binding protein is also reported to be low in children with protein-calorie malnutrition.

In prolonged starvation, a pseudo-Cushingoid syndrome exists; ACTH and plasma cortisol levels are elevated simultaneously. Some of the immunologic abnormalities of starvation have been attributed to this, although during refeeding there is no correlation between the time of return to normal of the cortisol plasma-binding protein levels and, for example, the reversal of the decrease in complement levels.

As to how the changes in cortisol metabolism may affect the metabolic response to starvation, glucocorticoids generally have a glucogenic function. Glucocorticoids given to experimental animals decrease protein synthesis by skeletal muscle and lead to augmented hepatic uptake and utilization of amino acids by increasing gluconeogenesis [234]. In the eviscerated rat, cortisol administration leads to increased levels of plasma amino acids, implicating the skeletal muscle as their source [235]. An in vitro study by Karl et al. [178] of muscle obtained from rats given cortisone for three days showed an increased alanine release (145%) and decreased glutamine release (37%); tissue alanine level remained unchanged, whereas that of glutamine decreased by 30% to 60%. Administration of dexamethasone to obese and nonobese fasting humans led to a rise in plasma alanine, whereas the plasma levels of other amino acids remain unchanged [236]. In line with this are experimental in vivo studies showing that administration of hydrocortisone leads to increases in intracellular hepatic and skeletal muscle alanine, exceeding that of all other amino acids.

The crossing over of gluconeogenic intermediates between pyruvate and phosphoenolpyruvate (PEP) observed in intact starved rats was not seen in adrenalectomized rats with constant serum insulin levels. This supports the concept that during starvation glucocorticoids enhance the rate of glucose production by the liver by permitting hepatic cAMP to stimulate the yet undefined mechanism(s) that controls the substrate flow between pyruvate and PEP [237].

Of interest is the observation that glucocorticoid administration increases glucagon secretion, indicating a multifactorial hormonal drive for the gluconeogenesis of starvation. Owen and Cahill [238] showed in obese subjects that the proteolytic effect of glucocorticoids disappears in long-term starvation. This supports the strong correlation between the tissue protein changes and the hormonal adaptations that occur in starvation.

Adrenal Medulla, Sympathetic Ganglia, Catecholamines

The roles of the catecholamines (epinephrine, norepinephrine) in the early and, especially, the late phases of starvation unaccompanied by stress are still largely unknown. The plasma norepinephrine level has been reported to fall early during starvation, whereas the plasma epinephrine level does not change or may increase.

A recent study of healthy fasting men showed that the urinary levels of adrenaline (epinephrine) levels decreased modestly but significantly [178]. The epinephrine released early in fasting can induce liver glycogenolysis and also can activate muscle phosphorylase via a cAMP mechanism. This would lead to enhancement of glycolysis and, if intense enough, to the point where pyruvate and lactate become main end products and contribute to acidosis and an oxygen debt. The pyruvate and lactate released into the blood enter liver pathways for gluconeogenesis, as already noted.

Fasting is associated with decreased rates of norepinephrine turnover in the heart, as demonstrated by Young and Landsberg [168] in rats fasted for two days. The fast-related suppression of norepinephrine turnover in the heart was found to occur also in the liver, pancreas, and spleen. These investigators interpret their data as indicating decreased catecholamine activity during early fasting. We have already mentioned the possible role of the decreased catecholamines in the lowered metabolic rate of starving people. Healthy young subjects starved for two days showed slight but statistically significant ($p < 0.01$) increased metabolic rate (+3.6%), and when epinephrine was infused intravenously, there was a decreased rise in plasma epinephrine but an increase in heart rate and blood glycerol; that is, the chronotropic, lipolytic, and thermogenic effects of the infused epinephrine were increased, despite lower levels of plasma epinephrine [239,240].

In later stages of food deprivation (but not total starvation), Shoemaker and Wurtman [241] found reduced brain tissue levels of norepinephrine and dopamine in protein-malnourished rats. In a small number of marasmic children, low urinary levels of metanephrines have been reported [242], whereas in those with kwashiorkor, elevated epinephrine and low dopamine urinary excretion have been reported [243].

Much more work is needed in the area of catecholamine function in starvation. Their calorigenic function and their role in the release of polypeptide hormones and in the control of various metabolic substrates are of major importance.

Sex Hormones

There is a paucity of studies regarding the behavior of the sex hormones during starvation, particularly in humans. A few short-term studies have been carried out in animals. In terms of the hypothalamic control mechanism, total starvation for 7 days of normal and castrated male rats did not affect the hypothalamic content of LH-releasing hormone [244]. Starvation in male hamsters did not affect pituitary weight or pituitary LH content, but serum LH levels fell significantly, as did seminal vesicle and testicular weights; in female hamsters, starvation decreased pituitary weight, while pituitary LH content increased and serum LH content remained unchanged; female hamsters also demonstrated decreased uterine weight, but no change in ovarian weight [60]. Serum LH levels fell after 10 days, while pituitary LH levels increased after 20 days in female rats subjected to 50% food restriction. In male rats similarly semistarved, serum testosterone decreased at 20 days, but serum and pituitary FSH levels were not affected [245].

Fasting of prepubertal heifers led to a significant decrease in serum prolactin levels, without blunting the prolactin response to arginine [246]. Decreased serum prolactin levels were also observed in starving rats [247].

Renal Function: Urinary Electrolyte and Uric Acid Excretion

Increased urinary excretion of sodium, potassium, and magnesium begins promptly early in starvation and continues elevated, although at lower levels. In contrast to the changes in starvation per se, sodium excretion decreases promptly after injury, while potassium excretion increases.

The basis for the early changes in sodium, potassium, and magnesium excretion in starvation is not known completely, although catabolism of tissue proteins with concomitant loss of intracellular cations has been implicated. Early studies by Gamble and his colleagues [248] showed that feeding small amounts of glucose (50 to 100 g daily) early in starvation led promptly to decreased excretion of sodium and potassium (Figure 20-21). Feeding a calorically equivalent amount of fat may increase the natriuresis and kaliuresis. Later investigators showed that plasma aldosterone and renin concentrations increase early in starvation [249–252]. Feeding carbohydrates led (as previously observed by others) to decreased urinary sodium excretion, but to no change in plasma renin activity or aldosterone levels. Aldosterone infusion had only 40% of the antinatriuretic effect it achieved before the fast, indicating a state of aldosterone resistance at the nephron. These observations are complemented by earlier studies by Schloeder and Stinebaugh [253], which demonstrated that fasting leads to increases in V/GFR and C_{H2O}/v, but to decreases in C_{H2O}/GFR, all of these changes being reversible by carbohydrate feeding. These changes reflect both maximal and distal nephron dysfunction and may be responsible in part for the natriuresis and aldosterone resistance of fasting. We have already pointed out the relationship between sodium excretion and plasma glucagon levels during fasting [184].

In the later phases of fasting, it has been suggested that the increased urinary excretions of sodium and potassium are to buffer the increased urinary ketones. Studies conducted by Sigler [254] of fasting obese women maintained on a fixed sodium intake showed a close correlation among urinary $Na^+ + K^+ + NH_4^+$ and urinary organic acid anions and H_2PO_4. Ammonium excretion rose and Na^+ excretion fell as the fast proceeded. Urinary excretion of Na^+ was greater than that of Cl^-. Glucose feeding led to the expected decrease in Na^+ excretion, and this correlated with a decrease in urinary organic acid anions. These data were interpreted by Sigler as indicating that obligatory cation coverage of the metabolically generated anions is a major mechanism responsible for the fasting natriuresis.

The mechanism of the carbohydrate action on urinary Na^+ and K^+ excretion is not completely understood but may be related to its roughly parallel effects in lessening protein catabolism; it does not appear to be due to secondary effects on certain hormones (aldosterone, renin, insulin, glucagon, glucocorticoids, and catecholamines).

Plasma sodium levels remain fairly stable for a long time, despite the high urinary losses, while plasma potassium levels fall [255]. In prolonged starvation, intracellular K^+ and Mg^+ fall. A relationship between K^+ and Mg^+ is evidenced by the following: erythrocyte K^+ levels were 5% to 9% below normal in patients demonstrating decreased plasma Mg^{2+} levels; administration of Mg^{2+} corrected the low erythrocyte K^+ levels. These observations are interpreted as showing an effect of extracellular Mg^{2+} on the ATP-ase system associated with the cell membrane Na^+-K^+ transfer mechanism in prolonged starvation.

Administration of KCl, 0.5 mmol/kg/day, to obese subjects undergoing prolonged starvation

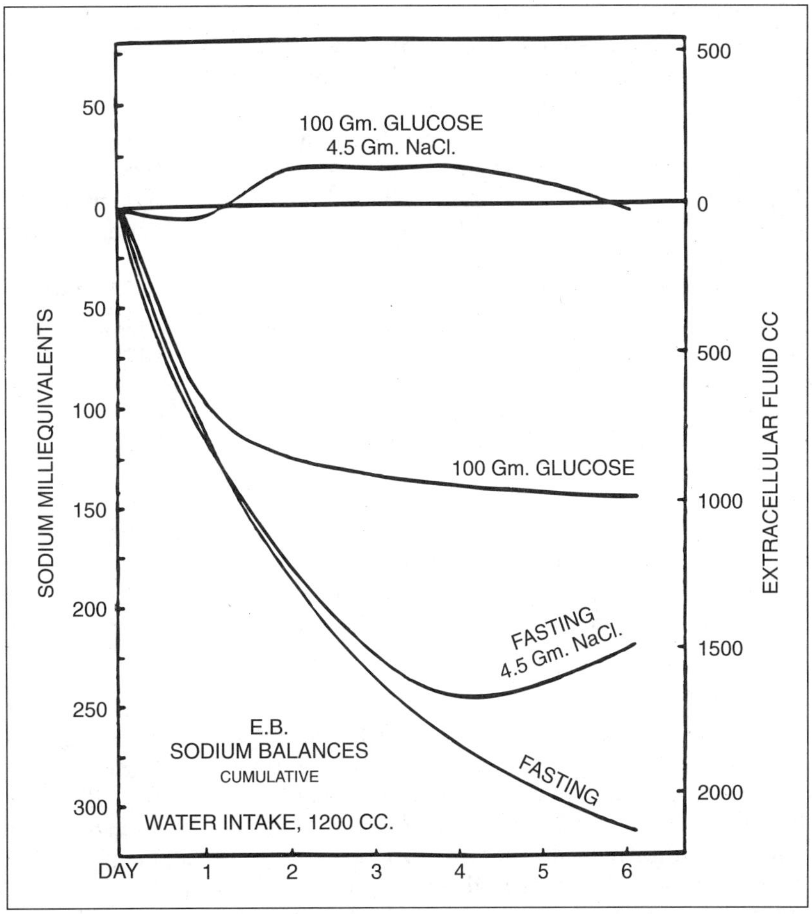

Figure 20-21. Cumulative sodium balances and water intake. (From JL Gamble. Physiological information gained from studies on life raft ration. *Harvey Lecture* 42:269, 1947.)

reduced daily urinary ammonium and β-hydroxybutyrate excretion by one-third, improved potassium balance, and increased chloride excretion [119]. Administration of $KHCO_3$, 0.5 mmol/kg/day, rather than KCl, led to a similar fall in ammonium excretion, but ketone body and bicarbonate excretion remained unchanged; potassium balance improved.

Urine pH fell significantly in both groups as the rate of excretion of urinary buffer (ammonium) decreased. The mechanism of the decrease in β-hydroxybutyrate excretion after potassium chloride administration is not apparent; however, because it was associated with increased chloride excretion, anion competition may be involved. When the $KHCO_3$ was increased to 1.5 to 2.0 mmol/kg/day, the urine was alkalinized, and ammonium excretion fell to negligible levels, resulting in nitrogen sparing of 2.0 g/day. Sapir et al. [117] interpret these findings as indicating that one-half of the increase in ammonium excretion observed in prolonged starvation is due to potassium deficiency. In their view, it is likely that nitrogen wastage caused by losses of urinary ammonium during starvation can be virtually eliminated by potassium supplementation and urinary alkalinization.

We have pointed out earlier in this chapter that potassium administration to fasting obese and nonobese subjects improves their glucose tolerance and leads to improved insulin secretion [170].

Sapir and Owen [118], in studies of fasting obese humans, found that there was no tubular maximal transport rate (reabsorption) for acetoacetate of β-hydroxybutyrate during the starvation ketonemia. They concluded that the reabsorption of ketones minimizes N loss (NH_4^+) and aids in maintaining ketonemia. Later, Reichard and colleagues [256] demonstrated a significant loss of acetone via expired air in starvation. This results in a significant saving of fixed base and NH_4^+.

Calcium and Phosphorus: Bone Hydroxyproline

Serum calcium levels fall gradually during starvation, reflecting a reduction in serum albumin and magnesium deficiency. The effect appears to be mediated by way of parathormone (secretion and/or tissue responsiveness). Fecal calcium is low because the amount of feces excreted is small (except late, when diarrhea may occur). Urinary calcium continues fairly high during starvation. The greatest urinary calcium excretion occurs when metabolic acidosis is well established. Significant loss of phosphate also occurs; the decrease in the ability of the kidney in starvation to excrete titratable acids is due in large measure to phosphate deficiency; administration of phosphate corrects this dysfunction.

Bone is the major source of the excreted calcium and phosphorus, but the relative loss of bone mass is less than that of many organs and tissues in starvation; significant osteomalacia is not seen except after prolonged starvation. Urinary hydroxyproline excretion increases during starvation, presumably reflecting collagenolysis of bone collagen and collagenolysis of subcutaneous supporting tissue as storage fat is catabolized.

Uric Acid

One of the characteristic biochemical changes in starvation is a rise in serum uric acid consequent to a decreased urinary excretion of uric acid. This latter is due primarily to a "blocking" effect (competitive inhibition) of uric acid tubular secretion by the increased serum and urinary levels of β-hydroxybutyrate, acetoacetate, and other keto or hydroxy acids; it may also be due to the low levels of urea in the glomerular filtrate.

Some Organ Changes in Starvation

Kidneys

The kidneys maintain function for a long time during starvation, despite their high metabolic requirement. Their continued function is possible because of their high blood supply (about 20% of cardiac output) and their ability to metabolize amino acids, lactate, pyruvate, glycerol, fatty acids, and β-hydroxybutyrate efficiently. Garcia-Salguero and Lupianez [257,258] found an increase in gluconeogenic flux in renal proximal tubules isolated from rats starved 16 to 48 hours, while in the distal tubules, glycolytic capacity decreased considerably. In contrast, neither proximal glycolytic nor distal gluconeogenic activity changed. As starvation goes on, as noted, gluconeogenesis by the kidney increases, so that after a while it is producing almost half the glucose, the rest being produced by the liver. There is a net uptake of glycine, alanine, and proline by the kidney, and a net release of serine. Angiotensin-converting enzyme activity decreases during fasting [259].

Polyuria, hyposthenuria, and proteinuria are common late in starvation. The decreased concentrative ability of the kidney is due in part to the decreased amounts of urea in the medulla, and thus lowering the medullary osmolar gradient. Infusions of urea to such subjects lead to the excretion of concentrated urine.

The kidneys of individuals dying of "uncomplicated" starvation show little in the way of morphologic changes, either grossly or histologically (light microscopy).

Liver

We have already discussed the rapid loss in liver weight that occurs in starved rats and some of the metabolic adaptations that occur in the liver during starvation. We have mentioned that the liver loses glycogen rapidly and gains fat. As starvation proceeds, liver fat decreases and liver protein is lost, but the number of hepatocytes seems unchanged for some time. Sorrentino and colleagues [260] found that the mechanism for cellular uptake of oleate in hepatocytes isolated from livers of rats starved for two days was preserved to a greater extent than the mechanisms for uptake of sulfobromophthalein, taurocholate, or glucose. Liver biopsies were found to be generally normal histologically in undernourished people who had lost 2 to 55 kg weight, although the liver cells sometimes contained considerable amounts of iron and chromolipoid pigment. Liver function, as judged by clinical liver function tests, is maintained for a considerable period of time.

Pancreas

Histologic studies of the pancreas in humans dead of starvation are hampered by the rapid postmortem autolysis that this organ undergoes. No specific abnormality in the islets has been reported, but pancreatic acinar atrophy and fibrosis have been found. These latter lesions are common in rats following prolonged calorie-protein deficiency.

Pituitary Gland

Half a century ago it was observed that the acidophils of the anterior pituitary were atrophied and degranulated in starved rats [261]. Findings in malnourished patients have been variable and are perhaps age dependent. For example, one study showed no changes in the pituitaries of infants dying from marasmus or kwashiorkor, or both [262], whereas another study of 101 malnourished patients (adults?) showed pituitary atrophy to be present in 49 of them. Degenerative lesions of the anterior lobe were present, including vacuolization, pycnosis, cellular atrophy, and calcification. The posterior lobe showed basophilic invasion [263]. Jung and associates [264] investigated the role of the dopaminergic system in the pituitary adaptation to energy deprivation. They concluded that factor(s) other than dopamine influence not only thyrotrophic activity but also other aspects of pituitary function during energy deprivation.

Gastrointestinal Tract

The gut is one of the more active organs metabolically, and so it is not surprising that it (especially the small intestine) decreases substantially in mass during starvation. Gastric emptying and intestinal transit times are prolonged. The rates of renewal and migration of the intestinal mucosal cells are slowed, but the composition of the cells seems unchanged (protein and RNA per unit DNA). Eventually there is a flattening of the villi and a reduction in absorptive surface area. The atrophic mucosa often has a lowered disaccharidase (especially lactase) activity. Digestion and absorption, particularly of fat and carbohydrate, may be impaired as a result of disturbance of small bowel mucosal cell functions and decreased activity of various pancreatic and gut mucosal enzymes, and gut permeability is increased [8,38,61,229,249,265–268]. The view has been advanced by Roediger [269] that depletion of luminal short-chain fatty acids during starvation leads to diminished cell membrane integrity, decreased absorption, and increased secretion and diarrhea, while Levin [270] has raised the possibility that glucagon is the major culprit. Terminally, there is generally severe diarrhea; postmortem examination has shown that the wall of the small intestine is so thin that it is almost transparent. A report that intussusception may occur in preadolescence secondary to starvation has appeared recently [271].

Little is known about the effects of starvation on the gut bacteria in humans. These bacteria influence mammalian metabolism and nutrition in important ways in health and disease [272], for example, the presence of the indigenous gut bacteria (the facultative anaerobes) increase metabolic rate by 15% to 20% without inducing an infectious disease. Body fat is greater in conventional rats than in germ-free rats; associated with this is a longer survival for conventional rats and mice than for their germ-free counterparts following starvation.

Respiratory and Cardiovascular Systems

Starvation of rats leads to decreased capacity of the lungs to synthesize protein, but the efficiency of synthesis is not reduced [273], and surface elastic forces are increased (decreased tissue elasticity?), leading to air-space enlargement [274]. These latter observations may be related to a decrease in lung lysyl oxidase activity, which falls dramatically in starved rats to 25% of control values after only 48 to 72 hours of starvation [275]. When young healthy women ate a limited diet, 40% of their normal caloric intake, for seven days, their ventilatory muscle strength and endurance were unchanged, although, as expected, their metabolic rate was lower and they were mildly hypoglycemic and ketotic [276].

Doekel et al. [277] had found earlier that feeding a 500-calorie carbohydrate diet to normal humans for 10 days led to a significant diminution in the hypoxic ventilatory response (42% of control); the hypercapnea ventilatory response was not significantly altered. The reason for the decreased hypoxic ventilatory response has not been determined. After five days of refeeding with a normal diet, the hypoxic ventilatory response returned to normal.

One normally thinks of the lungs and the kidneys as exerting primary regulatory influences on acid-base metabolism. The immediate and huge accumulation of organic acids that occurs with cardiac arrest serves to demonstrate the critical role the cardiorespiratory system normally plays in maintaining acid-base homeostasis. The major part of this role is related to the muscular activity of the heart, which results in perfusion of tissues with blood; maintenance of oxygen delivery and removal of CO_2 and acids resulting from tissue metabolism; delivery of lactate to the liver and kidney, which may recycle it to glucose; and delivery of hydroxybutyrate and acetoacetate to the brain and muscles (including the heart), where they are metabolized to $CO_2 + H_2O$, or to the lungs where, in addition to being metabolized to these latter compounds, the hydroxybutyrate and acetoacetate may be oxidized or provide the hydrogen ions that serve to drive the reaction $HCO_3^- + H^+ \rightarrow CO_2 + H_2O$ and thus participate in the respiratory compensation to metabolic acidosis. This respiratory mechanism, which serves to conserve fixed base and ammonia, may be one way in which keto acid oxidation spares nitrogen loss in starvation. The mechanism ultimately depends on the muscular work of the heart. The heart, in addition to its *muscular* work, carries out *metabolic* activities that regulate acid-base balance in the body.

The heart is a major consumer of acetoacetic acid in both well-nourished and starved states. The brain is the main consumer of ketoacids in starvation; depending on the rate of hepatic ketogenesis, the heart can use ketones not used by the brain. Because of the relatively high concentration of mitochondria in both of these organs, they are able to generate high levels of succinyl CoA. The brain and heart are thus able to activate acetoacetic acid.

$$\text{Acetoacetic acid} + \text{succinyl CoA} \longrightarrow \text{acetoacetyl CoA} + \text{succinate}$$
$$\text{acetoacetyl CoA} \searrow CO_2 + ATP + H_2O$$

Additionally, the heart has a unique metabolic action that influences acid-base balance. Consider the A-V differences in lactate for the heart and skeletal muscle:

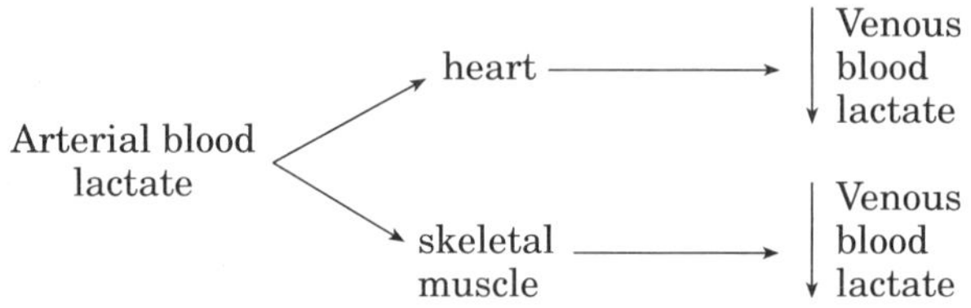

The *heart* is a *consumer* of lactate, which is normally oxidized completely by this tissue; it is the only organ that uses lactate as a direct energy source. *Skeletal muscle* is a *producer* of lactate. Liver and kidneys use lactate but mainly for glucose synthesis.

In the fed or fed-exercised state, the heart reduces acidosis by oxidizing lactate and permits maximal glucose utilization by skeletal muscle. In the postprandial state, glucose uptake by muscle is regulated by the blood levels of sugar and insulin. During exercise, muscle takes up additional glucose because of the increased circulation and metabolism. This is not true in the fasted state, in which blood insulin and glucose levels are both low. In the fasted state, muscle lactic dehydrogenase (LDH, M_4) activity decreases.

$NADH + H^+ + \text{pyruvate} \rightleftarrows \text{lactate} + NAD^+$ is a reversible reaction. However, because the K_m for pyruvate is low and its V_{max}(pyruvate lactate) high, muscle lactic dehydrogenase isoenzyme (LDH, M_4) is adapted to convert pyruvate to lactate at high rates. Rarely would it have occasion to work in the opposite direction because skeletal muscles import less lactate than they export. Additionally, in conditions in which glucose is completely oxidized by muscle, the LDH, M_4 would be nonfunctional because pyruvate would be converted to acetyl CoA and not to lactate. The LDH system in muscle is geared to provide lactate for export to the liver and kidneys for glucogenesis and to the heart for fuel, particularly during oxygen debt.

On the other hand, the lactic dehydrogenase isoenzyme in the heart (LDH, H) exerts an entirely different physiologic function. Whereas skeletal muscle is an exporter of lactate and its LDH, M_4 is adapted for this, the heart is an importer of lactate and its LDH, H isoenzyme is adapted for lactate oxidation. It has a high K_m for pyruvate and a low V_{max} for pyruvate reduction. As a result, pyruvate reduction is slower in the heart than in the muscle, but oxidation of lactate is much faster in the heart. When the fed individual exercises, the excess lactate produced by skeletal muscle can be used by the heart, thus sparing the liver the work of converting all the lactate to glucose, and decreasing the glucose requirement of the exercising heart. In contrast, in the starved resting individual, lactate production by skeletal muscle is limited. In starvation, the blood cells and brain release about 50 g of lactate/day, which is converted by the liver and kidneys to glucose for use again by the blood cells and brain. Concomitant with decreased lactate production by muscle in starvation are decreased levels of heart LDH, H and other heart enzymes connected with lactate and pyruvate metabolism. There is also a coincident loss of cofactors (magnesium, thiamine, potassium) for these enzymatic reactions; therefore, lactate utilization by the heart is decreased in starvation. It is not surprising, then, that cardiac function is impaired in starvation and cardiac failure late in starvation is common. Losses of intracellular and extracellular electrolytes not only affect heart muscle tone and contractility but influence its excitability as well. Sugden and Howard [138] have found recently in rats starved for up to 24 hours that cardiac lipoprotein lipase (LPL) activity increased promptly. Other data suggested that oxidation of fatty acids derived from plasma triglycerides via LPL substituted for carbohydrate oxidation at this time.

Prolonged caloric deficiency induces significant alterations in cardiac function and morphology [278–281] and in several cardiac lysosomal enzymes, particularly cathepsin D. Wildenthal and associates [282] speculate, from some studies of fetal mouse heart in culture, that this may be related to the prolonged low serum insulin and high concentrations of ketones and fatty acids in starvation. They had advanced the view that the altered cathepsin D activity might contribute to the net protein catabolism and cardiac atrophy of starvation. However, in a later study, Crie et al.

[283] showed that protein degradation of the hearts of starved rats was decreased as assessed in vitro, opposite in direction from what was predicted from the simultaneous changes in cathepsin D activity. Starvation has been reported to cause only a small decrease in the rate of protein synthesis by the heart, but because there is a progressive decrease in intrinsic cardiac proteolytic activity during starvation, the cardiac atrophy that occurs in starvation appears to result chiefly from the decrease in protein synthesis. Crie et al. [283] found cardiac alanine release to be significantly increased by starvation. Inhibition of pyruvate oxidation and consequent increased conversion of pyruvate to alanine seem to be important components of the process. The branched-chain amino acids were released to a lesser extent from the hearts of starved animals than would be explained on the basis of decreased protein degradation alone. Crie et al. [283] believe that increased oxidation of these compounds during starvation is the probable explanation for this finding.

Consolazio and associates [29] found changes in cardiac function of previously healthy men as early as 10 days after total nutrient deprivation other than water. When such men carried out submaximal work on the treadmill, their electrocardiograms promptly became abnormal (AVF and GRS axis changes), reflecting, in their view, "severe stress." In the study of semistarvation conducted by Keys and his associates (16), there were electrocardiographic changes in response to moderate exercise that were maximal at 12 weeks. These consisted of an increase of the Q-T interval, a continuous decrease in amplitudes at all deflections, and marked shifts to the right of the QRS and T wave axes.

As starvation goes on, the heart decreases progressively in size and function. Bradycardia, rhythm disturbances, a fall in blood pressure (both systolic and diastolic), decreased cardiac output, reduced sympathetic tone, elevated central venous pressure, and diminished ability to handle a fluid load all are characteristic [110,225]. Digoxin may show little inotropic effect at this time. Some of the psychological changes that may occur in starvation (decreased desire for muscular activity) may function indirectly to protect the heart.

Frank congestive failure consequent to the cardiac dysfunction, accentuated by anemia and excessive extracellular volume, may be a terminal event. Sudden death due to ventricular arrhythmias may occur. In humans dying from starvation, the heart is often atrophied to half its normal size and there may be myofibrillar degeneration.

Hematologic Changes

Progressive, but generally not severe, anemia (decreased erythrocyte formation and increased hemolysis) is common late in starvation. Early in starvation (10 days) there may be a relative increase in the circulating neutrophils, with a concomitant decrease in circulating lymphocytes, but later (after one to two months) neutropenia is characteristic. The neutrophils appear normal morphologically, and there is generally an increase in neutrophils in response to infection, even late in starvation. There are, however, abnormalities in neutrophil function, including impaired intracellular bactericidal and mobility defects, late in starvation [284]. Gelatinous transformation of the bone marrow and marrow cell necrosis have been observed in patients with anorexia and starved (involuntary) humans, many of whom were pancytopenic [285].

Starvation and Resistance to Infection

Clinicians have known for many years that malnutrition is associated often with a decreased resistance to certain infections, and considerable experimental evidence confirming and extending this has been obtained during the last 60 years. The period of food deprivation need not be long. Smith and Dubos [286] showed that when mice were starved for as short a time as 36 hours, their resistance to staphylococcal infections was markedly decreased. This was shown also to be true for tuberculous infection in mice starved for 30 hours or made protein-deficient by dietary restriction [287]. Elsewhere Dubos [288] states:

> Through a number of different mechanisms arrived at by revolutionary adaptation, man has achieved some sort of ecological equilibrium with the microorganisms that are ubiquitous in his environment. Indeed these microorganisms may be harbored in the body without causing disease, and establish relationships with the tissues—covering the whole gamut from the commensalism and symbiosis represented by the flora of the gut, to the various types of arrested or latent infections. The factors which determine whether the microbial agents are thus held in check, or undergo unrestrained multiplication, are, of course, highly complex. . . . I have presented the view that natural and acquired resistance depends more often upon the ability of the inflammatory response to create in and around the lesion a micro-environment inimical to the infectious agent.
>
> It is likely that disturbances in the general state of health often bring about qualitative and quantitative changes in the biochemical characteristics of the inflammatory area. These, in turn, may interfere with the processes which control the activities of micro-organisms within the lesion. As a result, the response of the body to infection and consequently the micro-environment in which the infectious process follows its

course, are under the control of factors which may be metabolic or psychic in origin. This concept accounts in part for the fact that susceptibility to infection can change independently of the immunological state of the infected individual. Since changes in susceptibility can occur rapidly, and be extremely transient, the intensity of exposure to an infectious agent may be less decisive than the physiological state of the exposed individual, in determining whether infection fails to take hold, becomes established, runs an abortive course, or evolves into overt disease.

In recent studies of mice subjected to short-term starvation (one to three days), Martinez et al. [289] found a disproportionate depletion of lymphoid tissue and a decrease in peripheral white blood cells (WBC), but no change in the peripheral differential count. Adoptive cell transfer experiments showed that immunocompetence of individual spleen immunocytes was *not* reduced by starvation. However, Pizzini et al. [290] found that mice, ingesting a commercial chow and then surviving starvation for five days (near death at that time), showed a significant decrease in spleen cell blastogenesis, both spontaneous and in response to concanavalin A.

Pulmonary surfactant obtained from rats starved for two days enhanced phagocytosis by alveolar macrophages [291].

Gianotti and associates [292] found that starvation of rats for 18 to 24 hours before burning led to increased bacterial translocation to mesenteric lymph nodes 4 hours after the burn, but bacterial killing was increased in the mesenteric lymph nodes, spleen, liver, and lungs.

Najjar et al. [293] reported elevated IgM levels in marasmic children; others have shown reduced levels of IgG globulin in such children [294]. In children with kwashiorkor, low, normal, and high levels of the immunoglobulins have been reported, but generally the levels have been found normal or elevated. Kwashiorkor complicated by overt infection led to a threefold increase in overall immunoglobulin synthesis. In fact, the initial high levels of immunoglobulins in kwashiorkor may reflect the subclinical infections common in such patients.

Law et al. [295] found no significant decrease in the levels of IgG, IgM, and IgA in adult patients who had undergone severe food deprivation, had suffered weight losses of at least 20 pounds, and had serum albumin levels below 3.2 g/100 ml. The patients were a mixed group with regard to diagnosis—dementia, heart disease, including some in congestive failure, and cerebrovascular accidents; none had malignant, hepatic, or primary immunologic diseases.

In contrast to the immunoglobulins, the serum levels of all complement proteins, except C_4, were markedly decreased in children with protein-calorie malnutrition; this may result in abnormal opsonification [296,297]. There was a rapid reversal of these changes following nutritional rehabilitation.

Although the levels of immunoglobulins are not reduced in starvation, the ability to synthesize antibodies is likely to be impaired. Cannon et al. [298] demonstrated many years ago that rabbits made hypoproteinemic by food protein deprivation had decreased antibody responses to *Escherichia typhosa* and *Salmonella paratyphi* vaccines. There is also clinical evidence that humans suffering from malnutrition or starvation may be unable to make circulating antibodies and interferon adequately in response to certain bacterial or viral antigens [299]. Thus, Coovadia et al. [300] showed that although the numbers of B lymphocytes isolated from the blood of children with marasmus or kwashiorkor were not significantly different from normal, the ability of these cells to produce antibodies 10 days after TAB (typhoid) vaccination was depressed. The specific cellular immunity response to smallpox vaccination is depressed in starvation [301].

Cellular aspects of the immune response have also been studied in starvation. It has long been known that malnutrition is frequently associated with atrophy of the lymphoid tissues and depression of cellular immunity. Thymic and lymph node atrophy, low total lymphocyte counts, diminished or absent delayed hypersensitivity responses, and abnormal in vitro lymphocytic function have all been described [268,294,296,302–304]. Cell-mediated cytotoxicity (CMC) was severely depressed in previously healthy animals after six days of a very low caloric diet and in patients with anorexia nervosa; the depression appeared to be reversible after refeeding [305].

There is evidence that the inflammatory response is depressed in starvation. As mentioned, decrease in the number and function of neutrophils is commonly observed in starvation. Guggenheim and Buechler [306] showed that peritoneal granulocytes obtained from rats subjected to protein and/or calorie malnutrition have decreased bactericidal activity. Yoshida and colleagues [307] showed that leukocytes from patients with protein-calorie malnutrition had depressed glycolytic activity; it is well known that normal phagocytic function depends on an intact glycolytic pathway. Subsequently, it was shown that malnutrition leads to motility defects in the granulocytes and an abnormality in intracellular bacterial activity [308]. Kendall and Nolan [284] found a highly significant difference in the function of polymorphonuclear cells of children below the third weight percentile and those of heavier children as assessed by nitro-blue tetrazolium staining and latex particles phagocytosis. Correlated with the depression of function of the inflammatory cells were changes in the histology of the bone marrow [309]. Bone marrow biopsies obtained from humans who had starved for prolonged periods showed fat atrophy, hypoplasia of hematopoietic cells, and gelatinous changes in the ground substance and cell necrosis. The gelatinous changes could also be reproduced in rabbits that had been undernourished for four months. In both humans and experimental animals, these changes were reversible with refeeding.

It is clear that part of the reduced capability of response of the starved organism to a variety of stimuli is reflected in its inability to mount adequate responses to challenges by various infectious agents. This is reflected both in the humoral and cellular components of the immune response and in nonimmune defense mechanisms. Nutritional rehabilitation reverses many of these alterations, although it is not known whether long-term malnutrition and starvation may leave some permanent insufficiencies in the immune responses and other defense reactions.

In recent years there has been increasing interest in possible adverse effects of malnutrition, primary and secondary, on the resistance of surgical patients to infection (chiefly bacterial and fungal). These matters are discussed at length elsewhere in this volume (Chapter 21).

Epilogue

A wide variety of metabolic changes and adaptations occur during starvation, all of which help animals and humans to survive a lack of exogenous nutrient supply in the face of continuing nutrient utilization for essential metabolic and physiologic processes.

These responses to food deprivation, per se, are different in many significant ways from the metabolic responses to severe injury and illness, although these latter are influenced in major ways by the nutrient intakes of the patients. As a result, the net physiologic and clinical consequences of injury and illness are conditioned importantly by the nutrient intakes of the patients. The nature of these effects, which are complex, additive, and at times synergistic, the ways in which they are brought about, and the methods of treating them are dealt with in other chapters of this volume.

This chapter has been concerned mainly with the ways in which the body adapts to conserve life in the absence of food intake. If the process has a purpose or subserves an important function in nature, it is not primarily to lengthen the period between the onset of starvation and death. The process is carried out in a singularly remarkable way, so that at almost any time, recovery, though not always complete, is possible, and fertility reestablished. This is possible because the integrity of some cells is maintained throughout starvation and because, even in those cells that are stripped of many structural and metabolically active features, the genetic material remains intact, as does the apparatus for expressing that material. Thanks to this fact, the remnants of starvation in Auschwitz, in Phnom Penh, and elsewhere, and their descendants survive and contribute importantly to the well-being of society. [*Editor's Note:* The interested reader is referred to the *Third Ross Conference on Medical Research: Nutrition and Sepsis,* JE Fischer (ed), 1982, which is available from Ross Laboratories, Columbus, Ohio. Although dated, there is much basic information here that can be read with profit.]

References

1. Hippocrates. *The Genuine Works of Hippocrates,* translated from Greek by Francis Adams. Baltimore: Williams & Wilkins, 1939.
2. Dubois EF. Metabolism in Fever and in Certain Infections. In LF Barker (ed), *Endocrinology and Metabolism,* Volume IV. New York: Appleton, 1922. P 94.
3. Benedict FGA. *Study of Prolonged Fasting.* Washington, DC: Carnegie Institute of Washington, 1915 Publication No. 280.
4. Cuthbertson DP. The disturbance of metabolism produced by bony and non-bony injury with notes on certain abnormal conditions of bone. *Biochem J* 24:1244, 1930.
5. Wolf AV. *Thirst.* Springfield, IL: Thomas, 1958.
6. Shils M, Olson J, Shike M (eds) *Modern Nutrition in Health and Disease* (8th ed.) Philadelphia: Lea & Febiger, 1995.
7. Klein PS, Forbes GB, Nader PR. Effects of starvation in infancy on subsequent learning disabilities. *J Pediatr* 87:8, 1975.
8. McCance RA, Widdowson EM. *The German Background: Studies of Undernutrition, Wuppertal 1946–1949.* London: Spec Rep Ser Med Res Coun, No. 275, 1951.
9. Benedict FG, et al. *Human Vitality and Efficiency under Prolonged Restrictions.* Washington, DC: Carnegie Institute of Washington, 1919. Publication No. 701.
10. Peters JP, Van Slyke DD. *Quantitative Clinical Chemistry Interpretations;* Volume 1. Baltimore: Williams & Wilkins, 1946.
11. Gamble JL, Ross GS, Tisdall J. Metabolism of fixed base during fasting. *J Biol Chem* 57:633, 1923.
12. Burger GCE, Drummond JC, Sandstead HR. *Malnutrition and Starvation in Western Netherlands.* September 1944–July 1945. The Hague: General State Printing Office, 1948.
13. Winick M (ed). *Nutrition, Pre- and Postnatal Development.* New York: Plenum, 1979.
14. Lindtjorn B. Famine in Ethiopia 1983–1985: Kwashiorkor and marasmus in four regions. *Ann Trop Paediatr* 7:1, 1987.

15. Bittles AH, McHugh JJ, Markov E. The Irish Famine and its sequel: Population structure changes in the Ards Peninsula, Co. Down, 1841–1911. *Ann Hum Biol* 13:473, 1986.
16. Keys A, et al. *The Biology of Human Starvation.* Minneapolis: University of Minnesota Press, 1950.
17. Bloom WL. Fasting as an introduction to the treatment of obesity. *Metabolism* 8:214, 1959.
18. Duncan GG, et al. Correction and control of intractable obesity: practical applications of intermittent periods of total fasting. *JAMA* 181:309, 1962.
19. Cahill GF Jr. Starvation in man. *N Engl J Med* 282:668, 1970.
20. Cahill GF Jr, et al. Hormone-fuel interrelationships during fasting. *J Clin Invest* 45:1751, 1966.
21. Owen OE, et al. Liver and kidney metabolism during prolonged starvation. *J Clin Invest* 48:574, 1969.
22. Owen OE, et al. Energy metabolism in feasting and fasting. *Adv Exp Med Biol* 111:169, 1979.
23. Felig P. The glucose-alanine cycle. *Metabolism* 22:179, 1973.
24. Felig P, Marliss EB, Cahill GF Jr. Metabolic response to human growth hormone during prolonged starvation. *J Clin Invest* 50:411, 1971.
25. Felig P, et al. Amino acid metabolism during prolonged starvation. *J Clin Invest* 48:584, 1969.
26. Waterlow JC. Metabolic adaptation to low intakes of energy and protein. *Ann Rev Nutr* 6:495, 1986.
27. Carlson MG, Snead WL, Campbell PJ. Fuel and energy metabolism in fasting humans. *Am J Clin Nutr* 60:29, 1994.
28. Lowry SF, et al. Whole-body protein breakdown and 3-methylhistidine excretion during brief fasting, starvation, and intravenous repletion in man. *Ann Surg* 202:21, 1985.
29. Consolazio CF, et al. Metabolic aspects of acute starvation in normal humans (10 days). *Am J Clin Nutr* 20:672, 1967.
30. Soares JM, Shetty PS. Basal metabolic rates and metabolic economy in chronic undernutrition. *Eur J Clin Nutr* 45:363, 1991.
31. Kinney JM, Gump FE, Long CL. Energy and tissue fuel in human injury and sepsis. *Adv Exp Med Biol* 33:401, 1972.
32. Cahill GF Jr. Starvation in man. *Clin Endocrinol Metab* 5(2):397, 1976.
33. Cahill GF Jr. Starvation: Some biological aspects. In JM Kinney, et al. *Nutrition and Metabolism in Patient Care.* Philadelphia: Saunders, 1988.
34. Kleiber M. *The Fire of Life. An Introduction to Animal Energetics.* New York: Wiley, 1961.
35. Garlick PJ, et al. Nutrition and protein turnover. *Biochem Soc Trans* 10:290, 1982.
36. Kark RM. Food hunger in a world of turmoil. *World Rev Nutr Diet* 6:1, 1966.
37. Schanberg S. *The New York Times.* February, 1975.
38. Porter A. *The Disease of the Madras Famine of 1877–1878.* Madras, India: Government Press, 1889.
39. Grande F. Energetics and weight reduction. *Am J Clin Nutr* 21:305, 1968.
40. Alpert SS. The energy density of weight loss in semistarvation. *Int J Obes* 12:533, 1988.
41. Kinney JM, et al. Carbohydrate and nitrogen metabolism after injury. *J Clin Pathol* 4:65, 1970.
42. Kinney JM, Long CL, Duke JH Jr. Carbohydrate Metabolism after Injury. In R Porter, J Knight (eds), *Energy Metabolism in Trauma.* London: Churchill, 1970. P 103.
43. Adibi SA. Metabolism of branched-chain amino acids in altered nutrition. *Metabolism* 25:1287, 1976.
44. Boyle JP, Shah SD, Cryer PE. Insulin, glucagon, and catecholamines in prevention of hypoglycemia during fasting. *Am J Physiol* 19:E651, 1969.
45. Gjedde A, Crone C. Induction processes in blood-brain transfer of ketone bodies during starvation. *Am J Physiol* 229:1165, 1975.
46. Hasselbalch SG, et al. Brain metabolism during short-term starvation in humans. *J Cereb Blood Flow Metab* 14:125, 1994.
47. Hawkins RA, Biebuyck JF. Ketone bodies are selectively used by individual brain regions. *Science* 205:325, 1979.
48. Henriksson J. The possible role of skeletal muscle in the adaptation to periods of energy deficiency. *Eur J Clin Nutr* 44:55, 1990.
49. Hoffer LJ. Starvation. In M Shils, J Olson, M Shike (eds), *Modern Nutrition Health and Disease* (8th ed). Philadelphia: Lea & Febiger, 1994. P 927.
50. Scornik OA. Role of protein degradation in the regulation of cellular protein content and amino acid pools. *Fed Proc* 435:1283, 1984.
51. Mortimore GE, Poso AR. Lysosomal pathways in hepatic protein degradation: Regulatory role of amino acids. *Fed Proc* 435:1289, 1984.
52. Ciechanover A, Finley D, Varshavsky A. The ubiquitin-mediated proteolyic pathway and mechanisms of energy-dependent intracellular protein degradation. *J Cell Biochem* 24:25, 1984.
53. Pfeifer U. Inhibition by insulin of the formation of autophagic vacuoles in rat liver. *J Cell Biol* 78:152, 1978.
54. Mortimore GE, Schworer CM. Induction of autophagy by amino acid deprivation in perfused rat liver. *Nature* 279:174–6, 1977.
55. Deter RL, Baudhuin P, deDuve C. Participation of lysosomes in cellular autophagy induced in rat liver by glucagon. *J Cell Biol* 35:C11, 1967.
56. Lowell BB, Ruderman NB. Regulation of myofibrillar protein degradation in rat skeletal muscle during brief and prolonged starvation. *Metabolism* 35:1121, 1986.
57. Li JB, Wassner SJ. Effects of food deprivation and refeeding on total protein and actomyosin degradation. *Am J Physiol* 246:E32, 1984.
58. Mortimore GE, Poso AR. Intracellular protein catabolism and its control during nutrient deprivation and supply. *Ann Rev Nutr* 7:539, 1987.
59. Tiao G, et al. Sepsis stimulates nonlysosomal, energy-dependent proteolysis and increases ubiquitin mRNA levels in rat skeletal muscle. *J Clin Invest* 94:2255, 1994.
60. Garlick PJ, et al. The effect of protein deprivation and starvation on the rate of protein synthesis in tissues of the rat. *Biochem Biophys Acta* 414:71, 1975.
61. McNurlan MA, Tomkins AM, Garlick PJ. The effect of starvation on the rate of protein synthesis in rat liver and small intestine. *Biochem J* 178:373, 1979.
62. Henshaw EC, et al. Control of protein synthesis in mammalian tissues through changes in ribosome activity. *J Biol Chem* 246:436, 1971.
63. Millward DJ, et al. Protein Turnover. In *Protein Metabolism and Nutrition* (EAAP Publication 16). London: University of London Press, 1976. P 49.
64. Mortimore GE, Ward WF. Behavior of the lysosomal sys-

tem during organ perfusion. An inquiry into the mechanism of hepatic proteolysis. *Front Biol* 45:157, 1976.

65. Garlick PJ, Millward DJ, James WP. The diurnal response of muscle and liver protein synthesis in vivo in meal-fed rats. *Biochem J* 136:935, 1973.
66. Millward DJ, et al. Relationship between protein synthesis and RNA content in skeletal muscle. *Nature* 241:204, 1973.
67. Ogata ES, Foung SK, Holliday MA. The effects of starvation and refeeding on muscle protein synthesis and catabolism in the young rat. *J Nutr* 108:759, 1978.
68. Stein TP, et al. Effect of nitrogen and calorie restriction on protein synthesis in the rat. *Am J Physiol* 230:1321, 1976.
69. Wassner SJ, Orloff S, Holliday MA. Protein degradation in muscle: Response to feeding and fasting in growing rats. *Am J Physiol* 233:E119, 1977.
70. Rannels DE, et al. Effect of starvation on initiation of protein synthesis in skeletal muscle and heart. *Am J Physiol* 235:E126, 1978.
71. Essen P, et al. Short-term starvation decreases skeletal muscle protein synthesis rate in man. *Clin Physiol* 12:287, 1992.
72. Wernerman J, von der Decken A, Vinnars E. Size distribution of ribosomes in biopsy specimens of human skeletal muscle during starvation. *Metabolism* 34:665, 1985.
73. Wernerman J, von der Decken A, Vinnars E. Polyribosome concentration in human skeletal muscle after starvation and parenteral or enteral feeding. *Metabolism* 35:447, 1986.
74. Jefferson LS, Li JB, Rannels SR. Regulation by insulin of amino acid release and protein turnover in the perfused rat hemicorpus. *J Biol Chem* 252:1476, 1977.
75. Jenkins AB, Whittaker M, Schoefield PJ. The starvation induced increase in muscle protein degradation is nonlysosomal in origin. *Biochem Biophys Res Commun* 86:1014, 1979.
76. Libby P, Goldberg AL. Leupeptin, a protease inhibitor, decreases protein degradation in normal and diseased muscles. *Science* 199:534, 1978.
77. Ord JM, et al. Mechanisms of degradation of myofibrillar and nonmyofibrillar protein in the heart. *Adv Myocardiol* 4:198, 1983.
78. Garber AJ, Karl IE, Kipnis DM. Carbon sources of alanine and glutamine released by skeletal muscle. *J Clin Invest* 52:31A, 1973.
79. Garber AJ, Karl IE, Kipnis DM. Alanine and glutamine synthesis and release from skeletal muscle. *Biol Chem* 251:826, 1976.
80. Waterlow JC, Stephen JML. Adaptation of the rat to a low-protein diet: The effect of a reduced protein intake on the pattern of incorporation of L-arginine. *Br J Nutr* 20:461, 1966.
81. Waterlow JC, Stephen JML. Use of carbon-14-labelled arginine to measure the catabolic rate of serum and liver proteins and the extent of amino-acid recycling. *Nature* 211:78, 1966.
82. Dice JF, et al. General characteristics of protein degradation in diabetes and starvation. *Proc Natl Acad Sci USA* 75:2093, 1978.
83. Smith DM, Sugden PH. Contrasting response of protein degradation to starvation and insulin as measured by N-methylhistidine or phenylalanine from the perfused rat heart. *Biochem J* 237:391, 1986.
84. Wannemacher RW Jr, Dinterman RE. Total body protein catabolism in starved and infected rats. *Am J Clin Nutr* 30:1510, 1977.
85. Albert JD, et al. Extremity amino acid metabolism during starvation and intravenous refeeding in humans. *Am J Physiol* 251:E604, 1986.
86. Albert JD, et al. Peripheral tissue metabolism in man with varied disease states and similar weight loss. *J Surg Res* 40:374, 1986.
87. Legaspi A, et al. Effect of starvation and total parenteral nutrition on electrolyte homeostasis in normal man. *JPEN* 12:109, 1988.
88. Legaspi A, et al. The effect of starvation and total parenteral nutrition on skeletal muscle amino acid content and membrane potential difference in normal man. *Surg Gynecol Obstet* 166:233, 1988.
89. Tracey KJ, et al. Protein and substrate metabolism during starvation and parenteral refeeding. *Clin Sci* 74:123, 1988.
90. Fong Y, et al. Starvation leads to decreased levels of mRNA for myofibrillar proteins. *J Surg Res* 46:457, 1989.
91. Young VR, et al. Potential use of 3-methylhistidine excretion as an index of progressive reduction in muscle protein catabolism during starvation. *Metabolism* 22:1429, 1973.
92. Henry CJK, Rivers JPW, Payne PR. Protein and energy metabolism in starvation reconsidered. *Eur J Clin Nutr* 42:543, 1988.
93. Consoli A, et al. Determination of Krebs cycle metabolic carbon exchange in vivo and its use to estimate the individual contributions of gluconeogenesis and glycogenolysis to overall glucose output in man. *J Clin Invest* 80:1303, 1987.
94. Sugden MC, Sharples SC, Randle PJ. Carcass glycogen as a potential source of glucose during short-term starvation. *Biochem J* 160:817, 1976.
95. Geiger SR (ed). *Handbook of Physiology.* Baltimore: Waverly, 1983.
96. Goldspink G. Biochemical Energetics for Fast and Slow Muscles. In L Bolis, HP Maddrell, K Schmidt-Nielsen (eds), *Comparative Physiology: Functional Aspects of Structural Materials.* Amsterdam: Elsevier, 1975.
97. Wendt IR, Gibbs CL. Energy production of rat extensor digitorum longus muscle. *Am J Physiol* 224:1081, 1973.
98. Russell DM, et al. Metabolic and structural changes in skeletal muscle during hypocaloric dieting. *Am J Clin Nutr* 39:503, 1984.
99. Essen B, Fohlin L, Saltin B. Skeletal muscle fiber types and sizes in anorexia nervosa patients. *Clin Physiol* 1:395, 1981.
100. Fang CH, et al. Differential expression of ubiquitin mRNA in red and white skeletal muscle reflects differences in sepsis-induced muscle proteolysis. *Surg Forum* 45:41, 1994.
101. Zamir O, et al. Muscle protein breakdown during endotoxemia in rats and after treatment with interleukin-1 receptor antagonist (IL-1ra). *Ann Surg* 216:381, 1992.
102. Hasselgren PO, Fischer JE. Recent advances on the regulation of muscle protein metabolism in catabolic states. With special reference to the role of cytokines and glucocorticoids for protein breakdown during sepsis. *RINPE* 10:72, 1992.
103. Ruderman NB, Schmahl FW, Goodman MN. Regulation of alanine formation and release in rat muscle in vivo: effect of starvation and diabetes. *Am J Physiol* 233:E109, 1977.
104. Ruderman NB, et al. Effect of starvation on muscle glucose metabolism: Studies with the isolated perfused rat hindquarter. *Fed Proc* 36:171, 1977.

105. Aoki TT, Finley RJ, Cahill RJ Jr. The Redox State and Regulation of Amino Acid Metabolism in Man. In PB Garland, CN Hales (eds), *Substrate Mobilization and Energy Provision in Man.* Biochemical Society Symposia No. 43, July 1977. London: The Biochemical Society, 1978. P 17.

106. Chua B, et al. Hormonal and Metabolic Control of Proteolysis. In PB Garland, CN Hales (eds), *Substrate Mobilization and Energy Provision in Man.* Biochemical Society Symposia No. 43, July 1977. London: The Biochemical Society, 1978. P 1.

107. Lehninger AL, Nelson DL, Cox MM. *Principles of Biochemistry* (2nd ed). New York: Worth, 1993.

108. Felig P, Wahren J. Amino acid metabolism in exercising man. *J Clin Invest* 50:2703, 1971.

109. Felig P, Wahren J. Protein turnover and amino acid metabolism in the regulation of gluconeogenesis. *Fed Proc* 33:1092, 1974.

110. Carlsten A, et al. Myocardial metabolism of glucose, lactic acid, amino acids in healthy human individuals at rest and at different work loads. *Scand J Clin Lab Invest* 13:418, 1961.

111. Felig P, Wahren J. Influence of endogenous insulin secretion on splanchnic glucose and amino acid metabolism in man. *J Clin Invest* 50:1702, 1971A.

112. Levenson SM, Crowley LV, Seifter E. Starvation. In W Ballinger, et al (eds), *Manual of Surgical Nutrition.* Philadelphia: Saunders, 1975. P 236.

113. Grey NJ, Karl I, Kipnis DM. Physiologic mechanisms in the development of starvation ketosis in man. *Diabetes* 24:10, 1975.

114. Pozefsky T, et al. Effect of brief starvation on muscle amino acid metabolism in non-obese man. *J Clin Invest* 57:444, 1976.

115. Bergstrom Y, et al. Intracellular free amino acid concentration in human muscle tissue. *J Appl Physiol* 36:693, 1974.

116. Walser M, et al. Evidence for an anabolic action of essential amino acid analogues in uremia and starvation. *Z Ernahrungswiss* 19:5, 1976.

117. Sapir DG, Chambers NE, Ryan JW. The role of potassium in the control of ammonium excretion during starvation. *Metabolism* 25:211, 1976.

118. Sapir DG, Owen OE. Renal conservation of ketone bodies during starvation. *Metabolism* 24:23, 1975.

119. Sapir DG, et al. Nitrogen sparing induced by a mixture of essential amino acids given chiefly as their keto-analogues during prolonged starvation in obese subjects. *J Clin Invest* 54:974, 1974.

120. Sapir DG, Walser M. Nitrogen sparing induced early in starvation by infusion of branched-chain ketoacids. *Metabolism* 26:301, 1977.

121. Buse MG, Reid SS. Leucine: a possible regulator of protein turnover in muscle. *J Clin Invest* 56:1250, 1975.

122. Marliss EB, et al. Muscle and splanchnic glutamine and glutamate metabolism in post-absorptive and starved man. *J Clin Invest* 50:814, 1971.

123. Matsutaka H, et al. Gluconeogenesis and amino acid metabolism: III. Uptake of glutamine and output of alanine and ammonia by non-hepatic splanchnic organs of fasted rats and their metabolic significance. *J Biochem* 74:1019, 1973.

124. Shulman G, et al. Adaptation of glucose production to a physiologic increment in glucagon. *Diabetes* 26:383, 1977.

125. Goldberg AL, St. John AC. Intracellular protein degradation in mammalian and bacterial cells. Part 2. *Ann Rev Biochem* 45:747, 1976.

126. Felig P, Wahren J, Raf L. Evidence of inter-organ amino acid transport by blood cells in humans. *Proc Natl Acad Sci USA* 70:1775, 1973.

127. Meister A. On the enzymology of amino acid transport. *Science* 180:33, 1973.

128. Korchak HM, Masoro EJ. Changes in the level of the fatty acid synthesizing enzymes during starvation. *Biochim Biophys Acta* 58:354, 1962.

129. Garber AJ, et al. Hepatic ketogenesis and gluconeogenesis in humans. *J Clin Invest* 54:981, 1974.

130. Apfelbaum TT. Choroba Glodowa. American Joint Committee, Warsaw 1946, as quoted by JR Dmochowski, FD Moore Choroba Glodowa. *N Engl J Med* 293:356, 1975.

131. Border JR. Metabolic response to short-term starvation, sepsis and trauma. *Surg Annu* 2:11, 1970.

132. Dietze G, Wicklmayer M, Mehnert H. Physiology of Metabolism During Starvation. In FW Ahnefeld, et al (eds), *Parenteral Nutrition.* Berlin: Springer, 1976. P 17.

133. McGarry JD, Foster DW. In support of the roles of malonyl-CoA and carnitine acyltransferase in the regulation of hepatic fatty acid oxidation and ketogenesis. *J Biol Chem* 254:8163, 1979.

134. McGarry JD, Foster DW. Regulation of ketogenesis and clinical aspects of the ketotic state. *Metabolism* 21:471, 1972.

135. Holness MJ, Snugden MC. Glucose utilization in heart, diaphragm, and skeletal muscle during the fed-to-starved-transition. *Biochem J* 270:245, 1990.

136. Ilian MA, Forsberg NE. A comparative study on gene expression of calpains, calpastatin, cathepsin D, and proteasome in tissue of fed and fasted rabbits. *J Nutr Biochem* 5:529, 1994.

137. Sugden MD, et al. Mechanisms involved in the coordinate regulation of strategic enzymes of glucose metabolism. *Adv Enzyme Regul* 33:71, 1993.

138. Sugden MC, Howard RM. Cardiac lipoprotein lipase activities in relation to glucose utilization during progressive starvation. *Biochem Soc Trans* 142S:21, 1993.

139. Randle PJ, Kerbey AL, Espinal J. Mechanisms decreasing glucose oxidation in diabetes and starvation: Role of lipid fuels and hormones. *Diabetes Metab Rev* 47:623, 1988.

140. Sherwin RS, Hendler RG, Felig P. Effect of ketone infusions on amino acid and nitrogen metabolism in man. *J Clin Invest* 55:1382, 1975.

141. Golden M, Waterlow JC, Picou D. Protein turnover, synthesis and breakdown before and after recovery from protein-energy malnutrition. *Clin Sci Mol Med* 53:473, 1977.

142. Golden M, Waterlow JC, Picou D. The relationship between dietary intake, weight change, nitrogen balance, and protein turnover in man. *Am J Clin Nutr* 30:1345, 1977.

143. Millward DJ. Protein deficiency, starvation, and protein metabolism. *Proc Nutr Soc* 38:77, 1979.

144. Campbell GA, et al. Effects of starvation in rats on serum levels of follicle-stimulating hormone, LH, thyrotropin, GH, and prolactin; response to LH-releasing hormone and thyrotropin-releasing hormone. *Endocrinology* 100:580, 1977.

145. Frexes-Steed M, et al. Role of insulin and branched-chain amino acids in regulating protein metabolism during fasting. *Am J Physiol* 258:E907, 1990.

146. Fryburg DA, et al. Effect of starvation on human muscle

protein metabolism and its response to insulin. *Am J Physiol* 259:E477, 1990.

147. Mansell PI, Macdonald IA. The effect of starvation on insulin-induced glucose disposal and thermogenesis in humans. *Metabolism* 39:502, 1990.

148. Nair KS, et al. Leucine, glucose, and energy metabolism after 3 days of fasting in healthy human subjects. *Am J Clin Nutr* 46:557, 1987.

149. Tsalikian E, et al. Increased leucine flux in short-term fasted human subjects: Evidence for increased proteolysis. *Am J Physiol* 247:E323, 1984.

150. Wolfe RR, et al. Effect of short-term fasting on lipolytic responsiveness in normal and obese human subjects. *Am J Physiol* 252:E189, 1987.

151. Clore JN, et al. Impaired modulation of hepatic glucose output overnight after a 72-h fast in normal man. *J Clin Endocrinol Metab* 70:865, 1990.

152. Klein S, et al. Effect of short and long term **B**-adrenergic blockade on lipolysis during fasting in humans. *Am J Physiol* 257:E65, 1989.

153. Nurjhan N, et al. Insulin dose-response characteristics for suppression of glycerol release and conversion to glucose in humans. *Diabetes* 35:1326, 1986.

154. Jensen MD, et al. Lipoysis during fasting. Decreased suppression by insulin and increased stimulation by epinephrine. *J Clin Invest* 79:207, 1987.

155. Elia M, et al. The energy cost of triglyceride-fatty acid recycling in nonobese subjects after an overnight fast and four days of starvation. *Metabolism* 36:251, 1987.

156. Lowell BB, Goodman MN. Protein sparing in skeletal muscle during prolonged starvation. Dependence on lipid fuel availability. *Diabetes* 36:14, 1987.

157. Rothschild MA, et al. Effects of a short term fast on albumin synthesis studies in vivo, in the perfused liver, and on amino acid incorporation by hepatic microsomes. *J Clin Invest* 47:2591, 1968.

158. James WPT, Hay AM. Albumin metabolism: Effect of the nutritional state and the dietary protein intake. *J Clin Invest* 47:1958, 1968.

159. Hoffenberg R, Black E, Brock JF. Albumin and gammaglobulin tracer studies in protein depletion states. *J Clin Invest* 45:143, 1966.

160. Gorozhanin VS, Lobkov VV. Hormonal and metabolic reactions in the human body during prolonged starvation. *Kosmicheskaia Biologiia i Aviakosmicheskaia Meditsina* 24:47, 1990.

161. Mirsky IA. The influence of insulin on the protein in metabolism of nephrectomized dogs. *Am J Physiol* 124:569, 1938.

162. Goodman MN, Ruderman NB. Insulin sensitivity of rat skeletal muscle: Effects of starvation and aging. *Am J Physiol* 236:E519, 1979.

163. Rudorff KH, Albrecht G, Staib W. Effect of insulin and proinsulin on the metabolism of alanine in the rat liver. *Horm Metab Res* 2:49, 1970.

164. Weinkove C. Insulin release and glucose tolerance in malnourished rats. Ph.D. Thesis, University of Cape Town. Cited by Pimstone B. Endocrine function in protein-calorie malnutrition. *Clin Endocrinol* 5:79, 1976.

165. Weinkove C, Weinkove EA, Pimstone B. Glucose tolerance and insulin release in malnourished rats. *Clin Sci Mol Med* 50:153, 1976.

166. Hedeskov CJ, Capito K. The pentose cycle and insulin release in isolated mouse pancreatic islets during starvation. *Biochem J* 152:571, 1975.

167. Rabinovitch A, et al. Insulin release and cyclic AMP accumulation in response to glucose in pancreatic islets of fed and starved rats. *J Clin Invest* 58:1209, 1976.

168. Young JB, Landsberg L. Suppression of sympathetic nervous system during fasting. *Science* 196:1473, 1977.

169. Abraira C, Lawrence AM. The Staub-Traugott phenomenon: III. Effects of starvation. *Am J Clin Nutr* 31:213, 1978.

170. Anderson JW, Herman RH, Newcomb KL. Improvement in glucose tolerance of fasting of obese patients given oral potassium. *Am J Clin Nutr* 22:1589, 1969.

171. Brodows RG. Starvation enhances the ability of insulin to inhibit its own secretion. *Metabolism* 34:53, 1985.

172. Stout RW, Henry RW, Buchanan KD. Triglyceride metabolism in acute starvation: The role of secretin and glucagon. *Eur J Clin Invest* 6:179, 1976.

173. Fisher M, et al. Kinetics of glucagon in man: Effects of starvation. *Proc Natl Acad Sci USA* 73:1735, 1976.

174. Lacy WW, et al. Control of plasma amino acids by glucagon and insulin. *Diabetes* 21:340, 1972.

175. Shoemaker WC, VanItallie TB. The hepatic response to glucagon in the unanesthetized dog. *Endocrinology* 66:260, 1960.

176. Marliss EB, et al. Glucagon levels and metabolic effects in fasting man. *J Clin Invest* 49:2256, 1970.

177. Mallette LE, Exton JH, Park CR. Control of gluconeogenesis from amino acids in the perfused rat liver. *J Biol Chem* 244:5713, 1969.

178. Karl IE, Garber AJ, Kipnis DM. Alanine and glutamine synthesis and release from skeletal muscle: III. Dietary and hormonal regulation. *J Biol Chem* 251:844, 1976.

179. Peterson RD, Beatty, C, Bocek RM. Effects of insulin and glucagon on carbohydrate and protein metabolism of adductor muscle and diaphragm. *Endocrinology* 72:71, 1963.

180. Arky RA, et al. Glucose and insulin response to intravenous glucagon during starvation. *Am J Clin Nutr* 23:691, 1970.

181. Hansen JDL. Cited by Pimstone B. Endocrine function in protein-calorie malnutrition. *Clin Endocrinol* 5:79, 1976.

182. Alleyene GAO, Scullard GH. Alterations in carbohydrate metabolism in Jamaican children with severe malnutrition. *Clin Sci* 37:631, 1969.

183. Walter RM, et al. The effect of adrenergic blockade on the glucagon responses to starvation and hypoglycemia in man. *J Clin Invest* 54:1214, 1974.

184. Saudek CD, Boulter PR, Arky RA. The natriuretic effect of glucagon and its role in starvation. *J Clin Endocrinol Metab* 36:761, 1973.

185. Pullman TN, Lavender AR, Aho I. Direct effect of glucagon on renal hemodynamics and excretion of inorganic ions. *Metabolism* 16:358, 1967.

186. Fichter MM, Pirke KM. Effect of experimental and pathological weight loss upon the hypothalamo-pituitary adrenal axis. *Psychoneuroendocrinology* 11:295, 1986.

187. Palmblad J, et al. Effect of total energy withdrawal (fasting) on the levels of growth hormone, thyrotropin, cortisol, adrenaline, noradrenaline, T^4, T^3, and rT^3 in healthy males. *Acta Med Scand* 201:15, 1977.

188. Merimee JJ, Fineberg SE. Growth hormone secretion in starvation: A reassessment. *J Clin Endocrinol Metab* 39:385, 1974.

189. Merimee JJ, Pulkkinen AJ, Burton CE. Diet-induced alterations of high secretion in man. *J Clin Endocrinol Metab* 42:931, 1976.

190. Smith SR, et al. Growth hormone in adults with protein calorie malnutrition. *J Clin Endocrinol Metab* 39:53, 1974.
191. Samuel AM, Deshpande UR. Growth hormone levels in protein calorie malnutrition. *J Clin Endocrinol Metab* 35:863, 1972.
192. Beas F, et al. Growth hormone in infant malnutrition: The arginine test in marasmus and kwashiorkor. *Br J Nutr* 26:169, 1971.
193. Pimstone B, et al. Growth hormone and protein-calorie malnutrition. Impaired suppression during induced hyperglycemia. *Lancet* 2:1333, 1967.
194. Pimstone B, et al. Studies in growth hormone secretion in protein-caloriemalnutrition. *Am J Clin Nutr* 21:482, 1968.
195. Milner RDG. Metabolic and hormonal responses to oral amino acids in infantile malnutrition. *Arch Dis Child* 46:301, 1971.
196. Tannenbaum GS, et al. Antiserum to somatostatin reverses starvation-induced inhibition of growth hormone but not insulin secretion. *Endocrinology* 102:1909, 1978.
197. Lunn PG, et al. Progressive changes in serum cortisol, insulin and growth hormone concentrations and their relationship to the distorted amino acid pattern during the development of kwashiorkor. *Br J Nutr* 29:399, 1973.
198. Schwarz F, et al. Influence of exogenous human growth hormone on the metabolism of fasting obese patients. *Metabolism* 21:297, 1972.
199. Jiang ZM, et al. Low-dose growth hormone and hypocaloric nutrition attenuate the protein-catabolic response after major operation. *Ann Surg* 210:513, 1989.
200. Grant DB, et al. Reduced sulfation faction in undernourished children. *Arch Dis Child* 48:596, 1973.
201. Daughaday WH, Kipnis DM. The growth-promoting and anti-insulin actions of somatotropin. *Recent Prog Horm Res* 22:49, 1966.
202. Phillips LS, Young HS. Nutrition and somatomedin: I. Effect of fasting and refeeding on serum somatomedin activity and cartilage growth activity in rats. *Endocrinology* 99:304, 1976.
203. Phillips LS, Vassilopoulou-Sellin R. Nutritional regulation of somatomedin. *Am J Clin Nutr* 32:1082, 1979.
204. Phillips LS, Vassilopoulou-Sellin R. Somatomedins. *N Engl J Med* 302:371, 1980.
205. Hintz RL, et al. Plasma somatomedin and growth hormone values in children with protein-calorie malnutrition. *J Pediatr* 92:153, 1978.
206. Salmon WD Jr. Interaction of somatomedin and a peptide inhibitor in serum of hypophysectomized and starved, pituitary-intact rats. *Adv Metab Disord* 8:183, 1975.
207. Van den Brande JL, DuCaju MVL. Plasma somatomedin activity in children with growth disturbances. Cited in Pimstone B. Endocrine function in protein-calorie malnutrition. *Clin Endocrinol* 5:79, 1976.
208. Godard C, Lemarchand-Beraud T. Plasma thyrotropin levels in severe infantile malnutrition. *Horm Res* 4:443, 1973.
209. Harland PSEG, Parkin JM. TSH levels in severe malnutrition. *Lancet* 2:1145, 1972.
210. Graham GG, et al. Thyroid hormonal studies in normal and severely malnourished infants and small children. *J Pediatr* 83:321, 1973.
211. Godard C. The endocrine glands in infantile malnutrition. *Helv Paediat Acta* 29:5, 1974.
212. Chopra IJ, Smith SR. Circulating thyroid hormones and thyrotropin in adult patients with protein calorie malnutrition. *J Clin Endocrinol Metab* 40:221, 1975.
213. Gardner DF, et al. Effect of triiodothyronine replacement on the metabolic and pituitary responses to starvation. *N Engl J Med* 300:579, 1979.
214. Harris ARC, et al. Effect of starvation on hypothalamic pituitary-thyroid function in rats. *Metabolism* 27:1074, 1978.
215. Harris ARC, et al. The role of sulfhydryl groups on the impaired hepatic 3,3′,5-triiodothyronine generation from thyroxine in the hypothyroid, starved, fetal, and neontal rodent. *J Clin Invest* 63:516, 1979.
216. Shimizu H, et al. Altered hormonal status in a female deprived of food for 18 days. *J Med Clin Exp Theory* 22:201, 1991.
217. Portnay GI, et al. The effect of starvation on the concentration and binding of thyroxine and triiodothyronine in serum and on the response to TRH. *J Clin Endocrinol Metab* 39:191, 1974.
218. Spaulding SW, et al. Effect of caloric restriction and dietary composition on serum T_3 in man. *J Clin Endocrinol Metab* 42:197, 1976.
219. Weissel M, Stummvoll HK, Kolbe H. T_3 metabolism in starvation [letter]. *N Engl J Med* 301:163, 1979.
220. Balsam A, Ingbar SH. Observations on the factors that control the generation of triiodothyronine from thyroxine in rat liver and the nature of the defect induced by fasting. *J Clin Invest* 63:1145, 1979.
221. Vagenakis AG. Thyroid Hormone Metabolism in Prolonged Experimental Starvation in Man. In RA Vigersky (ed), *Anorexia Nervosa*. New York: Raven, 1977. P 243.
222. Vagenakis AG, et al. Effect of starvation on the production and metabolism of thyroxine and triiodothyroninen euthyroid obese patients. *J Clin Endocrinol Metab* 45:1305, 1977.
223. Takagi A, et al. Serum concentrations, metabolic clearance rates, and production rates of reverse triiodothyronine, triidothyronine, and thyroxine in starved rabbits. *Endocrinology* 103:1434, 1978.
224. Chopra IJ, et al. Opposite effects of dexamethasone on serum concentrations of 3,3′,5-triiodothyronine (reverse T_3) and 3,3′,5-triiodothyronine (T_3). *J Clin Endocrinol Metab* 41:911, 1975.
225. Carter WJ, et al. Effect of thyroid hormone on metabolic adaptation to fasting. *Metabolism* 24:1177, 1975.
226. Wimpfheimer C, et al. Starvation-induced decreased sensitivity of resting metabolic rate to triiodothyronine. *Science* 205:1272, 1979.
227. Jung RT, et al. The role of catecholamines and thyroid hormones in the metabolic response to semistarvation. *Proc Nutr Soc* 38:17A, 1979.
228. Shetty PS, et al. The effect of catecholamine replacement on the metabolic response to semistarvation. *Proc Nutr Soc* 38:18A, 1979.
229. Chatterji A, Sen Gupta PC. Adrenals in malnourished infants. *Indian J Pathol Bacterial* 27:353, 1960.
230. Platt BS, Stewart RJC. Experimental protein deficiency: Histopathological changes in the endocrine glands of pigs. *J Endocrinol* 38:121, 1967.
231. Galvao-Teles A, et al. Free cortisol in obesity: Effect of fasting. *Acta Endocrinol* 81:321, 1976.
232. Smith SR, Bledsoe T, Chhetri MK. Cortisol metabolism and the pituitary-adrenal axis in adults with protein-calorie malnutrition. *J Clin Endocrinol Metab* 38:40, 1975.

233. Rao KSJ, Spikantia SG, Gopalan C. Plasma cortisol levels in protein-calorie malnutrition. *Arch Dis Child* 43:365, 1968.

234. Manchester KL. Site of Hormonal Regulation of Protein Metabolism. In HN Munro (ed), *Mammalian Protein Metabolism,* Volume IV. New York: Academic, 1970. P 229.

235. Smith OK, Long CNH. Effect of cortisol on the plasma amino nitrogen of eviscerated adrenalectomized diabetic rats. *Endocrinology* 80:561, 1967.

236. Wise JK, Hendler R, Felig P. Influence of glucocorticoids on glucagon secretion and plasma amino acid concentrations in man. *J Clin Invest* 52:2774, 1973.

237. Seitz HJ, et al. Physiologic significance of glucocorticoids and insulin in the regulation of hepatic gluconeogenesis during starvation in rats. *Metabolism* 25:1545, 1976.

238. Owen OE, Cahill GF Jr. Metabolic effects of exogenous glucocorticoids in fasted man. *J Clin Invest* 52:2596, 1973.

239. Mansell PI, Macdonald IA. Effects of underfeeding and of starvation on thermoregulatory responses to cooling in women. *Clin Sci* 77:245, 1989.

240. Mansell PI, Fellows IW, Macdonald IA. Enhanced thermogenic response to epinephrine after 48-h starvation in humans. *Am J Physiol* 258:R87, 1990.

241. Shoemaker WJ, Wurtman RJ. Prenatal undernutrition: Accumulation of catecholamines in rat brain. *Science* 171:1017, 1971.

242. Bourgeois B, Schmidt BJ, Bourgeois R. Some Aspects of Catecholamines in Under-Nutrition. In L Gardner, P Amacher (eds), *Endocrine Aspects of Malnutrition.* Proceedings of a Symposium Sponsored by the Kroc Foundation, 1973. P 163.

243. Hoeldtke RD, Wurtman RJ. Excretion of catecholamines and catecholamine metabolites in kwashiorkor. *Am J Clin Nutr* 26:205, 1973.

244. Root AW, et al. Effect of short term castration and starvation upon hypothalamic content of luteinizing hormone-releasing hormone in adult male rats. *Proc Soc Exp Biol Med* 150:602, 1975.

245. Howland BE. The influence of feed restriction and subsequent refeeding on gonadotrophin secretion and serum testosterone levels in male rats. *J Reprod Fertil* 44:429, 1975.

246. McAtee JW, Trenkle A. Effects of feeding, fasting, glucose and arginine on plasma prolactin levels in the bovine. *Endocrinology* 89:730, 1971.

247. Sirek AM, et al. Effect of starvation on pituitary growth hormone cells and blood growth hormone and prolactin levels in the rat. *Nutr Metab* 20:67, 1976.

248. Gamble JL. Physiological information gained from studies on the life raft ration. *Harvey Lect* 42:247, 1947.

249. Chinn RH, et al. The natriuresis of fasting: Relationship to changes in plasma renin and plasma aldosterone concentrations. *Clin Sci* 39:437, 1970.

250. Garnett ES, et al. The roles of carbohydrate, renin and aldosterone in sodium retention during and after total starvation. *Metabolism* 22:867, 1973.

251. Kolanowski J. Influence of glucose, insulin, and glucagon on sodium balance in fasting obese subjects. *Persp Biol Med,* Spring 1979. P 366.

252. Kolanowski J, Desmecht P, Crabbe J. Sodium balance and renal tubular sensitivity to aldosterone during total fast and carbohydrate refeeding in the obese. *Eur J Clin Invest* 6:75, 1976.

253. Schloeder FX, Stinebaugh BJ. Renal tubular sites of natriuresis of fasting and glucose-induced sodium conservation. *Metabolism* 19:1119, 1970.

254. Sigler MH. The mechanism of the natriuresis of fasting. *J Clin Invest* 55:377, 1975.

255. Stewart WK, Fleming LW. Relationship between plasma and erythrocyte magnesium and potassium concentrations in fasting obese subjects. *Metabolism* 22:535, 1973.

256. Reichard GA Jr, et al. Plasma acetone metabolism in the fasting human. *J Clin Invest* 63:619, 1979.

257. Garcia-Salguero L, Lupianez JA. Long term control of renal carbohydrate metabolism. I. Effect of starve-feed cycles on renal tubules gluconeogenesis. *Int J Biochem* 20:943, 1988.

258. Garcia-Salguero L, Lupianez JA. Metabolic adaptation of the renal carbohydrate metabolism. I. Effects of starvation on the gluconeogenic and glycolytic fluxes in the proximal and distal renal tubules. *Molec Cell Biochem* 83:167, 1988.

259. Butkus NE, Burman KD, Smallridge RC. Angiotensin-converting enzyme activity decreases during fasting. *Horm Metab Res* 19:76, 1987.

260. Sorrentino D, et al. Liver, pancreas, and biliary tract. The hepatocellular uptake of free fatty acids is selectively preserved during starvation. *Gastroenterology* 107:1415, 1994.

261. Jackson CM. The Effects of Inanition and Malnutrition upon Growth and Structure. Cited by BS Platt, et al (1925). In HN Munro, JB Allison (eds), *Mammalian Protein Metabolism,* Volume 2. New York: Academic, 1964. P 445.

262. Tejada C, Russfield AB. A preliminary report on the pathology of the pituitary gland in children with malnutrition. *Arch Dis Child* 32:343, 1957.

263. Zubiran S, Gomez-Mont F. Endocrine disturbances in chronic human malnutrition. *Vitam Horm* 11:97, 1953.

264. Jung RT, et al. Dopamine in the pituitary adaptation to starvation in man. *Postgrad Med J* 61:571, 1985.

265. Ecknauer R, Raffler H. Effect of starvation on small intestinal enzyme activity in germ-free rats. *Digestion* 18:45, 1978.

266. Elia M, et al. Effect of total starvation and very low calorie diets on intestinal permeability in man. *Clin Sci* 73:205, 1987.

267. Maxton DG, et al. Small-intestinal function during enteral feeding and starvation in man. *Clin Sci* 77:401, 1989.

268. Vint FW. Post-mortem findings in natives of Kenya. *East Afri Med J* 13:332, 1937.

269. Roediger WE. Famine, fiber, fatty acids, and failed colonic absorption: Does fiber fermentation ameliorate diarrhea? *JPEN* 18:4, 1994.

270. Levin RJ. The diarrhoea of famine and severe malnutrition: Is glucagon the major culprit? *Gut* 33:432, 1992.

271. Sarin YK, Sharma AK. Starvation a rare cause of intussusception in preadolescence. *Indian J Pediatr* 29:1168, 1992.

272. Levenson SM. The influence of the indigenous microflora on mammalian metabolism and nutrition. *JPEN* 2:75, 1978.

273. Rannels DE, Sahms RH, Watkins CA. Effects of starvation and diabetes on protein synthesis in lung. *Am J Physiol* 236:E421, 1979.

274. Sahebjami H, Vassallo CL. Effects of starvation and refeeding on lung mechanics and morphometry. *Am Rev Respir Dis* 119:443, 1979.

275. Madia AM, Rozovski SJ, Kagan HM. Changes in lung lysyl oxidase activity in streptozotocin-diabetes and in starvation. *Biochim Biophys Acta* 585:481, 1979.

276. Bender PR, Martin BJ. Ventilatory and treadmill endurance during acute semistarvation. *J Appl Physiol* 60:1823, 1986.

277. Doekel RC Jr, et al. Clinical semi-starvation: Depression of hypoxic ventilatory response. *N Engl J Med* 295:358, 1976.

278. Fisler JS. Cardiac effects of starvation and semistarvation diets: Safety and mechanisms of action. *Am J Clin Nutr* 56:230S, 1992.

279. Schocken DD, Holloway JD, Powers PS. Weight loss and the heart effects of anorexia nervosa and starvation. *Arch Intern Med* 149:877, 1989.

280. Smith AL. Effects of starvation on vaculolar apparatus of cardiac muscle tissue determined by electron microscopy, marker-enzyme assays and electrolyte studies. *Cytobios* 18:111, 1977.

281. Stokholm KH, Breum L, Astrup A. Cardiac contractility central haemodynamics and blood pressure regulation during semistarvation (published erratum appears in *Clin Physiol 1992 Mar*) 12(2):237. *Clin Physiol* 11:513, 1991.

282. Wildenthal K, et al. Dietary control of cardiac lysosomal enzyme activities. *Rec Adv Stud Cardiac Struct Metab* 8:519, 1975.

283. Crie JS, Sanford CF, Wildenthal K. Influence of starvation and refeeding on cardiac protein degradation in rats. *J Nutr* 110:22, 1980.

284. Kendall AC, Nolan R. Polymorphonuclear leukocytic activity in malnourished children. *Cent Afr J Med* 18:73, 1972.

285. Smith RR, Spivak JL. Marrow cell necrosis in anorexia nervosa and involuntary starvation. *Br J Haematol* 60:525, 1985.

286. Smith JM, Dubos RJ. The effect of nutritional disturbances on the susceptibility of mice to staphylococcal infections. *J Exp Med* 103:109, 1956.

287. Dubos RJ. Effect of metabolic factors on the susceptibility of albino mice to experimental tuberculosis. *J Exp Med* 101:59, 1955.

288. Dubos RJ. The micro-environment of inflammation or Metchnikoff revisited. *Lancet* 2:1, 1955.

289. Martinez D, et al. Immune mechanisms in leukemia: Suppression of cellular immunity by starvation. *J Natl Cancer Inst* 55:935, 1975.

290. Pizzini RP, et al. Dietary nucleotides reverse malnutrition and starvation induced immunosuppression. *Arch Surg* 125:86, 1990.

291. Sakai K, Ueyama A, Kishino Y. Pulmonary surfactant obtained from starved rats enhances phagocytosis of alveolar macrophages. *Cell Mol Biol* 37:475, 1991.

292. Gianotti L, et al. Role of early enteral feeding and acute starvation on postburn bacterial translocation and host defense: Prospective, randomized trials. *Crit Care Med* 22:265, 1994.

293. Najjar SS, Stephan M, Asfour RJ. Serum levels of immunoglobulins in marasmic infants. *Arch Dis Child* 44:120, 1969.

294. Chandra RK. Immunocompetence in undernutrition. *J Pediatr* 81:1194, 1972.

295. Law DK, Dudrick SJ, Abdou NI. Immunocompetence of patients with protein-calorie malnutrition. *Ann Intern Med* 79:545, 1973.

296. Neuman CG, et al. Immunologic responses in malnourished children. *Am J Clin Nutr* 28:89, 1975.

297. Sirisinha S, et al. Complement and C_3-proactivator levels in children with protein-calorie malnutrition and effect of dietary treatment. *Lancet* 1:1016, 1973.

298. Cannon PR, Chase WE, Wissler RW. The relationships of the protein reserves to antibody production. I. The effects of a low-protein diet and of plasmapheresis upon the formation of agglutinins. *J Immunol* 47:133, 1943.

299. Schlesinger L, et al. Decreased interferon production by leukocytes in marasmus. *Am J Clin Nutr* 29:758, 1976.

300. Coovadia HM, et al. An evaluation of factors associated with the depression of immunity in malnutrition and in measles. *Am J Clin Nutr* 27:665, 1974.

301. Saha K, et al. Under nutrition and immunity: Smallpox vaccination in chronically starved, undernourished subjects and its immunologic evaluation. *Scand J Immunol* 6:581, 1977.

302. Grace HJ, Armstrong D. Reduced lymphocyte transformation in protein-calorie manlnutrition. *South Afr Med J* 46:402, 1972.

303. Smythe PM, et al. Thymolymphatic deficiency and depression of cell mediated immunity in protein-calorie malnutrition. *Lancet* 2:939, 1971.

304. Watts T. Thymus weights in malnourished children. *J Trop Pediatr* 15:155, 1969.

305. Vaisman N, et al. The effect of different nutritional states on cell-mediated cytotoxicity. *Immunol Lett* 24:37, 1990.

306. Guggenheim K, Buechler E. Nutrition and resistance to infection. *J Immunol* 54:349, 1946.

307. Yoshida T, Metcoff J, Frenk S. Reduced pyruvic kinase activity, altered growth patterns of ATP in leukocytes and protein-calorie malnutrition. *Am J Clin Nutr* 21:162, 1968.

308. Selvaraj RJ, Bhat KS. Phagocytosis and leukocyte enzymes in protein-calorie malnutrition. *Biochem J* 127:255, 1972.

309. Tavassoli M, et al. Gelatinous transformation of bone marrow in prolonged self-induced starvation. *Scand J Haematol* 16:311, 1976.

21

Metabolic Response to Trauma and Infection

Palmer Q. Bessey

[T]here is a circumstance attending accidental injury which does not belong to disease . . . that the injury done has in all cases a tendency to produce both the disposition and the means of cure.
John Hunter, 1794 [1]

With this statement, the famed London anatomist and surgeon anticipated the recognition of a collection of characteristic physiologic and biochemical alterations that are seen in patients with trauma and critical illness. Hunter considered this "disposition and . . . means of cure" ultimately beneficial because it was associated with healing of the patient's wounds and ultimate recovery. More than a century later the Scottish biochemist, David Cuthbertson, began his systematic metabolic studies in patients with fractures, which were among the first to characterize the responses to injury [2,3]. He was particularly concerned with the problem of nonunion of fractures, all apparent failure of the "disposition and the means of cure," and his writings emphasized the catabolic and debilitating aspects of these alterations. In the United States, Francis Moore of Boston studied the responses to injury in the 1940s and '50s as a basis for understanding convalescence from surgery and improving perioperative care [4,5]. The demonstration of effective intravenous nutritional support by Dudrick, Wilmore, Vars, and Rhoads in 1967 [6,7] stimulated further interest in the metabolic responses to injury and critical illness because of the hope that the right amount and type of nutrition would prevent the wasting and mortality of catabolic illness. In the 1970s and '80s, several investigations expanded upon Moore's early studies of the hormonal regulation of these responses. It also became clear that the responses to infection and the responses to injury shared many similar features. When injured patients develop infections, their metabolic alterations would become more pronounced. This and the expansion of knowledge about growth factors, cytokines, and other inflammatory mediators in the last 10 to 15 years has emphasized the importance of inflammation as a common factor in these responses. Hunter's "disposition and . . . means of cure" is now subsumed in the general term, the metabolic responses to critical illness. These are encountered in patients with a variety of conditions, all of which involve an inflammatory response or focus of inflammatory tissue, including patients with mechanical trauma, burns, pancreatitis, adult respiratory distress syndrome (ARDS), and major infections.

Our understanding of the metabolic responses to injury and critical illness serves as the basis for current strategies for supportive care of critically ill patients. That understanding has advanced to the point where it is now possible to consider ways in which the responses might be altered to reduce the debility and death associated with critical illness. In this chapter, we shall first focus on the general features of these responses and the alterations in metabolism seen in critically ill patients. We shall next review several aspects of metabolic regulation that appear to influence these metabolic responses. Then we shall indicate how our understanding of these phenomena relate to the general clinical approach to a critically ill patient. Finally, we shall discuss some potential new strategies for the metabolic support of the critically ill.

Clinical Features

Time Course

An important feature of the metabolic responses to critical illness is that they evolve over time: they have a history. The priorities of care and the patient's response to therapy also change over time. In the United States, Francis Moore described four phases of convalescence from surgery [8]. The injury phase begins at the time of initiation of operation (injury) and lasts for one to two days following an elective procedure. During this time, the patient is somewhat withdrawn, avidly retains sodium and water, and seems ill. This is usually followed rather dramatically by a definite "turning point" when the patient begins to feel subjectively better and begins to take an interest in her or his surroundings and resumes participating in activities of daily living. At this point, a diuresis develops and the accumulated extracellular fluid is mobilized. The patient then begins to regain strength and stamina. There is restoration of both fat and protein mass. Cuthbertson identified two phases to the early responses to injury, which he dubbed the "ebb" and the "flow" phases (Table 21-1) [9]. The ebb phase occurs at and for a time after injury and is characterized by decreases in cardiac output, oxygen consumption, and body temperature as well as hyperglycemia and increased lactate concentrations. These changes are commonly associated with hypovolemia and inadequate cardiac performance. With successful resuscitation, the ebb evolves into a flow phase in which cardiac output, body temperature, and oxygen consumption are all elevated. In addition, there is an increased excretion of nitrogen in the urine reflecting an acceleration in net protein breakdown. Hyperglycemia persists and fatty acids may be elevated also. This phase may be prolonged and is associated with the presence of open wounds, infection, and other sites of inflammation.

The duration of these various responses depends on the nature of the initial insult. If the patient has an elective operation with minimal tissue injury, blood loss, and ischemia, then the responses are relatively mild and short-lived. The elective surgical patient can ambulate early, resume a diet, and has a short length of stay in hospital. The introduction of laparoscopic surgery has shortened these phases of convalescence even more. This appears to be not only because of more limited tissue injury, but also because of reduced

Table 21-1. Metabolic Responses to Injury and Critical Illness

	Ebb Phase	Flow Phase
Cardiac output	Reduced	Increased
Oxygen consumption	Reduced	Increased
Body temperature	Reduced	Increased
Nitrogen loss	—	Increased
Blood glucose	Increased	Increased
Glucose production	—	Increased
Lactate	—	Increased
Free fatty acids	Increased	Increased
Insulin	Normal or low	Elevated
Insulin resistance	Yes	Yes
Cathecholamines, glucagon, cortisol	Increased	Increased

pain [10]. In contrast, the patient sustaining severe multisystem trauma or a major burn will have the additional complications of shock and tissue ischemia. The sheer mass of cells affected, therefore, is huge compared to the patient having an elective operation. Patients may also have other insults that result in additional tissue inflammation such as the adult respiratory distress syndrome (ARDS) or any of a variety of infectious processes. The metabolic responses of these patients are accentuated and prolonged. The physiologic alterations that characterize these patients are those of the flow phase described by Cuthbertson. Because these are so prominent in many of the ICU patients and associated with foci of inflammation, they recently have been identified as the systemic inflammatory response syndrome (SIRS) [11].

The priorities of care in various phases of convalescence reflect the underlying abnormalities. Thus, in the ebb phase, the priorities are those of resuscitation: establishing an airway, assuring breathing and oxygenation, restoring and maintaining circulation, and tissue perfusion. In addition, restoration of tissue integrity, removal of necrotic debris, and control of infection are important surgical goals at this time. In the sense of the ebb phase, it is a time of damage control. In the following flow phase, it is a time for healing of wounds and resolution of acute inflammation. It is here that nutritional and metabolic support assume a high priority. Nutrition continues to be important later on in the restoration of muscle and fat mass.

Hypermetabolism

Metabolic rate is a measure of heat loss from the body. Because all physiologic and biochemical events ultimately depend on biochemical reactions and because these are inherently inefficient, resulting in a loss of free energy as heat, the metabolic rate is an indicator of the cellular activity of the body. When measured under carefully controlled "basal" conditions, the metabolic rate is reproducible and predictable based on age, sex, and body size [12]. When the metabolic rate of acutely ill patients is measured under similar conditions, it is usually greater than that predicted for the patient's age, sex, and body size. Acutely ill patients are thus "hypermetabolic."

Energy that is lost as heat from the body or any other biophysiologic system ultimately comes from the oxidation of organic fuels. These processes involve the consumption of oxygen (VO_2) and the production of carbon dioxide (VCO_2). These parameters may be determined by analysis of respiratory gas exchange. It is then possible to calculate the metabolic rate (MR) (heat loss) according to the equation originally defined by Weir [13,14].

$$\text{MR (kcal/m}^2\text{/h)} = \frac{[3.94 \times VO_2\ \text{(L/min)} + 1.11 \times VCO_2\ \text{(L/min)}] \times 60\ \text{(min/h)}}{\text{Body surface area (m}^2\text{)}}$$

There is also a correction commonly made for the heat generated by protein metabolism. It is a term related to the urinary nitrogen loss and is usually less than 3% to 5% of the total. Thus, if urinary nitrogen values are missing, the metabolic rate may still be calculated reliably.

The metabolic rate, or energy expenditure, is thus related to O_2 consumption and CO_2 production. Whole-body oxygen consumption is also related to cardiac output and by the Fick relationship:

$$VO_2 = CO_2\ \text{(L/min)} \times [O_2\ \text{content}_{\text{arterial}} - O_2\ \text{content}_{\text{pulmonary artery}}] \times 10$$

Oxygen consumption may be measured clinically either by an indirect calorimetry apparatus, often in the form of a portable metabolic cart, or it may be calculated from blood gas analyses and bedside measurements of cardiac output, usually by thermodilution. Hypermetabolic patients have an increased metabolic rate, increased oxygen consumption, and increased cardiac output. They also commonly require increased minute ventilation, in part to account for elevated CO_2 production.

The degree of hypermetabolism in patients is related to the underlying disease. In patients with burns, the proportion of the body surface area that is burned—along with age, and the presence or absence of inhalation injury and pneumonia—is the major determinant of survival [15]. Thus the size of the burn is a measure of its severity. There is also a close relationship between the proportionate increase in the metabolic rate measured under basal conditions and the extent of the body surface area burn [16]. The burn wound initially accounts for all of the inflammatory tissue the patient has. Hypermetabolism can thus be related to the total inflammatory mass. In other types of critically ill patients, the size of the inflammatory mass is less clearly quantitated, but the relationship between hypermetabolism and the mass of inflammatory tissue still appears to be valid. Survival in these patients, however, is related both to the magnitude of the inflammatory response and to a variety of other factors. Thus, various methods of quantitating the severity of a patient's critical illness—such as APACHE [17] or trauma and injury severity scores (TRISS) [18]—bear a strong relationship to survival but do not predict hypermetabolism with the same reliability as burn size does in burn patients (Table 21-2).

Other complications that may develop in critically ill patients such as ARDS and sepsis commonly lead to further increase in hypermetabolism. In most cases, this is associated with an expansion of the total mass of inflammatory tissue.

These observations emphasize the central importance of the size of the inflammatory mass in determining the intensity of the metabolic responses to critical illness. Recently a tetrad of clinical syndromes—systemic inflammatory response syndrome (SIRS), sepsis syndrome, sepsis, and septic shock—has been defined, reflecting this relationship and the aggravating role of infection [19].

Accelerated Nitrogen Loss and Muscle Wasting

Perhaps the component of the metabolic response to critical illness that has most significance in terms of its apparent effect on outcome is the alteration in protein metabolism. Cuthbertson was one of the first to demonstrate this marked increase of nitrogen loss associated with profound muscle wasting in patients' recovery from injuries [2,3]. On the basis of associated losses of phosphorous and sulfur, he concluded that skeletal muscle was the source [2]. In addition, he demonstrated that this nitrogen loss involved all muscles not just those close to the site of injury [20]. Thus, accelerated net skeletal muscle protein breakdown is a major debilitating component of the metabolic responses to injury and critical illness. This effect may be compounded by actual physical loss of tissue and body protein by inadequate food intake and by disuse atrophy of muscles that results from inactivity typically imposed by critical illness [21].

Table 21-2. Effect of Critical Illness on Basal Metabolism

Critical Illness	Stress Factor
Mild starvation	0.8–1.0
Elective operation	1.0–1.1
Peritonitis and other infections	1.05–1.25
Long-bone fracture	1.15–1.30
Multiple trauma, severe infection, head injury	1.3–1.55
Severe trauma, sepsis, ARDS, multiple organ system failure	1.5–1.7
Burns	
20%	1.16
30%	1.29
40%	1.43
50%	1.56
60%	1.69
70%	1.83

Source: Adapted from DW Wilmore. *The Metabolic Management of the Critically Ill.* New York: Plenum, 1977. P 14; PQ Bessey. Parenteral Nutrition and Trauma. In JL Rombeau, MD Caldwell (eds), *Parenteral Nutrition.* Philadelphia: Saunders, 1993. P 540; and DE Carlson et al. Resting energy expenditure in patients with thermal injuries. *Surg Gynecol Obstet* 174:270, 1992.

Increased nitrogen loss associated with critical illness usually demonstrates at a distinctive time course [3]. The nitrogen excretion typically peaks several days after the initial injury or other insult and gradually returns toward normal as the patients recover. This is well described for patients sustaining a variety of injuries and burns [22,23]. Furthermore, the intensity of the nitrogen loss also appears to be related to the severity of injury: the more severe the injury, the greater the degree of nitrogen loss.

These basic concepts came from early studies of nitrogen balance in critically ill patients. Differences in the total body nitrogen intake and loss was thought to reflect the net difference between protein synthesis and protein breakdown. More recent studies utilizing tracer quantities of amino acids labeled with an isotope of nitrogen (usually ^{15}N, the heavy isotope) have been consistent with balance studies [24]. Interpretation of these data involves the concept of a free amino acid pool to which amino acids are added both by protein breakdown and by protein intake and from which amino acids are removed both by excretion and by protein synthesis. If it is assumed that the size of the amino acid pool is constant, then the amount of amino acids flowing into and out from the pool, or turnover, reflects overall protein metabolic activity. (Protein turnover is typically increased following injuries.) By combining these measurements with nitrogen intake and loss, which can be measured, one may quantitate total body protein synthesis and total body protein breakdown. In patients with critical illness, both synthesis and breakdown may be increased [25].

Skeletal muscle protein breakdown may also be quantitated by measurements of the excretion of 3-methylhistidine (3-MH) [26]. This compound is formed from histidine when it is incorporated into the muscle proteins, actin and myosin. It is released with protein degradation and excreted unchanged in the urine. Increased excretion of 3-MH has been reported in patients with burns [27], trauma [28], and infections [29], indicating an increase in the rate of protein breakdown during these illnesses. Although the source of 3-MH is largely skeletal muscle it is also found in the smooth muscle of the gastrointestinal (GI) tract [30]. Thus, a portion of the 3-MH excreted may come from the GI tract, especially during periods of starvation and bowel rest.

The proteolytic response of muscle to critical illness may not be homogeneous. For example, Hasselgren and co-workers [31] found that protein breakdown associated with starvation and sepsis was greater in the extensor digitorum longus muscle (a fast-twitch muscle that functions intermittently to change limb position) than in the soleus (a slow-twitch red fiber muscle that maintains position). In addition, the contractile myofibrillar proteins, actin and myosin, appear to be proportionately more labile than other protein constituents. Accentuated proteolytic responses of fast-twitch muscles and myofibrillar protein to burns have also been observed by other investigators [32]. These phenomena may be responsible in part for the rapid development of weakness and debility in patients with critical illness.

Metabolic Alterations

Amino Acid Metabolism

Although concentrations of free amino acids are most conveniently measured in the plasma, intracellular pools of free amino acids are thought to be more closely related to protein synthesis and degradation. Quantitatively, the intracellular pool is the most important. As much as 80% of the body's free amino acid pool is found in skeletal muscle, and the concentrations of amino acids can be as much as 30 times greater than those in plasma [33,34]. Interestingly, the relative concentrations are not the same as would be expected from the amino acid composition of protein. Essential amino acids constitute only 8.4% of the total intracellular amino acid pool. Glutamine, glutamate, and alanine constitute approximately 79%, and the single nonessential amino acid glutamine represents 61% of the total [34]. Glutamine and usually total amino acid concentrations fall after trauma [35,36], sepsis [37], elective operation [38], inactivity, and starvation [35]. Concentrations of other specific amino acids such as phenylalanine, tyrosine, alanine, and the branched-chain amino acids (BCAA) may increase [39–41]. The fall in intracellular glutamine concentration appears to be a typical response to critical illness or to any condition in which there is a net loss of skeletal muscle protein [37,39], and it also appears to be graded, that is, related to severity of critical illness (Figure 21-1) [42]. Intracellular glutamine concentrations are closely related to overall cellular amino acid balance. It has been proposed that glutamine is in fact a regulator of intracellular protein metabolism [43–45].

The fall in intracellular glutamine is usually associated with the net release of amino acids from muscle. The amino acids glutamine and alanine are most important in this regard in that they may account for as much as 70% of the total amino acids released [46]. This implies that in the process of protein breakdown there is intracellular transformation of other amino acids to form alanine and glutamine. In a study of patients with major burns, Aulick and Wilmore [47] found that amino acid release from the lower extremities were five times greater than in control subjects. In this study, only 10 amino acids were actually measured, and of these alanine was the only single amino acid whose release was significantly differ-

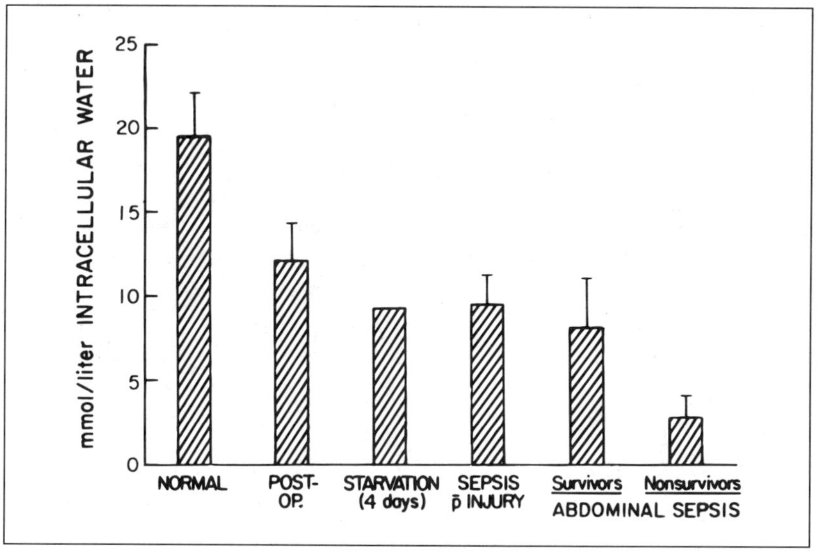

Figure 21-1. The reduction in intracellular skeletal muscle glutamine appears to be related to the severity of critical illness. (From DW Wilmore, PR Black, F Muhlbacher. Injured man: Trauma and sepsis. In RW Winters (ed), *Nutritional Support of the Seriously Ill Patient.* New York: Academic, 1983. P 40.)

ent between the two groups. Glutamine was not measured. The degree of alanine release was not related to the extent of the burn on the leg, but rather to the total burn size and to oxygen consumption. Thus, amino acid release from muscle in vivo appears to be a graded response, as are many other of the metabolic responses to critical illness. In further studies of burn patients, the uptake of amino acids across the splanchnic bed was three to four times greater than in postabsorptive normal controls [48]. In addition, the increased splanchnic uptake corresponded to the increased peripheral release. Increased splanchnic amino acid uptake has also been demonstrated in septic patients. This increased uptake is associated with an increase in hepatic protein synthesis (especially the so-called acute-phase proteins) [49, 50] and with an increased rate of glucose production by the liver.

A variety of amino acids may be utilized for gluconeogenesis, but alanine is quantitatively the most important. In that process, of course, the amino group from alanine and other amino acids will be split off, ultimately to form urea, which is then transported to the kidney and excreted. Glutamine also serves as a major pathway for nitrogen excretion. Glutamine can be metabolized in the kidney to produce ammonia, which is an important buffering mechanism for excreted acid loads [51]. The carbon atoms also have gluconeogenic potential through conversion to Krebs cycle intermediates. In the past several years, it has become apparent that glutamine is an important respiratory fuel for the GI tract and other cell populations that undergo rapid proliferation such as inflammatory and epithelial cells and cells that proliferate in wounds [52,53]. Under conditions of catabolic illness, glutamine is actively absorbed by the GI tract and converted to alanine and ammonia [54]. The alanine then passes to the liver, where it can be used for gluconeogenesis and acute-phase protein synthesis. The ammonia formed in the GI tract and the urea formed by the conversion of alanine to glucose are both ultimately excreted. This is the irreversible, final step of protein breakdown.

In summary, critical illness is associated with an accelerated net loss of amino acids from peripheral tissue, particularly skeletal muscle. Most of the nitrogen is carried as glutamine and alanine. The glutamine can be utilized primarily by the GI tract, but also by wounds and other foci of inflammation, as a respiratory fuel, metabolized to alanine and ammonia. The alanine from this process and the alanine released from muscle are taken up by the liver and utilized largely for gluconeogenesis. The nitrogen is lost as ammonia and urea, which are excreted. The clinical impact for the patient is accelerated erosion of muscle mass and worsening debility.

Carbohydrate Metabolism

Blood glucose concentrations are normally maintained within a very narrow range by adjustments in both glucose uptake and glucose production. During critical illness, patients demonstrate hyperglycemia and glucose intolerance. Glucose tolerance tests in patients early after injury—in the ebb phase—reveal elevated concentrations of glucose that return toward normal slowly (Figure 21-2). Because insulin is a major determinant of

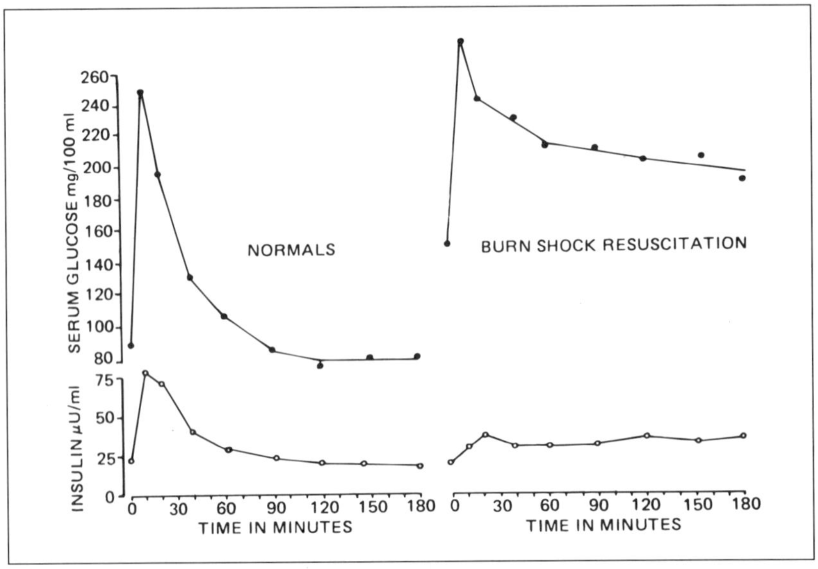

Figure 21-2. Intravenous glucose tolerance test of normal subject and patient during burn shock resuscitation (ebb phase). Glucose intolerance is related primarily to reduced elaboration of insulin. (From DW Wilmore. *The Metabolic Management of the Critically Ill.* New York: Plenum, 1977. P 95.)

glucose tolerance, insulin concentrations are usually monitored during tests of glucose tolerance. Relative to normal controls, insulin concentrations are typically reduced early following injury, suggesting that the β cell response to glucose is impaired. Later during the flow phase, even though glucose intolerance persists, insulin concentrations are normal or high [55]. Fasting, basal blood glucose, and insulin concentrations in patients satisfactorily recovering from moderate trauma are both elevated compared with control, but the increase in insulin is proportionately much greater (Table 21-3). This suggests an altered relationship between insulin and glucose in patients recovering from critical illness.

Black and his associates [56] characterized this altered relationship between glucose and insulin by utilizing glucose clamp techniques in patients recovering from moderate trauma and age-matched controls. Under conditions of fixed hyperglycemia, normal subjects demonstrated continuous increases in both insulin concentration and whole-body glucose disposal. Under the same conditions, patients had limited glucose disposal despite increasing insulin concentrations, which were more abundant than in controls. When hyperinsulinemia was maintained with an insulin infusion and glucose "clamped" at normal levels, the patients had lower glucose disposal rates at all insulin doses and concentrations studied (50 to 500 U/ml). Thus, the patients had insulin resistance. Based on the dose-response relationship, it appeared that this was a postreceptor defect [56].

Wolfe and his colleagues [57,58] studied glucose oxidation in patients following major elective abdominal surgery and following burns. They found that there was an apparent upper limit for glucose oxidation in both groups, which was much lower than the rates for normals. Collectively, these reports suggest that there is a limitation to glucose utilization in patients with critical illness and that this response, like many others, is a graded one—related to the severity of injury (Table 21-4).

Table 21-3. Basal Concentrations of Glucose and Insulin

	Plasma Glucose (mg/dl)	Serum Insulin (μU/ml)
Normal subjects	98 ± 1	12 ± 1
Recovering trauma patients	104 ± 2	17 ± 2

Glucose concentration is the result of the balance between the rate of glucose uptake and excretion and the rate of glucose production, absorption, and administration. Glucose production is elevated in stable patients following injury [59]. In studies of burn patients, the increase in glucose production was strongly related to the degree of hypermetabolism and, thus, to injury severity [60]. Under normal conditions, glucose production is suppressed by insulin. In critically ill patients, however, this suppression is blunted. Black [56] observed that glucose production was elevated in recovering trauma patients and incompletely suppressed even at high concentrations of insulin. This relatively nonsuppressible endogenous glucose production contributes to the glucose intolerance observed during the flow phase.

If glucose production is increased during critical illness and glucose uptake in insulin-sensitive tissues—principally muscle and fat—is reduced, then there must be increased uptake of glucose in other tissues not influenced by insulin, as long as glucose concentrations are relatively stable. Wilmore and associates [61] studied regional metabolic alterations in patients with major burns. The presence of a healing wound on an extremity was associated with an increase in blood flow to the extremity, which was directed to the surface wound [62]. There was also an increase in glucose uptake across the extremity that was matched by an increase in lactate release. There was no difference in oxygen consumption between extremities that had large burn wounds or small ones. Oxygen consumption was related to the patient's total burn size. Studies of fibroblasts from wounds demonstrate increased enzymatic capacity for glycolysis [63]. In critically ill patients, therefore, the

Table 21-4. Maximal Rates of Glucose Oxidation or Disposal

	mg/kg · min	g/kg · day	kcal/day (70 kg)
Postoperative	7	10.1	2400
Moderate injury	6	8.6	2050
Severe burn	5	7.2	1710

Source: Data from RR Wolfe et al. Investigation of factors determining optimal glucose infusion rate in total parenteral nutrition. *Metabolism* 29:892, 1980; PR Black et al. Mechanisms of insulin resistance following injury. *Ann Surg* 196:420, 1982; and RR Wolfe et al. Glucose metabolism in severely burned patients. *Metabolism* 28:1031, 1979.

wound or mass of inflammatory tissue is a major site of glucose uptake. Much of this is not oxidized, but partially metabolized to lactate and released back into the circulation. Glucose fuels the healing wound. [*Editor's Note:* This may not be completely correct. Some of the diverse cellular elements in a healing wound may use other substrates.]

Lipid Metabolism

Adipose tissue is the largest fuel reserve in the body accounting for some 20% of the body weight in a healthy adult of normal body composition. The lipolysis of fat reserves to form glycerol and free fatty acids provides a source of energy for most cells in the body, except for those that specifically require glucose. Under normal conditions, fasting mobilizes fat stores, and glucose suppresses lipolysis. Under conditions of critical illness, lipolysis is a major source of energy and is not suppressed when exogenous glucose is administered. Plasma free fatty acids are typically elevated. This is usually associated with increased turnover of fatty acids also. Galster and associates [64] measured fatty acid turnover in patients with uncomplicated burns. They found that free fatty acid concentration and turnover correlated and were directly related to the size of the burn, that is, to the severity of injury. In elegant studies of lipid metabolism in trauma patients, Shaw and Wolfe [65] found that glycerol turnover was more than doubled in patients as compared with normal controls. There is also a doubling of the free fatty acid (FFA) oxidation rate, but only a 30% increase in FFA turnover. This suggested that when triglycerides were hydrolyzed some of the free fatty acids were oxidized directly in the cells and did not pass into the circulation as did glycerol.

Infection

Infection is a common component of critical illness. It may be part of the patient's primary disease as in perforated diverticulitis, or it may develop secondarily, complicating some other primary inflammatory process, as in pneumonia developing in a patient with multiple trauma. The metabolic alterations that develop in response to infection are clinically similar to those that accompany trauma. Wilmore [48] observed that hypermetabolic burn patients that developed bacteremia became even more hypermetabolic: they had increased O_2 consumption and glucose production. Patients that developed bacteremia and organ failure, however, had decreased metabolic rate and glucose production. Aulick [66] demonstrated the additive effect of infection and wounds in an animal model. Animals with burn wounds colonized with bacteria were more hypermetabolic than animals whose wounds were treated with topical antimicrobial agents.

Patients with infection manifest hypermetabolism, accelerated net skeletal muscle protein loss, glucose tolerance, and a variety of other alterations, including fever, leukocytosis, increased hepatic production of the so-called acute-phase proteins, and decreases in the concentrations of several trace minerals. These have been grouped together in the term *acute-phase response* [66]. This response, however, is not specific for infection and is seen in patients with a wide variety of inflammatory processes, although particularly marked fever and leukocytosis are usually associated with uncontrolled infection.

Role of the Gut

Since the first edition of this text was published in 1983, our conceptions of the GI tract during critical illness have changed markedly. We used to believe that the gut was fairly inert during critical illness, unless stress bleeding or an intraluminal infection developed. Since then a great deal of work has been done (much of it is chronicled in other chapters of this book), so now the gut is viewed as playing a central amplifying role in many of the responses to critical illness observed in patients [67]. In 1984, Mochizuki and Alexander [68] reported an important series of studies they had performed in animals. They placed gastrostomies in guinea pigs and then subjected the animals to a standard scald burn on the back. Some of the animals began to receive gastrostomy feedings immediately after the burn during resuscitation. Others were fasted during the resuscitation period and allowed to resume an oral diet 36 to 48 hours postburn. Early feedings preserved the mass and integrity of the intestinal mucosa, whereas the period of fasting resulted in marked atrophy of the mucosa and superficial erosions. In addition, the animals receiving early enteral feedings had less intense metabolic responses than the controls. When nutritional support was provided intravenously, mucosal changes similar to those in fasted animals were still seen [69]. Although these studies can be viewed as supporting the benefits of early nutritional support, equally important was the association between preservation of the gut mucosal integrity and a reduction in the intensity of the metabolic responses. Animals who had received early gastrostomy feedings had lower cortisol levels (a stress hormone) and had much less of a reduction in muscle weight than those animals treated with initial bowel rest. They hypothesized that preservation of the GI mucosal integrity triggered less of a catabolic response and reduced the metabolic cost of critical illness.

Another important study was one carried out by O'Dwyer [70], who measured intestinal permeability in normal subjects given a small dose of endotoxin. Lactulose and mannitol, two high-molecular-weight sugars, were administered to the volunteers, and the amounts of these sugars excreted in the urine over the next several hours was determined. These compounds have a high molecular weight, and under normal conditions they are neither metabolized nor absorbed to a large degree so that an increase in urinary excretion indicates a change in permeability of the GI tract. As seen in Table 21-5, endotoxin increased the amount of sugar detectable in the urine, and this was associated with higher peak norepinephrine concentration, an indicator of the intensity of metabolic responses. In addition, the work of Deitch and Berg [71–73] described the phenomenon of bacterial translocation following a variety of noxious stimuli in animals. The importance of bacterial translocation as a source of portal or systemic bacteremia is not clear [74], but alterations in GI permeability may alter bacterial clearance and the absorption or release of endotoxin.

Since the first edition of the book, it has also been well established that the amino acid glutamine is a major respiratory fuel for the GI tract [52,53]. Under conditions of stress or critical illness, the GI tract actively absorbs glutamine from the circulation. Because circulating glutamine concentrations are low during critical illness and because standard nutritional support may provide little or no glutamine, GI integrity may be further compromised by relative nutritional deficiency.

Patients with critical illness often have some insult to their GI tracts early in the course of their disease either because of bowel rest, or operation, or injury. If endotoxin gains access to the circulation from clearance of bacteria associated with an intravenous device or pneumonia, then the patient may develop an accentuation of some of the clinical responses to critical illness, and the permeability of the GI tracts may be increased. This may lead to enhanced bacterial clearance or endotoxin absorption from the GI tract, which will further accentuate clinical symptoms and lead to further permeability alterations. The GI tract thus may participate in a vicious cycle of events that amplify clinical responses to critical illness and magnify the metabolic cost of disease [67].

Integrated Metabolic Responses to Critical Illness

The organ systems and tissues that appear to play major roles in the metabolic responses to critical illness include liver, muscle, gut, kidneys, and wound. In addition, the heart provides the force behind the increased circulatory needs of the critically ill patient. Enhanced blood flow serves to increase transport of various substrates and other compounds between organs (Figure 21-3). The wound consumes glucose and also has increased requirements for amino acids to support protein synthesis and cellular proliferation. Glucose is metabolized to lactate, which can then be released back into the circulation. Lactate is taken up by the liver and reprocessed to glucose via the Cori cycle. Thus, glucose is cycled between the liver and the wound. The muscle appears to be a major source of amino acids, which are released largely as glutamine and alanine. Glutamine is a primary fuel for the GI tract and cells, such as inflammatory cells [75]. Glutamine may also be taken up by the kidneys and used to buffer an increased acid load from accelerated lean tissue proteolysis. Glutamine is metabolized to ammonia and alanine in the gut and then transported to the liver, where ammonia is excreted and the alanine can be utilized to form new glucose. The liver also produces acute-phase proteins. All these processes require energy and are a source of increased heat production.

Regulation

The regulation of these interrelated metabolic alterations has been an active area of investigation

Table 21-5. Effects of Endotoxin in Humans

	Control	Endotoxin
Lactulose excretion (mg/12 hr)	145 ± 19	263 ± 36
Mannitol excretion (mg/12 hr)	4.9 ± 0.3	5.7 ± 0.3
Peak norepinephrine (pg/ml)	137 ± 8	430 ± 70
Peak cortisol (μg/dl)	10 ± 1	29 ± 2
Leukocyte count (10^3/mm^2)	6.2 ± 0.4	10.0 ± 1.0

Source: Data from ST O'Dwyer et al. A single dose of endotoxin increases intestinal permeability in healthy humans. *Arch Surg* 123:1459, 1988.

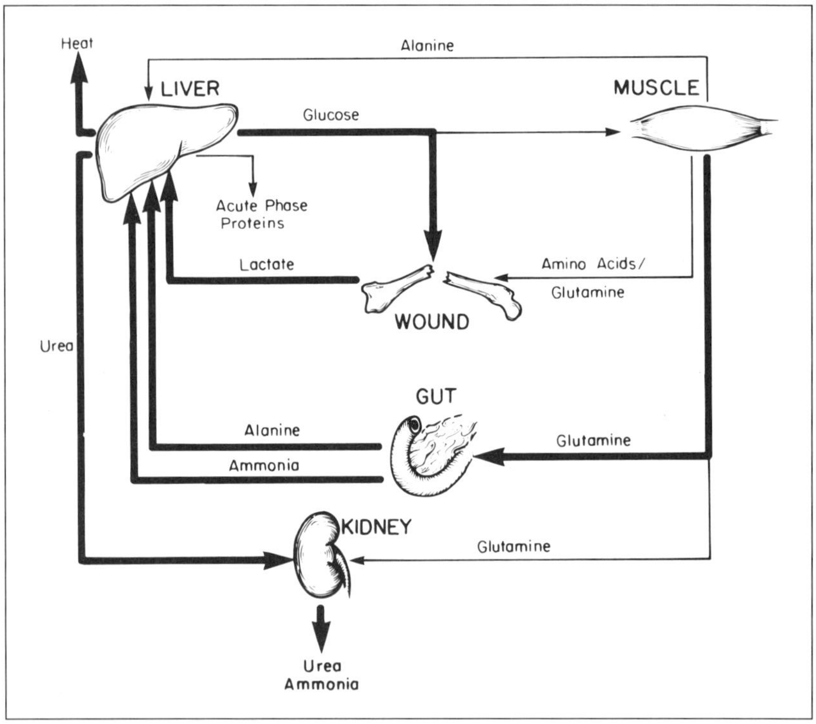

Figure 21-3. The metabolic responses to critical illness involve alterations in the function of several organ systems. The movement of substrates between regional tissue beds is supported by enhanced blood flow. (From PQ Bessey. Parenteral nutrition and trauma. In JL Rombeau, MD Caldwell (eds), *Clinical Nutrition: Parenteral Nutrition.* Philadelphia: Saunders, 1993. P 546.)

for many years. Although a clear understanding of the characteristics of these responses may serve as a basis for supportive care, elucidation of regulatory mechanisms may point to opportunities to modify the nature of these responses to the net benefit of the patient, and so reduce the overall metabolic cost of critical illness. Regulation of the responses involves both neuroendocrine and inflammatory mechanisms. It is useful to think of the responses as part of a reflex arc. This includes an afferent limb consisting of all the various signals indicating the presence of an injury or an infection and an efferent limb consisting of signals that alter the function of specific organs and tissues.

Ebb Phase

In a series of classic experiments, Hume and Egdahl [76] demonstrated that an intact nervous system up to the level of the midbrain is essential for initiating the early responses to injury. They measured the concentration of corticosteroids in the adrenal venous blood in response to the standard injury to an extremity. The usual increase in steroid concentrations could be obliterated by section of the peripheral nerve or spinal cord. These studies indicated that neural afferent signals (presumably pain) and the central nervous system (CNS) were major components in the neuroendocrine reflex arc. In another group of experiments, Egdahl [77] removed the cortex, thalamus, and hypothalamus in various combinations. The change in corticosteroid concentration in response to injury was seen in all groups except those in which the hypothalamus had been removed.

These studies emphasize the important coordinating role played by the central nervous system, specifically the hypothalamus. The hypothalamus is the highest level of integration for autonomic functions. When brain structures superior to the hypothalamus are removed, most autonomic functions are preserved [78]. Autonomic functions integrated at the level of the hypothalamus include food intake, water intake, and temperature control. In addition, the hypothalamus has connections to the anterior pituitary and regulates the concentrations of a variety of pituitary hormones including adrenotropic hormone (ACTH), thyroid-stimulating hormone (TSH), growth hormone (GH), prolactin luteotropic hormone, and follicle-stimulating hormone. In addition, the hypothalamus is a source of the posterior pituitary hormone, antidiuretic hormone (ADH).

Several neural afferent signals may influence the hypothalamus (Figure 21-4). Pain is a major indicator of injury even during general anesthesia and operative procedures. Thus, patients with paraplegia and those with neural blockade with epidural or spinal anesthesia, or even local anesthesia to some extent, manifest reduced early injury responses [79]. In addition, local tissue

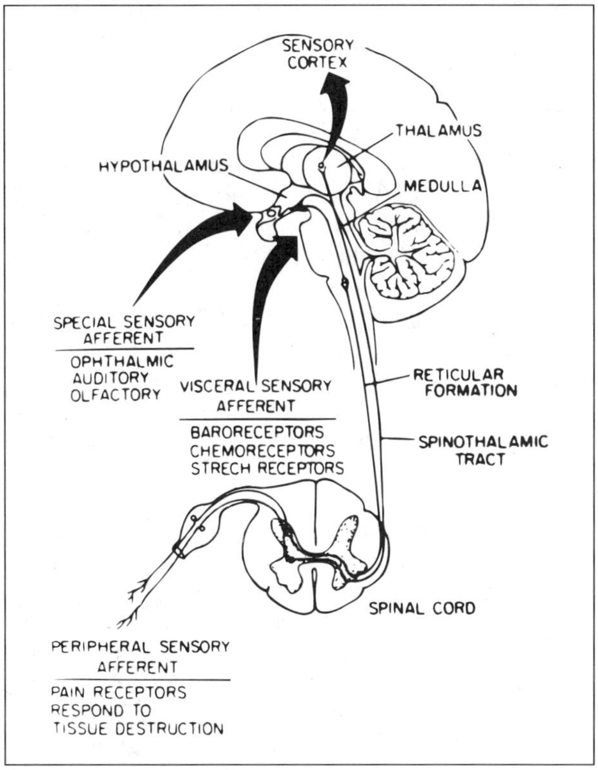

Figure 21-4. Afferent neurologic pathways by which the central nervous system is altered to the immediate presence of an injury. (From MB Popp, MF Brennan. Metabolic response to trauma and infection. In JE Fischer (ed), *Surgical Nutrition* [1st ed]. Boston: Little, Brown, 1983. P 481.)

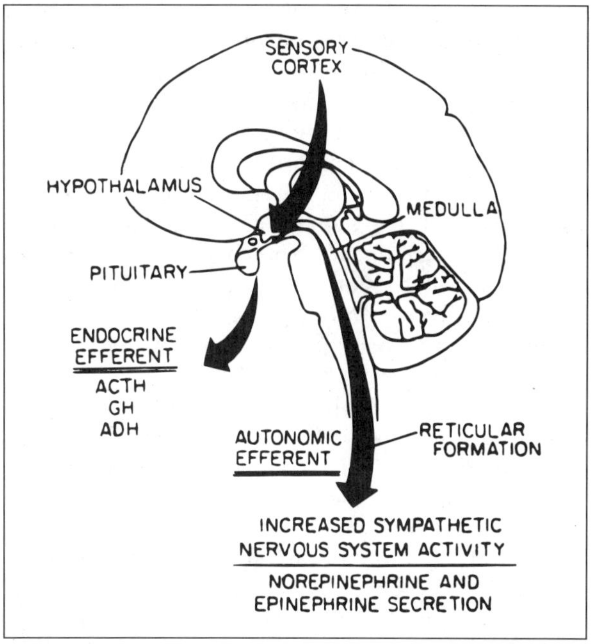

Figure 21-5. Efferent pathways that influence the neuroendocrine response to injury and critical illness. (From MB Popp, MF Brennan. Metabolic response to trauma and infection. In JE Fischer (ed), *Surgical Nutrition* [1st ed]. Boston: Little, Brown, 1983. P 481.)

damage may release proteolytic enzymes and other mediators that may stimulate specific peripheral nerves, which then transmit signals to the CNS. These signals project onto the cortex via the thalamus and thus produce subjective sensation of pain.

Other neural afferent signals may come from feedback control systems important in maintaining homeostasis. Hypovolemia will affect neural signals that arise from the atrial stretch receptors and are then integrated in the hypothalamus [80]. Baroreceptors in the aortic arch and the carotid bulb are sensitive to changes in blood pressure. These two systems enable subjects to compensate quickly for acute hypovolemia [81]. Vasoconstriction in the periphery and in the splanchnic bed shifts the distribution of blood flow. If volume loss is not too excessive, blood pressure and pulse rate will be minimally affected [82,83]. A variety of chemoreceptors may be affected by hypoxia and changes in glucose concentration [84, 85].

The hypothalamus influences end organ function by both the autonomic nervous system and the pituitary axis (Figure 21-5). The autonomic nervous system is divided into sympathetic and parasympathetic divisions. All blood vessels and organ systems are innervated by one or both of these divisions, which under normal conditions influence vasomotor tone and most organ function. The sympathetic division of the autonomic nervous system appears to be the major effector pathway for acute responses to a variety of stressful situations including operation, trauma, burns, myocardial infarction, cold, and anxiety. The classic work of Cannon [86] emphasized the importance of the sympathetic division of the autonomic nervous system in the response to stressful situations. He demonstrated that the sympathetic ganglia were composed of a few preganglionic fibers synapsed with multiple nerves to the periphery. The central signals were thus multiplied and distributed to a wide variety of target tissue. This provided an explanation for the earlier observation that oblation of parts of the sympathetic nervous system could abolish or modify many of the clinical features seen in response to stress such as tachycardia, peripheral vasoconstriction, piloerection, and diaphoresis. It was also appreciated that hyperglycemia was a typical response to stress. Over a century ago, Claude Bernard [87] demonstrated that stimulation of the hypothalamus increased blood sugar concentrations.

The adrenal medulla is a component of the sympathetic nervous system. The secretion of the hormone epinephrine results from sympathetic stimulation of the adrenal medulla. Epinephrine then distributes this autonomic signal throughout the body via the circulation. Measurements of blood catecholamines and urinary catecholamine excretion further document the role of the sympathetic nervous system in the acute response to stress [88–92]. Norepinephrine is thought to appear in the circulation from an overflow or leak from sympathetic nerve endings. Norepinephrine has primarily α-adrenergic effects, whereas epinephrine exerts primarily β-adrenergic effects at physiologic concentrations [93].

Infusion of norepinephrine or epinephrine results in an increase in glucose and free fatty acid concentrations [94]. In part, this is mediated by a decrease in insulin concentration [95]. The studies of Porte [94,95] have characterized adrenergic influences on the pancreatic β cell. Alpha-adrenergic stimulation by norepinephrine or high-dose epinephrine appears to inhibit insulin release, whereas β stimulation permits an exaggerated insulin response to increasing blood sugar concentrations. In addition, Bessey [96] demonstrated that an infusion of epinephrine caused insulin resistance acutely. Thus, as the result of a variety of mechanisms, stimulation of the sympathoadrenal axis results in a rapid increase in the blood glucose concentration. This serves as a readily available source of energy for exercising muscle and the central nervous system.

In addition to catecholamines, other hormones are elevated acutely following injury. Glucagon is a peptide hormone elaborated by the pancreatic α cell. Its major role is to promote gluconeogenesis by the liver. The release of glucagon from the pancreatic α cell also appears to be under sympathoadrenal control and is promoted by β-adrenergic stimuli [97,98]. Glucagon, thus, would appear to contribute to the hyperglycemic response to injury and acute stress.

Certain pituitary hormones are also elevated acutely following injury. Elevations of the circulating concentrations of cortisol are commonly seen following trauma, burns, and operation [99–101]. The secretion of cortisol is under the control of ACTH from the anterior pituitary. The presence of cortisol appears to be important for the early responses to injury and stress because adrenalectomized animals do not tolerate shock or injury unless maintenance glucocorticoids are administered [102]. Thus, cortisol has been viewed as having a permissive role in the early stress response rather than exerting direct effects [103]. Sherwin and his associates [104,105] studied the effects of cortisol and the other counterregulatory hormones of glucagon and epinephrine on glucose homeostasis both in humans and in animals. Any one of the hormones resulted in only a modest and/or transient increase in blood sugar concentration, but when all three hormones were administered together at doses that achieved physiologic elevations, there was a marked increase in glucose concentration, which persisted throughout the several hours of the experiment (Figure 21-6). Thus, cortisol appears not merely to permit other hormones to exert their influence but is itself essential for the full development of clinical responses seen in acutely ill patients.

Flow Phase

Neuroendocrine Mediators

With resuscitation and stabilization, the clinical ebb phase evolves into the flow phase. As discussed, these alterations primarily include hypermetabolism, accelerated net muscle protein breakdown, glucose intolerance, and insulin resis-

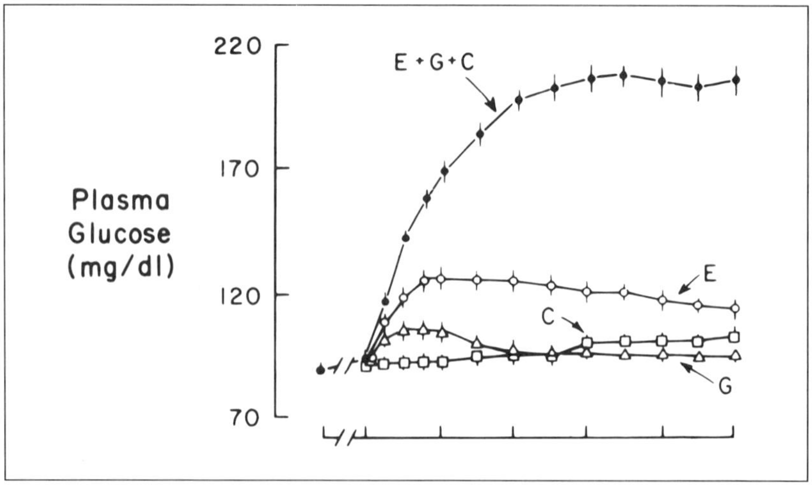

Figure 21-6. Synergistic influence of the stress hormones—cortisol, glucagon, epinephrine—on blood glucose concentration. The three hormones together result in hyperglycemia that is greater than that produced by any one of the hormones alone, and the effect is sustained. (From HM Shamoon, R Hendler, RS Sherwin. Synergistic interactions among the anti-insulin hormones in the pathogenesis of stress hyperglycemia in humans. *J Clin Endocrinol Metab* 52:1240, 1981.)

tance. In addition, there is an acute-phase response consisting of fever and leukocytosis. These appear to be graded responses that are related to the size of the wound or the mass of inflammatory tissue. They resolve as the wounds heal and inflammation subsides.

The role of neural input as an afferent signal is less clear in the flow phase than it is in the ebb phase. For example, hypermetabolic burn patients whose wounds are treated with topical anesthetics remained hypermetabolic [106]. The brain, however, appears to continue to play an important coordinating role. Thus, morphine, general anesthetics, and sedatives reduce hypermetabolism [107–109]. Several endocrine hormones appear to influence metabolic alterations in the flow phase. Cortisol, glucagon, and the catecholamines are increased in concentration in the early phases of the injury response and persist to varying degrees later [110]. The degree of hypermetabolism is related to urinary catecholamine excretion and to the concentrations of cortisol and glucagon following severe injury [101,111,112]. Based on the studies of Sherwin and his associates cited above, Bessey and co-workers [113] administered an infusion of hydrocortisone, glucagon, and epinephrine to normal volunteers to achieve and sustain physiologic elevations of counterregulatory hormone concentration. This simple manipulation of the hormonal environment resulted in many of the physiologic alterations characteristic of critical illness (Table 21-6). Some of the subjects also received infusions of epinephrine or cortisol alone. Results of those studies suggested that the effects of the hormones combined reflected different types of interactions between them. For example, the increase in metabolic rate appeared to reflect additive effects of the individual hormones. Glucose intolerance and insulin resistance appeared to represent primarily an effect of cortisol. The increase in nitrogen excretion, however, seemed to represent a synergistic interaction between all three hormones; any of the hormones individually had only a small effect on nitrogen excretion relative to control. Though the infusion of counterregulatory hormones increased whole-body nitrogen loss and muscle protein catabolism determined by isotopic techniques, increased net skeletal muscle protein breakdown after 3 days of the infusion was not observed [114]. Thus, the increase in stress hormone concentration does not appear to be a sufficient stimulus by itself to account for the clinical features of critical illness as encountered in patients.

The role of insulin during these hypermetabolic responses bears consideration. The best appreciated effect of insulin is its influence on glucose uptake by peripheral tissue that is sensitive to insulin, specifically muscle, fat, and liver. Insulin interacts with specific insulin receptors located in the plasma membrane [115]. Once bound, insulin acts in part by stimulating phosphorylation of tyrosine kinase. The uptake of glucose appears to involve the action of a specific regulatable glucose transporter protein, which is translocated from the center of the cell to the plasma membrane [116]. These interactions then permit the passage of glucose across the membrane into the cell along a concentration gradient. The glucose transporter protein regulatable by insulin is known as Glut-4. Other glucose transporter proteins do not depend on insulin and are found in other cells. In critically ill patients, insulin-mediated glucose uptake is impaired. This

Table 21-6. Metabolic Effects of Stress Hormone Infusion

	Control	Hormone Infusion
Cortisol (μg/dl)	12 ± 1	40 ± 84
Glucagon (pg/ml)	79 ± 14	507 ± 65
Epinephrine (pg/ml)	22 ± 5	417 ± 52
Metabolic rate (kcal/m²·hr)	32.2 ± 1.1	38.4 ± 1.3
Nitrogen balance (g/day)	−0.2 ± 0.4	−3.2 ± 0.4
Protein breakdown (g nitrogen/day)	38.4 ± 1.9	46.5 ± 2.5
Muscle amino acid nitrogen (mmol/L intracellular H_2O)	43.5 ± 0.6	37.6 ± 1.5
Plasma glucose (mg/dl)	94 ± 2	133 ± 4
Glucose production (mg/kg·min)	2.08 ± 0.06	2.55 ± 0.06
Serum insulin (μU/ml)	8 ± 1	22 ± 3
C-peptide excretion (μg/day)	44.0 ± 6.4	141.3 ± 16.9
Insulin-mediated glucose disposal (mg/kg·min)	8.62 ± 0.51	3.22 ± 0.51
Insulin-mediated forearm glucose uptake (mg/100ml·min)	1.03 ± 0.09	0.48 ± 0.12

Source: Adapted from PQ Bessey et al. Combined hormonal infusion simulates the metabolic response to injury. *Ann Surg* 200:264, 1984; and PQ Bessey et al. Post-traumatic skeletal muscle proteolysis: The role of the hormonal environment. *World J Surg* 13:465, 1989.

would appear to be a postreceptor defect that may involve the alterations of intracellular movement of Glut-4.

Under normal conditions, insulin reduces net skeletal muscle protein breakdown. It appears to do this primarily by alternating the rate of protein breakdown rather than affecting the rate of protein synthesis [117,118]. This ability of insulin to reduce net muscle catabolism appears to be preserved in stable patients recovering from trauma, even though insulin-mediated glucose uptake is impaired [119,120].

Infusion of hydrocortisone, glucagon, and epinephrine did not appear to increase net skeletal muscle protein breakdown in normal volunteers, but it did increase concentrations of glucose and insulin, similar to clinical findings during the flow phase [113,114]. At the onset of critical illness in the ebb phase, however, insulin is normal or suppressed. Studies of muscle protein breakdown in vitro have demonstrated that insulin can abrogate the catabolic effects of glucocorticoids if present in the incubation medium at the outset [121]. When added after the cortisol effect had been established, however, insulin reduced but did not abolish the increased rate of net breakdown. To test whether or not the suppression of insulin in the ebb phase might influence later catabolic effects of counterregulatory hormones, Bessey and Lowe [122] administered the somatostatin analogue during the first day of a 72-hour infusion of counterregulatory hormones. The early insulin response to hyperglycemia was blunted, and this was associated with a further increase in whole-body nitrogen excretion. There was no effect on net skeletal muscle protein breakdown after 24 hours of somatostatin and triple hormone infusions. Forty-eight hours later, however, when the insulin response in both studies was not impaired, net skeletal muscle protein breakdown was significantly increased. Thus, the inhibition of the insulin response early during stress hormone infusion modified the ultimate catabolic effects of the hormones. The results of these studies also suggest that the early loss of nitrogen may come from a central source, presumably the splanchnic bed [123]. The increase in muscle protein breakdown would then be a secondary phenomenon that may serve to mobilize amino acids from the periphery to replete splanchnic amino acid pools.

Other hormones may exert anabolic effects in the critically ill patient. Growth hormone, or somatotropin, is a group of related polypeptides synthesized by the somatotrophic cells in the anterior pituitary [124]. Growth hormone release is stimulated by a releasing factor elaborated in the hypothalamus. Growth hormone promotes amino acid uptake, protein synthesis, and growth. With nutritional support it enhances the efficiency of protein assimilation [125]. There also appears to be a synergistic interaction with insulin [126]. Growth hormone acts in part by stimulating the elaboration of insulin-like growth factor (IGF-1) located primarily in the liver and muscle. Isotopic studies indicate that growth hormone may specifically stimulate protein synthesis, whereas IGF-1 appears to reduce protein breakdown [127,128]. Growth hormone also induces some degree of insulin resistance and is associated with diminished glucose tolerance and enhanced lipolysis [129]. IGF-1 and insulin share many common metabolic effects [130]. IGF-1 secretion is under the control of growth hormone, and IGF-1 receptors are present in the plasma membrane of the same cells that appear to produce IGF-1 in response to growth hormone. Thus, IGF-1 may work in an autocrine manner stimulating the growth of the same cell type by which it is synthesized.

Inflammatory Mediators—Cytokines

Although endocrine mediators appear to play an important role in the regulation of metabolic events during critical illness, they alone do not account for the clinical alterations observed in many critically ill patients. Other mechanisms must also participate. Growth in understanding the role of cytokines and other inflammatory mediators has been especially important in this regard. These developments are detailed elsewhere in this book, but some discussion here is warranted.

Early studies indicated that a circulating factor elaborated by white cells, later identified as interleukin-1 (IL-1), stimulated muscle protein breakdown and involved the prostaglandin cascade [131,132]. Later studies confirmed the involvement of the prostaglandin cascade but did not demonstrate a direct proteolytic effect either in vitro or in vivo [133]. Watters [134] created sterile inflammation in normal subjects by injections of steroidal compound etiocholanolone. This resulted in fever, leukocytosis, and alterations of acute-phase proteins. It had little effect, however, on nitrogen excretion. In contrast, elevations of counterregulatory hormone concentrations induced a variety of metabolic alterations, including increased nitrogen excretion, but it did not produce an appreciable change in body temperature or in acute-phase proteins. In additional studies, Watters [135] administered etiocholanolone in normal volunteers during an infusion of counterregulatory hormones. The subjects manifested both an acute-phase response and a moderate degree of hypermetabolism. These combined alterations appeared to reproduce all of the metabolic derangements seen in patients with acute clinical disease [136]. Thus, both endocrine and inflammatory mediators appear to be responsible for clinical alterations seen in critically ill patients. No one mechanism predominates.

IL-1 is a protein or family of proteins that appears to have an important role in the acute-phase response [137]. It was one of the first cytokines to be identified. IL-1 induces fever when administered intravenously. A much smaller amount injected intrathecally will produce the same febrile response, indicating that IL-1 acts via a central mechanism [138]. IL-1 immunoreactivity has been demonstrated in the hypothalamus of humans, suggesting that IL-1 may serve as a central modulating signal [139].

Tumor necrosis factor (TNF) has a variety of local and systemic effects that appear to be dose dependent. Endotoxin is a strong stimulus for TNF elaboration. When they gave endotoxin in small doses, Michie and associates [140] observed a sharp rise in TNF concentration approximately one and one-half hours after the endotoxin. The TNF was cleared rapidly and preceded the appearance of symptoms, fever, and leukocytosis. Some of the responses appeared to be mediated by prostaglandins because cyclo-oxygenase blockade ameliorated symptoms but did not affect the rise of TNF and the development of leukocytosis following endotoxin. Tracey and Lowry [141] provided dramatic evidence of the importance of TNF as a mediator of the responses to endotoxin. When lethal doses of endotoxin were administered to experimental animals, death could be prevented by the prior administration of an antibody against TNF. TNF is the first in a cascade of cytokines that are elaborated in response to endotoxin [142]. IL-1 follows TNF, and then IL-6 and IL-8 appear. IL-6 is the principal mediator of the acute-phase response in the sense that it plays a major role in increasing hepatic protein synthesis [143].

The mechanisms by which cytokines are related to the metabolic alterations seen in patients and how they interact with other mediators has not been fully characterized. For example, an inverse relationship between hypercortisolemia and TNF has been observed in critically ill burn patients [144]. Barber and her associates [145] demonstrated that cortical infusion could blunt the TNF response to endotoxin in humans and suppress the development of symptoms; however, this effect was dependent. When the cortisol was administered six hours prior to endotoxin, there was suppression of TNF appearance, but there was no effect on the development of symptoms, and there was an enhancement of the hypercortisolemia induced by endotoxin. Recently it has become apparent that there are other endogenous compounds that neutralize the effects of several of the cytokines. These include soluble receptors for TNF and IL-2, each of which can bind to its specific circulating cytokine, and an IL-1 receptor antagonist that competitively inhibits IL-1 binding. These compounds seem to appear in the circulation in a characteristic sequence following trauma [146], much as do the cytokines in response to endotoxin.

Michie [147] administered prolonged infusions of TNF to animals and humans. Negative nitrogen balance developed in all cases, but it was related to the onset of anorexia and reduced food intake rather than to the development of hypermetabolism. In animals that had adrenalectomies, TNF did not increase nitrogen loss [148]. Hasselgren and colleagues [149] could prevent the increase in myofibrillar protein breakdown in muscle in an animal model of intraabdominal sepsis by administering a steroid antagonist. When glucocorticoids were administered alone, however, they observed little effect on increased total and myofibrillar muscle protein breakdown [150]. TNF by itself also had only a small effect, but when administered concomitantly with glucocorticoids, it amplified the steroid effect by a factor of two [151]. TNF appears to have little if any direct influence on muscle protein breakdown. Rather, it may potentiate the glucocorticoid effect.

Interleukin-1, on the other hand, may have a direct effect on net muscle protein metabolism. Zamir and his associates [152] administered recombinant IL-1α (rIL-1α) and observed an increase in myofibrillar protein breakdown in muscle harvested subsequently. This effect was not reduced by administration of the IL-1 receptor antagonist, and it occurred in animals with adrenalectomies. In other studies, IL-1 receptor antagonist prevented the increase in muscle proteolysis in a septic model [153].

Zamir and Hasselgren [154] proposed that at least two different mechanisms accelerate proteolysis in sepsis. One involves stimulation of the pituitary adrenal axis and elaboration of glucocorticoids. This process may be amplified by TNF. IL-1, however, appears to increase muscle protein breakdown by a glucocorticoid-independent pathway. Tiao and associates [155] provided data to elucidate these mechanisms further. One pathway also involves lysosomes. The other is nonlysosomal but is energy-dependent and requires the presence of a polypeptide, ubiquitin, which is found in all eukaryotic cells [155]. This ubiquitin pathway appears to be the major route for proteolysis in sepsis [156]. In addition, Tiao and his colleagues [157] have demonstrated that the glucocorticoid receptor antagonist not only decreased the proteolysis associated with sepsis but also blocked the usual sepsis-induced increase in ubiquitin messenger RNA. Thus, the mechanism whereby glucocorticoids accelerate muscle proteolysis in sepsis involves the synthesis of ubiquitin.

Strategies of Treatment

Contemporary treatment of critically ill patients reflects our understanding of the many physiologic responses to their acute disease. The ebb phase can be viewed as a type of "damage control." Blood flow is redirected to organs most essential to short-term survival; vasoconstriction may limit hemorrhage; multiple mechanisms increase blood glucose and free fatty acid concentrations, thereby assuring a supply of fuel for working cells. Clinical care of patients during the ebb phase is ultimately directed to establishing tissue oxygen delivery that is adequate to support cellular needs. The ABCs of resuscitation must be assured, hemorrhage controlled, and tissue integrity restored. In cases of bacteremia and septicemia, the infection must be controlled with antibiotics and appropriate drainage or debridement.

The flow phase is associated with the healing of wounds and resolution of foci of inflammation. The goals of patient care are to promote these processes and prevent the development of conditions that might exacerbate or prolong catabolic responses. Aggressive treatment of the primary disease remains an important metabolic therapy. Fixation of fractures, debridement of necrotic tissue, surgical closure of wounds, and appropriate treatment of infection should be accomplished expeditiously.

Hypermetabolism is a consistent feature of the metabolic responses to critical illness, particularly during the flow phase after resuscitation. Above-normal cardiac output, oxygen consumption, and energy expenditure are the rule. The intensity of the hypermetabolic response appears to be dependent on the size of the wound or the mass of the inflammatory tissue. There are several lines of evidence suggesting that this is in fact a beneficial and thus desirable response. Several years ago, Clowes and Del Guercio [158] reported improved survival in patients following major operations if cardiac output was elevated. Shoemaker [159] found that an above-normal cardiac output was associated with a favorable outcome in critically ill patients. More recently, Moore and colleagues [160] aggressively resuscitated patients following severe multisystem trauma. Those who had an above-normal cardiac index and oxygen consumption had a markedly lower incidence of multiple organ failure and death than those patients whose hemodynamic variables were in the "normal" range (Table 21-7). Wilmore studied the effect of the ambient temperature on hypermetabolism in burn patients [16]. Hypermetabolism was sensitive to the ambient temperature and increased as the temperature was reduced. As the temperature was lowered, some patients were unable to increase their metabolic rates. In those cases, metabolic rate actually fell and catecholamine excretion increased. Those patients subsequently died. Recently, Shiozaki and associates [161] studied burn patients who could not restore their body temperature quickly after skin grafting. They were unable to increase their metabolic rates in response to cold and had a high mortality. Thus, the ability to increase cardiac output and oxygen consumption has survival benefit. Cardiac output in the high normal or supranormal range (cardiac index of 3.5 to 4.5 $l/m^2 \cdot min$) is an appropriate therapeutic goal. Aggressive early resuscitation and stabilization, including maintenance of circulating volume and pharmacologic support of the heart as needed, should be accomplished as expeditiously as possible.

A myriad of signals may initiate catabolic responses. The development of these during a period of recovery also may perpetuate and exacerbate ongoing responses. Pain control, sedation, precautions against infection, maintenance of intravascular volume and hemodynamic performance, and maintenance of a warm environment are all important components in the general care of the critically ill patient.

More specific strategies based on our under-

Table 21-7. Cardiovascular Performance 12 Hours After Trauma and Multiple Organ Failure

Number of patients	16	24
O_2 consumption ($ml/m^2 \cdot min$)	<150	>150
Cardiac index ($l/m^2 \cdot min$)	3.7 ± 0.3	4.6 ± 0.2
Number developing multiple organ failure	12	4

Source: Data from FA Moore et al. Incommensurate oxygen consumption in response to maximal oxygen availability predicts postinjury multiple organ failure. *J Trauma* 33:58, 1992.

standing of critical illness also have been proposed to minimize or limit catabolic signals. Ibuprofen and other cyclo-oxygenase inhibitors may ameliorate some of the clinical responses to endotoxin and other early inflammatory events involving cytokines [162]. For example, ibuprofen markedly reduced the toxic side effects of IL-2 therapy given to patients with malignancy [163]. The use of these agents either routinely or to limit the development of fever may have potential benefit in limiting catabolic responses during critical illness. Hypoperfusion or shock is commonly encountered, particularly near the onset of a critical illness in the ebb phase. Ischemia may lead to the depletion of ATP and other high-energy compounds in cells, which will then contribute to the generation of toxic oxygen free radicals when perfusion is restored [164]. In addition, bacterial killing by leukocytes involves the generation of oxygen radicals [165]. These toxic oxygen radicals are a potential source of additional injury to tissues. Thus, the administration of high doses of vitamins with antioxidant properties, vitamins A, C, and E, has been advocated in critically ill patients [166]. In the past there has been concern that extremely hypermetabolic states may result in some injury to the myocardium, potentially related to high catecholamine secretion [167]. Herndon and associates [168] administered the β-blocker, propranolol, to children with extensive burns. They were able to reduce cardiac work during the period of recovery without apparently adversely affecting clinical outcome. More recent work has compared the effects of the selective β_1-blocking agent, metoprolol, and the mixed β_1, β_2 agent, propranolol, in a series of burned children [169]. Both agents decreased cardiac work. In addition, the β_1 and β_2 blocking agent reduced lipolysis. There was no effect on protein metabolism. This strategy would have the most benefit for critically ill patients with limited cardiac reserve, but studies in that population need to be completed. Selective decontamination of the GI tract has been proposed as a strategy for reducing infectious complications and death in critically ill patients. Although there appears to be a reduction in the incidence of gram-negative pneumonias, a true clinical benefit has yet to be demonstrated [170]. Finally, attempts to neutralize endotoxin or interfere with the cytokine cascade have shown some potential beneficial effects both in animal experiments and preliminary human trials. Unfortunately, none of these approaches has proven to be beneficial in more rigorous testing [171,172]. As more is learned about the responses to critical illness and the mechanisms that perpetuate or exacerbate the initial insults, new proposals for therapy to limit catabolic signals will be forthcoming.

The increased metabolic rate and accelerated nitrogen loss in hypermetabolic patients affects their nutritional requirements. They require additional energy substrate and protein to support the healing of wounds and resolution of inflammatory processes. The increased nutritional requirements in most patients are modest, as shown in Figure 21-7. Markedly heightened nutrition requirements are typically seen only in patients with excessive burns or severe sepsis and organ failure. Exogenous nutrition support may be necessary to meet a patient's needs, but overfeeding should be avoided. If an excess amount of energy substrate is administered to normal subjects, they will increase their CO_2 production in relation to their O_2 consumption (RQ, respiratory quotient) [173]. This is considered to indicate that the subjects are generating ATP through oxidation of carbohydrate alone. If RQ is greater than one, that indicates that carbohydrate is being converted to fat. When

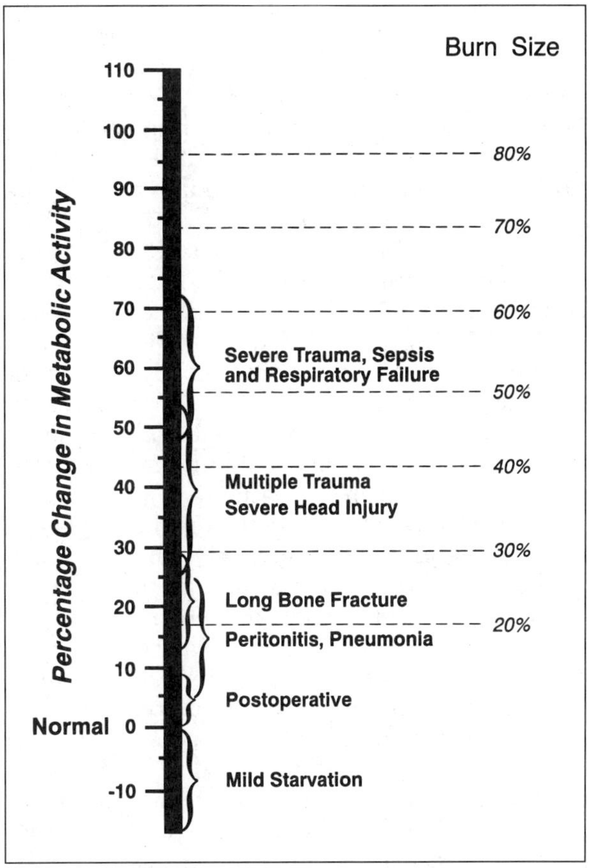

Figure 21-7. Elevations in resting metabolic activity due to critical illness. In most cases, the increase in energy expenditure in patients receiving contemporary care is modest. Large burns still result in the most intense hypermetabolism seen in clinical medicine. (Adapted from DW Wilmore. *The Metabolic Management of the Critically Ill.* New York: Plenum, 1977. P 14; PQ Bessey. Parenteral nutrition and trauma. In JL Rombeau, MD Caldwell (eds), *Clinical Nutrition: Parenteral Nutrition.* Philadelphia: Saunders, 1993. P 540; and DE Carlson et al. Resting energy expenditure in patients with thermal injuries. *Surg Gynecol Obstet* 174:270, 1992.)

critically ill patients are given excess amounts of nutrition, especially carbohydrate, both their CO_2 production and O_2 consumption increase. By driving O_2 consumption, nutritional support adds to the patient's hypermetabolic response. Thus, excessive nutritional support becomes a factor exacerbating the patient's critical illness. Nutritional support is best provided via the GI tract, as is emphasized often in this text. The provision of at least 40% of protein needs via the enteral route has a marked positive impact on the course of the patient's critical illness [174]. This may help to preserve the integrity of the mucosal barrier and thus neutralize the potential amplifying effect of the GI tract on the metabolic responses to critical illness. [*Editor's Note:* I have often reacted with some wonderment to the equation of beneficial effects of gut feeding on mucosal integrity. Surely there are other explanations, including increased hepatic protein synthesis.]

Our growing understanding of the mechanisms involved in the metabolic responses to critical illness and their regulation has led to the proposal of a variety of therapeutic strategies that may modify the responses to critical illness, rather than merely support them. The branched-chain amino acids (BCAA)—leucine, isoleucine, and valine—were thought to have an important benefit in the nutritional support of critically ill patients. Unlike most amino acids, BCAA are metabolized primarily in muscle. Cerra [175] reported that BCAA-enriched intravenous feedings led to an earlier restoration of positive nitrogen balance in critically ill patients. A subsequent randomized prospective study by Bower and associates [176], however, demonstrated relatively small biochemical benefits and could find no impact on the clinical course of the patients.

Recent work has focused on the importance of glutamine as a fuel for rapidly dividing cells, such as the cells in wounds and those of the GI tract. Glutamine is the principal carrier of nitrogen from muscle and may have a role in the regulation of overall muscle protein metabolism [43,44]. Glutamine is not normally present in commercially available amino acid preparations because of its instability during heat sterilization. Thus, standard nutritional support, deficient in glutamine, might contribute to the exacerbation or perpetuation of the responses to critical illness by inadequately supporting the gut and thereby potentiating the deleterious influence of the gut on catabolic responses and/or by failing to maintain intracellular glutamine concentration and thus promoting protein breakdown. Ziegler and associates [177] reported a recent experience with glutamine-enriched intravenous feedings in patients following bone marrow transplantation. Glutamine was added to the intravenous feedings at the time of compounding utilizing cold sterilization techniques. Glutamine enrichment was associated with an improved nitrogen balance, decreased incidence of infectious complications, and shortened hospital stay. Another tactic for increasing the amount of glutamine in intravenous solutions has been proposed by Tremel and his associates [178]. They added a dipeptide containing glutamine to the intravenous nutrition of patients following major elective operation and observed an improvement in nitrogen balance compared with isonitrogenous standard regimens. Several commercial products for enteral nutrition are now available that contain substantial amounts of glutamine. Further experience should help to clarify under what conditions glutamine-enriched nutritional preparations may be an effective nutritional strategy.

Although the responses to critical illness are generally considered to be catabolic, wound healing and other anabolic processes do occur in this setting. Wounds heal, infections abate, and inflammation subsides. Growth hormone is typically increased after injury [179]. Exogenous human growth hormone was administered to burn patients over 20 years ago [180]. It promoted nitrogen uptake as long as nutritional intake was satisfactory. Growth hormone was only available as a biologic preparation at that time, and it had many associated side effects limiting its applicability. With the development of recombinant human growth hormone, however, the incidence of adverse side effects has been reduced. Manson [181] studied the effects of human growth hormone on human volunteers receiving intravenous feedings. The feedings provided a normally sufficient amount of nitrogen but were hypocaloric. During control studies, the subjects were consistently in negative nitrogen balance, but during growth hormone administration, nitrogen balance was positive. Jiang and colleagues [182] administered growth hormone to patients who had major upper abdominal elective operations and intravenous feedings. The feedings were hypocaloric but contained a sufficient amount of amino acids to meet the daily requirement for nitrogen. Growth hormone was administered daily, and intravenous feedings began preoperatively and continued for one week postoperatively. Both groups of patients had negative nitrogen balance immediately surrounding the time of surgery. The group receiving growth hormone, however, quickly achieved positive nitrogen and potassium balance. The control group returned to a positive balance much more slowly. At the end of two weeks, both groups had lost weight. Based on bioelectric impedance assessment of body composition, the control subjects had lost a combination of protein, fat, and water, whereas those receiving growth hormone had lost only fat. In addition, patients receiving growth hormone maintained hand-grip strength throughout the perioperative period. Thus, growth hormone altered the efficiency of nitrogen retention and preserved muscle mass and function.

Herndon [183] utilized growth hormone in the management of severely burned children. The patients receiving growth hormone had more rapid healing of donor sites than control patients. This was associated with increased concentrations of IGF-1. Because the donor sites could be reharvested sooner, patients receiving growth hormone had a shortened hospital stay. Additional recent studies attempted to characterize some of the mechanisms responsible for this beneficial effect of growth hormone on wound healing [184]. Burn patients receiving daily doses of human growth hormone demonstrated increased concentration of IGF-1 receptors in the healing epidermis. In addition, type VII collagen, a major component of the anchoring fibrils involved in the adhesion of the epidermis and dermis, was increased. Knox and associates [185] administered growth hormone to adult patients with major burns and compared them with a similar group of patients who had identical therapy but no growth hormone. Growth hormone reduced the mortality by a factor of three.

In spite of insulin resistance in regard to glucose uptake, insulin remains an important anabolic hormone and can enhance muscle amino acid balance [119]. Insulin is also known to have properties as a growth factor, perhaps by binding to the IGF-1 receptor [186]. Thus, moderately high insulin concentrations may serve to reduce skeletal muscle wasting and to stimulate cellular proliferation and differentiation in the wound. Inculet [187] demonstrated improved nitrogen balance in patients receiving intravenous feedings following major elective surgery. In addition, insulin administered early in the course of critical illness may reduce whole-body nitrogen loss and muscle protein breakdown [122]. Because there is enhanced glucose production, hyperglycemia, and insulin resistance during critical illness, there is an additional margin of safety to insulin administration in this setting. Close control of blood glucose (110 to 160 mg/ml) with exogenous insulin may have metabolic benefit.

Conclusion

The metabolic responses to critical illness consist of a broad array of biochemical and physiologic alterations. They may be initiated by a variety of conditions and insults, and they are perpetuated by the presence of inflammatory tissue—that is, a wound. These responses appear to have survival value and provide, in John Hunter's words, a "disposition and means of cure." Wounds heal, and patients recover. But there is a cost. Lean tissue is rapidly eroded in an attempt to provide fuel and amino acids for the biochemical support of the healing wound. If the process is intense or prolonged, organ failure and death may ensue. The most effective anticatabolic therapy is early and aggressive attention to the wound. Pus should be drained, dead tissue debrided, tissue integrity restored, and the wound closed. The sooner this can occur, the sooner the patient's metabolic activity may return toward normal, and the lower will be the metabolic cost. Support of the patient includes maintaining adequate cardiac performance and oxygen delivery, avoiding additional stresses or developments that could exacerbate existing catabolic responses, and providing nutritional support in amounts sufficient to meet nutritional needs using the GI tract whenever possible. Additional therapies that modify the metabolic responses themselves may also benefit the host. The provision of glutamine in nutritional support and the administration of growth hormone appear promising in this regard.

References

1. Hunter J. *A Treatise on the Blood, Inflammation, and Gun-Shot Wounds*. London: George Nicol, 1794. Facsimile edition, Birmingham, AL: Gryphon, 1985.
2. Cuthbertson DP. The disturbance of metabolism produced by bony and non-bony injury, with notes on certain abnormal conditions of bone. *Biochem J* 24:1244, 1930.
3. Cuthbertson DP. Observations on disturbance of metabolism produced by injury to the limbs. *Q J Med* 25:233, 1932.
4. Moore FD, Ball MR. *The Metabolic Response to Surgery*. Springfield, IL: Thomas, 1952.
5. Moore FD. Metabolism in trauma: The meaning of definitive surgery—the wound, the endocrine glands, and metabolism. *Harvey Lect,* 1958. P. 74.
6. Dudrick SJ, et al. Long-term oral parenteral nutrition with growth, development, and positive nitrogen balance. *Surgery* 64:134, 1986.
7. Wilmore DW, Dudrick SJ. Growth and development of an infant receiving all nutrients exclusively by vein. *JAMA* 203:860, 1968.
8. Moore FD. Getting well: The biology of surgical convalescence. *Ann NY Acad Sci* 73:387, 1958.
9. Cuthbertson DP. Post-shock metabolic response. *Lancet* 1:433, 1942.
10. Mealy K, et al. Physiological and metabolic responses to open and laparoscopic cholecystectomy. *Br J Surg* 79: 1061, 1992.
11. American College of Chest Physicians, Society of Critical Care Medicine Consensus Conference. Definitions for sep-

sis and organ failure and guidelines for the use of innovative therapies in sepsis. *Crit Care Med* 20:864, 1992.

12. DuBois EF. *Basal Metabolism in Health and Disease.* Philadelphia: Lea & Febiger, 1936. P 163.
13. Weir JB deV. New methods for calculating metabolic rate with special reference to protein metabolism. *J Physiol (London)* 109:1, 1949.
14. Ben-Porat M, Sideman S, Burstein S. Energy metabolism rate equation for fasting and postabsorptive subjects. *Am J Physiol* 244:R764, 1983.
15. Shirani KZ, Pruitt BA, Mason AD. The influence of inhalation injury and pneumonia on burn mortality. *Ann Surg* 205:82, 1987.
16. Wilmore DW, et al. Catecholamines: Mediator of the hypermetabolic response to thermal injury. *Ann Surg* 180: 653, 1974.
17. Knaus WA, et al. APACHE—acute physiology and chronic health evaluation: A physiologically based classification system. *Crit Care Med* 9:591, 1981.
18. Boyd CR, Tolson MA, Copes WS. Evaluating trauma care: The TRISS method. *J Trauma* 27:370, 1987.
19. Rangel-Frausto MS, et al. The natural history of the systemic inflammatory response syndrome (SIRS): A prospective study. *JAMA* 273:117, 1995.
20. Cuthbertson DP, McGirr JL, Robertson JSM. The effect of fracture of bone on the metabolism of the rat. *Q J Exp Physiol* 29:13, 1939.
21. Cuthbertson DP. The physiology of convalescence after injury. *Br Med Bull* 3:96, 1945.
22. Wilmore DW. Nutrition and metabolism following thermal injury. *Clin Plast Surg* 1:603, 1974.
23. Kinney JM. Energy Deficits in Acute Illness and Injury. In AP Morgan (ed), *Proceedings of a Conference on Energy Metabolism and Body Fuel Utilization.* Cambridge: Harvard University Press, 1966.
24. Picou D, Taylor-Roberts T. The measurement of total protein synthesis and catabolism and nitrogen turnover in infants on different amounts of dietary protein. *Clin Sci* 36:283, 1969.
25. Kien CL, et al. Increased rates of whole body protein synthesis and breakdown in children recovering from burns. *Ann Surg* 187:383, 1978.
26. Young VR, Munro HN. N^{τ}-Methylhistidine (3-methylhistidine) and muscle protein turnover: An overview. *Fed Proc* 37:2291, 1978.
27. Bilmazes C, et al. Quantitative contributors by skeletal muscle to elevated rates of whole-body protein breakdown in burned children as measured by 3-methylhistidine output. *Metabolism* 27:671, 1978.
28. Williamson DH, et al. Muscle protein catabolism after injury in man as measured by urinary excretion of 3-methylhistidine. *Clin Sci Molec Med* 52:527, 1977.
29. Long CL, et al. Muscle protein catabolism in the septic patient as measured by 3-methylhistidine excretion. *Am J Clin Nutr* 30:1349, 1977.
30. Wassner SJ, Li JB. N^{τ}-methylhistidine release: Contributions of rat skeletal muscle, GI tract, and skin. *Am J Physiol* 243:E293, 1982.
31. Hasselgren PO, et al. Total and myofibrillar protein breakdown in different types of rat skeletal muscle: Effects of sepsis and regulation by insulin. *Metabolism* 38:634, 1989.
32. Downey RS, et al. Protein dynamics in skeletal muscle after trauma: Local and systemic effects. *Surgery* 99:265, 1986.
33. Munro HN. Free Amino Acid Pools and Their Role in Regulation. In HN Munro (ed), *Mammalian Protein Metabolism,* vol. 4. New York: Academic, 1970.
34. Bergstrom J, et al. Intracellular free amino acid concentration in human muscle tissue. *J Appl Physiol* 36:693, 1974.
35. Askanazi J, et al. Muscle and plasma amino acids after injury: The role of inactivity. *Ann Surg* 188:797, 1978.
36. Fuerst P, et al. Influence of amino acid supply on nitrogen and amino acid metabolism in severe trauma. *Acta Chir Scand* 494(S):136, 1979.
37. Askanazi J, et al. Muscle and plasma amino acids following injury: Influence of intercurrent infection. *Ann Surg* 792:78, 1980.
38. Vinnars E, Bergstrom J, Fuerst P. Influence of the postoperative state on the intracellular free amino acids in human muscle tissue. *Ann Surg* 182:665, 1975.
39. Askanazi J, et al. Muscle and plasma amino acids after injury: Hypocaloric glucose vs. amino acid infusion. *Ann Surg* 191:465, 1980.
40. Wedge JH, et al. Branched chain amino acids, nitrogen excretion and injury in man. *Clin Sci Molec Med* 50:393, 1976.
41. Everson TC, Fritschel MJ. The effect of surgery on the plasma levels of the individual essential amino acids. *Surgery* 31:226, 1952.
42. Wilmore DW, Black PR, Muhlbacher F. Injured Man: Trauma and Sepsis. In RW Winters (ed), *Nutritional Support of the Seriously Ill Patient.* New York: Academic, 1983.
43. Rennie MJ, et al. Characteristics of a glutamine carrier in skeletal muscle have important consequences for nitrogen loss in injury, infection and chronic disease. *Lancet* 2:1008, 1986.
44. Johnson DJ, et al. Branched chain amino acid uptake and muscle free amino acid concentrations predict postoperative muscle nitrogen balance. *Ann Surg* 204:513, 1986.
45. Smith RJ. The role of skeletal muscle in interorgan amino acid exchange. *Fed Proc* 45:2172, 1986
46. Garber AJ, Karl IE, Kipnis DM. Alanine and glutamine synthesis and release from skeletal muscle. I. Glycolysis and amino acid release. *J Biol Chem* 251:826, 1976.
47. Aulick LH, Wilmore DW. Increased peripheral amino acid release following burn injury. *Surgery* 85:560, 1979.
48. Wilmore DW, et al. Effect of injury and infection on visceral metabolism and circulation. *Ann Surg* 192:491, 1980.
49. Miller LL, et al. The dominant role of the liver in plasma protein synthesis. *J Exp Med* 94:431, 1951.
50. Kushner I. The acute phase response: An overview. *Methods Enzymol* 163:373, 1988.
51. Pitts RF. Renal Regulation of Acid Base Balance. In *Physiology of Kidney and Body Fluids (3rd ed).* Chicago: Year Book, 1974.
52. Souba WW, et al. The role of glutamine in maintaining a healthy gut and supporting the metabolic response to injury and infection. *J Surg Res* 48:383, 1990.
53. Zielke HR, et al. Reciprocal regulation of glucose and glutamine utilization by cultured human diploid fibroblasts. *J Cell Physiol* 95:41, 1978.
54. Souba WW, Wilmore DW. Postoperative alteration of arteriovenous exchange of amino acids across the gastrointestinal tract. *Surgery* 94:342, 1983.
55. Allison SP, Hinton P, Chamberlain MJ. Intravenous glucose-tolerance, insulin, and free fatty acid levels in burned patients. *Lancet* 2:1113, 1968.

56. Black PR, et al. Mechanisms of insulin resistance following injury. *Ann Surg* 196:420, 1982.
57. Wolfe RR, et al. Investigation of factors determining optimal glucose infusion rate in total parenteral nutrition. *Metabolism* 29:892, 1980.
58. Wolfe RR, et al. Glucose metabolism in severely burned patients. *Metabolism* 28:1031, 1979.
59. Long CL, et al. Carbohydrate metabolism in man: Effect of elective operations and major injury. *J Appl Physiol* 31:110, 1971.
60. Wilmore DW, Mason AD, Pruitt BA Jr. Alterations in glucose kinetics following thermal injury. *Surg Forum* 26:81, 1975.
61. Wilmore DW, et al. Influence of the burn wound on local and systemic responses to injury. *Ann Surg* 186:444, 1977.
62. Aulick LH, et al. Muscle blood flow following thermal injury. *Ann Surg* 188:778, 1978.
63. Im MJC, Hoopes JE. Energy metabolism in healing skin wounds. *J Surg Res* 10:459, 1970.
64. Galster AD, et al. Plasma palmitate turnover in subjects with thermal injury. *J Trauma* 24:938, 1984.
65. Shaw JHF, Wolfe RR. An integrated analysis of glucose, fat, and protein metabolism in severely traumatized patients. *Ann Surg* 209:63, 1989.
66. Aulick LH, et al. Effects of infection on oxygen consumption and core temperature in experimental thermal injury. *Ann Surg* 204:48, 1986.
67. Wilmore DW, et al. The gut: A central organ after surgical stress. *Surgery* 104:917, 1988.
68. Mochizuki H, et al. Mechanism of prevention of postburn hypermetabolism and catabolism by early enteral feeding. *Ann Surg* 200:297, 1984.
69. Saito H, Trocki O, Alexander JW. The effect of route of nutrient administration on the nutritional state, catabolic hormone secretion, and gut mucosal integrity after burn injury. *JPEN* 11:1, 1987.
70. O'Dwyer ST, et al. A single dose of endotoxin increases intestinal permeability in healthy humans. *Arch Surg* 123:1459, 1988.
71. Berg RD. Translocation of Indigenous Bacteria from the Intestinal Tract. In DJ Hentges (ed), *Human Intestinal Microflora in Health and Disease.* New York: Academic 1983.
72. Deitch EA, Winterton J, Berg R. Thermal injury promotes bacterial translocation from the gastrointestinal tract in mice with impaired T-cell-mediated immunity. *Arch Surg* 121:97, 1986.
73. Baker JW, et al. Hemorrhagic shock induces bacterial translocation from the gut. *J Trauma* 28:896, 1988.
74. Moore FA, et al. Gut bacterial translocation via the portal vein: A clinical perspective in patients with major torso trauma. *J Trauma* 31:629, 1991.
75. Ogle CK, et al. Effect of glutamine on phagocytosis and bacterial killing by normal and pediatric burn patient neutrophils. *JPEN* 18:128, 1994.
76. Hume DM, Egdahl RH. The importance of the brain in the endocrine response to injury. *Ann Surg* 150:697, 1959.
77. Egdahl RH, Story JL, Melby JC. Effect of progressive removal of the brain on adrenal cortical hypersecretion due to operative trauma. *Fed Proc* 17:435, 1958.
78. Koizumi K, McBrooks C. The Autonomic Nervous System and Its Role in Controlling Visceral Activities. In *Medical Physiology* (13th ed), St. Louis: Mosby, 1974.
79. Bromage PR, Shibata HR, Willoughby HW. Influence of prolonged epidural blockade on blood sugar and cortisol responses to operations upon the upper part of the abdomen and the thorax. *Surg Gynecol Obstet* 132:1051, 1971.
80. Oberg B, White S. Circulatory effects of interruption and stimulation of cardiac vagal afferents. *Acta Physiol Scand* 80:383, 1970.
81. Frye R, Braunwald E, Cohen E. Studies on Starling's law of the heart: I. The circulatory response to acute hypervolemia and its modification by ganglionic blockade. *J Clin Invest* 39:1043, 1960.
82. Skillman JJ, et al. The hemodynamic effect of acute blood loss in normal man, with observations on the effect of the Valsalva maneuver and breath holding. *Ann Surg* 166:713, 1967.
83. Watkins GM, et al. Bodily changes in repeated hemorrhage. *Surg Gynecol Obstet* 139:161, 1974.
84. Guyton AC, et al. Arterial pressure regulation: Overriding dominance of the kidneys in long-term regulation and in hypertension. *Am J Med* 52:584, 1972.
85. Sakata KS, Hayano S, Sloviter HA. Effect on blood glucose concentrations of changes in availability of glucose to the brain. *Am J Physiol* 204:1127, 1963.
86. Cannon WB. *The Wisdom of the Body.* New York: Norton, 1939.
87. Frohman LA, Bernardis LL. Effect of hypothalamic stimulation on plasma glucose, insulin, and glucagon levels. *Am J Physiol* 221:1596, 1971.
88. Franksson C, Gemzell CA, von Euler US. Cortical and medullary adrenal activity in surgical and allied conditions. *J Clin Endocrinol Metab* 14:608, 1954.
89. Goodall McC, Stone C, Haynes BW. Urinary output of adrenaline and noradrenaline in severe thermal burns. *Ann Surg* 145:479, 1957.
90. Davies CL, et al. The relationship between plasma catecholamines and severity of injury in man. *J Trauma* 24:99, 1984.
91. Jaattela A, et al. Plasma catecholamines in severely injured patients: a prospective study on 45 patients with multiple injuries. *Br J Surg* 62:177, 1975.
92. Groves AC, et al. Plasma catecholamines in patients with serious postoperative infection. *Ann Surg* 178:102, 1973.
93. Furchgott RI. The receptors for epinephrine and norepinephrine (adrenergic receptors). *Pharmacol Rev* 11:429, 1959.
94. Porte D Jr, et al. The effect of epinephrine on immunoreactive insulin levels in man. *J Clin Invest* 45:228, 1966.
95. Porte D Jr, Robertson RP. Control of insulin secretion by catecholamines, stress, and the sympathetic nervous system. *Fed Proc* 32:1792, 1973.
96. Bessey PQ, et al. Epinephrine acutely mediates skeletal muscle insulin resistance. *Surgery* 94:172, 1983.
97. Wilmore DW. *The Metabolic Management of the Critically Ill.* New York: Plenum 1977. P 101.
98. Iverson J. Adrenergic receptors and the secretion of glucagon and insulin from the isolated, perfused canine pancreas. *J Clin Invest* 52:2102, 1973.
99. Meguid MM, et al. Hormone-substrate interrelationships following trauma. *Arch Surg* 109:776, 1974.
100. Vaughan GM, et al. Cortisol and corticotrophin in burned patients. *J Trauma* 22:263, 1982.
101. Hume DM, Bell CC, Bartter F. Direct measurement of adrenal secretion during operative trauma and convalescence. *Surgery* 52:174, 1962.
102. Selye H. The general adaptation syndrome and the diseases of adaptation. *J Clin Endocrinol Metab* 6:117, 1946.

103. Ingle DJ. The permissive actions of hormones. *J Clin Endocrinol Metab* 14:1272, 1954.
104. Ferrannini E, DeFronze RA, Sherwin RS. Transient hepatic response to glucagon in man: Role of insulin and hyperglycemia. *Am J Physiol* 242:E73, 1982.
105. Shamoon HM, Hendler R, Sherwin RS. Synergistic interactions among the anti-insulin hormones in the pathogenesis of stress hyperglycemia in humans. *J Clin Endocrinol Metab* 52:1235, 1981.
106. Wilmore DW, et al. Central Nervous System Function Following Thermal Injury. In AW Wilkinson, DP Cuthbertson (eds), *Metabolism and the Response to Injury.* Chicago: Year Book, 1976. P 274.
107. Taylor JW, et al. The effect of central nervous system narcosis on the sympathetic response to stress. *J Surg Res* 20:313, 1976.
108. Dempsey DT, et al. Energy expenditure in acute trauma to the head with and without barbiturate therapy. *Surg Gynecol Obstet* 160:128, 1985.
109. Fried RC, et al. Barbiturate therapy reduces nitrogen excretion in acute head injury. *J Trauma* 29:1558, 1989.
110. Wilmore DW. Nutrition and metabolism following thermal injury. *Clin Plast Surg* 1:603, 1974.
111. Harrison TS, Seaton JF, Feller I. Relationship of increased oxygen consumption to catecholamine excretion in thermal burns. *Ann Surg* 165:169, 1967.
112. Wilmore DW, et al. Hyperglucagonaemia after burns. *Lancet* 1:73, 1974.
113. Bessey PQ, et al. Combined hormonal infusion simulates the metabolic response to injury. *Ann Surg* 200:264, 1984.
114. Bessey PQ, et al. Post-traumatic skeletal muscle proteolysis: The role of the hormonal environment. *World J Surg* 13:465, 1989.
115. Lee J, Pilch PF. The insulin receptor: Structure, function, and signaling. *Am J Physiol* 262:C319, 1994.
116. Mueckler M. Family of glucose-transporter genes: Implications for glucose homeostasis and diabetes. *Diabetes* 39:6, 1990.
117. Gelfand RA, Barrett EJ. Effect of physiologic hyperinsulinemia on skeletal muscle protein synthesis and breakdown in man. *J Clin Invest* 80:1, 1987.
118. Fryburg DA, et al. Effect of starvation on human muscle protein metabolism and its response to insulin. *Am J Physiol* 259:E477, 1990.
119. Brooks DC, et al. Insulin stimulates branched chain amino acid uptake and diminishes nitrogen flux from skeletal muscle of injured patients. *J Surg Res* 40:395, 1986.
120. Brooks DC, et al. Post-traumatic insulin resistance in uninjured skeletal muscle. *J Surg Res* 37:100, 1984.
121. Tischler ME, et al. Metabolic Response of Muscle to Trauma: Altered Control of Protein Turnover. In *Clinical Nutrition and Metabolic Research Proc,* 7th Congress of ESPEN, Munich, 1985. Basel: Karger, 1986. P 40.
122. Bessey PQ, Lowe KA. Early hormonal changes affect the catabolic response to trauma. *Ann Surg* 218:476, 1993.
123. Hourani H, et al. Effect of insulin-induced hypoglycemia on protein metabolism in vivo. *Am J Physiol* 259:E342, 1990.
124. Strobl JS, Thomas MJ. Human growth hormone. *Pharm Rev* 46:1, 1994.
125. Manson J, McK, Smith RJ, Wilmore DW. Growth hormone stimulates protein synthesis during hypocaloric parenteral nutrition: Role of hormonal-substrate environment. *Ann Surg* 208:136, 1988.
126. Wolf RF, et al. Growth hormone and insulin combine to improve whole-body and skeletal muscle protein kinetics. *Surgery* 112:284, 1992.
127. Fryburg DA, Gelfand RA, Barrett EJ. Growth hormone acutely stimulates forearm muscle protein synthesis in normal humans. *Am J Physiol* 260:E499, 1991.
128. Russell-Jones DL, et al. Use of a leucine clamp to demonstrate that IGF-1 actively stimulates protein synthesis in normal humans. *Am J Physiol* 267:E591, 1994.
129. Ziegler TR, et al. Metabolic effects of recombinant human growth hormone in patients receiving parenteral nutrition. *Ann Surg* 208:6, 1988.
130. Boulware SD, et al. Comparison of the metabolic effects of recombinant human insulin-like growth factor-1 and insulin: Dose-response relationships in healthy young and middle-aged adults. *J Clin Invest* 93:1131, 1994.
131. Baracos V, et al. Stimulation of muscle protein degradation and prostaglandin E_2 release by leukocytic pyrogen (interleukin-1): A mechanism for the increased degradation of muscle proteins during fever. *N Engl J Med* 308:553, 1983.
132. Clowes GHA, et al. Muscle proteolysis induced by a circulating peptide in patients with sepsis or trauma. *N Engl J Med* 308:545, 1983.
133. Moldawer LL, et al. Interleukin-1 and tumor necrosis factor do not regulate protein balance in skeletal muscle. *Am J Physiol* 253:766, 1987
134. Watters JM, et al. The induction of interleukin-1 in humans and its metabolic effects. *Surgery* 98:298, 1985.
135. Watters JM, et al. Both inflammatory and endocrine mediators stimulate host responses to sepsis. *Arch Surg* 121:179, 1985.
136. Coleman W, DuBois EF. Calorimetric observations on the metabolism of typhoid patients with and without food. *Arch Int Med* 15:887, 1915.
137. Dinarello CA. The interleukin-1 family: 10 years of discovery. *FASEB J* 8:1314, 1994.
138. Turchik JB, Bornstein OL. Role of the central nervous system in acute-phase responses to leukocyte progress. *Infect Immunol* 30:439, 1980.
139. Breder CD, Dinarello CA, Saper CB. Interleukin-1 immunoreactive innervation of the human hypothalamus. *Science* 240:321, 1988.
140. Michie HR, et al. Tumor necrosis factor and endotoxin induce similar metabolic responses in human beings. *Surgery* 104:280, 1988.
141. Tracey KJ, et al. Anti-cachectin/TNF monoclonal antibodies prevent septic shock during lethal bacteremia. *Nature* 330:662, 1987.
142. Fong Y, Lowry SF. Cytokines and the Cellular Response to Injury and Infection. In JL Meakins (ed), *Surgical Infections: Diagnosis and Treatment.* New York: Scientific American, 1994. P 65.
143. Koj A. The role of interleukin-6 as the hepatocyte stimulating factor in the network of inflammatory cytokines. *Ann NY Acad Sci* 557:1, 1989.
144. Marano MA, et al. Serum cachectin/tumor necrosis factor in critically ill patients with burns correlates with infection and mortality. *Surg Gynecol Obstet* 170:32, 1990.
145. Barber AE, et al. Glucocorticoid therapy alters hormonal and cytokine responses to endotoxin in man. *J Immunol* 150:1999, 1993.
146. Cinat M, et al. Soluble cytokine receptors and receptor antagonists are sequentially released after trauma. *J Trauma* 39:112, 1995.

147. Michie HR, et al. Chronic TNF infusion causes anorexia but not accelerated nitrogen loss. *Ann Surg* 209:19, 1989.

148. Mealy K, et al. Are the catabolic effects of tumor necrosis factor mediated by glucocorticoids? *Arch Surg* 125:42, 1990.

149. Hall-Angeras M, et al. Effects of the glucocorticoid receptor antagonist RU38486 on muscle protein breakdown in sepsis. *Surgery* 109:468, 1991.

150. Hall-Angeras M, et al. Corticosterone alone does not explain increased muscle proteolysis in septic rats. *J Surg Res* 48:368, 1990.

151. Hall-Angeras M, et al. Interaction between corticosterone and tumor necrosis factor stimulated protein breakdown in rat skeletal muscle, similar to sepsis. *Surgery* 108:460, 1990.

152. Zamir O, et al. The effect of interleukin-1 and the glucocorticoid receptor blocker RU38486 on total and myofibrillar protein breakdown in skeletal muscle. *J Surg Res* 50:579, 1991.

153. Zamir O, et al. Muscle protein breakdown during endotoxemia in rats after treatment with interleukin-1 receptor antagonist (IL-1ra). *Ann Surg* 216:381, 1992.

154. Zamir O, et al. Tumor necrosis factor (TNF) and interleukin-1 (IL-1) induce muscle proteolysis through different mechanisms. *Mediat Inflam* 1:247, 1992.

155. Tiao G, et al. Sepsis stimulates nonlysosomal, energy-dependent proteolysis and increases ubiquitin mRNA levels in rat skeletal muscle. *J Clin Invest* 94:2255, 1994.

156. Finely D, Chau V. Ubiquitination. *Annu Rev Cell Biol* 7:25, 1991.

157. Tiao G, et al. Blockade of the glucocorticoid receptor inhibits sepsis-induced muscle proteolysis and transcription of the ubiquitin gene. Presented at the 28th meeting of the Association for Academic Surgery, Albuquerque, NM. November 1994.

158. Clowes GHA Jr, Del Guercio LR. Circulatory response to trauma of surgical operations. *Metabolism* 9:67, 1960.

159. Bland R, Shoemaker WC, Shabot MM. Physiologic monitoring goals for the critically ill patient. *Surg Gynecol Obstet* 147:833, 1978.

160. Moore FA, et al. Incommensurate oxygen consumption in response to maximal oxygen availability predicts post-injury multiple organ failure. *J Trauma* 33:58, 1992.

161. Shiozaki T, et al. Recovery from postoperative hypothermia predicts survival in extensively burned patients. *Am J Surg* 165:326, 1993.

162. Revhaug A, et al. Inhibition of cyclooxygenase attenuates the metabolic response to endotoxin in humans. *Arch Surg* 123:162, 1988.

163. Eberlein TJ, et al. Ibuprofen causes reduced toxic effects of interleukin-2 administration in patients with metastatic cancer. *Arch Surg* 124:542, 1989.

164. Grace PA. Ischaemia-reperfusion injury. *Br J Surg* 81: 637, 1994.

165. Roos D. The involvement of oxygen radicals in microbicidal mechanisms of leukocytes and macrophages. *Klin Wochenschr* 69:957, 1991.

166. Maderazo EG, et al. A randomized trial of replacement antioxidant vitamin therapy for neutrophil locomotory dysfunction in blunt trauma. *J Trauma* 31:1142, 1991.

167. Joshi VV. Effects of burns on the heart. *JAMA* 211:2130, 1970.

168. Herndon DN, et al. Effect of propranolol administration on hemodynamic and metabolic responses of burned pediatric patients. *Ann Surg* 208:484, 1988.

169. Herndon DN, et al. Lipolysis in burned patients is stimulated by the β_2 receptor for catecholamines. *Arch Surg* 129:1301, 1994.

170. Van Saene HKF, Stoutenbeek CC, Stoller JK. Selective decontamination of the digestive tract in the intensive care unit: Current status and future prospects. *Crit Care Med* 20:691, 1992.

171. Bone RC. Sepsis, sepsis syndrome, and the systemic inflammatory response syndrome (SIRS): Gulliver in Laputa. *JAMA* 273:155, 1995.

172. Baue AE. Multiple organ failure, multiple organ dysfunction syndrome, and the systemic inflammatory response syndrome: Where do we stand? *Shock* 2:385, 1994.

173. Wilmore DW. *The Metabolic Management of the Critically Ill*. New York: Plenum, 1977. P 14.

174. Border JR, et al. The gut origin septic states in blunt multiple trauma (ISS = 40) in the ICU. *Ann Surg* 206:427, 1987.

175. Cerra FB, et al. Branched chains support postoperative protein synthesis. *Surgery* 92:192, 1982.

176. Bower RH, et al. Branched chain amino acid-enriched solutions in the septic patient: A randomized, prospective trial. *Ann Surg* 203:13, 1986.

177. Ziegler TR, et al. Clinical and metabolic efficacy of glutamine-supplemented parenteral nutrition after bone marrow transplantation: A randomized double blind, controlled study. *Ann Intern Med* 116:821, 1992.

178. Tremel H, et al. Glutamine dipeptide-supplemented parenteral nutrition maintains intestinal function in the critically ill. *Gastroenterology* 107:1595, 1994.

179. Jeevanandam M, et al. Decreased growth hormone levels in the catabolic phase of severe injury. *Surgery* 111:495, 1992.

180. Wilmore DW, et al. Anabolic effects of growth hormone and high caloric feedings following thermal injury. *Surg Gynecol Obstet* 138:875, 1974.

181. Manson JM, Wilmore DW. Positive nitrogen balance with human growth hormone and hypocaloric intravenous feeding. *Surgery* 100:188, 1986.

182. Jiang Z-M, et al. Low-dose growth hormone and hypocaloric nutrition attenuate the protein-catabolic response after major operation. *Ann Surg* 210:513, 1989.

183. Herndon DN, et al. Effects of recombinant human growth hormone on donor-site healing in severely burned children. *Ann Surg* 212:424, 1990.

184. Herndon DN, et al. Characterization of growth hormone enhanced donor site healing in patients with large cutaneous burns. *Ann Surg,* in press.

185. Knox J, et al. Increased survival after major thermal injury: The effect of growth hormone therapy in adults. Presented at the 54th Annual Meeting of the Association for the Surgery of Trauma, San Diego, CA. September 29, 1994.

186. Hill DJ, Milner RD. Insulin as a growth factor. *Pediatr Res* 19:879, 1985.

187. Inculet RI, et al. Insulin decreases muscle protein loss after operative trauma in man. *Surgery* 99:752, 1986.

Selected Readings

The metabolic response to injury and critical illness has intrigued many investigators over the centuries. Many "classic" references are included in the main reference list. I list here a select few of the sources that have been particularly important in my understanding of the subject.

Cuthbertson DP. Post-shock metabolic response. *Lancet* 1:433, 1942.

David Patton Cuthbertson was a lecturer in physiologic chemistry at the University of Glasgow. He was the first to study the metabolic responses to injury in this century utilizing relatively modern chemical techniques. His keen clinical observations and the results of his systematic studies formed the framework for all subsequent investigations. This reference is his Arris and Gayle lecture, given at the Royal College of Surgeons in London at the height of World War II. In it he describes the ebb and flow periods and summarizes many of his investigations.

Moore FD, Ball MR. *The Metabolic Response to Surgery.* Springfield, IL: Thomas, 1952.

Frances D. Moore and his indomitable research associate, Margaret (Peggy) Ball, contributed greatly to our knowledge of the metabolism of the surgical patient and of convalescence. They combined imagination, observation, and analysis of clinical and laboratory data, and they began to dissect the different aspects of the responses to injury and surgery. This book presents some remarkable observations and the authors' early attempts to reproduce the metabolic responses in normal, healthy subjects by a variety of nontraumatic manipulations.

Watters JM, et al. Both inflammatory and endocrine mediators simulate host responses to sepsis. *Arch Surg* 121:179, 1985.

This study was conducted just as the identification and study of the cytokines was becoming a major theme in the literature. These investigators were attempting to simulate the responses to injury and critically ill patients in normal subjects. This study demonstrated that there was no simple mechanism that could account for the metabolic alterations observed in sick patients. Multiple mechanisms, in this case a variety of endocrine interactions as well as mediators of inflammation, resulted in the clinical presentation of surgical patients.

Wilmore DW. *The Metabolic Management of the Critically Ill.* New York: Plenum, 1977.

This little book presents a wonderfully readable account of the metabolism and nutritional support of sick patients. Even though some of the material is a bit dated, it is still a superb general summary of the field. Unfortunately, only one edition of this book was ever published, and it may be difficult to locate.

Wilmore DW, et al. Influence of the burn wound on local and systemic responses to injury. *Ann Surg* 186:444, 1977.

This is but one of several landmark studies by these authors who were at the Brooke Army Burn Unit in the 1970s. It is of particular interest to me because of the ingenious study design, the wealth of data, and the insight into the dynamic relationship between regional responses to a wound and systemic alteration.

22

Nutrition and Neoplasia

John M. Daly
Alex C. Cech

Malnutrition is a prevalent problem among all hospitalized patients, but particularly in those with cancer. Bistrian [1] and Willcutts [2] estimated that 10% to 30% of all hospitalized patients suffer from malnutrition. A syndrome of severe, involuntary weight loss and wasting is seen in cancer patients and is termed cancer cachexia. A majority of patients have evidence of malnutrition at the first diagnosis of malignancy, with nearly all manifesting cachexia at the time of death. An association between malnutrition at the time of cancer diagnosis and eventual poor outcome has been well documented. Whether reversing malnutrition can restore normal function and improve outcome is still controversial. This chapter will focus on the syndrome of cancer cachexia: its causes, effects, and the role of nutritional support.

Cancer cachexia is a paraneoplastic syndrome marked by findings of weight loss, anorexia, asthenia, atrophy of muscle mass and visceral organs, and abnormal energy metabolism. The primary abnormality is a net negative energy balance in the host. More energy is expended by the host and tumor combined than the host is able to ingest, leading to marked weight loss. This has been termed relative hypophagia.

Malnutrition is very commonly associated with malignancy. DeWys et al. [3] found that 50% of patients have lost weight at the time of diagnosis, with a subset of patients losing more than 10% of their premorbid body weight. Nixon et al. [4] found that 88% of hospitalized patients with cancer have a low creatinine/height ratio, a measure of malnutrition. Furthermore, 42% of the patients also had decreased triceps skinfold thickness, a measure of body fat stores. In a study of cancer patients undergoing major surgical procedures, Buzby et al. [5] defined a degree of protein-calorie malnutrition in 55% of patients. Weight loss, however, is not a universal feature of malignancies. Camoriano et al. [6] examined weight changes in 646 women with node-positive breast cancer that were either being observed or receiving chemotherapy; weight gain for all patients was 1.8 kg over 60 weeks, with greater gains in the treated group.

Patients clearly do worse if they are malnourished at the time of cancer diagnosis [7,8]. Chlebowski et al. [9] studied patients with non-small cell carcinoma of the lung and found that malnutrition at the time of presentation correlated with a poor outcome. The Eastern Cooperative Oncology Group survey of over 3000 cancer patients also demonstrated that a loss of as little as 6% of body weight correlated with a significantly decreased length of survival in patients with a variety of tumors, despite both groups receiving similar treatments [3]. In rare subgroups of patients, this correlation is not true; in the study by Camoriano et al. [6], a greater weight gain was actually associated with greater risk of relapse and risk of death.

Nutritional status also affects the tumor response to therapy in patients with a variety of tumors and animal tumor models. Chlebowski et al. [9] found that patients with weight loss had a worse response to therapy, a finding corroborated by the Eastern Cooperative Oncology Group study [3]. Shamberger et al. [10] found a similar pattern in patients with sarcoma. Numerous animal studies also support these findings. Cachectic and tumor-bearing animals, when compared to a well-nourished tumor-bearing group, had a diminished response to treatment with doxorubicin [11]. Popp et al. [12] found a similarly poor response to treatment in a rat model of lymphoma with cachexia. Nutritional status also affects the host response to surgical resection of tumor. Moley et al. [13] found a decreased survival in animals undergoing tumor resection if they were also malnourished. Hickman et al. [14] found that the level of serum albumin was a predictor of postoperative course in patients undergoing resection.

Not only does malnutrition predict a poor response to therapy and eventual outcome, but progressive wasting is responsible for as many as two-thirds of all deaths due to cancer [15–17]. In 22% of patients dying from cancer, the only other abnormality found at autopsy was malnutrition [15]. Therefore, many believe that there is a theoretical advantage to supplemental nutrition. It has long been hoped that malnutrition and the resultant deficiencies could be easily reversed with feeding. The experimental results, however, are variable.

In animal studies, TPN has at best only reversed some of the changes in cachectic animals [18,19]. In human studies, TPN has failed to restore lean body mass in cancer patients [20,21]. Most significantly, the ultimate goal of prolonging survival has not been met by giving TPN to cancer patients [18,22]. Nonetheless, some animal studies suggest that the addition of hormones [23] or exercise [24] to feeding regimens can preserve lean body mass in tumor-bearing animals. TPN has also been shown to improve measures of whole-body protein kinetics [25]. The immediate goal of nutritional support in the cancer patients remains the preservation of lean body mass [26].

Mechanisms

Cancer cachexia is a paraneoplastic phenomenon characterized by a constellation of symptoms including anorexia, unintentional weight loss, asthenia, tissue wasting, and organ dysfunction. Although the mechanisms causing cancer cachexia remain unclear, they are likely multifactorial. A large variety of tumors in many locations can cause cancer cachexia, but the site of a malignancy has been shown to be important. Fong et al. [27] demonstrated that the site of a tumor is important in determining its metabolic effects. They implanted tumors either subcutaneously or into the liver and showed that a similar degree of anorexia was caused when the liver tumor was only 1% of total body weight while the subcutaneous tumor had to be 10% of body weight. They suggested that proximity to competent tissue macrophages that could produce cytokines such as TNF was a critical difference [27]. There is also no consistent correlation between tumor size, histology, disease duration, or stage and cancer cachexia [28–30]. However, the cachexia is clearly due to the tumor. In animal models, a tumor must be present to cause weight loss [13]. Many have also shown that an animal is able to restore its weight and reverse abnormalities in metabolism after tumor removal [31]. Norton et al. [32] have shown that cachexia can be transferred from a tumor-bearing to a normal animal across shared circulation. Cancer cachexia bears many similarities to the weight loss seen in other chronically and critically ill patients. Patients undergoing radiation, with chronic infections, debilitating diseases, and acute injuries including trauma, demonstrate a similar pattern of weight loss and wasting. This suggests that cachexia may be a common response to stressful states [7].

Hypophagia

Regardless of other mechanisms involved, central to the weight loss of cancer cachexia is an energy imbalance. The host and tumor combined expend more energy than the host is able to assimilate. This has been termed "relative hypophagia" in that the host, for a variety of reasons, fails to increase intake to meet the increased expenditure [7]. Anorexia is both common in cancer patients [33] and fundamental to cancer cachexia [34,35]. Normal animals will increase food intake in situations demanding increased energy expenditure, while both tumor-bearing animals [36–39] and cancer patients decrease their intake [7,8, 33–35,40]. Some have suggested that reduced food intake and starvation may be the sole cause of cancer cachexia [41]. This would not explain why nutrition support is unable to reverse the weight loss and all of its associated effects. TPN has been able to improve but not completely reverse the abnormalities in cancer cachexia [18,22], including only partial restoration of lean body mass [20,21]. Obeid et al. [42] pair-fed rats with or without a transplantable Leydig cell tumor that caused anorexia, weight loss, and muscle wasting. They concluded that the rate of loss of body fat was greater than could be explained by anorexia alone [42].

Clearly, hypophagia is essential to the entire syndrome of cancer cachexia, but it alone is inadequate to account for all its manifestations. It is necessary to account for its prevalence among tumors of varying stages, anatomic locations, and histologies. In turn, the causes of anorexia in the cancer patient are also multifactorial. They include mechanical, central, psychological, and iatrogenic causes.

Cancer cachexia is a particularly common problem in patients with head and neck tumors. Due to their location, these tumors have a propensity to obstruct the gastrointestinal tract early in their course. Similarly, upper gastrointestinal tumors such as esophageal and pancreatic tumors are prone to cause mechanical obstructions. In some of these patients, the mechanical obstruction is clearly the primary cause of the cancer cachexia. Burt et al. [43] demonstrated that in patients with esophageal cancer, TPN can reverse the weight loss and other metabolic derangements associated with the tumor. Obstruction of the biliary or pancreatic systems by tumor can also lead to impaired absorption of nutrients. Other tumors may cause bowel obstructions, blind loops, or colonic fistulas. Tumors may also cause functional obstructions by interfering with normal bowel motility. Rats were implanted with the Walker 256 carcinoma, and food intake was measured daily. The rats were fasted overnight, fed a bolus of liquid food by gavage, and residual gastric contents were measured three hours later. Tumor growth was associated with a progressive decline in voluntary food intake. The percentage of gastric contents cleared in three hours was unchanged despite tumor growth [44].

Pain, whether related to feeding or not, can also significantly reduce food intake. Postprandial pain with upper GI malignancy can result in a food aversion with significant weight loss. Tumors of the GI tract can also cause early satiety or gastric outlet obstruction with significant reduction in total food intake.

Central Mechanisms

There are numerous central mechanisms by which nutrient intake is reduced in the cancer patient. Nausea and a lack of appetite are centrally mediated and can have profound effects on oral intake. Critical components of appetite are a normal sense of taste and smell. Alterations in these senses are a common cause of anorexia [33,40]. Taste perception, in turn, is altered in as many as one-third of all patients with tumors. The changes include an elevated threshold for sensing sweets and a reduced threshold for bitter and salty tastes [45]. The cause of altered taste and smell is not clear but may involve zinc deficiency. Russ et al. [46] have also made the interesting observation that supplemental nutrition may help restore these senses to normal. Although changes in taste and smell are well documented, there is poor correlation with weight loss.

Other central mechanisms include direct effects on the appetite center in the lateral hypothalamus. Masumo et al. [47] have shown that a tumor-derived substance directly injected into the lateral ventricle of rats decreases food intake. Elevated levels of certain neurotransmitters, particularly dopamine, serotonin, and its precursor tryptophan, have been associated with anorexia. Chance et al. [48] measured regional brain levels of various neurotransmitters in food-deprived, partially refed, or satiated rats. Dopamine and its metabolites were elevated in the corpus striatum and nucleus accumbens in satiated rats. All animals that had been food-deprived had elevated levels of the serotonin metabolite, 5-hydroxyindolacetic acid, in most brain areas whether they were refed or not. Dopamine levels were associated with satiety and serotonin levels with overall nutritional status [48].

Patients with extensive hepatic involvement by tumor may become nauseated due to the high levels of lactate produced by the anaerobic metabolism of the tumor. Chance et al. [49] again showed that blood ammonia levels were increased (113%) in rats five days after hepatoma-induced anorexia. Giving ammonia to normal rats to achieve similar blood levels also induced anorexia [49]. Chance et al. [50] hypothesized that a sarcoma causes anorexia by consuming glutamine and producing ammonia, which goes on to affect neurotransmitter levels; these changes were rapidly reversed by tumor resection. They found elevated plasma ammonia levels in tumor (sarcoma)-bearing rats before the onset of anorexia, which continued to rise as the tumor grew and anorexia progressed. Associated findings included elevated brain glutamine and large neutral amino acid levels along with increases in dopamine metabolite levels in the corpus striatum, nucleus accumbens, hypothalamus, and amygdala. Serotonin metabolite levels were increased in the brains of anorectic and nonanorectic tumor-bearing animals [51]. [*Editor's Note:* More recent work from this group [52] has proposed a mechanism involving NPY, a central neurotransmitter, the most powerful orexigenic agent known.]

Cytokines associated with cancer cachexia have effects on the central nervous system. Intracerebroventricular microinfusions of recombinant human tumor necrosis factor (rhTNF) and recombinant human interleukin-1β (rhIL-1β) significantly suppress food intake in rats. rhTNF and rhIL-1β specifically suppress the activity of glucose-sensitive neurons in the lateral hypothalamic area; glucose-insensitive neurons are not affected. These results suggest that TNF and IL-1β act directly in the central nervous system to suppress appetite, and this effect may be operative during acute and chronic disease [53]. Bernstein et al. [54] found that lesions in the area postrema attenuate the anorectic effects of TNF, a finding also described for tumor-associated anorexia. However, in this model a rapid tolerance to the anorectic effects of TNF developed [54]. Recent investigations have drawn attention to the paracrine actions of TNF that predominate when it is produced locally in the brain or other organs. For instance, when compartmentalized production of TNF occurs in the central nervous system, it directly mediates fever, anorexia, and altered whole-body metabolism. Because these changes are mediated within the neural network, they occur independent of simultaneously sampled serum TNF levels. These paracrine actions may differ markedly from the hormone-like actions associated with systemic cytokine release. TNF may be beneficial in some diseases, yet injurious in others [55].

Other proposed mediators of cachexia also have central mechanisms. Toxohormone-L, a polypeptide extracted and purified from ascites of patients with hepatoma and suggested to cause anorexia, was infused into the third cerebroventricle of rats. Food intake decreased on the first day after infusion, and the suppressive effect on feeding was dose-dependent in linear fashion ($p < 0.05$). These findings suggest that anorexia and cachexia produced in cancer patients may essentially be due to the central suppressive effect of toxohormone-L on food intake [56].

IL-1, a polypeptide hormone produced by activated monocytes or macrophages or both, stimulates the release of hypothalamic corticotrophin-releasing factor (CRF). Because CRF acts centrally in the brain to reduce food intake, it was hypothesized that IL-1 might induce anorexia through this central action of CRF. This study showed that IL-1, both endogenously released and exogenously administered, induces the suppression of food intake in rats and that endogenous CRF in the brain is involved in the IL-1-induced anorexia. Lipopolysaccharide (LPS), a potent stimulant of the release and production of endogenous IL-1, caused anorexia in a dose-related manner, and this effect was significantly blocked by pretreatment with glucocorticoid hormones that inhibited the production of endogenous IL-1 by LPS. In addition, intraperitoneal injection of IL-1 resulted in a dose-related suppression of food intake. Finally, anorexia induced by IL-1 was diminished by the immunoneutralization of endogenous CRF in the brain. This connection between IL-1 and CRF may represent a mechanism by which anorexia results from the activation of the immune system by such immunologic challenges as acute infectious diseases [57].

Henkin et al. [58] also suggested that the psychological effects of having cancer may significantly reduce food intake. Depression and a sense of hopelessness are common in patients following the diagnosis of cancer [59], but many patients present with weight loss prior to a diagnosis of malignancy. Symptoms of cancer may precede the diagnosis by several months. Some patients may become depressed due to the fear of malignancy precipitated by an early symptom. Psychological causes often reflect anxiety about cancer and its possible progression, depression, anticipatory phenomena, and learned food aversions. Preexisting psychiatric disorders, especially anorexia nervosa or paranoid states, may substantially complicate cancer treatment. Learned food aversions, which can further restrict limited intake, have been demonstrated in children receiving chemotherapy and may also contribute to aversions of specific foods seen among adult patients after chemotherapy or radiation. Optimal management often involves use of a combination of modalities: psychotherapeutic, behavioral, and/or pharmacologic supplemented by education, counseling, and support [60].

Iatrogenic Mechanisms

Although etiologies of cancer cachexia derive from the tumor directly, there are also many iatrogenic mechanisms [61]. Radiation therapy may cause severe nutritional deficits. The field of irradiation and the total dose are critical factors in determining the effects of radiation on nutrition. The rapidly dividing cells of the mucosa throughout the gastrointestinal tract are particularly sensitive to the effects of radiation. When the head and neck are targeted, radiation therapy may cause xerostomia and severe mucositis [62]. Irradiation of bowel may similarly cause ulcerations with subsequent decreased oral intake as well as malabsorption of what little food is eaten.

Chemotherapy commonly leads to decreased oral intake for a variety of reasons. Chemotherapeutic drugs sometimes affect the rapidly dividing cells of the gastrointestinal tract, leading to ulcerations, stomatitis, and ultimately malabsorption. Cancer chemotherapy may also affect the host's appetite and nutritional intake by directly stimulating the chemoreceptor trigger zone, causing nausea. A randomized study of patients receiving chemotherapy for testicular cancer demonstrated that patients not receiving any nutritional support developed negative nitrogen and total energy balance [63]. Patients receiving TPN remained in positive nitrogen balance while getting TPN but developed negative balance when TPN was discontinued.

Energy Utilization

The degree of malnutrition is often out of proportion to the decreased oral intake. Although decreased intake clearly contributes to the weight loss, there are other factors that increase the energy demands or decrease the utilization of nutrients. Moley et al. [26] have demonstrated that anorectic patients with tumors lose more weight than patients with anorexia due to other causes.

Freund et al. [64] assessed the resting energy expenditure of 30 free-feeding control and methylcholanthrene-induced sarcoma-bearing rats prior to and following surgical removal of the tumor. Tumor-bearing rats demonstrated carcass wasting and massive tumor growth. The resting energy expenditure was not affected by the presence and growth of a tumor or its removal [64]. Cancer patients ($n = 106$) and noncancer subjects ($n = 96$) were classified as weight-stable ($n = 70$) or weight-losing ($n = 132$). Cancer patients had elevated resting energy expenditure (REE) compared with either weight-losing (23.6 ± 0.4 vs. 20.5 ± 0.5 kcal/kg/day) or weight-stable controls (22.0 ± 0.6 vs. 17.9 ± 0.4 kcal/kg/day). Cancer patients had increased fat oxidation irrespective of weight loss [65].

Many studies have shown that tumors affect the resting energy expenditure of the tumor-bearing host. Different types of tumors seem to either increase or decrease REE. Bozzetti et al. [66] studied 65 patients with cancer and found that 60% had an increased REE that correlated with weight loss. Similarly, Lindmark et al. [67] found REE increased only in cancer patients with weight loss. Others have shown a more mixed response. Knox et al. [68] used the Harris-Benedict formula to predict REE and then measured it in patients with cancer. They found that 26% were hypermetabolic, but 42% were normal, and 36% were actually hypometabolic. Dempsy et al. [69] studied 173 patients with gastrointestinal malignancies and found similar results: 22% were hypermetabolic, 42% were normal, and 36% were hypometabolic. The site of the tumor was important in that patients with gastric tumors were more likely to be hypermetabolic than patients with hepatobiliary tumors. Similarly, Buzby et al. [5] found that patients with pancreatic cancer were hypometabolic. Merrick et al. [70] studied 21 patients with colorectal cancer and found their REE to be at predicted levels. REE, body cell mass, and body fat were measured in 6 male and 7 female volunteers and in a homogeneous group of noncachectic patients with sarcoma ($n = 7$). The patients all had large localized tumors, without either history or clinical evidence of decreased food intake or weight loss, and had received no prior treatment for cancer. The REE corrected for body surface area was similar in male and female controls but was 25% greater in male sarcoma patients than in male controls ($p < 0.05$). This difference was doubled when REE was corrected for body cell mass ($p < 0.01$) [71]. REE was measured in 104 patients with newly detected gastric or colorectal cancer and was compared with healthy subjects. REE in gastric or colorectal cancer patients was not significantly different from REE in control subjects. No significant differences in REE were found when patients with liver metastases were compared with patients without metastases. There were no differences in REE between gastric and colorectal cancer patients. However, the decrease in energy expenditure, which normally occurs during starvation and weight loss in healthy men and women, was not demonstrated in weight-losing, gastric, or colorectal cancer patients [72]. These data correlate with the clinical finding that patients with colon cancer do not become cachectic until late in their course. The failure to decrease REE as anorexia develops may contribute to, but does not cause, the cachexia.

In patients with tumor-associated hypermetabolism, treatment may markedly improve the abnormality. Curative tumor resection in patients has been shown to return REE to normal, while a palliative resection only partially improved it [31]. Despite these varied reports, a consensus has developed that REE increases in most patients with cancer. Others have suggested that using the Harris-Benedict formula to define normal REE is inappropriate in the starved patient. Because the normal response to semistarvation is a decrease in REE, a "normal" REE may be very abnormal [68,73].

Metabolism

In a subset of patients, energy expenditure is clearly increased. The causes of the increase are not clear. Some suggest the tumor acts like an "energy sink." Solid tumors have been demonstrated to excessively take up glucose [74] and amino acids [75]. Tumors may also induce the host to expend more energy to cope with metabolic by-products of the tumor [76]. Cori's cycle suggested that the host expends excessive amounts of energy in recycling lactic acid produced by anaerobic tumor metabolism back into glucose to be used by the tumor again.

The tumor has many other effects on host metabolism. To some extent, the changes in energy metabolism may represent a normal stress response of rerouting nutrients from the periphery to the liver. Chronically, this results in abnormalities of protein, lipid, and carbohydrate metabolism. Conlon et al. [77] examined extremity metabolism in a rabbit model with a peripherally implanted tumor (VX-2). Tumor-bearing rabbits were hypophagic and had systemic hypoinsulinemia, elevated plasma triglycerides, and altered plasma amino acid levels. Hind-limb efflux from tumor-bearing limbs was elevated for lactate and most amino acid levels. These alterations were not just due to the hypophagia in the tumor-bearing animals because they were significantly different from both normally fed, non-tumor-bearing controls as well as non-tumor-bearing animals pair-fed to the tumor-bearing rabbits [77].

Glucose

In 1919, glucose intolerance became the earliest recognized metabolic abnormality in cancer patients. Prior to the development of severe malnutrition, colon, gastric, sarcoma, endometrial, prostate, localized head, neck, and lung cancer, patients had many of the metabolic abnormalities of type II (non-insulin-dependent) diabetes mellitus. These metabolic abnormalities include glucose intolerance, an increase in both hepatic glucose production and glucose recycling, and insulin resistance. In a study of over 600 cancer patients, a diabetic pattern of glucose intolerance was noted in over one-third of the patients. A possible stimulus for the increase in hepatic glucose production could be the glucose needs of the tumor. Abnormally high glucose utilization rates in small amounts of tumor tissue have recently been described, suggesting that small tumors may have large needs for glucose calories. An increase in anaerobic glycolysis in the tumor tissue can increase lactate production in the tumor-bearing human, thus supplying substrate to the liver to increase glucose production rates [78].

Abnormal glucose metabolism is found in tumor-bearing animals and patients early in the tumor-bearing state before the onset of cachexia [79,80]. Peripheral utilization of glucose, hepatic gluconeogenesis, and consequently glucose turnover are all abnormal. Whole-body glucose consumption is increased in tumor-bearing patients [81]. In tumor-bearing hosts, there is also increased conversion of alanine and lactate to glucose [76,79,82], suggesting that the tumors may be consuming large amounts of glucose. Animals bearing a cachexia-inducing tumor, the MAC16 adenocarcinoma, showed a progressive decrease in blood glucose levels with increasing weight loss, while animals bearing a histologically similar tumor, the MAC13 adenocarcinoma, showed no change in either body weight or blood glucose levels with growth of the tumor [83]. Glucose utilization by the MAC13 tumor was significantly higher than by the MAC16 tumor, and in animals bearing tumors of either type, the tumor was the second major consumer of glucose after the brain [84].

Gastrointestinal tumors have also been shown to increase the basal rate of hepatic gluconeogenesis. Blumberg et al. [85] studied glucose synthesis by hepatocytes from normal and sarcoma-bearing rats. Hepatocytes in tumor-bearing animals made significantly more glucose from both alanine and lactate than normal cells. This increased production was partially inhibited by tolbutamide. Shaw et al. [86] demonstrated a direct correlation between the extent of the tumor and the increase in production of glucose. In patients with the largest tumors, glucose production failed to be suppressed even with intravenous infusions of glucose. This may contribute to the glucose intolerance often seen not only in the cancer patient but also in the critically ill patient [87]. The increased glucose synthesis serves the tumor, which primarily consumes glucose and produces lactate [88]. This concept was popularized by Gold [89], who also suggested inhibiting gluconeogenesis as a potential therapy. Inhibition of phosphoenolpyruvate carboxykinase (by hydrazine sulfate) in patients with non-small cell lung cancer increased food intake and subsequently improved the tumor response to therapy [9].

Insulin resistance occurs in cachectic cancer patients and is also seen experimentally with TNF-α administration. Insulin sensitivity and energy metabolism were measured in 11 patients with gastrointestinal cancer and 10 controls, using the euglycemic glucose clamp and indirect calorimetry. Patients with cancer were significantly more insulin-resistant than controls ($p < 0.01$) and in such patients insulin resistance correlated with serum TNF-α level ($rs = 0.74$, $p < 0.01$). Fasting insulin levels also correlated inversely with insulin sensitivity ($rs = 0.62$, $p = 0.003$) [90]. Emery et al. [91] examined postprandial lipid and glycogen synthesis in tumor-bearing animals. The rate of glycogen synthesis was increased twofold in tumor-bearing animals compared to normal controls. Pair-fed, non-tumor-bearing animals actually decreased their rate of glycogen synthesis compared to normal controls. Tumor-bearing animals did not increase the rate of lipid synthesis, as did normal controls, while pair-fed, non-tumor-bearing animals increased it. Therefore, tumor-bearing animals failed to show the normal adaptive response to reduced nutritional intake [91].

Abnormalities in glucose metabolism have led others to consider the role of insulin in cancer cachexia. Cersosimo et al. [92] examined the effects of insulin on glucose turnover in 5 cancer-bearing patients and 5 controls. Total body glucose use was diminished in the cancer patients, consistent with a state of insulin resistance. The impaired action of insulin on peripheral glucose use was associated with an increased peripheral lactate release [92]. Chance et al. [93] examined the effects of a sarcoma on glucose metabolism in rats. In anorectic tumor-bearing rats, plasma levels of insulin were decreased while glucagon and lactate levels were increased. Daily injections of insulin in the tumor-bearing rats corrected the anorexia and increased the animals' body weight. Insulin therapy also decreased plasma levels of glucagon and lactate, and abnormal plasma concentrations of several amino acids were corrected toward normal. Tumor growth was not affected [93]. Adding insulin to TPN in tumor-bearing animals demonstrated an increased survival with resection [13] and even without resection of the tumor [94]. Tumor-bearing animals receiving insulin had an increase in body protein mass [23]. Insulin administration also improved animal tolerance of and response to chemotherapy [11]. Fraker et al. [95] have also shown that insulin may reverse some of the effects of TNF. Massive tumors, particularly sarcomas, can absorb large quantities of glucose. Instituting TPN may lead to lactic acidosis in such patients as large amounts of glucose are suddenly made available to the tumor, but such results are rare [96].

Protein

The cachectic cancer patient has lost the ability to regulate protein synthesis and breakdown normally. In cases of short-term fasting, increased muscle breakdown provides amino acids for eventual conversion to glucose in the liver. In chronic fasting, an otherwise normal person will eventually decrease muscle breakdown and switch to fat stores to conserve lean body mass [97]. Chronic malnutrition in a normal person causes a decrease in whole-body protein synthesis, decreased catabolism, and decreased protein turnover [98]. This adaptation to fasting is lost in the tumor-bearing host because whole-body protein turnover and synthesis are increased, as are protein catabolism and liver protein synthesis [99,100]. The liberated amino acids are converted to glucose and synthesized into acute-phase proteins in the liver [7,8].

Although serum albumin levels decrease with malignancy, liver synthesis of albumin is increased [101,102]. In children with leukemia, the accelerated rates of protein turnover correlate with an increased energy expenditure [103], while Fearon et al. [35] also found an increase in protein turnover without an increase in REE in adults with colon cancer. Early and severe loss of body weight associated with pronounced tissue changes developed in rats transplanted with a fast-growing ascites hepatoma (Yoshida AH-130). Skeletal muscle protein content showed an early and marked decrease, while in the liver it transiently increased 4 days after implantation and then declined to values lower than in control animals. Protein loss in gastrocnemius muscle and liver result mainly from enhancement of protein catabolism [104].

The effects of progressive cachexia on protein metabolism in skeletal muscle has been investigated in mice bearing the MAC16 adenocarcinoma, which produces cachexia with tumor burdens of <1% of the host weight. Weight loss was accompanied by loss of whole-body nitrogen in proportion to the overall loss of body mass. Using L-[^{3}H]phenylalanine to label proteins in gastrocnemius muscle, a significant depression (60%) in protein synthesis occurred in animals with a weight loss between 15% and 30% accompanied by an increase in protein degradation, which grew larger with increasing weight loss between 15% and 30% [105]. The increased whole-body protein turnover results in the eventual loss of host muscle mass while net tumor protein synthesis is increased [106].

Shaw et al. [86] demonstrated that infusions of glucose in patients with gastrointestinal malignancies no longer suppress protein catabolism, as seen in normal individuals. Jeevanandam et al. [107] have shown that TPN can reduce protein catabolism in cachectic patients both with and without tumors. Using ^{15}N to trace protein turnover, they found that 10 days of TPN decreased whole-body protein catabolism by 50% in cancer patients and 59% in noncancer patients. This accompanied similar decreases in protein synthesis of 21% and 33% respectively [107].

Most investigators have observed increased rates of whole-body protein turnover, synthesis, and catabolism in both weight-stable and weight-losing cancer patients. Some studies have suggested a relationship between the extent of disease and the degree of aberration in amino acid kinetic parameters. Investigators have attempted to reverse some of these alterations by provision of substrate (nutritional support) or administration of specific pharmacologic or anabolic agents such as hydrazine sulfate, insulin, growth hormone, and β_2 agonists.

The role of TPN in cancer and its effects on protein and amino acid kinetics and tumor growth have been reviewed, as well as the possible benefits of specific amino acid nutritional formulations with increased branched-chain amino acids (BCAAs), arginine, and glutamine. Although many of these approaches appear promising, a significant impact on clinically definable parameters remains to be demonstrated [108]. Belizario et al. [109] found circulating levels of a skeletal muscle proteolysis-inducing factor (PIF) in 25 of 50 cancer patients. The plasma of these patients was ultrafiltered to retain molecules 0-25kDa, coincubated with an indicator muscle, and monitored for tyrosine release. None of the plasma obtained from normal individuals contained any detectable activity. Indomethacin and anti-IL-1 antibodies abrogated the proteolysis activity in some but not all of the specimens from cancer patients [109].

Insulin plays a major role in the regulation of BCAA metabolism. Six cachectic patients with localized gastrointestinal malignancies and 5 controls underwent 120-minute euglycemic insulin infusions [110]. An infusion of D-[^{3}H]glucose was used to quantify endogenous glucose production. Total body glucose uptake was decreased in patients with cancer compared with control subjects, consistent with a state of insulin resistance. Progressive euglycemic insulin infusion induced a decrease in arterial plasma BCAA concentrations in both patients with cancer and control subjects. There was no change in postabsorptive forearm BCAA flux with progressive hyperinsulinemia. Insulin-induced BCAA hypoaminoacidemia is unimpaired in this group of patients, manifesting resistance to insulin action on glucose metabolism. Peripheral BCAA flux is not affected by systemic insulin infusion, suggesting that skeletal muscle is not a major site of BCAA disposal during insulin-mediated hypoaminoacidemia [110].

Lipid

Lipid metabolism is closely linked to carbohydrate and protein metabolism and is also affected by malignancy. Cancer cachexia is accompanied by a loss of body fat stores. This occurs despite an increase in serum triglycerides and total lipids [34,38,40]. Transport of triglycerides into adipocytes for storage requires lipoprotein lipase. Decreased levels of this enzyme have been found in cancer patients [7].

This model of a transplantable Leydig cell tumor in rats showed the same characteristics as human cancer cachexia, including anorexia, weight loss, and muscle wasting. Comparison with pair-fed controls showed that the rate of loss of body fat was greater than could be explained by anorexia alone. The rate of lipogenesis tended to decrease during the later stages of tumor growth, particularly in the liver. There was a significant decrease in plasma glucose concentration by day 10. In contrast, LPL activity in adipose tissue was depressed from the earliest stage of tumor growth, and this is likely to be a major cause of lipid depletion in cancer. There was no difference in adipose tissue LPL activity between the fed and postabsorptive states in the tumor-bearing rats, indicating that the normal response to nutrient intake was impaired [42]. The decreased enzyme levels correlate with loss of body fat and may provide a mechanistic explanation. Thus, in vitro lipolysis was correlated with the in vivo loss of total carcass lipids induced by the presence of the same tumor. This study identified and isolated this "lipolysis-promoting" factor (LPF), released into the extracellular environment (conditioned media) by the human A375 melanoma cell line. The mechanism of "lipolysis promotion" by LPF appears to be by the induction of cellular lipase activity [111].

Briddon et al. [112] studied plasma levels of free fatty acids, triglycerides, and tissue levels of lipoprotein lipase in colon adenocarcinoma (MAC16)-bearing mice. They noted extensive mobilization of host body fat reserves, but in this case plasma triglyceride levels were reduced. Plasma-free fatty acid levels were first decreased and then increased to a peak around a 2 g weight loss, then declined again. Lipoprotein lipase in adipose tissue rose until a weight loss of 2.5 g was reached and then declined [112].

The effect of cancer cachexia on the oxidative metabolism of lipids has been studied in mice transplanted either with the MAC16 adenocarcinoma, which induces profound loss of body weight and depletion of lipid stores, or the MAC13 adenocarcinoma, which is the same histologic type, but which grows without an effect on host body weight or lipid stores. While oxidation of D-[U-^{14}C]glucose did not differ between animals bearing tumors of either type and non-tumor-bearing controls, oxidation of [^{14}C]triolein administered by intragastric intubation was significantly ($p < 0.05$) higher in animals bearing the MAC16 tumor than in either non-tumor-bearing controls or in animals bearing the MAC13 tumor. The level of tumor lipids was also higher in the MAC16 than in the MAC13 tumor [113].

The mouse NC tumor, a subcutaneously transplanted adenocarcinoma originally of mammary origin, was also studied. Measurements per gram of tissue were made of 17 fatty acids, the combined amounts of ω-3, ω-6, saturated, unsaturated, and total fatty acids, and of various fatty acid ratios in the tumor, mammary tissue, spleen, liver, and plasma. Compared with mammary tissue from normal mice, tumors of vehicle-treated controls had less than 7 of the fatty acids [114].

The increase in serum triglycerides seen in the tumor-bearing animal model can be reversed by tumor resection [38]. The increased serum lipid levels may be due in part to lipolysis caused by a circulating factor found in tumor-bearing animals [115]. Beck et al. [116] have described a factor in the urine and plasma of mice and humans with cancer cachexia that is not present in normal patients or simply acutely starved subjects and that has lipid mobilizing activity. This suggests that this lipid mobilizing factor may be responsible for catabolism of host adipose tissue in cancer cachexia [116]. Some have tried to exploit this increase in serum lipid levels to detect cancer. Fossel et al. [117] have been able to screen patients with and without cancer based on elevated plasma lipid levels as detected by nuclear magnetic resonance (NMR). Other investigators, though, have failed using these screening procedures but have found an increased incidence of abnormally elevated plasma lipids in cancer patients [118,119].

Using radiolabeled tracer studies to follow glycerol and fatty acids, Shaw et al. [120] demonstrated an increased turnover of lipids in patients with cancer and weight loss. Wilson et al. [121] have shown that lipid clearance is also abnormal in patients with colon cancer. They noted an increased clearance of intravenously administered fat in 15 of 21 patients with tumors. In 14 of those 15, the fat clearance returned to normal 12 weeks after curative resections. There is also a loss of the ability to regulate lipid metabolism. In otherwise normal semistarved people, there is accelerated lipid mobilization, but an infusion of a preferred fuel such as glucose will suppress this increase in mobilization. This suppression of lipid mobilization in the presence of a preferred fuel is lost in cancer patients [120].

Circulating Factors

Theologides [122] first suggested that circulating factors may be responsible for the constellation of abnormalities seen in cancer cachexia. Illig et al. [123] demonstrated that a cachexia-causing factor circulates in the bloodstream of some tumor-bearing hosts. Plasma was collected in a sterile fashion from terminally cachectic rats previously implanted with a sarcoma. Control plasma was collected in similar fashion. Plasma from tumor-bearing (TBP) or non-tumor-bearing rats (NTBP) was continuously infused for 4 days into 20 normal rats. Rats receiving TBP demonstrated an immediate and profound anorexia compared with those receiving NTBP. The total decline in body weight was greater in the TBP group as compared with the NTBP group (-35.2 ± 3.4 vs. -14.6 ± 4.0, $p < 0.001$). Mean daily nitrogen balance during treatment was negative in the rats receiving TBP (-14.5 ± 20.1 mg) while remaining highly positive in the rats receiving NTBP (110.7 ± 19.3, $p < 0.002$). Finally, cardiac and gastrocnemius muscle masses were decreased, while hepatic mass was unaffected (-35.2 ± 3.4 vs. -14.6 ± 4.0, $p < 0.001$) [123]. This was substantiated by elegant experiments done by Mordes et al. [124] and later by Norton et al. [32], which demonstrated that cachexia could be transmitted from a tumor-bearing host to a normal animal across a parabiotic anastomosis. Others had shown even earlier that other effects could also be transmitted including a decrease in liver catalase activity [125]. The search for the circulating factor responsible for cancer cachexia has led to not a single agent, but rather to a number of different factors that combine to create cancer cachexia in its fullest degree.

Chance et al. [50] hypothesized that a sarcoma causes anorexia by consuming glutamine and producing ammonia, which goes on to affect neurotransmitter levels; these changes were rapidly reversed by tumor resection. Elevated (150%) plasma levels of ammonia were noted in sarcoma-bearing anorectic rats. There was a 20-fold increase in ammonia levels in the blood draining from these sarcomas. Infusing comparable levels of ammonia into otherwise normal rats produced anorexia and changes in brain neurotransmitter levels comparable to tumor-bearing animals [126].

There are several potential sources for circulating factors including the tumor itself or normal host factors produced in response to a tumor load. These host-derived factors may be either abnormal products or normal factors synthesized by the host in its attempt to control the tumor that are now synthesized in abnormally large quantities or that have new access to the circulation. This later model of normal host factors causing cachexia when produced or released inappropriately suggests a paradigm for understanding the similarities between cancer cachexia and the weight loss seen in chronic infections or acute illnesses. A common patterned response may be elicited by these various stresses to the host leading to the programmed release of similar signals, causing cachexia.

No single tumor-derived factor has been isolated that would account for cancer cachexia. Nonetheless, different tumors produce various agents with similar effects. Masumo et al. [47] have described a tumor-derived factor, toxohormone-L, which can mediate hypophagia through its central action. Toxohormone-L, a polypeptide extracted and purified from ascites of patients with hepatoma, was infused into the rat third cerebroventricle. Food intake decreased on the first day after infusion. The suppressive effect on feeding was dose-dependent in linear fashion ($p < 0.05$). These findings suggest that anorexia and cachexia produced in cancer patients may essentially be due to the suppressive effect of toxohormone-L on food intake [56]. Belizario et al. [109] found circulating levels of a skeletal muscle proteolysis-inducing factor (PIF) in 25 of 50 cancer patients. Plasma was ultrafiltered to retrain molecules 0-25kDa and coincubated with an indicator muscle and monitored for tyrosine release. None of the 18 normal patients' plasma contained any detectable activity. Indomethacin and anti-IL-1 antibodies abrogated the activity in some but not all of the specimens [109].

A different molecule termed lipolytic factor has been isolated from MAC16 adenocarcinoma and causes progressive weight loss [115]. Beck et al. [116] described a factor in the urine and plasma of mice and humans with cancer cachexia that is not present in normals or simply acutely starved subjects and that has lipid mobilizing activity. They suggest this lipid mobilizing factor may be responsible for catabolism of host adipose tissue in cancer cachexia [116]. Mori et al. [127] have described yet another factor derived from melanomas that inhibits lipoprotein lipase. Lipoprotein lipase is necessary for the transport of triglycerides into adipocytes for storage as fat. Thus, an inhibitor of lipoprotein lipase may contribute to the loss of fat stores seen in cancer cachexia. Other potential candidates for circulating factors that cause cancer cachexia include calcitonin, bombesin, serotonin, neuropeptide Y, and cytokines.

Cytokines

The normal host response to numerous stresses including injury, infection, and tumor includes an immune component. Many of the effects of the immune system are mediated via cytokines that are normal products of leukocytes. Leukocyte-derived mediators of the immune system were originally classified as lymphocyte-derived lymphokines and macrophage-derived cytokines. It has become clear that not only do the actions of many lymphokines and cytokines overlap and complement each other, but also many of these factors can be produced by both lymphocytes and macrophages, and even by other nonimmune cells such as fibroblasts and vascular endothelial cells. As a result, the nomenclature has been simplified and all are now classified as cytokines. Cytokines derived from leukocytes were originally termed interleukins to differentiate them from products of nonimmune cells. However, as the common features of various cytokines were appreciated and nonimmune cell sources of traditional interleukins were discovered, interleukins were more appropriately grouped with a large family of cytokines. Nonetheless, the nomenclature has preserved interleukin (IL) as a common designation.

Anorexia and degradation of skeletal and connective tissue protein, as well as increases in hepatic protein synthesis and energy expenditure, can be reproduced by the administration of activated macrophage products. During inflammatory states, including active tumor growth, increased production of some cytokines, including IL-1 and TNF-α (cachectin), have been observed [128]. The strongest evidence for a causal role for cytokines in cancer cachexia has come from rodent studies in which tumor-bearing animals have been passively immunized with antibodies directed against individual cytokines. However, there has been no consistent finding that one cytokine is universally involved in cancer cachexia in histologically distinct tumor models.

One ominous finding in several tumor models has been that the endogenous production of cytokines appears to support tumor growth. Such findings raise the intriguing possibility that these cytokines, while contributors to tissue wasting and anorexia, may also serve the tumor as either direct or indirect cell growth factors [129]. Because a similar profile of cytokines is produced in response to a variety of insults, many of which result in weight loss similar to that seen in cancer cachexia, cytokines may be the common shared mechanism. Furthermore, it is likely that a number of cytokines interact to together orchestrate the body's response to numerous insults. Cytokines have overlapping physiologic activities, which makes it likely that no single substance is the sole cause of cachexia in most cancer patients [130]. Therefore, it may be difficult to dissect the effects of any single cytokine from the syndrome caused by the cytokine cascade seen in response to an insult. With this in mind, the evidence suggesting a role for TNF, IL-1, and IL-6 in causing tumor-associated cachexia will be examined.

Tumor Necrosis Factor (TNF)

Caswell et al. [131] demonstrated that the serum of BCG-treated mice had potent antitumor properties. They subsequently purified the factor and called it tumor necrosis factor (TNF). The macrophage was found to produce TNF. In work done later and independently, Cerami et al. [132] found that rabbits infected with trypanosomiasis suffered severe weight loss and had elevated serum lipid levels. These abnormalities were associated with a decrease in the activity of lipoprotein lipase, an enzyme necessary for the transport of triglycerides into adipocytes where they can be converted to fat stores. The same group of investigators also found a substance in the serum of endotoxin-treated mice with similar activity. It was later recognized that endotoxin-stimulated macrophages were a source of this agent, called cachectin. Ultimately, both cachectin and TNF were sequenced and found to be identical [133], and are now called alternatively cachectin/TNF or just simply TNF.

TNF has been found to reproduce many aspects of cancer cachexia when administered in small doses, but in larger doses it reproduces many of the changes seen in septic shock [134]. Socher et al. [135] gave a continuous infusion of TNF by minipump and showed a dose-dependent induction of anorexia, weight loss, and changes in body composition. Twice-daily bolus administration of TNF at the same total daily dose did not cause these changes. Furthermore, in the absence of TNF administration, pair-feeding animals to the same amount as the TNF-treated group did not cause cachexia.

Rats treated with recombinant human TNF, 100 μg/kg intraperitoneally twice daily for 5 consecutive days, demonstrated a decrease in food intake, nitrogen balance, and body weight gain vs. saline-treated controls [95]. Concurrent insulin administration of 2 U/100 g subcutaneously twice daily reversed all of these changes to control levels. Llovera et al. [136] examined the effects in rats of an 8-day TNF-α treatment on overall protein metabolism in the liver, diaphragm, heart, and hind-leg muscles. Groups consisted of TNF-α-treated and control female Wistar rats. TNF was administered in twice daily injections for 8 days. All rats were radioactively labeled with $NaH^{14}CO_3$ 24 hours prior to TNF-α treatment. At 0, 1, 2, 4, and 8 days during TNF-α treatment, 5 rats per group were killed to measure the radioactive decay of labeled protein in specific tissues to estimate fractional protein turnover. TNF-α treatment resulted in a transient decrease in food intake and body weight 24 hours after the beginning of the TNF-α treatment. In all types of tissues studied, TNF-α treatment resulted in increases in both protein synthesis and protein degradation, with a greater increase in the protein degradation that resulted in a reduced protein accumulation following TNF-α treatment. This reduction in protein accumulation was directly associated with a decreased soleus muscle mass on day 8 of the treatment [136]. Daily administration of an escalating dose of TNF to mice caused a progressive loss of body weight, representing 12% of the original weight over a 6-day period. Weight loss was associated with decreased food intake, and pair-fed controls exhibited a weight loss of similar magnitude to that caused by TNF-α. However, weight loss in animals bearing a murine adenocarcinoma (MAC16) occurred without a change in energy intake and thus differed from that produced by TNF-α. Anti-TNF-α monoclonal antibodies at levels capable of protecting mice against lethal endotoxemia were ineffective in reversing weight loss in animals bearing the MAC16 tumor and had no effect on the increase in tumor volume [137].

Clinical trials have been conducted administering TNF to cancer patients. In these studies, TNF was found to cause anorexia and abnormal elevations in serum triglyceride levels [138,139]. However, in these studies no weight loss was documented, possibly because the doses of TNF were small.

In an elegant set of experiments, tumors were transfected with the TNF gene and inoculated into animals. These transfected tumors were shown to produce large amounts of TNF in vivo. Animals inoculated with the TNF-secreting tumors developed anorexia and depletion of fat stores leading to weight loss, and ultimately they died earlier when compared to animals inoculated with the nonsecreting tumor [37].

The role of TNF in mediating cancer cachexia is further suggested by the ability of antibodies against TNF to reverse hypophagia and weight loss in tumor-bearing animals. Antibodies reversed the cachexia seen in mice with MCA-induced sarcomas and Lewis lung adenocarcinomas [140,141]. Gelin et al. [140] administered anti-TNF monoclonal antibodies to tumor-bearing mice. The antibody inhibited tumor growth at the end of 11 days of therapy. It also significantly improved food intake, but whole-body fat-free weight did not change while body lipid content showed a trend toward improvement. The acute-phase response was not affected [140]. Sherry et al. [141] transplanted both MCA sarcomas and Lewis lung adenocarcinomas to mice and immediately began administering anti-TNF antibodies to achieve a passive immunity. Anti-TNF antibodies reversed the hypophagia, weight loss, and depletion of body lipid and protein stores caused by the MCA sarcoma. The Lewis lung adenocarcinoma caused depletion of body lipid stores, and anti-TNF antibodies also partially reversed this effect. When anti-TNF antibodies were started much later in the course of disease, once animals had already begun to lose weight, others failed to show a similar efficacy of anti-TNF antibodies [142].

Costelli et al. [143] examined protein metabolism in Yoshida ascites hepatoma-bearing rats. Protein degradation was increased in gastrocnemius muscle, heart, and liver, while synthesis rates were similar to non-tumor-bearing controls. TNF was detected in the plasma of tumor-bearing animals, and the administration of anti-TNF antibodies to the tumor-bearing rats attenuated early perturbations in insulin and corticosterone levels and decreased protein degradation. The antibody treatment, however, did not affect total body weight [143].

Administration of low doses of TNF over several days induces tolerance to TNF. The mechanism of TNF tolerance is not well understood but may involve alterations of the cell surface TNF receptor or the transcriptional regulation of genes related to TNF toxicity. TNF-tolerant animals appear to be protected from subsequent tumor-associated cachexia [144]. Sheppard et al. [145] were able to induce tolerance to TNF in rats already bearing a tumor and showed that, even at this late stage, tolerance to TNF could prevent the cachexia seen in TNF-sensitive, tumor-bearing rats. Tolerance to TNF not only improved food intake in these tumor-bearing rats but also prolonged survival [144,145].

The question remains why the host does not develop a tolerance through continuous exposure to tumors that either normally produce TNF or induce the host to release it. Tracey et al. [146] were able to overcome tolerance to TNF by administering increasing doses of TNF. These rats, initially tolerant to low doses of TNF, developed anorexia, weight loss, and depletion of body lipid and protein stores when escalating doses of TNF were administered. This would parallel the clinical setting in which an increasing tumor burden would likely be associated with increased secretion of TNF, therefore never allowing the host to become fully tolerant to the effects of TNF.

Serum levels of TNF do not correlate with clinical findings of cachexia in cancer patients or tumor-bearing animals. It has been easier to demonstrate elevated TNF levels in patients with chronic infections or sepsis than in those with malignancies [147–150]. Balkwill et al. [151] found elevated serum TNF levels in only 50% of patients with detectable disease. Serum TNF levels also elevated in 18% of patients in whom the cancer was in remission. Ardizzoia et al. [152] screened 48 cancer patients compared to 40 controls for serum TNF levels. Elevated TNF levels were seen in 27 of the 48 (56%) with mean levels higher in cancer patients than in controls. Within the cancer group, the highest levels were in those with metastatic disease [152]. TNF may be difficult to detect in serum if it is normally secreted in a cyclic fashion. An active membrane-bound receptor has been described that could make detection of serum levels difficult [153]. Circulating TNF receptor has also been described, derived from the proteolytic cleavage of the transmembrane form, which may bind circulating TNF and make it more difficult to measure. Even in patients receiving an infusion of TNF with obvious physiologic effects, serum levels can be undetectable [154].

The mechanisms by which TNF causes cachexia are poorly understood. TNF may act centrally through effects on the satiety center in the hypothalamus [155]. Bernstein et al. [54] found that lesions in the area postrema can attenuate the anorectic effects of TNF, a finding also described for tumor-associated anorexia. In this model, a rapid tolerance to the anorectic effects of TNF developed [54]. Others suggest that TNF causes anorexia by reducing gastric emptying [156]. In Sherry's studies, anti-TNF antibodies blocked some of the cachectic effects of a tumor [141]. In those same animals, administration of anti-TNF antibodies was associated with a reduced tumor mass. One could imagine that the primary effect of the antibodies was to reduce the tumor mass, and the reversal of tumor-associated cachexia was only secondary to the decreased tumor mass. This is unlikely to be the mechanism because it was shown that tolerating animals to TNF also reduced the cachectic effects of a tumor without affecting the tumor size [144,145].

Interleukin-1 (IL-1)

IL-1 is an inflammatory cytokine produced by macrophages. Evidence suggests that it may be a central mediator of septic shock because its intravenous administration causes increased cardiac output, decreased systemic vascular resistance, and hypotension [157]. In addition to activating T and B lymphocytes, IL-1 induces several hematologic and metabolic changes typical of host responses to infection and injury. When administered to animals, IL-1 causes hypotension, systemic vascular resistance, and a decrease in central venous pressure, while cardiac output and heart rate increase. When the dose of IL-1 or TNF was reduced to 1 μg/kg, no hemodynamic changes were observed; however, the combination of these low doses of both cytokines resulted in a profound shock-like state [157].

Alexander et al. [158] protected mice from a lethal dose of lipopolysaccharide (LPS) by administering IL-1 receptor antagonists after LPS. Serum levels of TNF after LPS were not altered by IL-1ra, suggesting that IL-1 may mediate the lethal effects of LPS [158]. Others have shown that much smaller doses of IL-1 than those required to cause hemodynamic changes can cause anorexia [159]. IL-1 has been shown to be more potent than even TNF in causing anorexia [160]. As little as 10% of the pyrexia-causing dose of IL-1 will cause hypophagia and alterations in hepatic metabolism in mice [128]. Dinarello et al. [161] showed that a single injection of IL-1 in meal-fed rats would reduce food intake by 40% and that chronic administration slowed normal weight gain.

Gelin et al. [140] administered anti-IL-1R antibodies to tumor-bearing mice. The anti-IL-1R Ab had no agonist activity. Tumor growth was inhibited at the end of 11 days of therapy, and food intake was significantly improved. Whole-body fat-free weight did not change, while body lipid content showed a trend toward improvement [140].

As with TNF, circulating plasma levels of IL-1 have been difficult to correlate with cancer cachexia. IL-1 has been more readily found in the serum of infected patients than in those with malignancies. Moldawer et al. [162] found detectable plasma levels in only 1 of 23 patients with cancer, compared with 5 of 6 bacterially infected patients. Measurement of circulating levels of IL-1 is made more difficult by the presence of plasma inhibitors of IL-1, which can interfere with the measurement of IL-1 bioactivity [163].

Although plasma levels of IL-1 have been difficult to measure, a role for IL-1 in cancer cachexia is suggested by the findings of Jensen et al. [164]. Their group demonstrated the induction of the IL-1 gene in the livers of cachectic, tumor-bearing rats, while the plasma levels of IL-1 were simultaneously undetectable.

The mechanisms of IL-1 action remain unclear, but in part seem to include effects on the central nervous system [165]. Direct intracerebroventricular injection of IL-1 causes significant anorexia [53]. Uehara et al. [57] have suggested that IL-1 causes anorexia through the stimulation of CRF release by the hypothalamus. They have shown that IL-1 administered intraperitoneally causes anorexia, while the simultaneous injection of CRF antiserum into the cerebral ventricles prevents this effect. Another mechanism of IL-1 action is through prostaglandins. Pretreatment of animals with ibuprofen prior to an IL-1 infusion completely blocked its anorexic effects, and a fish oil-based diet abolished it in comparison to corn oil or chow diets. Chronic daily administration of IL-1 caused persistent inhibition of food intake for 7 of 17 days in chow- and corn oil-fed rats, but had no effect in fish oil-fed rats [159].

Interleukin-6 (IL-6)

IL-6 is another inflammatory cytokine produced by macrophages and fibroblasts. IL-6, like TNF and IL-1, has been implicated as a mediator of sepsis. IL-6 is the most consistently elevated cytokine detectable after various stresses, including elective surgery, trauma, and sepsis [166]. Elevated plasma IL-6 levels have also been correlated with poor outcome following meningococcal sepsis [166].

Circulating levels of IL-6 have also been easier to detect in tumor-bearing hosts. Increased levels have been found in mice bearing a variety of different tumors [167]. Serum concentrations of IL-6 progressively increased in mice bearing a transplantable MCA-induced sarcoma. In transplantable colon-26 adenocarcinoma-bearing mice, tumor size correlated with serum IL-6 and transforming growth factor beta (TGF-β) concentrations in serum [168]. Elevated IL-6 concentrations were also positively correlated with increased serum concentrations of the hepatic acute-phase reactant protein, amyloid P [169]. Jablons et al. [170] also found circulating levels of IL-6 that correlated with tumor burden. The sera of untreated TB mice contained levels of IL-6 that paralleled the extent of tumor burden. The detection of de novo IL-6 was also confirmed in animals bearing tumors of different histologies (MCA102 sarcoma, MCA38 adenocarcinoma, and B16 melanoma) [167]. Untransfected Lewis lung carcinoma (LLC), or LLC-IL-6 cells containing an expression vector for huIL-6 with documented in vitro secretion were transplanted into C57BL/6 mice subcutaneously. Mean survival times of these mice were significantly shorter for the IL-6 secreting tumors compared with controls. The mean survival time of LLC-IL-6 cell-transplanted mice was significantly shorter than that of LLC cell-transplanted mice, without a measurable difference of tumor size. Plasma concentrations of IL-6 steadily increased in LLC-IL-6 cell-transplanted mice. Mean body weight and serum albumin levels were significantly lower in LLC-IL-6 cell-transplanted mice than in LLC cell-transplanted mice. IL-6 caused a state similar to cachexia without a detectable increase of IL-1α and TNF-α in the plasma [171]. Rats were implanted subdermally with tumor tissue fragments. Ad libitum- and pair-fed controls were sham-incised. Bioassays for TNF and IL-6 were performed on serial plasma samples. Tumor growth induced significant anorexia, weight loss, and a decline in motor activity corresponding to an increase in mean plasma IL-6 levels, independent of reduced food intake or weight loss alone as shown in pair-fed controls [172]. This model of cachexia fulfills the criteria of an early effect with a small tumor mass not related to the growth rate of the tumor and progressive wasting of muscle and fat without a detectable loss of appetite.

C-26.IVX is a cell line derived from murine colon-26 adenocarcinoma that retains the transplantability of the original tumor and induces true cachexia in syngeneic hosts. Increasing levels of IL-6 in C-26.IVX-bearing mice correlate with the development of cachexia. When the primary tumors were resected, mice gained weight and the levels of IL-6 in the serum were reduced significantly. Moreover, monoclonal antibody to murine IL-6 (but not anti-TNF antibody) was able to significantly suppress the development of key parameters of cachexia in tumor-bearing mice [173]. Administration of a relatively high amount of LPS to mice induced a transient weight loss, hypoglycemia, hypertriglyceridemia and an increase in the hepatic acute-phase reactant, fibrinogen. Pretreatment of mice with the rat anti-murine IL-6 antibody, but not with a control antibody, resulted in a significant improvement of LPS-induced hypoglycemia and weight loss as well as a significant decrease of plasma fibrinogen levels. Anti-IL-6 antibody had no effect on LPS-induced hypertriglyceridemia. On the other hand, pretreatment of mice with anti-murine TNF (TN3.19) antibody was able to completely inhibit elevation of triglycerides and modestly improve LPS-induced weight loss, although it had no effect on hypoglycemia and fibrinogen production. Taken together, these results suggest that IL-6 plays a role in some of the metabolic changes associated with both an acute (i.e., LPS challenge) and chronic (C-26 cachexia) inflammatory conditions [174].

Others have suggested a causative role for IL-6 in tumor-induced metabolic changes. Gelin et al. [169] found that elevated plasma levels of IL-6 correlated with the induction of acute-phase protein synthesis. This is consistent with the findings that IL-6 is a potent agent in triggering hepatic synthesis of acute-phase proteins [175].

IL-6 reduces adipose lipoprotein lipase (LPL) activity and may contribute to the loss of body fat stores associated with some cases of cancer cachexia. Because TNF increases circulating IL-6, some of its effects may be mediated or potentiated by IL-6. LPL activity in adipose tissue of mice decreased after administration of IL-6 or TNF and in cultured adipocytes after addition of these cytokines. Injection of IL-6 intraperitoneally reduced adipose tissue LPL activity by 53% within 4.5 to 5.5 hours. Injection of TNF elevated serum IL-6 levels and reduced adipose tissue LPL activity by 70% [176].

Gamma-Interferon (IFN-γ)

Langstein et al. [177] noted that administration of repetitive sublethal doses of recombinant murine IFN-γ to non-tumor-bearing rats caused a significant decline in food intake and body weight. Rats maintained persistent diminished food intake and diminished body weight gain while receiving recombinant murine IFN-γ. Passive immunization against recombinant rat IFN-γ allowed cachectic tumor-bearing rats to eat more food, have a lesser decline in body weight, live longer, and tolerate larger tumors than similar tumor-bearing rats given nonspecific control antibody. Tumor-bearing rats treated with an antisera to recombinant murine TNF, which was 100% protective when given to non-tumor-bearing rats 6 hours before a lethal endotoxin challenge, did not differ significantly from tumor-bearing rats treated with control antibody with respect to food intake, body weight, survival, or tumor size. Serum levels of TNF or IFN-γ were not detectable in cachectic tumor-bearing rats. The administration of exogenous IFN-γ can simulate cachexia in non-tumor-bearing rats and that passive immunization against it can partially reverse the cachectic changes associated with cancer and prolong survival. These findings suggest that IFN-γ may be an important mediator of cachexia in this rat tumor model [177].

Mice were inoculated with a line of Chinese hamster ovary tumor cells that had been genetically engineered to produce murine IFN-γ. Severe cachexia, as evident from body weight loss and reduced food intake, occurred in these mice, but not in those injected with control cells, i.e., the original, non-IFN-γ-producing line. Monoclonal antibodies against IFN-γ, given prior to injection of the tumor cells, prevented cachexia. In addition to IFN-γ, the presence of the tumor cells was also required for cachexia to develop. As evident from pair-feeding experiments, reduced food intake could only partially account for the rapid and extensive body weight loss [178].

C57BL/6N mice bearing Lewis lung tumors were treated with anti-IFN-γ monoclonal antibodies. Early (but not late) treatment inhibited tumor growth, suggesting that endogenous IFN-γ promotes initial tumor cell proliferation. Tumor development was associated with failure to gain weight or with progressive weight loss. Anti-IFN-γ given early or late counteracted this wasting syndrome. Fat loss was enhanced by IFN-γ and antagonized by anti-IFN-γ [179].

Specific Nutrients That May Enhance Immune Function

When patients with malignant disease are given nutritional support, the potential for stimulating tumor growth is an obvious concern. Although numerous animal studies demonstrate significant acceleration of tumor growth during nutritional repletion, gross tumor stimulation by exogenous nutrient provision has not been clearly documented in humans. Mullen et al. [180] demonstrated no difference in protein synthesis rates of upper gastrointestinal cancers in 25 patients receiving TPN compared with patients nourished orally. Tumor fractional protein synthesis rates were identical in the two groups of patients despite a substantial increase in protein calorie intake in parenterally nourished patients. Nixon et al. [181] noted no direct clinical or biochemical evidence of tumor stimulation with TPN for patients with metastatic colon cancer compared with patients fed orally. Thus, in the clinical situation, use of nutritional support is not contraindicated by concerns regarding tumor growth stimulation. [*Editor's Note:* I am not certain that the view held by the authors is universally accepted. Increased protein synthesis in head and neck tumors extirpated from patients receiving preoperative TPN was reported by Baron et al. [182]. While Nixon et al. [181] did not report any *direct* evidence of tumor growth, their report did cause a stir by suggesting that patients on TPN demonstrated a decreased survival interval as compared with patients not receiving TPN. Discussion centered on whether the two groups were comparable, with some suggesting that the group receiving TPN had a heavier tumor burden. No such ambiguity existed in the report by Shamberger et al. [10] of decreased recurrence-free interval in lymphoma patients treated with TPN in a randomized prospective trial. In my opinion, although data are difficult to achieve [183], there is cause for concern.]

Arginine

Arginine is an amino acid that is not considered essential for adult mammals, as it can be synthesized in vivo via urea cycle intermediates. Arginine plays an important role in protein synthesis, urea cycle metabolism, and the synthesis of the high-energy compounds creatine and creatine phosphate. Two pathways of arginine metabolism have been identified as potential sources of critical mediators of arginine immunomodulatory actions in vivo. The so-called arginase pathway, in which arginine is converted to urea and ornithine, generates polyamines by the action of ornithine decarboxylase on the latter compound. This route of polyamine synthesis was proposed as the mechanism whereby arginine augments lymphocyte mitogenesis [184]. Induction of arginase was also proposed as the effector pathway in arginine-dependent macrophage-mediated tumor cell cytotoxicity [185]. A second, more recently described pathway of arginine metabolism leads to the generation of reactive nitrogen intermediates, principally nitric oxide and its peroxynitrite derivatives. These reactive nitrogen intermediates are derived from arginine through the action of nitric oxide synthase. It is postulated that macrophage-mediated tumor cytotoxicity and fungistasis are mediated through this pathway [186].

Arginine supplementation in the tumor-bearing host may inhibit tumor growth and reduce metastatic spread in immunogenic tumors [187]. Reynolds et al. [188] showed that arginine supplementation in mice bearing either immunogenic or nonimmunogenic tumors resulted in enhanced splenocyte mitogenesis and IL-2 production in comparison to control mice on regular diets. However, tumor growth was inhibited only in the immunogenic tumor model, suggesting augmentation of antitumor immunity with arginine supplementation. In contrast, Yeatman et al. [189] reported beneficial effects of dietary arginine depletion on liver metastases in a murine model. This effect was attributed to the dependence of this particular tumor model on arginine for optimal growth in vitro and in vivo.

In clinical trials, supplemental arginine in normal human volunteers led to significant increases in peripheral blood lymphocyte proliferation to mitogens and in the T-helper/T-suppressor cell ratio [190,191]. To determine the clinical effect of supplemental arginine, Daly et al. [192], in a controlled randomized trial, studied arginine-supplemented versus glycine-supplemented enteral nutrition via jejunostomy in cancer patients undergoing major surgery. Mean lymphocyte proliferation and T-helper subsets were significantly elevated in the arginine-supplemented group. A subsequent study showed that this effect was dependent on the administration of arginine with other amino acids and calories because administration of arginine as the sole amino acid source did not augment T-cell function. This finding implied a complex pattern for the immunomodulatory role in arginine, including interaction with other dietary elements to mediate the observed immunologic effects [193]. Clearly, arginine has great potential as an immunomodulator and may prove useful in catabolic conditions such as severe sepsis and postoperative stress.

Glutamine

Glutamine is quantitatively the most abundant amino acid in the circulation and in the intracellular free amino acid pool. Rose [194] determined in 1938 that glutamine can be synthesized de novo in the body and hence was a nonessential amino acid. Eagle [195] had earlier reported that glutamine was required in high concentration in tissue culture media for optimal growth of cultured mammalian cells, a practice that continues today. Research in our laboratory has shown that macrophage superoxide, nitric oxide production, *Candida* killing, and tumor cytotoxicity are enhanced with increasing glutamine concentration in vitro.

In rats, glutamine-supplemented TPN has been found to improve peritoneal and alveolar macrophage function [196]. In a model of orthotopic small bowel transplantation, rats receiving glutamine-supplemented TPN had improved gut structure and glucose absorption and a decrease in bacterial translocation compared with control animals [197]. Following radiotherapy or chemotherapy for tumors, glutamine supplementation has been shown experimentally to improve the response to therapy and reduce treatment-related intestinal mucosal damage [198,199].

In the tumor-bearing host, it has been postulated that glutamine may represent an anabolic substrate that enhances tumor growth [200]. Although in vitro tumor cell growth can be stimulated with glutamine supplementation, in vivo animal studies have failed to confirm this phenomenon. Studies utilizing sarcoma and mammary adenocarcinoma models in rats have demonstrated that glutamine supplementation can improve host nutritional status without enhancing tumor growth [201,202]. [*Editor's Note:* Again, a note of caution. Our own studies of experimental tumors [126] indicate that glutamine is *the* principal nitrogen source, as measured by arteriovenous differences across tumors.]

Glutamine-supplemented TPN in postoperative patients can preserve the intracellular glutamine pool and improve nitrogen balance in the supplemented group compared to controls [203]. The most comprehensive trial of glutamine efficacy in a clinical setting is that of Ziegler et al. [204]. In a randomized double-blind prospective study, bone marrow transplant patients receiving glutamine-supplemented TPN were compared to patients receiving standard TPN. The glutamine-supplemented group demonstrated a significant improvement in nitrogen balance, significantly shorter hospital stay, and a significant reduction in infectious complications. Although most enteral feeding formulas contain a significant amount of glutamine, parenteral glutamine supplementation remains limited. Glutamine is not included in commercially available TPN solutions, primarily due to the relative instability of glutamine in such solutions. Glutamine analogues or innovative parenteral formulations may overcome this problem in the future and enable glutamine to be included as an integral component of TPN regimens. [*Editor's Note:* The two studies thus far available utilizing glutamine peptides in perioperative TPN patients [205,206] demonstrated statistical but not likely biologic improvement in nitrogen balance in the glutamine-supplemented groups.]

Conclusion

Despite the numerous investigations performed over the last two decades, the place of nutritional support in the management of malignant disease remains ill defined, although some generalizations can be made. The conventional indication for providing supplemental nutrition has been to increase body weight and muscle mass and to reduce mortality and morbidity in the patient with cancer undergoing surgery. The evidence suggests that perioperative nutritional support, if given for at least 10 days, may reduce morbidity and mortality in some patients. Although this subgroup has not been fully characterized, it probably represents those patients with biochemical evidence of severe malnutrition, manifest as low serum albumin concentration and excessive weight loss. [*Editor's Note:* It is of interest that the only studies in perioperative TPN in patients with cancer to show efficacy are those patients with upper gastrointestinal cancer. The significance of this finding is not clear.]

References

1. Bistrian BR, et al. Prevalence of malnutrition in general medical patients. *JAMA* 235:1567, 1976.
2. Willcutts HD. Nutritional assessment of 1000 surgical patients in an affluent suburban community hospital. *JPEN* 1:25, 1977.
3. DeWys WD, Begg D, Lavin PT. Prognostic effect of weight loss prior to chemotherapy in cancer patients. *Am J Med* 69:491, 1980.
4. Nixon DW, et al. Protein-calorie undernutrition in hospitalized cancer patients. *Am J Med* 68:683, 1980.
5. Buzby GP, et al. Prognostic nutritional index in gastrointestinal surgery. *Am J Surg* 139:160, 1980.
6. Camoriano JK, et al. Weight change in women treated with adjuvant therapy or observed following mastectomy for node-positive breast cancer. *J Clin Oncol* 8:1327, 1990.
7. Langstein HN, Norton JA. Mechanisms of cancer cachexia. *Hematol Oncol Clin North Am* 5:103, 1991.
8. Norton JA, Peacock JL, Morrison SD. Cancer cachexia. *Crit Rev Oncol Hematol* 7:289, 1987.
9. Chlebowski RT, et al. Hydrazine sulfate influence on nutritional status and survival in non-small-cell lung cancer. *J Clin Oncol* 8:9, 1990.
10. Shamberger RC, et al. A prospective, randomized study of adjuvant parenteral nutrition in the treatment of sarcoma: Results of metabolic and survival studies. *Surgery* 96:1, 1984.
11. Peacock JL, Gorschboth CM, Norton JA. Impact of insulin on doxorubicin-induced rat host toxicity and tumor regression. *Cancer Res* 47:4318, 1987.
12. Popp MB, Morrison SD, Brennan MF. Total parenteral nutrition in a methylcholanthrene-induced rat sarcoma model. *Cancer Treat Rep* 65(suppl 5):137, 1981.
13. Moley JF, Morrison SD, Norton JA. Preoperative insulin reverses cachexia and decreases mortality in tumor-bearing rats. *J Surg Res* 43:21, 1987.
14. Hickman DM, et al. Serum albumin and body weight as predictors of postoperative course in colorectal cancer. *JPEN* 4:314, 1980.
15. Warren S. The immediate cause of death in cancer. *Am J Med Sci* 184:610, 1932.
16. Harnett WL. *A Survey of Cancer in London.* London: British Empire Cancer Campaign, 1952. P. 26.
17. Lawson DH, et al. Metabolic approaches to cancer cachexia. *Ann Rev Nutr* 2:277, 1982.
18. Brennan MF. Total parenteral nutrition in the cancer patient. *N Engl J Med* 305:375, 1981.
19. McGeer AJ, Detsky AS, O'Rourke K. Parenteral nutrition in patients receiving cancer chemotherapy. *Ann Intern Med* 110:734, 1989.
20. Cohn SH, et al. Body composition and dietary intake in neoplastic disease. *Am J Clin Nutr* 34:1997, 1981.
21. Nixon DW, et al. Hyperalimentation of the cancer patient with protein calorie undernutrition. *Cancer Res* 41:2038, 1981.
22. Koretz RL. Parenteral nutrition: Is it oncologically logical? *J Clin Oncol* 2:534, 1984.
23. Moley JF, et al. Body composition changes in rats with experimental cancer cachexia: Improvement with exogenous insulin. *Cancer Res* 48:2784, 1988.
24. Norton JA, Lowry SF, Brennan MF. Effects of work-induced hypertrophy on skeletal muscle of tumor and non-tumor bearing rats. *J Appl Physiol* 46:654, 1979.
25. Shaw JHF, Wolfe RR. Whole-body protein kinetics in patients with early and advanced gastrointestinal cancer: The response to glucose infusion and total parenteral nutrition. *Surgery* 103:148, 1988.
26. Moley JF, et al. Body cell mass in cancer-bearing and anorexic patients. *JPEN* 11:219, 1987.
27. Fong Y, et al. Tumor location influences local cytokine production and host metabolism. *Surg Oncol* 1:65, 1992.
28. Dewys WD. Anorexia in cancer patients. *Cancer Res* 37:2354, 1977.
29. Theologides A. Cancer cachexia. *Cancer* 43:2004, 1979.
30. Shils ME. Nutritional problems induced by cancer. *Med Clin North Am* 63:1009, 1977.
31. Luketich ID, et al. Ablation of abnormal energy expenditure in cancer patients after curative tumor resection. *Arch Surg* 125:337, 1990.
32. Norton JA, et al. Parabiotic transfer of anorexia/cachexia in male rats. *Cancer Res* 45:5547, 1985.
33. Balducci L, Hardy C. Cancer and nutrition: A review. *Compr Ther* 13:60, 1987.
34. Beutler B. Cachexia: A fundamental mechanism. *Nutr Rev* 46:5919, 1988.
35. Fearon KCH, et al. Influence of whole body protein turnover rate on resting energy expenditure in patients with cancer. *Cancer Res* 48:2590, 1988.
36. Bibby MC, et al. Characterization of a transplantable adenocarcinoma of the mouse colon producing cachexia in recipient animals. *J Natl Cancer Inst* 78:539, 1987.
37. Oliff A, et al. Tumors secreting human TNF/cachectin induce cachexia in mice. *Cell* 50:555, 1987.
38. Stovroff MC, Fraker DL, Norton JA. Cachectin activity in the serum of cachectic, tumor-bearing rats. *Arch Surg* 124:94, 1989.
39. Svaninger G, Isaksson O, Lundholm K. Growth hormone

and experimental cancer cachexia. *J Natl Cancer Inst* 79:1359, 1987.

40. Kern KA, Norton JA. Cancer cachexia. *JPEN* 12:286, 1988.
41. Brennan MF. Uncomplicated starvation versus cancer cachexia. *Cancer Res* 37:2359, 1977.
42. Obeid OA, Emery PW. Lipid metabolism in cachectic tumor-bearing rats at different stages of tumor growth. *Nutr Cancer* 19:87, 1993.
43. Burt ME, Brennan MF. Nutritional support of the patient with esophageal cancer. *Semin Oncol* 11:127, 1984.
44. McCarthy DO, Daun IM. The role of gastric stasis in tumor-induced anorexia in rats. *Cancer* 70:1601, 1992.
45. Dewys WD. Changes in taste sensation and feeding behavior in cancer patients: A review. *J Hum Nutr* 32:447, 1978.
46. Russ J, Dewys WD. Correction of taste abnormality of malignancy with intravenous hyperalimentation. *Arch Intern Med* 138:799, 1977.
47. Masumo H, Yamasak N, Okuda H. Purification and characterization of a lipolytic factor (toxohormone-L) from cell free fluid of ascites sarcoma 180. *Cancer Res* 41:284, 1981.
48. Chance WT, et al. Neurotransmitter alterations associated with feeding and satiety. *Brain Res* 416:228, 1987.
49. Chance WT, et al. Hyperammonemia and anorexia in Morris hepatoma-bearing rats. *Physiol Behav* 50:397, 1991.
50. Chance WT, et al. Reversal of neurochemical aberrations after tumor resection in rats. *Am J Surg* 155:124, 1988.
51. Chance WT, et al. Possible role of ammonia in experimental cancer anorexia. *Brain Res* 486:316, 1989.
52. Chance WT, Balasubramaniam A, Fischer JE. Neuropeptide Y and the development of cancer anorexia. *Ann Surg,* in press.
53. Plata-Salaman CR, Oomura Y, Kai Y. Tumor necrosis factor and interleukin-1 beta: Suppression of food intake by direct action in the central nervous system. *Brain Res* 448:106, 1988.
54. Bernstein IL, Taylor EM, Bentson KL. TNF-induced anorexia and learned food aversions are attenuated by area postrema lesions. *Am J Physiol* 260:R906, 1991.
55. Tracey KJ, Cerami A. Tumor necrosis factor in metabolism of disease: Hormonal actions versus local tissue effects. *Nouv Rev Fr Hematol* 34:S37, 1992.
56. Okabe Y, et al. Anorexia induced by toxohormone-L isolated from ascites fluid of patients with hepatoma. *Physiol Behav* 52:333, 1992.
57. Uehara A, et al. Anorexia induced by interleukin-1: Involvement of corticotropin-releasing factor. *Am J Physiol* 257:R613, 1989.
58. Henkin RI, Mattes-Kulig D, Lynch RA. Taste and smell acuity in patients with cancer. *Fed Proc* 42:550, 1983.
59. Plumb MJ, Holland J. Comparative studies of psychological function in patients with advanced cancer: I. Self-related depressive symptoms. *Psychosom Med* 39:264, 1977.
60. Lesko LM. Psychosocial issues in the diagnosis and management of cancer cachexia and anorexia. *Nutrition* 5:114, 1989.
61. McAnena OJ, Daly IM. Impact of antitumor therapy on nutrition. *Surg Clin North Am* 66:1213, 1986.
62. Chencharick JD, Mossman KL. Nutritional consequences of the radiotherapy of head and neck cancer. *Cancer* 51:811, 1983.
63. Drott C, et al. Total parenteral nutrition as an adjuvant to patients undergoing chemotherapy for testicular carcinoma: Protection of body composition—a randomized, prospective study. *Surgery* 103:499, 1988.
64. Freund HR, et al. Resting energy expenditure of host and tumor is similar in rats with methylcholanthrene-induced sarcoma. *Arch Surg* 122:1151, 1987.
65. Hyltander A, et al. Elevated energy expenditure in cancer patients with solid tumours. *Eur J Cancer* 27:9, 1991.
66. Bozzetti F, Pagnoni AM, DelVecchio M. Excessive caloric expenditure as a cause of malnutrition in patients with cancer. *Surg Gynecol Obstet* 150:229, 1980.
67. Lindmark L, et al. Resting energy expenditure in malnourished patients with and without cancer. *Gastroenterology* 87:402, 1984.
68. Knox LS, et al. Energy expenditure in malnourished cancer patients. *Ann Surg* 197:152, 1983.
69. Dempsy DT, et al. Energy expenditure in malnourished cancer patients. *Cancer* 53:1265, 1984.
70. Merrick HW, et al. Energy requirements for cancer patients and the effects of total parenteral nutrition. *JPEN* 12:8, 1988.
71. Peacock JL, et al. Resting energy expenditure and body cell mass alterations in noncachectic patients with sarcomas. *Surgery* 102:46, 1987.
72. Fredrix EW, et al. Resting energy expenditure in patients with newly detected gastric and colorectal cancers. *Am J Clin Nutr* 53:1318, 1991.
73. Morrison SD. Control of food intake in cancer cachexia: A challenge and a tool. *Phys Behav* 17:705, 1976.
74. Alexander HR, et al. Substrate alterations in sarcoma-bearing rat model: Effect of tumor growth and resection. *J Surg Res* 48:471, 1990.
75. Norton JA, Burt ME, Brennan MF. In vivo utilization of substrate by human sarcoma-bearing limbs. *Cancer* 45:2934, 1980.
76. Inculet RI, et al. Gluconeogenesis in the tumor-influenced rat hepatocyte: Importance of tumor burden, lactate, insulin, and glucagon. *J Natl Cancer Inst* 79:1039, 1987.
77. Conlon KC, et al. Extremity metabolism in the cachectic, VX-2 carcinoma-bearing rabbit. *J Surg Res* 55:330, 1993.
78. Tayek JA. A review of cancer cachexia and abnormal glucose metabolism in humans with cancer. *J Am Coll Nutr* 11:445, 1992.
79. Burt ME, et al. Metabolic alterations in a noncachetic animal tumor system. *Cancer* 47:2138, 1981.
80. Copeland GP, et al. Glucose metabolism in patients with gastrointestinal malignancy but without excessive weight loss. *Eur J Surg Oncol* 13:11, 1987.
81. Holroyde CP, et al. Glucose metabolism in cachectic patients with colorectal cancer. *Cancer Res* 44:5910, 1984.
82. Waterhouse C. Lactate metabolism in patients with cancer. *Cancer* 33:66, 1974.
83. McDevitt TM, Tisdale MJ. Tumour-associated hypoglycaemia in a murine cachexia model. *Br J Cancer* 66:815, 1992.
84. Mulligan HD, Tisdale MJ. Metabolic substrate utilization by tumour and host tissues in cancer cachexia. *Biochem J* 277:321, 1991.
85. Blumberg D, et al. Tolbutamide inhibits gluconeogenesis in the tumor-influenced hepatocyte. *J Surg Res* 55:565, 1993.
86. Shaw JHF, Humberstone DM, Wolfe RR. Energy and protein metabolism in sarcoma patients. *Ann Surg* 207:283, 1988.

87. Norton JA, et al. Glucose intolerance in sarcoma patients. *Cancer* 54:3022, 1984.

88. Cori CF, Cori GT. The carbohydrate metabolism of tumors. II: Changes in the sugar, lactic acid, and CO_2-combining power of blood passing through a tumor. *J Biol Chem* 66:397, 1925.

89. Gold J. Proposed treatment of cancer by inhibition of gluconeogenesis. *Oncology* 22:185, 1968.

90. McCall IL, Tuckey JA, Parry BR. Serum tumour necrosis factor alpha and insulin resistance in gastrointestinal cancer. *Br J Surg* 79:1361, 1992.

91. Emery PW, Carpenter TT, Obeid OA. Alterations in postprandial glycogen and lipid synthesis in cachectic tumorbearing rats. *Nutr Cancer* 20:231, 1993.

92. Cersosimo E, et al. The effect of graded doses of insulin on peripheral glucose uptake and lactate release in cancer cachexia. *Surgery* 109:459, 1991.

93. Chance WT, et al. Reversal of tumor-induced biochemical abnormalities by insulin treatment in rats. *J Natl Cancer Inst* 77:497, 1986.

94. Peacock JL, Norton JA. Impact of insulin on survival of cachectic tumor-bearing rats. *JPEN* 12:260, 1988.

95. Fraker DL, Merino MJ, Norton JA. Reversal of the toxic effects of cachectin by concurrent insulin administration. *Am J Physiol* 256:E725, 1989.

96. Goodgame JR, Pizzo P, Brennan MF. Iatrogenic lactic acidosis association with hypertonic glucose administration in a patient with cancer. *Cancer* 42:800, 1978.

97. Cahill GF. Starvation in man. *N Engl J Med* 282:668, 1970.

98. Norton JA, Stein TP, Brennan MF. Whole body protein synthesis and turnover in normal man and malnourished patients with and without cancer. *Ann Surg* 123:1981, 1981.

99. Fearon KCH, et al. Cancer cachexia: Influence of systemic ketosis on substrate levels and nitrogen metabolism. *Am J Clin Nutr* 47:42, 1988.

100. Jeevanandam M, et al. Cancer cachexia and protein metabolism. *Lancet* 1:1423, 1984.

101. Karlberg HI, Kern KA, Fischer JE. Albumin turnover in sarcoma bearing rats in relation to cancer anorexia. *Am J Surg* 145:95, 1983.

102. Karlberg I, et al. Reutilization of amino acids in relation to albumin turnover in nongrowing mice with sarcoma. *Cancer Res* 42:2284, 1982.

103. Kien CL, Carmitta BM. Close association of accelerated rates of whole body protein turnover (synthesis and breakdown) and energy expenditure in children with newly diagnosed acute lymphocytic leukemia. *JPEN* 11:129, 1987.

104. Tessitore L, Bonelli G, Baccino FM. Early development of protein metabolic perturbations in the liver and skeletal muscle of tumor bearing rats: A model system for cancer cachexia. *Biochem J* 241:153, 1987.

105. Smith KL, Tisdale MJ. Increased protein degradation and decreased protein synthesis in skeletal muscle during cancer cachexia. *Br J Cancer* 67:680, 1993.

106. Tayek JA, Blackburn GL, Bistrian BR. Alterations in whole body, muscle, liver, and tumor tissue protein synthesis and degradation in Novikoff and Yoshida sarcoma tumor growth studied in vivo. *Cancer Res* 48:1554, 1988.

107. Jeevanandam M, et al. Effects of total parenteral nutrition on whole body protein kinetics in cachetic patients with benign or malignant disease. *JPEN* 12:229, 1988.

108. Pisters PW, Pearlstone DB. Protein and amino acid metabolism in cancer cachexia: Investigative techniques and therapeutic interventions. *Crit Rev Clin Lab Sci* 30:223, 1993.

109. Belizario JE, et al. Bioactivity of skeletal muscle proteolysis-inducing factors in the plasma proteins from cancer patients with weight loss. *Br J Cancer* 63:705, 1991.

110. Pisters PW, et al. Insulin action on glucose and branched-chain amino acid metabolism in cancer cachexia: Differential effects of insulin. *Surgery* 111:301, 1992.

111. Taylor DD, et al. Identificatian of a human tumor-derived lipolysis-promoting factor. *Cancer Res* 52:829, 1992.

112. Briddon S, Beck SA, Tisdale MJ. Changes in activity of lipoprotein lipase, plasma free fatty acids and triglycerides with weight loss in a cachexia model. *Cancer Lett* 57:49, 1991.

113. Mulligan HD, Beck SA, Tisdale MJ. Lipid metabolism in cancer cachexia. *Br J Cancer* 66:57, 1992.

114. Yazici Z, et al. Changes in tissue fatty acid composition in murine malignancy and following anticancer therapy. *Br J Cancer* 65:163, 1992.

115. Beck SA, Tisdale MJ. Production of lipolytic and proteolytic factors by a murine tumor-producing cachexia in the host. *Cancer Res* 47:5919, 1987.

116. Beck SA, Tisdale MJ. Lipid mobilising factors specifically associated with cancer cachexia. *Br J Cancer* 63:846, 1991.

117. Fossel ET, Carr JM, McDonagh J. Detection of malignant tumors by nuclear magnetic resonance spectroscopy of plasma. *N Engl J Med* 316:1415, 1987.

118. Engan T, et al. Proton nuclear magnetic resonance spectroscopy of plasma from healthy subjects and patients with cancer. *N Engl J Med* 322:949, 1990.

119. Okunieff P, et al. Lack of efficacy of water-suppressed proton nuclear magnetic resonance spectoscopy of plasma for the detection of malignant tumors. *N Engl J Med* 322:953, 1990.

120. Shaw JHF, Wolfe RR. Fatty acid and glycerol kinetics in septic patients and in patients with gastrointestinal cancer: The response to glucose infusion and parenteral feeding. *Ann Surg* 205:958, 1987.

121. Wilson AW, Kirk CJC, Goode AW. The effects of weight loss, operation and parenteral nutrition on fat clearance in patients with colorectal cancer. *Clin Sci* 73:489, 1977.

122. Theologides A. Pathogenesis of cachexia in cancer. *Cancer* 29:484, 1972.

123. Illig KA, Maronian N, Peacock JL. Cancer cachexia is transmissible in plasma. *J Surg Res* 52:353, 1992.

124. Mordes JP, Rossini AA. A tumor-induced anorexia in the Wistar rat. *Science* 213:565, 1981.

125. Herzfeld A, Greengard O, Warren S. Tissue enzyme changes in parabiotic rats with subcutaneous lymphoma or fibrosarcoma. *J Natl Cancer Inst* 60:825, 1978.

126. Chance WT, et al. Hyperammonemia in anorectic tumorbearing rats. *Life Sci* 43:67, 1988.

127. Mori M, Yamaguchi K, Kaoru R. Purification of a lipoprotein lipase-inhibiting protein produced by melanoma cell line associated with cancer cachexia. *Biochem Biophys Res Comm* 160:1085, 1989.

128. Moldawer LL, Georgieff M, Lundholm K. Interleukin 1, tumour necrosis factor-alpha (cachectin) and the pathogenesis of cancer cachexia. *Clin Physiol* 7:263, 1987.

129. Moldawer LL, Rogy MA, Lowry SF. The role of cytokines in cancer cachexia. *JPEN* 16:43S, 1992.

130. McNamara MJ, Alexander HR, Norton JA. Cytokines and their role in the pathophysiology of cancer cachexia. *JPEN* 16:50S, 1992.

131. Caswell EA, Old LJ, Kassel RL. An endotoxin-induced serum factor that causes necrosis of tumors. *Proc Natl Acad Sci USA* 72:3666, 1975.

132. Cerami A, Beutler B. The role of cachectin/TNF in endotoxic shock and cachexia. *Immunol Today* 9:28, 1988.

133. Beutler B, Cerami A. Cachectin and tumor necrosis factor as two sides of the same biological coin. *Nature* 320:584, 1986.

134. Tracey KJ, Lowry SF, Cerami A. Physiologic responses to cachectin. In *Tumor Necrosis Factor and Related Endotoxins.* New York: CIBA, 1987. P 88.

135. Socher SM, Friedman A, Martinez D. Recombinant human tumor necrosis factor induces acute reduction in food intake and body weight in mice. *J Exp Med* 167:1957, 1988.

136. Llovera M, Lopez-Soriano FJ, Argiles JM. Effects of tumor necrosis factor-alpha on muscle-protein turnover in female Wistar rats. *J Natl Cancer Inst* 85:1334, 1993.

137. Mulligan HD, et al. Weight loss in a murine cachexia model is not associated with the cytokines tumour necrosis factor-alpha or interleukin-6. *Cancer Lett* 65:239, 1992.

138. Abbruzzese JL, Levin B, Ajani JA. Phase I trial of recombinant human gamma interferon and recombinant human tumor necrosis factor in patients with advanced gastrointestinal cancer. *Cancer Res* 49:4057, 1989.

139. Blick M, Sherwin SA, Rosenblum M. Phase I study of recombinant tumor necrosis factor in cancer patients. *Cancer Res* 47:2986, 1987.

140. Gelin J, et al. Role of endogenous tumor necrosis factor alpha and interleukin 1 for experimental tumor growth and the development of cancer cachexia. *Cancer Res* 51:415, 1991.

141. Sherry BA, et al. Anticachectin/tumor necrosis factor-α antibodies attenuate development of cachexia in tumor models. *FASEBJ* 3:1956, 1989.

142. Langstein HN, et al. The roles of interferon-gamma and tumor necrosis factor in an experimental rat model of cachexia. *Cancer Res* 51:2302, 1991.

143. Costelli P, et al. Tumor necrosis factor-alpha mediates changes in tissue protein turnover in a rat cancer cachexia model. *J Clin Invest* 92:2783, 1993.

144. Stovroff MC, et al. Cachectin/tumor necrosis factor: A possible mediator of cancer anorexia in the rat. *Cancer Res* 48:2784, 1988.

145. Sheppard BC, et al. Prolonged survival of tumor-bearing rats with repetitive low-dose recombinant tumor necrosis factor. *Cancer Res* 50:3928, 1990.

146. Tracey KJ, et al. Cachectin/tumor necrosis factor induces cachexia, anemia, and inflammation. *J Exp Med* 167: 1211, 1988.

147. Aderka D, et al. Cachectin/tumour-necrosis-factor production by cancer patients [letter]. *Lancet* 2:1190, 1985.

148. Scuderi P, et al. Raised serum levels of tumor necrosis factor in parasitic infections. *Lancet* 2:1364, 1986.

149. Socher SH, et al. Tumor necrosis factor not detectable in patients with clinical cancer cachexia. *J Natl Cancer Inst* 80:595, 1988.

150. Waage A, Espevik T, Lamik J. Detection of tumor necrosis factor like cytotoxicity in serum from patients with septicemia but not untreated cancer patients. *Scand J Immunol* 24:739, 1986.

151. Balkwill F, et al. Evidence for tumor necrosis factor/cachectin production in cancer. *Lancet* 2:1229, 1987.

152. Ardizzoia A, et al. Tumor necrosis factor in solid tumors: Increased blood levels in the metastatic disease. *J Biol Regul Homeost Agents* 6:103, 1992.

153. Kriegler M, et al. A novel form of TNF/cachectin is a cell surface cytotoxic transmembrane protein: Ramifications for the complex physiology of TNF. *Cell* 53:45, 1988.

154. Darling G, et al. Cachetic effects of recombinant human necrosis factor in rats. *Cancer Res* 50:4008, 1990.

155. Tracey KJ, et al. Metabolic effects of cachectin/tumor necrosis factor are modified by site of production. *J Clin Invest* 86:2014, 1990.

156. Patton JS, et al. Development of partial tolerance to the gastrointestinal effects of high doses of recombinant tumor necrosis factor-alpha in rodents. *J Clin Invest* 80:1587, 1987.

157. Okusawa S, et al. Interleukin 1 induces a shock-like state in rabbits. Synergism with tumor necrosis factor and the effect of cyclooxygenase inhibition. *J Clin Invest* 81:1162, 1988.

158. Alexander HR, et al. A recombinant human receptor antagonist to interleukin-1 improves survival after lethal endotoxemia in mice. *J Exp Med* 173:1029, 1991.

159. Hellerstein MK, et al. Interleukin-1-induced anorexia in the rat. Influence of prostaglandins. *J Clin Invest* 84:228, 1989.

160. Moldawer LL, et al. Regulation of food intake and hepatic protein synthesis by recombinant-derived cytokines. *Am J Physiol* 254:G450, 1988.

161. Dinarello CA, et al. Interleukin-1, anorexia, and dietary fatty acids. *Ann NY Acad Sci* 587:332, 1990.

162. Moldawer LL, Drott C, Lundholm K. Monocytic production and plasma bioactivities of interleukin-1 and tumour necrosis factor in human cancer. *Eur J Clin Invest* 18:486, 1988.

163. Larrick IW. Native interleukin 1 inhibitors. *Immunol Today* 10:61, 1989.

164. Jensen JC, et al. Enhanced hepatic cytokine gene expression in cachectic tumor bearing rats. *Surg Forum* 41:469, 1990.

165. Carter DB, et al. Purification, cloning, expression and biological characterization of an interleukin-1 receptor antagonist protein. *Nature* 344:633, 1990.

166. Waage A, et al. The complex pattern of cytokines in serum from patients with meningococcal septic shock. Association between interleukin 6, interleukin 1, and fatal outcome. *J Exp Med* 169:333, 1989.

167. McIntosh JK, et al. In vivo induction of IL-6 by administration of exogenous cytokines and detection of de novo serum levels of IL-6 in tumor-bearing mice. *J Immunol* 143:162, 1989.

168. Tanaka M, et al. Detection of serum cytokine levels in experimental cancer cachexia of colon 26 adenocarcinoma-bearing mice. *Cancer Lett* 72:65, 1993.

169. Gelin J, et al. Appearance of hybridoma growth factor/interleukin-6 in the serum of mice bearing a methylcholanthrene-induced sarcoma. *Biochem Biophys Res Commun* 157:575, 1988.

170. Jablons DM, et al. Induction of interferon-beta$_2$/interleukin-6 (IL-6) by cytokine administration and detection of circulating interleukin-6 in the tumor-bearing state. *Ann NY Acad Sci* 557:157, 1989.

171. Ohe Y, et al. Interleukin-6 cDNA transfected Lewis lung carcinoma cells show unaltered net tumour growth rate but cause weight loss and shorten survival in syngenic mice. *Br J Cancer* 67:939, 1993.

172. Smith BK, Conn CA, Kluger MJ. Experimental cachexia: Effects of MCA sarcoma in the Fischer rat. *Am J Physiol* 265:R376, 1993.

173. Strassmann G, et al. Evidence for the involvement of interleukin 6 in experimental cancer cachexia. *J Clin Invest* 89:1681, 1992.

174. Strassmann G, et al. The role of interleukin-6 in lipopolysaccharide-induced weight loss, hypoglycemia and fibrinogen production, in vivo. *Cytokine* 5:285, 1993.

175. Wong GG, Clark SC. Multiple actions of interleukin 6 within a cytokine network. *Immunol Today* 9:137, 1988.

176. Greenberg AS, et al. Interleukin 6 reduces lipoprotein lipase activity in adipose tissue of mice in vivo and in 3T3-L1 adipocytes: A possible role for interleukin 6 in cancer cachexia. *Cancer Res* 52:4113, 1992.

177. Langstein HN, et al. The roles of gamma-interferon and tumor necrosis factor alpha in an experimental rat model of cancer cachexia. *Cancer Res* 51:2302, 1991.

178. Matthys P, et al. Severe cachexia in mice inoculated with interferon-gamma-producing tumor cells. *Int J Cancer* 49:77, 1991.

179. Lundholm K, Hyltander A, Sandstrom R. Nutritional support in cancer treatment. *Curr Opin Oncol* 3:621, 1991.

180. Mullen JL, et al. Protein synthesis dynamics in human gastrointestinal malignancies. *Surgery* 87:331, 1980.

181. Nixon DW, et al. Total parenteral nutrition as an adjunct to chemotherapy of metastatic colorectal cancer. *Cancer Treat Rep* 65(suppl):121, 1981.

182. Baron PL, et al. Effects of parenteral nutrition on cell cycle kinetics of head and neck cancer. *Arch Surg* 121: 1282, 1986.

183. Fischer JE. Editorial: Adjuvant parenteral nutrition in the patient with cancer. *Surgery* 96:578, 1984.

184. Klein D, Morris D. Increased arginase activity during lymphocyte mitogenesis. *Biochem Biophys Res Commum* 81:100, 1978.

185. Currie GA. Activated macrophages kill tumor cells by releasing arginase. *Nature* 273:758, 1978.

186. Hibbs JB, Traintor RR, Vavrin Z. Macrophage cytotoxicity: Role for L-arginine deiminase and imino nitrogen oxidation to nitrite. *Science* 235:473, 1987.

187. Tachibana K, et al. Evaluation of the effect of arginine enriched amino acid solution on tumor growth. *JPEN* 9:428, 1985.

188. Reynolds JV, et al. Arginine as an immunomodulator. *Surg Forum* 38:415, 1987.

189. Yeatman TJ, Risley G, Brunson M. Depletion of dietary arginine inhibits growth of metastatic tumor. *Arch Surg* 126:1376, 1991.

190. Barbul A, et al. Arginine enhances wound healing and lymphocyte immune responses in humans. *Surgery* 108:331, 1990.

191. Barbul A. The role of arginine as an immune modulator. In *Nutrient Modulation of the Immune Response.* New York: Marcel Dekker, 1993.

192. Daly JM, et al. Immune and metabolic effect of arginine in the surgical patient. *Ann Surg* 208:122, 1988.

193. Siga R, et al. Parenteral arginine infusion in patients: Nutrient substrate or pharmacologicagent. *JPEN* 16:423, 1992.

194. Rose WC. The nutritive significance of amino acids. *Physiol Rev* 18:109, 1938.

195. Eagle H. Nutritional needs of mammalian cells in tissue cultures. *Science* 122:501, 1935.

196. Shou J, et al. Total parenteral nutrition, bacterial translocation and host immune function. *Am J Surg* 167:145, 1994.

197. Zhang W, et al. Improvement of structure and function in orthotopic small bowel transplantation in the rat by glutamine. *Transplantation* 56:512, 1993.

198. Fox AD, et al. Effect of a glutamine supplemented enteral diet on methotrexate-induced enterocolitis. *JPEN* 12:325, 1988.

199. Klimberg VS, et al. Prophylactic glutamine protects the intestinal mucosa from radiation injury. *Cancer* 66:62, 1990.

200. Kovacevic Z, Morris HP. The role of glutamine in the oxidative metabolism of malignant cells. *Cancer Res* 32:326, 1972.

201. Austgen TR, et al. The effects of glutamine enriched total parenteral nutrition on tumor growth and hot tissues. *Ann Surg* 215:107, 1992.

202. Klimberg VS, et al. Glutamine enriched diets support muscle glutamine metabolism without stimulating tumor growth. *J Surg Res* 48:319, 1990.

203. Hammarqvist F, et al. Addition of glutamine to total parenteral nutrition after elective abdominal surgery spares free glutamine in muscle, counteracts the fall in muscle protein synthesis, and improves nitrogen balance. *Ann Surg* 209:455, 1989.

204. Ziegler TR, et al. Clinical and metabolic efficacy of glutamine-supplemented parenteral nutrition after bone marrow transplantation. *Ann Intern Med* 116:821, 1992.

205. Hammarqvist F, et al. Addition of glutamine to total parenteral nutrition after elective abdominal surgery spares free glutamine in muscle, counteracts the fall in muscle protein synthesis, and improves nitrogen balance. *Ann Surg* 209:455, 1989.

206. Stehle P, et al. Effect of parenteral glutamine peptide supplements on muscle glutamine loss and nitrogen balance after major surgery. *Lancet* 1:231, 1989.

Selected Readings

Brennan MF. Total parenteral nutrition in the cancer patient. *N Engl J Med* 305:375, 1981.

An excellent review of the metabolic abnormalities in the cancer patient. Results of clinical trials are presented.

Buzby GP, et al. Prognostic nutritional index in gastrointestinal surgery. *Am J Surg* 139:160, 1980.

This retrospective study demonstrates the correlation between nutritional parameters such as serum proteins, body fat composition and cellular immune function with morbidity after operation.

Kern KA, Norton JA. Cancer cachexia. *JPEN* 12:286, 1988.

A superb review of the mechanisms of cachexia in patients with neoplastic disease.

Langstein HN, Norton JA. Mechanisms of cancer cachexia. *Hematol Oncol Clin North Am* 5:103, 1991.

Cancer cachexia is a significant problem in patients with malignant disease. The etiologies are multifactorial and may be due to cytokines, biochemical by-products, psychological causes, and physiologic alterations.

McAnena OJ, Daly JM. Impact of antitumor therapy on nutrition. *Surg Clin North Am* 66:1213, 1986.

Surgery, chemotherapy, and radiation treatment impact adversely on nutrient intake and nutritional status.

23

Changes in Immunologic Function

Gordon P. Buzby
John C. Kucharczuk

Physicians have long attempted to use nutritional therapy to change the clinical outcome of their patients. Unfortunately, when viewed retrospectively, these early attempts were often not based on scientific principles or even common sense. During the nineteenth century, it was common practice for physicians to deprive febrile patients of both food and water. Their rationale for this popular approach was not clear, and it was not until 1914 that Warren Coleman and Eugene DuBois used the Benedict "universal respiration apparatus" to show that the metabolic rate of typhoid patients actually exceeded that of normal individuals by 40% [1]. This work scientifically confirmed the earlier notion of Graves that, contrary to the prevailing belief of the time, it was important to "feed a fever" [2].

In 1932, Cuthbertson contributed further evidence that ill or injured patients may have supranormal nutrient requirements when he observed that urinary nitrogen excretion increases in patients with injury to the limbs and suggested a relationship between the extent of injury and the rate of protein catabolism [3]. By 1936, Studley had reviewed a series of patients who died after operations for chronic peptic ulcer disease and found that the percentage of preoperative weight loss correlated well with mortality rates [4]. This observation caught the attention of surgeons, but it was not until 1944 that immune dysfunction was recognized as a possible factor contributing to poor surgical outcome in undernourished patients. In that year, Cannon and his colleagues demonstrated the relationship between protein deficiency and increased surgical infections. Cannon was well received. He presented his observation to the American Surgical Association meeting in Chicago on May 3, 1944, and it was later published in the Annals of Surgery [5]. [*Editor's Note:* In contrast to the work of DuBois, Cuthbertson, and Studley, each of which is widely appreciated, Cannon's contribution has not received the credit it deserves.] In large part, this paper marks the beginning of the era of surgical interest in using nutritional manipulation to decrease the rate of postoperative infections and thereby improve surgical outcome.

The last 50 years has seen a dramatic increase in both our understanding of the impact of nutritional status on immune function and our appreciation of the importance of this impact on the ultimate success or failure of our surgical interventions. This half-century of nutritional and surgical investigation into the workings of the immune system may be loosely viewed as having three overlapping but somewhat distinct phases. The first phase was primarily observational and consisted mainly of epidemiologic studies examining the impact of chronic undernutrition on immune function. This phase can be called the Observational Phase and was largely dominated by nutrition scientists working in underdeveloped countries where protein undernutrition in children was endemic and large numbers of patients with kwashiorkor could be studied in detail. These studies contributed immensely to our understanding of the defects that occur in specific components of the immune response in malnourished subjects, but their relevance to surgical practice was largely unappreciated. Subsequent epidemiologic studies, this time in hospitalized surgical [6] and medical patients [7], demonstrated a heretofore unrecognized high incidence of nutritional deficiencies in these populations similar in some respects to those observed in chronically undernourished children. [*Editor's Note:* The studies referred to here were carried out in an urban setting in an indigent population. The rates of malnutrition reported are probably higher than in other hospital settings, but the point is well taken.] Detailed studies of immune function in these malnourished patients, often using techniques developed by nutritionists working in third-world countries, revealed surprisingly similar patterns of immune dysfunction. It became apparent that even previously well-nourished patients can rapidly develop a state of relative malnutrition when a traumatic injury or surgical insult leads to a catabolic stress, and with this will often come a compromise in immune defenses [8]. It became clear that severe trauma or infection alters substrate metabolism and immune function at both systemic and tissue levels [9]. The importance of a high level of nutritional awareness to the surgical practitioner had become evident.

The second phase of the surgeon's interest in nutritional immunology is ongoing and can be termed the Classic Interventional Phase. The moving force in this phase has been primarily physician-scientists (largely surgeons), many with concurrent and complementary clinical and scientific expertise. In this phase, nutrients are viewed primarily as either substrates that provide energy (fats and carbohydrates), building blocks that are incorporated into structural and functional proteins (amino acids), or catalysts and cofactors that facilitate biochemical reactions (vitamins, trace elements). In this view, malnutrition occurs when the supply of exogenous nutrients is inadequate or the organism cannot effectively utilize these nutrients. Endogenous stores are utilized and eventually depleted, resulting in the classic pattern of weight loss, body cell mass erosion, and protein catabolism. Because a variety of functional proteins and biochemical reactions are essential to normal immune function, defects in immune function will eventually ensue.

In the Classic Interventional Phase, the goal of nutritional support is to provide adequate substrates, building blocks, cofactors, and catalysts so that normal metabolic processes can proceed unimpaired. With the development of total parenteral nutrition (TPN) in 1968 [10], the goal of providing adequate exogenous nutrients can be achieved in virtually any patient even if the gastrointestinal tract is unavailable. The impact of this on patient survival cannot be overstated, and classic nutritional support has been and remains a highly successful modality. Over the 25 years since the introduction of TPN, the ability to salvage critically ill patients continues to improve. Nevertheless, surgeons remain frustrated by patients who survive initial events, only to succumb later to sepsis or systemic inflammatory syndromes despite being provided advanced critical care and optimal nutritional support by currently available techniques. Frustration in caring for this group of patients has led to questions regarding the role of nutrition in critically ill patients and to interest in whether nutritional modulation can be used to further improve clinical outcome. As the "molecular" effects of critical illness are elucidated, it is probable that further improving patient outcome will depend on manipulation of the balance between the beneficial and harmful effects of a wide range of inflammatory mediators. Recently, critical care medicine has been said to be entering an era of "nutriceutical therapy" [11].

This new term describes current attempts at modulating cytokine responses, improving wound healing, and reducing infection by the manipulation of nutrient intake. Nutritional therapy has moved from its traditional supportive roles to a new role as a pharmacologic agent, and with this we have entered the third phase of surgical-nutritional immunology: the Molecular Phase. [*Editor's Note:* Dr. J. Wesley Alexander should be credited, I believe, with the term nutritional pharmacology—the phrase we are currently using. I hope we are able to proudly claim the term Molecular Phase.]

This chapter summarizes the immunologic consequences of malnutrition as characterized during the Observational Phase and describes the impact of nutritional support on immune function as currently practiced in the Classic Interventional Phase. We include discussion of the orchestration of the immune response at the tissue level and the effects of immune mediators on metabolism that form the foundation of the Molecular Phase. Finally, we include a review of the effects of specific nutrients on immune function, including glutamine, arginine, dietary nucleotides, and omega-3 fatty acids, perhaps the first clinically important forays into the era of molecular nutrition.

Impact of Malnutrition on Immune Function

The effect of nutritional deficiencies on immune function is complex. Undernutrition in some circumstances may be protective. Famine has been observed to suppress the activity of malarial infection in humans with reactivation following refeeding [12]. In mice, caloric restriction (50% of normal) may improve survival after a challenge with *Salmonella* peritonitis, while severe protein restriction (1% and 5% of diet) impairs survival in the same model [13]. In general, chronic protein-calorie malnutrition is associated with impaired rather than enhanced function in most components of the immune system.

Lymphocyte Function

T-cell function may be particularly sensitive to protein-calorie deprivation. Skin test anergy, a crude measure of T-cell function, is commonly observed in children with chronic protein-calorie malnutrition, and T-cell-dependent regions of thymic and peripheral lymphoid tissues are depleted [14]. Similarly, anergy is frequently seen in malnourished surgical patients [15]. The presence of anergy correlates with other measures of chronic undernutrition in hospitalized patients, including hypoalbuminemia and depressed serum transferrin levels [16], and anergic patients suffer more complications after surgery than their well-nourished counterparts [16,17]. The mechanism or mechanisms underlying impaired T-cell function in malnourished subjects is not known, but the presence of immunosuppressive serum factors [18] or changes in immunoregulatory signals (for example, IL-1 and PGE_2) [19] have been suggested as possible factors.

B-cell-mediated humoral immunity may be less sensitive to protein-calorie deprivation. Although germinal centers may be atrophic, and circulating populations of B-cells may be reduced in size, serum immunoglobulin levels are normal or elevated in chronically undernourished children, perhaps in response to repeated infections [20]. Starvation does not impair the level of antibody titers generated in response to vaccination in animals [21]. Similarly, in surgical patients, levels of circulating immunoglobulins (IgA, IgG, and IgM) are usually normal even when measures of T-cell function (T-rosette formation, skin test anergy) or nutritional status (serum albumin, serum transferrin, creatinine height index, anthropometrics) are markedly abnormal [16]. Although early postnatal malnutrition may be associated with profound and persistent depression in levels of circulating immunoglobulins [22], undernutrition beyond infancy appears to depress cell-mediated immunity (CMI) to a greater extent than humoral immunity [19].

Neutrophil and Macrophage Function

Circulating neutrophils, macrophages (blood monocytes), and fixed-tissue macrophages participate in the immune response by ingesting and killing pathogens directly and by processing pathogens for presentation to lymphocyte-mediated mechanisms of pathogen elimination (CMI). Neutrophils from undernourished children [23] or patients with anorexia nervosa [24] have a diminished capacity to kill bacteria, and neutrophil migration is frequently impaired in malnourished surgical patients but does not correlate with surgical complications in these patients [16]. Attempts to better characterize this defect have been frustrated by lack of a good animal model.

Similarly, the impact of malnutrition on the ability of macrophages to process foreign antigens is not clear. Monocyte phagocytosis of latex particles and antibody-coated erythrocytes is preserved in vitro in cells derived from children with kwashiorkor [25]. Similarly, both phagocytosis and degranulation appear qualitatively normal in macrophages from undernourished rats [26]. Although these relatively crude measures of macrophage function fail to consistently demonstrate nutrition-related defects, regulation of macrophage function in vivo is complex and may be altered by changes in activity of cytokines and eicosanoids (IL-1, IL-6, TNF, and PGE_2) and various macrophage-activating (interferon-γ) and inhibiting factors. A particularly important role for interferon-γ has been suggested in the up-regulation of macrophage phagocytic function and microbial killing [27]. The role of cytokines is discussed in greater detail in a subsequent section of this chapter.

Complement

Alterations in levels of several components of serum complement have been described in chronically undernourished children [28] and in marasmic animals [29]. However, serum levels of C3 and C4 were usually normal in a series of malnourished surgical patients despite significant abnormalities in other measures of immune function (neutrophil migration, CMI, etc.), and levels of complement did not correlate with surgical complications [16]. To date, no pivotal role for malnutrition-induced alterations in complement nor their correction with nutritional therapy has been identified in surgical or critically ill patients.

Vitamin and Mineral Deficiencies

Deficiencies in vitamins, minerals, and other micronutrients are rarely seen in current clinical practice. This is largely due to the ease and safety with which "all-in-one" preparations can be administered. Nevertheless, it is important to recognize the clinical manifestations of these deficiencies when they occur and to have an awareness of the potential immunologic consequences. Below, we provide a brief description of vitamins and minerals with recognized effects on immune function. Readers interested in additional information on vitamins and trace metals are directed to Chapters 9 and 10, respectively.

Vitamin A

Vitamin A is a fat-soluble vitamin stored in the liver, usually in large quantities. Vitamin A deficiency may alter antibody production in some models [30] and may also impair phagocytosis in animals [31]. Although increased susceptibility to infection is a prominent feature of avitaminosis A, the greater direct relevance of vitamin A to the surgeon may relate to its role in wound healing, collagen synthesis and cross-linking, and maintenance of epithelial barriers.

Vitamin B

Riboflavin (B_2) and pantothenic acid may participate indirectly in protection against microbial invasion through their roles in maintenance of epithelial barrier function, but any clinically important direct impact on immune function appears unlikely. Deficiencies of vitamin B_{12} and pyridoxine B_6 may impact more directly on immune function. Vitamin B_{12} is required for normal erythrocyte and neutrophil development. Patients with vitamin B_{12} deficiency have megaloblastic anemia, macrocytic neutrophils with hypersegmented nuclei, and depressed neutrophil function [32]. Pyridoxine deficiency is also associated with impaired neutrophil function in some animal models as well as abnormalities in antibody formation and CMI [33,34].

Vitamin C

Vitamin C is a water-soluble vitamin that holds special interest from an historical perspective. Egyptians recognized scurvy as early as 1500 B.C. During the eighteenth century, British sailors realized that eating citrus fruits could prevent scurvy during long journeys at sea. Deficiencies of vitamin C may impair chemotaxis of inflammatory cells and alter macrophage function, but the greater relevance of vitamin C to surgical infections probably relates to its role in wound healing and the inflammatory response. A further role for vitamin C in critically ill patients has recently been suggested, in that its participation in the antioxidant effect of vitamin E could theoretically be of value to ameliorate free radical damage to normal tissues in severely stressed patients. Although intriguing, the potential clinical value of this observation remains unexplored [35].

Vitamin E

Vitamin E is a fat-soluble vitamin whose major function is as an antioxidant. In low-birth-weight infants, vitamin E deficiency may lead to hemolytic anemia, probably due to oxidation of the lipid membrane of erythrocytes. Similarly, in burn patients, serum concentrations of vitamin E are decreased, perhaps due to their consumption by oxygen radicals. As noted above, the role of vitamin E either with or without vitamin C in reducing tissue injury due to free radicals released in severely stressed patients is of great potential interest. From the point of view of immune function, vitamin E is probably of less importance. Vitamin

E deficiency in mice may actually be protective against death due to *Plasmodium berghei* [36].

Minerals

As with vitamins, deficiencies in minerals are rarely recognized as important contributors to immune defects in surgical patients. Although appropriate levels of zinc are required for normal macrophage function in vitro [37] and magnesium-deficient rats exhibit an impaired specific antibody response [38], it is questionable whether these observations are relevant to clinical practice. Perhaps the most important observation to the surgeon was the demonstration that increasing iron concentrations potentiate bacterial infectious capacity and worsen bacterial infection [39]. Supplemental iron should probably be avoided in patients with active bacterial infections or patients likely to experience a bacterial challenge (for example, an operation involving the gastrointestinal tract) in the near future.

The Impact of Nutritional Support on Immune Function

Nutritional support, whether it be by the enteral or parenteral route, will correct immunologic dysfunction in many patients. As noted previously, classic nutritional support provides substrates, protein precursors, cofactors, and catalysts in quantities thought appropriate to meet ongoing needs and replete stores. The success of this approach depends on the premise that in many patients, malnutrition and immune dysfunction result from inadequate nutrient intake relative to demands, and if exogenous nutrients are provided in adequate quantities, they will be metabolized appropriately and effectively. Fortunately, this premise is true for many of our patients, and nutritional support as currently practiced is highly (although not universally) effective. A subset of patients remain catabolic despite optimal nutritional support, implying that their ongoing catabolism is not the result of nutrient deprivation but rather disordered metabolism, precluding appropriate utilization of nutrients even when they are present. These challenging patients are the subject of a subsequent section of this chapter. First, however, we will review the impact of current methods of nutritional support on immune function.

Refeeding will correct many of the previously discussed alterations in immune function seen in malnourished patients. Skin test anergy is probably the most extensively studied marker of immune function in surgical patients vis-à-vis the impact of nutritional support. [*Editor's Note:* It is very important that as anergy is discussed, the technique of skin injection or placing antigens be defined, as results may be different.] As early as 1976, it was apparent that TPN could correct skin test anergy in malnourished cancer patients [40]. [*Editor's Note:* Anergy in cancer may be different: A positive response by skin test may follow resection of the tumor, without any nutritional intervention.] Further, critically ill patients who responded to TPN with correction of preexisting anergy experienced improved survival relative to those who remained anergic [41]. Similarly, patients who showed improvement in nutritional status during TPN as measured by an increase in serum transferrin also experienced fewer postoperative infections (5% infection rate) than patients whose transferrin remained low (60% infection rate) despite TPN [42]. Whether this represents improved outcome due to a nutritional effect or due to increased iron binding and a resultant decreased bacterial virulence is not known.

As a result of studies such as these, there was great enthusiasm during the early 1980s for the expanded use of TPN in surgical patients. Many nonrandomized studies suggested reduced infection rates in surgical patients treated with TPN prior to operations, further supporting this enthusiasm. A few studies, however, suggested a more cautious enthusiasm. For example, nearly at the same time that reversal of anergy with TPN had been demonstrated and associated with improved outcome, a similar result was achieved with levamisole, a nonspecific immune stimulant [43]. These observations suggested that immune dysfunction and malnutrition might occur simultaneously in the same patient with no cause-and-effect relationship. If this was true, then nutritional support of malnourished patients might not consistently correct their concurrent immune dysfunction (as might be true in neoplastic disease).

The impact of nutritional repletion on immune function has never been evaluated in human patients in a systematic fashion. Further, nutritional support has not been evaluated in a prospective randomized study to specifically identify its impact on immune function independent of other clinical variables and other concurrent forms of treatment. It is clear that patients who ultimately do well usually show improvement in nutritional status and immune function with nutritional support, and those who do poorly do not show improvement in either. It seems likely that immune dysfunction in some surgical patients probably relates to nutritional factors and can be corrected with nutritional therapy, while immune dysfunction in others is independent of nutritional factors (even though they might be present) and will be refractory to nutritional support.

The Impact of Nutritional Support on Surgical Infections and Morbidity

Despite few studies evaluating the impact of nutritional support on immune function specifically, several studies have evaluated the effect of nutritional support on outcome in surgical patients and have secondarily reported its effect on rates of infection. These studies have produced inconsistent results. Viewed individually, many of these studies were too small to provide meaningful results. However, in 1987, a review paper was published in which a meta-analysis was used to evaluate the results of all available trials of perioperative TPN (as listed in the MEDLINE database from 1966 to August 1986) [44]. In this meta-analysis, results of 19 studies were reviewed and the results of 11 that met criteria for adequate design were pooled. A small improvement in operative outcome with TPN was suggested, but the 95% confidence interval for rates of complications was wide, ranging from 12.8 percentage points better for TPN-treated patients to 2.3 percentage points worse. The authors concluded that any possible benefit of perioperative TPN in well-nourished patients must be small and is probably not clinically important, while the efficacy in mildly or severely malnourished patients may be greater but requires further confirmation. This study was useful, but the efficacy of perioperative TPN in reducing surgical complications in the large population of patients with degrees of malnutrition ranging from mild to severe remained uncertain.

A Veterans Affairs (VA) multi-institutional trial published in 1991 provides data that may clarify the impact of TPN on surgical infections in this large population [45,46]. Four hundred and fifty-nine patients for this study were recruited from a population of adult veterans requiring nonemergent laparotomy or thoracotomy. Patients were randomly assigned to receive either TPN for 7 to 15 days prior to operation or to receive no perioperative TPN. For 90 days after the operation, patients were monitored for complications. Rates of major complications (TPN group: 25.5%; control group: 24.6%) and mortality (TPN group: 13.4%; control group: 10%) were similar. Of interest, more infectious complications occurred in the TPN group (14.1% vs. 6.4%; $p = 0.01$), but more noninfectious complications occurred in the control group (22.2% vs. 16.7%; $p = 0.20$). The response to TPN (beneficial or deleterious) was dependent on the baseline nutritional status of the patient. The increased rate of infections was confined to patients identified as either well nourished or only mildly malnourished. Severely malnourished patients (only 5% of all surgical admissions to hospitals participating in the study) experienced significantly fewer noninfectious complications with TPN (5% vs. 43%; $p = 0.03$) with a reduction in overall major complications (21% vs. 47%) approaching statistical significance ($p = 0.11$).

The increased infection rate in TPN-treated patients was not explained simply by the presence of a catheter (catheter sepsis or unexplained bacteremia) but reflected a higher frequency of common postoperative infections (especially pneumonia and wound infections). Likewise, differences in the type of operations performed did not readily explain this observation, with procedures usually associated with increased risk of infection (open colon procedures) being performed with somewhat greater frequency in control patients.

It is unclear whether the TPN was causally related to this increased rate of infection. TPN-treated patients were hospitalized on average five days longer prior to operation than control patients, perhaps providing greater opportunity for colonization with resistant pathogens. Alternatively, TPN per se may have in some way predisposed to clinically apparent infection as a result of the route of feeding, the energy source, the quantity of calories provided, or the decreased oral intake associated with parenteral feeding.

A possible role for lipids in this process was suggested by results of a study by Muller et al. [47]. In that study, patients receiving TPN in which lipid supplied 50% of the caloric intake experienced more major operative complications and deaths than controls and significantly more deaths than patients receiving lipid-free TPN. In the VA study [46], all patients received a portion of their calories as long-chain triglycerides (500 kcal/day), less than but similar to the lipid load in the Muller study. Alternatively, TPN-associated hyperglycemia may be a factor predisposing to infection. Patients in the VA study who experienced one or more episodes of hyperglycemia (defined as serum glucose >300 mg/dl) in the preoperative period suffered postoperative infections with twice the frequency of those who experienced no hyperglycemia (31% vs. 15%) [48].

Results of the VA study [46] suggest that parenteral refeeding prior to operation does not produce clinically important improvement in immune function in most patients and may actually impair immune function in some. This finding should not be extrapolated to all patient populations. As previously noted, patients with demonstrable immune dysfunction (for example, anergy) show improved survival when anergy is corrected with TPN [41]. Likewise, some patient populations may be especially at risk for clinically important immune dysfunction on a nutritional basis and would be especially responsive to nutritional support. Patients with severe liver disease may be one such population. In a recent randomized study of patients undergoing hepatectomy for hepatocellular carcinoma, branched-chain amino acid–enriched TPN was provided to half of the patients for seven days prior to operation; control patients received a regular oral diet [49]. TPN-fed patients experienced fewer complications (34% vs. 55%; relative risk, 0.66; 95% confidence interval 0.45 to 0.96) predominantly because of fewer septic complications (17% vs. 37%; relative risk, 0.57; 95% confidence interval 0.34 to 0.96). The beneficial effect of TPN was most marked for patients with cirrhosis or normal livers and was not seen in patients with chronic active hepatitis who actually experienced more morbidity when given preoperative TPN (50% vs. 25%, NS). This study suggests a particularly important role for refeeding in patients with liver disease but also demonstrates the variability of the response depending on the nature of the underlying disease.

The Impact of Route of Feeding: Enteral Versus Parenteral

The studies discussed above have all evaluated the effect of parenteral feeding on immune function and rates of infection. It is becoming increasingly apparent that the route of nutrient administration (enteral or parenteral) may be as important as the nature and/or amounts of nutrients provided in determining the impact of nutritional support on immune function. In 1970, Boeckman and Krill [50] noted increased rates of bacterial and fungal infectious complications in children receiving TPN for extended periods of time. Shortly after this observation, TPN was shown to be associated with atrophy of the villous structures of the gastrointestinal tract of rats [51], and later animal studies demonstrated increased rates of bacterial translocation with TPN [52]. These observations generated enthusiasm for the hypothesis that gastrointestinal tract translocation of bacteria or endotoxin may be responsible for many of the immunologic and metabolic abnormalities seen in critically ill patients. The fact that this hypothesis may be overly simplistic was demonstrated in a study of patients with major torso trauma in which endotoxin was rarely measurable in portal venous samples, even though patients went on to develop severe metabolic and immunologic derangements [53]. Recent experimental evidence in dogs suggests an alternative pathway for translocation via the thoracic duct [54]. This pathway could deliver endotoxin and/or enteric bacteria directly to the pulmonary circulation where it would encounter the elaborate immune surveillance in the lung, leading to production of a wide range of inflammatory mediators. Further study is needed to determine the clinical relevance of this potential alternate pathway in the development of the systemic inflammatory syndrome and multiple organ failure.

Despite the inability to define a precise mechanism, enteral feeding has been documented to reduce infection rates relative to TPN. Although many studies comparing enteral and parenteral feeding have insufficient statistical power to yield strong conclusions, Moore et al. [55] have reported a meta-analysis of eight studies comparing enteral and parenteral nutrition in high-risk surgical patients. Their analysis concludes that enteral nutrition results in a reduced incidence of infection (18% vs. 35%; $p = 0.01$) as well as a decreased incidence of sepsis. Similarly, Kudsk and colleagues [56] showed in a prospectively, randomized trial that after blunt and penetrating abdominal trauma, enterally nourished patients have a reduced incidence of pneumonia, intraabdominal abscess, and line sepsis as compared with TPN-fed patients.

Interestingly, the route of nutrition can also have an effect on cytokine production. Lowry has shown that normal healthy volunteers who receive seven days of TPN have higher peak TNF-α (tumor necrosis factor-alpha) concentrations after endotoxin challenge than do normal subjects [57]. This finding suggests that perhaps appropriate enteral feeding could attenuate the immunologic and metabolic abnormalities seen in critically ill patients by blunting production of the proximal cytokine TNF. (The impact of TNF and other cytokines on immune function is discussed in greater detail in a subsequent section in this chapter.) In contrast, Santos and colleagues [58] recently reported a study of the effects of intravenous endotoxin challenge on healthy volunteers after receiving either two days of enteral or seven days of parenteral feedings. While they did not demonstrate a significant difference in levels of TNF, the parenterally fed subjects did demonstrate an attenuated response in the release of interleukin-6. They suggest that this blunted response may be due to increased cortisol levels seen after parenteral feeding.

Regardless of the mechanism, it is clear that enteral feeding is associated with fewer clinically important infections than is parenteral feeding.

Whether this is due to more effective treatment of malnutrition-induced immune dysfunction, less disruption of normally functioning components of the immune system, or less activation of inflammatory mediators is not known.

Nutritional Immunology: The Molecular Phase

To this point we have discussed the impact of malnutrition on immune function and the successes and limitations of classic nutritional support in correcting immune dysfunction. Although life-saving in many patients, currently available techniques for parenteral and enteral feeding fall short in many patients in whom catabolism persists and infectious morbidity progresses to death despite "optimal" treatment. For nutritional support to further improve outcome in these patients, the roles of specific nutrients in modulating the complex biochemical disorders responsible for their clinical deterioration must be better understood. This is the focus of great interest today as we enter what we have termed the Molecular Phase of surgical nutrition. In the remainder of this chapter we consider some of the more promising early work in this area. We begin with a brief review of the impact of stress and critical illness on the immune system and conclude with a discussion of several interventions that may prove clinically useful to ameliorate this impact.

Alterations of Immune Function During Stress

The Classic Stress Hormones

Numerous factors interact during stress and injury to produce alterations in immune function that only recently are being clarified. Early investigations focused on the effects of the "classic" stress hormones on metabolism and the immune system. Bessey et al. [59] investigated the role of three classic stress hormones in an attempt to simulate the metabolic derangements found during the catabolic state in critically ill patients. They selectively infused cortisol, glucagon, or epinephrine, alone and in combination, into nine normal healthy volunteers. When infused together, these hormones caused many of the signs of catabolic illness such as hypermetabolism, negative nitrogen balance, insulin resistance, and sodium retention. They did not, however, produce the fever or consistent alterations in acute-phase proteins characteristically seen in septic or critically ill patients. Clearly a number of other mediators were playing an active role. Recently it has become apparent that cytokines and eicosanoids are of pivotal importance in this regard and may be of special relevance to immune function. Further, their levels and/or activity may be amenable to dietary manipulation.

Cytokines: TNF, IL-1, IL-6, INF-γ

The cytokines are a group of soluble polypeptides involved in orchestration of immune function and metabolism. These peptides have impact on the effector phases of both innate and acquired immunity. Although cytokines can be produced by all nucleated cells (mast cells, fibroblasts, endothelial cells, keratinocytes, smooth muscle cells, and malignant cells), it is production by effector cells of the immune system that may have the most profound effects on critically ill patients.

Cytokines act by binding to receptors on cell membranes. Once bound to the receptor, their signal is transduced to the nucleus of the target cell and leads to changes in gene expression. These changes are manifest by production of mRNA and subsequent protein synthesis. The secretion of cytokines by effector cells is often brief and self-limited. Cytokines are not stored by effector cells but rather manufactured in short, rapid bursts when needed.

Unfortunately, detection of cytokines and understanding of their action is difficult. Under normal conditions, cytokines act at the tissue level in a paracrine or autocrine fashion. They are not usually detected in high levels in systemic circulation unless they are dysfunctional. Furthermore, cytokines have both pleotrophic and redundant properties. They are pleotrophic because they can act on many different cell types, and they are redundant because actions initially attributed to a particular cytokine are often found to be elicited by other cytokines. It is therefore difficult to clearly elucidate the function of a particular cytokine and equally difficult to select a given cytokine target for possible intervention. Nevertheless, clinical trials are under way evaluating the impact of blocking specific cytokines, and it appears likely that dietary manipulation of cytokine production may be possible. Early work with four of the well-described cytokines—TNF, IL-1, IL-6, and interferon-γ—appears particularly promising from the perspective of immune modulation.

Tumor necrosis factor (TNF) is a "proximal" cytokine made primarily by macrophages. The term proximal refers to the fact that it is produced early in an amplifying cascade and induces production of other cytokines. TNF was identified as a powerful immune agent in 1975 by Carswell et al. [60] who found that endotoxin induced a serum factor that could cause necrosis of sarcoma and other transplanted malignancies in mice. The relevance of this observation to stress metabolism was not immediately apparent. However, in the late 1970s and early 1980s attention focused on a substance called cachectin, which was secreted by stimulated macrophages and had the ability to suppress lipoprotein lipase [61,62]. In 1985, TNF and cachectin were identified as the same protein [63]. This protein, produced by macrophages, has effects on both the immune system and metabolism. By 1991, Van Der Poll and colleagues [64] had shown that TNF mimics the metabolic response to infection in humans.

The physiologic response to TNF is dose-related. At low concentration, TNF acts in a paracrine and autocrine fashion to up-regulate expression of endothelial adhesion molecules (important for immune function), activate phagocytic cells, and stimulate production of other cytokines. At higher levels, TNF acts as an endocrine hormone causing fever (endogenous pyrogen), activation of the coagulation system, suppression of bone marrow (immune suppression), cachexia, and, in conjunction with IL-6, acute-phase protein production by the liver.

IL-1 is another proximal cytokine. Like TNF, it can be produced by a variety of cell types; however, the activated monocyte/macrophage appears to be the major producer. IL-1 release can be stimulated directly by endotoxin or by TNF. IL-1 has been identified as an endogenous pyrogen, regulating fever through its action on prostaglandin synthesis in the hypothalamus [65]. IL-1 is a powerful pro-inflammatory mediator involved in systemic inflammatory responses. It has been shown in a nonhuman primate model that IL-1 infusion replicates the hemodynamic and some of the metabolic changes elicited by endotoxin [66]. In addition to causing fever, IL-1 infusion also causes increases in acute-phase proteins [67]. Thus, like TNF, IL-1 appears to be involved in the interface between the immune system and metabolic control.

Although there are many similarities between TNF and IL-1, there is one major difference: the existence of a naturally occurring IL-1 receptor antagonist (IL-1ra). IL-1ra is produced by mononuclear phagocytes and binds to IL-1 receptors where it is biologically inactive. To date, IL-1 is the only cytokine for which an endogenous competitive inhibitor has been identified. IL-1ra has been shown to decrease mortality from sepsis in pretreated experimental animals [68].

IL-6 is a cytokine produced in response to TNF or IL-1. IL-6 has many functions including its role as a growth factor for activated B lymphocytes. From a metabolic point of view, its most interesting function may be its induction of production of acute-phase proteins by the liver, including fibrinogen [69]. It is elevated levels of fibrinogen that cause red blood cells to form rouleaux and that form the basis for measurement of the erythrocyte sedimentation rate.

Interferon-γ (INF-γ) is a cytokine produced by T-lymphocytes and natural killer cells. Its production is stimulated directly by antigen and enhanced by IL-2 (produced by T-helper cells). A major function of INF-γ appears to be its potent activation of monocytes and macrophages. Koerner et al. [70] demonstrated that although INF-γ alone does not induce TNF expression, in combination with endotoxin-stimulated macrophages, it potentiates the cytoplasmic accumulation of mRNA for TNF. Thus, through INF-γ the cellular immune system can up-regulate TNF production.

The Eicosanoids

It is clear that fat metabolism and dietary fat intake can influence immune function [71]. The omega-3 polyunsaturated fatty acids (ω-3) and omega-6 polyunsaturated fatty acids (ω-6) are essential fatty acids. They are components of the cell membrane and the substrate for a group of lipid mediators called the eicosanoids. Eicosanoids are a class of highly active metabolic products of arachidonic acid. These products include the leukotrienes, the prostaglandins (PGE), and the thromboxanes. Some eicosanoids, including PGE_2, have been shown to suppress leukocyte function in vitro [72], and suppression of their production theoretically could be associated with improved immune function.

Dietary Manipulation of Immune Function

Given this background, we now consider several approaches to nutritional support designed with specific intent to improve immune function. Some approaches may capitalize on the previously described interactions between inflammatory mediators and immunity, whereas others either do not or the mechanisms are not clear.

Arginine

Arginine is a dibasic amino acid with potent immune stimulatory and metabolic regulatory properties. It causes secretion of insulin, prolactin, and growth hormone. Arginine is usually considered a nonessential amino acid; however, because it is required during stress states, it is better referred to as a semiessential amino acid [73]. Dietary supplementation with arginine has been shown to impart survival advantage to animals with 30% body-surface burns [74] as well as animals challenged with intraperitoneal bacterial inoculates

[75]. Similar results have been demonstrated in humans. Daly and colleagues [76] conducted a randomized trial in which patients received either standard or arginine-supplemented enteral feeding postoperatively. They found increased T-cell mitogenesis, improved nitrogen balance, decreased infectious complications, and decreased wound complications in patients receiving the supplemented feeding.

The precise mechanism of immune enhancement by arginine remains unclear. At the cellular level, arginine improves T-lymphocyte function and increases the number of T-helper cells [77]. On the molecular level, L-arginine is a substrate for nitric oxide production [78], which may be important because of the role of nitric oxide as a final common mediator in cell regulation and cell-to-cell communication.

Nitric oxide initially was identified as the mediator accounting for the biologic activity of endothelial-derived relaxing factor produced by endothelial cells [79]. From an immunologic perspective, it is of interest that nitric oxide produced from arginine is required for optimal DNA synthesis in human lymphocytes [80]. Further, nitric oxide synthesis in macrophages alters their antimicrobial activity against both bacteria and parasites [81]. Because inducible calcium-independent forms of nitric oxide synthetase are substrate-limited, dietary arginine manipulation offers a potential for modulation of nitric oxide production.

For further discussion about the role of arginine and nitric oxide, the reader is referred to Chapters 14 and 16, respectively.

Glutamine

Glutamine is the most abundant amino acid in the body and the most in demand during states of critical illness. Glutamine represents a major fuel source for the enterocyte [82] and is important in maintaining gut barrier function. Glutamine is also required for nucleotide synthesis and may thereby play an important role in the production of rapidly proliferating effector cells of the immune system. During periods of catabolic stress, glutamine requirements are met by increased efflux of glutamine from skeletal muscle. Both the supply and demand of glutamine is probably controlled by cytokines at the tissue level. IL-1 activity decreases enterocyte uptake of glutamine [83]. This decrease may be important in sparing circulating glutamine for use by cells of the immune system undergoing rapid proliferation. In addition, glutamine supplementation appears to directly enhance T-cell function. A recent study determined the effect of five days of glutamine-supplemented TPN on postoperative T-cell response and cytokine production in patients undergoing colorectal surgery [84]. In that study TPN administration was associated with an increase in T-cell DNA synthesis, but it had no effect on IL-2 or IL-6 production, perhaps suggesting a clinical role for glutamine supplementation as a nutritional method to enhance T-cell function. Another recent study suggests a clinical benefit for intravenous glutamine from a reduced infection perspective. In a randomized, double-blind study, bone marrow transplant patients receiving glutamine-supplemented TPN had fewer episodes of infection and decreased hospital stays [85]. Most commercially available enteral formulas contain glutamine. Intravenous amino acid solutions, however, do not contain glutamine because of its instability.

Omega-3 Fatty Acids

A great deal of interest was generated in the ω-3 fatty acids when it was noted that guinea pigs had improvement in immune and metabolic function after burn injury if fed enteral diets based on ω-3 fatty acids [86]. In the normal diet, fat is provided from both plant and animal sources. Most currently available enteral support diets, however, derive lipid calories only from vegetable oils containing ω-6 polyunsaturated fats. This may lead to an imbalance in the ω-6/ω-3 ratio in the cell membrane. Metabolism of ω-6 fatty acid leads to production of thromboxane A2 (which causes vasoconstriction and platelet aggregation) and PGE_2 (an immunosuppressive). Metabolism of ω-3 fatty acids, on the other hand, produces PGE_3 (a markedly less potent immunosuppressive than PGE_2) and thromboxane A3 (a markedly less potent procoagulant than thromboxane A2).

As with the cytokines, the eicosanoids have powerful effects on both the immune system and metabolism. It appears possible that by supplying less ω-6 fatty acids and more ω-3 fatty acids, nutritional therapy might be effective in limiting the production of harmful mediators while augmenting the production of beneficial ones. There are, however, some potential pitfalls with ω-3 fatty acid supplementation, particularly the question of toxicity due to free radical generation from fish oils containing ω-3 fatty acids [87]. The role of ω-3 fatty acids is further discussed in Chapter 18.

Dietary Nucleotides

In 1983, Van Buren et al. [88] noted that renal transplant patients receiving TPN required less immunosuppression than patients on normal diets. Subsequent animal studies showed that this immunosuppression may be caused partly by nucleotide restriction. In mice, for example, specific antibody production to T-cell-dependent antigens is attenuated after a three-week nucleotide-free diet [89]. T-cell-dependent antibody production can be returned rapidly (within one week) to normal levels, however, with nucleotide supplementation.

The exact immunologic mechanism of dietary nucleotide function remains unclear. It is known that during certain phases of the cell cycle, lymphocytes cannot produce nucleotides and must rely on de novo synthesis by the liver [90]. If, during a condition of stress, the demand for nucleotides is so greatly exaggerated that it exceeds the liver's capacity for production, exogenous nucleotides may be required to maintain immune function. Human studies to evaluate this hypothesis have not been published.

Conclusion

It is clear that nutritional status has a profound impact on immune function. Currently available methods to provide nutritional support effectively treat or prevent malnutrition and will correct immune dysfunction when it is due to macronutrient, vitamin, or mineral deficiency. In many critically ill and severely stressed patients, however, additional factors contribute to immune dysfunction. In these patients, nutritional deficits and immune dysfunction coexist, but correction of the former has little impact on the latter. Successful treatment of these patients must await better clarification of the role of various inflammatory mediators and the impact of specific nutrients on their activity.

References

1. Coleman W, DuBois E. The influence of high calorie diet on the respiratory exchanges in typhoid fever. *Arch Intern Med* 14:168, 1994.
2. Graves R. *Lectures on the Practice of Medicine.* Dublin: New Sydenham Society, 1884.
3. Cuthbertson D. Observations on the disturbance of metabolism produced by injury to the limbs. *Q J Med* 25:233, 1932.
4. Studley H. Percentage of weight loss: A basic indicator of surgical risk in patients with chronic peptic ulcer. *JAMA* 106:458, 1936.
5. Cannon P, Wissler R, Woolridge R. The relationship of protein deficiency to surgical infection. *Ann Surg* 120:514, 1944.
6. Bistrian B, et al. Protein status of general surgical patients. *JAMA* 230:858, 1974.
7. Bistrian B, et al. Prevalence of malnutrition in general medical patients. *JAMA* 235:1567, 1976.
8. Wilmore D. Catabolic illness: Strategies for enhancing recovery. *N Engl J Med* 325:695, 1991.
9. Goldstein S, Elwyn D. The effects of injury and sepsis on fuel utilization. *Annu Rev Nutr* 9:445, 1989.
10. Dudrick S, Wilmore D, Rhoads J. Long-term parenteral nutrition with growth, development, and positive nitrogen balance. *Surgery* 64:134, 1968.
11. Zaloga G. Frontiers in critical care nutrition. *New Horizons* 2:121, 1994.
12. Murray J, Murray S. Suppression of infection by famine: A paradox? *Perspect Biol Med* 20:471, 1977.
13. Peck MD, Babcock GF, Alexander JW. The role of protein and calorie restriction on outcome from *Salmonella* infection in mice. *JPEN* 16:561, 1992.
14. Smythe PM, et al. Thymolymphatic deficiency and depression of cell-mediated immunity in protein-calorie malnutrition. *Lancet* 2:939, 1971.
15. Meakins JL, et al. Delayed hypersensitivity: Indicator of acquired failure of host defenses in sepsis and trauma. *Ann Surg* 186:241, 1977.
16. Mullen JL, et al. Implications of malnutrition in the surgical patient. *Arch Surg* 114:121, 1979.
17. Buzby GP, et al. Prognostic nutritional index in gastrointestinal surgery. *Am J Surg* 139:160, 1980.
18. Beatty W, Dowdle EB. Deficiency in kwashiorkor serum of factor required for optimal lymphocyte transformation in vitro. *Clin Exp Med* 35:433, 1979.
19. Bell RC, Hoffman-Goetz L, Keir R. Monocyte factors modulate in vitro T-lymphocyte mitogenesis in protein malnutrition. *Clin Exp Immunol* 63:194, 1986.
20. Chandra RK. Interactions of nutrition, infection and immune response. Immunocompetence in nutritional deficiency, methodological considerations and interventional strategies. *Acta Paediatr Scand* 68:137, 1979.
21. Narayanan RB, et al. The effect of undernutrition on immunologic response to BCG, and TAB vaccines in mice maintained on a natural diet. *Bulletin WHO* 56:781, 1978.
22. Aref GH, Badr El Din MK, Hassan AI. Immunoglobulins in kwashiorkor. *J Trop Med Hyg* 73:186, 1970.
23. Seth V, Chandra RK. Opsonic activity, phagocytosis, and bactericidal capacity of polymorphs in undernutrition. *Arch Dis Child* 47:282, 1972.
24. Gotch FM, et al. Reversible granulocyte killing defect in anorexia nervosa. *Clin Exp Immunol* 21:244, 1975.
25. Douglas SD, Schopfer K. Phagocytic function in protein calorie malnutrition. *Clin Exp Immunol* 7:121, 1974.
26. Keusch GT, et al. Antibacterial functions of macrophages in experimental protein-calorie malnutrition. I. Description of the model, morphological observations, and macrophage surface IgG receptors. *J Infect Dis* 138:125, 1978.
27. Murray HW. Interferon-gamma: The activated macrophage and host defense against microbial challenge. *Ann Int Med* 108:595, 1988.
28. Chandra RK. Serum complement and immunoconglutinin in malnutrition. *Arch Dis Child* 50:225, 1975.
29. Wonder JA, Stinnett JD, Alexander JW. The effects of malnutrition on variables of host defense in the guinea pig. *Surgery* 84:542, 1978.
30. Worthington BS. Effect of nutritional status on immune phenomena. *J Am Diet Assoc* 65:123, 1974.
31. Krishan S, Krishan AD, Mustafa AS. Effect of vitamin A and undernutrition on the susceptibility of rodents to malarial parasite *Plasmodium berghei. J Nutr* 106:784, 1976.
32. Kaplan S, Basford R. Effect of vitamin B_{12} and folic acid deficiencies on neutrophil function. *Blood* 47:801, 1976.
33. Axelrod AE. Immune processes in vitamin deficiency states. *Am J Clin Nutr* 24:265, 1971.

34. Axelrod AE, Hojper S. Effects of pantothenic acid, pyridoxine, and thiamine deficiencies upon antibody formation to influenza virus PR-8 in rats. *J Nutr* 72:325, 1960.
35. Grant JD. Nutritional support in critically ill patients. *Ann Surg* 220:610, 1994.
36. Eckman J, Eaton JW, Jacob HS. Role of vitamin E in regulating malaria expression. *Clin Res* 24:480A, 1976.
37. Chvapil M, et al. Effect of zinc on peritoneal macrophages in vitro. *Infect Immunol* 16:367, 1977.
38. McCoy JH, Kenney MA. Depressed immune response in the magnesium-deficient rat. *J Nutr* 105:791, 1975.
39. Weinberg ED. Iron and susceptibility to infectious disease. *Science* 184:952, 1974.
40. Copeland EM, MacFadyen BV, Dudrick SJ. Effect of intravenous hyperalimentation on established delayed hypersensitivity in the cancer patient. *Ann Surg* 184:60, 1976.
41. Christou NV, Meakins JL. Delayed hypersensitivity: A mechanism for anergy in surgical patients. *Surgery* 86:78, 1979.
42. Smale BF, et al. Prognostic value of serum transferrin in the surgical patient. *Surg Forum* 32:112, 1981.
43. Meakins JL, et al. Anergy in surgical patients: Therapeutic approaches. *Ann Surg* 190:286, 1979.
44. Detsky AS, et al. Perioperative parenteral nutrition: A meta-analysis. *Ann Intern Med* 107:195, 1987.
45. Buzby GP, et al. Study protocol: A randomized clinical trial of total parenteral nutrition in malnourished surgical patients. *Am J Clin Nutr* 47:366, 1988.
46. Buzby GP, et al. (The Veterans Affairs Total Parenteral Nutrition Cooperative Study Group). Perioperative total parenteral nutrition in surgical patients. *N Engl J Med* 325:525, 1991.
47. Muller JM, Keller HW, Brenner U. Indications and effects of preoperative parenteral nutrition. *World J Surg* 10:53, 1987.
48. Knox LS. A secondary analysis of factors associated with postoperative infection in malnourished surgical patients. Unpublished PhD dissertation.
49. Fan ST, Lo CM, Lai ECS. Perioperative nutritional support in patients undergoing hepatectomy for hepatocellular carcinoma. *N Engl J Med* 331:1547, 1994.
50. Boeckman C, Krill C. Bacterial and fungal infections complicating parenteral alimentation in infants and children. *J Pediatr Surg* 5:117, 1970.
51. Johnson L, et al. Structural and hormonal alterations in the gastrointestinal tract of parenterally fed rats. *Gastroenterology* 68:1177, 1975.
52. Alverdy J, Aoys E, Moss G. Total parenteral nutrition promotes bacterial translocation from the gut. *Surgery* 104:185, 1988.
53. Moore F, et al. Gut bacterial translocation via the portal vein: A clinical perspective with major torso trauma. *J Trauma* 31:629, 1991.
54. Shnaper A, et al. Translocating gut bacteria reach the pulmonary artery by means of the thoracic duct during hemorrhagic shock. *Surg Forum* 45:72, 1994.
55. Moore F, et al. Early enteral feeding, compared with parenteral, reduces postoperative septic complications: The results of a meta-analysis. *Ann Surg* 216:172, 1992.
56. Kudsk K, et al. Enteral versus parenteral feeding: Effects on septic morbidity after blunt and penetrating abdominal trauma. *Ann Surg* 215:503, 1992.
57. Lowry S. Modulating the metabolic response to injury and infection. *Proc Nutr Soc* 51:267, 1992.
58. Santos A, et al. Does the route of feeding modify the inflammatory response? *Ann Surg* 220:115, 1994.
59. Bessey P, et al. Combined hormonal infusion simulates the metabolic response to injury. *Ann Surg* 200:264, 1984.
60. Carswell L, et al. Endotoxin-induced serum factor that causes necrosis of tumors. *Proc Natl Acad Sci USA* 72:3666, 1975.
61. Kawakami M, et al. Studies of endotoxin-induced decrease in lipoprotein lipase activity. *J Exp Med* 154:631, 1981.
62. Kawakami M, et al. Lipoprotein lipase suppression in 3T3-L1 cells by an endotoxin-induced mediator from exudate cells. *Proc Natl Acad Sci USA* 79:912, 1982.
63. Beutler B, et al. Identity of tumor necrosis factor and the macrophage-secreted factor cachectin. *Nature* 316:522, 1985.
64. Van Der Poll T, et al. Tumor necrosis factor mimics the metabolic response to acute infection in healthy human. *Am J Physiol* 261:E457, 1991.
65. Endres S, Van Der Meer J, Dinarello C. Interleukin-1 in the pathogenesis of fever. *Eur J Clin Invest* 17:469, 1987.
66. Fischer E, et al. Comparison between effects of interleukin-1α administration and sublethal endotoxemia in primates. *Am J Physiol* 261:R442, 1991.
67. Dinarello C. Interleukin-1 and interleukin-1 antagonism. *Blood* 8:1627, 1991.
68. Ohlsson K, et al. Interleukin-1 receptor antagonist reduces mortality from endotoxic shock. *Nature* 348:550, 1990.
69. Gauldie J, et al. Interferon B-2: B-cell stimulating factor and type 2 shares identity with monocyte-derived hepatocyte-stimulating factor and regulates the major acute-phase protein response in liver cells. *Proc Natl Acad Sci USA* 84:7251, 1987.
70. Koerner T, Adams D, Hamilton T. Regulation of tumor necrosis factor expression: Interferon-gamma enhances the accumulation of mRNA for TNF induced by lipopolysaccharide in murine peritoneal macrophages. *Cell Immunol* 109:437, 1987.
71. Kinsella J, et al. Dietary polyunsaturated fatty acids and eicosanoids: potential effects on the modulation of inflammatory and immune cells—an overview. *Nutrition* 6:24, 1990.
72. Goodwin J, Ceuppens J. Regulation of the immune response by prostaglandins. *J Clin Immunol* 3:295, 1983.
73. Barbul A. Arginine and immune function. *Nutrition* 6:53, 1990.
74. Saito H, et al. Metabolic and immune effects of dietary arginine supplementation after burn. *Arch Surg* 122:748, 1987.
75. Madden H, et al. Stimulation of T cell immunity enhances survival in peritonitis. *J Surg Res* 30:175, 1981.
76. Daly J, et al. Enteral nutrition with supplemental arginine, RNA, and omega-3 fatty acids in patients after operation: Immunologic, metabolic and clinical outcome. *Surgery* 112:56, 1992.
77. Daly J, et al. Immune and metabolic effects of arginine in the surgical patient. *Ann Surg* 208:512, 1988.
78. Modcada S, Palmer R, Higgs E. Biosynthesis of nitric oxide from L-arginine: A pathway for the regulation of cell function and communication. *Biochem Pharmacol* 38:1709, 1989.
79. Palmer R, Ferrige A, Moncada D. Nitric oxide release accounts for the biologic activity of endothelium-derived relaxing factor. *Nature* 257:524, 1987.
80. Efron D, et al. Nitric oxide generation from L-arginine is

essential for optimal human peripheral blood lymphocyte DNA synthesis. *Surgery* 110:327, 1991.

81. Nathan C, Hibbs J. Role of nitric oxide synthesis in macrophage antimicrobial activity. *Curr Opin Immunol* 3:65, 1992.
82. Souba W. Glutamine: A key substrate for the splanchnic bed. *Ann Rev Nutr* 11:285, 1991.
83. Austgen T, et al. Cytokine regulation of intestinal glutamine utilization. *Am J Surg* 163:174, 1991.
84. O'Riordain M, et al. Glutamine-supplemented total parenteral nutrition enhances T-lymphocyte responses in surgical patients undergoing colorectal resection. *Ann Surg* 220:212, 1994.
85. Ziegler T, et al. Clinical and metabolic efficacy of glutamine-supplemented parenteral nutrition after bone marrow transplantation: A randomized, double-blind, controlled study. *Ann Intern Med* 116:821, 1992.
86. Alexander J, et al. The importance of lipid type in the diet after burn injury. *Ann Surg* 20:1, 1986.
87. Peck M. Omega-3 polyunsaturated fatty acids: Benefit or harm during sepsis? *New Horizons* 2:230, 1994.
88. Van Buren C, et al. The influence of dietary nucleotides on cell-mediated immunity. *Transplantation* 36:350, 1983.
89. Jyonouchi H. Nucleotide actions on humoral immune responses. *J Nutr* 124:138S, 1994.
90. Rudolph F, et al. Role of RNA as a dietary source of pyrimidines and purines in immune function. *Nutrition* 6:45, 1990.

Selected Readings

Buzby GP, et al. (The Veterans Affairs Total Parenteral Nutrition Cooperative Study Group). Perioperative total parenteral nutrition in surgical patients. *N Engl J Med* 325:526, 1991.

A large (459 patients) prospective randomized study to determine if perioperative TPN decreases serious complications after major abdominal or thoracic surgery in malnourished patients. The results demonstrate that preoperative TPN should be limited to a subgroup of severely malnourished patients. Patients who were classified as borderline or mildly malnourished had increased rates of infectious complications with preoperative TPN.

Chandra RK (1990 McCollum Award Lecture). Nutrition and immunity: Lessons for the past and new insights into the future. *Am J Clin Nutr* 53:1087, 1990.

A broad-reaching review of the effects of malnutrition and infection on health and survival. The author focuses particular attention on pediatric populations in underdeveloped countries. This presentation includes a review of host defense systems, epidemiologic observations on malnutrition, and the effects of micronutrient deficiencies. He promotes preventive nutritional measures to improve the development and survival of underprivileged children.

Grant JP. Nutritional support in critically ill patients. *Ann Surg* 220:610, 1994.

This is a current review on nutritional substrates for use in critically ill patients. It includes discussion of agents under investigation in addition to those currently in clinical use. The newer nutritional substrates are evaluated according to a classic nutritional viewpoint (that is, nutritional substrates as building blocks) as well as a molecular viewpoint (that is, nutritional substrates as pharmacologic agents).

Lowry SF, Thompson WA. Nutrient modification of inflammatory mediator production. *New Horizons* 2:164, 1994.

This article reviews evidence suggesting that nutritional manipulation may influence production of inflammatory mediators. It includes sections on cytokines and classic hormone interactions, role of gastrointestinal barrier function, effect of the route of alimentation on inflammatory mediator production, and the influence of specific nutrients on the stress response in critically ill patients. The article suggests that controlled clinical trials are needed to elucidate the beneficial or detrimental effects of nutrient modulation on the inflammatory response.

Mainous MR, Deitch EA. Nutrition and infection. *Surg Clin North Am* 74(3):659, 1994.

This article reviews the consequences of malnutrition on surgical and posttraumatic patients. The main focus is on the indications for nutritional support, importance of timing/route of support, and methods for estimating a patient's nutritional requirements.

24

Nutritional Support in Hepatic Failure

Josef E. Fischer
Gregory M. Tiao

Among the most complex problems in patient management are those that involve failure of one of the metabolically active organs, such as the liver or kidney. The liver, which is the primary metabolic factory of the body, clears nutrients (as well as toxins) from the portal blood, processing and preparing them for distribution to the periphery in response to endocrine, neural, or cytokine stimuli. Management of hepatic failure is complicated by the myriad processes that normally take place in the liver, as well as by its central role in managing metabolism. The liver is thought to house at least 600 enzymes, and support of all of these processes is clearly not possible.

In general, the options in management of organ failure are:

1. Organ transplantation.
2. Employment of an extracorporeal device that assumes temporary or permanent function.
3. General supportive measures allowing for recovery of organ function.

The advent and development of successful orthotopic liver transplantation has markedly changed the outcome of patients with liver failure. Successful liver organ transplantation has improved the prognosis of patients with fulminant liver failure [1,2] and end-stage cirrhosis [3]. Organ availability, however, limits the use of hepatic transplantation as a primary therapy [2].

There are several recently developed therapeutic alternatives employing extracorporeal devices. The most promising option entails the recently described bioartificial liver—a hollow-fiber dialysis cartridge containing living hepatocytes. The hepatocytes are derived from either porcine liver [4] or a well-differentiated hepatoblastoma cell line [5]. These devices are being evaluated in clinical trials [4,5]. Another extracorporeal option involves ex vivo pig-liver perfusion as a bridge to transplantation [6]. This alternative has been considered intermittently over the past 30 years [7]; however, recent advances in the understanding of molecular biology has made possible the development of transgenic animals whose livers synthesize human proteins and enzymes. The livers from these animals in turn could be used as xenographic donors [8]. Either approach, along with the more "traditional" concept of charcoal hemoperfusion [9], may only provide temporary support by acting as a bridge to either natural recovery or transplantation. Both of these options require further study.

Despite these new forms of therapy, general supportive measures remain the major form of therapy for patients in hepatic failure. This is due in large part to the capacity of the liver to regenerate. Therapy in hepatic failure is often a play for time until the powers of regeneration allow return of normal function. Some of the many influences on hepatic failure and hepatic regeneration have been known for many years, including the combination of insulin and glucagon (although the ideal stoichiometric relationship is still not clear). Others, such as hepatocyte growth factor, have only recently been identified [10]; still others are permissive, such as steroids, growth hormone, and triiodothyronine. Few such influences, however, are as manageable as nutrition.

In discussing nutritional support in hepatic failure, it is reasonable to define the circumstances under which such support may be useful. Hepatic failure can be defined as either acute or chronic, with some middle ground for mixed disease. Fulminant hepatic failure, usually secondary to viral or toxic hepatitis, involves a patient with prior normal nutrition and liver function. The course is progressive and acute, with outcome decided within weeks. Nutritional support in this setting may be helpful as an adjunct to the extracorporeal forms of therapy described above. Nutritional support may also be potentially helpful prior to transplantation as it may reduce protein depletion, resulting in improved immunologic status post-transplant.

In chronic conditions such as alcoholic hepatitis, elements of acute necrosis are usually superimposed on chronic liver damage. In our experience, this often fatal condition requires prolonged nutritional support to improve survival [11]. In a group of patients with alcoholic hepatitis less ill than those that we have seen, survival has been improved by an aggressive program of nutritional support [12].

Acute-on-chronic hepatic failure occurs in the patient with preexistent liver disease, usually cirrhosis, who has sustained an acute insult secondary to gastrointestinal bleeding, infection, starvation, or surgical intervention. It is primarily these patients with whom this chapter deals and for whom nutritional support is most beneficial.

Multisystem organ failure is increasingly being recognized as a cause of death in surgical patients. Sustained gluconeogenesis at the expense of structural and functional protein in essential organs, particularly the liver, in response to prolonged and excessive stress, especially sepsis, may be at least one etiology of this condition [13]. The management of septic patients, therefore, does not differ markedly from the management of patients with acute-on-chronic hepatic failure and requires vigorous and aggressive nutritional support.

Pathophysiology of Acute Hepatic Failure

Normal Flow and Architecture

Under normal circumstances, the major source of blood supply to the liver is portal blood, containing both nutrient and toxic substances absorbed from the gut and representing between 65% and 80% of total hepatic blood flow. It is nutrient-rich and relatively oxygen-poor, although the venous oxygen content of the afferent blood is not so low as other venous effluents from other parts of the body. Portal blood mixes at the level of the hepatic sinusoid with arterial blood, relatively nutrient-poor and oxygen-rich, which in turn comprises between 20% and 35% of normal hepatic blood flow.

Flow originates at the periphery of the hepatic lobule, the portal triad, which contains the hepatic artery, portal vein, and bile canaliculus surrounded by a small amount of fibrous tissue containing lymphocytes and macrophages. Mixed portal and arterial blood flows centripetally, perfusing single plates of hepatocytes in an orderly progression. Presumably, not all cells function simultaneously; as many as two-thirds may be "resting" at any given time. Possibly there exists a continuum of functional capacity that diminishes in a centripetal fashion; indeed, those cells at the periphery of the lobule are relatively oxygen- and nutrient-rich, whereas those at the central portion may be marginal with respect to oxygen and nutrient supply.

Genesis of Portal Hypertension

The continued evolution of chronic liver disease with repeated insults to the liver, usually on the basis of alcohol and malnutrition, results in distortion of the lobular architecture as a result of piecemeal necrosis, bridging necrosis, collapse of the fine reticular framework, and replacement by fibrous tissue. Nodules of regenerating hepatocytes derive their blood supply largely from the hepatic artery. The portal vein has little role in their perfusion, thus depriving them of a major source of nutrients. These hepatocytes are particularly vulnerable because hepatic artery flow is responsive to sympathetic tone, and dehydration, anesthesia, shock, or sepsis may rapidly compromise hepatic artery flow, resulting in acute deterioration. In addition, the cirrhotic architecture distorts the orderly access of single plates of hepatocytes to both arterial and portal flow [14].

Hepatocytes in regenerating nodules are of varying functional capacity. Depending on the activity of the disease, they may manifest any degree of normal function, dysfunction, or necrosis. Intrahepatic shunts form in fibrous septa as a result of the regenerative process. These shunts, as well as compression of the hepatic venous radicles and sinusoids by regenerating nodules, result in increased resistance to portal flow. Portal pressure in turn rises, leading to the formation of extrahepatic portasystemic shunts. Initially, these low-resistance extrahepatic shunts reduce portal pressure toward normal; conceivably, some of the extrahepatic shunts may then close. With further disruption of hepatic architecture, intrahepatic shunting increases and portal pressure continues to rise, resulting in greater flow through extrahepatic shunts; this then progresses toward hepatofugal flow. When the percentage of shunting is small, clearance of a particular portal substance (for example, glucose, amino acids, insulin, glucagon, or endotoxin) is probably not significantly affected. The shunted substance, with subsequent circulation through the splanchnic circuit, may eventually be cleared; in addition, there would be prolonged exposure to peripheral tissues. Overall, concentration is likely to remain at or near normal. As the percentage of shunting progressively increases toward hepatofugal flow, a critical value is reached and systemic plasma concentrations of the substance rise to a new steady-state level.

It is important to keep in mind that portal hypertension represents a homeostatic process, that is, an attempt on the part of the liver to maintain flow in the face of increased resistance. The associated plasma volume expansion, probably secondary to increased aldosterone and ADH and decreased sensitivity to atrial natriuretic factor [15], may be viewed teleologically as an attempt to increase perfusion pressure and thus flow. Consequently, although normalizing portal pressure may be advantageous or even life-saving in the instance of variceal bleeding, the concomitant decrease in hepatic flow may be ultimately deleterious and probably contributes to the long-term hepatic failure that may follow shunting procedures. In addition, nutritional restriction secondary to encephalopathy results in further damage to the liver, as sufficient protein and calories for healing of the damaged parenchyma are no longer available [16,17]. This in turn contributes to a vicious cycle of decreased hepatic function.

An important adaptive mechanism is hepatic vascular autoregulation: When portal flow is diminished, hepatic arterial flow increases. Following end-to-side portacaval shunt, patients who are capable of autoregulation seem to fare better [18, 19]. However, cause and effect are difficult to establish here. The ability to autoregulate may merely indicate the severity of liver disease; patients who compensate may simply have a less advanced form of the disease and therefore tolerate shunting better. Our patients with central splenorenal shunts who, after a time, show diminished portal flow, also tend to manifest enormous hypertrophy of the hepatic artery and continue to do well [20].

Alterations in Various Metabolic Processes

It is beyond the scope of this chapter to discuss the various derangements of metabolic function in hepatic failure. However, a brief review of the disorders in carbohydrate, fat, and protein metabolism is necessary to any discussion of nutritional support.

Alterations in Carbohydrate Metabolism

The hormonal milieu underlying carbohydrate metabolism involves the storage hormone insulin and the catabolic hormone glucagon. There is widespread evidence that diminished degradation of glucagon and insulin results in persistent elevation of both of these hormones in compromised hepatic function [21–23]. Hyperglucagonemia has been correlated with portasystemic shunting [21], and it is likely that hyperinsulinemia results by the same mechanism [22]. The net result, however, is an effectively decreased insulin-glucagon ratio due to glucagon predominance and/or cellular insensitivity to insulin, which results in cirrhosis in a tendency toward catabolism in the classic glucagon-insulin imbalance scenario [23]. In experimental animals, the decreased insulin-glucagon ratio becomes more prominent as the liver continues to fail [24]. Soon after portasystemic shunting, for example, insulin is mildly elevated and glucagon is elevated somewhat. As hepatic failure and hepatic coma supervene, glucagon increases precipitously, whereas insulin either remains the same or falls. Similar data have been obtained in humans by Ziparo and associates [25]. In their studies, true alpha-cell hyperfunction suppressible by somatostatin occurs in post-shunt patients, especially those with hepatic encephalopathy.

The source of hyperglucagonemia is not entirely clear. Teleologically, one may argue that it is directed at increasing glucose production by a failing liver or mobilizing and releasing hepatic fat for peripheral calories. Glucagon is responsive to a number of influences, including ammonia [26] and a number of amino acids, including the aromatic amino acids, which are present in excess concentration in the blood. The combination of hyperglucagonemia against the background of increased epinephrine and increased steroids (probably in turn due to decreased degradation) provokes a state of sustained gluconeogenesis, as Sherwin and co-workers have proposed [21].

The cirrhotic liver fails to store glucose; chronic hyperglucagonemia presumably results in depletion of glycogen. Despite this, fasting hypoglycemia is rare. Hepatic gluconeogenesis is active and, as in prolonged starvation, is probably assisted by renal gluconeogenesis. Other energy sources also lessen the requirement for glucose production. Lipolysis liberates glycerol (which contributes to gluconeogenesis) as well as fatty acids, which are utilized directly or oxidized to ketones, although this latter pathway may be impaired [27]. Skeletal muscle proteolysis liberates branched-chain amino acids; at least one carbon atom is oxidized locally while the amino groups and possibly some of the carbon skeleton [28] are contributed to pyruvate to form alanine (glucose-alanine cycle).

Postprandial hyperglycemia, however, is characteristic of cirrhosis. This glucose intolerance occurs after both intravenous and oral glucose and is associated with an exaggerated insulin response. The latter is probably due to shunting; however, the hyperglycemia may be multifactorial. Shunting of glucose probably contributes little to this hyperglycemia. Peripheral cellular uptake of glucose is insulin-dependent and, although hepatocellular uptake of glucose is independent of insulin, hepatocellular metabolism of glucose is also insulin-dependent. The decreased insulin-glucagon ratio may therefore account for this hyperglycemia.

The primary hepatic responsibilities in carbohydrate metabolism are: (1) glucose storage, (2) glucose production, and (3) maintaining a steady fuel concentration and therefore a steady plasma osmolarity. In summary, the cirrhotic liver fails only in the first of these, maintaining adequate capacity for the remaining functions. However, with superimposed acute deterioration, gluconeogenesis may ultimately fail, resulting in hypoglycemia. When hypoglycemia becomes profound, this is usually a sign of fatal outcome. Hepatic uptake of substrates for this pathway ceases, resulting in gross hyperaminoacidemia and lactic acidemia.

Alterations in Lipid Metabolism

The abnormalities in metabolism extend to the treatment of fatty acids. Under normal circumstances, lipolysis is a major source of energy, accounting for approximately 75% to 85% of normal energy expenditure during resting starvation. The liver plays a central role in the metabolism of relatively long-chain fatty acids to ketone bodies, a major source of peripheral energy, as well as maintaining normal plasma concentrations of relatively short-chain fatty acids.

The issue of fatty acid metabolism is somewhat controversial. Although short-chain fatty acids, together with ammonia and methane thiols, occupy a relatively prominent place in one of the current hypotheses of hepatic encephalopathy [29], some investigators have given relatively large amounts of these substances without deleterious effects [30]. Moreover, in conditions in which short-chain fatty acids have been implicated, in the coma of congenital disorders or those involving hypoglycin A [31,32], the concentrations of short-chain fatty acids are literally hundreds of times higher than those seen in patients with hepatic encephalopathy.

Nonesterified fatty acids circulate in the bloodstream at least partially bound to albumin. Their importance with respect to hepatic encephalopathy is their displacement of bound tryptophan from albumin [33]. With lipid mobilization and increased nonesterified fatty acids within the circulation, unbound tryptophan increases, thus becoming more available for transport across the blood-brain barrier [34]. The overall effect of the failing liver on lipid metabolism is to deprive the body of a major source of energy, thus making the organism turn to gluconeogenesis as a primary source.

Alterations in Nitrogen Metabolism

The cirrhotic tendency toward gluconeogenesis requires an equal capacity for ureagenesis in order to prevent hyperammonemia. A wide range of hepatocellular dysfunction may be present in chronic cirrhotic failure; the reserve capacity for glucose production is adequate (at least initially), but the reserve capacity for ureagenesis may be less well preserved.

It is difficult to distinguish the hyperammonemia resulting from a diminished ureagenic capacity from that resulting from shunting of ammonia of gut origin. Gut gluconeogenesis from glutamine is active; ammonia from this source, as well as from intraluminal deamination of amino acids, requires successful transport to the liver for urea synthesis. Shunting of a critical portion of portal blood would result in persistent elevation of plasma ammonia concentrations.

Of greater importance is the particular amino acid pattern that characterizes cirrhosis and acute-on-chronic failure. The branched-chain amino acids (BCAA)—leucine, isoleucine, and valine—are usually below normal, whereas phenylalanine, tyrosine, free tryptophan, methionine, glutamate, aspartate, and, to a lesser extent, histidine, are usually elevated [35].

The BCAA are unique in their partial utilization as an energy source by tissues other than the liver; relatively little oxidation occurs in the liver. They represent between 60% and 100% of the splanchnic clearance of amino acids, as well as between 60% and 100% of peripheral nitrogen accumulation in patients in energy and nitrogen balance [36]. In circumstances in which the production or utilization of the usual energy substrates (glucose, fatty acids, ketones) is impaired, the BCAA may be expected to contribute a greater percentage of energy needs, perhaps up to 30% or 40%. Enhanced peripheral consumption thus provides a reasonable explanation for the diminished plasma levels in acute-on-chronic failure. In fulminant hepatic failure, BCAA levels remain relatively normal despite gross elevation of all other amino acids, and their concentration is maintained largely by the periphery with little effect by the liver [35,37].

Tryptophan is unique in being albumin-bound. In acute-on-chronic failure, although the total concentration of tryptophan remains normal or diminished, the unbound fraction is elevated [33, 34,38,39]. Tryptophan appears to be displaced by nonesterified fatty acids or bilirubin [39], both of which are present in high concentration. Associated hypoalbuminemia may further compound this competitive process.

The elevations of phenylalanine, tyrosine, methionine, glutamate, aspartate, and histidine are not explained as easily. Why these particular amino acids are elevated, while others are relatively normal, is not immediately obvious. As mentioned earlier in regard to hyperammonemia, distinguishing the effects of hepatocellular dysfunction from those of shunting is often difficult. The conversion of phenylalanine to tyrosine has been found to be impaired in cirrhosis, and seems to correlate well with the estimation of portal-systemic shunting [40].

It has been demonstrated that the hepatic uptake of each amino acid upon single circulatory passage through the liver varies quite dramatically [41]. Histidine, aspartate, glutamate, and the aromatic amino acids are at the upper end of this spectrum; that is, between 80% and 100% of these amino acids are cleared on initial passage through a normally functioning liver. Others such as alanine, lysine, proline, and arginine demonstrate only 20% to 40% clearance. This may shed some light on the selective elevations in cirrhosis and acute-on-chronic failure. The plasma concentrations of those amino acids with particularly high uptake indices on initial passage may be most seriously affected if shunting alone were to deny their direct access to the sinusoids. However, a particular problem at the hepatocellular membrane, impeding uptake, could conceivably account for these selective elevations as well.

It is interesting that phenylalanine, tyrosine, histidine, methionine, and tryptophan have been implicated in the control of flux of other amino acids through the hepatocyte membrane in vitro [42]. The liver serves as the principal site of catabolism of these amino acids via enzymes that are inducible by and normally responsive to sharply increased concentrations in the circulation.

The common clinical setting of acute-on-chronic failure often involves a combination of starvation, surgical or traumatic insult, and sepsis resulting in extensive skeletal muscle proteolysis. Amino acids from this source, as well as from the gastrointestinal tract (secondary to blood degradation), only tend to exacerbate the abnormal pattern that existed prior to the insult.

As an indicator of the abnormalities in protein metabolism during liver disease, we use the plasma ratio of BCAA to aromatic amino acids as a guide in the clinical therapy of these patients:

$$\text{Ratio} = \frac{\text{Valine} + \text{Leucine} + \text{Isoleucine}}{\text{Phenylalanine} + \text{Tyrosine}}$$

In a normal individual, this ratio is 3.5 to 4.0. In hepatic disease, the ratio falls below 2.5; in hepatic coma it drops below 1.2; and in profound coma it is less than 0.8. Some have found this ratio useful as a prognostic index.

Hypotheses of Hepatic Encephalopathy

From the foregoing discussion, it is clear that the dramatic abnormalities in nitrogen metabolism constitute a major handicap in providing nutritional support to patients with hepatic failure. Hepatic coma, with its intolerance to protein, imposes a severe dietary restriction in these patients. Moreover, because protein is the essential component for protein synthesis and hepatic regeneration, as well as the metabolic substrate for immunologic host defense [43], it is clear that protein restriction carried out beyond a certain point is deleterious. Thus, the provision of adequate protein without provoking hepatic encephalopathy is critical in nutritional support.

The difficulties with ammonia as the principal etiologic agent in hepatic encephalopathy are well known. Although a detailed description of the theories and hypotheses of hepatic encephalopathy is beyond the scope of this chapter, a few comments should suffice. Hepatic encephalopathy in its various presentations is a subtle disease. Mood swings and subtle disturbances in judgment, day-night rhythm, and posture indicate a disorder that is not toxic but neurotransmissive in nature. The lack of correlation between ammonia and the grade of encephalopathy is well known, but the excuses that ammonia cannot be measured accurately (after six decades!) begin to wear thin. In addition, it is relatively easy both in experimental animals and in man to dissociate blood levels of ammonia and symptomatology. Monoamine oxidase inhibitors, for example, decrease blood ammonia, but patients become more symptomatic [44]. Glutamine synthetase inhibitors, such as methionine sulfoximine, increase brain ammonia yet decrease its toxicity in experimental animals [45]. Clearly, ammonia in and of itself does not explain hepatic encephalopathy.

Others have speculated that ammonia, mercaptans, methane thiols, and short-chain fatty acids in combination may be the source of symptomatology [29]. Aside from the fact that this is but another toxic hypothesis, it has been difficult for other laboratories to confirm these hypotheses because of difficulties in measurement. Furthermore, it is not clear how the failing liver allows the accumulation of these compounds. Short-chain fatty acids have been administered by some investigators to patients with a history of encephalopathy, without provoking the symptom complex [30].

The role of the GABA-ergic system in the pathogenesis of hepatic encephalopathy has also received significant attention. In 1982, it was proposed that gut-derived GABA (gamma-aminobutyric acid) may contribute to hepatic encephalopathy [46]. This was based on the observations that plasma levels of GABA were increased in patients in hepatic coma [47] and in a rabbit model of fulminant hepatic failure [48]. It was hypothesized that the increased GABA occurred due to decreased clearance of GABA secondary to liver dysfunction and to shunting of blood around the liver. As GABA is an inhibitor of neurotransmission, excessive GABA could alter neurotransmission. Subsequent studies failed to correlate plasma [49] or cerebrospinal fluid (CSF) [50] concentration and hepatic encephalopathy. More recent reports demonstrated that GABA levels [51] and GABA receptors [52] were not changed in patients who died in hepatic coma. This evidence makes it less likely that abnormalities in GABA concentration per se induce hepatic encephalopathy.

Recently, it has been found that "endogenous" benzodiazepine-like substances are elevated in the CSF of patients with hepatic encephalopathy [53]. It has been suggested that binding of these "endogenous" benzodiazepines to GABA-related receptors may facilitate GABA-ergic transmission. The identity of the endogenous benzodiazepines, ligands, has yet to be determined. Clinical studies utilizing benzodiazepine antagonists have been reported with some benefit; however, sample sizes are small and the specific role in the etiology of chronic hepatic encephalopathy is still not clear. The GABA hypothesis, if applicable, is likely to be applicable to fulminant hepatic failure.

There is also recent evidence suggesting that glutamatergic dysfunction may contribute to hepatic encephalopathy. In vitro studies showed increased glutamate release from brain slices taken from portacaval-shunted rats as compared to sham-operated rats [54]. In vivo studies using microdialysis have shown that there is increased brain glutamate release in animals with hepatic encephalopathy [55]. Glutamate receptor binding studies show decreased receptor densities in two different animal models of hepatic encephalopathy, suggesting down-regulation by the increased extracellular levels of glutamate [56,57]. Further study in humans is needed to clarify the role of glutamatergic dysfunction in hepatic encephalopathy.

Unified Hypothesis of Hepatic Encephalopathy

The current concept of the etiology of hepatic encephalopathy, known as the unified hypothesis, implies a multifactorial nature in which ammonia is merely an indicator of disturbed nitrogen metabolism [58].

The clinical manifestation is considered to be a disturbance in central and peripheral neurotransmitters, particularly in the aminergic system. This phylogenetically primitive midline system comprises less than 5% of the neurons in the central nervous system but has tremendous ramifications and feedback circuits throughout. The locus ceruleus, for example, situated under the fourth ventricle, is largely noradrenergic in nature; although it consists of only 1500 neurons, it has associations with the entire nervous system. Indeed, no central nervous system neuron seems to be distant from the ramifications of the aminergic system, suggesting a neuroregulatory function. The anatomic relationship between aminergic neurons also suggests a regulatory function; the axons and dendrites usually end free in the matrix instead of forming classic synapses [59].

The unified hypothesis points to the amino acid imbalance characteristic of cirrhosis and acute-on-chronic failure as the etiology of this aminergic disturbance. Phenylalanine, tyrosine, unbound tryptophan, methionine, and histidine, as well as the BCAA, are all neutral pH. Blood-brain barrier transport of these neutral amino acids is via system-L [60,61]. Presumably a common carrier is involved that each amino acid competitively employs. Increased brain concentrations of phenylalanine, tyrosine, unbound tryptophan, methionine, and histidine result directly from their high plasma concentrations, as well as indirectly from diminished competition from low plasma BCAA concentrations. An intrinsic alteration involving the velocity of transport across system-L may also be involved [62].

Phenylalanine, tyrosine, tryptophan, methionine, and histidine are all precursors of aminergic neurotransmitters. The crux of the hypothesis is the imbalance of aminergic products that results from excessive brain concentrations of these amino acids. Studies in both experimental animals and humans suggest that decreased norepinephrine and dopamine [63,64], as well as increased serotonin [34,39,65–67] and the phenylethylamines (tyramine, octopamine, and phenylethanolamine) [64,68–72], correlate closely with the presence of hepatic encephalopathy. The presence of 5-hydroxyindoleacetic acid and homovanillic acid in CSF of patients with hepatic encephalopathy also supports this concept of aminergic derangement [49,73].

How does ammonia fit into this hypothesis? As mentioned earlier, hyperammonemia stimulates the release of glucagon [26], thereby further promoting gluconeogenesis and the requirement for comparable ureagenesis. In the brain, however, ammonia is represented as glutamine, the product of a small, rapidly turning-over pool of glutamate [74]. It has been known for some time that CSF glutamine in patients correlates very well with the level of hepatic encephalopathy [75]. Studies in experimental animals have provided evidence of an excellent correlation between CSF glutamine and the concentrations of phenylalanine, tyrosine, and tryptophan [76]. Glutamine, being of neutral pH, also traverses the blood-brain barrier via system-L. If the brain were to export glutamine in blood-brain fashion, the system-L carrier would then be free to exchange at an increased rate for the neutral amino acids [58]. This concept, which is supported by a series of experiments carried out both in experimental animals and in isolated brain capillaries from shunted and normal animals [38], may also explain why the toxicity of ammonia is decreased when methionine sulfoximine, an inhibitor of glutamine synthetase, is given to experimental animals [45]; methionine sulfoximine inhibits the transport of neutral amino acids, possibly because of decreased glutamine within the brain [77].

The relationship between amino acid concentrations in plasma and brain in animals following portacaval shunt also lends support to this hypothesis. Simultaneous determination of plasma and brain neutral amino acids suggests that the brain accumulates neutral amino acids against a gradient. If the penetration of neutral amino acids across the blood-brain barrier is by facilitated diffusion, the brain concentrations of amino acids should not be higher than plasma unless another factor is at work.

One can predict the brain concentrations of various neutral amino acids from plasma competition ratios as calculated from the equations of Fernstrom and Faller [78]. The concentrations of neutral amino acids in brains of animals with liver disease are in considerable excess of predicted concentrations but seem to follow linear correlations as if subjected to another influence. If, however, glutamine is exchanged across the blood-brain barrier for other neutral amino acids, the excess of observed over predicted values may be correlated with brain glutamine. In fact, the correlation is excellent; only animals with normal brain glutamine have normal brain neutral amino acids [77, 79]. Moreover, isolated brain capillaries preloaded with glutamine and incubated with ammonia, or capillaries from shunted animals, manifest similar increases in capillary neutral amino acid uptake. Blocking synthesis of glutamine with methionine sulfoximine inhibits the increased in vitro uptake of neutral amino acids stimulated by ammonia. For further details, which are beyond the scope of this chapter, the interested reader is referred to Samuels, et al. [77] and Buse and Reid [79].

Thus, if one examines the current unified concept of hepatic encephalopathy, there is provision for ammonia, the disturbed hormonal balance of insulin and glucagon, increased plasma concentrations of phenylalanine, tyrosine, unbound tryptophan, methionine, and histidine, as well as decreased plasma concentrations of their blood-brain barrier competitors, the BCAA. Furthermore, this hypothesis explains the reported beneficial clinical effects of such diverse compounds as L-dopa [80,81], bromocriptine [82], and the BCAA as well as neomycin and lactulose.

Nutritional Support in Hepatic Encephalopathy

Since the initial report by Alexander and colleagues in 1980 [43], it has been recognized that enteral nutrition is physiologically superior to parenteral support in reducing the hypermetabolism of injury. Unfortunately, patients with liver failure, because of liver dysfunction and the subsequent risk of encephalopathy, often cannot tolerate enteral protein loads. Parenteral support is thus called on.

Parenteral nutrition consisting of individual amino acids is better tolerated than equivalent amounts of oral protein. In our clinical experience, even patients with grade 1 encephalopathy will sufficiently normalize their plasma amino acid pattern due to decreased catabolism and increased protein synthesis, so that 50% to 60% will tolerate standard parenteral formulas. However, to deliver sufficient protein equivalent to patients who are catabolic, a special formulation is often necessary.

Beneficial Effects of the Branched-Chain Amino Acids (BCAA)

The use of BCAA-enriched solutions in patients with liver failure is perhaps the earliest example of nutritional pharmacology. There are nine metabolic reasons why BCAA-enriched solutions may be beneficial.

1. BCAA are a useful energy source. Patients with hepatic encephalopathy begin with fewer stores of glycogen and less fat reserves; they are highly catabolic and glucose resistant; and ketogenesis and the utilization of fatty acids are probably decreased because of the impairment of the hepatic mechanism that makes ketone bodies from fatty acids. Under normal circumstances, BCAA comprise only about 6% to 7% of the energy needs. On a theoretical basis, because they do not go through glucose, they conceivably could supply over 30% of the energy needs because there is a glucose resistance, hypermetabolism, and decreased ketogenesis. BCAA may be utilized directly by the muscle, heart, liver, and brain and possibly elsewhere.
2. BCAA decrease the efflux of other amino acids through the myocyte membrane, thus decreasing the aromatic amino acids in the circulation.
3. Leucine decreases muscle proteolysis and increases protein synthesis [52,83–85].
4. Hepatic protein synthesis is apparently increased by all amino acids in humans. In humans, there is evidence that leucine may be the most potent in this regard [86].
5. Administration of BCAA normalizes the plasma amino acid pattern secondary to decreased muscle protein breakdown [36] and increased protein synthesis, thus utilizing the aromatic amino acids. A caloric source of glucose appears better than fat, perhaps because of the influence of insulin [87].
6. The neutral amino acids, including the aromatic amino acids and the BCAA, compete for entry through system-L across the blood-brain barrier. Under normal circumstances, the BCAA provide the bulk of competition. Increasing plasma BCAA concentrations will not only decrease aromatic amino acid plasma levels, as mentioned above, but will also prevent their penetration across the blood-brain barrier by direct competition.
7. In hepatectomized animals, the administration is hypercatabolic of BCAA increases the reduced brain norepinephrine in three of seven regions [88].
8. On a theoretical basis, peripheral catecholamine synthesis will be normalized by having a more normal precursor pool.
9. BCAA increase the metabolism of ammonia by muscle. The BCAA probably donate the amino group for glutamine synthesis [89,90].

Given these benefits, BCAA-enriched, aromatic amino acid–deficient solutions have been available for the past 20 years. A series of clinical trials have been published testing their efficacy in the treatment of hepatic encephalopathy.

Human Trials with BCAA-Enriched Solutions

Anecdotal Studies

The first study demonstrating the benefits of BCAA-enriched solutions was reported in 1976 [91]. There are a number of other anecdotal studies in which various solutions enriched with BCAA have been utilized in the treatment of liver failure and hepatic encephalopathy [92–96]. The results from these first anecdotal studies were positive, and from them several conclusions can be made:

1. In patients who are intolerant to conventional solutions or to oral protein and who have a history or presence of hepatic encephalopathy, up to 125 g of BCAA-enriched solutions are well tolerated [11].
2. Instead of aggravating hepatic encephalopathy with the high amino acid load, hepatic encephalopathy is actually ameliorated, with the patient's mental status improving.
3. BCAA-enriched solutions are designed for the treatment of acute-on-chronic hepatic failure and not fulminant hepatitis, in which the plasma amino acid pattern is quite different from that of acute-on-chronic hepatic failure. Massive hyperaminoacidemia occurs in fulminant hepatitis, reflecting a dying liver. There are reports, however, suggesting a beneficial effect in fulminant hepatitis [92].
4. Hepatic failure is hypercatabolic [11,97], with a doubling of normal amino acid requirements from 0.55 g/kg/day to 1.1 g/kg/day in liver failure patients given a caloric source of 30 to 35 kcal/kg/day. Only with near-positive nitrogen balance will the full benefits of the BCAA on brain aromatic amino acids levels and the resulting effect on hepatic encephalopathy be apparent.

Randomized Prospective Trials

Early anecdotal reports stimulated significant interest in BCAA-enriched solutions, resulting in seven properly carried out randomized prospective trials in the treatment of hepatic encephalopathy [98–105], all of which differed in design and execution (Table 24-1). Unfortunately, while all agree it would have been desirable to compare the BCAA-enriched solutions to standard amino acid solutions, limitations imposed by the FDA in some of these trials prevented inclusion of an amino acid control group. In the only trial that attempted to compare two amino acid solutions [102], the "conventional" amino acid mixture was extensively modified from standard solutions, containing more BCAA and less aromatic amino acids. In all but two trials [98–101,103,105], the principal caloric source was hypertonic glucose. All of these trials demonstrated a positive effect of BCAA solutions. In the remaining two trials [102,104], lipid was used as the primary caloric source; although the results showed no benefit, this may reflect the energy source and not the amino acid solutions used.

The beneficial effects of the BCAA-enriched solutions can be put into three categories: (1) "wake-up" time, (2) nutritional effects, and (3) outcome and survival.

"Wake-up" Time. Wake-up from hepatic encephalopathy was at least as good and more rapid in patients receiving BCAA-enriched solutions as compared to the standard medical treatment of lactulose/neomycin, and significantly better than the control group receiving hypertonic dextrose alone (Table 24-2). In the U.S. multicenter trial [98], wake-up to grade 1 encephalopathy was 77% as opposed to 26% in the neomycin control group. In the Danish prospective trial [101] in which concurrent therapy was utilized for patients who had remained in hepatic encephalopathy for 4 days, improvement from encephalopathy was at least twice as fast in patients receiving BCAA-

Table 24-1. Trial Design, Groups, and Therapy

Lead author	Arm 1	Arm 2	Arm 3
Rossi-Fanelli [103]	Lactulose + $D_{20}W$	$D_{20}W$ + BCAA	
Fiaccadori [100]	Lactulose + $D_{30}W$ (A)	$D_{30}W$ + FO80 (B)	A + B
Michel [102]	Conventional amino acid formula	FO80 (glucose and fat)	
Wahren [104]	D_5W (+ 30 cal/kg/day glucose and fat)	BCAA (+ 30 cal/kg/day glucose and fat)	
Cerra [99]	Neomycin + $D_{25}W$	$D_{25}W$ + FO80 + placebo	
Gluud [101]	$D_{30}W$	$D_{25}W$ + FO80	
U.S. multicenter [98]	Neomycin + $D_{25}W$	$D_{25}W$ + FO80 + placebo	
Strauss [105]	Neomycin + $D_{25}W$	$D_{25}W$ + FO80	

Table 24-2. Wake-up Rate (to Grade 0/0–1) from Hepatic Encephalopathy

	Wake-up rate (%)		Time interval to wake-up	
Lead author	Control	Study	Control	Study
Rossi-Fanelli [103]	47	70	31.5 hr	27.6 hr
Fiaccadori [100]	56	94-100*	—	—
Michel [102]	25	35	—	—
Wahren [104]	48	56	—	—
Cerra [99]	25	56*	—	—
Gluud [101]	60	70	4 days	2 days*
U.S. multicenter [98]	17 (26)	53* (77)	—	5-6 days
Strauss [105]	67	93	71 hr	33 hr

*$p < 0.05$. Figures in parentheses represent wake-up to grade 1.

enriched solutions (26% BCAA/patient/24 hr) as compared to hypertonic glucose (12.5%/patient/24 hr). In the Italian trial reported by Rossi-Fanelli et al. [103], 70% of patients treated with BCAA and hypertonic dextrose were awake at the end of 48 hours, versus only 47% of those treated with lactulose alone. In the other Italian trial reported by Fiaccadori et al. [100], BCAA either alone or with lactulose resulted in wake-up rates of 94% and 100%, respectively, at the end of the treatment period as opposed to 56% with lactulose alone. In the Brazilian trial reported by Strauss et al. [105], patients treated with BCAA-enriched solutions had a mean wake-up time of 33 hours as opposed to 71 hours in the neomycin control group. Although statistical significance was not achieved in some of these studies (due to small sample size), a recent meta-analysis combining these trials [106] has demonstrated the overall effectiveness of BCAA-enriched solutions in the treatment of hepatic encephalopathy when glucose is used as the caloric source.

Nutritional Effects. One of the major objectives of any form of nutritional support is to limit the catabolism of illness and to maintain protein stores. One measure of the effectiveness of the nutritional intervention is nitrogen balance. As mentioned above, patients in hepatic failure are hypercatabolic, requiring 1.1 g protein/kg/24 hr. Unfortunately, nitrogen balance was measured in only a few of these trials. In only the U.S. multicenter trial [98] did patients receiving BCAA-enriched solutions come close to achieving nitrogen equilibrium. In contrast, the report by Michel et al. [102] showed patients with nitrogen balance of −10 g/24 hr despite nutritional support. This may explain some of the discrepancies between the positive results obtained from the U.S. multicenter trial as compared with some of the other trials.

Outcome and Survival. Patients with hepatic encephalopathy are critically ill, and it is unlikely that the differences accrued from nutritional intervention are to be greater than 10% to 15% given the severity of illness. In only the U.S. multicenter trial [98] and the Italian trial reported by Fiaccadori et al. [100] were sufficient numbers of patients enrolled to demonstrate this level of difference in survival between the two groups. It is of interest therefore that only in these two trials did survival improve with BCAA-enriched solutions (Table 24-3). In the U.S. multicenter trial [98], statistically improved survival was seen with BCAA as compared to neomycin, while in the Italian trial [100], statistically improved survival was observed with the BCAA as compared to lactulose. In all of the other studies, statistically significant differences between treatment groups were not obtained. This again may reflect the small numbers of patients in each individual study.

Table 24-3. Survival from Hepatic Encephalopathy

	Mortality (%)	
Lead author	Control	Study
Rossi-Fanelli [103]	29	23
Fiaccadori [100]	46	3
Michel [102]	25	30
Wahren [104]	20 (70)*	40 (70)*
Cerra [99]	25 (40)*	0 (17)*
Gluud [101]	10	20
U.S. multicenter [98]	55 (69)*	17 (27)*
Discharged alive	26	55
Strauss [105]	13	13

*Figures in parentheses represent overall in-hospital mortality.

Additional evidence for the efficacy of a 35% branched chain–enriched, aromatic amino acid–deficient solution with hypertonic dextrose was recently published by Fan and associates at the University of Hong Kong [107]. In a prospective trial, 124 patients undergoing resection of hepatocellular carcinoma were randomized for half of the patients to receive only oral nutrition and the other half to receive perioperative intravenous nutritional support using the aforementioned solution. A lipid emulsion and dextrose were used as the caloric sources, with medium-chain triglycerides comprising 50% of the lipids. There was a statistically significant reduction in the overall postoperative morbidity rate in the perioperative nutrition group as compared to the control group (34% vs. 55%, $p < 0.05$), predominantly because of fewer septic complications (17% vs. 37%, $p < 0.05$). In addition, there was a lower incidence of the necessity for using diuretic agents to control ascites (25% vs. 50%, $p < 0.05$), less weight loss (0 kg vs. 1.4 kg, $p = 0.01$), and less deterioration of liver function as measured by the change in rate of indocyanine green clearance (−2.8% vs. 4.8%, $p < 0.05$). However, the difference in mortality (5 of 64 in the perioperative nutrition group and 9 of 60 in the control group) was not statistically significant. Thus, in patients with cirrhosis undergoing a significant hepatic resection, the outcome can be improved considerably by perioperative parenteral nutrition, as shown in this study of patients who were treated 7 days preoperatively and 7 days postoperatively for 12 hours overnight. Whether a larger group of patients or different measurements would have resulted in a statistically significant improvement in mortality is not clear from this study.

Oral Trials

BCAA-enriched solutions have also been tested in enteral nutritional formulations in the treatment of patients with chronic hepatic encephalopathy. Several studies with small sample sizes did not show a beneficial effect of BCAA solutions. However, in studies with larger patient sample sizes (greater than 20), BCAA-enriched solutions improved hepatic encephalopathy and nitrogen balance [108–111].

Based on these trials, the efficacy of the BCAA-enriched solutions, in conjunction with glucose as the caloric source, in the treatment of hepatic encephalopathy has been established. It would also appear that the BCAA-enriched solutions have a positive effect in terms of outcome during hepatic encephalopathy.

Criteria for the Institution of BCAA-Enriched Solutions

We use BCAA-enriched solutions according to the following criteria:

1. Hepatic encephalopathy of grade 2 or higher.
2. BCAA-aromatic amino acid ratio less than 2.5 in a patient with preexisting liver dysfunction.
3. A patient with known hepatic dysfunction whose mental status is indeterminable (for example, because the patient is intubated).
4. Intolerance to greater than 40 to 50 g of a commercially available amino acid mixture. As previously mentioned, approximately half of patients requiring parenteral nutrition will tolerate standard amino acid mixtures. Because 40 to 50 g of protein is insufficient for long-term nutritional support, changing to a BCAA-enriched solution is indicated.

Whenever possible, we utilize the enteral route using Hepatic-Aid, the BCAA-enriched enteral formulation. If enteral nutrition is contraindicated, parenteral access is obtained and Hepatamine, the BCAA-enriched parenteral formulation, is administered.

Hepatamine contains 4% amino acids and 25% hypertonic glucose. Patients are begun at a rate of 40 ml/hr, and the rate is increased by 20 ml/hr/day until the targeted caloric requirement is reached. This invariably results in greater than 75 to 80 g amino acids/day. If glucose intolerance is present, a 15% glucose solution is utilized.

Liver Failure in Patients with Sepsis and Multisystem Organ Failure

Although the efficacy of BCAA-enriched parenteral solutions has not been clearly established in patients with sepsis, patients who are septic and have altered mental status and liver dysfunction can be supported with Hepatamine because some of the metabolic abnormalities that occur during sepsis are comparable to the changes that occur during liver failure, including glucose resistance and decreased utilization of fat as a caloric source. This combination explains the excessive protein degradation that occurs during sepsis, that is, amino acids are again being used as a source of energy. If sepsis continues unabated, the syndrome of multisystem organ failure can result, with the liver being the central organ involved. Once this process begins, the similarity to hepatic failure becomes even more pronounced. Freund et al. [112] noted that the distinctive plasma amino acid pattern in sepsis and septic encephalopathy has many similarities to the amino acid profile of liver failure. Plasma levels of the amino acids phenylalanine, tyrosine, methionine, and cysteine are elevated; however, BCAA levels are low-normal to normal rather than decreased as in hepatic encephalopathy. Based on a number of studies, septic encephalopathy and survival can be predicted from amino acid patterns [113].

Combined Hepatic and Renal Failure

A frequent dilemma is how to treat a patient with the hepatorenal syndrome, that is, combined liver and renal failure. This is an extraordinarily difficult circumstance in which there are few readily available solutions. Each solution exacts a price, and one must select which complication seems most manageable. If for some reason a patient in renal failure will not readily tolerate dialysis, usually because of decreased peripheral resistance, Nephramine or a similar hypertonic dextrose-essential amino acid solution can be used. These solutions, however, usually consist largely of the aromatic amino acids, with fewer BCAA. While the rise in blood urea nitrogen (BUN) will be diminished if hepatic encephalopathy is present, as is usually the case in the hepatorenal syndrome, this will aggravate the encephalopathy. If one chooses to treat the encephalopathy with a BCAA-enriched, aromatic amino acid–deficient hypertonic dextrose solution, this is usually effective, at least temporarily, from the standpoint of hepatic encephalopathy. Unfortunately, the BUN elevation rises rapidly. One can be comforted by the fact, and indeed this is small comfort, that the disease is usually fatal, and it is usually not possible to salvage patients with hepatorenal syndrome unless there is improvement in hepatic function. Thus, any improvement in survival of these patients results from the improvement in hepatic function, not from whatever treatment we may choose.

Summary

Nutritional support in patients with liver failure has undergone significant improvement over the past 25 years with the development and proven efficacy of BCAA-enriched amino acid solutions. This, along with the development of Nephramine, represents the inception of nutritional pharmacology. As the nutritional needs of patients become better understood from the standpoint of molecular biology, nutritional pharmacology may become the basis for all future nutritional support.

References

1. Brems J, et al. Fulminant hepatic failure: The role of liver transplantation as primary therapy. *Am J Surg* 154:137, 1987.
2. Chapman R, et al. Liver transplantation for acute hepatic failure? *Lancet* 335:32, 1990.
3. Iwatsuki K, et al. Liver transplantation in the treatment of bleeding esophageal varices. *Surgery* 104:697, 1988.
4. Rozga J, et al. A bioartificial lever to treat severe acute liver failure. *Ann Surg* 219:538, 1994.
5. Sussman N, et al. Reversal of fulminant hepatic failure using an extracorporeal liver device. *Hepatology* 16:60, 1992.
6. Chari RS, et al. Brief report: Treatment of hepatic failure with ex vivo pig liver perfusion followed by liver transfusion. *N Engl J Med* 331:234, 1994.
7. Eisman B, Liem D, Raffucci F. Heterologous liver perfusion in treatment of hepatic failure. *Ann Surg* 162:329, 1965.
8. Platt H, et al. Transplantation of discordant xenografts: A review of progress. *Immunol Today* 11:450, 1990.
9. O'Grady J, et al. Controlled trials of charcoal hemoperfusion and prognostic factors in fulminant hepatic failure. *Gastroenterology* 94:1186, 1988.
10. Nakamura T, et al. Molecular cloning and expression of human hepatocyte growth factor. *Nature* 342:440, 1989.
11. Freund H, et al. Infusion of branched-chain amino acid solution in patients with hepatic encephalopathy. *Ann Surg* 196:209, 1982.
12. Nasrallah SM, Galambos JT. Amino acid therapy in alcoholic hepatitis. *Lancet* 2:1276, 1980.
13. Sax H, Talamini M, Fischer JE. Clinical use of branched-chain amino acids in liver disease, sepsis, trauma and burns. *Arch Surg* 121:358, 1986.
14. Sherlock S. *Diseases of the Liver and Biliary System.* Oxford: Blackwell, 1975. P 427.
15. Brunkhorst R, et al. Renal effects of atrial natriuretic peptide in cirrhotic rats with and without captopril pretreatment. *Nephron* 64:275, 1993.
16. Baldessarini RJ, Fischer JE. S-adenosyl-methionine following portacaval anastomoses. *Surgery* 62:311, 1967.
17. Fischer JE. Portal hypertension and bleeding esophageal varices. *Am J Surg* 140:337, 1980.
18. Burchell AR, et al. Hepatic artery flow improvement after portacaval shunt: A single hemodynamic clinical correlate. *Ann Surg* 184:289, 1976.
19. Parke WF, Rousselot LM, Burchell AR. A sixteen year experience with end-to-side portacaval shunt for variceal hemorrhage. Analysis of data and comparison with other types of portosystemic anastomoses. *Ann Surg* 168:957, 1968.
20. Fischer JE, et al. Comparison of distal and proximal splenorenal shunts: A randomized prospective trial. *Ann Surg* 194:531, 1981.
21. Sherwin R, et al. Hyperglucagonemia in Laennec's cirrhosis: The role of portal-systemic shunting. *N Engl J Med* 290:239, 1974.
22. Eigler N, Sacca L, Sherwin RS. Synergistic interactions of physiologic investment of glucagon, epinephrine and cortisol in the dog. A model for stress-induced hyperglycemia. *J Clin Invest* 63:114, 1979.
23. Soeters PB, Fischer JE. Insulin, glucagon, amino acid imbalance, and hepatic encephalopathy. *Lancet* 2:880, 1976.

24. Soeters PB, et al. Insulin, glucagon, portal-systemic shunting, and hepatic failure in the dog. *J Surg Res* 23:183, 1977.
25. Fischer JE, et al. A unified hypothesis on hepatic encephalopathy. In Orloff MJ, Stipa S, Ziparo V (eds), *Medical and Surgical Problems of Portal Hypertension,* Vol 34. London: Academic, 1980.
26. Strombeck DR, Rogers Q, Stern JS. Effects of intravenous ammonia infusion on plasma levels of amino acids, glucagon, and insulin in dogs [Abstract]. *Gastroenterology* 74:1165, 1978.
27. Biebuyck JF, et al. Neurochemistry of hepatic coma: Alterations in putative transmitter amino acids. In Williams R, Murray-Lyons IM (eds), *Artificial Liver Support* (Proceedings of an International Symposium on Artificial Support Systems for Acute Hepatic Failure). London: Pittman, 1974. P 51.
28. Felig P. The glucose alanine cycle. *Metabolism* 22:179, 1973.
29. Zieve FJ, et al. Synergism between ammonia and fatty acids in the production of coma: Implications for hepatic coma. *J Pharmacol Exp Ther* 191:10, 1974.
30. Morgan MH, et al. Medium chain triglycerides and hepatic encephalopathy. *Gut* 15:180, 1974.
31. Budd MA, et al. Isovaleric acidemia: Clinical features of a new genetic defect of leucine metabolism. *N Engl J Med* 277:321, 1967.
32. Tanaka K, Isselbacher KF, Shih V. Isovaleric and alphamethylbutyric acidemias induced by hypoglycin A: Mechanism of Jamaican vomiting sickness. *Science* 175:69, 1972.
33. McMenamy RH, Oncley JL. The specific binding of L-tryptophan to serum albumin. *J Biol Chem* 233:1436, 1958.
34. Cummings MG, et al. Regional brain study of indoleamine metabolism in the rat in acute hepatic failure. *J Neurochem* 27:741, 1976.
35. Fischer JE, et al. Plasma amino acids in patients with hepatic encephalopathy: Effects of amino acid infusions. *Am J Surg* 127:40, 1974.
36. Felig P. Amino acid metabolism in man. *Annu Rev Biochem* 44:936, 1975.
37. Rosen HM, et al. Plasma amino acid patterns in hepatic encephalopathy of differing etiology. *Gastroenterology* 72:483, 1977.
38. Cardelli-Cangiano P, et al. Uptake of amino acids by brain microvessels isolated from rats after portacaval anastomosis. *J Neurochem* 36:627, 1981.
39. Ono J, et al. Tryptophan and hepatic coma. *Gastroenterology* 74:196, 1978.
40. Levine RJ, Conn HO. Tyrosine metabolism in patients with liver disease. *J Clin Invest* 46:2012, 1967.
41. Pardridge WM, Jefferson LS. Liver uptake of amino acids and carbohydrates during a single circulatory passage. *Am J Physiol* 228:1155, 1975.
42. Jeejeebhoy KN, Phillip RJ. Isolated mammalian hepatocytes in culture. *Gastroenterology* 71:1086, 1976.
43. Alexander JW, et al. Beneficial effects of aggressive protein feeding in severely burned children. *Ann Surg* 192:505, 1980.
44. Dawson AM, Sherlock S. Effect of an amine oxidase inhibitor in liver disease. *Lancet* 1:1332, 1957.
45. Warren KS, Schenker S. Effect of an inhibitor of glutamine synthesis (methionine sulfoximine) on ammonia toxicity and metabolism. *J Lab Clin Med* 64:442, 1964.
46. Schafer DF, Jones EA. Hepatic encephalopathy and the gamma-aminobutyric system. *Lancet* 1:18, 1982.
47. Ferenci P, et al. Changes in the status of neurotransmitter receptors in a rabbit model of hepatic encephalopathy. *Hepatology* 4:186, 1984.
48. Ferenci P, et al. Serum levels of gamma-aminobutyric acid-like activity in acute and chronic hepatocellular disease. *Lancet* 1:811, 1983.
49. Levy LJ, Losowsky MS. Plasma gamma aminobutyric acid concentrations provide evidence of different mechanisms in the pathogenesis of hepatic encephalopathy in acute and chronic liver disease. *Hepatogastroenterology* 36:494, 1989.
50. Moroni F, et al. Hepatic encephalopathy: Lack of changes of gamma aminobutyric acid content in plasma and cerebrospinal fluid. *Hepatology* 7:816, 1987.
51. Lavoie J, et al. Amino acid changes in autopsied brain tissue from cirrhotic patients with hepatic encephalopathy. *J Neurochem* 49:692, 1987.
52. Butterworth RF, et al. Affinities and densities of high affinity [^{3}H]muscimol (GABA-A) binding sites and of central benzodiazepine receptors are unchanged in autopsied brain tissue from cirrhotic patients with hepatic encephalopathy. *Hepatology* 8:1084, 1988.
53. Olasmaa M, et al. Endogenous benzodiazepine receptor ligands in human and animal hepatic encephalopathy. *J Neurochem* 55:2015, 1990.
54. Butterworth RF, et al. Effect of portacaval anastomosis on electrically stimulated release of glutamate from rat hippocampal slices. *J Neurochem* 56:1481, 1991.
55. Tossman U, et al. Brain cortical amino acids measured by intracerebral dialysis in portacaval shunted rats. *Neurochem Res* 12:265, 1987.
56. Peterson C, et al. Selective loss of N-methyl-D-aspartate-sensitive L-[^{3}H]glutamine binding sites in rat brain following portacaval anastomosis. *J Neurochem* 55:386, 1990.
57. Maddison JE, et al. Alterations in cortical [^{3}H]kainate and α-[^{3}H]amino-3-hydroxy-5-methyl-4-isoxazolepropionic acid binding in a spontaneous canine model of chronic hepatic encephalopathy. *J Neurochem* 56:1881, 1991.
58. James JH, et al. Hyperammonemia, plasma amino acid imbalance, and blood-brain amino acid transport: A unified theory of portalsystemic encephalopathy. *Lancet* 2:772, 1979.
59. Dismukes K. New look at the aminergic nervous system. *Nature* 269:557, 1977.
60. Oldendorf WH. Brain uptake of radiolabelled amino acids, amines and hexoses after arterial injection. *Am J Physiol* 221:1629, 1971.
61. Pardridge WM, Oldendorf WH. Kinetic analysis of blood-brain barrier transport of amino acids. *Biochim Biophys Acta* 401:128, 1975.
62. James JH, Escourrou J, Fischer JE. Blood-brain neutral amino acid transport activity is increased after portacaval anastomosis. *Science* 200:1395, 1978.
63. Dodsworth JM, et al. Depletion of brain norepinephrine in acute hepatic coma. *Surgery* 75:811, 1974.
64. Faraj BA, Camp VM, Ansley JD. Evidence for central hypertyraminemia in hepatic encephalopathy. *J Clin Invest* 67:395, 1981.
65. Baldessarini RJ, Fischer JE. Serotonin metabolism in

rat brain after surgical diversion of the portal venous circulation. *Nature (New Biol)* 254:25, 1973.

66. Curzon G, et al. Effects of chronic portacaval anastomosis on brain tryptophan, tyrosine and 5-hydroxytryptamine. *J Neurochem* 24:1065, 1975.
67. Fischer JE. False neurotransmitters and hepatic coma. *Res Publ Assoc Res Nerv Ment Dis* 53:53, 1974.
68. Fischer JE, Baldessarini RJ. False neurotransmitters and hepatic failure. *Lancet* 2:75, 1971.
69. Lam KC, et al. Role of a false neurotransmitter, octopamine, in the pathogenesis of hepatic and renal encephalopathy. *Scand J Gastroenterol* 8:465, 1973.
70. Manghani KK, et al. Urinary and serum octopamine in patients with portal-systemic encephalopathy. *Lancet* 2:943, 1975.
71. Nespoli A, et al. The role of false neurotransmitters in the pathogenesis of hepatic encephalopathy and hyperdynamic syndrome in cirrhosis. *Arch Surg* 116:1129, 1981.
72. Rossi-Fanelli F, et al. Phenylethanolamine and octopamine in hepatic encephalopathy. In Mosnaim AD, Wolf ME (eds), *Noncatecholic Phenylethylamines*. New York: Dekker, 1980. P 231.
73. Knell AJ, et al. Dopamine and serotonin metabolism in hepatic encephalopathy. *Br Med J* 1:549, 1974.
74. Berl S, et al. Metabolic compartments in vivo: Ammonia and glutamic acid metabolism in brain and liver. *J Biol Chem* 237:2562, 1962.
75. Hourani BT, Hamlin EM, Reynolds TB. Cerebrospinal fluid glutamine as a measure of hepatic encephalopathy. *Arch Intern Med* 127:1033, 1971.
76. Smith AR, et al. Alterations in plasma and CSF amino acids, amines and metabolites in hepatic coma. *Ann Surg* 187:343, 1978.
77. Samuels S, Fish F, Freedman LS. Effect of gammaglutamyl cycle inhibitors on brain amino acid transport and utilization. *Neurochem Res* 3:619, 1978.
78. Fernstrom JD, Faller DV. Neutral amino acids in brain: Changes in response to food ingestion. *J Neurochem* 30:1531, 1978.
79. Buse MG, Reid M. Leucine, a possible regulation of protein turnover in muscle. *J Clin Invest* 56:1250, 1975.
80. Fischer JE, James JH. Treatment of hepatic coma and hepatorenal syndrome. Mechanism of L-dopa and aramine. *Am J Surg* 123:222, 1972.
81. Parkes JD, Sharpstone P, Williams R. Levodopa in hepatic coma. *Lancet* 2:1341, 1970.
82. Morgan M, Jacobovitz A, Ellithorn A. Successful use of bromocriptine in the treatment of patients with chronic portasystemic encephalopathy. *N Engl J Med* 296:793, 1977.
83. Chua B, Siehl D, Morgan H. A role for leucine in regulation of protein turnover in working rat hearts. *Am J Physiol* 239:E510, 1980.
84. Chua B, Siehl D, Morgan H. Effect of leucine and metabolites of branched chain amino acids on protein turnover in heart. *J Biol Chem* 54:8358, 1979.
85. Odessy R, Goldberg AL. Oxidation of amino acids by diaphragm from fed and fasted rats. *Am J Physiol* 223:1384, 1972.
86. Bower RH, Fischer JE. Hepatic indications for parenteral nutrition. In Rombeau J, Caldwell M (eds), *Clinical Nutrition: Parenteral Nutrition*. Philadelphia: Saunders, 1986. P 602.
87. Gelfand RA, Hendler RS, Sherwin RS. Dietary carbohydrate and metabolism of ingested protein. *Lancet* 1:65, 1979.
88. Herlin P, et al. Effect of total hepatectomy and administration of branched chain amino acids on regional norepinephrine, dopamine, and amino acids in rat brain. *Ann Surg* 198:172, 1983.
89. Lockwood AH, et al. The dynamics of ammonia metabolism in man: Effect of liver disease and hyperammonemia. *J Clin Invest* 63:449, 1979.
90. Riggio O, et al. Influence of ammonia on leucine utilization in muscle and adipose tissue in vitro. *Surg Forum* 35:95, 1984.
91. Fischer JE, et al. The effect of normalization of plasma amino acids on hepatic encephalopathy in man. *Surgery* 80:77, 1976.
92. Fryden A, Weiland O, Martensson J. Successful treatment of hepatic coma with balanced solution of amino acids. *Scand J Infect Dis* 14:180, 1982.
93. Higashi T, et al. Effect of branched chain amino acid infusion on alterations on CSF neutral amino acids and their transport across the blood-brain barrier in hepatic encephalopathy. In Walser M, Williamson R (eds), *Metabolism and Clinical Implications of Branched Chain Amino and Ketoacids*. New York: Elsevier, 1981. P 465.
94. Holm E, et al. Amino acid solutions for parenteral nutrition and for adjuvant treatment of encephalopathy in liver cirrhosis: Studies concerning 120 patients. In Walser M, Williamson R (eds), *Metabolism and Clinical Implications of Branched Chain Amino and Ketoacids*. New York: Elsevier, 1981. P 513.
95. Okada A, et al. Treatment of hepatic encephalopathy with BCAA-enriched amino acid mixtures. In Walser M, Williamson R (eds), *Metabolism and Clinical Implications of Branched Chain Amino and Ketoacids*. New York: Elsevier, 1981. P 447.
96. Watanabe A, et al. Serum amino acids in hepatic encephalopathy: Effects of branched chain amino acid solutions on serum amino gram. *Acta Hepatogastroenterology* 26:346, 1979.
97. Marchesni G, et al. Anticatabolic effects of branched-chain amino acid enriched solutions in patients with liver cirrhosis. *Hepatology* 2:420, 1982.
98. Cerra FB, et al. Disease-specific amino acid solution (F080) in hepatic encephalopathy: A prospective, randomized, double-blind, controlled study. *JPEN* 9:288, 1985.
99. Cerra FB, et al. Cirrhosis, encephalopathy and improved results with metabolic support. *Surgery* 94:612, 1983.
100. Fiaccadori F, et al. Branched chain amino acid enriched solutions in the treatment of hepatic encephalopathy: A controlled trial. In Capocaccia L, Fischer JE, Rossi-Fanelli F (eds), *Hepatic Encephalopathy in Chronic Liver Failure*. New York: Plenum, 1984. P 333.
101. Gluud C, et al. Preliminary treatment results with balanced amino acid infusion to patients with hepatic encephalopathy [Abstract]. *Scand J Gastroenterol* 18(Suppl 86):19, 1983.
102. Michel H, et al. Treatment of hepatic encephalopathy by infusion of a modified amino acid solution: Results of a controlled study of 47 cirrhotic patients. In Capocaccia L, Fischer JE, Rossi-Fanelli F (eds), *Hepatic Encephalopathy in Chronic Liver Failure*. New York: Plenum, 1984. P 301.
103. Rossi-Fanelli F, et al. Branched chain amino acid vs. lactulose in the treatment of hepatic coma: A controlled study. *Dig Dis Sci* 27:929, 1982.

104. Wahren J, et al. Is intravenous administration of branched chain amino acids effective in the treatment of hepatic encephalopathy? A multicenter study. *Hepatology* 3:475, 1983.

105. Strauss E, et al. A randomized controlled clinical trial for the evaluation of the efficacy of an enriched branched chain amino acid solution compared to neomycin in hepatic encephalopathy. *Hepatology* 3:862, 1983.

106. Naylor CD, et al. Parenteral nutrition with branched-chain amino acids in hepatic encephalopathy: A meta-analysis. *Gastroenterology* 97:1033, 1989.

107. Fan S-T, et al. Perioperative nutritional support in patients undergoing hepatectomy for hepatocellular carcinoma. *N Engl J Med* 331:1547, 1994.

108. McGhee A, et al. Comparison of the effects of Hepatic-Aid and a casein modular diet on encephalopathy, plasma amino acids and nitrogen balance in cirrhotic patients. *Ann Surg* 197:288, 1983.

109. Egberts SH, et al. Branched chain amino acids in the treatment of latent portosystemic encephalopathy: A double-blind placebo-controlled crossover study. *Gastroenterology* 88:887, 1985.

110. Horst D, et al. Comparison of dietary protein with an oral branched-chain enriched amino acid supplement in chronic portal-systemic encephalopathy: A randomized controlled trial. *Hepatology* 4:279, 1984.

111. Marchesni G, et al. Long-term oral branched-chain amino acid treatment in chronic hepatic encephalopathy: A randomized double-blind casein-controlled trial. *J Hepatology* 11:92, 1990.

112. Freund H, Ryan JA, Fischer JE. Amino acid derangements in patients with sepsis: Treatment with branched chain amino acid enriched infusions. *Ann Surg* 188:423, 1978.

113. Freund H, et al. Plasma amino acids as predictors of the severity and outcome of sepsis. *Ann Surg* 190:571, 1979.

Selected Readings

Cerra FB, et al. Disease-specific amino acid solution (F080) in hepatic encephalopathy: A prospective, randomized, double-blind, controlled study. *JPEN* 9:288, 1985.

This paper presents the results of the U.S. multicenter trial on the effects of intravenous BCAA-enriched solutions on hepatic encephalopathy. In conjunction with other studies, this study demonstrates the benefits of BCAA on hepatic encephalopathy and mortality.

Egberts SH, et al. Branched chain amino acids in the treatment of latent portosystemic encephalopathy: A double-blind placebo-controlled crossover study. *Gastroenterology* 88: 887, 1985.

In this paper, the beneficial effects of oral BCAA-enriched solutions on a series of psychomotor functions are presented. This paper, in conjunction with other studies, demonstrates the benefits of BCAA when given orally in hepatic encephalopathy.

Naylor CD, et al. Parenteral nutrition with branched-chain amino acids in hepatic encephalopathy: A meta-analysis. *Gastroenterology* 97:1033, 1989.

This paper presents a meta-analysis of all current BCAA studies, showing the clear benefits of BCAA in hepatic encephalopathy.

25

Nutritional Management in Acute Renal Failure

Tory A. Meyer
Gary W. Raff
Josef E. Fischer

Studies suggest that as many as 5% of hospitalized patients develop a deterioration in renal function and that 20% of these go on to fulminant acute renal failure [1,2]. Acute renal failure is most often (50%–60%) secondary to poor renal perfusion on the basis of hypotension, hypovolemia, or cardiac failure [3], with sepsis playing a role in 20% of cases. The hypermetabolic response to injury and acute renal failure has been shown to be associated with significant morbidity, including impaired wound healing [4], immunosuppression [5], and loss of essential protein stores [6–8]. The mortality of these patients is also high, with estimates of 40% to 70% mortality [9]. In both experimental models and clinical trials, nutritional support has been found to aid in renal recovery or nitrogen balance [10–14] and to reduce morbidity and mortality in surgical patients [12,14,15]. Although other studies refute the efficacy of specific formulations, careful consideration of nutritional requirements is an essential part of comprehensive patient care.

This chapter will discuss the many metabolic abnormalities that occur in acute renal failure, their implications for nutritional treatment before and after the institution of dialysis, and the prospects for future therapies for this disease.

Editor's Note: I originally asked Dr. Ronald Abel to write this chapter. He and Dr. Gary Raff began the chapter, but it could not be completed because of Dr. Abel's tragic death. Dr. Meyer and I completed the chapter.

Metabolic Abnormalities

The metabolic derangements of acute renal failure are often difficult to distinguish from the effects of the inciting trauma or infection. However, both conditions are characterized by catabolism and altered metabolism of proteins and their constituents, carbohydrates, lipids, vitamins, minerals, and electrolytes [2].

Protein

Muscle catabolism is a primary feature of the metabolic response to both injury and acute renal failure. As renal failure alone may be responsible for losses of 150 to 200 g/day of protein [16], this response may be devastating in an already injured hypermetabolic patient. In experiments of starvation in animals, death was associated with as little as 25% depletion of protein stores [17]. A variety of factors in renal failure are believed to drive this catabolic response.

Insulin is an important mediator of amino acid transport into skeletal muscle. Although hyperinsulinemia is characteristic of patients with injury or infection as well as acute renal failure, peripheral resistance to insulin is seen both in uremia [18] and after injury [19]. Increased peripheral resistance to insulin has been demonstrated in an animal model of acute renal failure to cause a decrease in amino acid uptake and insulin-mediated protein synthesis [20].

Other hormones that have been implicated in this catabolic response include glucagon and parathyroid hormone. Glucagon has been found to be elevated in patients with renal failure [21,22]. Intravenous administration of glucagon has been shown to result in a profound increase in urea production, presumably secondary to release of stores of glucogenic amino acids for the process of gluconeogenesis [23]. Parathyroid hormone excretion has been found to be elevated in acute renal failure [24] and is a known stimulant of muscle catabolism [25]. It has thus been proposed as a mediator of protein loss, as unlikely as it seems. In an in vitro rat muscle preparation, parathyroid hormone was found to cause a dose-dependent increase in amino acid release [25]. However, studies in uremic patients after parathyroidectomy have failed to show metabolic effects, casting doubt on the role of this hormone in renal failure [26].

It is far more likely that other substances such as cytokines are involved in the catabolic response. Tumor necrosis factor (TNF) and interleukin-1 (IL-1), often elevated in patients with sepsis or trauma, have been shown to induce muscle proteolysis [27,28]. The process of hemodialysis itself is believed to exacerbate cytokine production, as monocyte activation with release of TNF and IL-1 may occur from contact with the dialysis membrane [29]. Synthetic membranes appear to induce less inflammatory reactions and offer potential benefits in this regard [30].

In addition to increased breakdown of protein into urea, there is evidence that patients with renal failure have impaired protein synthetic activity. The accumulation of urea and several other nitrogenous metabolites, such as phenolic acid, guanidines, and middle molecules, have been found to interfere with protein metabolism [31]. Delaporte and coworkers have also shown that these presumed "uremic toxins" from plasma dialysates of uremic patients decrease protein synthesis in vitro [32,33]. By examining the effect of plasma on protein synthesis from patients before and after hemodialysis, they have shown that these inhibitory substances may be dialyzed and are absent once patients undergo renal transplant. The patient with renal failure complicating sepsis is likely to be particularly prone to this inhibition of protein synthesis, as plasma from septic patients has also been shown to inhibit protein synthesis in vitro [8]. Because TNF and IL-1 inhibit protein synthesis in addition to promoting muscle catabolism [28], these cytokines and others may be playing a role in this metabolic response.

Urea

The major nitrogenous end product of protein metabolism is urea. Because the hypermetabolism of the underlying sepsis or trauma is characterized, at least in part, by glutamine and alanine release with conversion to urea, hypermetabolic patients with renal failure and a decreased capacity to excrete urea are especially prone to become uremic. Work by Lacy [34] has shown that acute uremia in rats stimulates hepatic urea production, mainly by conversion of gluconeogenic amino acids into glucose and urea. Similarly, Frohlich and coworkers demonstrated that rats rendered acutely uremic by nephrectomy had higher rates of gluconeogenesis and ureagenesis compared to control and sham-operated animals [35]. Evidence that the source of these amino acids is catabolized muscle is seen in experiments of isolated muscle from uremic mice in which higher rates of alanine and glutamine release are noted versus pair-fed control animals [36]. This endogenous proteolytic rather than dietary source of urea has been supported in studies of patients with renal failure who are given no nitrogen intake but who have maintained concomitant high urea nitrogen appearance [16]. Patients with rhabdomyolysis or sepsis and renal failure have the highest degree of protein breakdown, and in one study urea nitrogen appearance was approximately 12 g/day, nearly four times that of other patients in renal failure [16].

The increase in urea nitrogen appearance in patients with renal failure does not appear to have nutritional value. Although early experiments with low-protein diets were interpreted as showing nutritional utilization of urea, presumably by intestinal breakdown to ammonia that was subsequently absorbed and utilized, later studies have shown otherwise. In experiments using isotopically labeled urea, Varcoe and coworkers found that only 0.13% of albumin nitrogen was produced from urea in normal subjects and only 2.57% of albumin in patients in chronic renal failure [37]. Furthermore, studies by Mitch et al. [38,39] in which intestinal ureolysis was inhibited with nonabsorbable antibiotics showed that the nitrogen yielded from degraded urea was not being used for amino acid synthesis but was being recycled into urea. Protein balance actually improved when urea production was inhibited, strongly suggesting that urea nitrogen was not contributing to protein production. From these studies, it would seem that there is no nutritional benefit to the elevated urea of renal failure, and the physiologic significance of this increased urea production in uremia remains unclear.

The Aminogram

An examination of the plasma amino acid profile of patients with acute renal failure reveals abnormalities very similar to patients with chronic renal failure or nutritional depletion [2]. There is an overall decrease in the total concentration of essential amino acids and branched chain amino acids (valine, leucine, and isoleucine), although quantities of phenylalanine may be slightly increased [2,16]. Plasma clearance of phenylalanine has been found to be decreased in both acute and chronic renal failure. While impaired conversion of phenylalanine to tyrosine has been described in chronic renal failure, this does not appear to occur in acute renal failure, as tyrosine levels are appropriate with the administration of phenylalanine [40,41]. These findings may indicate that impairment of conversion from phenylalanine to tyrosine, with an obligate buildup of other phenylalanine metabolites, is a relatively late phenomenon in renal failure. It is not a function of hepatic impairment, as might be hypothesized.

Conversely, histidine clearance is increased in both chronic and acute renal failure [2,16]. In patients in chronic renal failure, nitrogen balance was improved following supplementation with histidine, and a clinical syndrome of wasting, abnormal erythropoesis, and skin lesions has been described in patients with histidine-deficient diets [42]. These findings indicate that histidine is an essential amino acid in these patients, and it is now thought that arginine and histidine are semi-essential amino acids and that their rate of synthesis may be insufficient in stress situations. Ultimately, however, in the case of histidine as with the other amino acids, the physiologic impact of their specific deviation from normal levels is poorly understood.

Carbohydrate

Carbohydrate metabolism is adversely affected by both acute renal failure itself as well as the underlying infection or trauma, in a fashion similar to protein metabolism. Because most experimental data has been accumulated in patients with chronic renal failure, extrapolation to the patient with acute renal failure should be applied cautiously. Nevertheless, both acute renal failure and the sepsis or trauma that frequently precipitates renal dysfunction are characterized by problems with decreased peripheral utilization of glucose and increased glucose production.

In a series of studies in chronically uremic men, DeFronzo et al. [18,43] demonstrated that the basis for the glucose intolerance in these patients is a loss of sensitivity to insulin, which is more likely secondary to a postreceptor or membrane transport problem rather than a prereceptor defect. It is probable that this decreased sensitivity to insulin is exacerbated by increased hepatic gluconeogenesis. Frohlich et al. [44] demonstrated increased hepatic gluconeogenesis in experimental models of uremia, largely secondary to serine dehydratase activity. Similarly, trauma patients without renal dysfunction have been shown to have peripheral insulin resistance on the basis of a postreceptor defect [19], and septic patients have been found to have an increase in hepatic gluconeogenesis largely as a result of alanine breakdown [45].

A number of circulating factors in this patient population have been implicated as effective antagonists of the action of insulin, including growth hormone, parathyroid hormone, glucagon, cortisol, and the catecholamines [26,44,46,47]. Sherwin et al. [48] have shown that the increased tissue sensitivity to glucagon seen in renal failure is decreased following dialysis. This may be one reason why dialysis improves glucose tolerance. Although the serum levels of these hormones are generally elevated in acute renal failure patients, no studies have been able to show a clear relationship between these substances and the insulin resistance of acute renal failure [22,26,44,47].

The diabetic patient with acute renal failure poses the opposite problem of clinical management. Due to the abrupt decrease in kidney degradation of insulin, requirements for insulin may be dramatically reduced. If insulin doses are not decreased concomitantly with the onset of renal failure, severe hypoglycemia may result. Regular monitoring of blood glucose is essential in the prevention of hypoglycemia in these patients.

Lipids

The lipid profile of patients with acute renal failure is characterized by hypertriglyceridemia with a predominance of low and very low density lipoproteins (LDL and VLDL) [49]. Both LDL and HDL cholesterol content is markedly reduced. In an animal model of chronic uremia, the increase in triglycerides was not believed to be secondary to increased endogenous production [50], and it is speculated that a circulating lipoprotein lipase inhibitor may cause a decrease in VLDL removal and the hypertriglyceridemia seen in acute renal failure [51].

Post-heparin lipolytic activity is decreased in patients with acute renal failure secondary to inhibited hepatic triglyceride lipase activity [49]. In a test of the ability to clear parenterally administered fat emulsions, patients exhibited a 50% decrease in the fractional elimination rate. These defects in lipid metabolism occur in the first few days of acute renal failure and are not affected by the degree of renal insufficiency or the presence of oliguria [49].

Fluids and Electrolytes

The acute decrease or cessation of glomerular filtration can have rapid effects on volume status, pH, and plasma electrolyte composition. Conditions in which there is tissue damage or large shifts in fluid, such as is seen in rhabdomyolysis, trauma, or burn injury, may result in an enormous release of intracellular potassium, phosphate, or other ions. For these reasons, the patient in acute renal failure represents a great challenge in fluid and electrolyte management and may require dialysis to correct these abnormalities acutely.

Acidosis occurs in these patients for several reasons. In addition to the release of hydrogen ions and organic acids from damaged tissue, hypercatabolism results in increased acid production. Vigorous amino acid repletion intended to promote anabolism may instead exacerbate the problem. Similarly, nutritional therapy with excessive amounts of carbohydrate, which may yield an increased respiratory quotient (RQ) and CO_2 production, can precipitate respiratory acidosis. Should this latter complication of nutritional support arise, more fat may be used as an alternative source of calories. Perhaps most important in the etiology of acidosis in these patients is the decreased or absent capacity of the kidney to excrete both the obligate acid load and any of the above sources of acid.

The effect of this metabolic acidosis is to further impair protein metabolism. In animal studies of chronic uremia, acidosis has been shown to induce an increase in net protein loss that was independent of insulin or glucocorticoid production [52]. Work by May et al. [53] has also demonstrated that acidosis stimulates glucocorticoid production, which in turn activates branched-chain keto-acid dehydrogenase. Because this enzyme is the rate-limiting step for branched-chain amino acid breakdown, the net result is protein catabolism.

The most common and acutely dangerous electrolyte abnormality of acute renal failure is hyperkalemia, which occurs due to both the increased release of intracellular potassium, as mentioned above, and decreased excretion. The acidemia of acute renal failure also serves to increase serum potassium as intracellular potassium is released in exchange for hydrogen ions. Because potassium excretion in the distal renal tubule is flow-dependent, maintainence of urine output greater than 1000 cc/day is not usually associated with hyperkalemia.

Similarly, hyperphosphatemia may occur secondary to decreased phosphate excretion and increased release of intracellular stores. This electrolyte abnormality may be complicated by hypocalcemia, especially in cases of rhabdomyolysis or radiation/chemotherapy of tumors.

Sources of Protein

In the early 1960s, Giovannetti found that uremic patients treated with an energy-rich diet containing only 6 to 11 g/day of protein, plus essential amino acids or proteins of high biologic value, were brought into positive or neutral nitrogen balance [54]. Other investigators used this type of diet and found that patients had slower renal decline, lived longer, and had fewer symptoms attributable to their renal failure [55–57]. The finding that protein restriction decreases the progression of renal failure may be due to several mechanisms, the most likely of which is referred to as the hyperfiltration hypothesis [58]. This theory is based on the fact that increased protein intake causes an increase in overall and single nephron filtration. With a reduced number of nephrons functioning in renal failure, hyperfiltration is exacerbated by "normal" quantities of protein, and the increased pressure and flow induce glomerulosclerosis, proteinuria, and progressive renal deterioration [58, 59]. Diets with a higher concentration of essential amino acids or proteins of high biologic value may enable patients to maintain nitrogen balance with less overall protein intake and slower progression of renal failure. Thus, it is apparent that the composition of nutrition administered to patients in renal failure should include proteins of high biologic value so as to optimize nitrogen balance, minimize progression of disease, and even promote renal recovery [10].

Efficacy of Essential Versus Combined Essential and Nonessential Amino Acid Solutions

Since Giovannetti and Giordano first described the improvements seen in chronically uremic patients after administration of essential amino acids [54,60], clinicians have sought to determine the most efficacious proportions of glucose and essential and nonessential amino acids in acute renal failure. The goals of nutritional therapy have been to deter nitrogen loss and maintain renal function. Abel et al. [12] conducted a prospective randomized trial of 53 patients in acute renal failure and compared infusion of glucose alone with glucose plus essential amino acids. They found that compared to patients who received glucose alone, those given essential amino acids had a lower mortality (75% vs. 44%), fewer complications, and a trend toward earlier return to normal serum creatinine [12]. The difference in survival was even more striking in patients with infections or other complications of acute renal failure, as well as patients in oliguric renal failure. This trial followed earlier work demonstrating that administration of essential amino acids lowered blood urea nitrogen (BUN), potassium, phosphorus, and magnesium levels in patients who developed acute renal failure after aortoiliac surgery [61]. Likewise, in a study of 20 patients with acute renal failure, Leonard et al. [62] showed that patients given glucose with essential amino acids had a reduced rate of BUN elevation compared to patients given glucose alone, although no change in mortality was observed. Baek et al. [14] compared a predominantly essential amino acid solution plus glucose versus glucose alone in a study of 129 postoperative patients in acute renal failure and found a small decrease in mortality and hyperkalemia in patients given the amino acid solution.

Both animal and human studies have demonstrated that nonessential amino acids are beneficial to the normal growth of the young [63,64] and may be useful in promoting nitrogen balance [65], prompting their use in this patient population. In a prospective randomized trial of 30 patients with acute renal failure, Feinstein et al. [16] compared isocaloric solutions of glucose alone, glucose plus essential amino acids, and glucose plus a mixture of essential and nonessential amino acids. This study demonstrated no statistically significant improvement in mortality, recovery of renal function, or nitrogen balance among any of the three treatment groups. Nevertheless, there did seem to be a trend in the data. Patients treated with glucose and essential amino acids rather than a mixture of essential and nonessential amino acids had lower urea nitrogen appearance (6.7 vs. 14.0), lower net protein degradation (49.0 vs. 98.9), lower end-of-trial serum creatinine and BUN (5.5 vs. 6.1 and 46 vs. 73, respectively), higher rates of renal recovery (63% vs. 25%), and nearly one-half the mortality (45% vs. 75%). A follow-up study by this same group examining larger quantities of nonessential amino acids (11.3 g/day) also showed that although urea nitrogen appearance was lower in the essential amino acid group, there was no advantage in terms of protein balance, renal recovery, or survival [66]. However, this study may be a manifestation of a type II statistical error, in that the groups are so small that any beneficial effect would likely not be detected.

In an attempt to resolve the controversy over whether essential amino acids were beneficial in the treatment of acute renal failure, Naylor et al. [67] performed a meta-analysis of the four major randomized clinical trials. Upon pooling of the data, they found that use of essential amino acids was associated with an absolute increase in initial survival of 24% compared to glucose alone. However, when the data were reanalyzed using a quality factor, no statistical significance was found between treatment groups. A clear answer to the question of benefit awaits further trials with larger numbers of patients. Nonetheless, from the data available, essential amino acids would appear to be an important component in the nutritional management of these patients.

Effects of Dialysis

The nutritional requirements of a patient in acute renal failure who is undergoing dialysis are quite different from those of the pre-dialysis patient. Conventional hemodialysis machines remove many undesirable substances such as urea and "uremic toxins"; however, amino acids, peptides, and proteins are also removed by the process. It is estimated that at least 6 to 8 g of free amino acids plus 3 to 4 g of protein-bound amino acids are removed during each session of hemodialysis [68]. Larger pore size on the dialyzer membranes and low glucose content of the dialysate are both associated with even greater amino acid losses [69]. Protein losses are exacerbated by glucose losses that promote further gluconeogenesis and protein breakdown [70]. Glucose inclusion in the dialysate may promote intracellular movement of amino acids, thereby making less amino acid available for removal [67]. Fortunately, this is becoming less of a problem as most dialysis centers include glucose in their dialysate. The inclusion of 450 mg/dL of glucose will reduce the amino acid loss by 50% [71]. With this in mind, once a patient in renal failure is being dialyzed, protein administration should be increased accordingly.

Water-soluble vitamins (most notably B_6, folic acid, and C) are also removed by dialysis, and in a previously malnourished patient with acute renal failure, even a short course of this procedure may significantly worsen their deficiency. Inadequate stores of B_6 are known to cause impaired immunologic activity and neurologic function, and therefore daily administration of at least 10 mg of pyridoxine hydrochloride is recommended in the patient undergoing repeated dialysis [40].

Therapy

Enteral nutrition is advocated over parenteral therapy whenever possible because of its lower cost, lower risk to the patient, ease of initiation, and recent findings that immediate enteral feeding after injury may decrease septic complications, promote gut metabolic and immunologic functions, and diminish the adverse metabolic response seen in these patients [72,73]. A list of several of the currently available enteral and parenteral solutions for renal failure patients is shown in Table 25-1.

Determining Needs

Acute renal failure in and of itself may not be associated with an increase in energy expenditure, but it is generally believed that the underlying sepsis or injury accounts for the hypermetabolism seen in these patients [74]. Clear evidence to this effect is the absence of an increased metabolic rate in the resting energy expenditure of patients in renal failure secondary to drug toxicity [75].

Most patients with acute renal failure on the basis of infection, ischemia, or trauma have multiple indications for the initiation of nutritional support. Nonetheless, a nutrition history and physical exam are important for determining extent and area of compromise. For example, patients with a history of cirrhosis or recent weight loss secondary to cancer may already be severely malnourished, while those with a history of alcohol abuse or gastrointestinal bleeding will be at greater risk of developing B_{12}/folate or iron deficiency, respectively. The physical exam may also demonstrate signs of malnutrition or vitamin deficiency such as loss of fat reserve or the pale sclera of iron deficiency anemia. Extensive anthropometric tests have been described for the assessment of nutritional status [76]; however, these tests may be less meaningful in an ICU patient who is sedated, on a ventilator, or swollen with significant edema.

In the nutritional assessment of a patient, clinicians often examine the levels of plasma proteins such as albumin, prealbumin, retinol-binding protein, and transferrin as a measure of recent and long-term nutritional status. These indices are less useful in acute renal failure for two reasons. First, the majority of patients with acute renal failure and sepsis or trauma will have enormous fluid shifts due to capillary leak syndrome, making interpretation of these serum protein concentrations very difficult. Second, many of these proteins are excreted renally, and thus changes in their serum levels are multifactorial. Nonetheless, decreased levels of albumin, transferrin, and some complement proteins, and increased levels of prealbumin and retinol-binding protein have been documented in patients with acute renal failure [16,66,76].

Calories

The preferred method of determining caloric needs or resting energy expenditure is that of indirect calorimetry, which measures oxygen consumption and carbon dioxide production and directly calculates energy expenditure. This is a simple procedure using a metabolic cart and can easily be connected into a ventilator circuit. Because this procedure is performed in a resting patient, the results may be multiplied by an activity factor (1.1–1.3) to determine total energy expenditure. The respiratory quotient can also be derived from a metabolic cart, and this aids in assessment of substrate utilization. When this is not possible or unnecessary, a rough approximation of caloric needs may be determined by using the Harris-Benedict equation for basal energy expenditure:

Table 25-1. Renal Failure Formulations

Parenteral Amino Acid Formulas[a]	NephrAmine (5.4%)	Aminosyn-RF (5.2%)	Aminess (5.2%)
Nitrogen (g/dl)	0.65	0.79	0.66
Amino acid concentration	0.054	0.052	0.052
Essential amino acids (mg/dl)			
Isoleucine	560	462	525
Leucine	880	726	825
Lysine	640	535	600
Methionine	880	726	825
Phenylalanine	880	726	825
Threonine	400	330	375
Tryptophan	200	165	188
Valine	640	528	600
Histidine	250	429	412
Nonessential amino acids (mg/dl)			
Arginine	0	600	0
Cysteine	<20	0	0
Electrolytes (mEq/l)			
Sodium	5	0	0
Potassium	0	5.4	0
Chloride	<3	0	0
Acetate	44[b]	105[b]	50
Enteral Formulas[c]		**Nepro**	**Suplena**
Cal/l		2000	2000
G protein/l		70	30
G carbohydrate/l		216	255
G fat/l		96	95.6
Nonprotein cal:nitrogen		153:1	395:1
mOsm/kg H_2O		635	615
Sodium (mEq/l)		36	34
Potassium (mEq/l)		27	28.6
Calcium (mg/l)		1358	1370
Phosphorus (mg/l)		679	721

[a]Data from Intravenous Nutritional Therapy. In BR Olin (ed), *Facts and Comparisons.* St. Louis: Lippincott, 1995, with permission.
[b]Approximate values.
[c]From University of Cincinnati Hospital Nutrition Services, adult enteral formulary, June 1994.

$$\text{Basal energy expenditure (kcal/day)} =$$

$$66.5 + 13.7\,(\text{weight in kg}) + 5\,(\text{height in cm}) - 6.8\,(\text{age})\ [\text{males}]$$

$$655.1 + 9.56\,(\text{weight in kg}) + 1.85\,(\text{height in cm}) - 4.68\,(\text{age})\ [\text{females}]$$

This number should then be multiplied by an activity and stress factor to determine the total energy expenditure:

$$\text{Total energy expenditure} = \text{basal energy expenditure} \times \text{activity factor} \times \text{stress factor}$$

The activity factor = 1.25 for a hospitalized patient, although no activity factor is necessary for paralyzed or heavily sedated patients on a ventilator. The stress factor may be read from one of any number of published tables of estimated increases in metabolic work according to the specific clinical circumstances (Table 25-2). Stress factors may overestimate caloric needs in some patients.

From the above calculations, the typical patient in acute renal failure will have a total energy expenditure of 35 to 50 kcal/kg/day. This is consistent with measured energy expenditures of patients in acute renal failure as determined by indirect calorimetry in a study by Mault et al. [77].

Protein

Because the proportion of nitrogen in mixed proteins is constant, and urea is the major nitrogenous product of protein metabolism, net protein

Table 25-2. Stress Factors

Clinical Circumstance	Stress Factor
Mild starvation	0.85–1.0
Post-op (no complications)	1.0–1.05
Cancer*	1.10–1.45
Peritonitis*	1.05–1.25
Multitrauma/infection*	1.3–1.55
Burn*	1.5–1.7

* = proportional to extent of disease.
Source: From KN Apelgren, DW Wilmore. Nutritional care of the critically ill patient. *Surg Clin North Am* 63:597, 1983.

loss or gain may be determined from urea nitrogen appearance. Urinary nitrogen appearance may be calculated as follows, with all values expressed as g/day [78]:

$$\text{Urinary nitrogen appearance} = \text{urinary urea nitrogen} + \text{dialysate urea nitrogen} + \text{change in body urea nitrogen}$$

The change in body urea nitrogen may be calculated by the following formula over a 24-hour period:

$$\begin{aligned}\text{Change in body urea nitrogen} &= [\text{change in serum urea nitrogen (g/L)}] \\ &\times [\text{initial body weight (kg)} \times 0.6 \text{ L/kg}] \\ &+ [\text{change in body weight (kg/day)}] \\ &\times [\text{initial serum urea nitrogen} \times 1 \text{ L/kg}]\end{aligned}$$

This formula should be applied in the interdialytic time period and assumes that all weight gain is secondary to water weight. The factor of 0.6 L/kg is an estimation of percentage of water body weight in normal people and must be increased if there is evidence of edema. The conversion from urea nitrogen appearance to net protein degradation can be estimated by multiplying the urea nitrogen appearance by 6.75 and then adding in the amount of protein lost in feces and shed skin (roughly 3 to 6 g/day):

$$\text{Net protein breakdown (g/day)} = [\text{urea nitrogen appearance} \times 6.75] + 4.5$$

Protein intake and net protein degradation will be roughly equivalent in a patient in zero nitrogen balance. The administration of protein to septic or injured patients with acute renal failure may be liberalized once dialysis or hemofiltration has been instituted, in order to achieve a more favorable calorie-nitrogen ratio.

Alternative Sources of Protein

Two other sources of protein have been used with some success in the nutritional support of patients with hypermetabolism and renal failure: branched-chain amino acids (BCAAs) and keto-acid analogs. BCAAs have been shown to reduce post-injury catabolism [79,80], increase hepatic protein synthesis [81], and are known to be oxidized by skeletal muscle and adipose tissue without the intervention of glucose [81]. Their use in hypercatabolic patients has been found to increase nitrogen balance in a dose-dependent fashion [82], with the maximal nitrogen retention noted with a 50% BCAA solution, the highest concentration tested in this study. Excretion of 3-methylhistidine was unaffected by BCAA administration, supporting the finding that BCAAs work through stimulation of protein synthesis rather than decreased proteolysis [82]. The protein-sparing effect of these amino acids, however, is present only for the first seven days of therapy. The other potential advantage of this specialized amino acid formulation in patients in acute renal failure is its inhibitory effect on ureagenesis. In a study of septic ICU patients comparing high BCAA solutions to standard amino acid solutions, Bower et al. [83] found a lower elevation of blood urea nitrogen with the high BCAA solutions, but only with the solution enriched with leucine. While there was a trend toward higher nitrogen retention in the BCAA group, the difference was not statistically significant. However, BCAAs may be useful adjuncts in selected renal failure patients with protein restriction.

Keto-acid analogs have also been used in the treatment of patients with chronic renal failure. Animal studies by Goldberg and Tischler [84] demonstrated that leucine stimulated protein synthesis and inhibited protein degradation in a rat diaphragm preparation. However, when an inhibitor of leucine amino acid transaminase was added, no inhibition of protein degradation was seen, suggesting that one of the metabolites of leucine was affecting protein degradation. The addition of one of the keto-acid metabolites, α-ketoisocaproate, again induced inhibition of protein degradation [84]. Human trials have since been performed [85–88] demonstrating that a low-protein diet (0.3 g/kg/day) with keto-acid analog administration significantly slowed progression of renal failure, as estimated by the slope of the inverse creatinine or radioisotopically determined glomerular filtration rate. In one study [88], the keto-acid supplement was found to slow progression of disease by approximately 50%. Further studies are needed to determine if keto-acids are efficacious in the treatment of acute renal failure. The principal difficulty is in supplying enough of these substances because of solubility and ionic problems.

Carbohydrates

Carbohydrate should make up approximately 60% to 70% of total calories given. This percentage may need to be increased to nearly 100% in patients requiring severe protein restriction and/or who have lipid intolerance. The two untoward effects of overadministration of carbohydrates are hyperglycemia and respiratory acidosis due to an increased respiratory quotient, although this latter complication occurs far less frequently than the attention paid to it. Because patients with trauma or sepsis and acute renal failure manifest glucose intolerance, administration of exogenous insulin may be required. Close monitoring of the blood sugar is an important part of preventing this problem. Once the proper insulin-glucose ratio is established, it is our policy to add insulin to the TPN solution so that alterations in the rate of glucose administered are automatically reflected in the amount of insulin delivered. If insulin is given separately from the TPN solution, slow increases or decreases in the rate of TPN or tube feedings help minimize wide fluctuations in blood sugar.

Lipids

Due to the relative hypertriglyceridemia seen in acute renal failure, it is advisable to check serum triglyceride levels prior to the initiation of nutrition with lipids. If these levels are acceptable, lipids may be added to the formulation. Fat should comprise approximately 20% of the caloric regimen, as hepatic protein synthesis seems optimal at this level. Higher amounts of fat are appropriate if less glucose calories are desired because of hyperglycemia or difficulty weaning from the ventilator.

Fluids and Electrolytes

Estimation of the composition of all fluid losses is essential to the volume and electrolyte management of patients with impaired renal function. Nasogastric aspirates, fistula output, diarrhea, and urine (if patients are non-oliguric) should be quantitated and analyzed for electrolyte composition. Insensible losses are usually approximated at 400 to 600 ml/day in many patients. However, the presence of fever, large open wounds, or burns are associated with much greater evaporative losses. Burn-related evaporative loss (in ml/hr) may be estimated by adding 25 to the percent total body surface area burn and multiplying by the body surface area (in m^2) [89]. Losses due to fever may be calculated by adding 15% of basal requirements per hour per degree of temperature above 37°C [90].

Optimally, total volume intake and output are equivalent in these patients, although capillary leak syndrome with resulting edema and intravascular depletion frequently mandate the further administration of crystalloid or colloid. Daily weight measurements are very useful for the approximation of total body fluid status.

The management of electrolyte and acid-base status also relies on close monitoring of intake and output. The administration of bicarbonate for correction of acidosis may be limited by its effect on volume status. If parenteral nutrition has been instituted, substitution of phosphate salts by sodium acetate may decrease acidosis. Hyponatremia is treated with salt and water restriction in the well-hydrated patient. Hyperkalemia may be temporarily treated with intravenous bicarbonate or glucose and insulin, causing potassium to shift into the intracellular space; however, this therapy does nothing to correct whole-body excess of potassium, and swift recurrence is likely. TPN with essential amino acids and hypertonic dextrose manifests a rather more permanent hypokalemic effect [61]. Kayexalate, a sodium-potassium exchange resin, may be given in a mannitol suspension, either orally per nasogastric tube or as an enema, and will result in lowering of total body potassium. In a cardiac emergency, intravenous calcium should be given.

Patients with hypocalcemia and hyperphosphatemia on the basis of rhabdomyolysis-induced acute renal failure frequently have calcium deposits in many peripheral tissues. Administration of further calcium or even vitamin D may result in further calcium deposition and worsening renal failure. Lowering of phosphate levels by means of phosphate binders will simultaneously improve calcium levels, as precipitation is prevented.

The malnourished patient who is started on parenteral nutrition may have different electrolyte abnormalities, especially if the patient's etiology of renal failure is not a hypermetabolic cause. The increased anabolism seen with refeeding a malnourished patient is associated with an intracellular movement of potassium, phosphorus, and magnesium, and these ions may require vigorous supplementation [61].

Prospects for Advances in Therapy

For several decades the nondialytic therapy for acute renal failure has included the use of diuretics, volume expanders such as mannitol, and vasoactive drugs [91]. Recently, several new therapies have arisen that have implications both for improved nutritional support of these patients and for the patients' overall survival.

Renal Replacement Therapy

Continuous arteriovenous hemofiltration was popularized in the early 1980s as a means of filtering blood in a more physiologic manner than conventional dialysis. Its advantages include the ability to remove large quantities of fluid (10–20 L/day) without an adverse effect on blood pressure, to control blood urea nitrogen despite aggressive administration of parenteral amino acids [92], and to deliver any desired quantity of carbohydrate via a countercurrent dialysate (hemodiafiltration) [93]. In one study, the procedure was found to remove 24 g/day of nitrogen, 60% to 70% of which was urea [94]. In a study of hypercatabolic patients with liberal protein administration, nitrogen balance was achieved in 6 of 19 patients while maintaining control of uremia [94]. Although clinical trials comparing this modality with hemodialysis are still forthcoming, it seems likely that this more physiologic blood-filtering mechanism, in conjunction with nutritional support, may improve nitrogen balance in these patients.

Insulin-Like Growth Factor

Insulin-like growth factor-1 (IGF-1) is a peptide synthesized and secreted in the glomeruli and distal and collecting tubules (among other tissues). IGF-1 binds to receptors found in glomeruli and proximal tubules [95]. This growth factor is believed to play a role in the regulation of glomerular filtration rate and renal tubular regeneration after ischemic injury, as shown by experiments both in rats and man [96,97]. Administration of recombinant IGF-1 or analogs of IGF-1 to rats with experimentally induced renal failure has been shown to have several remarkable effects, including increased glomerular filtration rate to the level of normal controls, decreased nitrogen loss enabling positive nitrogen balance, and maintained or increased body weight [97]. In other experiments, recombinant IGF-1 was found to not only increase DNA synthesis in glomeruli and renal tubules, but to reduce overall body protein catabolism as evidenced by increased protein synthesis and decreased protein degradation in epitrochlearis muscles [98]. This peptide shows promise for promoting renal recovery and metabolic equilibrium in patients with acute renal failure.

Growth Hormone

Growth hormone has long been known to act as an anabolic factor, with administration causing positive nitrogen balance and growth [99,100]. Recent studies, however, suggest that this hormone is intimately involved in glutamine metabolism by decreasing glutamate utilization and enabling glutamine production [101]. Similarly, in a phase I trial in humans, recombinant growth hormone was administered with TPN to 18 trauma or burn patients, with resulting decreases in nitrogen excretion (1356 mmol/day to 899 mmol/day), BUN, potassium and phosphorus excretion for several weeks of administration. Not surprisingly, circulating IGF-1 (which is normally stimulated by growth hormone) was also elevated, which may explain some or all of the effects of growth hormone [102]. This protein-sparing effect of growth hormone has been demonstrated in other trials as well, including a prospective randomized trial of post-gastrectomy or colectomy patients who were fed hypocaloric nutrition with or without growth hormone. Patients receiving growth hormone maintained lean body mass and strength, had significantly less weight loss, and showed increased uptake of amino acids and protein synthesis [103]. Further studies in patients with renal failure appear warranted.

Erythropoeitin

Erythropoeitin has been used in chronic renal failure patients for several years, primarily for its salutary effect on the anemia often seen in these patients. Although some claim that its use is associated with normalization of the aminogram in patients with chronic renal failure [104], these findings have not been confirmed [105]. Other investigators have found that in rats with cisplatin-induced renal failure, administration of recombinant human erythropoeitin was associated with significantly greater renal functional recovery as well as increased tubular regeneration assessed by ^{3}H-thymidine incorporation [106]. These effects were not found to be associated with increased erythrocyte mass, blood pressure, or renal iron content.

Summary

The injured or septic patient with acute renal failure continues to represent a challenge in both nutritional management and overall survival. Although profound advances in the therapy of these patients have not been realized recently, use of essential amino acids and hypertonic dextrose appears to offer some improvement in survival, especially in patients with severe renal failure. Newer therapies such as hemofiltration, IGF-1, and growth hormone hold some promise for these patients, but more likely better elaboration of the network of mediators leading to hypercatabolism will be essential to enable earlier intervention and improved patient outcome.

References

1. Hou SH, et al. Hospital acquired renal insufficiency: A prospective study. *Am J Med* 74:243, 1983.
2. Takala J. Nutrition in acute renal failure. *Crit Care Clin* 3:155, 1987.
3. Balslov, JT, Jorgenson HE. A survey of 499 patients with acute anuric renal insufficiency. *Am J Med* 34:753, 1963.
4. Windsor JA, Knight GS, Hill GL. Wound healing response in surgical patients: Recent food intake is more important than nutritional status. *Br J Surg* 75:135, 1988.
5. Gorse GJ, Messner RL, Stephens ND. Association of malnutrition with nosocomial infections. *Infect Control Hosp Epidemiol* 10:194, 1989.
6. Windsor JA, Hill GL. Grip strength: A measure of the proportion of protein loss in surgical patients. *Br J Surg* 75:880, 1988.
7. Hasselgren PO, et al. Total and myofibrillar muscle protein breakdown in different types of rat skeletal muscle: Effect of sepsis and regulation with insulin. *Metabolism* 38:634, 1989.
8. Clowes GH, et al. Muscle proteolysis induced by circulating peptide in patients with sepsis and trauma. *N Engl J Med* 308:545, 1983.
9. Bluemle LW, Webster GD, Elkinton JR. Acute tubular necrosis. *Arch Intern Med* 104:190, 1959.
10. Toback FG. Amino acid enchancement of renal regeneration after acute tubular necrosis. *Kidney Int* 12:193, 1977.
11. Toback FG, et al. Amino acid administration enhances renal protein metabolism after acute tubular necrosis. *Nephron* 33:238, 1983.
12. Abel RM, et al. Improved survival from acute renal failure after treatment with intravenous essential L-amino acids and glucose. *N Engl J Med* 288:695, 1973.
13. Berlyne GM, et al. The dietary treatment of acute renal failure. *Q J Med* 36:59, 1967.
14. Baek SM, et al. The influence of parenteral nutrition on the course of acute renal failure. *Surg Gynecol Obstet* 141:405, 1975.
15. Mullen JL, et al. Reduction of operative morbidity and mortality by combined preoperative and postoperative nutritional support. *Ann Surg* 192:604, 1980.
16. Feinstein EI, et al. Clinical and metabolic responses to parenteral nutrition in acute renal failure. *Medicine* 60:124, 1981.
17. Montemurro DG, Stevenson JA. Survival and body composition of normal and hypothalamic obese rats in acute starvation. *Am J Physiol* 198:757, 1960.
18. DeFronzo RA, Alvestrand A. Glucose intolerance in uremia: Site and mechanism. *Am J Clin Nutr* 33:1438, 1980.
19. Black PR, et al. Mechanisms of insulin resistance following injury. *Ann Surg* 196:420, 1982.
20. Clarke AS, Mitch WE. Muscle protein turnover and glucose uptake in rats with acute uremia. *J Clin Invest* 72:836, 1983.
21. Bilbrey GL, et al. Hyperglucagonemia of renal failure. *J Clin Invest* 53:841, 1974.
22. Bilbrey GL, et al. Hyperglucagonemia in uremia: Reversal by renal transplantation. *Ann Intern Med* 82:525, 1975.
23. Marliss EB, et al. Glucagon levels and metabolic effects in fasting man. *J Clin Invest* 49:2256, 1970.
24. Massry SG, Arieff AL, Coburn JW. Divalent ion metabolism in patients with acute renal failure: Studies on the mechanism of hypocalcemia. *Kidney Int* 5:437, 1974.
25. Garber AJ. Effects of parathyroid hormone on skeletal muscle protein and amino acid metabolism in the rat. *J Clin Invest* 71:1806, 1983.
26. Amend WJ, et al. The influence of serum calcium and parathyroid hormone upon glucose metabolism in uremia. *J Lab Clin Med* 86:435, 1975.
27. Zamir O, et al. Tumor necrosis factor (TNF) and interleukin-1 (IL-1) induce muscle proteolysis through different mechanisms. *Mediators of Inflammation* 1:247, 1992.
28. Zamir O, et al. Effect of tumor necrosis factor or interleukin-1 on muscle amino acid uptake and the role of glucocorticoids. *Surg Gynecol Obstet* 177:27, 1993.
29. Dinarello CA. Interleukin-1: Its multiple biological effects and its association with hemodialysis. *Blood Purif* 6:164, 1988.
30. Bergstrom J. Factors causing catabolism in maintenance hemodialysis patients. *Mineral Electrolyte Metab* 18:280, 1992.
31. Kopple JD. Abnormal amino acid and protein metabolism in uremia. *Kidney Int* 4:340, 1978.
32. Delaporte C, Gros F. In vitro inhibition of protein synthesis by dialysates of plasma from uremic patients. *Eur J Clin Invest* 11:139, 1981.
33. Delaporte C, Gros F, Anagnostopolous T. Inhibitory effects of plasma dialysate on protein synthesis in vitro: Influence of dialysis and transplantation. *Am J Clin Nutr* 33:1407, 1980.
34. Lacy WW. Effect of acute uremia on amino acid uptake and urea production by perfused rat liver. *Am J Physiol* 216:1300, 1969.
35. Frohlich J, et al. The effect of acute uremia on gluconeogenesis in isolated perfused rat livers. *Eur J Clin Invest* 4:453, 1974.
36. Garber AJ. Skeletal muscle protein and amino acid metabolism in experimental chronic uremia in the rat: Accelerated alanine and glutamine formation and release. *J Clin Invest* 62:623, 1978.
37. Varcoe R, et al. Efficiency of utilization of urea nitrogen for albumin synthesis by chronically uremic and normal man. *Clin Sci Mol Med* 48:379, 1975.
38. Mitch WE, Leitman P, Walser M. Effect of oral neomycin and kanamycin in chronic uremic subject: I. Urea metabolism. *Kidney Int* 11:116, 1977.
39. Mitch WE, Walser M. Effect of oral neomycin and kanamycin in chronic uremic subject: II. Nitrogen balance. *Kidney Int* 11:122, 1977.
40. Kopple JD, et al. Amino acid and protein metabolism in renal failure. *Am J Clin Nutr* 31:1532, 1978.
41. Druml W, et al. Phenylalanine-tyrosine metabolism in acute and chronic renal failure. Abstract, 7th Congress of the European Society of Parenteral and Enteral Nutrition, Munich, Federal Republic of Germany, Sept. 9–11, 1985.
42. Kopple JD, Swenseid ME. Evidence that histidine is an essential amino acid in normal and chronically uremic man. *J Clin Invest* 55:881–891, 1975.

43. DeFronzo RA, Tobin JD, Andres R. The glucose clamp technique: A method for quantifying insulin secretion and resistance. *Am J Physiol* 237:E214, 1979.
44. Frohlich J, Schollmeyer P, Gerok W. Carbohydrate metabolism in renal failure. *Am J Clin Nutr* 131:1541, 1978.
45. Hasselgren PO, et al. Current concepts of protein turnover and amino acid transport in liver and skeletal muscle during sepsis. *Arch Surg* 123:992, 1988.
46. Bilbug GL, et al. Hyperglucagonemia of renal failure. *J Clin Invest* 53:841, 1974.
47. Samaan NA, Freeman RM. Growth hormone levels in severe renal failure. *Metabolism* 19:102, 1970.
48. Sherwin RS, et al. Influence of uremia and hemodialysis on the turnover and metabolic effects of glucagon. *J Clin Invest* 57:722, 1976.
49. Druml W, et al. Lipid metabolism in acute renal failure. *Kidney Int* 24:S123, 1983.
50. Bagdade JB, et al. Hyperlipidemia in renal failure: Studies of plasma lipoprotein, hepatic triglyceride production and tissue lipoprotein lipase in a chronically uremic rat model. *J Lab Clin Med* 91:176, 1978.
51. Murase T, et al. Inhibition of lipoprotein lipase by uremic plasma, a possible cause of hypertriglyceridemia. *Metabolism* 52:875, 1975.
52. May RC, Kelly RA, Mitch WE. Mechanisms for defects in muscle protein metabolism in rats with chronic uremia: The influence of metabolic acidosis. *J Clin Invest* 79:1099, 1987.
53. May RC, et al. Branched-chain amino acid metabolism in rat muscle: Abnormal regulation in acidosis. *Am J Physiol* 252:E712, 1987.
54. Giovannetti S, Maggiore Q. A low nitrogen diet with proteins of high biological value for severe chronic uraemia. *Lancet* 1:1000, 1964.
55. Berlyne GM, Shaw AB, Nilwarangkur S. Dietary treatment of chronic renal failure: Experiences with a modified Giovannetti diet. *Nephron* 2:129, 1965.
56. Lonergan ET, Lange K. Use of specia protein-restricted diet in uremia. *Am J Clin Nutr* 21:595, 1968.
57. Hood CEA, et al. Dialysed egg as nitrogen source in dietary control of chronic renal failure. *Lancet* 1:479, 1969.
58. Brenner BM, Meyr TW, Hostetter TH. Dietary protein intake and the progressive nature of kidney disease: The role of hemodynamically mediated glomerular injury in the pathogenesis of progressive glomerular sclerosis in aging, renal ablation, and intrinsic renal disease. *N Engl J Med* 307:652, 1982.
59. Kleinknecht, Laouari K, Hinglais N. Protein intake and deterioration renal function in rats: Experimental data and hypothetical mechanism. *Contrib Nephrol* 60:135, 1988.
60. Giordano C. Use of exogenous and endogenous urea for protein synthesis in normal and uremic man. *J Lab Clin Med* 62:231, 1963.
61. Abbott WM, Abel RM, Fischer JE. Treatment of acute renal insufficiency after aortoiliac surgery. *Arch Surg* 103:590, 1971.
62. Leonard CD, Luke RG, Siegel RR. Parenteral essential amino acids in acute renal failure. *Urology* 6:154, 1975.
63. Pennisi AJ, Wang M, Kopple JD. Effects of protein and amino acid diets in chronically uremic and control rats. *Kidney Int* 13:472, 1978.
64. Swendseid ME, Kopple JD. Amino acid requirement and non-specific nitrogen. *Infusionstherapie* 2:203, 1975.
65. Anderson HL, Heindel MB. Effect of nitrogen balance of adult man of varying source of nitrogen and level of caloric intake. *J Nutr* 99:82, 1969.
66. Feinstein EI, et al. Total parenteral nutrition with high or low nitrogen intakes in patients with acute renal failure. *Kidney Int* 26:S319, 1983.
67. Naylor CD, et al. Does treatment with essential amino acids and hypertonic glucose improve survival in acute renal failure? A meta-analysis. *Ren Fail* 10:141, 1988.
68. Apelgren KN, Wilmore DW. Nutritional care of the critically ill patient. *Surg Clin North Am* 63:597, 1983.
69. Kopple JD. Dietary requirements. In SG Massry and AL Sellers (eds), *Clinical Aspects of Uremia and Dialysis.* Springfield, IL: Thomas, 1976. P 453.
70. Wathen RL, et al. The metabolic effects of hemodialysis with and without glucose in the dialysate. *Am J Clin Nutr* 31:1870, 1978.
71. Kopple JD, et al. The free and bound amino acids removed by hemodialysis. *Trans Am Soc Artif Intern Organs* 19:309, 1973.
72. Kudsk KA, et al. Enteral versus parenteral feeding: Effects on septic morbidity after blunt and penetrating trauma. *Ann Surg* 215:503, 1992.
73. Moore EE, Jones TN. Benefits of immediate jejunostomy feeding after major abdominal trauma: A prospective randomized study. *Trauma* 26:874, 1986.
74. Soop M, et al. Energy expenditure in postoperative multiple organ failure with acute renal failure. *Clin Nephrol* 32:139, 1989.
75. Schneeweiss B, et al. Energy metabolism in acute and chronic renal failure. *Am J Clin Nutr* 52:596, 1990.
76. Blumenkrantz MF, et al. Methods for assessing nutritional status of patients with renal failure. *Am J Clin Nutr* 33:1567, 1980.
77. Mault JR, et al. Starvation: A major contribution to mortality in acute renal failure? *Trans Am Soc Artif Intern Organs* 29:390, 1983.
78. Kopple JD, Cianciaruso B. Nutritional management of acute renal failure. In JE Fischer (ed), *Surgical Nutrition* (1st ed). Boston: Little, Brown, 1983. P 576.
79. Cerra FB, et al. Branched chains support postoperative protein synthesis. *Surgery* 92:192, 1982.
80. Blackburn GL, et al. Branched chain amino acid administration and metabolism during starvation, injury and infection. *Surgery* 86:307, 1979.
81. Freund HR, James HJ, Fischer JE. Nitrogen sparing mechanisms of singly administered branched chain amino acids in injured rats. *Surgery* 90:237, 1981.
82. Cerra F, Mazusky J, Teasley K. Nitrogen retention in critically ill patients is proportional to branched chain amino acid load. *Crit Care Med* 11:775, 1983.
83. Bower RH, et al. Branched chain amino acid-enriched solutions in the septic patient: A randomized, prospective trial. *Ann Surg* 203:13, 1986.
84. Goldberg AL, Tischler ME. Regulatory effects of leucine on carbohydrate and protein metabolism. In M Walser, JR Williamson (eds), *Metabolism and Clinical Implications of Branched Chain Amino and Ketoacids.* New York: Elsevier/North-Holland, 1981. P 205.
85. Lucas PA, et al. The risks and benefits of a low protein-essential amino acid-keto acid diet. *Kidney Int* 29:995, 1986.
86. Mitch WE, et al. The effect of a keto acid-amino acid supplement to a restricted diet on the progression of chronic renal failure. *N Engl J Med* 311:623, 1984.

87. Walser M, et al. Progression of chronic renal failure in patients given ketoacids following amino acids. *Kidney Int* 32:123, 1987.

88. Walser M, Hill S, Ward L. Progression of chronic renal failure on substituting a ketoacid supplement for an amino acid supplement. *J Am Soc Nephrol* 2:1178, 1992.

89. Goodwin CW, Finkelstein JL, Madden MR. Burns. In S Schwartz (ed), *Principles of Surgery* (6th ed.) New York: McGraw-Hill, 1994. P. 238.

90. Hiyama DT (ed), Fluids and electrolytes. In *The Mont Reid Surgical Handbook* (2nd ed). St. Louis: Mosby 1990. P 14.

91. Puschett JB. Non-dialytic therapy of acute renal failure. *Int J Artif Organs* 8:249, 1985.

92. Bellomo R, et al. Use of continuous haemodiafiltration: An approach to the management of acute renal failure in the critically ill. *Am J Nephrol* 12:240, 1992.

93. Bellomo R, Martin H, Parkin G, et al. Continuous arteriovenous haemodiafiltration in the critically ill: Influence on major nutrient balances. *Intensive Care Med* 17:399, 1991.

94. Chima CS, et al. Protein catabolic rate in patients with acute renal failure on continuous arteriovenous hemofiltration and total parenteral nutrition. *J Am Soc Nephrol* 3:1516, 1993.

95. Grone HJ, Neumann P, Fuchs E. Localization and characterization of IGF-1 receptors in fetal and adult human kidneys. *Miner Electrolyte Metab* 18:256, 1992.

96. Guler HP, et al. Insulin-like growth factor 1 increases glomerular filtration rat and plasma flow in man. *Acta Endocrinol* 121:101, 1989.

97. Martin AA, et al. Effect of insulin-like growth factor-1 peptides in rats with acute renal failure. *J Endocrinol* 140:23, 1994.

98. Ding H, et al. Recombinant human insulin-like growth factor-1 accelerates recovery and reduces catabolism in rats with ischemic acute renal failure. *J Clin Invest* 91:2281, 1991.

99. Vittis T, Vukmirovich R, Gaebler O. Utilization of ammonia nitrogen, administered by intragastric intraperitoneal and subcutaneous routes: Effects of growth hormone. *Arch Biochem Biophys* 106:475, 1964.

100. Kostyo J, Nutting DF. Growth hormone and protein metabolism. In *Handbook of Physiology.* Baltimore: American Physiological Society, 1974, Section 7, Volume IV (2). P 187.

101. Welbourne TC, Horton K, Cronin MJ. Growth hormone and renal glutamine and glutamate handling. *J Am Soc Nephrol* 2:1171, 1992.

102. Ziegler TR, et al. Use of human growth hormone combined with nutritional support in a critical care unit. *JPEN* 14:574, 1990.

103. Jiang SM, et al. Low-dose growth hormone and hypocaloric nutrition attenuate the protein-catabolic response after major operation. *Ann Surg* 210:513, 1989.

104. Riedel E, et al. Correction of amino acid metabolism by recombinant human erythropoeitin therapy in hemodialysis patients. *Kidney Int* 36:S216, 1989.

105. Garibotto G, Guerri G, Robaudo C. Erythropoeitin treatment and amino acid metabolism in hemodialysis patients. *Nephron* 65:533, 1993.

106. Vaziri ND, Zhou XJ, Liao SY. Erythropoeitin enhances recovery from cisplatin-induced acute renal failure. *Am J Physiol 266:F360,* 1994.

Selected Readings

Abel RM, et al. Improved survival from acute renal failure after treatment with intravenous essential L-amino acids and glucose. *N Engl J Med* 288:695, 1973.

A classic randomized prospective trial of the treatment of patients in acute renal failure given essential amino acids and hypertonic dextrose versus hypertonic dextrose alone. The results clearly demonstrate the superiority of essential amino acids and hypertonic dextrose in decreasing mortality and morbidity in patients with acute renal failure. More rapid recovery was also demonstrated in the essential amino acid group.

Kopple JD. Abnormal amino acid and protein metabolism in uremia. *Kidney Int* 14:340, 1978.

Kopple JD, et al. Amino acid and protein metabolism in renal failure. *Am J Clin Nutr* 31:1532, 1978.

These articles provide an in-depth discussion of amino-acid and protein-metabolism abnormalities in uremia.

Mirtallo JM, Kudsk KA, Ebbert ML. Nutritional support of patients with renal disease. *Clin Pharm* 3:253, 1984.

This article provides a good overview of the assessment and management of patients in chronic renal failure.

Seidner DL, Matarese LE, Steiger EZ. Nutritional care of the critically ill patient with renal failure. *Semin Nephrol* 14:53, 1994.

A discussion of the metabolic and immune response to injury and acute renal failure and the nutritional therapy of these patients.

26

Nutrition of Heart and Lung

Herbert R. Freund

There is an obvious functional relationship between the closely linked cardiovascular and pulmonary systems. The primary goal of the cardiorespiratory system is to provide adequate amounts of oxygen to the tissues to meet their metabolic demands and to remove carbon dioxide. To achieve these goals, the lungs and heart cooperate in four major functions:

1. Gas exchange between the atmosphere and the lung alveoli.
2. Exchange of oxygen and carbon dioxide between the alveoli and the blood.
3. The right heart pumps the blood through the lungs to facilitate exchange of oxygen and carbon dioxide between the alveoli and the blood.
4. The left heart, governed by the heart's rhythmical control system, pumps the blood through the peripheral organs, to transport oxygen to the various cells.

Oxygen delivery is a function of arterial oxygen content (CaO_2) and cardiac output. Alterations in both CaO_2 and cardiac output occur routinely during various pulmonary and/or cardiac disease states. Either cardiovascular instability or respiratory insufficiency can be life-threatening, and only an understanding of these functional and metabolic interactions enables the restoration of cardiopulmonary homeostasis and stability.

The care of the critically ill surgical patient often involves support for multisystem derangements or failure. These metabolic derangements occur in the various affected organs in response to a similar line of mediators like cytokines, prostaglandins, nitric oxide, hormones, and free radicals. This stereotypic chain of events gives rise to serious speculations about the close functional and metabolic relationship between health and disease and between the various organs, particularly between closely linked ones like the heart and lungs. Nutritional care of these patients constitutes a complicated problem and requires a challenging effort. Attention must be paid to both the heart and the lungs. Specialized nutritional requirements must be considered and then satisfied, possibly by specialized formulations tailored to the metabolism and needs of these anatomically and functionally related systems.

The Respiratory System

This section will correlate pulmonary biology, physiology, and metabolism in health and disease and will analyze the role of nutritional support for the respiratory system in these states. The respiratory mechanism consists of two metabolically important components: the respiratory muscles and the lung itself with its various and diverse systems and mechanisms.

Ventilatory Muscle Function

Under normal circumstances, respiratory muscles require 50 cal/day (3% of resting energy expenditure [REE]) and follow similar enzymatic profile, contractile behavior, and fatigue responses as that of the heart or skeletal limb musculature trained for endurance. Under various clinical states, the work of ventilation may approach up to 50% of total energy expenditure. The human diaphragm consists of approximately three-quarters slow-twitch and one-quarter fast-twitch fibers. The diaphragm depends almost equally on oxidation of glycogen and lipids for its energy requirements during activity.

Energy demands of respiratory muscles are determined by the work of breathing, muscle strength, and muscle efficiency, while energy availability is governed by blood flow and oxygen content, blood substrate levels, energy stores in muscles, and the ability to extract these energy sources.

The depletion of muscle glycogen was found to be linearly related to the intensity and duration of respiratory load, with more fast-twitch glycolytic fibers being depleted of glycogen than slow-twitch oxidative fibers. In one study, intramuscular triglycerides were totally consumed during acute loaded breathing and did so much earlier than did glycogen [1]. The diaphragm seems to be less dependent on anaerobic metabolism than are nonrespiratory skeletal muscles. Even when there is evidence of diaphragmatic muscle fatigue, there is no change in the lactate-pyruvate ratio.

Protein-calorie malnutrition resulting from catabolism and hypermetabolism does not spare the respiratory muscles. In both animal and humans models, losses of body weight and of diaphragm mass are similar following acute and chronic illnesses, indicating that diaphragm muscle mass is not spared and changes with nutritional status in a similar way to skeletal muscles [2]. In the undernourished hamster the maximal tetanic tension was found to be reduced to the same extent as the reduction in diaphragm muscle mass, indicating the cause of respiratory muscle weakness to be the loss of contractile elements. Similarly, nutritionally depleted patients also exhibited significant reductions in respiratory muscle strength as assessed by maximal static inspiratory and expiratory pressures [3]. Maximal voluntary ventilation and vital capacity were also reduced in direct proportion to the degree of weakness of the respiratory muscles. In another study, a direct relationship was found between the body cell mass and maximal inspiratory pressures [4].

The loss of muscle mass results from a starvation-induced decrease in protein synthesis and increase in protein degradation [5,6]. During this time, the diaphragm avidly oxidizes branched-chain amino acids to provide energy, produces alanine and glutamine for gluconeogenesis, and by a regulatory effect stimulates muscle protein synthesis and reduces muscle protein degradation [6,7]. Another stimulus reducing protein degradation in both skeletal and diaphragmatic muscle is work-induced muscle hypertrophy.

Protein synthesis per unit of muscle DNA and RNA remains normal, indicating the starvation-induced reduction in muscle protein synthesis to be due to reduced synthetic capacity. Increased protein degradation appears to be associated with cytokine-induced activity of proteolytic enzymes.

Although malnutrition affects all muscle fiber types, its major effect is on fast-twitch glycolytic fibers; this effect is potentiated by the stress-induced increase in the counter-regulatory hormones. Malnutrition has less effect on the slow-twitch high oxidative fibers. Thus, endurance of respiratory muscles is relatively well maintained, but maximal inspiratory and expiratory strength is not. The latter results in a higher percentage of generated-to-total available force being used, possibly resulting in increased muscle fatigue and respiratory failure [8].

In patients with no previous malnutrition and pulmonary compromise, a limited catabolic event will have only a marginal functional effect on respiration. However, in the presence of previous malnutrition and pulmonary compromise, as in chronic lung disease, such changes may result in acute respiratory failure, pulmonary infections, difficulty in weaning from mechanical ventilation, and a life-threatening situation.

The Pulmonary Parenchyma

Fasting and starvation in experimental animals cause decreases in both wet and dry lung weight that are less severe than the loss of body weight [9]. Lung weight tends to return to normal following refeeding. These changes are accompanied by the decreased production of surfactant, decreased protein and collagen production, and increased proteolysis. The net result is an increase in surface active forces and decreased tissue elasticity, leading to a tendency of the lungs to collapse, and a decrease in the percentage of volume retained at a given transpulmonary pressure [9]. Structurewise, partial starvation also resulted in air-space enlargement with minimal alveolar wall destruction and reduced internal surface area. These emphysema-like changes are similar to naturally occurring emphysema.

Short-term fasting has resulted in a significant reduction in protein synthesis by lung slices with reduction of total lung protein, RNA content, and RNA-DNA ratio in lung tissue [10]. Longer starvation has resulted in a 27% reduction in the protein content of lung tissue and a 50% reduction in lung RNA content, with no change in DNA content, indicating that the number of cells was not altered but that cell size was reduced or connective tissue protein and fat were lost [9]. The continued reduction of various connective tissue components like elastin is apparently responsible for the loss of lung tissue elasticity, with possible permanent damage to air spaces architecture. Refeeding reverses these changes to normal with cellular hyperplasia and increased cell synthetic activity, return of hydroxyproline to normal levels, and complete restoration of surfactant.

Very few, albeit conflicting, animal studies suggest that the release of proteinases is responsible for lung injury. Neutrophils, monocytes, and alveolar macrophages are supposedly the major source of endogenous elastase and other proteinases. The destructive activity of elastase and other proteinases is checked by an antiproteinase system, mainly α_1-antitrypsin. An intact antioxidant system is crucial for maintaining the balance between proteinases and antiproteinases in the lung. It is unclear whether malnutrition will induce α_1-antitrypsin deficiency. However, the lung's antioxidant system might be affected and thus be hampered in its ability to inactivate elastase [10]. Nutritional depletion of copper, iron, selenium, ceruloplasmin, and vitamins C and E might also impair the integrity and function of the lung's antioxidant defense mechanism. Biochemically, fast and starvation cause changes in lung collagen composition (increased ultrafilterable hydroxyproline peptides and soluble collagen) coupled with a high proteinolytic activity, suggesting continuous collagen breakdown and repair. Others have found decreased crude connective tissue and reduced hydroxyproline, elastin, and protein in starved-growth–retarded young rats.

Although not conclusive, and sometimes even conflicting, it can be safely stated that nutrition plays an important role in the damage and repair process of normal as well as diseased lungs.

Surfactant

The lung surfactant is secreted by type II pneumocytes and consists of dipalmitoyl lecithin bound to apoprotein. Its primary role is to prevent alveolar collapse at end expiration and to reduce the work of breathing required to reexpand alveoli by decreasing surface tension during expiration and by increasing surface tension during inspiration.

Surfactant and its breakdown products also serve as a chemotactic stimulus for pulmonary macrophages and as food for the macrophages.

Short- or long-term food deprivation decreases the dipalmitoyl phosphatidyl-choline content, the incorporation of phosphorus, and the pulmonary phospholipid content in the lung leading to a reduced rate of surfactant synthesis, inadequate tissue stores, reduced release into alveoli, and inadequate alveolar levels. The effect of surfactant depletion on lung mechanics has been variable. Some have shown normal alveolar stability despite a reduced alveolar pool of surfactant in starvation. Others have reported an increase in recoil forces as a result of increased surface tension or elastic forces. Compared with control animals, the inflation air-pressure volume curve in chronically fasted rats required higher pressures to attain equal lung volumes, implying an increased work of breathing in starved animals secondary to increased surface elastic forces. Refeeding reversed these deranged pressure-volume curves.

The decreased surfactant activity of starvation is secondary to a significant decrease in volume density of lamellar bodies of the pneumocyte in which surfactant is synthesized and stored. Furthermore, the volume density of mitochondria in granular pneumocytes is also decreased, implying decreased energy production by mitochondria for surfactant synthesis and secretion. Another factor involved would be a decrease in enzyme activity necessary for synthesis of phospholipids.

Pulmonary Defense Mechanisms

Pulmonary defense mechanisms depend on the integrity of the respiratory epithelium and its protecting layers and its immune system.

The alveolar macrophage is the main defensive instrument of the lung and acts mainly by phagocytosis and subsequent killing of trapped particles by oxygen radicals and proteases [11]. The macrophage is attracted to the interstitial area of the lung and alveoli by surfactant. There is a close relationship and interaction between the alveolar macrophage, T-lymphocytes, IgG, IgA, complement, fibronectin, and surfactant with its breakdown products.

In addition to the alveolar macrophage, pulmonary cell defense is also mediated via T-lymphocytes and lymphokine-mediated reactions [11].

Humoral and cell-mediated immune responses also take part in lung defense via IgA, IgG, microbial neutralizing and opsonizing antibodies, and macrophage-stimulating T-lymphocytes.

Humoral mechanisms are mediated via IgA, which is the major immunoglobulin of the respiratory system and acts as a barrier to viruses and bacteria. IgG plays its main function in the lower respiratory tract and can also neutralize toxins, viruses, and gram-negative bacteria.

Nutritional deficiency is associated with an increased number of lymphatic cells in alveolar and bronchial washings, reduction of T-helper to T-suppressor cell ratio, decrease in ciliary movement, and increase of bacterial adherence to epithelial cells. Specific deficiencies that impair immunocompetence include deficiency of vitamin A, pyridoxine, and zinc; deficiencies of copper, selenium, iron, vitamin E, carotene, and ascorbic acid impair antioxidant protective mechanisms. The possible role of glutamine for the immune system will be discussed under a separate heading.

Starvation-induced protein-calorie malnutrition impairs lung phagocytic antibacterial defenses. However, in some studies, although fewer alveolar macrophages were obtained, they still maintained normal phagocytic activity. Others found a depressed phagocytic activity with well-maintained bactericidal activity. A recent clinical study was able to correlate nutritional impairment with increased colonization of the lower respiratory tract with pseudomonas [12].

Control of Ventilation

Ventilation is controlled in the respiratory center of the medulla oblongata by hydrogen ions and CO_2. Nutrition can also affect control of ventilation. The metabolic rate and the hypoxic drive can change significantly in response to nutrients. Fasting or starvation can reduce oxygen consumption, basal metabolic rate, minute ventilation, mean inspiratory flow rate, and ventilatory response to hypoxia in normal volunteers, mediated by sympathetic suppression of the neural ventilatory drive. Both metabolic rate and hypoxic drive were increased following ingestion of a 1000 kcal meal of either carbohydrate or protein. Subjects fed daily a 500 kcal carbohydrate or a 550 kcal amino acids diet displayed decreased metabolic rate and decreased hypoxic ventilatory drive, possibly mediated by thyroid hormone and catecholamines. Neither of the previously experimental diets altered the ventilatory response to hypercarbia except for a 1000 kcal protein meal or parenteral amino acids, which increased the hypercapnic drive.

Recently, the branched-chain amino acids were found to exert a special enhancement of the ventilatory response to hypoxia and particularly to hypercarbia. This will be discussed under the heading of amino acids and respiratory failure.

The Effect and Role of Various Nutrients in Respiratory Failure

Acute respiratory failure often results from or accompanies injury and sepsis, which lead to catabolism and hypermetabolism. The ensuing protein-calorie malnutrition can be complicated further in the critically ill patient with chronic lung disease, with or without chronic nutritional depletion. This chapter will not deal with the general guidelines and specifics of nutritional support but rather with the issues and problems that are unique to respiratory failure. For general principles and techniques of parenteral and enteral nutrition, the reader is referred to the appropriate chapters in this book.

Amino Acids

In addition to serving as substrate for protein synthesis, amino acids were reported to increase minute ventilation, oxygen consumption, and ventilatory response to hypoxia and hypercarbia [13, 14]. In eight patients with weight loss greater than 10%, infused 7.5 mg or 15 mg of nitrogen/kcal resting energy expenditure, the higher dose of nitrogen infused caused a significant reduction in arterial carbon dioxide tension ($PaCO_2$) with increased sensitivity and enhanced ventilatory response to carbon dioxide [15]. The effect of protein on minute ventilation (VE) and carbon dioxide production (VCO_2) during weaning from mechanical ventilation was studied in patients with acute respiratory failure due to COPD. A high protein intake during weaning was associated with a higher VE, higher VCO_2, and lower $PaCO_2$, suggesting an increase in ventilatory sensitivity to CO_2 by high protein intake and possibly enhanced weaning [16].

It was recently reported that the infusion of branched-chain amino acids (BCAA) in normal volunteers caused a major increase in ventilatory response to CO_2 inhalation, which was not evoked by a standard amino acid mixture [17]. The difference in the ventilatory responses between the regular and the BCAA solutions seems to be of unlikely clinical significance in patients with normal ventilatory reserves. However, it might turn out to be either beneficial or detrimental in critically ill patients with marginal or severely deranged pulmonary function. Unfortunately, no such studies have been undertaken as yet.

Glutamine and the Lungs

Glutamine is the most abundant free amino acid, both in the circulation as well as in the free amino acid pool of the body. Glutamine is the precursor for synthesis of amino acids, proteins, nucleotides, and other biologically active molecules. It is the most important precursor for ammoniagenesis in the kidney, the major end product of ammonia-trapping pathways in the liver, a substrate for gluconeogenesis, and an oxidative substrate in rapidly proliferating cells and tissues like enterocytes, white blood cells, and fibroblasts.

The principal organs of glutamine synthesis and release are the skeletal muscle (40% to 45%), the lungs (55% to 60%), and, to a much smaller degree, the brain and heart. Actually, the lungs are the most important organ of glutamine release in the postabsorptive state. The lungs, similar to skeletal muscle, play an important role in regulating glutamine metabolism during catabolic states by the accelerated release of glutamine. Net lung glutamine and alanine release doubled following the administration of dexamethasone and increased even further in endotoxin-treated rats and in septic patients. Dexamethasone also increased both glutamine synthetase activity and mRNA release [18–20].

Both endothelial cells in the lung as well as type II alveolar cells play a role in lung glutamine metabolism [21–23]. Glutamine released by skeletal muscle and the lung is avidly taken up and consumed by the gastrointestinal tract and the kidneys. In the gut, glutamine serves as the major source of energy for the enterocyte and as energy for lymphatic tissue and macrophages. In the kidneys, glutamine supports ammoniagenesis. Other consumers of glutamine are the liver, cells of the immune system (mainly macrophages and lymphocytes), and fibroblasts.

Lung glutamine release is also accelerated during sepsis [24,25]. Within one hour of an intravenous bolus of endotoxin, net lung glutamine efflux is increased, but this augmented output immediately follows the onset of sepsis and is short-lived. Subsequent development of pulmonary failure eliminates this augmented response. The apparent reversion to net glutamine balance may be due to the simultaneous increase in glutamine uptake by pulmonary endothelial cells. This is supported by the increased transport of glutamine in lung endothelium in response to tumor necrosis factor (TNF) [26] and interleukin-1 (IL-1) [27]. In general, endothelial cells together with hepatocytes, lymphocytes, and macrophages are the major consumers of glutamine following a septic insult.

Recent interest in the role of glutamine in the immune system might shed further light on the role and effects of glutamine in the lung via its pulmonary defense mechanisms. A high activity of glutaminase and a high rate of glutamine utilization has been found in a variety of lymphoid tissues examined and in macrophages [28–31]. These high rates of glutamine consumption suggest that glutamine plays an important role in these cells, but what role exactly is not yet elucidated. Some have suggested energy generation while others have suggested provision of intermediates for the biosynthesis of purine and pyrimidine nucleotide for the synthesis of DNA and mRNA. Another hypothesis has suggested that glutaminolysis provides optimal conditions for the precise rate regulation of purine and pyrimidine nucleotide synthesis at specific times of the cell cycle (metabolic control logic). Whatever its role, the high rate of glutamine utilization by lymphocytes and macrophages suggests glutamine to be important for immune function. As the alveolar macrophage is the main defensive instrument of the lung, it is logical to assume that the provision of glutamine would prove beneficial in states of injury and sepsis by also boosting the defense mechanism of the lungs.

Carbohydrate

Hypocaloric amounts of glucose administered to normal volunteers resulted in a low metabolic rate, decreased minute ventilation, and decreased response to hypoxia. The administration of glucose to cover resting energy expenditure increased minute ventilation in proportion to the increase in carbon dioxide production [32] and increased the ventilatory response to hypoxia [14]. This increased respiratory work in response to the increased carbon dioxide production caused by carbohydrate oxidation is one of the major reasons for the current common practice of using mixed glucose-fat fuel in the critically ill patient, particularly when mechanically ventilated for respiratory failure. Excessive carbohydrate intake in mechanically ventilated patients was reported to result in the accumulation of excess carbon dioxide and difficulty in weaning off the respirator [33].

It is yet unclear whether the increased CO_2 production from high carbohydrate loads is of any clinical significance in patients without preexisting respiratory failure. In a study of eucapnic COPD and severe hypercapnic COPD patients, both groups, who were not injured or septic, were able to dispose of the excess CO_2 produced as a result of a high carbohydrate meal. The problem exists, if at all, only in very few critically ill or septic patients with previous pulmonary problems and marginal respiratory function or reserve to whom a sudden and excessive carbohydrate load is administered.

A recent study comparing a mixed energy source with dextrose only in patients with a mean measured REE of 1.2 times the calculated basal energy expenditure demonstrated no difference between patients with normal or previous pulmonary disease when measuring oxygen consumption (VO_2), carbon dioxide production (VCO_2), and respiratory quotient (RQ). Carbohydrate loading (1.5 to 2.25 times REE) significantly increased $PaCO_2$ compared to mixed fuel administration. However, in patients fed only 1.5 times the REE, with no overfeeding, the mean RQ never exceeded 1, stressing the adverse effects of overfeeding, rather than the mere fact of using carbohydrates [34].

Lipids

Intravenous fat emulsions were reported to cause impairment of pulmonary function in healthy adults, premature infants, patients with preexisting pulmonary disease, and experimental animals. The lung function abnormalities usually involve increased diffusion capacity inequalities. More recent studies have claimed that intravenously administered lipid emulsions did not interfere with pulmonary diffusion capacity even in critically ill patients. An eight-hour infusion of 500 ml of a 20% fat emulsion caused decreases in PO_2/FiO_2, increases in mean pulmonary arterial pressure and shunting, and increases in pulmonary vascular resistance, more so in septic patients [35]. Patients with adult respiratory distress syndrome (ARDS) had significant decreases in PO_2/FiO_2 during four- or eight-hour infusion periods of 500 ml of a 10% fat emulsion, consistent with increases in the oxygen gradient and shunting. However, these changes seem to be infusion-rate related, so that oxygenation problems observed with intravenous fat emulsions may probably be eliminated completely with slower infusion rates [36].

Fat emulsions cause vasoactive changes that seem to be associated with prostaglandin production from linoleic acid via the cyclo-oxygenase pathway. The vasodilatory effects of prostaglandins alter pulmonary blood volume or the pulmonary capillary surface area for gas exchange, resulting in increased shunting and decreased diffusion capacity. Indomethacin administered to animals was reported to ameliorate these effects of lipid infusion with no change in hypertriglyceridemia.

One study has even indicated that the use of lipid emulsions improves pulmonary mechanical properties and surfactant production in the injured rat [37]. Moreover, extensive work from Kinney's group has indicated that intravenous fat emulsions are a preferred fuel source for the injured and septic patient [38,39]. Intravenous fat emulsions have also been implicated in causing impaired polymorphonuclear cell function and in reducing survival in various experimental animal models. A cumulative dose response reticuloendothelial system impairment was reported with intravenous lipid administration. Recently introduced middle-chain triglycerides (MCT) emulsions were reported not to impair the reticuloendothelial clearance of bacteria as much as long-chain triglycerides (LCT) emulsions. Combined LCT-MCT emulsions are currently commercially available. As a further development, structured lipids that are rearranged triglycerides with linoleic acid and MCT on the same glycerol molecule were recently shown not to impair the reticuloendothelial system function. Dietary fatty acid composition also affects eicosanoid metabolism, and, although not yet specifically looked at in lung function and metabolism, the composition of fat administered will certainly affect surfactant metabolism and pulmonary defense mechanisms.

Nutritional Support for Respiratory Failure, Mechanical Ventilation, and Weaning

Surgical patients in need of mechanical ventilation are undernourished as a result of their primary affliction, with or without an additional acute injury or stress leading to the process of metabolic response to injury with its ensuing catabolic and hypermetabolic consequences. Undernutrition, with or without added catabolism and hypermetabolism, results in muscle weakness and involves respiratory muscles and immune function derangements also. Nutritional therapy should aim at the maintenance and repletion of lost muscle mass and function with subsequent earlier and easier weaning of surgical patients from mechanical ventilation. Ventilator dependence has been related to a paradoxical breathing pattern, which is the result of respiratory muscle fatigue and decreased efficiency, to decreased respiratory drive, and to anxiety.

The general principles for treating respiratory muscle failure include: (1) Rest the fatigued muscle, namely, mechanically ventilate the patient; (2) remove noxious insults like hypoxia, deranged pH, electrolyte imbalance, deficiency states, hypovolemia, infection, sepsis, and other conditions that mechanically impede breathing; and (3) rebuild respiratory musculature by nutritional repletion and by general and respiratory muscle training.

Within the scope of this chapter, we will limit the discussion to nutritional intervention and the nutritional aspects of weaning patients from mechanical ventilation only. There is ample data concerning nutritional derangements and repletion of patients with chronic obstructive pulmonary diseases. Unfortunately, relatively little research has been accomplished on acute pulmonary failure, particularly in the surgical patient population. Results of nutritional intervention are scarce and so far, only retrospective data exist to support the role of nutritional intervention in weaning patients from mechanical ventilation.

In starved rats, short-term nutritional repletion normalized surfactant concentrations with no change in tissue elasticity and airspace abnormalities [40]. Nutritional support was reported to improve peripheral muscle function well before repletion of muscle mass [41]. One month of TPN in 11 youngsters with cystic fibrosis significantly improved their nutritional status as well as their maximum inspiratory and expiratory pressures, with no improvement in other pulmonary function indices [42]. Other studies in cystic fibrosis patients offer conflicting results. Keys et al. [43] observed decreased vital capacity and respiratory efficiency after 12 and 24 weeks of semistarvation in human volunteers. Twelve weeks of refeeding resulted in a slow reversal to control levels.

A few retrospective studies reported beneficial effects like an 86% weaning and extubation rate in patients receiving TPN compared to only 22% in patients treated with routine glucose-electrolyte therapy [44]. Eight out of 14 (57%) unweanable medical ICU patients were ultimately weaned following a prolonged course of parenteral or enteral nutrition. In a similar retrospective study, only 36.3% of surgical ICU patients receiving routine intravenous fluid therapy were weaned compared to 90.9% similar patients receiving nutritional support as TPN or enteral tube feeding [34]. Another study reported that patients' ability to breathe spontaneously was dependent on their nutritional intake; with increasing caloric intake, the percentage of spontaneously breathing patients increased from 11% to 79% [45]. Kelly et al. [4] demonstrated that in 21 of 29 critically ill patients receiving TPN for 2 weeks, both inspiratory muscle strength as well as body cell mass improved significantly and in a highly correlated manner. High protein intake was associated with significantly higher carbon dioxide production (VCO_2) and smaller increases in $PaCO_2$ during weaning compared to moderate protein intake, suggesting that for mechanically ventilated patients, high-protein nutrition may be beneficial in enhancing weaning from mechanical ventilation [16].

These results, although indicating that malnutrition negatively affects respiratory muscle function and that nutritional support improves maximal inspiratory pressure, do not yet establish the role of nutrition in weaning from mechanical ventilation and do not indicate whether nutritional support affects morbidity and outcome of ventilated surgical patients. At present, it seems logical to offer nutritional support; however, there is insufficient data to offer definite recommendations regarding its optimal form for patients with impaired respiratory function.

Patients with pulmonary insufficiency share many of the problems encountered in cardiac patients, mainly the need for sodium and volume restriction. As interactions between nutrients and respiration have been repeatedly suggested, special care should be taken in selecting the amounts and composition of nutrients to be infused in the catabolic patient with compromised respiratory function. As mentioned earlier, the ventilatory response to hypoxia and particularly to hypercarbia is enhanced with an increasing intake of amino acids. These effects seem to be even more enhanced when using BCAA. This stimulation of respiratory function might well have beneficial effects by improving the ventilatory efficiency. However, it might also turn out to be detrimental, inducing muscle fatigue and difficulty in weaning. These potential advantages and disadvantages of amino acid infusions need further study. Thus, the amount of protein supplied should be advanced slowly and its possible beneficial or detrimental effect on respiration closely monitored. In general, a daily nitrogen intake of 200 to 450 mg/kg body weight seems adequate to restore body cell mass in depleted-catabolic patients.

Recent publications indicated a cytokine-mediated increased glutamine uptake by pulmonary endothelium, probably in support of pulmonary structural integrity and lung glutamine balance [27]. Furthermore, the addition of glutamine to cultured pulmonary artery endothelial cells significantly increased ATP synthesis and improved survival following hydrogen peroxide injury [26]. Thus, glutamine might prove in further animal and clinical studies to be a useful therapeutic agent for the injured lung.

A similar situation exists regarding the supply of calories to this type of patient. In general, the catabolic patient in need of ventilatory support should receive up to 1.5 times resting energy expenditure while the respiratory rate, vital capacity, minute ventilation, and blood gases are carefully monitored. Nonprotein calories should be provided as a mixture of about 60% carbohydrate and 40% fat, in an attempt to avoid excessive carbon dioxide production as a result of excess glucose, while protecting the reticuloendothelial system from high lipid infusion rates. It was recommended to limit glucose intake to a maximum of 4 to 5 mg/kg/min [46], although even this amount and rate might prove excessive in patients with limited respiratory reserve. In an attempt to make weaning easier, it was also recommended to reduce the caloric intake to about 50% of needed calories in patients with marginal respiratory function, although this has not been proven in a clinical study. This reduction in protein and caloric intake fits well with the need for a gradual return to normal of the sodium pump, which is deranged by malnutrition [47]. With excessive refeeding of malnourished patients, large amounts of sodium shift from the intracellular into the extracellular compartment, contributing to the development of edema with possible further difficulty in weaning. Thus, it is important, at least at the early stage of refeeding, to limit protein, calories, fluids, and sodium. Once the patient has been weaned off mechanical ventilation, caloric and protein intake should be gradually increased to the fully desired nutritional support regimen, attempting to achieve positive balance and repletion.

The Heart*

Three main topics are of major interest when discussing nutrition and the heart. The first aspect is basic cardiac metabolism and its adaptation to states of ischemia and reperfusion. The second, and most interesting to the scholar and practitioner of surgical nutrition, is the pathophysiology and effects of protein-calorie malnutrition on the heart and possible means of correcting these derangements. The third aspect, which will not be discussed in this chapter, is the dietary effects and implications on the etiology and development of atherosclerotic cardiovascular disease.

Energy for the myocardium is derived from free fatty acids, glucose, ketone bodies, lactate, pyruvate, and amino acids. Under resting conditions cardiac metabolism is essentially a process of aerobic oxidative phosphorylation via the Krebs cycle [48]. In the fasting state free fatty acids play the major role in the oxidative metabolism of the heart. Plasma free fatty acids are transported to the heart as albumin-bound fatty acids and taken up by the myocardium by a single-pass extraction rate of 40% to 60%. It was recently suggested that the influx of fatty acids into human myocardium is facilitated by a fatty acid binding protein located in the membrane of cardiac capillary endothelial cells [49]. In the fed state, when glucose and insulin levels are high, the contribution of glucose to oxidative metabolism becomes dominant. During fasting or diabetes, when circulating free fatty acid levels are high, cardiac glucose oxidation is inhibited and glycogen is formed and stored.

Cardiac glycogen level increases as the result of the inhibition of glucose oxidation, so that glucose taken up forms glycogen rather than passing along the glycolytic pathway. When circulating fatty acids are low, as in the fed state, then the inhibiting effects of fatty acids on glycolysis are removed. Glycolytic flux from glucose is then regulated by the rate of glucose transport across cell membrane, which in turn depends on circulating glucose and insulin concentrations. Circulating glucose and insulin levels act as a signal linking the rate of glycolysis in the heart and the rate of lipolysis in adipose tissue. Under conditions of ischemia or hypoxia the heart becomes dependent on anaerobic metabolism, with glycolysis being its major pathway. Under both aerobic and anaerobic conditions, breakdown of ATP and its resynthesis serve as the fuel for the contractile cycle of the heart.

The major sites of metabolic regulation of cardiac glycolysis are the rate of glucose transport across the cell membrane and the activity of the enzyme phosphofructokinase. Additional sites of regulation are enzyme levels of hexokinase, glyceraldehyde phosphate dehydrogenase, and pyruvate dehydrogenase. All these sites are inhibited by fatty acid oxidation, thus explaining the preferential use of fatty acids when available. In

*Parts of this section, although completely revised and rewritten, are based on Dr. Ronald M. Abel's Nutrition and the Heart. In JE Fischer (ed), *Surgical Nutrition*. Boston: Little, Brown, 1983.

the fed state, when circulating free fatty acid levels are low, then the inhibition imposed by free fatty acids on glycolysis is removed. Conversely, high circulating glucose and insulin levels will act as a signal for the activation of glycolysis and will inhibit free fatty acid release from adipose tissue.

Decades of intensive research elucidated the complicated sequence of messengers involved in cardiac metabolism in health and disease. Catecholamine stimulation so common in myocardial ischemia, due to the combination of painful stimuli, other associated stressful events and reflex stimulation from the ischemic heart, causes increased cyclic adenosine monophosphate (AMP) levels in ischemic myocardial tissue. The excess of cyclic AMP could promote accumulation of fatty acids and their metabolites, thus explaining the increased free fatty acid levels during myocardial ischemia and their deleterious effects on arrhythmias and ventricular function. Moreover, cyclic AMP as the second messenger activates a protein kinase A, which in turn liberates its catalytic subunit to phosphorylate and activates phospholamban. The end result is enhanced calcium channel activity and uptake of calcium into the sarcoplasmic reticulum. The increased rate of calcium uptake results in the positive inotropic effect of catecholamines. To help maintain the increased mitochondrial activity that accompanies the positive inotropic effect, enhanced transfer of calcium across the inner mitochondrial membrane is thought to act directly by stimulation of the citric acid cycle, which in turn promotes the rate of oxidative phosphorylation and rate of adenosine triphosphate (ATP) production.

ATP is the crucial energy source for contraction and for maintenance of transmembrane ion gradients. However, it is not the critical level of ATP per se that is important. Rather, it is the turnover rate of ATP, especially ATP derived from glycolytic flux, that is crucial for maintenance of viability. When ATP breaks down, as a result of vigorous heart work, hypoxia or ischemia, counter-regulatory mechanisms are set in motion by the formation of its breakdown products like adenosine diphosphate (ADP), AMP, adenosine, and inorganic phosphate. Because ATP is replenished from phosphocreatine, its level may stay unchanged, yet its breakdown products in the tissue will rise.

AMP and inorganic phosphate will stimulate phosphofructokinase and glycolysis. Adenosine produced in the myocyte will diffuse to the extracellular space and act on arterioles to cause coronary vasodilatation and opening of cardiac ATP-dependent potassium channels, as well as inhibition of myocardial calcium channels. Because the concentration of adenosine required to alter channel regulation are in the micromolar range compared with the millimolar range of cytosolic ATP, breakdown of a small fraction of ATP will significantly increase the activity of adenosine to act as coronary vasodilator without any measurable change in ATP concentration. Adenosine in micromolar amounts can enhance the opening of the potassium channels during ischemia and thus counter-regulate the severity of ischemia. Adenosine also inhibits the calcium current by counteracting the ischemia-mediated opening of calcium channels. Furthermore, it can inhibit the atrioventricular node from producing tachyarrhythmias, so common during ischemia. The effect of adenosine is also often apparent as a reduced heart rate.

Metabolism of Ischemia and Reperfusion Injury

Ischemia produces two major metabolic derangements: those consequent to decreased oxygen delivery to the tissue and those due to decreased washout of metabolites. During ischemia, a decrease in oxidative phosphorylation occurs, and a four- to five-fold increase in glycolysis with pyruvate being converted to lactate to maintain the beating of the anaerobic heart takes its place. Fatty acid utilization is depressed and the decrease in β-oxidation leads to free fatty acid accumulation with their attendant risk of arrhythmias and depressed contractility. Lactate production is the end point of anaerobic glycolysis, with proton production resulting chiefly from the turnover of ATP by its continuous glycolytic synthesis and subsequent breakdown. Proton accumulation can inhibit cardiac contraction and glycolysis at the levels of certain key enzymes.

Cellular calcium overload seems to be the direct cause of the pathological alterations that occur during ischemia and reperfusion. Calcium overload inhibits the glycolytic flux with fall in the production of glycolytic ATP and possible cell death. Current evidence points toward the turnover rate of ATP, rather than its critical tissue level, to be crucial in maintenance of tissue viability, especially the ATP derived from glycolytic flux. When ATP breaks down, counter-regulatory mechanisms are set in motion by its breakdown products like ADP, AMP, adenosine, and inorganic phosphate. Another detrimental aspect of ischemia is a sequence of events entitled reperfusion injury. Reperfusion injury includes: stunning, arrhythmias, cell necrosis, and microvascular injury. The suggested mechanisms for reperfusion damage include formation of free radicals, intracellular cytosolic calcium overload, or both. Not only may free radicals lead to an increase of cytosolic calcium, but the increased calcium may in turn lead to increased formation of free radicals.

In addition, recent discoveries identified two endogenous vasoactive substances, both released from endothelium. One is nitric oxide, which is the active vasodilator component of the endothelium-derived relaxation factor (EDRF). The other is the vasoconstrictor polypeptide, endothelin. Nitric oxide is formed from arginine and vasodilates by stimulating guanylate cyclase and the production of vasodilator cyclic guanosine monophosphate. Endothelin, which is formed during prolonged ischemia, is a strong vasoconstrictor acting by a combination of calcium channel stimulation and inositol triphosphate. Exercise, increased coronary flow, and acetylcholine will promote release of nitric oxide to mediate vasodilatation. Prolonged ischemia, hemorrhage, and reperfusion will release endothelin and the vasoconstrictor regulatory mechanisms.

Starvation, Malnutrition, and the Heart

Not long ago, the heart was believed to be spared during starvation. Two major human studies performed during World War II, only one of which was voluntary, changed this view. Reported in individuals who died of starvation during the Warsaw Ghetto uprising was cardiac atrophy with an average heart weight of only 220 to 275 g and "brown atrophy" with loss of epicardial fat. In a classic series of experiments on normal volunteers, Keys and co-workers [43,50] prospectively studied the precise effects of starvation and semistarvation in man. They subjected 32 volunteers to hypocaloric diets, which resulted in the loss of approximately 25% of initial body weight within six months; the patients then received a suitable period of nutritional rehabilitation. They noted a decrease in heart size in all dimensions, and the hearts assumed more of a vertical position in the chest following weight loss. Arterial and venous pressure fell, reductions in stroke volume, cardiac output and cardiac index were noted, and heart rate frequently diminished to extreme levels of bradycardia. An attempt to provide rapid nutritional repletion frequently resulted in early signs of congestive heart failure during the rehabilitative phase of these experiments [51].

Several investigators have confirmed that total protein-calorie deprivation may cause myocardial atrophy and myofibrillar degeneration with a 20% to 30% decrease in myofibrillar diameter. Morphometry revealed dilatation of the myocyte T-system, exocytosis of intracellular components into the extracellular space of the T-system, and the ratio of mitochondria to myofibrils decreased progressively during starvation, possibly compromising cellular energy supply [52]. Gelfand et al. [53] discussed the development of "microcardia" resulting from malnutrition in a group of patients in whom tropical sprue played an important factor in the development, and later the maintenance, of malnutrition.

There has also been an unfortunate experience with self-induced marasmus. Garnett et al. [54] reported the sudden and unexpected death in an otherwise healthy, but morbidly obese, young woman subjected to 30 weeks of therapeutic total starvation to obtain rapid weight reduction. Cardiac death occurred as a result of refractory ventricular fibrillation. Autopsy examination revealed a dilated, atrophied heart of 250 g; ultrastructural examination confirmed the presence of atrophy and destruction of myofibrils. In 1977, the Center for Disease Control reported that at least 58 young women ingesting so-called liquid protein diets died in the United States. In an attempt to control morbid obesity by limiting all nutrient intake to commercial products containing protein with no additional supplemental calories, these women developed sudden cardiac death without prior evidence of heart disease. Although many of the terminal arrhythmias (primarily ventricular tachycardia and fibrillation, which were unresponsive to ordinary therapeutic endeavors) could have been associated with electrolyte abnormalities, there were a number of deaths documented in which electrolyte patterns appeared normal [55]. The autopsy material from this group of patients confirmed the presence of starvation-induced myocardial atrophy.

In a series of experiments in a dog model of protein-calorie malnutrition (42% body weight loss) and refeeding, Abel et al. [56,57] used the isovolumetric left heart preparation on total cardiopulmonary bypass. They found the malnourished hearts to be edematous, atrophied, and low on glycogen content. All these changes were reversed to control levels on refeeding. Histologically, they observed edema and a 20% reduction in the mean myofibrillar diameter. Myocardial atrophy and interstitial edema were also reported by others [56,57]. The hemodynamic changes in Abel's study included persistent and significant depression of left ventricular (LV) function, reflected as a decrease in peak LV dp/dt at similar LV volumes compared with controls. A decrease in LV compliance (Figure 26-1) was observed in malnourished animals compared with controls; refed animals demonstrated some improvement

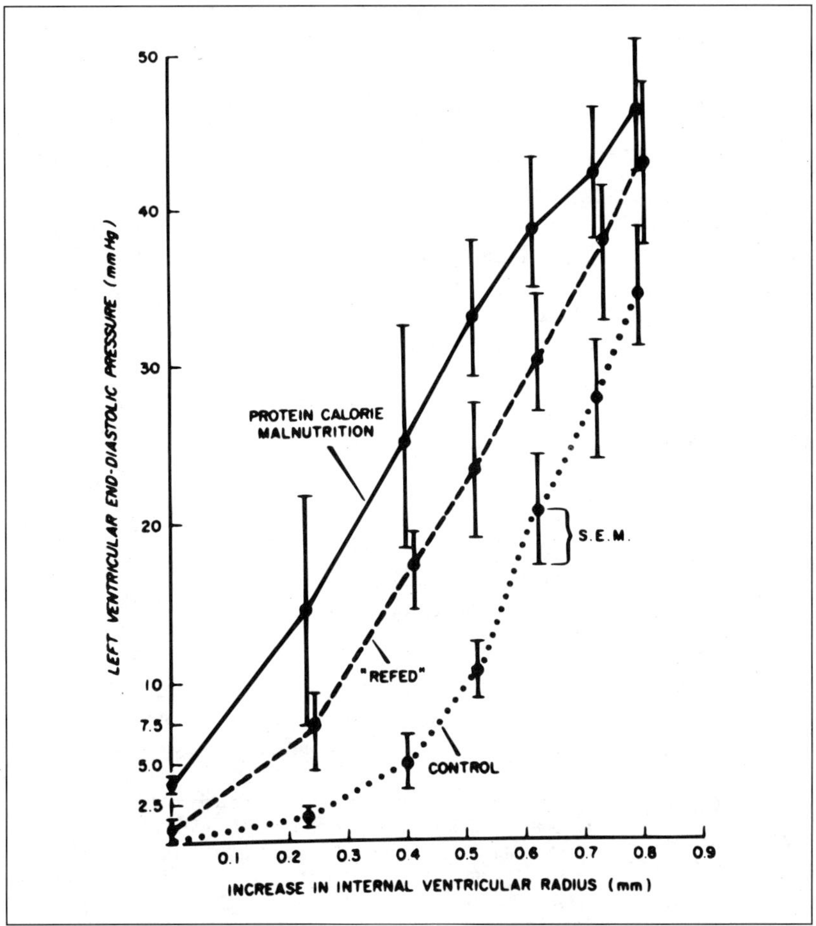

Figure 26-1. Significant depression of left ventricular function in protein-calorie malnourished dogs reflected as a decrease in peak left ventricular systolic pressure and left ventricular dp/dt at similar left ventricular volumes, compared with controls. These changes are only partially reversed in the refed dogs. (From RM Abel. Nutrition and the heart. In JE Fischer (ed), *Surgical Nutrition* [1st ed]. Boston: Little, Brown, 1983, with permission.)

in this decreased compliance but did not return to control values. Following a short-term nutritional convalescence, refed animals demonstrated persistent abnormalities of LV function, including decreases in LV compliance and in maximum developed LV dp/dt (see Figure 26-1). Others reported reduction in left ventricular compliance, force velocity, peak developed pressure, cardiac contractility, and stroke volume as well as chamber volume reduction, which was proportionate to body weight loss [58]. Our own studies in the Lagendorff preparation of the rat demonstrated that developed force and force velocity decreased progressively during six weeks of protein malnutrition. These changes were significantly more pronounced at higher heart rates and returned to normal following refeeding [59]. Recently, four weeks of experimental food restriction were reported to result in a 23% reduction of ventricular ATP levels with no change in phosphocreatine. Furthermore, a loss of creatine-kinase activity and ATPase activity were found, suggesting predominantly a myofibrillar damage [106].

Nutritional Repletion of the Heart

In the cardiac patient, clinicians might encounter two different states of malnutrition. The first is the classic cardiac cachexia seen in patients with long-standing congestive heart failure. In the etiology of cardiac cachexia, several factors were named, including anorexia, an elevated metabolic rate, cellular hypoxia due to hypoperfusion and impaired delivery of nutrients to the tissues, deranged removal of cellular waste products, and possibly increased urinary and fecal nutrient losses [60]. The second form of malnutrition is iatrogenic as the result of complicated cardiac surgery or any other type of complicated major surgery in the cardiac patient.

Considerations of nutritional support are very different in these two types of cardiac cachexia. In the first form, we are dealing with patients in long-standing congestive heart failure, due mainly to rheumatic valvular disease or congenital heart malformations, who need corrective cardiac surgery. In the second group of patients, which is certainly more common in recent years, we are dealing with an excessive metabolic response to major surgery and ensuing postoperative complications in patients who initially presented in a satisfactory nutritional status. These are mainly patients undergoing coronary artery bypass grafts for ischemic heart disease or patients with ischemic heart disease undergoing any other noncardiac major surgical intervention. A third but much smaller group would be patients with a severe myocardial infarction, undergoing resuscitation, and subsequently developing cardiac failure, renal failure, and the need for mechanical ventilation.

Forty percent of patients awaiting open-heart surgery for valve replacement manifested significant reductions of lean body mass. These depleted patients had longer hospital stays and increased mortality following valvuloplasty [61]. In a study of 44 malnourished patients undergoing cardiac surgery, Abel et al. [62] observed higher rates of sepsis and respiratory failure, longer stays in the intensive care unit, greater hospital costs, and increased mortality compared to normally nourished operated controls. This incidence of complications and higher mortality rate were not improved by a postoperative five-day course of TPN. However, reduced morbidity was reported in three patients undergoing triple-valve replacement following three weeks of preoperative TPN [63]. Heymsfield et al. [58] reported reversal of anergy and positive nitrogen balance following preoperative alimentation in cardiac cachexia. Keys et al. [43,50], in their classic experiments, reported a prolonged period of disability following nutritional repletion in starving normal volunteers. Animal data from Abel's group [56,57] suggested that despite nutritional repletion of malnourished dogs, significant depression of ventricular performance still existed. Our own data in the Langendorff preparation of a rat model of starvation and refeeding demonstrated that although a constant heart-body weight ratio was maintained during both starvation and refeeding, developed force and force velocity decreased during protein malnutrition as compared to control rats. These changes were less obvious at low heart rates but became very significant at elevated heart rates of 300 and 400 beats/min (Figure 26-2). These experimental protein malnutrition-induced derangements in myocardial function, in particular at times of increased demands as during higher heart rates, reversed almost completely to normal on prolonged refeeding [59].

Similar considerations exist in infants with congenital heart diseases. Failure to thrive and growth retardation delay the surgical correction of their anomalies and, in a vicious cycle, impedes

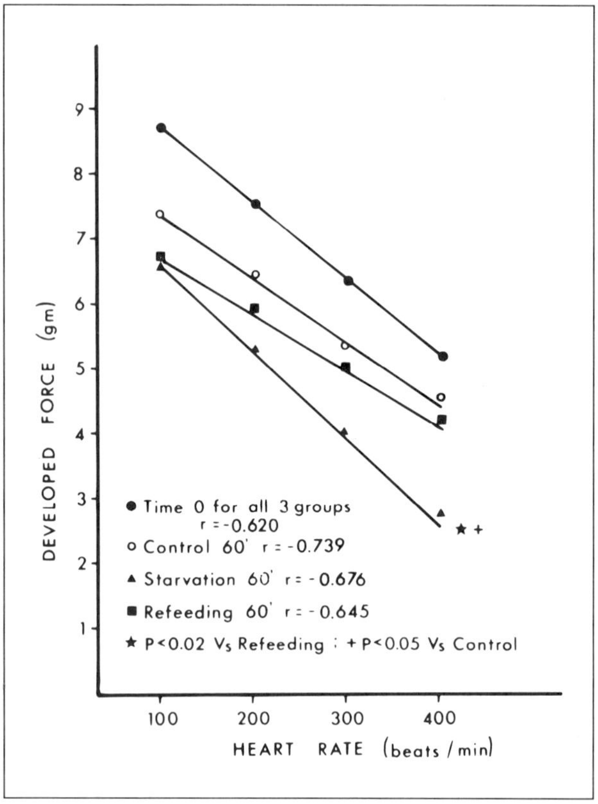

Figure 26-2. Correlation of developed force and heart rate in control, starving, and refed isolated rat hearts at time zero (same line for all three groups) and after 60 minutes of Langendorff perfusion. Note the stronger decline in developed force of starving animals compared to the control and the refed groups ($p < 0.02$–0.05) indicating the stronger effect of starvation in higher heart rates and increased cardiac work. (From HR Freund, J Holyrode. Cardiac function during protein malnutrition and refeeding in the isolated rat heart. *JPEN* 10:470, 1986, with permission.)

catch-up growth due to the development of pulmonary hypertension. Moreover, prolonged nutritional deficits and growth retardation increase surgical risk and delay recovery in those infants with complex defects not correctable during the neonatal period. Schwartz et al. [64] found, in a randomized five-month study, that infants with congenital cardiac defects complicated by malnutrition manifest increased nutrient requirements for growth and weight gain (mean 147 kcal/kg/day), and that continuous, 24-hour nasogastric alimentation is the most effective method to satisfy these needs. Bougle et al. [65] treated 13 children for 40 days with enteral feeding via nasogastric tubes at 137 kcal/kg/day and were able to show weight gain and growth, and to safely accomplish cardiac surgery in 9 of these patients. A similar report was published by Vanderhoof et al. [66], allowing for earlier and safer surgical intervention in 11 tube-fed infants.

In another interesting study, preoperative nutritional manipulations were attempted in 312 patients who were to undergo elective coronary artery bypass surgery. It was possible to alter myocardial glycogen stores and thus offer better myocardial protection by the preoperative supplementation of a combination of oral fat and intravenous hypertonic glucose [67].

Nutritional Support and Specific Nutrient Requirements and Considerations

The following section will deal only with specific issues relating to the nutritional support of cardiac patients. The broader and more explicit guidelines, techniques, and practice of nutritional support in general are discussed in other appropriate chapters of this book.

Amino Acids

Abel et al. [56] determined the cardiovascular effects of a commercially available infusion of amino acids in the canine isovolumetric heart preparation. Within five minutes following initiation of a crystalline amino acid infusion, consistent improvements in left ventricular (LV) function were noted in all animals as evidenced by an increased peak developed LV pressure and LV dp/dt max. Furthermore, the force-velocity relationships of the LV demonstrated consistent positive isotropic effects of this infusion.

Later work with the use of branched-chain amino acids (BCAA) in the septic [68,69] and ischemic [70–72] rat heart suggested new insight into possible nutritional and metabolic manipulations of the heart. Protein turnover in cardiac as well as skeletal muscle is affected by the provision of amino acids, particularly the BCAA. This effect on cardiac and skeletal muscle is related not only to the BCAA role as an energy substrate via oxidation and gluconeogenesis, but also involves their ability to regulate turnover by accelerating protein synthesis and inhibiting protein degradation [73–78]. The effects on protein turnover are particularly apparent under conditions of elevated BCAA concentration, and even metabolites of the BCAA modify protein turnover in cardiac and skeletal muscle [79]. In vivo studies in a rat injury model [80–82] and some other clinical studies [83–86] confirmed these nitrogen-sparing effects of BCAA, although in general, the results in septic patients are rather disappointing.

It is generally agreed that myocardial depression and ultimately failure occurs in sepsis [87, 88]. Suggested causes for the heart failure observed in sepsis include structural damage to the myocardium [88,89], increased circulatory requirements resulting in hypotension and inadequate coronary perfusion [89], intracardiac fluid and ionic disturbances [57], or a toxic phenomenon in the form of a myocardial depressant factor [90, 91]. In our series of experiments with the isolated rat heart Langendorff preparation [68,69], significant reductions of both developed force and force velocity of the heart were demonstrated during sepsis (Figure 26-3). These deranged systolic properties improved during perfusion with a variety of glucose and amino acid formulations, suggesting a mechanical washout effect of a "toxic" substance. Furthermore, a distinct improvement in systolic properties was apparent when utilizing an amino acid formulation containing 42% BCAA, suggesting that a significant and important improvement in cardiac function can be achieved by supplying balanced BCAA-enriched amino acid solutions [69, 92].

Subsequently, we looked into the myocardial protecting effects of BCAA during ischemia and reperfusion of the Langendorff and working heart preparations [70–72]. Perfusion with BCAA resulted in prolongation of the time to initiation of ischemic contracture and improvement of postischemic pressure recovery [70]. A phosphorous-31 magnetic resonance study revealed higher ATP levels in the BCAA group that coincided with the improved recovery of systolic and diastolic functions, indicating that BCAA protect from myocardial ischemic injury, decrease depletion of ATP during ischemia, and enhance postischemic hemodynamic function. However, the most striking beneficial effects were observed in the ischemic energy-depleted working heart where an oxygenated BCAA containing cardioplegic solution was able to enhance cardiac protection. The recovery of aortic flow, coronary flow, cardiac output, aortic pressure, stroke volume, and minute work was significantly better with the addition of BCAA (Figure 26-4). During reperfusion, recovery of ATP and creatine-phosphate was enhanced, and release of purine nucleotide catabolites and LDH were decreased with BCAA. Thus, during global ischemia in the energy-depleted heart, BCAA, as part of the cardioplegia solution, enhanced myocardial protection [71,72]. Beneficial effects on myocardial function were also reported for various other amino acids.

In both animal and human studies, glutamate and aspartate had been shown to exert cardioprotection during ischemia and reperfusion. In pigs, the supply of both these amino acids reduced myocardial infarct size [93]. In patients with stable angina, improvement in ischemia was reported. Low-output failure following open-heart surgery improved following the administration of glutamate with improved cardiac and stroke indices. Suggested mechanisms of action improve the al-

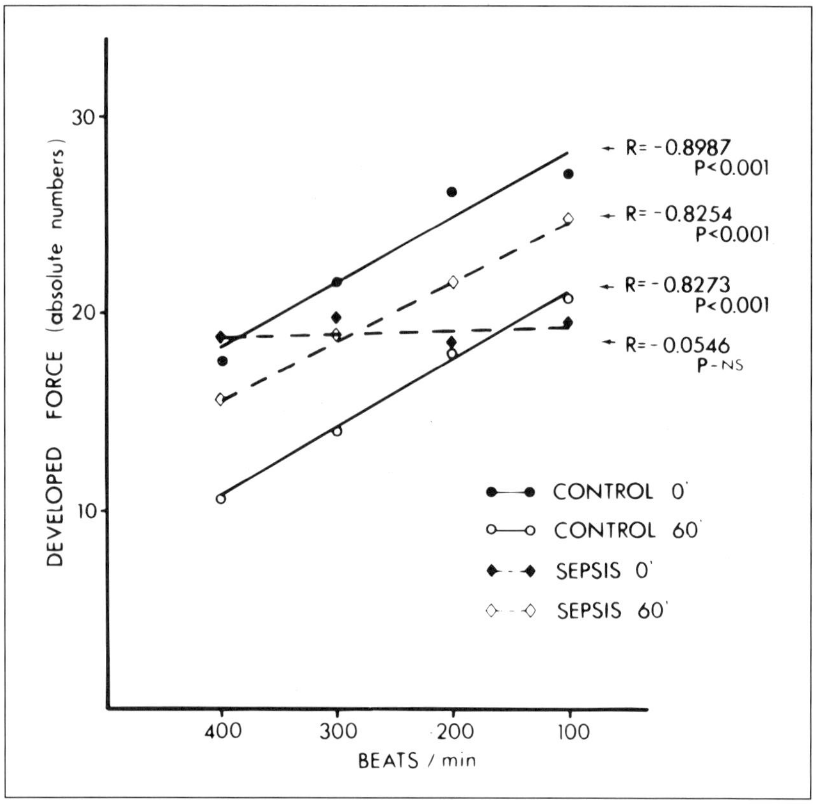

Figure 26-3. Regression lines for developed force and heart rate in control and septic animals at time zero and after 60 minutes of Langendorff perfusion. Note similar slopes for control animals at time zero and 60 minutes while septic animals exhibited significantly ($p < 0.05$) different slopes. At time zero in septic animals, developed force did not decrease with increasing heart rate as observed in control animals. After 60 minutes of perfusion, septic animals regained this negative linear correlation of developed force and heart rate ($p < 0.001$), with developed force being significantly improved at 60 minutes compared with time zero. (From HR Freund, et al. The effect of branched-chain amino acids on systolic properties of the normal and septic isolated rat heart. *Arch Surg* 120:488, 1985. Copyright 1985, American Medical Association, with permission.)

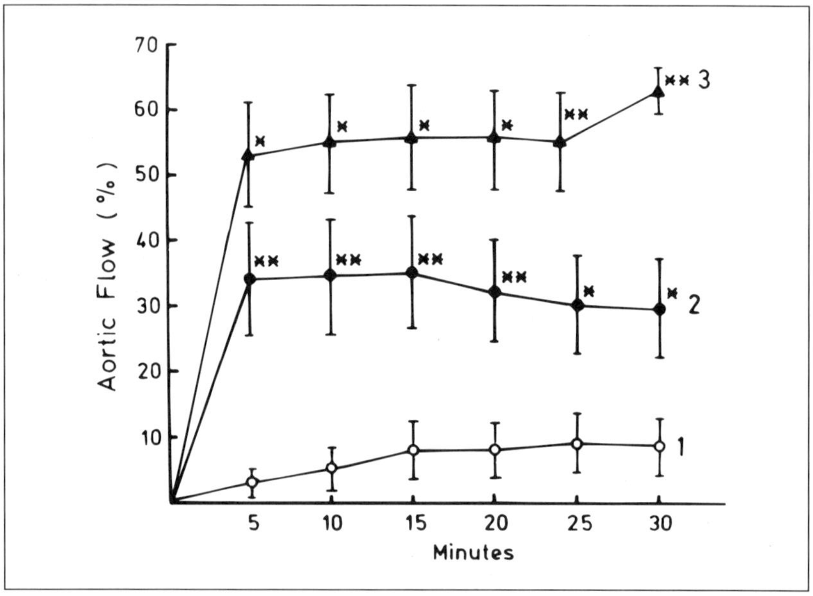

Figure 26-4. Aortic flow recovery, expressing cardiac output of the working heart, during postischemic reperfusion with: (1) Cardioplegic solution without glucose; (2) Cardioplegic solution with glucose; (3) Cardioplegic solution with glucose and branched-chain amino acids (BCAA). The addition of BCAA significantly enhanced cardiac protection with improved recovery of aortic flow, coronary flow, cardiac output, aortic pressure, stroke volume, and minute work. Recovery of ATP, creatine phosphate (CP), purine nucleotide catabolites, and LDH release were also improved.
*$p < 0.05$.
**$p < 0.01$.
(From H Schwalb, et al. The effect of amino acids on the ischemic heart. *J Thorac Cardiovasc Surg* 98:551, 1989, with permission.)

tered glucose and fatty acid metabolism in the ischemic and reperfused heart [94]. Four weeks of 5% arginine-enriched diet resulted in preservation of the endothelium-derived relaxation factor levels and reduction in the loss of myocardial creatine kinase activity in the ischemic and reperfused rat heart [95], thus suggesting cardioprotective effects of arginine.

Glucose

Catecholamine activity, the severity of myocardial infarction, and plasma free fatty acid levels are strongly linked, leading to the conclusion that increased concentrations of free fatty acids are harmful to the acute myocardial infarction process, whereas provision of glucose could be beneficial [48]. Hypertonic glucose [96], a carbohydrate-amino acid mixture [56], and insulin [97,98], were all reported to exert positive inotropic effects. Provision of glucose with the consequent release of insulin did in fact reduce the adverse effects of free fatty acids in myocardial infarction and led to the experimental use of glucose-insulin-potassium (GIK). However, conflicting results were published, and GIK is still in need of a properly controlled study in acute myocardial infarction. Our own experimental results in the Langendorff preparation of the normal rat heart indicate that neither insulin nor glucagon affected the function of the normal heart. However, insulin, and to a lesser degree glucagon, exerted positive inotropic effects on the isolated septic rat heart [99].

Fat

Grimes and Abel [100] reported that a 10% concentration of intravenous fat emulsion produced consistently negative effects on canine myocardium. Furthermore, significant decreases in systemic vascular resistance repeatedly occurred following Intralipid infusion in the same preparation. However, these observations were not confirmed in patients recovering from coronary bypass surgery in whom no adverse hemodynamic changes occurred with the infusion of relatively high doses of fat [101]. Only enormous amounts of fat (5.25 mg/kg/min), which are never used in clinical practice, resulted in the depression of myocardial contractility [102]. Thus, there seems to be no contraindication to the use of fat emulsions in the cardiac patient, either as part of the glucose system or as part of the "all-in-one" system.

The long-chain polyunsaturated ω-3 fatty acids (PUFA) found in fish oil are long known to possess beneficial effects on the cardiovascular system. More recently, their effect on the regulation of platelet-vessel wall interaction was appreciated. PUFA can influence the balance between arachidonic acid metabolites: thromboxane A_2 (platelet aggregation and vasoconstriction properties) and prostacycline (antiplatelet aggregation and vasodilatory). Administration of dietary fish oils reduces TXA_2 and LTB_4 synthesis with no change in PGI_2 and PGI_3 formation, thus positively affecting coronary blood flow, endothelium integrity and platelet activity and thrombosis. The net result is a reduction of myocardial ischemia and infarction [103].

Recommendations for Nutritional Support in Cardiac Patients

There are really only minor modifications in the nutritional management of cardiac patients compared to ordinary patients in need of nutritional support. The major difference is the need to often restrict total volume (to approximately 1500 ml/day) and sodium (to approximately 1.5 g/day) administration. Other minor considerations are that diuretic therapy might bring about the need for additional potassium, magnesium, and possibly zinc supplementation. Additional potassium might also be needed to support the process of anabolism.

Most patients will tolerate fluid and gas exchange loads imposed by continuous enteral or parenteral nutrition. However, some patients, particularly those who are severely malnourished with limited cardiac and/or pulmonary reserve, might develop the "refeeding syndrome" [43,50, 104]. These patients may develop dyspnea, hypercapnia, tachycardia, elevated venous pressure, congestive heart failure, or even cardiac arrest. It thus seems necessary not only to closely monitor volume and electrolyte intake and balance, but also to carefully adjust caloric input and source, and rate of nutritional repletion.

Because no prospective randomized studies have ever been performed to settle the question of to whom, how much, and for how long nutritional support is needed to decrease morbidity and mortality in depleted patients undergoing cardiac surgery, there are really no valid guidelines to select patients for whom perioperative nutritional support would be advantageous and would outweigh the potential risks and the delay of surgery. More general definitive proof exists, however, in the perioperative Veterans Administration study that did not include cardiac patients and that concluded that perioperative nutritional support is beneficial only in the very depleted group of patients [105]. [*Editor's Note:* This is complicated by the fact that only severely malnourished patients were helped, but the duration of preoperative TPN was from 7 to 10 days. Experimental and the few clinical studies that exist suggest that reversing protein-calorie malnutrition of the heart takes from 4 to 6 weeks.]

Neither is there enough data to recommend a distinct and specific nutritional support regimen for the cardiac patient. As already proven in the early days of TPN, cardiac patients manage well with regular amino acid formulations. However, although clinically not tested, there is some animal data to suggest the use of BCAA in cardiac patients, particularly during sepsis, ischemia, and reperfusion. Arginine was also claimed to offer some cardioprotection in animal studies and deserves further clinical studies. The heart, being an organ of glutamine synthesis, might well be similarly affected as skeletal muscle and the lung, and turn out to be in need of exogenous glutamine administration during injury and sepsis.

As free fatty acids are harmful to the myocardium, high concentrations of glucose calories seem to be warranted during nutritional support of the cardiac patient. However, there seems to be no contraindication to the administration of intravenous fat emulsions in the cardiac patient. The use of long-chain polyunsaturated ω-3 fatty acids, which showed some beneficial effects in animals, awaits further studies in humans, particularly during or following ischemia.

Special consideration should be afforded to electrolytes, minerals, vitamins, and trace elements that have paramount effects on heart metabolism and function, like potassium, calcium, magnesium, vitamin B, and selenium.

References

1. Haddad GG, Akabas SR. Adaptation of respiratory muscles to acute and chronic stress. *Clin Chest Med* 7:79, 1986.
2. Arora NS, Rochester DF. Effect of body weight and muscularity on human diaphragm muscle mass, thickness, and area. *J Appl Physiol* 52:64, 1982.
3. Arora NS, Rochester DF. Respiratory muscle strength and maximal voluntary ventilation in undernourished patients. *Am Rev Respir Dis* 126:5, 1982.
4. Kelly SM, et al. Inspiratory muscle strength and body composition in patients receiving total parenteral nutrition therapy. *Am Rev Respir Dis* 130:33, 1984.
5. Fulks RM, Li JB, Goldberg AL. Effects of insulin, glucose and amino acids on protein turnover in rat diaphragm. *J Biol Chem* 250:290, 1975.
6. Goldberg AL, Odessey R. Oxidation of amino acids by diaphragm from fed and fasted rats. *Am J Physiol* 223:1384, 1972.
7. Odessey R. Amino acid and protein metabolism in the diaphragm. *Am Rev Respir Dis* 119:107, 1979.
8. Lewis MJ, Belman MJ. Nutrition and the respiratory muscles. *Clin Chest Med* 9:337, 1988.
9. Sahebjami H. Nutrition and the pulmonary parenchyma. *Clin Chest Med* 7:111, 1986.
10. Wilson DO, Rogers RM, Hoffman RM. Nutrition and chronic lung disease. *Am Rev Respir Dis* 132:1347, 1985.
11. Sibille Y, Reynolds HY. Macrophages and polymorphonuclear neutrophils in lung defense and injury. *Am Rev Respir Dis* 141:471, 1990.
12. Niederman MS, et al. Nutritional status and bacterial binding in the lower respiratory tract in patients with chronic tracheostomies. *Ann Intern Med* 100:795, 1984.
13. Wilson DO, Rogers RM, Hoffman RM. Nutrition and chronic lung disease. *Am Rev Respir Dis* 132:1347, 1985.
14. Zwillich CW, Sahn SA, Weil JV. Effects of hypermetabolism upon respiratory gas exchange in normal man. *J Clin Invest* 66:900, 1977.
15. Askanazi J, et al. Effect of protein intake on ventilatory drive. *Anesthesiology* 60:106, 1984.
16. Van den Berg B, Stam H, Hop WCJ. Effect of dietary protein in content on weaning from the ventilator. *Clin Nutr* 8:207, 1989.
17. Takala J, et al. Changes in respiratory control induced by amino acid infusions. *Crit Care Med* 16:465, 1988.
18. Ardawi MSM. Glutamine-synthesizing activity in lungs of fed, starved, acidotic, diabetic, injured, and septic rats. *Biochem J* 270:829, 1990.
19. Sarantos P, Howard D, Souba WW. Dexamethasone regulates glutamine synthetase expression in rat lung. *Metabolism* 42:795, 1993.
20. Souba WW, et al. Effects of glucocorticoids on lung glutamine and alanine metabolism. *Surgery* 108:213, 1990.
21. Hautamaki RD, Green B, Souba WW. Characterization of L-glutamine transport by type II alveolar cells. *Am J Physiol* 262:L459, 1992.
22. Herskowitz K, et al. Characterization of L-glutamine transport by pulmonary artery endothelial cells. *Am J Physiol* 260:L241, 1991.
23. Leighton B, et al. Maximum activities of some key enzymes of glycolysis, glutaminolysis, Kreb Cycle and fatty acid utilization in bovine pulmonary endothelial cells. *FEBS Lett* 225:93, 1987.
24. Austgen TA, et al. Glutamine metabolism by the endotoxin-injured lung. *J Trauma* 31:1068, 1991.
25. Plumley DA, et al. Accelerated lung amino acid release in hyperdynamic septic surgical patients. *Arch Surg* 125:57, 1990.
26. Hinshaw DB, Burger JM. Protective effect of glutamine on endothelial cell ATP in oxidant injury. *J Surg Res* 49:222, 1990.
27. Souba WW, et al. Cytokine modulation of glutamine transport by pulmonary artery endothelial cells. *Surgery* 110:295, 1991.
28. Ardawi MSM, Newsholme EA. Intracellular localization and properties of phosphate-dependent glutaminase in rat mesenteric lymph nodes. *Biochem J* 127:289, 1984.
29. Ardawi MSM. Glutamine and glucose metabolism in human peripheral lymphocytes. *Metabolism* 37:99, 1988.
30. Ardawi MSM, Newsholme EA. Glutamine metabolism in lymphocytes of the rat. *Biochem J* 212:835, 1983.
31. Newsholme P, Gordon S, Newsholme EA. Rates of utilization and fates of glucose, glutamine, pyruvate, fatty acids and ketone bodies by mouse macrophages. *Biochem J* 242:631, 1987.
32. Rodriguez JL, et al. Ventilatory and metabolic effects of glucose infusions. *Chest* 88:512, 1985.
33. Askanazi J, et al. Respiratory changes induced by the large glucose loads of total parenteral nutrition. *JAMA* 243:1444, 1980.
34. Delafosse B, et al. Respiratory changes induced by parenteral nutrition in postoperative patients undergoing inspiratory pressure support respiration. *Anesthesiology* 66:393, 1987.
35. Venus B, et al. Hemodynamic and gas exchange alterations during intralipid infusion in patients with ARDS. *Chest* 95:1278, 1989.
36. Hwang TL, Huang SL, Chen MF. Effects of intravenous fat emulsion on respiratory failure. *Chest* 97:934, 1990.
37. Bahrami S, et al. Mechanical properties of the lungs of post-traumatic rats are improved by including fat in total parenteral nutrition. *JPEN* 11:560, 1987.
38. Askanazi J, Carpentier YA, Elwyn DH. Influence of total parenteral nutrition on fuel utilization in injury and sepsis. *Ann Surg* 191:40, 1980.
39. Robin AP, et al. Influence of parenteral carbohydrate on fat oxidation in surgical patients. *Surgery* 95:608, 1984.
40. Sahebjami H, Vassallon CL. Effects of starvation and refeeding on lung mechanics and morphometry. *Am Rev Respir Dis* 119:443, 1979.
41. Russell DM, et al. Metabolic and structural changes in skeletal muscle during hypocaloric dieting. *Am J Clin Nutr* 39:503, 1984.

42. Mansell AL, Andersen JE, Muttart CR. Short-term pulmonary effects of total parenteral nutrition in children with cystic fibrosis. *J Pediatr* 104:700, 1984.
43. Keys A, et al. *The Biology of Human Starvation.* Minneapolis: The University of Minnesota Press, 1950.
44. Mattar JA, et al. Parenteral nutrition as a useful method for weaning patients from mechanical ventilation. *JPEN* 2:50, 1978.
45. Laaban JP, et al. Influence of caloric intake on the respiratory mode during mandatory minute volume ventilation. *Chest* 87:67, 1985.
46. Burke JF, et al. Glucose requirements following burn injury. *Ann Surg* 190:274, 1979.
47. Patrick J, Golden MHN. Leukocytes, electrolytes and sodium transport in protein-energy malnutrition. *Am J Clin Nutr* 30:1478, 1977.
48. Opie LH. Cardiac metabolism: Emergence, decline and resurgence. Parts I & II. *Cardiovasc Res* 26:721 & 817, 1992.
49. Vyska K, et al. Fatty acid uptake in normal human myocardium. *Circ Res* 69:857, 1991.
50. Keys A, Henschel A, Taylor HL. The size and function of the human heart in semistarvation and in subsequent rehabilitation. *Am J Physiol* 50:153, 1947.
51. Dimondon R, Henschel A, Keys A. The electrocardiogram of man in semistarvation and subsequent rehabilitation. *Am Heart J* 35:584, 1948.
52. Vandewoude MFJ, Buyssens N. Effect of aging and malnutrition on rat myocardium: the myocyte. *Virchows Arch [A]* 421:179, 1992.
53. Gelfand M, Jones JJ, Thomas GE. Nutritional microcardia, recovery of heart size and function with treatment. *Cent Afr J Med* 21:107, 1975.
54. Garnett ES, et al. Gross fragmentation of cardiac myofibrils after therapeutic starvation for obesity. *Lancet* 1:914, 1969.
55. Michiel RR, et al. Sudden death in a patient on a liquid protein diet. *N Engl J Med* 298:1005, 1978.
56. Abel RM, Subramanian VA, Gay WA, Jr. Effects of an intravenous amino acid nutrient solution on left ventricular contractility in dogs. *J Surg Res* 23:201, 1977.
57. Abel RM, et al. Biochemical, adverse hemodynamic and ultra-structural changes in dog hearts subjected to protein-calorie malnutrition. *Am Heart J* 97:733, 1979.
58. Heymsfield SB, et al. Cardiac abnormalities in cachectic patients before and during nutritional repletion. *Am Heart J* 95:584, 1978.
59. Freund HR, Holyrode J. Cardiac function during protein malnutrition and refeeding in the isolated rat heart. *JPEN* 10:470
60. Heymsfield SB, Smith J, Redd S, et al. Nutritional support in cardiac failure. *Surg Clin North Am* 61:635, 1981.
61. Walesby RK, Goode AW, Bental HH. Nutritional status of patients undergoing valve replacement by open heart surgery. *Lancet* 1:76, 1978.
62. Abel RM, et al. Malnutrition in cardiac surgical patients: results of a prospective randomized evaluation of early postoperative parenteral nutrition. *Arch Surg* 111:45, 1976.
63. Blackburn GL, et al. Nutritional support in cardiac cachexia. *J Thorac Cardiovasc Surg* 73:489, 1977.
64. Schwartz SM, et al. Enteral nutrition in infants with congenital heart disease and growth failure. *Pediatrics* 86:368, 1990.
65. Bougle D, et al. Nutritional treatment of congenital heart disease. *Arch Dis Child* 61:799, 1986.
66. Vanderhoof JA, et al. Continuous enteral feedings: an important adjunct to the management of complex congenital heart disease. *Am J Dis Child* 136:825, 1982.
67. Lolley D, et al. Clinical experience with preoperative myocardial nutrition management. *J Cardiovasc Surg* 26: 236, 1985.
68. Freund HR. Effects of malnutrition and sepsis on systolic properties of isolated rat heart. In JM Kinney, PR Borum (eds), *Perspectives in Clinical Nutrition.* Baltimore/Munich: Urban & Schwarzenberg, 1989. P. 43.
69. Freund HR, et al. The effect of branched-chain amino acids on systolic properties of the normal and septic isolated rat heart. *Arch Surg* 120:483, 1985.
70. Schwalb H, Freund HR, Uretzky G. Role of amino acids in myocardial protection during ischemia and reperfusion. In JM Kinney, PR Borum (eds), *Perspectives in Clinical Nutrition.* Baltimore/Munich: Urban & Schwarzenberg, 1989. P. 57.
71. Schwalb H, et al. The protective effect of enriched branched-chain amino acid formulation in the ischemic heart. *J Mol Cell Cardiol* 19:991, 1987.
72. Schwalb H, et al. The effect of amino acids on the ischemic heart. *J Thorac Cardiovasc Surg* 98:551, 1989.
73. Buse MG, Reid SS, Leucine. A possible regulator of protein turnover in muscle. *J Clin Invest* 56:1250, 1975.
74. Fulks RM, Li JB, Goldberg AL. Effects of insulin, glucose and amino acids on protein turnover in rat diaphragm. *J Biol Chem* 250:290, 1975.
75. Odessey R. Amino acid and protein metabolism in the diaphragm. *Am Rev Respir Dis* 119:107, 1979.
76. Chua BHL, Siehl DL, Morgan HE. Effect of leucine and metabolites of branched-chain amino acids on protein turnover in heart. *J Biol Chem* 254:8358, 1979.
77. Chua BHL, Siehl DL, Morgan HE. A role for leucine in regulation of protein turnover in working rat hearts. *Am J Physiol* 239:510, 1980.
78. Morgan HE, Chua BHL, Boyd TA. Branched-chain amino acids and the regulation of protein turnover in heart and skeletal muscle. In M Walser, RJ Williamson (eds), *Metabolism and Clinical Implications of Branched-Chain Amino and Keto-Acids.* New York: Elsevier/North-Holland, 1981. P. 217.
79. Tischler ME, Desautels M, Goldberg AL. Does leucine, leucyl tRNA, or some metabolite of leucine regulate protein synthesis and degradation in skeletal and cardiac muscle? *J Biol Chem* 257:1613, 1982.
80. Freund HR, et al. The role of the branched-chain amino acids in decreasing muscle catabolism in vivo. *Surgery* 83:611, 1978.
81. Freund HR, Yoshimura N, Fischer JE. The effect of branched-chain amino acids and hypertonic glucose infusions on post injury catabolism in the rat. *Surgery* 87:401, 1980.
82. Freund HR, James JH, Fischer JE. Nitrogen sparing mechanisms of singly administered branched chain amino acids in the injured rat. *Surgery* 90:237, 1981.
83. Cerra FB, et al. The effect of stress level, amino acid formula and nitrogen dose on nitrogen retention in traumatic and septic stress. *Ann Surg* 205:282, 1987.
84. Cerra FB, et al. Branched-chains support postoperative protein synthesis. *Surgery* 92:192, 1982.
85. Freund HR, et al. Infusion of the branched-chain amino acids in postoperative patients: Anti-catabolic properties. *Ann Surg* 190:18, 1979.
86. Freund HR, Ryan JA, Fischer JE. Amino acid derangements in patients with sepsis: treatment with branched-chain amino acid rich infusions. *Ann Surg* 188:423, 1978.

87. Hinshaw LB. Myocardial function in endotoxin shock. *Circ Shock* 1:43, 1979.

88. Postel J, Schloerb PR. Cardiac depression in bacteremia. *Ann Surg* 186:74: 1977.

89. Siegel JH, et al. Physiological and metabolic correlations in human sepsis. *Surgery* 86:163, 1979.

90. Goldfarb RD, Weber P, Eisenman J. Isolation of a shock-induced circulating cardio-depressant substance. *Am J Physiol* 237:168, 1979.

91. Lefer AM. Role of a myocardial depressant factor in the pathogenesis of circulatory shock. *Fed Proc* 29:1836, 1978.

92. Markovitz LJ, et al. The different effects of leucine, isoleucine and valine on systolic properties of the normal and septic isolated heart. *J Surg Res* 38:231, 1985.

93. Engelman RM, et al. Reduction of infarct size by systemic amino acid supplementation during reperfusion. *J Thorac Cardiovasc Surg* 101:855, 1991.

94. Pisarenko OI, Lepilin MG, Ivanov VE. Cardiac metabolism and performance during L-glutamic acid infusion in postoperative cardiac failure. *Clin Sci* 70:7, 1986.

95. Aoki N, et al. Protection of the coronary endothelium and the myocardium from ischemia-reperfusion injury by arginine. *Circulation* 84 (Suppl II):1093, 1991.

96. Ko KK, Paradise RR. The effects of substrate on contractility of rat atria depressed with halothane. *Anesthesiology* 31:532, 1969.

97. Farah AE, Alousi AA. The actions of insulin on cardiac contractility. *Life Sci* 29:975, 1981.

98. Kao RL, et al. The effect of insulin and anoxia on the metabolism of isolated mature rat cardiac myocytes. *Arch Biochem Biophys* 203:587, 1980.

99. Markovitz LJ, Hasin Y, Freund HR. The effect of insulin and glucagon on systolic properties of the normal and septic isolated rat heart. *Basic Res Cardiol* 80:377, 1985.

100. Grimes JB, Abel RM. Acute hemodynamic effects of intravenous fat emulsion in dogs. *JPEN* 3:40, 1979.

101. Fisch D, Abel RM. Hemodynamic effects of intravenous fat emulsions in patients with heart disease. *JPEN* 5:402, 1981.

102. Abel RM, Fisch D, Grossman ML. Hemodynamic effects of intravenous 20% soy oil emulsion following coronary bypass surgery. *JPEN* 7:534, 1983.

103. Leaf A, Weber PC. Cardiovascular effects of ω-3 fatty acids. *N Engl J Med* 318:549, 1988.

104. Heymsfield SB, Caspar K, Funfar J. Physiologic response and clinical implications of nutrition support. *Am J Cardiol* 60:75G, 1987.

105. Buzby GP, et al (Veterans Affairs Total Parenteral Nutrition Cooperative Study Group). Perioperative total parenteral nutrition in surgical patients. *N Engl J Med* 325:525, 1991.

106. Kirsch A, Savabi F. Effect of food restriction on the phosphocreatine energy shuttle components in rat heart. *J Mol Cell Cardiol* 24:821, 1992.

Selected Readings

Abel RM, et al. Malnutrition in cardiac surgical patients: Results of a prospective, randomized evaluation of early postoperative parenteral nutrition. *Arch Surg* 111:45, 1976.

An early prospective randomized study to evaluate the role of nutritional support in malnourished patients undergoing open-heart surgery. It was clearly demonstrated that patients judged to be malnourished preoperatively had less satisfactory results and a higher mortality rate following cardiac surgery compared to similar but nonmalnourished patients. Five to six days of postoperative total parenteral nutrition was unable to reverse these untoward effects of malnutrition. This study not only demonstrated the increased morbidity and mortality of malnutrition but also failed to demonstrate any beneficial effects of nutritional support, probably due to the very limited period of nutritional support offered in this study. Amazingly, this effort was never repeated by any other group of researchers.

Goldberg AL, Odessey R. Oxidation of amino acids by diaphragm from fed and fasted rats. *Am J Physiol* 223:1384, 1972.

This is one of a group of excellent papers originating from Dr. Goldberg's group at Harvard elucidating the amino acid metabolism and regulation in skeletal muscle and the diaphragm, with special emphasis on the role and effects of branched-chain amino acids in muscle metabolism.

Keys A, Henschel A, Taylor HL. The size and function of the human heart in semi-starvation and in subsequent rehabilitation. *Am J Physiol* 50:153, 1947.

An early pioneering and prospective human classic series of experiments on the effects of prolonged starvation and refeeding in young volunteers. Hypocaloric diets offered for 12 to 24 weeks resulted in the loss of approximately 25% of initial body weight, a decrease in heart size, decreased arterial and venous pressures, reduced cardiac performance, and diminished heart rate. Too-rapid nutritional repletion frequently resulted in early signs of congestive heart failure during the rehabilitative phase. These early observations were repeatedly confirmed by later investigators.

Opie LH. Cardiac metabolism: Emergence, decline and resurgence. Part I and II. *Cardiovasc Res* 26:721, 1992.

This extensive and comprehensive review of Professor Opie, who contributed extensively during many decades of cardiac metabolism research, covers the field of cardiac metabolism from the early days of Ringer in London to today's modern concepts of cardiac metabolism, involving electrophysiology, ischemia, reperfusion, cardioplegia, calcium and potassium channels, and the therapy of ischemia.

Rochester D. Malnutrition and the respiratory muscles. *Clin Chest Med* 7:91, 1986.

Malnutrition is a leading cause of impaired respiratory muscle contractility, affecting both strength and endurance. In this review, Dr. Rochester, who contributed extensively to the research of respiratory muscle function, summarizes data dealing with respiratory muscle function during injury and infection, in patients on mechanical ventilation because of respiratory failure, and those with chronic destructive pulmonary disease. Not less important, an attempt is made to evaluate the effects of nutritional repletion on respiratory muscles in these states.

Sahebjami H. Nutrition and the pulmonary parenchyma. *Clin Chest Med* 7:111, 1986.

This is an excellent summary of extensive research relating to the question whether malnutrition affects the structure and function of the lung. This review by Dr. Sahebjami, whose group contributed greatly to this topic, offers a comprehensive review of the effects of fasting and starvation on lung parenchyma in humans and experimental animals.

27

Special Needs of the Pediatric Patient

Brad W. Warner

Nutritional management of the pediatric patient is unique and cannot be based on the naive assumption that "children are small adults." Immature enzyme systems, impaired motility, and underdeveloped gastrointestinal host defense mechanisms all restrict the administration and advancement of enteral feeding. Parenteral nutrition is also associated with a variety of distinctive complications, probably due to many of these same factors.

Differences in body composition between premature, term, and older infants dictate an understanding of essential substrates, vitamins, minerals, and energy requirements. The impact of growth and how this influences the utilization of energy, protein, and fat is important because caloric and substrate deprivation during periods of rapid brain growth and development can be associated with irreversible neurologic injury or developmental delay [1].

The period of most rapid change in the functional gastrointestinal tract of the human appears to be during the last trimester of gestation. The gastrointestinal tract of the premature infant may therefore need to assume a role for which it is not well prepared. An understanding of the capabilities of the gastrointestinal tract at various levels of development is essential for rational nutritional support.

Functional Development of the Gastrointestinal Tract

A thorough understanding of functional gastrointestinal tract development in the human has been restricted due to the relative unavailability of human tissue for analysis. Although a large body of information has been derived from animal studies, several major differences make direct application to humans inappropriate. For example, newborn rats and mice are deficient in many gastrointestinal tract enzymes that have already fully developed in other mammals in utero [2]. Further, postnatal ontogenic changes within the gastrointestinal tract in these animals appear to be more highly coordinated and predictable than in humans.

Motility

By the 16th to 17th week of gestation, swallowing begins to occur in the human fetus [3,4]. At this time, the daily volume of swallowed amniotic fluid is in the range of 2 to 7 ml and increases to roughly 50% of the amniotic fluid volume (400–450 ml) by the time the infant is at term [3,4]. The direct relationship between coordination of sucking and swallowing and gestational age is important as it relates to expectations for oral feeding. Gryboski has defined both immature and mature suck-swallow patterns in premature infants [5]. The mature suck-swallow pattern is rarely seen prior to 34 weeks gestation. Enteral feeding prior to this gestational age therefore must be provided by way of a tube.

Esophageal motility is impaired in the premature infant. In a group of premature infants and term infants less than 12 hours of age, Gryboski documented many biphasic peristaltic waves and simultaneous contractions thought to represent uncoordinated response of the esophagus to deglutition and neuronal immaturity [6]. In that study, the decreased resting tone of the lower esophageal sphincter mechanism was confirmed. This observation partially explains the high incidence of gastroesophageal reflux that is well known to occur in the premature infant population. In another study, the resting pressure of the lower esophageal sphincter was found to correlate more closely with postnatal age, suggesting a fair degree of postnatal maturation [7].

Although there are no systematic studies that address the ontogeny of gastric emptying in the premature infant, clinical experience suggests that emptying is abnormal. The need for transpyloric feeding tubes is therefore commonplace. As in adults, gastric emptying in premature infants decreases as the caloric density of the formula increases [8]. Intragastric pressures generated during spontaneous antral contractions are found to increase in direct correlation with gestational age [9].

Manometric studies show that fasting of the small intestine of adults and term infants occurs in a cycle and consists of three phases: a period of quiescence, irregular activity, and a regular phasic propagating activity (migrating motor complex; MMC). In premature infants, the latter MMC phase was found to be absent and the timing of its appearance was found to directly correlate with gestational age [10]. Despite these findings in the fasting state, no differences were detected in motility between term infants and premature infants in response to enteral feeding [11]. Early (postnatal days 3–5) enteral feeding of premature infants was found to be associated with earlier maturation of intestinal motility, faster tolerance of full oral nutrition, and fewer hospital days compared with a matched group of premature infants whose enteral feeding was begun late (postnatal days 10–14) [12]. In that study, early-fed infants were also found to have significantly higher plasma concentrations of gastrin and gastric inhibitory peptide. The data from these studies would support the notion that early enteral feeding of premature infants is beneficial. This must be interpreted with caution, however, because early enteral feeding of the premature infant is regarded by some as a risk factor for the development of neonatal necrotizing enterocolitis [13,14].

Little is known about motility development within the colon. Meconium aspiration results from in utero defecation in response to stress and occurs almost entirely in term or post-term infants. Failure to pass meconium in a term infant beyond 24 to 48 hours after delivery should raise a suspicion for mechanical obstruction (for example, atresia, stenosis, meconium ileus, etc.) or a motility disorder of the colon such as Hirschsprung's disease or small left-colon syndrome as seen with infants of diabetic mothers.

Secretion

The secretion of digestive and absorptive enzymes and their time of appearance is depicted in Table 27-1. A lingual lipase has been detected in the suckling infant and is felt to be important in the digestion of milk triglycerides [15]. This enzyme is well suited for hydrolysis in the stomach because it is active in the absence of bile salts and has a low pH optimum. Salivary amylase is also present at birth, but in quantities less than adult levels.

Gastric acid secretion is generally immature in the newborn infant relative to older children and adults. Production of both gastric acid and pepsinogen is less than 50% of adult levels for the first three months of life and does not become fully developed until after two years of age [16].

Table 27-1. Digestion and Absorption

Factors	First Detectable (weeks gestation)	Term Neonate (% of adult)
Protein		
H^+	At birth	<30
Pepsin	16	<10
Trypsinogen	20	10–60
Chymotrypsinogen	20	10–60
Procarboxypeptidase	20	10–60
Enterokinase	26	10
Peptidases (brush border and cytosol)	<15	>100
Amino acid transport	Unknown	>100
Macromolecular absorption	Unknown	>100
Fat		
Lingual lipase	30	>l00
Pancreatic lipase	20	5–10
Pancreatic colipase	Unknown	Unknown
Bile acids	22	50
Medium-chain triglyceride uptake	Unknown	100
Long-chain triglyceride uptake	Unknown	10–90
Carbohydrate		
Alpha amylases		
Pancreatic	22	0
Salivary	16	10
Lactase	10	>100
Sucrase-isomaltose	10	100
Glucoamylase	10	50–100
Monosaccharide absorption	11–19	<100 (unknown)

Source: E Lebenthal, PC Lee, LA Heitlinger. Impact of development of the gastrointestinal tract on infant feeding. *J Pediatr* 102:1–9, 1983. Used with permission.

Serum gastrin levels are extremely high in infants [17] and although gastrin receptors have not been measured in the human stomach, it is likely that they are less well developed as has been shown in the rat [18]. It has been suggested that low acid and pepsinogen early in life may be important for immunoglobulins to be active and for antigens to be recognized in the gastrointestinal tract [19].

Despite adult levels of pancreatic trypsin and roughly half of the adult levels of chymotrypsin, the human infant is immature with regard to protease activity [20]. Secretion of these enzymes are minimally stimulated by pancreozymin [20], which may play a role for the enhanced absorption of intact proteins by human infants during the first several months of life [21].

In newborns, bile acid synthesis is maximal and ileal reabsorption is inefficient [22]. This leads to a reduction in the bile acid pool size and intraluminal concentration of bile acids. The bile acid pool size in a premature of 32 weeks gestation has been estimated to be only 50% of that in a full-term infant [22]. This probably accounts for the malabsorption of 10% to 20% of fat intake noted to occur in the formula-fed premature infant [22].

Digestion and Absorption

Carbohydrate

In the neonate, small intestine hydrolytic activities are largely restricted to the components of maternal milk. Carbohydrate intake during infancy comprises 35% to 55% of the total calories of the diet. Lactose is the predominant carbohydrate in human milk, and its corresponding hydrolytic enzyme lactase is a relatively late developing enzyme in the fetus. At 28 weeks gestation, only 30% of the activity of lactase is present compared with term infants [23]. In contrast, sucrase and isomaltose activities at the same gestation are at 70% term levels [23]. Clinically, some premature infants may be lactose-intolerant, and special formulas have been designed that contain only 50% of the total carbohydrate as lactose or that contain no lactose at all.

The capacity of disaccharide hydrolysis per day has been measured by Auricchio et al. [24]. Between 2 and 3 months gestation, 2.05 g maltose, 0.02 g sucrose, 0.02 g isomaltose, and 0.01 g lactose can be hydrolyzed. By month 8 of gestation, a significant rise is noted as 60 g maltose, 34 g sucrose, 21.3 g isomaltose, and 5.8 g lactose can be hydrolyzed. At term, the infant should be able to hydrolyze 107 g maltose, 72 g sucrose, 46 g isomaltose, and 60 g lactose in 24 hours.

Improved methods of fetal dating and enzyme activity suggest that lactase levels may actually be present at 50% adult levels as early as 14 weeks gestation [25]. Many premature infants have been noted to tolerate lactose-containing formulas. Therefore the widespread practice of avoiding lactose in the very premature infant may not be justified.

The period from infancy to childhood is characterized by three phases, each with a different major source of dietary carbohydrate [26]. The initial phase is characterized by lactose and sucrose, which are the main carbohydrates of human milk and formula in the absence of solids. In the transitional phase, solid foods are introduced and various polysaccharides, namely starches, are added. In the final phase, the shift to solid food is complete and polysaccharides predominate. Lactase activity declines with age and is never as high as in the mature newborn.

Protein

Hydrolysis and absorption of protein normally occurs in gastric, pancreatic, and intestinal phases. In the preterm or term infant, the relative reduced gastric acid production and decreased pepsin activity make the gastric component contribute less to protein hydrolysis than it will later in life. Despite this, protein absorption in the infant is relatively efficient and occurs primarily in the proximal small intestine depending on both pancreatic proteases (to a limited extent) and intestinal peptidases.

Although enterokinase has only 10% activity compared with adult levels, the efficiency of protein absorption does not seem to be affected [23]. The concentration of trypsin in the duodenal lumen is near adult levels in the preterm and term infant [27]. Except for amino-peptidases, brush-border and cytosolic peptidases are well developed even in preterm babies [28].

In clinical studies, adequate protein absorption despite limited digestive capacities has been demonstrated [29]. Ten-day-old infants can completely digest and absorb 1.3% protein in cow's milk (roughly 1.95 g/kg/day) whereas infants 4 to 6 months old can completely digest and absorb 2.5% protein in cow's milk (about 3.75 g/kg/day) [30].

The neonatal mammalian small intestine has a capacity to ingest macromolecules by an endocytotic mechanism [21]. It is likely that this phenomenon is greater in the newborn period and decreases as the child grows older. This is supported by the observation that premature and term infants can absorb greater quantities of ingested food antigen than older infants or adults [31]. Clinically, adverse reactions to cow's milk protein becomes progressively less common during the first year of life [19]. Further, Eastham et al. [32] detected a larger percentage of serum samples with antibodies to food antigens in infants less than three months compared with infants exposed to antigen after three months of age, a finding that suggests a greater ability of food proteins to be absorbed prior to three months of age. There is evidence to suggest that the absorption of intact proteins continues to a limited extent in older children and adults [33,34]. It has been suggested that there are several clinical conditions in which the gastrointestinal mucosal barrier may be immature and thus have a greater capacity to absorb ingested antigens [21]. These diseases include neonatal necrotizing enterocolitis, toxigenic diarrhea, malabsorption, dermatitis, sudden infant death syndrome, and gastrointestinal allergy.

Fat

The ability of the preterm infant to absorb fat is less compared with term infants. Several factors account for this, including low levels of pancreatic lipase in the duodenum [20]. This low concentration may be due to a lack of secretion, synthesis, or both by the exocrine pancreas. Further, intraluminal bile acid concentration within the small intestine of the premature infant is below the critical micellar concentration for sufficient solubilization of lipids and their hydrolytic products. As discussed above, this is likely due to immaturity of bile acid reabsorption with exaggerated fecal and urinary losses rather than insufficient hepatic bile acid synthesis. The average intraduodenal bile acid concentration of the premature infant was found to be less than 2 mmol/L, compared with 5 mmol/L in the term infant and 8 mmol/L in the adult [35,36]. Alternative pathways for lipid digestion exist in the neonate and are likely of considerable importance in face of lower pancreatic lipase excretion. These include a lingual lipase, a possible gastric lipase, and a mother's milk lipase (mammary lipase).

The composition of dietary lipid greatly influences digestibility and absorption. Term and preterm infants tolerate fats from human milk better than from cow's milk, possibly due to the lipases present in the former [37]. Vegetable fats are absorbed more efficiently than animal fats [38], and saturated fatty acids are not as well utilized as unsaturated fatty acids. In neonates, portal transport seems to be efficient while lymphatic transport is incomplete. Short- and medium-chain fatty acids are therefore absorbed and transported more readily than long-chain fatty acids [39].

Functional Development of the Liver

In the developing fetus, the liver accounts for roughly 10% of total body volume and decreases to 5% of the body weight at the time of birth. In contrast, in adults the liver accounts for 2% of body weight. In the postnatal period, liver growth occurs in proportion to height, weight, and age [40].

Bile secretion begins at approximately the 12th week of gestation with the relative concentrations of the major components of bile varying throughout development. Fetal serum bile acid levels stay at low levels due to placental transport and maternal excretion [41]. In the intestinal lumen of newborns, total bile acids are low and bacterially derived secondary bile acids are absent [42]. Developmental changes in various components of bile acid metabolism is depicted in Figure 27-1. The physiologic components of the enterohepatic circulation of bile acids are well defined, and there appears to be an age-related impairment of many of the processes [43].

Hepatic metabolic function, as reflected in bilirubin physiology, is immature in the newborn. Activity of the rate-limiting enzyme in bilirubin excretion, UDP-glucuronyltransferase, is decreased [44]. Rapid postnatal development of this enzyme in preterm infants compared with slower in utero development suggests that birth-related rather than age-related factors are important for the emergence of this enzyme [44]. This is but one of the many functional impairments (Table 27-2) responsible for the common occurrence of unconjugated hyperbilirubinemia seen during infancy [16].

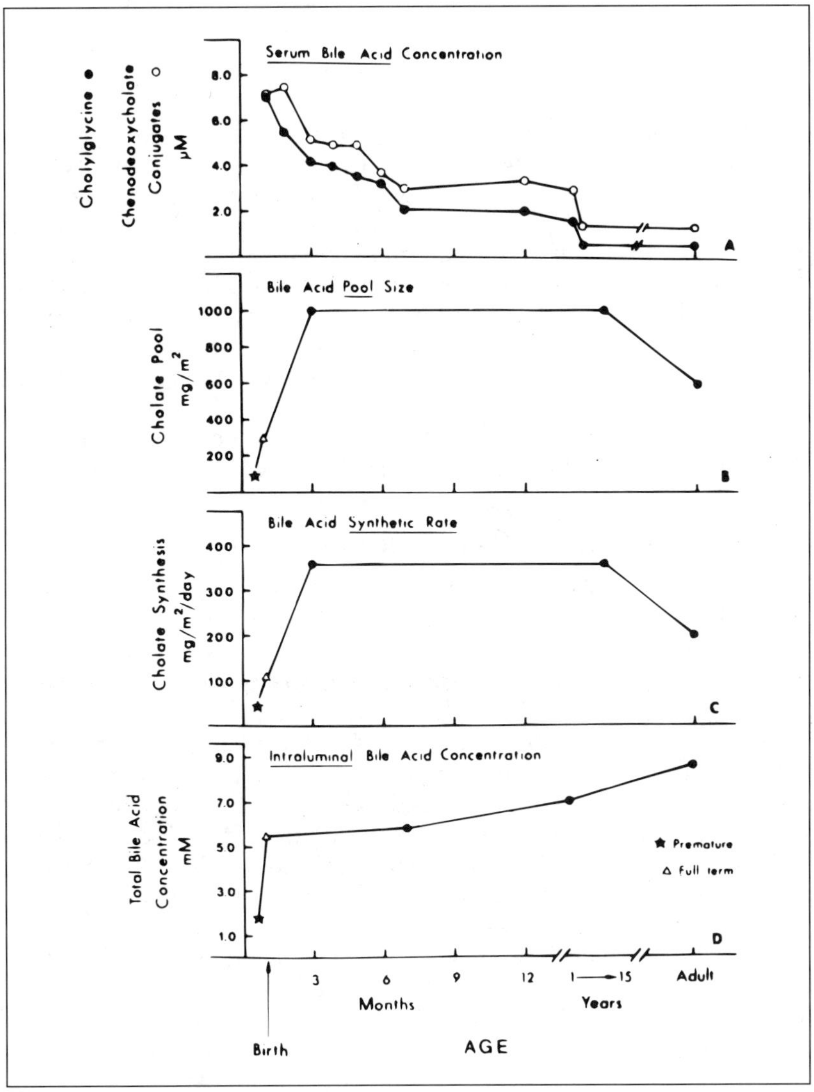

Figure 27-1. Graphic depiction of compiled data regarding developmental changes in various aspects of bile acid metabolism in humans. (**A**) Progressive decline in the serum concentration of the primary bile acids, cholyglycine (●) and conjugated chenodeoxycholate (○), with age. (**B**) and (**C**) Bile acid kinetics studied by isotopic dilution reflected in bile acid pool size and bile acid synthetic rate. (**D**) Total bile concentration in duodenal samples. (From WF Balistreri, JE Heubi, FJ Suchy. Immaturity of the enterohepatic circulation in early life: Factors predisposing to "physiologic" maldigestion and cholestasis. *J Pediatr Gastroenterol Nutr* 2:346, 1983, with permission.)

Table 27-2. Alterations in Bilirubin Transport and Metabolism Responsible for Elevated Serum Concentrations of Unconjugated Bilirubin in Early Life

1. Cessation of placental transport and maternal detoxification
2. Dynamic status of hepatic blood flow, bilirubin shunted away from the sinusoid
3. Bilirubin production rates high in neonates due to:
   - large red-cell mass
   - short red-cell life span
   - inefficient erythropoiesis
   - increased heme oxygenase activity
4. Less efficient albumin binding in newborn due to:
   - lower serum albumin concentration
   - decreased albumin-binding capacity
   - stress (e.g., sepsis, acidosis, hypoxia)
5. ↓ uptake and ↓ intracellular binding by hepatocytes (decreased Y protein)
6. Decreased conjugation (↓ activity of glucuronyl transferase)
7. Impaired bile secretion
8. Altered enterohepatic circulation of bilirubin:
   - ↓ bacterial flora, thus ↓ formation of urobilinogen
   - hydrolysis of conjugated bilirubin to unconjugated bilirubin by way of intestinal β-glucuronidase with subsequent reabsorption
   - human milk β-glucuronidase mediating deconjugation

Source: WF Balistreri. Anatomic and biochemical ontogeny of the gastrointestinal tract and liver. In RC Tsang, BC Nichols (eds), *Nutrition in Infancy.* Philadelphia: Hanley & Belfers, 1988. Pp 35–57. Used with permission.

With regard to carbohydrate metabolism, the term infant is born with liver glycogen stores that become exhausted within 12 hours of delivery [45]. The ability to synthesize glucose from lactate, pyruvate, and amino acids is low in the fetus and develops rapidly after birth [46]. Gluconeogenic enzymes—which include pyruvate carboxylase, mitochondrial phosphoenolpyruvate carboxykinase (PEPCK), fructose-1,6-biphosphatase, and glucose-6-phosphatase—are at 50% to 100% adult values in the liver of near-term fetuses. In comparison, cytosolic PEPCK levels are extremely low (0–25% adult levels), and this enzyme is therefore considered to be the rate-limiting enzyme for gluconeogenesis [46]. It seems that the process of birth and not the developmental stage is the important factor that induces liver PEPCK because premature delivery results in a rapid rise in activity of this enzyme. This is probably due, in part, to a rise in plasma levels of glucagon [46]. For the glycolytic enzymes phosphofructokinase-1 and pyruvate kinase, levels are lower in fetal livers compared with pediatric and adult samples [47]. Of interest is the detection of a relative fall in glycolytic enzyme activity compared with a rise in gluconeogenic enzyme activity during the last weeks of gestation—a teleologically important transition towards the gluconeogenic role that is required after birth [47].

Biochemical immaturity of protein synthetic processes within the liver may have a significant influence upon nutritional management. Cystathionase activity, important in the conversion of methionine to cysteine, is immature in the preterm infant [48]. In contrast, decarboxylase enzyme levels that are rate-controlling in the biosynthesis of polyamines are much higher in the fetal liver than in the mature state [49]. The synthesis of physiologically important polyamines may be directly related to the metabolism of RNA and the modulation of rapid growth. As the placenta does not contribute significantly to the plasma proteins of the fetus, the fetal liver is capable of synthesizing all plasma proteins except gammaglobulin [50].

Body Composition

An understanding of body composition of the preterm and term neonate is important as it relates to caloric reserve during periods of starvation as well as the composition of body weight gain during growth. Body fat deposition is one of the most remarkable changes to occur during late fetal development (Figure 27-2). In the preterm infant, the relatively reduced amount of body fat is detrimental as the relative lack of insulation renders the infant more susceptible to cold stress-induced hypermetabolism. Further, as fat is a major energy source, starvation of the preterm infant for long periods of time is poorly tolerated. Considering a 70 kg adult, fat reserves amount to roughly 141,000 kcal. A term infant (assuming that 15% of the body weight is adipose tissue) has a fat reserve of 4800 kcal. In contrast, the 1000 gm

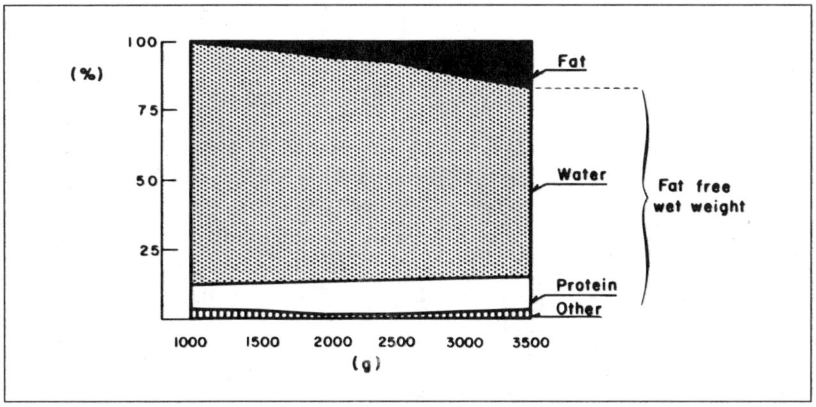

Figure 27-2. Changes in body composition as a function of fetal weight and gestational age. (From WC Heird, RW Winters. Total parenteral nutrition: State of the art. *J Pediatr* 86:6, 1975, with permission.)

preemie has a fat reserve of only 200 kcal [51], barely enough for 96 hours of starvation.

During growth, the energy cost of protein deposition is estimated to be 8.66 kcal/g and of fat is 12 kcal/g [52]. The energy cost of weight gain can be thus calculated from the knowledge of the body compositional changes during growth (Table 27-3). The most dramatic changes in the composition of body weight gain during growth occurs during the first 4 months of life when body fat is rapidly deposited [53]. Energy requirements per gram of body weight therefore appear to directly relate to the proportion of fat synthesized and deposited during late fetal development and early infancy [52].

Indications

The indications for nutritional support of the pediatric patient are similar to those for the adult patient. The enteral route is generally preferred because it is more physiologic, safe, and less expensive. Multiple situations exist in the pediatric patient, however, whereby the gastrointestinal tract cannot be used and parenteral support is indicated.

Low-birth-weight infants account for the largest percentage of pediatric patients that require parenteral nutrition [54]. Pediatric surgical disorders in which parenteral nutrition is routinely used include congenital disorders that prevent the use of the gastrointestinal tract. Examples of these include gastroschisis, esophageal atresia with or without tracheoesophageal fistula, intestinal atresia, or meconium ileus. The role of parenteral nutrition in these cases is for support of growth until the condition is corrected.

Short-bowel syndrome results from the inability of the gastrointestinal tract to absorb sufficient nutrients to sustain life. This results from either a deficiency of intestinal absorptive surface area (for example, after massive resection) or functional disorders that impair motility (intestinal aganglionosis, pseudo-obstruction) and/or absorption (chronic diarrhea of infancy). Neonatal necrotizing enterocolitis accounts for the majority of cases of short-bowel syndrome in the pediatric population, followed by intestinal atresias, midgut volvulus, gastroschisis, and aganglionosis [55]. The minimum length of bowel necessary for survival in neonates was traditionally thought to be 40 cm without the presence of the ileocecal valve [56]. However, since the advent of parenteral nutrition, survivors with as little as 11 to 20 cm have been reported [57,58]. Multiple remedial surgical procedures may need to be performed on the gastrointestinal tract to allow discontinuation or reduction in the amount of parenteral nutrition [59].

Necrotizing enterocolitis (NEC) is one of the most serious acquired gastrointestinal disorders encountered during the neonatal period. It is recognized clinically as abdominal distention, bloody stools, feeding intolerance, and radiographic evidence of pneumatosis intestinalis. The overall incidence of NEC in neonatal intensive care units is in the range of 1% to 5% [60]. Prematurity and birth weight seem to be the only consistent risk factors [61]. The association between prematurity and NEC suggests an immaturity of the gastrointestinal tract as playing a role in the pathogenesis. Steroid administration accelerates the maturation of fetal tissues and was shown to reduce the incidence of NEC in premature infants that received antenatal maternal glucocorticoids [62].

Roughly one-half of the infants that develop NEC can be managed conservatively using nasogastric decompression and antibiotics. Surgery is often required for clinical deterioration and/or evidence for intestinal perforation. Bowel resection is often indicated with the creation of intestinal stomas. Because over 90% of infants with NEC have received some type of enteral feeding, the current standard of care is to discontinue all enteral nutrition in these patients once the diagnosis

Table 27-3. Body Composition of Reference Children

						Components of Fat-Free Body Mass (% of Body Weight)						
			Fat				Water			Minerals		
Age	Length (cm)	Weight (g)	g	%	Fat-Free Body Mass	Protein	Total Body	Extracellular	Cellular	Osseous	Nonosseous	Carbohydrate
Boys												
Birth	51.6	3545	486	13.7	3059	12.9	69.6	42.5	27.0	2.6	0.6	0.5
1 mo	54.8	4452	671	15.1	3781	12.9	68.4	41.1	27.3	2.6	0.6	0.5
2 mo	58.2	5509	1095	19.9	4414	12.3	64.3	38.0	26.3	2.4	0.6	0.5
3 mo	61.5	6435	1495	23.2	4940	12.0	61.4	35.7	25.8	2.3	0.6	0.5
4 mo	63.9	7060	1743	24.7	5317	11.9	60.1	34.5	25.7	2.3	0.5	0.4
5 mo	65.9	7575	1913	25.3	5662	11.9	59.6	33.8	25.8	2.3	0.5	0.4
6 mo	67.6	8030	2037	25.4	5993	12.0	59.4	33.4	26.0	2.3	0.5	0.4
9 mo	72.3	9180	2199	24.0	6981	12.4	60.3	33.0	27.2	2.3	0.6	0.5
12 mo	76.1	10150	2287	22.5	7863	12.9	61.2	32.9	28.3	2.3	0.6	0.5
18 mo	82.4	11470	2382	20.8	9088	13.5	62.2	32.3	29.9	2.5	0.6	0.5
24 mo	87.2	12590	2456	19.5	10134	14.0	62.9	31.9	31.0	2.6	0.6	0.5
3 yr	95.3	14675	2576	17.5	12099	14.7	63.9	31.1	32.8	2.8	0.6	0.5
4 yr	102.9	16690	2656	15.9	14034	15.3	64.8	30.5	34.2	2.9	0.6	0.5
5 yr	109.9	18670	2720	14.6	15950	15.8	65.4	30.0	35.4	3.1	0.6	0.5
6 yr	116.1	20690	2795	13.5	17895	16.2	66.0	29.6	36.4	3.2	0.6	0.5
7 yr	121.7	22850	2931	12.8	19919	16.5	66.2	29.1	37.1	3.3	0.6	0.5
8 yr	127.0	25300	3293	13.0	22007	16.6	65.8	28.3	37.5	3.4	0.6	0.5
9 yr	132.2	28130	3724	13.2	24406	16.8	65.4	27.6	37.8	3.5	0.6	0.5
10 yr	137.5	31440	4318	13.7	27122	16.8	64.8	26.7	38.0	3.5	0.6	0.5
Girls												
Birth	50.5	3325	495	14.9	2830	12.8	68.6	42.0	26.7	2.6	0.6	0.5
1 mo	53.4	4131	668	16.2	3463	12.7	67.5	40.5	26.9	2.5	0.6	0.5
2 mo	56.7	4989	1053	21.1	3936	12.2	63.2	37.1	26.1	2.4	0.6	0.5
3 mo	59.6	5743	1366	23.8	4377	12.0	60.9	35.1	25.8	2.3	0.6	0.5
4 mo	61.9	6300	1585	25.2	4715	11.9	59.6	33.8	25.8	2.3	0.5	0.4
5 mo	63.9	6800	1769	26.0	5031	11.9	58.8	33.0	25.9	2.2	0.5	0.4
6 mo	65.8	7250	1915	26.4	5335	12.0	58.4	32.4	26.0	2.2	0.5	0.4
9 mo	70.4	8270	2066	25.0	6204	12.5	59.3	32.0	27.3	2.3	0.5	0.4
12 mo	74.3	9180	2175	23.7	7005	12.9	60.1	31.8	28.3	2.3	0.5	0.5
18 mo	80.2	10780	2346	21.8	8434	13.5	61.3	31.4	29.8	2.4	0.6	0.5
24 mo	85.5	11910	2433	20.4	9477	13.9	62.2	31.5	30.8	2.4	0.6	0.5
3 yr	94.1	14100	2606	18.5	11494	14.4	63.5	31.3	32.2	2.5	0.6	0.5
4 yr	101.6	15960	2757	17.3	13203	14.8	64.3	31.2	33.1	2.5	0.6	0.5
5 yr	108.4	17660	2949	16.7	14711	15.0	64.6	31.0	33.6	2.5	0.6	0.5
6 yr	114.6	19520	3208	16.4	16312	15.2	64.7	30.8	34.0	2.6	0.6	0.5
7 yr	120.6	21840	3662	16.8	18178	15.2	64.4	30.3	34.1	2.5	0.6	0.5
8 yr	126.4	24840	4319	17.4	20521	15.2	63.8	29.6	34.2	2.5	0.6	0.5
9 yr	132.2	28460	5207	18.3	23253	15.1	63.0	28.9	34.1	2.5	0.6	0.5
10 yr	138.3	32550	6318	19.4	26232	15.0	62.0	28.1	33.9	2.5	0.6	0.5

Source: SJ Foman, et al. Body composition of reference children from birth to age 10 years. *Am J Clin Nutr* 35:1169, 1982. Used with permission. © Am J Clin Nutr, American Society for Clinical Nutrition.

has been made. Parenteral nutrition therefore becomes critically important during the period of conservative management (10–14 days) or after intestinal resection in the immediate postoperative period.

Requirements

Energy

Energy requirements during the neonatal and early infancy periods are at levels higher than any

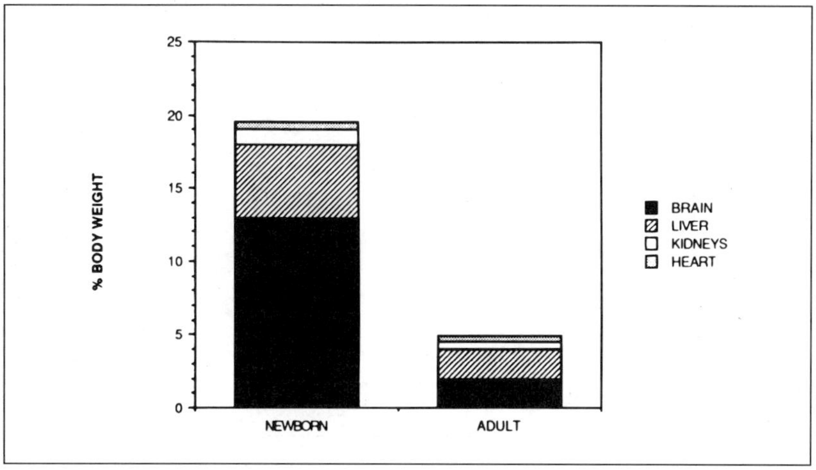

Figure 27-3. Contribution of the four most metabolically active organs to body weight in newborns and adults. (From SC Denne. Energy requirements. In RA Polin, WW Fox [eds], *Fetal and Neonatal Physiology.* Philadelphia: Saunders, 1992, pp. 215–223, with permission.)

other time during life. Several factors contribute to the differences between neonates, older children, and adults and include the effects of body composition, growth, and higher rates of energy expenditure.

When energy metabolism is expressed as kcal/kg body weight, the metabolic rate of neonates is roughly twice that of normal adults (50 versus 25 kcal/kg/day). This may be partially explained by the contribution of the four most metabolically active organs (brain, liver, kidneys, heart) to overall body weight of the neonate when compared with the adult (Figure 27-3). It is estimated that these organs alone account for approximately two-thirds of total energy expenditure [63].

Energy intake and hence caloric requirements are determined by the energy that is excreted, stored, or expended (Figure 27-4). These latter two components are considered metabolizable energy. Measured basal metabolic rates for term infants vary depending on methodology and range from 43 to 60 kcal/kg/day [64,65]. These measurements are similar to those reported for preterm infants (47 kcal/kg/day) [66]. The thermic effect of feeding (diet-induced thermogenesis or specific dynamic action) represents the energy expended to absorb and assimilate nutrients and accounts for roughly 10% of the daily energy expenditure.

The environmental temperature at which oxygen consumption and metabolic rate are at their lowest is described as the critical temperature or neutral thermal environment [67]. Temperatures below this point result in increased energy expenditure in the infant that is proportionate to the fall in the environmental temperature. In preterm infants, the response to cold stress is dependent on gestational age, weight, and postnatal age.

Because neonates sleep 80% to 90% of the day, energy expended for physical activity is a much smaller component of total energy expenditure when compared with adults. Activity represents an increasing component of the daily energy expenditure as the infant grows. In contrast, activity levels of preterm infants are quite low with the component of energy expenditure for activity reported to be approximately 3% [66].

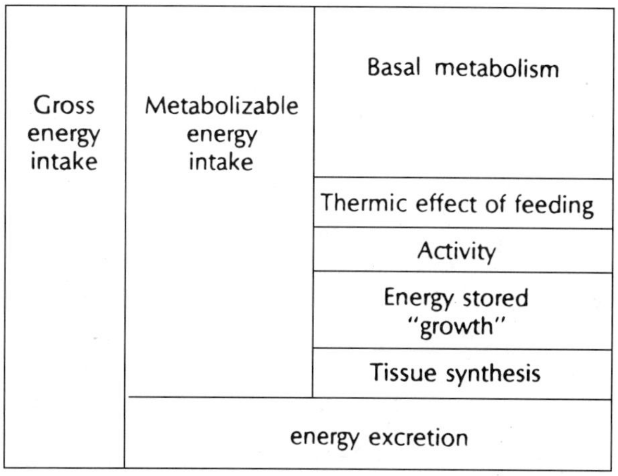

Figure 27-4. Partitioning of the energy requirements during infancy. (From NF Butte. Energy requirements during infancy. In RC Tsang, BL Nichols [eds], *Nutrition During Infancy.* Philadelphia: Hanley & Belfers, 1988, pp. 86–99, with permission.)

Growth is an important component of total energy needs of the neonate and is greatest during the first 2 to 12 weeks of extrauterine life. Approximately 40% of total energy utilized by the 2-week-old term infant is delegated to growth, and this percentage falls off rapidly to levels of 1% to 2% by 24 months of age (Figure 27-5) [68]. In preterm infants, the percentage of energy allocated for growth is in the range of 60% [66]. Energy requirements for maintenance take priority over growth. If energy intake is below maintenance levels, growth will be halted.

Estimates of energy requirements for enteral

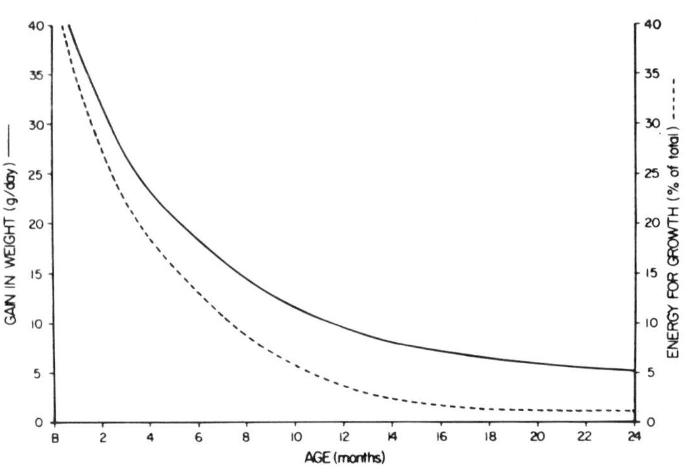

Figure 27-5. Daily gain in body weight and percentage of energy intake utilized for growth at two weeks to two years of age. B = birth; solid line = weight gain (grams/day); dotted line = energy for growth (%). (From TA Anderson. Nutritional needs as a function of age: Birth through 24 months. In AM Rudolph [ed], *Pediatrics* [17th ed]. Norwalk, CT: Appleton-Century-Crofts, 1982, pp. 169–172, with permission.)

Table 27-4. Average Energy Requirement by Age

Age (mo)	Average Energy Requirement* (kcal/kg/d)
0–1	124.0
1–2	116.0
2–3	109.0
3–4	103.0
4–5	99.0
5–6	96.5
6–7	95.0
7–8	94.5
8–9	95.0
9–10	99.0
10–11	100.0
11–12	104.5

*Based on measured intakes.
Source: GH Beaton. Nutritional needs during the first year of life: Some concepts and perspectives. *Pediatr Clin North Am* 32(2):277, 1985.

feeding during the first year of life for term infants are depicted in Table 27-4. The small rise in energy requirements during the last part of this year probably reflect increasing physical activity. A discrepancy between these estimates for required energy intakes and actual measured intakes of breast-fed infants suggests that these estimates may be too great [69]. In preterm infants, The American Academy of Pediatrics Committee on Nutrition has recommended that sufficient calories should be delivered to approximate in utero weight gain [70]. The recommended 15 g/day of weight gain for the preterm infant is generally achieved with a total energy intake of 120 kcal/kg/day. Guidelines for caloric requirements in older children are shown in Table 27-5.

Table 27-5. Caloric Requirements on Total Parenteral Nutrition

Age (yr)	Caloric Requirement (cal/kg/d)
0–1	90–120
1–7	75–90
7–12	60–75
12–18	30–60

Source: JA Kerner Jr. Fat requirements. In JA Kerner (ed), *Manual of Pediatric Parenteral Nutrition*. New York: Wiley, 1983. P 65.

Fewer calories are required when nutrition is delivered intravenously, and adequate growth in neonates has been documented with parenteral intakes in the range of 88–90 kcal/kg/day [71,72]. In a study of 22 preterm infants, nitrogen retention was minimally affected by parenteral infusion of greater than 70 kcal/kg/day (at constant nitrogen intake), suggesting that basal metabolic needs were probably met at this level [73].

Carbohydrate

Glucose is the sole carbohydrate available for parenteral nutrition. Minimum glucose infusion rates are critical as hypoglycemia may precipitate seizures and subsequent permanent neurologic injury [74]. Hypoglycemia during the first three days of life has been defined for full-term and preterm infants as less than 30 mg/dl and less than 20 mg/dl, respectively [75]. For infants older than three days, hypoglycemia is defined as less than 40 mg/dl for term infants and less than 20 mg/dl in preterm infants. Glucose infusion rates should therefore be known for each infant. The minimum infusion rate for the prevention of hypoglycemia is 4 mg/kg/min.

From a practical standpoint, infusion rates are begun at 6 mg/kg/min and advanced by 2 mg/kg/min each day until levels of 11 to 12 mg/kg/min are tolerated. This may take several days to achieve. Higher rates of infusion may be required but should be slowly increased as endogenous insulin production allows for maintenance of normoglycemia. Dextrose concentrations above 12.5% are poorly tolerated by peripheral infusion and mandate central venous access.

Hyperglycemia (>125 mg/dl) is more common in the preterm infant and may be associated with significant morbidity. The resultant increase in serum osmolality may result in brain cell dehydration, capillary dilatation, and intracranial hemorrhage [76]. Further, significant hyperglycemia produces glycosuria with an attendant osmotic diuresis and dehydration. The fragile nature of glucose metabolism in infants of very low birth weight (1100 g or less) was underscored by the frequent occurrence of hyperglycemia (36 of 50 infants) when glucose infusion rates exceeded 6 mg/kg/min [77]. This is likely due to decreased or abnormal responsiveness of insulin receptors [78].

If hyperglycemia prevents the administration of sufficient calories, insulin may be added to the parenteral solution. A word of caution regarding insulin is in order because the infant's response may be extremely unpredictable [78]. A very small dosage of insulin may result in profound hypoglycemia, seizures, and permanent neurologic impairment. The same dose in another similar infant may have no effect on blood sugar. A repeat dose may result in hypoglycemia.

Fat

The administration of fat is an important component in the optimal nutritional management of the neonate. Fats are vital for normal growth and development and are the main energy source of the newborn infant [79]. In human milk and most infant formulas, approximately 40% to 50% of the energy is derived from fat. Fats have a high caloric content and are isotonic, thus allowing for parenteral administration by peripheral vein.

Benefits to the parenteral administration of fat plus glucose rather than glucose alone as the source of nonprotein calories include more optimal nitrogen retention. Nose et al. [80] reported lower basal metabolic rates and respiratory quotients along with higher nitrogen retention rates in infants and children that received more physiologic levels of fat (32% of total energy intake) plus glucose compared with those that received a high glucose solution containing minimal fat (5% of total energy intake). Other investigators have confirmed higher metabolic rates and respiratory quotients in infants receiving glucose alone as the sole nonprotein energy source [81,82]. Rates of CO_2 production may be critically important for preterm infants with bronchopulmonary dysplasia and inability to wean from mechanical ventilation. The lower respiratory quotient afforded by the combination of fat and glucose as opposed to glucose alone may therefore be very important.

An additional benefit to the administration of fat includes the prevention of essential fatty acid deficiency (EFAD). Requirements for essential fatty acids in the neonate are fairly high due to rapid growth and poor tissue stores. Up to 4% of total fat intake should consist of polyunsaturated fats of the ω6 family [83]. The Committee on Nutrition of the American Academy of Pediatrics has recommended intakes of 3.3 g fat/100 kcal, of which 300 mg should be ω6 fatty acids [70]. Requirements for preterm infants are probably greater, as four-fold greater intake of linoleic acid was necessary to prevent the development of an elevated plasma triene-tetraene ratio [84]. While clinical evidence for EFAD may take several weeks to months to develop in adults, signs may be evident as early as 1 week in infants [85].

Some difficulties exist in the parenteral administration of fat to preterm and term infants that must be considered. The ability to clear the infused lipid is inversely related to gestational age and tolerance of increasing doses improves with infant maturation [86,87]. Lipoprotein lipase levels are lower in preterm infants [88] and may be augmented by addition of heparin (as low as 1 U/ml) to the parenteral nutrition solution [89]. A significantly greater increase in serum free fatty acid levels and lipoprotein lipase activity was observed when higher dosages of heparin were given (137 U/day) [90]. Because free fatty acid levels rise in the infants that receive the heparin, it is likely that the free fatty acids are produced in excess of the infant's ability for their catabolism [79]. Heparin is currently not routinely administered to enhance the clearance of intravenous lipid.

Unconjugated hyperbilirubinemia ("physiologic jaundice") is common in the preterm infant. Fatty acids competitively bind to albumin and can displace the unconjugated bilirubin leading to an increased risk for kernicterus [91,92]. Displacement occurs when the molar ratios of free fatty acid to albumin exceed 6 [93]. Hyperbilirubinemia, therefore, is not an absolute contraindication to the administration of lipids, providing that this ratio is carefully monitored.

Carnitine is important in the mitochondrial oxidation of free fatty acids. To be metabolized, free fatty acids must undergo activation to acyl-

CoA. The inner mitochondrial membrane is impermeable to acyl-CoA, and carnitine is the carrier by which long-chain fatty acids are able to be transported via an enzymatic reaction involving carnitine acyltransferase I, carnitine acyltransferase II, and carnitine translocase [94]. The body supply of carnitine derives from endogenous synthesis as well as dietary sources. While human breast milk contains carnitine, soy-based infant formulas and parenteral nutrition solutions do not. Without exogenous intake, blood and tissue carnitine levels fall in preterm and term infants due to limited endogenous synthesis [95–97]. These observations have led to the assumption that carnitine is an essential component of the diet of newborn infants.

Although a characteristic clinical syndrome of carnitine deficiency induced by insufficient intake has not yet been reported, there is evidence to suggest that L-carnitine supplementation of the diet may be important. In a group of preterm infants receiving parenteral nutrition, Schmidt-Sommerfeld and co-workers demonstrated increased plasma acylcarnitine levels and lower free fatty acid to β-hydroxybutyrate ratios in response to supplementation with L-carnitine [98]. In some studies of L-carnitine supplemented patients, enhanced ketone body production was demonstrated [99,100]. In other studies, L-carnitine supplementation had no effect on ketone body production [101,102]. The reasons for these disparate results may be due to the concomitant administration of glucose and amino acids that influence fatty acid oxidation. Because glucose is known to be the preferred energy source, fatty acid oxidation is suppressed in direct correlation with the rate of glucose infusion. Although it would appear that L-carnitine supplementation may theoretically improve fatty acid oxidation and ketogenesis in preterm infants or neonates requiring long-term administration of carnitine-free nutrition, conclusive evidence is currently lacking.

Lipid infusions are begun at a dose of 0.5 g/kg/day and advanced in increments of 0.25 to 0.5 g/kg/day to 3 g/kg/day. The 20% soybean oil emulsion (Intralipid; Kabi-Vitrum; Franklin, OH) appears to be better tolerated than the 10% emulsion, perhaps because of a lower phospholipid-triglyceride ratio of the 20% solution [103]. If the rate of lipid administration exceeds the rate of clearance, then visible lactescence and hyperlipidemia result. Simple visual inspection of the plasma for turbidity is unreliable for monitoring patients receiving intravenous fat [104]. Serum triglyceride levels should be maintained below 150 mg/dl [105]. As opposed to short infusion periods, a 20- to 24-hour infusion period is recommended to avoid significant lipemia [79]. Lipemia may interfere with oxygenation [106], perhaps through prostaglandin-mediated changes in pulmonary vascular tone and increased intrapulmonary shunting [107] or lipid microemboli [108].

Protein

The optimal amount and quality of protein to administer to preterm infants is not completely understood. The American Academy of Pediatrics Committee on Nutrition endorses the concept that protein requirements should be determined by the intake necessary to duplicate intrauterine rates of weight gain (15 g/kg/day) and nitrogen accretion (300 mg/kg/day) [70]. Others believe that the inadequate protein content of human milk is outweighed by the other nonnutritive benefits such as protection from infection. Further, while this concept may be appropriate for minimal rates of weight gain, others feel that greater weight gain and protein accretion should be the goal during the first two to four weeks of life [109].

The minimal enteral intake of protein that results in rates of weight gain and nitrogen retention that are similar to intrauterine rates appears to be roughly 2.8 g/kg/day [110]. Greater intakes of protein in excess of intrauterine rates (3.8 g/kg/day) resulted in greater rates of weight gain and nitrogen retention. Although levels of amino acids and blood urea nitrogen were mildly greater in the higher protein intake groups, it is unclear whether this is beneficial. One advantage may be a reduced length of hospitalization due to the more rapid achievement of a prescribed discharge weight [110]. Most preterm formulas provide approximately 3 to 3.6 g/kg/day of protein, which allows for rates of weight gain and nitrogen retention in excess of intrauterine rates [111,112]. In contrast, parenteral protein requirements are roughly 10% greater (3.0 g/kg/day) than enteral protein requirements [73]. This difference appears to be due to greater urinary nitrogen losses with parenteral versus enteral nutrition.

Specific amino acid requirements of the preterm infant are more difficult to define. Estimated requirements for each amino acid may be deduced from knowledge of the amount that accumulates during normal intrauterine development assuming a constant rate of growth (15 g/kg/day) (Table 27-6). Estimated requirements for each amino acid may be deduced based on the assumption that 70% of the ingested intake is absorbed and retained. Another way to estimate specific amino acid requirements is to assume that the requirements can be met by an intake of protein that results in a normal plasma amino acid pattern [113]. Normal

Table 27-6. Amino Acid Requirements (mg/kg/day) of the Low-Birth-Weight Infant as Predicted from Fetal Rates of Amino Acid Accretion

Amino Acid	Accretion Rate, 0.9–2.4 kg[a]	Estimated Requirement[b]
Isoleucine	52	74
Leucine	113	161
Lysine	108	154
Methionine	30	43
Cyst(e)ine	—	—
Phenylalanine	62	89
Tyrosine	44	63
Threonine	62	89
Tryptophan	—	—
Valine	71	101
Histidine	39	55
Arginine	115	164
Alanine	109	156
Aspartate	136	194
Glutamate	196	280
Glycine	178	254
Proline	127	181
Serine	66	94
Total Nitrogen	242	346[c]

[a]Data concerning total accretion rate of cyst(e)ine and tryptophan as well as asparagine and glutamine are not available.
[b]Equivalent to a protein intake of 2.2 g/kg/day (i.e., 346 mg × 6.38).
[c]Accretion rate/0.7, based on the assumption that 70% of the intake is retained.
Source: WC Heird, S Kashyap. Protein and amino acid requirements. In RA Polin, WW Fox (eds), *Fetal and Neonatal Physiology.* Philadelphia: Saunders, 1992. P 450. Used with permission.

plasma amino acid levels for preterm, term, and older children are depicted in Table 27-7. Based on the plasma concentrations of most amino acids in preterm infants fed 2 g/kg/day of bovine milk protein, the intake of each amino acid provided by this intake has been assumed to be the minimum requirement. More recent data on the optimal amount of protein (2.8 g/kg/day) [110] probably makes these requirements underestimated.

Due to immature enzyme systems, several amino acids may need to be supplemented as they are considered conditionally essential or acquired essential during alimentation of the preterm infant. These amino acids include histidine, cysteine, tyrosine, and taurine [114]. Breast milk contains high concentrations of cysteine and taurine while standard parenteral amino acid formulations are low in or devoid of these amino acids. Histidine deletion from the diet of a group of healthy infants resulted in failure to grow (as measured by weight gain) with the development of an eczematous rash [115]. These symptoms resolved when histidine was reintroduced in the diet.

Due to the reduced levels of cystathionase in term and preterm infants the ability of these infants to convert methionine to cysteine is impaired. Cysteine (and its dimer cystine) is therefore considered to be an essential component of the diet of preterm infants. Infusion of glucose and electrolytes to a group of preterm and term infants resulted in low plasma cystine levels that did not change after addition of synthetic L-amino acids containing high concentrations of methionine [116]. In contrast, no significant improvement in nitrogen retention was observed in a group of appropriate-size-for-gestational-age infants when cysteine hydrochloride was added to the parenteral nutrition solution [117]. Cysteine is normally unstable in aqueous solution but may be added as cysteine hydrochloride to the parenteral nutrition at the time the infusate is prepared. Unfortunately, the lower pH of the infusate results in the development of metabolic acidosis [118].

Taurine is thought to be an important amino acid for the developing preterm infant and is not present in most synthetic infant formulas. Although taurine may be necessary for functional aspects of brain, retina, heart, and liver, its exact role in preterm infant nutrition is not clear. While taurine levels in plasma, blood cells, and urine of children on long-term parenteral nutrition are low and correlate with the duration of therapy [119], a clinical picture of taurine deficiency has yet to be described. Further, supplementation of infant formula with taurine has not demonstrated enhanced growth, fat absorption, or production of taurine-conjugated bile acids [120–123].

While more conventional parenteral amino acid solutions are based on the composition of high-quality dietary protein (egg yolk), they do not take into account the special protein needs of the growing infant. Several solutions have been designed especially for low-birth-weight infants and have been based on the composition of human milk protein or mathematically designed to mimic the plasma amino acid pattern of normal term infants on a diet of breast milk. Table 27-8 shows how the amino acid patterns of several of these specialized formulations compare to those in the protein deposited by the developing fetus.

At present, it is not totally clear that these solutions justify their significantly greater cost. Increased weight gain and improved nitrogen balance were not demonstrated in a group of postsurgical preterm infants using one of these special formulations when compared with a standard for-

Table 27-7. Normal Plasma Amino Acid Values[a]

Amino Acid	Premature First Day[b]	Newborn before First Feeding[c]	16 day–4 month	9 month–2 year
Taurine	105–255	101–181	—	14–91
OH-Proline	0–80	0	—	—
Aspartic	0–20	4–12	17–21	0–9
Threonine	155–275	196–238	141–213	33–128
Serine	195–345	129–197	104–158	24–172
Asp + Glut	655–1155	623–895	—	46–290
Proline	155–305	155–305	141–245	51–185
Glutamic	30–100	27–77	—	—
Glycine	185–735	274–412	178–248	56–308
Alanine	325–425	274–384	239–345	99–313
Valine	80–180	97–175	123–199	57–262
Cystine 1/2	55–75	49–75	33–51	—
Methionine	30–40	21–37	15–21	3–29
Isoleucine	20–60	31–47	31–47	26–94
Leucine	45–95	55–89	56–98	45–155
Tyrosine	20–220	53–85	33–75	11–122
Phenylalanine	70–110	64–92	45–65	23–69
Ornithine	70–110	66–116	37–61	10–107
Lysine	130–250	154–246	117–163	45–144
Histidine	30–70	61–93	64–92	24–112
Arginine	30–70	37–71	53–71	11–65
Tryptophan	15–45	15–45	—	—
Citrulline	8.5–23.7	10.8–21.1	—	—
Ethanolamine	13.4–105	32.7–72	—	—
α-Amino-*n*-butyric	0–29	8.7–20.4	—	—

[a]Values in μmol/liter, range for ± 1 SD from the mean.
[b]JC Dickinson, H Rosenblum, PB Hamilton. Ion exchange chromatography of the free amino acids in the plasma of infants under 2,500 g at birth. *Pediatrics* 45:606, 1970.
[c]JC Dickinson, H Rosenblum, PB Hamilton. Ion exchange chromatography of the free amino acids in the plasma of the newborn infant. *Pediatrics* 36:2, 1965.
Source: Reprinted with permission from S Meites (ed), *Pediatric Clinical Chemistry*. American Association for Clinical Chemistry, 1977. P 29–30.

mulation [124]. Alternatively, no differences in nitrogen retention, weight gain, or biochemical parameters were found in a group of infants and children that received either the specialized pediatric formulation or a traditional mixture [125]. Further, net protein gain and rates of protein synthesis and breakdown were similar in a group of infants receiving a parenteral nutrition regardless of whether the amino acid formulation was based on breast milk or egg protein [126].

Fluids, Electrolytes, and Minerals

The greater body surface area per unit of body weight in the infant results in increased sensible and insensible water loss. Transepithelial water losses are an important component of insensible losses because the skin and subcutaneous tissues are more permeable in the preterm infant. Factors affecting fluid requirements are shown in Table 27-9. It is important to realize that excessive fluid administration may be harmful and is associated with patent ductus arteriosus, necrotizing enterocolitis, intraventricular hemorrhage, and bronchopulmonary dysplasia [127]. For parenteral fluids, the standard formula of 100 ml/kg for the first 10 kg of body weight, 50 ml/kg for the second 10 kg, and 20 ml/kg for the third 10 kg of body weight is a reasonable starting point. These requirements may increase by 20% when infants are placed under phototherapy lights or even higher when under radiant warmers. Beyond 30 kg of body weight, it is more prudent to use body surface area (2000 ml/M^2) as a means of calculating fluid requirements. A 30 kg patient can be considered to be roughly 1 M^2. With regard to enteral fluid

Table 27-8. Amino Acid Pattern of Pediatric Parenteral Amino Acid Mixtures and of the Developing Fetus

Amino Acid	Aminosyn-PF (mg/g)	Trophamine (mg/g)	Neopham (mg/g)	Fetal Protein (mg/g)
Isoleucine	76	82	49	35
Leucine	119	140	110	75
Lysine	68	82	83	72
Methionine	18	33	20	20
Cyst(e)ine	0	3	0	—
Phenylalanine	43	48	42	41
Tyrosine	6	23	8	29
Threonine	52	42	56	41
Tryptophan	18	20	22	—
Valine	64	78	56	47
Histidine	32	48	33	26
Arginine	123	122	64	77
Alanine	70	53	99	72
Aspartate	53	32	64	90
Glutamate	82	50	111	130
Glycine	38	37	33	118
Proline	82	68	88	84
Serine	50	38	60	41

Source: WC Heird, S Kashyap. Protein and amino acid requirements. In RA Polin, WW Fox (eds), *Fetal and Neonatal Physiology.* Philadelphia: Saunders, 1992. P 459.

Table 27-9. Factors Affecting Pediatric Fluid Requirements

Factors increasing requirements:
- Radiant warmers
- Conventional single-walled incubators
- Phototherapy
- Ambient temperature above neutral thermal range
- Respiratory distress
- Any hypermetabolic problem
- Elevated body temperature
- Diuretic treatment
- Diarrhea
- Glycosuria (with associated osmotic diuresis)
- Intravenous alimentation
- Renal tubular defects
- Fistulas, stomas

Factors decreasing requirements:
- Heat shields
- Thermal blankets
- Double-walled incubators
- Placing infant in relatively high humidity
- Use of warm, humidified air via endotracheal tube
- Oliguria

Source: M Marian. Pediatric nutrition support. *Nutr Clin Pract* 8:199–209, 1993.

administration, a volume of 180 ml/kg/day is necessary to meet caloric goals (120 kcal/kg) using standard infant formulas (20 kcal/oz).

General guidelines for electrolyte and mineral requirements for infants and children are depicted in Table 27-10. Actual requirements for each individual patient must be considered in light of status of hydration, medications, renal function, and ongoing losses. The immature kidneys of the preterm infant are not able to effectively concentrate and result in excessive urinary losses of sodium and water. Significant sources of sodium intake that are not often considered include peripheral intravenous and arterial lines infused with normal saline or certain antibiotics.

Substantial amounts of calcium and phosphorus are required to support rapid skeletal bone development and prevent the development of rickets. To match in utero accretion rates, preterm infants would require 5 to 7.5 mEq/kg/day of elemental calcium and 1 to 2 mm/kg/day of phosphate salts [127]. Unfortunately, these intakes are usually impossible to achieve with either parenteral or enteral feeding. While the solubility of these ions in aqueous solution is improved by lowering the pH of the solution [128], precipitation can occur if the solubility coefficient is exceeded in an attempt to meet the needs of the preterm infant. Other factors that contribute to precipitation include low amino acid or glucose content and prolonged exposure of the intravenous tubing to the

Table 27-10. Recommended Daily Intake of Electrolytes and Minerals for Parenteral Nutrition Solutions

Element	Daily Amount
Sodium	2–4 mEq/kg
Potassium	2–3 mEq/kg
Chloride	2–3 mEq/kg
Magnesium	0.2–0.50 mEq/kg
Calcium gluconate*	100–500 mg/kg
Phosphorus	1–2 mmol/kg

*Gluconate is the recommended calcium salt for use in parenteral nutrition solutions.
Source: RL Poole. Electrolyte and mineral requirements. In JA Kerner (ed), *Manual of Pediatric Parenteral Nutrition*. New York: Wiley, 1983. P 130.

high temperatures of the infant incubator [129]. Whereas phosphorus requirements are generally based on the amount required to maintain normal serum levels, serum calcium levels remain normal even in the presence of significant bone demineralization [130]. Calcium should therefore not be removed from the parenteral nutrition solution in the presence of normal serum levels. Clinically, bone demineralization is inferred by noting an increase in serum levels of alkaline phosphatase. The cause for this elevation may be difficult to determine because high levels are seen with parenteral nutrition-associated cholestasis as well as rapid growth. Fractionation of the alkaline phosphatase into heat-stable (liver) and heat-labile (bone) components may be useful.

Magnesium is important for many enzymatic reactions, and low levels are associated with hypokalemia and hypocalcemia. Low serum magnesium levels may be seen in infants with DiGeorge's syndrome, neonatal hepatitis, biliary atresia, and infants of diabetic mothers [131]. Hypomagnesemia may also be acquired through significant diarrheal or ostomy output as well as diuretic use.

Vitamins

The Nutrition Advisory Group of the American Medical Association first suggested the need for separate adult and pediatric vitamin formulations for parenteral nutrition in 1979 [132]. This was approved by the United States Food and Drug Administration in 1981, and new guidelines were proposed in 1988 [133]. A summary of these suggested modifications is shown in Table 27-11.

The fat-soluble vitamins (A, D, E, and K) differ in several respects from the water-soluble vitamins with regard to the pediatric population. Fat-soluble vitamins are stored in body tissues, the potential for overdosage and toxicity exist, and requirements are dependent on age and degree of

Table 27-11. Suggested Intakes of Parenteral Vitamins in Infants and Children

Vitamin	Term Infants and Children (dose/d)	Preterm Infants*: Current Suggestions (dose/kg body weight)	Preterm Infants*: Best Estimate for New Formulation (dose/kg body weight)
Lipid soluble			
A (μg)	700	280	500
E (mg)	7	28	2.8
K (μg)	200	80	80
D (μg)	10	4	4
(IU)	400	160	160
Water Soluble			
Ascorbic acid (mg)	80.0	32.0	25.0
Thiamin (mg)	1.2	0.48	0.35
Riboflavin (mg)	1.4	0.56	0.15
Pyridoxine (mg)	1.0	0.4	0.18
Niacin (mg)	17.0	6.8	6.8
Pantothenate (mg)	5.0	2.0	2.0
Biotin (μg)	20.0	8.0	6.0
Folate (μg)	140.0	56.0	56.0
Vitamin B_{12} (μg)	1.0	0.4	0.3

*Maximum not to exceed term infant dose.
Source: Modified from HL Greene, et al. Guidelines for the use of vitamins, trace elements, calcium, magnesium, and phosphorus in infants and children receiving total parenteral nutrition. *Am J Clin Nutr* 48:1324, 1988.

maturation. On the other hand, due to transplacental transport, the neonate is born with sufficient levels of most water-soluble vitamins. Because the water-soluble vitamins are not appreciably stored in the body, urinary losses and diminished intake set the stage for the development of vitamin deficiency [134].

Vitamin A

In the adult, hepatic stores of vitamin A will not become depleted for over one year in the absence of a dietary source. In contrast, growing children have only a few weeks' storage [135], and preterm infants have virtually no hepatic reserves. This latter group is at extremely high risk for the development of a clinical deficiency [136]. Clinically, vitamin A deficiency is most often recognized in children [137], and the signs are primarily ocular. The earliest signs include night blindness followed by involvement of the cornea and conjunctiva as a result of the normal loss of epithelial differentiation [137]. Other signs include anorexia, slowed growth, increased susceptibility to infections, and disturbances of the reproductive system. Bronchopulmonary dysplasia (BPD) has been associated with low plasma retinol levels in the preterm infant [138,139], and supplementation resulted in increased plasma levels and a significant reduction in BPD [140]. Further work in this area is indicated. Vitamin A toxicity is manifest clinically by dermatitis, irritability, cheilosis, and gingivitis.

Vitamin D

The primary role of vitamin D is in the stimulation of calcium and phosphorus absorption from the gastrointestinal tract. Vitamin D also works to promote calcium reabsorption from the kidneys and bone. Vitamin D deficiency is manifested clinically as rickets, which includes craniotabes, rachitic rib rosary, bowed legs, and muscle weakness. The mandated addition of vitamin D to milk has virtually eliminated the occurrence of vitamin D-deficient rickets in the United States. Vitamin D intoxication leads to hypercalcemia resulting in vomiting, constipation, and growth retardation.

Human milk contains less than 40 IU/L of vitamin D [141] and is dependent on maternal intake of vitamin D [142] and sunshine exposure [143]. Infants fed breast milk alone may therefore be at risk for the development of vitamin D deficiency. Most infant formulas and whole cow's milk contain roughly 400 IU/L of vitamin D.

Vitamin E

The primary and perhaps only function for vitamin E is as a biologic antioxidant, protecting membrane polyunsaturated fatty acids (PUFAs) from peroxidation. Because iron also catalyzes the peroxidation of cell membranes, addition of iron to infant formulas also increases the requirement for vitamin E [144]. Vitamin E deficiency can be recognized as two distinct patterns of presentation. The first is in children with fat malabsorption due to biliary atresia, cystic fibrosis, or abetalipoproteinemia and presents as a progressive sensory and motor neuropathy within the first decade of life [145,146]. The second pattern of deficiency is one of hemolytic anemia in preterm infants within the first two months of life. This was first recognized in a group of preterm infants fed a formula containing high levels of PUFAs and low levels of vitamin E [147]. In this group of infants, all clinical and hematologic abnormalities corrected after the initiation of oral vitamin E therapy.

Administration of vitamin E to preterm infants is not without significant risk because a syndrome of pulmonary deterioration, thrombocytopenia, liver and renal failure, and death has been described [148]. Further, the incidence of necrotizing enterocolitis has been reported to be greater in infants receiving oral and/or parenteral vitamin E supplementation [149,150].

Vitamin K

Plasma clotting factors II, VII, IX, and X are dependent on vitamin K for their synthesis. The vitamin K-dependent factor levels are directly related to the gestational age of the neonate and are low in comparison to adult levels. The infant is born with inadequate vitamin K stores and because of the many reports of intracranial hemorrhage in infants not supplemented, vitamin K prophylaxis is given as an intramuscular injection at the time of birth. Although controversial, a hemorrhagic disease of the newborn may develop in unsupplemented newborns as ecchymoses, gastrointestinal hemorrhage, and excessive bleeding at the umbilical stump or following circumcision. The newborn infant appears to be especially susceptible to the toxic effects of the synthetic water-soluble vitamin K compounds manifested as hemolysis, hyperbilirubinemia, and kernicterus. The toxicity appears to be dose-dependent and at dosages greater than 1 mg/kg [151].

Vitamin C (Ascorbic Acid)

Vitamin C participates in a wide variety of hydroxylation reactions: the metabolism of tyrosine, carnitine, norepinephrine, and collagen. In the preterm infant, the activity of the immature hepatic enzyme *p*-hydroxyphenylpyruvic acid oxidase, responsible for the catabolism of tyrosine, is enhanced by ascorbic acid. Concern for the neurodevelopmental risks of elevated tyrosine levels has been considered the main rationale for ascorbic acid supplementation in the newborn period [141]. Ascorbic acid deficiency is known as scurvy. In the infantile form, scurvy is characterized by irritability, tenderness, swelling, and pseudoparalysis of the lower extremities. In preterm infants, sepsis and failure to thrive are associated with ascorbic acid deficiency [152]. Hemorrhagic manifestations may follow with bleeding at tooth eruption sites, diarrhea, epistaxis, or ocular bleeding. Ascorbic acid toxicity is rare as it is cleared rapidly by the kidneys.

Vitamin B_1 (Thiamine)

Thiamine functions as a cofactor in oxidative decarboxylation reactions involving carbohydrate. Thiamine needs are therefore directly proportional to carbohydrate intake. Thiamine deficiency results in beriberi, which consists of high-output congestive heart failure, lactic acidosis, and peripheral neuropathy. While thiamine deficiency has not been reported in breast-fed infants of well-nourished mothers, infantile beriberi can occur in infants of mothers who are alcoholic or malnourished. The most reliable marker of thiamine deficiency is the activity of erythrocyte transketolase.

Riboflavin

Riboflavin coenzymes are essential components of several enzymes involved in electron transport. Riboflavin deficiency is characterized by angular stomatitis, glossitis, cheilosis, seborrheic dermatitis around the nose and mouth, and changes in the eye that include reduced tearing, photophobia, corneal vascularization, and cataracts. Riboflavin is extremely sensitive to ultraviolet light, and biochemical evidence for riboflavin deficiency has been observed in breast-fed infants receiving phototherapy for hyperbilirubinemia [153]. Despite these concerns, no deficiency states have been described in infants receiving vitamin-supplemented parenteral nutrition.

Vitamin B_6 (Pyridoxine)

A deficiency of vitamin B_6 is rare and characterized clinically by a hypochromic microcytic anemia, gastrointestinal disturbances, failure to thrive, irritability, and seizures. No deficiency states have been reported in parenterally fed infants.

Niacin

Niacin refers to both nicotinic acid and nicotinamide and participates in a variety of metabolic reactions including fat synthesis, tissue respiration, and glycolysis. Pellagra is the deficiency state and includes diarrhea, dermatitis, and dementia. No deficiency states have been reported in parenterally fed infants receiving vitamin supplementation.

Pantothenic Acid

Although deficiency of pantothenic acid has been observed in several animal species, in humans it has been described only under extraordinary circumstances such as extreme malnutrition. Clinically, deficiency is seen as the "burning feet" syndrome and is associated with insomnia, gastrointestinal disturbances, headache, and muscle weakness.

Biotin

Until recently, parenteral vitamin preparations in the United States did not contain biotin. Due to its ubiquitous nature in food and the fact that it is synthesized by intestinal bacteria, deficiency states are extremely rare. A clinical syndrome of biotin deficiency was described in a child with short-bowel syndrome consisting of an exfoliative dermatitis, alopecia, pallor, irritability, and lethargy [154]. Deficient states might develop in unsupplemented infants in whom intestinal absorption is impaired or bacterial synthesis is reduced due to antibiotic administration.

Folic Acid

Tetrahydrofolate is the coenzyme form of folic acid and is a donor and acceptor of single carbon units in amino acid and nucleotide metabolism. Folic acid deficiency is one of the most common nutritional vitamin deficiencies in humans and is most common under conditions that are associated with increased folic acid requirements such as rapid growth of the preterm infant and severe hemolytic disease of the newborn. Folic acid requirements are approximately 10 times that of adults on the basis of body weight. The manifestations of dietary folate deficiency include hypersegmentation of neutrophils, megaloblastic changes on the blood smear, and poor growth [155]. Folic acid deficiency has been reported to develop in infants fed formulas based on heated or boiled evaporated milk, a practice that inactivates folate [156].

Vitamin B_{12}

Dietary B_{12} is usually present in considerable excess over requirements. One exception to this is in the infant who is entirely breast-fed by a vegetarian mother who consumes no eggs or dairy products [157]. Vitamin B_{12} deficiency is important despite its rarity due to the danger of irreversible neurologic injury unless it is diagnosed and treated early and due to the fact that most nutritional deficiencies of B_{12} require therapy throughout life [158]. B_{12} also needs to be supplemented in infants who have undergone surgical resection of the terminal ileum for such pediatric surgical diseases as atresia, midgut volvulus, or necrotizing enterocolitis.

Trace Elements

Although trace elements constitute less than 0.01% of total body weight, they play a pivotal role in growth and development. In preterm infants, the normal placental transfer of trace elements has been interrupted, and without supplementation deficiency states may rapidly develop. Recommended intakes for several trace elements are shown in Table 27-12.

Zinc is an essential component of various enzyme reactions and extremely important for growth. In fact, the earliest sign of zinc deficiency in an infant is a decline in growth velocity. With more severe depletion, the infant may become irritable, lethargic, and develop a characteristic rash, diarrhea, and alopecia. Factors to consider in the development of zinc deficiency are the increased zinc losses seen with persistent diarrhea or through high-output ostomies or gastrocutaneous fistulas [159,160].

There are substantial hepatic stores of copper in the term neonate despite relatively low serum levels. The lower serum levels are probably due to limited ceruloplasmin synthesis [133]. Early features of copper deficiency include osteoporosis, neutropenia, and an iron-resistant microcytic anemia. In preterm infants, neurologic abnormalities, anorexia, failure to thrive, and hepatomegaly may become evident. Because 80% of absorbed copper is excreted by the biliary system, one of the main considerations in copper replacement is hepatic function. Copper toxicity may develop in supplemented patients with impaired bile excretion (biliary atresia, parenteral nutrition-associated cholestasis). For the same reason, manganese should also be withheld in patients with cholestasis. While liver failure should result in the withholding of copper and manganese, renal failure should limit the replacement of selenium, chromium, and molybdenum.

Techniques

Parenteral

The ability to secure reliable and safe access to either peripheral or central veins in children can be extremely challenging. The choice as to whether to use peripheral or central access is best determined by the anticipated duration of therapy [161]. Long-term maintenance of peripheral veins in small children is extremely difficult. The dextrose concentration of the parenteral solution for peripheral veins should not exceed 12.5% due to vein sclerosis, and this may limit the number of calories to be administered.

In children with an anticipated prolonged need for parenteral nutrition and normal life ex-

Table 27-12. Recommended Intravenous Intakes of Trace Elements[a]

Element	Infants: Preterm[b] (μg · kg⁻¹ · d⁻¹)	Infants: Term (μg · kg⁻¹ · d⁻¹)	Children (μg · kg⁻¹ · d⁻¹)	Children [maximum μg/d]
Zinc	400	250 < 3 mo 100 > 3 mo	50	[5000]
Copper[c]	20	20	20	[300]
Selenium[d]	2.0	2.0	2.0	[30]
Chromium[d]	0.20	0.20	0.20	[5.0]
Manganese[c]	1.0	1.0	1.0	[50]
Molybdenum[d]	0.25	0.25	0.25	[5.0]
Iodide	1.0	1.0	1.0	[70]

[a]When total parenteral nutrition is only supplemental or limited to < 4 wk, only zinc need be added. Thereafter, addition of the remaining elements is advisable.
[b]Available concentrations of manganese and molybdenum are such that dilution of the manufacturer's product may be necessary.
[c]Omit in patients with obstructive jaundice.
[d]Omit in patients with renal dysfunction.
Source: Modified from HL Greene, et al. Guidelines for the use of vitamins, trace elements, calcium, magnesium, and phosphorus in infants and children receiving total parenteral nutrition. Report of the Subcommittee on Pediatric Parenteral Nutrient Requirements from the Committee on Clinical Practice Issues of The American Society for Clinical Nutrition. *Am J Clin Nutr* 48:1324, 1988. Revised reprint December 1990. © Am J Clin Nutr, American Society for Clinical Nutrition.

pectancy (short-bowel syndrome, pseudo-obstruction, aganglionosis, etc.), the choice of central vein for catheter placement becomes critical. Every effort should be made to avoid ligating major tributary vessels. This employs the use of percutaneous central venous cannulation whenever possible or a cutdown onto smaller branches of main vessels (facial vein, external jugular, etc.). Because children are less cooperative than adults and the risk of technical misadventure combined with the risk of sedation are great, placement of central venous catheters are usually performed in the operating room using general anesthesia. Exceptions to this rule are in small infants who are already on a ventilator [162] or in the placement of catheters into the saphenous or femoral vein via a formal cutdown using local anesthesia [163]. There appear to be no major differences in infectious, thrombotic, or mechanical complications in catheters placed in the operating room versus those that are placed in the nursery. Fluoroscopy is liberally used during placement of central venous catheters in children. The position of the guide wire (if used) is confirmed before the larger peel-away sheath and introducer are inserted over the wire as well as the final catheter position. For small catheters (less than 5 Fr) contrast material may be injected through the catheter to allow for visualization during fluoroscopy. No more than 1 to 2 ml is usually needed. The catheter is secured to the skin with a nonabsorbable suture and left in place until tissue ingrowth into the catheter cuff has occurred. As in adults, the best place for externalization of the catheter is the anterior chest because this allows for a flat surface to apply an occlusive dressing.

Available sizes for Broviac catheters in children include 2.7 Fr, 3.0 Fr, 4.2 Fr, 5.0 Fr, 6.5 Fr, and 7 Fr. In children with long-standing central lines and clinically apparent thromboses, ultrasound of the great veins may be useful to document patency. Magnetic resonance imaging (MRI) may also be employed. In light of these two relatively noninvasive tests and concerns about minimization of radiation exposure, venography is performed less frequently than in the past.

In comparison with adults, central venous catheters in the pediatric population are associated with a somewhat higher incidence of catheter-related sepsis, depending on the patient population studied. We discovered a catheter sepsis rate of 9% in a group of preterm infants under 1000 g [164]. In a large study of infants and children, septic complications were reported at 4% [165]. In pediatric oncology patients, rates of infection are reported to occur in the range of 18% to 55% [166,167].

Mechanical complications requiring catheter removal are fairly common and include catheter breaks, occlusion, and dislodgement. Catheter repair kits afford the opportunity to maintain large-bore catheters; however, smaller catheters (2.7 Fr or 3.0 Fr) are more easily injured and do not withstand repair as well as larger catheters. Similarly, smaller catheters are occluded more readily and were the reason for catheter removal in 4% of catheters in a group of pediatric oncology patients [167]. Catheter dislodgement may occur with greater frequency in younger children and appears to be directly related to the distance between the cuff of the catheter and the catheter exit site [167]. Malposition of the tip of the catheter may also occur. We recently reported a noninvasive method to reposition the catheter tip without the need for reoperation or catheter replacement [168]. A burst of saline that is injected through the catheter has been successful in repositioning these catheters in a fair percentage of patients.

Peripherally inserted central venous catheters (PCVC) are emerging as another option for access to the central venous circulation. While these catheters may not provide the same long-term access afforded by standard central catheters, their advantages are that they do not require an operating room or anesthesia and nonsurgical physicians are capable of line placement. On the other hand, a sizable peripheral vein must be present. Further, the small, floppy catheter must be guided into a central position from a fair distance and this is not always successful. Finally, we have recently experienced the fracture and embolization of a PCVC into the pulmonary artery of a young child receiving home antibiotics [169]. The safety of these catheters for use in the pediatric population for home therapy has not definitively been established.

Enteral

The techniques and routes of feeding access to the gastrointestinal tract in children is not unlike that in adults. Enteral feeding is preferred to parenteral feeding whenever possible. Nasogastric or nasoenteric feeding is common during periods of hospitalization. However, these routes are impractical for long-term home management. An exception would be for small infants, in which parents may be taught to insert nasogastric tubes for bolus feeding during the day and/or continuous drip feeding during the night. Nasoenteric tubes are at significant risk for dislodgement and are easily clogged due to medications, both of which limit their utility.

Gastrostomy tubes are standard routes by which enteral feeding may be delivered to the infant or child and are usually well tolerated. Although the standard technique for gastrostomy tube placement remains as an open procedure performed in the operating room, a fair experience has accumulated with the percutaneous endoscopic method that is at least as safe [170]. The advantages of this method in children are not completely accepted because general anesthesia is usually required. Access to either the stomach or jejunum may also be achieved using fluoroscopy and interventional radiologic techniques [171].

Jejunostomy tubes are infrequently used in children due to the limited tube size that does not occlude to the lumen of the bowel. Further, these small tubes frequently clog following the administration of medications. We have used the soft, Silastic Broviac catheter as a route of feeding into the mucus fistula end of the small bowel to promote adaptation following multiple resections and anastomoses for multiple intestinal atresias [172].

A frequently encountered pediatric surgical problem is enteral feeding of the neurologically impaired child. This patient population typically has a very high incidence of gastroesophageal reflux (GER), and placement of a simple gastrostomy may set the stage for severe reflux problems such as esophagitis, aspiration pneumonia, and apnea. These children should therefore be studied preoperatively to determine if GER is present. An upper gastrointestinal series should first be performed to exclude congenital (duodenal web, pyloric stenosis) or acquired (duodenal ulcer or hematoma) lesions associated with gastric outlet obstruction and to confirm normal gastric anatomy. A 12- or 24-hour pH probe should then be performed to determine whether pathologic GER is present. Because it has been shown that gastrostomy placement alone in this population can cause GER [173], some have advocated the performance of an antireflux procedure in addition to the gastrostomy in all neurologically impaired patients regardless of the preoperative reflux status [174]. This, however, is not the predominant approach.

Complications

The technical, septic, and metabolic complications of enteral and total parenteral nutrition (TPN) are well described elsewhere in this text and, with the exceptions previously outlined, are similar in adults and children. One major complication of TPN that presents in a unique manner in the pediatric patient compared with the adult is cholestasis. In children, TPN-related cholestasis may lead to cirrhosis with end-stage liver failure and death. The liver dysfunction related to TPN in adults, however, seldom progresses beyond fatty infiltration. The hepatobiliary complications of TPN are characterized by three distinct clinical syndromes [175]. The first syndrome is seen primarily in adults and is characterized by hepatic steatosis, steatoheopatitis, and the infrequent occurrence of cholestasis. The second pattern is seen primarily in infants and characterized predominantly by cholestasis. The third constellation of signs is common to both age groups and consists of the gallbladder-related problems of sludge formation and stones.

The true incidence of hepatic dysfunction associated with TPN is difficult to define but is seen primarily in premature infants. In a group of mostly preterm infants, 34% were noted to develop an elevated bilirubin within 2 weeks of the initiation of TPN [176]. This was noted to resolve in the majority of infants 4 weeks following the discontinuation of the TPN. In a more recent series, a direct serum bilirubin of greater than 1.5 mg/dL was seen in 7.4% of a group of 624 infants [177]. The actual incidence may be greater, as it has been suggested that serum levels of γ glutamyl transpeptidase or bile acids may be more sensitive indicators of TPN-related hepatic injury [178].

Other factors thought to play a role in TPN-cholestasis include prematurity, low birth weight, sepsis, lack of enteral nutrition, and gastrointestinal conditions that require operative intervention [175]. The physiology of bile secretion in the preterm infant may be important because bile salt pool size, synthesis, and intestinal concentration are all low in comparison to term infants [22]. Gestational age has been shown to be inversely related to peak serum bilirubin levels in parenterally fed infants [179]. Fasting (with accompanying reduced hormonal and neural stimulation of bile flow) and sepsis may compound the effect of TPN [178].

Excess or deficiency of various amino acids have been implicated in the pathogenesis of TPN-cholestasis. Jaundice occurred more rapidly and to a greater extent in infants receiving TPN solutions containing a higher protein content (3.6 g/kg/day vs. 2.3 g/kg/day) [180]. In an animal study comparing two different amino acid formulations, impaired bile flow was noted only in the group receiving the formulation deficient in serine [181]. Deficiency of taurine has also been considered because it is not present in most parenteral amino acid formulations, is considered a conditionally essential amino acid in the preterm infant, and is the principal bile acid conjugate in the neonate promoting bile flow and preventing lithocholate toxicity [182]. Taurine supplementation has been shown to promote bile acid secretion in low-birth-weight infants [183]. In another trial, however, taurine supplementation did not alter biochemical tests of hepatic toxicity [184].

Interference with the enterohepatic circulation of bile salts may contribute to liver injury. Colonization of the gut with colonic-type bacteria due to intestinal stasis results in increased production of lithocholic acid, which has been shown to impair bile flow and induce cholestasis [185]. The pattern of hepatic injury induced by lithocholate is similar to that seen with TPN-cholestasis [186,187]. Further, pretreatment of patients with either oral metronidazole [188] or gentamicin [189] resulted in a reduced incidence of TPN-related dysfunction. The beneficial effect of antibiotic administration may also be related to reducing the number of bacteria or bacterial by-products (for example, endotoxin) translocating across the gut mucosa and into the portal circulation. The light and electron microscopic pattern of liver injury associated with TPN is very similar to that following endotoxin administration [190].

Contamination of TPN solutions has also been implicated in liver injury. The degradation of tryptophan by solutions contaminated with sodium bisulfite may produce cholestasis [191]. Aluminum contamination of the TPN solution has also been suggested as a cause of cholestasis [192]. In modern-day parenteral solutions, it is unlikely that these contaminants are present.

It is important to emphasize that the diagnosis of TPN-induced cholestasis should be one of exclusion. The differential diagnosis of hyperbilirubinemia in the neonate is extensive. Sepsis from any cause should be ruled out and noninvasive imaging using ultrasound, radionuclide scanning, and liver biopsy should be performed. In a large group of patients referred for evaluation of TPN-related liver disease, 10% were noted to have jaundice from other causes [193]. A word of caution concerning the interpretation of radionuclide scans in fasted patients receiving TPN is in order. The gallbladder does not visualize in up to 36% of patients [194]. The diagnosis of cholecystitis in these young patients may therefore be extremely difficult.

After the diagnosis of TPN-related cholestasis has been established, the best therapy is to begin or increase enteral feeding and wean the TPN as much as possible. Indeed, established evidence of periportal fibrosis, portal-portal bridging, and frank cirrhosis has been described in a group of infants receiving TPN for greater than 60 days [195]. Other maneuvers include reducing the amount of protein and decreasing the calorie-nitrogen ratio to roughly 150 [193]. In cases of severe chronic liver disease, transplantation of the liver with or without the small bowel has been successful in selected cases [196,197].

References

1. Winick M. Early nutrition and brain development. In WC Heird (ed), *Nutritional Needs of the Six to Twelve Month Old Infant.* New York: Raven, 1991.
2. Henning SJ. Functional development of the gastrointestinal tract. In LR Johnson (ed), *Physiology of the Gastrointestinal Tract* (2nd ed). New York: Raven, 1987.
3. Abramovich DR. Fetal factors influencing amniotic fluid volume and composition of liquor amni. *J Obstet Gynaecol Br Commonwealth* 77:865, 1970.
4. Pritchard JA. Fetal swallowing and amniotic fluid volume. *Obstet Gynecol* 28:606, 1966.
5. Gryboski JD. Suck and swallow in the premature infant. *Pediatrics* 43:96, 1969.
6. Gryboski JD. The swallowing mechanism of the neonate: I. Esophageal and gastric motility. *Pediatrics* 35:445, 1965.
7. Boix-Ochoa J, Canals J. Maturation of the lower esophagus. *J Pediatr Surg* 11:749, 1976.
8. Siegel M. Gastric emptying time in premature and compromised infants. *J Pediatr Gastroenterol Nutr* 2(Suppl. 1):136, 1983.
9. Bisset WM, et al. Ontogeny of fasting small intestinal motor activity in the human infant. *Gut* 29:483, 1988.
10. Berseth CL. Gestational evaluation of small intestine motility in preterm and term infants. *J Pediatr* 115:646, 1989.
11. Berseth CL. Neonatal small intestinal motility: Motor responses to feeding in term and preterm infants. *J Pediatr* 117:777, 1990.
12. Berseth CL. Effect of early feeding on maturation of the preterm infants' small intestine. *J Pediatr* 120:947, 1992.
13. Brown EG, Sweet AY. Preventing necrotizing enterocolitis in neonates. *JAMA* 240:2452, 1978.
14. Goldman HI. Feeding and necrotizing enterocolitis. *Am J Dis Child* 134:553, 1980.
15. Hamosh M, et al. Lipids in milk and the first steps in their digestion. *Pediatrics* 75(Suppl.):146, 1984.
16. Agunod M, et al. Correlative study of hydrochloric acid, pepsin, and intrinsic factor secretion in newborns and infants. *Am J Dig Dis* 14:400, 1969.
17. Auricchio S. Recent advances in pediatric gastroenterology. *Pediatr Res* 11:997, 1977.
18. Takeuchi K, Peitsch W, Johnson LR. Mucosal gastrin receptor: V. Development in newborn rats. *Am J Physiol* 240:G163, 1981.
19. Lebenthal E, Leung YK. Feeding the premature and compromised infant: Gastrointestinal considerations. *Pediatr Clin North Am* 35:215, 1988.
20. Lebenthal E, Lee PC. Development of junctional response in human exocrine pancreas. *Pediatrics* 66:556, 1980.
21. Walker WA. Absorption of protein and protein fragments in the developing intestine: Role of immunologic/allergic reactions. *Pediatrics* 75(Suppl.):167, 1985.
22. Watkins JB. Role of bile acids in the development of the enterohepatic circulation. In E Lebenthal (ed), *Textbook of Gastroenterology and Nutrition in Infancy.* New York: Raven, 1981.

23. Antonowicz I, Lebenthal E. Developmental patterns of small intestinal enterokinase and disaccharidase activities in the human fetus. *Gastroenterology* 72:1299, 1977.

24. Auricchio S, Rubino A, Murset G. Intestinal glycosidase activities of the human embryo, fetus and newborn. *Pediatrics* 35:944, 1965.

25. Lacroix B, et al. Early organogenesis of human small intestine: Scanning electromicroscopy and brush border enzymology. *Gut* 25:925, 1984.

26. Lebenthal E, Lee PC, Heitlinger LA. Impact of development of the gastrointestinal tract on infant feeding. *J Pediatr* 102:1, 1983.

27. Borgstrom B, Lindquist B, Lundh G. Enzyme concentration and absorption of protein and glucose in duodenum of premature infants. *Am J Dis Child* 99:338, 1960.

28. Auricchio S, Stellato A, DeVizia B. Development of brush border peptidases in human and rat small intestine during fetal and neonatal life. *Pediatr Res* 15:991, 1981.

29. Feinstein MS, Smith CA. Digestion of protein by premature infants, as indicated by nitrogen absorption from whole versus hydrolyzed protein. *Pediatrics* 7:19, 1951.

30. Hirata Y, Matsuo P, Kobubu H. Digestion and absorption of milk proteins in infants' intestine. *Kobe J Med Sci* 11:103, 1965.

31. Grusky FL, Cooke RE. The gastrointestinal absorption of unaltered protein in normal infants and in infants recovering from diarrhea. *Pediatrics* 16:763, 1969.

32. Eastham EJ, et al. Antigenicity of infant formulas: Role of immature intestine on protein permeability. *J Pediatr* 93:561, 1978.

33. Korenblat RE, et al. Immune response of human adults after oral and parenteral exposure to bovine serum albumin. *J Allergy* 41:226, 1968.

34. Wilson SJ, Walzer M. Absorption of undigested proteins in human beings. *Am J Dis Child* 50:49, 1935.

35. Watkins JB, Ingall D, Szczepanik P. Bile salt metabolism in the newborn. *N Engl J Med* 288:531, 1973.

36. Watkins JB, et al. Bile salt metabolism in the human premature infant: Preliminary observations of pool size and synthesis rate following prenatal administration of dexamethasone and phenobarbitol. *Gastroenterology* 69:706, 1975.

37. Fomon SJ, et al. Excretion of fat by normal full-term infants fed various milks and formulas. *Am J Clin Nutr* 23:1299, 1970.

38. Hanna FM, Navarrete DH, Hsu FA. Calcium-fatty acid absorption in term infants fed human milk and prepared formulas simulating human milk. *Pediatrics* 45:216, 1970.

39. Roy CC, et al. Correction of the malabsorption of the preterm infant with a medium chain triglyceride formula. *Pediatrics* 86:446, 1975.

40. Coppoletta JM, Wolbach SB. Body length and organ weights of infants and children: A study of body length and normal weights of the more important vital organs of the body between birth and twelve years of age. *Am J Pathol* 9:55, 1933.

41. Itoh S, et al. Foetal maternal relationships of bile acid pattern estimated by high-pressure liquid chromatography. *Biochem J* 204:1411, 1982.

42. Colombo C, et al. Biliary bile acid composition of the human fetus in early gestation. *Pediatr Res* 21:197, 1987.

43. Balistreri WF. Anatomic and biochemical ontogeny of the gastrointestinal tract and liver. In RC Tsang, BL Nichols (eds), *Nutrition during Infancy.* Philadelphia: Hanley & Belfus, 1988.

44. Kawade N, Onishi S. The prenatal and postnatal development of UDP-glucuronyl-transferase activity towards bilirubin and the effect of premature birth on this activity in the human liver. *Biochem J* 196:257, 1981.

45. Shelly HJ. Glycogen reserves and their changes at birth and in anoxia. *Br Med Bull* 17:137, 1961.

46. Girard J. Gluconeogenesis in late fetal and early neonatal life. *Biol Neonate* 50:237, 1986.

47. Sadava D, et al. Development of enzymes of glycolysis and gluconeogenesis in human fetal liver. *Biol Neonate* 62:89, 1992.

48. Gaull G, Sturman JA, Raiha NC. Development of mammalian sulfur metabolism: Absence of cystothionase in human fetal tissues. *Pediatr Res* 6:538, 1972.

49. Janne J, Holtta E, Guha SK. Polyamines in mammalian liver during growth and development. In H Popper, F Schaffner (eds). *Progress in Liver Diseases.* New York: Grune & Stratton, 1976.

50. Dancis J, Braverman N, Lind J. Plasma protein synthesis in the human fetus and placenta. *J Clin Invest* 36:398, 1957.

51. Zlotkin SH, Stalling VA, Pencharz PB. Total parenteral nutrition in children. *Surg Clin North Am* 32:381, 1985.

52. Forbes GB. Fetal growth and body composition: Implications for the premature infant. *J Pediatr Gastroenterol Nutr* 2(Suppl. 1):S52, 1983.

53. Fomon SJ, et al. Body composition of reference children from birth to age 10 years. *Am J Clin Nutr* 35:1169, 1982.

54. Heird WC, Kashyap S, Gomez MR. Parenteral alimentation of the neonate. *Semin Perinatol* 15:493, 1991.

55. Warner BW, Ziegler MM. Management of the short bowel syndrome in the pediatric population. *Pediatr Clin North Am* 40(6):1335, 1993.

56. Wilmore DW. Factors correlating with successful outcome following extensive intestinal resection in newborn infants. *J Pediatr* 80:88, 1972.

57. Galea MH, Carachi R, Kapila C. Short bowel syndrome: A collective review. *J Pediatr Surg* 27:592, 1992.

58. Kurz R, Sauer H. Treatment and metabolic findings in extreme short bowel syndrome with 11 cm jejunal remnant. *J Pediatr Surg* 18:257, 1983.

59. Warner BW, Chaet MS. Nontransplant surgical options for management of the short bowel syndrome. *J Pediatr Gastroenterol Nutr* 17:1, 1993.

60. Ryder RW, Shelton JD, Guinan ME. Necrotizing enterocolitis: A prospective multicenter investigation. *Am J Epidemiol* 112:113, 1980.

61. Kleigman RM, et al. Epidemiological study of necrotizing enterocolitis among low-birth-weight infants. *J Pediatr* 100:440, 1982.

62. Bauer CR, et al. A decreased incidence of necrotizing enterocolitis after prenatal glucocorticoid therapy. *Pediatrics* 73:682, 1984.

63. Holliday MA, et al. The relation of metabolic rate to body weight and organ size. A review. *Pediatr Res* 1:185, 1967.

64. Benedict FG, Talbot FB. Metabolism of growth from birth to puberty, in Carnegie Institution of Washington, Publication 302. Washington, DC: Carnegie Institute, 1921, P 1–213.

65. Karlberg P. Determination of standard energy metabolism (basal metabolism) in normal infants. *Acta Paediatr Scand* 89(Suppl.):41, 1952.

66. Reichman BL, et al. Partition of energy metabolism and energy cost of growth in the very low-birth-weight infant. *Pediatrics* 69:446, 1982.

67. Hill JR. The development of thermal stability in the newborn baby. In JHP Jonxis, HKA Visses, JA Traelstra (eds), *The Adaption of the Newborn Extrauterine Life.* Leiden: Stenfert Kroese NV, 1964. P 223–228.

68. Anderson, TA. Birth through 24 months. In AM Rudolph (ed), *Pediatrics* (18th ed) Norwalk, CT: Appleton & Lange, 1987.

69. Garza C, Butte NF. Energy intakes of human milk-fed infants during the first year. *J Pediatr* 117:S124, 1990.

70. American Academy of Pediatrics, Committee on Nutrition: Nutritional needs of low-birth-weight infants. *Pediatrics* 75:976, 1985.

71. Cashore WJ, Sedaghatian MR, Usher RH. Nutritional supplements with intravenously administered lipid, protein hydrolysate and glucose in small premature infants. *Pediatrics* 56:88, 1975.

72. Coran AG. The long-term total intravenous feeding of infants using peripheral veins. *J Pediatr Surg* 8:801, 1973.

73. Zlotkin SH, Bryan MH, Anderson GH. Intravenous nitrogen and energy intakes required to duplicate in utero nitrogen accretion in prematurely born human infants. *J Pediatr* 99:115, 1981.

74. Anderson JM, Milner RDG, Stritch SJ. Effects of neonatal hypoglycemia on the nervous system: A pathological study. *J Neurol Neurosurg Psychiatry* 30:295, 1967.

75. Sann L. Neonatal hypoglycemia. *Biol Neonate* 58(Suppl. 1):16, 1990.

76. Finberg L. Dangers to infants caused by changes in osmolal concentrations. *Pediatrics* 40:1031, 1967.

77. Dweck HS, Cassady G. Glucose intolerance in infants of very low birth weight:I. Incidence of hyperglycemia in infants of birth weights 1,000 grams or less. *Pediatrics* 53:189, 1974.

78. Goldman SL, Hirata T. Attenuated response to insulin in very low birth weight infants. *Pediatr Res* 14:50, 1980.

79. Hamosh M. Lipid metabolism in premature infants. *Biol Neonate* 52(Suppl. 1):50, 1987.

80. Nose O, Tipton JR, Ament ME, et al. Effect of the energy source on changes in energy expenditure, respiratory quotient, and nitrogen balance during total parenteral nutrition in children. *Pediatr Res* 21:538, 1987.

81. Sauer P, Van Aerde J, Smith J, et al. Substrate utilization of newborn infants fed intravenously with or without a fat emulsion [Abstract]. *Pediatr Res* 18:804, 1984.

82. Van Aerde J, Sauer P, Smith J, et al. Contribution of glucose and fat to the energy expenditure of parenterally fed neonates [Abstract]. *Pediatr Res* 19:322A, 1985.

83. Leichty EA. Fat metabolism and requirements, In FA Polin, WW Fox (eds), *Fetal and Neonatal Physiology.* Philadelphia: Saunders, 1992.

84. Farrell PM, et al. Essential fatty acid deficiency in premature infants. *Am J Clin Nutr* 48:220, 1988.

85. Friedman Z, et al. Rapid onset of essential fatty acid deficiency in the newborn. *Pediatrics* 58:640, 1976.

86. Andrew G, Chan G, Schiff D. Lipid metabolism in the neonate: I. The effects of intralipid infusion on plasma trigylceride and free fatty acid concentrations in the neonate. *J Pediatr* 88:273, 1976.

87. Sherman AT, Bryan MH, Angel A. The effect of gestational age on intralipid tolerance in newborn infants. *J Pediatr* 91:134, 1977.

88. Dhanireddy R, et al. Postheparin lipolytic activity and intralipid clearance in very low birth weight infants. *J Pediatr* 98:617, 1981.

89. Rovamo L, et al. Postheparin plasma lipoprotein and hepatic lipase in preterm neonates. *Pediatr Res* 18:1104, 1984.

90. Spear ML, et al. Effect of heparin dose and infusion rate on lipid clearance and bilirubin binding in premature infants receiving intravenous fat emulsions. *J Pediatr* 112:94, 1988.

91. Starinsky R, Shafrir E. Displacement of albumin-bound bilirubin by free fatty acids: Implications for neonatal hyperbilirubinemia. *Clin Chim Acta* 29:311, 1970.

92. Thiessen H, Jacobsen J, Brodersen R. Displacement of albumin bound bilirubin in fatty acids. *Acta Paediatr Scand* 61:285, 1972.

93. Andrew G, Chan G, Schiff D. Lipid metabolism in the neonate: II. The effect of intralipid on bilirubin binding in vitro and in vivo. *J Pediatr* 88:279, 1976.

94. Rubaltelli FF, et al. Carnitine and the premature. *Biol Neonate* 52(Suppl. 1):65, 1987.

95. Penn D, et al. Effect of nutrition on tissue carnitine concentrations in infants of different gestational age. *Biol Neonate* 47:130, 1985.

96. Penn D, Schmidt-Sommerfeld E, Pascu F. Decreased tissue of carnitine levels in newborn infants receiving total parenteral nutrition. *J Pediatr* 98:976, 1981.

97. Schiff D, et al. Plasma carnitine levels during intravenous feeding of the neonate. *J Pediatr* 95:1043, 1979.

98. Schmidt-Sommerfeld E, Penn D, Wolf H. Carnitine deficiency in premature infants receiving total parenteral nutrition: Effect of L-carnitine supplementation. *J Pediatr* 102:931, 1983.

99. Helms RA, et al. Enchanced lipid utilization in infants receiving oral L-carnitine during long-term parenteral nutrition. *J Pediatr* 109:984, 1986.

100. Orzali A, et al. Effect of carnitine on lipid metabolism in the newborn: I. Carnitine supplementation during total parenteral nutrition in the first 48 hours of life. *Biol Neonate* 43:186, 1983.

101. Melegh B, et al. Feeding pre-term infants with L-carnitine supplemented formula. *Acta Paediatr Hung* 30:27, 1989.

102. Orzali A, et al. Effect of carnitine on lipid metabolism in the neonate: II. Carnitine addition to lipid infusion during prolonged total parenteral nutrition. *J Pediatr* 104:436, 1984.

103. Haumont D, et al. Plasma lipid and plasma lipoprotein concentrations in low birth weight infants given parenteral nutrition with 20% compared to 10% intralipid. *J Pediatr* 115:787, 1989.

104. Schreiner RL, et al. An evaluation of methods to monitor infants receiving intravenous lipids. *J Pediatr* 94:197, 1979.

105. American Academy of Pediatrics, Committee on Nutrition: Use of intravenous fat emulsions in pediatric patients. *Pediatrics* 68:738, 1981.

106. Pereira GR, et al. Decreased oxygenation and hyperlipanemia during intravenous fat infusions in premature infants. *Pediatrics* 66:26, 1980.

107. Hageman JR, et al. Intralipid alternations in pulmonary prostaglandin metabolism and gas exchange. *Crit Care Med* 11:794, 1983.

108. Puntis JWL, Rushton DI. Pulmonary intravascular lipid in neonatal necropsy specimens. *Arch Dis Child* 66:26, 1991.

109. Heird WC, Kashyap S. Protein and amino acid requirements. In RA Polin, WW Fox (eds), *Fetal and Neonatal Physiology.* Philadelphia: Saunders, 1992.

110. Kashyap S, et al. Growth, nutrient retention, and metabolic response in low birth weight infants fed varying intakes of protein and energy. *J Pediatr* 113:713, 1988.

111. Gross SJ. Growth and biochemical response of preterm infants fed human milk or modified infant formula. *N Engl J Med* 308:237, 1983.

112. Shenai JP, Reynolds JW, Babson SG. Nutritional balance studies in very-low-birth-weight infants: Enhanced nutrient retention rates by an experimental formula. *Pediatrics* 66:233, 1980.

113. Snyderman SE. The protein and amino acid requirements of the premature infant. In JHP Ionxix, HKA Vissy, D Troelstra (eds), *Metabolic Processes in the Foetus and Newborn Infant.* Leiden: Stenfert Kroese, 1971.

114. Laidlaw SA, Kopple JD. Newer concepts of the indispensable amino acids. *Am J Clin Nutr* 46:593, 1987.

115. Snyderman SE, et al. The histidine requirement of the infant. *Pediatrics* 31:786, 1963.

116. Pohlandt F. Cystine: A semi-essential amino acid in the newborn infant. *Acta Paediatr Scand* 63:801, 1974.

117. Zlotkin SH, Anderson GH. Sulfur balances in intravenously fed infants: Effects of cysteine supplementation. *Am J Clin Nutr* 36: 862, 1982.

118. Laine L, et al. Cysteine usage increases the need for acetate in neonates who receive total parenteral nutrition. *Am J Clin Nutr* 54:565, 1991.

119. Vinton NE, et al. Taurine concentrations in plasma, blood cells, and urine of children undergoing long-term total parenteral nutrition. *Pediatr Res* 21:399, 1987.

120. Jarvenpaa AL. Feeding the low-birth-weight infant: IV. Fat absorption as a function of diet and duodenal bile acids. *Pediatrics* 72:684, 1983.

121. Jarvenpaa AL, et al. Feeding the low-birth-weight infant: I. Taurine and cholesterol supplementation of formula does not affect growth metabolism. *Pediatrics* 71:171, 1983.

122. Jarvenpaa AL, et al. Preterm infants fed human milk attain intrauterine weight gain. *Acta Paediatr Scand* 72:239, 1983.

123. Jarvenpaa AL, et al. Feeding the low-birth-weight infant: III. Diet influences bile acid metabolism. *Pediatrics* 72:677, 1983.

124. Helms RA, et al. Comparison of pediatric versus standard amino acid formulation in pre-term neonates requiring parenteral nutrition. *J Pediatr* 110:466, 1987.

125. Coran AG, Drongowski RA. Studies on the toxicity and efficacy of a new amino acid solution in pediatric parenteral nutrition. *JPEN* 11:368, 1987.

126. Mitton SG, Garlick PJ. Changes in protein turnover after the introduction of parenteral nutrition in premature infants: Comparison of breast milk and egg protein-based amino acid solutions. *Pediatr Res* 32:447, 1992.

127. ASPEN Board of Directors: Guidelines for the use of parenteral and enteral nutrition in adult and pediatric patients. Section VII: Nutrition support for low-birth-weight infants. *JPEN* 17:335A, 1993.

128. Eggert LD, et al. Calcium and phosphorus compatibility in parenteral nutrition solutions for neonates. *Am J Hosp Pharm* 39:49, 1982.

129. Venkataraman PS, Brissie EO, Tsang RC. Stability of calcium and phosphorus in neonatal parenteral nutrition solutions. *J Pediatr Gastroenterol Nutr* 2:640, 1983.

130. Rose J, et al. Nutrient needs of the preterm infant. *Nutr Clin Proc* 8:226, 1993.

131. Tsang RC. Neonatal magnesium disturbances. *Am J Dis Child* 124:282, 1972.

132. American Medical Association Department of Foods and Nutrition: Multivitamin preparations for parenteral use: A statement by the Nutrition Advisory Group. *JPEN*

133. Greene HL, et al. Guidelines for the use of vitamins, trace elements, calcium, magnesium, and phosphorus in infants and children receiving total parenteral nutrition: Report of the Subcommittee on Pediatric Parenteral Nutrient Requirements from the Committee on Clinical Practice Issues of the American Society for Clinical Nutrition. *Am J Clin Nutr* 48:1324, 1988.

134. Greene HL. Water soluble vitamin. In E Lebenthal (ed), *Textbook of Gastroenterology and Nutrition in Infancy.* New York: Raven, 1981.

135. Olson JA, Gunning DB, Tilton RA. Liver concentrations of vitamin A and carotenoids as a function of age and other parameters of American children who died of various causes. *Am J Clin Nutr* 39:903, 1984.

136. Shenai JP, et al. Plasma vitamin A and retinol binding protein in premature and term neonates. *J Pediatr* 99:302, 1981.

137. Underwood BA. Vitamin A in animal and human nutrition. In MB Sprn, AB Roberts, DS Goodman (eds), *The Retinoids.* Orlando: Academic, 1984.

138. Hustead VA, et al. Relationship of vitamin A (retinol) status to lung disease in the preterm infant. *J Pediatr* 105:610, 1984.

139. Shenai JP, Chytil F, Stahlman MT. Vitamin A status of neonates with bronchopulmonary dysplasia. *Pediatr Res* 19:185, 1985.

140. Shenai JP, et al. Clinical trial of vitamin A supplementation in infants susceptable to bronchopulmonary dysplasia. *J Pediatr* 111:269, 1987.

141. Moran JR, Greene HL. Vitamin requirements. In RA Polin, WW Fox (eds), *Fetal and Neonatal Physiology.* Philadelphia: Saunders, 1992.

142. Specker BL, Tsang RC, Hollis BW. Effect of race and diet on human milk vitamin D and 25-hydroxyvitamin D. *Am J Dis Child* 139:1134, 1985.

143. Specker BL, et al. Sunshine exposure and serum 25-hydroxy-vitamin D concentrations in exclusively breast-fed infants. *J Pediatr* 107:372, 1985.

144. Williams ML, et al. Role of dietary iron and fat on vitamin E deficiency anemia of infancy. *N Engl J Med* 292:887, 1975.

145. Miller DP, Lloyd JK, Wolff OH. Vitamin E and neurologic function: Abetalipoproteinemia and other disorders of fat absorption. *CIBA Found Symp* 101:106, 1983.

146. Sokol RJ, et al. Vitamin E deficiency with normal serum vitamin E concentrations in children with chronic cholestasis. *N Engl J Med* 310:1209, 1984.

147. Oski FA, Barness LA. Vitamin E deficiency: A previously unrecognized cause of hemolytic anemia in the premature infant. *J Pediatr* 70:211, 1967.

148. Bove KE, et al. Vasculopathic hepatotoxicity associated with e-ferol syndrome in low-birth-weight infants. *JAMA* 254:2422, 1985.

149. Finer NN, et al. Vitamin E and necrotizing enterocolitis. *Pediatrics* 73:387, 1984.

150. Johnson L, et al. Relationship of prolonged pharmocologic serum levels of vitamin E to incidence of sepsis and necrotizing enterocolitis in infants with birth weight 1,500 grams or less. *Pediatrics* 75:619, 1985.

151. Meyer TC, Angus J. The effect of large doses of "Synkavit" in the newborn. *Arch Dis Child* 31:212, 1956.

152. Ingalls TH. Ascorbic acid requirements in early infancy. *N Engl J Med* 218:872, 1938.

153. Hovi L, Hekali R, Siimes MA. Evidence of riboflavin depletion in breast-fed newborns and its further acceleration during treatment of hyperbilirubinemia by phototherapy. *Acta Paediatr Scand* 68:567, 1979.

154. Mock DM, et al. Biotin deficiency: An unusual complication of parenteral alimentation. *N Engl J Med* 304:820, 1981.

155. Matoth Y, et al. Folate nutrition and growth in infancy. *Arch Dis Child* 54:271, 1979.

156. Strelling MK, Blackledge DG, Goodall HB. Diagnosis and management of folate deficiency in low-birth-weight infants. *Arch Dis Child* 54:271, 1979.

157. Dallman PR. Nutritional anemia of infancy: Iron, folic acid and vitamin B_{12}. In RC Tsang, BL Nichols, (eds), *Nutrition During Infancy.* Philadelphia: Henley & Belfus, 1988.

158. Meyers PA, Miller DR. Megaloblastic anemias. In DR Miller, RL Baehner, CW McMillan (eds), *Blood Diseases of Infancy and Childhood.* St. Louis Mosby, 1984.

159. Ruz M, Solomons N. Fecal zinc excretion during oral rehydration therapy for acute infectious diarrhea [Abstract]. *Fed Proc* 46:748, 1987.

160. Wolman SL, et al. Zinc in total parenteral nutrition: Requirements and metabolic effects. *Gastroenterology* 76:458, 1979.

161. Ziegler MM, et al. Route of pediatric parenteral nutrition: Proposed criteria revision. *J Pediatr Surg* 15:472, 1980.

162. Lally KP, et al. Broviac catheter insertion: Operating room or neonatal intensive care unit. *J Pediatr Surg* 22:823, 1987.

163. Hogan L, Pulito AR. Broviac central venous catheters inserted via the saphenous or femoral vein in the NICU under local anesthesia. *J Pediatr Surg* 27:1185, 1992.

164. Warner BW, et al. Multiple purpose central venous access in infants less than 1,000 grams. *J Pediatr Surg* 22:820, 1987.

165. Goutail-Flaud MF, et al. Central venous catheter-related complications in newborns and infants: A 587 case survey. *J Pediatr Surg* 26:645, 1991.

166. LaQuaglia MP, et al. A prospective analysis of vascular access device-related infections in children. *J Pediatr Surg* 27:840, 1992.

167. Weiner ES, et al. The CCSG prospective study of venous access devices: An analysis of insertions and causes for removal. *J Pediatr Surg* 27:155, 1992.

168. Warner BW, Ryckman FC. A simple technique to redirect malpositioned silastic central venous catheters. *JPEN* 16:473, 1992.

169. Linz DN, Bisset GN, Warner BW. Fracture and embolization of a peripherally-inserted central venous catheter. *JPEN* (in press).

170. Gauderer MW. Percutaneous endoscopic gastrostomy: A 10-year experience with 220 children. *J Pediatr Surg* 26:288, 1991.

171. Albanese CT, et al. Percutaneous gastrojejunostomy versus Nissen fundoplication for enteral feeding of the neurologically impaired child with gastroesophageal reflux. *J Pediatr* 123:371, 1993.

172. Chaet MS, Warner BW, Sheldon CA. Management of multiple jejuno-ileal atresias with an intraluminal silastic stent. *J Pediatr Surg* 29(12):1604, 1994.

173. Mollit DL, Golladay S, Seibert JJ. Symptomatic gastroesophageal reflux following gastrostomy in neurologically impaired patients. *Pediatrics* 75:1124, 1985.

174. Jolley SG, Smith EI, Tunell WP. Protective antireflux operation with feeding gastrostomy: Experience with children. *Ann Surg* 201:736, 1985.

175. Quigley EMM, et al. Hepatobiliary complications of total parenteral nutrition. *Gastroenterology* 104:286, 1993.

176. Postuma R, Trevenen CL. Liver disease in infants receiving total parenteral nutrition. *Pediatrics* 63:110, 1979.

177. Bell RL, et al. Total parenteral nutrition-related cholestasis in infants. *JPEN* 10:356, 1986.

178. Whitington PF. Cholestasis associated with total parenteral nutrition in infants. *Hepatology* 5:693, 1985.

179. Pereira GR, et al. Hyperalimentation-induced cholestasis: Increased incidence and severity in premature infants. *Am J Dis Child* 135:842, 1981.

180. Vileisis RA, Inwood RJ, Hunt CE. Prospective controlled study of parenteral nutrition-associated cholestatic jaundice: Effect of protein intake. *J Pediatr* 96:893, 1980.

181. Belli DC, et al. Total parenteral nutrition-associated cholestasis in rats: Comparison of different amino acid mixtures. *JPEN* 11:67, 1987.

182. Belli DC, et al. The effect of taurine on the cholestatic potential of sulfated lithocholate and its conjugates. *Liver* 11:162, 1991.

183. Okamoto E, et al. Role of taurine in feeding the low birth-weight infant. *J Pediatr* 104:936, 1984.

184. Cooke RJ, Whitington PF, Kelts D. Effect of taurine supplementation on hepatic function during short-term parenteral nutrition in the premature infant. *J Pediatr Gastroenterol Nutr* 3:234, 1984.

185. Palmer RH, Hruban Z. Production of bile acid duct hyperplasia and gallstones by lithocholic acid. *J Clin Invest* 45:1255, 1964.

186. Kakis G, Yousef IM. Mechanism of cholic acid protection in lithocholate-induced intrahepatic cholestasis in rats. *Gastroenterology* 78:1402, 1980.

187. Palmer RH. Bile acids, liver injury and liver disease. *Arch Intern Med* 130:606, 1972.

188. Kubota A, et al. The effect of metronidazole on TPN-associated liver dysfunction in neonates. *J Pediatr Surg* 25:618, 1990.

189. Spurr SG, Grylack LJ, Mehta NR. Hyperalimentation-associated neonatal cholestasis: Effect of oral gentamicin. *JPEN* 13:633, 1989.

190. Utili R, Abernathy CO, Zimmerman HJ. Cholestatic effects of *Escherichia coli* endotoxin on the isolated perfused rat liver. *Gastroenterology* 70:248, 1976.

191. Merritt RJ, et al. Cholestatic effect of intraperitoneal administration of tryptophan to suckling rat pups. *Pediatr Res* 18:904, 1984.

192. Klein GL, et al. Hepatic abnormalities associated with aluminum loading in piglets. *JPEN* 11:293, 1987.

193. Farrell MK, Balistreri WF. Parenteral nutrition and hepatobiliary dysfunction. *Clin Perinatol* 13:197, 1986.

194. Warner BW, et al. The value of hepatobiliary scans in fasted patients receiving total parenteral nutrition. *Surgery* 102:595, 1987.

195. Benjamin DR. Hepatobiliary dysfunction in infants and children associated with long-term total parenteral nutrition: A clinicopathologic study. *Am J Clin Pathol* 76:276, 1981.

196. Grant D, et al. Experimental clinical intestinal transplantation: Initial experience of a Canadian center. *Transplant Proc* 22:2497, 1990.

197. Williams JW, et al. Splanchnic transplantation: An approach to the infant dependent on parenteral nutrition who develops irreversible liver disease. *JAMA* 261:1458, 1989.

Selected Readings

Henning SJ. Functional development of the gastrointestinal tract. In LR Johnson (ed), *Physiology of the Gastrointestinal Tract* (2nd ed). New York: Raven, 1987.

An excellent review of gastrointestinal tract development by one of the noted authorities in this field.

Lebenthal E, Lee PC, Heitlinger LA. Impact of development of the gastrointestinal tract on infant feeding. *J Pediatr* 102:1, 1983.

Presents a nice discussion of developmental aspects of the gastrointestinal tract as it relates to nutritional support.

Quigley EMM, et al. Hepatobiliary complications of total parenteral nutrition. *Gastroenterology* 104:286, 1993.

A concise and up-to-date review of TPN-cholestasis in infants. This also presents a nice discussion of TPN-liver dysfunction in adults and contrasts the differences between the two age groups.

Reichman BL, et al. Partition of energy metabolism and energy cost of growth in the very low-birth-weight infant. *Pediatrics* 69:446, 1982.

A classic reference that presents a breakdown of the energy needs of the growing infant.

Warner BW, Chaet MS. Nontransplant surgical options for management of the short bowel syndrome. *J Pediatr Gastroenterol Nutr* 17:1, 1993.

A review of all known surgical options for management of the short-bowel syndrome.

V

Specific Modes of Therapy

28

Parenteral Nutrition

Michael S. Nussbaum
Scott M. Berry

A problem that has challenged physicians throughout the history of medicine has been the inability to provide adequate calories to malnourished or catabolic patients when the intestinal route was nonfunctional or inaccessible. [*Editor's Note:* In actuality, throughout most of recent history, physicians were adding to catabolism by bleeding, purging, leeching, and "starving a fever."]

Since 1968, the provision of intravenous nutrition has developed from a rare and complicated clinical intervention into a routine and safe therapy that is commonplace in almost all clinical settings. The technology on which parenteral nutrition is based can be traced back over 300 years to animal experiments performed by Sir Christopher Wren. In 1656 Wren successfully administered intravenous wine, opium, and other substances to dogs. This was over 150 years before Blundell reported the first successful attempts at intravenous therapy in humans (blood transfusions) in 1818. Subsequently, in 1831 Latta successfully treated cholera patients with intravenous infusion of saline. In 1843 Claude Bernard safely infused a variety of nutrients including sugar solutions, egg whites, and milk into animals.

Over the course of the next 50 years, multiple reports detailed successful subcutaneous, intravenous, and rectal administration in animals and humans of a variety of nutrients including fat, milk, glucose, whole protein, and protein hydrolysates [1]. What followed was the development of combination solutions containing dextrose and protein components, which, when administered in adequate amounts, were capable of maintaining normal nutrition in dogs. Such treatments were made possible by placing cannulas directly into the superior vena cava in these dogs [2]. However, the large volume and high concentrations of solution required to provide the needed calories limited the clinical applicability of these treatments. With the introduction of safe and effective diuretics, Rhoads was able to provide enough calories to achieve a positive nitrogen balance by infusing at least 5 liters of solution per day as 10% dextrose and hydrolyzed proteins [3]. Unfortunately, the response to diuretics was not always predictable, leading to complications of acute volume overload and pulmonary edema in some patients. The concentration of solution that could be infused via peripheral veins was limited due to the high incidence of phlebitis and thrombosis of peripheral veins with infusion of hypertonic dextrose solutions. In 1968, Dudrick adapted the technique of subclavian venipuncture, first described in 1952 by Aubaniac [4], and demonstrated that hypertonic dextrose and amino acid solutions could be safely administered to humans via this route with minimal complications [5]. This breakthrough marked the beginning of the modern era of parenteral nutrition therapy through which total caloric needs could be safely provided for a prolonged time via a central venous catheter in a reasonable volume of solution.

The multiple recent advances in overall nutritional management of patients who cannot eat for prolonged periods of time have improved the clinician's ability to successfully provide essential nutrients for patients who otherwise might have died. An understanding of the nutritional and metabolic derangements and requirements have played a central role in the care of these patients. The hypermetabolic response to major illness or injury is a generalized response initiated by a variety of stimuli such as shock, severe inflammation, and the extensive tissue injury associated with major burns and traumatic injury. Regardless of the underlying nutritional status of the patient before the illness or injury, this marked hypercatabolic response can rapidly lead to severe wasting of lean body mass, impairment of vital organ function, and a delayed or diminished response to inflammatory and infectious processes. Therefore, it is clear that in nutritionally depleted and critically ill patients some nutritional intervention will be required. Such intervention is necessary to maintain and support these individuals' metabolic needs during their illnesses and recoveries until they are able to meet these needs on their own.

Early during acute illnesses, individuals often have a multitude of complex physical and physiologic derangements that take precedence over their metabolic needs. Emergent operative intervention and stabilization of the patient's ventilatory, hemodynamic, acid-base, and fluid-electrolyte status remain the priorities of initial management. Nutritional intervention should be considered only once these factors have been optimized and adequate cardiopulmonary function and tissue oxygenation have been restored, thus allowing for optimal delivery and utilization of the supplemental nutrients. Generally, these derangements can be addressed rapidly, and the prompt initiation of nutrition support, when indicated, is almost always possible within the first 24 to 48 hours.

Nutrition support by the total parenteral route (TPN) has been the traditional mainstay of nutritional therapy for postoperative, critically ill, or injured patients who could not eat. Clearly, parenteral nutrition is required in patients whose gastrointestinal tracts are nonfunctional or in whom bowel rest is desired. However, the early institution of enteral nutrition is generally safe, effective, and appears to improve the overall outcome in this population of patients. Although still controversial, there appears to be a significantly lower incidence of septic morbidity in patients fed enterally after severe injury [6]. Enteral nutrition is considerably less expensive than parenteral and may also prevent atrophy of the gastrointestinal villi. Mucosal atrophy of the gastrointestinal tract is theoretically linked to a loss of the barrier function of the intact intestinal mucosa, a concept that has yet to be demonstrated in humans in clinical circumstances. [*Editor's Note:* As stated elsewhere, it may be that a small amount of translocation of bacteria or their products is not only normal but desirable from an immunologic surveillance advantage. Some evidence supporting this view is the increased translocation observed after furnishing of glutamine, presumably an energy source [7]. Massive translocation and breakdown of the intestinal barrier, if it occurs, is injurious.]

Although gastric and colonic motility is often impaired during critical illness and in the early postoperative period, small intestinal motility and absorption is usually intact. Small-bore nasoenteric feeding tubes can usually be placed in a fluoroscopy suite or at the bedside to take advantage of this fact. Nevertheless, due to complications that limit the amount of nutrients that can be delivered, it is often difficult to adequately meet the metabolic needs of some patients via the gastrointestinal tract. Mechanical problems with the delivery system, gastrointestinal dysfunction, interruptions of feeding in preparation for operative procedures and diagnostic tests, and metabolic complications may limit the effectiveness of enteral therapy [8,9]. Therefore, concomitant parenteral nutrition is frequently required if the patient is intolerant of enteral nutrition or until enteral feedings can be advanced to meet the individual's needs [10,11]. The advantages of enteral feeding may be unrelated to total nutrient intake, and any amount of enteral feeding may be better than no enteral feeding at all, even when TPN provides the majority of caloric intake [12]. The exact amount of enteral feeding that may exert a beneficial effect is not known, but it may be as little as 10% to 20% of total caloric needs.

The effective and appropriate delivery of parenteral nutrition requires a detailed understanding of the techniques for accurately determining the metabolic requirements of the patient, the specific components utilized in the formulations, and the indications for the initiation of nutrition support. Specific disease states and organ dysfunction often demand that the nutritional formulation be tailored to meet specific needs and restrictions. Safe and effective techniques for gaining access to the central venous system and maintaining sterility for that access in a nosocomially hostile environment are essential in all cases in which central parenteral nutrition is indicated. Finally, understanding the potential mechanical and metabolic complications associated with TPN is important to avoid or promptly recognize these potentially serious morbidities.

Determination of Energy Requirements

The goal of parenteral nutrition support in the acute setting should be weight maintenance rather than weight gain throughout the course of illness. This approach generally avoids complications of overfeeding while assuring optimal nutrient metabolism. These patients demand very careful assessments of their caloric and nutrient needs, often requiring specific tailoring of the rate of delivery and formulation of the parenteral solutions. Basal energy requirements (BEE) can be initially estimated using the Harris-Benedict equations, which are based on the patient's age, sex, height, and weight (Table 28-1) [13]. Additional adjustments for stress and activity are made by multiplying the basal values by Long's activity and stress factors, which generally range from 1.2 to 2.1 (see Table 28-1) [14]. Another method for estimating energy requirements is based on providing 30 to 35 kcal/kg/day. These rules of thumb can be used to identify approximate needs when initiating nutrition support and are quite accurate in uncomplicated situations. However, these methods are often inaccurate in complicated critical illness [15]. The formulas commonly underestimate the energy needs of mechanically ventilated surgical [16], injured [17], or chronic obstructive pulmonary disease (COPD) patients [18], whereas the activity factors often overestimate the caloric requirements in other mechanically ventilated, sedated patients [15]. In addition to the problems of underfeeding such catabolic patients, a major advance in recent years has been the recognition of excessive feeding as a complication that manifests its most severe effects in critically ill patients. Therefore, although these formulas and stress factors are sufficient for assessing the uncomplicated nonintensive care unit (ICU) patient and for initiating nutrition support in the critically ill, they only accurately predict an

Table 28-1. Formulas for Estimating Energy Expenditure

Harris-Benedict Equation[a]

Males: BEE (kcal) = 66.5 + [13.8 × weight (kg)] + [5 × height (cm)] − [6.8 × age(yr)]

Females: BEE (kcal) = 655.1 + [9.6 × weight (kg)] + [1.8 × height (cm)] − [4.7 × age(yr)]

Activity and Stress Factors[b]

Total estimation of energy requirements = BEE × activity factor × stress factor

Activity factor:	Confined to bed = 1.2	Out of bed = 1.3
Stress factor:	Minor operation = 1.2	Skeletal trauma = 1.35
	Major sepsis = 1.6	Major thermal injury = 2.1

Calculation of Metabolic Rate (in patients with thermodilution pulmonary artery catheter)

Metabolic Rate (kcal/hr) = VO_2 (ml/min) × 60 min/hr × 1 L/1000 ml × 4.83 kcal/L

VO_2 (ml/min) = Cardiac Output (L/min) × [Arterial Oxygen Content (CaO_2, ml/L) − Mixed Venous Oxygen Content ($CmvO_2$, ml/L)] utilizing canopy measurements

[a]Source: Modified from JA Harris, FG Benedict. Biometric studies of basal metabolism in man. Carnegie Institute of Washington, Publication #279, 1979.

[b]Source: Modified from Long CL, et al. Metabolic response to injury and illness: Estimation of energy and protein needs from indirect calorimetry and nitrogen balance. *JPEN* 3:452, 1979.

individual's needs about one-third of the time in the ICU setting.

The majority of complex and/or critically ill patients who require nutrition support will benefit from assessment by indirect calorimetry. Actual measurement of the patient's oxygen consumption and carbon dioxide production utilizing an automated metabolic cart is useful in determining energy expenditure in the resting, fed patient. This allows for an accurate prediction of the patient's actual resting energy expenditure (REE) and respiratory quotient (RQ) during the period of measurement (Figure 28-1) [19]. Such measurements are most accurate and reproducible in patients who are endotracheally intubated. However, carefully conducted measurements can be performed in a cooperative normally breathing (nonintubated) patient. For many years these devices were subject to large errors that limited their clinical use, but recent improvements in equipment and technique have led to much wider applicability, particularly in the critical care setting [20,21]. In general, candidates for indirect calorimetric measurement include patients with multiple risk and stress factors that may considerably skew Harris-Benedict results and patients who fail to respond adequately to estimated nutritional needs.

More specifically, the metabolic cart measurement should include but is not restricted to a variety of patient populations. Patients who benefit from indirect calorimetry are those with multiple nutritional risk and stress factors or in whom the disease state affects energy and nutrient requirements, making the Harris-Benedict or other energy equations less accurate. These include patients with neurologic trauma or major neurologic disease, amputations, paralysis, cancer with residual tumor burden, acute pancreatitis, COPD, and multiple trauma. Other clinical situations in which REE measurement is likely to improve the accurate determination of energy requirements include patients in whom height and weight cannot be accurately obtained; patients who fail to respond sufficiently to provision of estimated nutritional needs; all ICU patients who remain in critical care units for 5 days or longer; serial measurements for severely hypermetabolic or hypercatabolic patients; all liver transplant patients and other transplant patients as deemed necessary; and morbidly obese patients. Although usually accurate, there are certain clinical scenarios in which metabolic cart analysis will not reflect the patient's true needs. These include patients on high frequency ventilation; patients in whom canopy measurements are inappropriate (for example, claustrophobics); canopy-measured patients who are at significant risk of nosocomial infection (for example, neutropenia, AIDS, reverse isolation); patients with chest tubes and a significant air leak; patients with incompetent tracheal cuffs; patients in whom the FiO_2 is greater than 60% when open circuit measurement systems are utilized; and patients in whom dialysis is in progress (defer measurement until postdialysis) [22].

Metabolic carts have become more commonplace in most medical centers and large ICUs where many complex patients are cared for. In addition, newer methods are on the horizon for the continuous measurement of oxygen consumption by replenishment techniques or by mass spectrophotometer [20,21,23–25]. These will allow more accurate determination of the patient's continuous energy expenditure as opposed to the "snapshot" that the current technology affords us. These advanced technologies are not available in all settings. Another method for determining the REE is to calculate the metabolic rate from measurements of oxygen consumption (VO_2). This requires the placement of a thermodilution pulmonary artery catheter which many critically ill patients already have in place for hemodynamic monitoring (see Table 28-1).

Substrate Requirements

Carbohydrate

Once a patient's energy requirements have been determined, it is important to provide these calories in a substrate formulation that can be utilized most efficiently. Glucose is the primary source of calories; however, the optimal dietary intake of carbohydrate is not known. The maximum rate of glucose oxidation is approximately 5 mg/kg/min (7.2 g/kg/day) [26]. A portion of this glucose will be provided by ongoing gluconeogenesis. In the unstressed patient, gluconeogenesis is inversely related to plasma insulin concentration and is responsive to glucose administration. In contrast, in the critically ill or septic patient, gluconeogenesis is much higher than normal and is related to an increased anaerobic use of glucose in healing and inflammatory tissue. This leads to increased lactate production, which is transported to the liver and recycled back to glucose. Normally, gluconeogenesis decreases with increasing glucose intake, but in the critically ill patient, it is only completely suppressed at intakes of greater than 600 g/day [27]. Gluconeogenesis is stimulated primarily by glucagon, and, therefore, the suppressive effect of glucose administration is diminished in catabolic and septic patients. To an extent, this effect may

UNIVERSITY OF CINCINNATI MEDICAL CENTER
NUTRITION SUPPORT DIAGNOSTICS
INDIRECT CALORIMETRIC MEASUREMENT

Brief Diagnosis/Indication:

Nutrition Therapy During Testing: [ ] TPN Formula_____[ ] Lipids___ Rate____
[ ] IVF____________________ Rate_______
[ ] TF Formula______________ Rate_______
[ ] PO Diet__________________________

Activity Profile: Bed Rest_________
Ambulatory_________ **PT**____________
Other__________**Temperature**_________
Medications______________________
Canopy_____**Mask**______**Ventilator**____
Settings: FIO$_2$_____**V$_E$**_____**Freq**______
V$_T$_________**FECO$_2$**_______**PaCO$_2$**__________

MEASUREMENT RESULTS

$\dot{V}CO_2$__________mL/min
$\dot{V}O_2$__________mL/min
RQ__________
REE__________

	Estimated Energy Expenditure	Measured Energy Expenditure	Current Total qd Intake
5000 –			
4000 –			
3000 –			
2000 –			
1000 –			

Special considerations:______________________________
Interpretation:______________________________
____
Recommendations:______________________________
____

Date:___/___/___

Time:__________

____
Operator

____
Nutrition Support Attending

	Transaction Code:		Description:
	NSSR	CART	12934
	RESP	CART	02934

White - Medical Record **Yellow** - MD **Pink** - Billing **Goldenrod** - Department

Figure 28-1. Form used for reporting of indirect calorimetric measurement and assessment at the University of Cincinnati Medical Center. (From the Department of Parenteral and Enteral Nutrition, University of Cincinnati Medical Center. Reproduced with permission.)

be overcome by the administration of insulin with nearly normal glucose uptake by all tissues except in the presence of sepsis [28]. With ongoing sepsis, maximal glucose uptake is only approximately 50% of normal, even with insulin administration. In addition to stimulating peripheral glucose uptake, the rate of protein breakdown and lipolysis is suppressed by insulin administration, even in the presence of critical illness or sepsis [29]. Therefore, a reasonable starting point would be to provide approximately 5 g (20 kcal) of glucose/kg/day. Glucose has a known protein-sparing effect [30,31]; however, critically ill patients often tolerate large glucose loads poorly due to the insulin resistance described above, with concomitant glucose intolerance, excess carbon dioxide production, and hepatic dysfunction [32,33].

Fat

The polyunsaturated fatty acids linoleic and linolenic are essential for growth and maintenance of health. These fatty acids are important precursors in the synthetic pathways of prostaglandins and leukotrienes. Many intravenous fat emulsion solutions were tried in experimental and clinical situations between the 1920s and 1960s. Most caused serious adverse reactions including nausea, vomiting, back pain, and fever. Many explanations were offered, the most commonly accepted being that lipid particles given parenterally did not possess a protein coat comparable to that of natural chylomicrons [34]. However, this theory was disproved by Harvel [35] and Carlsson [36], who independently demonstrated that the parenterally infused lipids of an artificial intravenous emulsion receive apoproteins from existing lipoproteins circulating in plasma. Furthermore, the metabolism of parenteral lipid is indistinguishable from enterally absorbed fats and occurs via hydrolysis by lipoprotein lipase with apoprotein transfer to form chylomicrons.

The probable cause of this lipid reaction was not uncovered until the 1960s. Before that time, studies of lipid infusions done in a canine laboratory model showed that an infusion rate of 3 g/kg/day was well tolerated. This lipid infusion rate was well below toxic levels for dogs because of their high metabolic rates. However, when human studies at similar infusion rates were performed, lipid toxicity occurred. When corrections for metabolic rate were made and upper limits of lipid infusion for humans were established, it became clear that lipids could be provided parenterally without serious sequelae. Lipid preparations could then be compared based on their composition.

An additional factor that may have contributed to the toxicity observed with early lipid preparations was the emulsifying agent used in the preparation process. Certain emulsifiers, which were previously thought inert, were shown to have severe toxic effects. Modern preparations have eliminated these types of emulsifiers and their subsequent severe side effects, thus making routine lipid infusions safe. Long-chain fatty acids have been the mainstay of parenteral lipid provision, with most parenteral lipid emulsions being made from soybean or safflower oil. These emulsions consist of fat in the form of long-chain triglycerides (LCT): three fatty acids containing 16 to 18 carbons attached to a glycerol backbone (Figure 28-2). The fatty acids contained in these emulsions

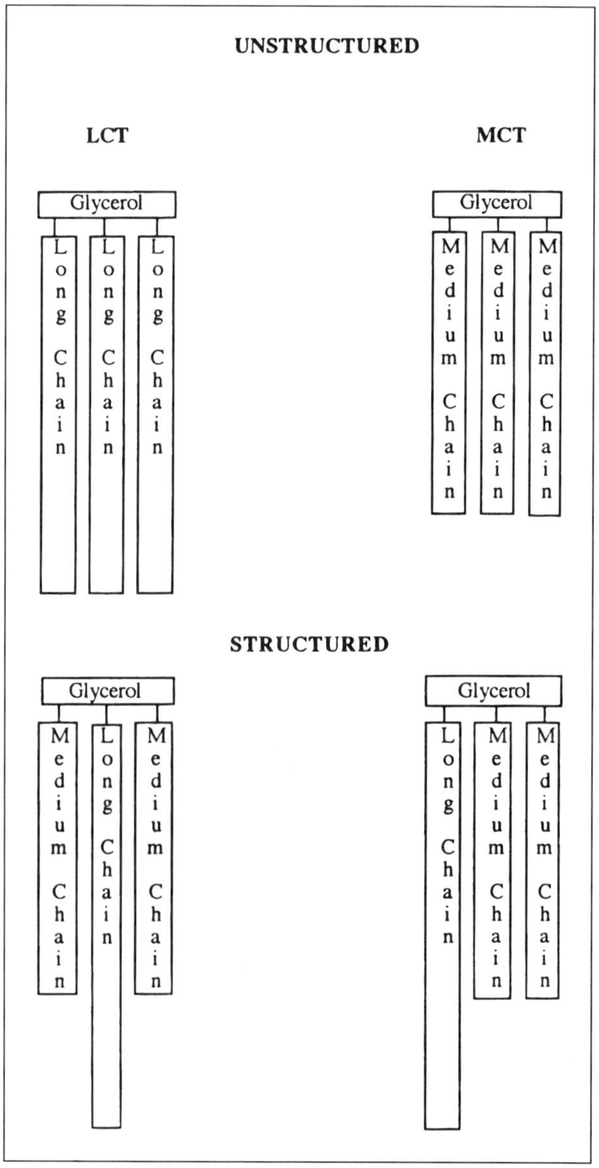

Figure 28-2. Unstructured and structured triglycerides.

are usually linoleic (18 : 2 ω-6), oleic (18 : 1 ω-9), palmitic (16 : 0), α-linolenic (18 : 3 ω-3), and stearic (18 : 0) (Figure 28-3). They represent a highly concentrated energy source and prevent essential fatty acid deficiency when provided as 2% to 6% of total calories. However, during stress long-chain fatty acids are oxidized less well [37] and are associated with reticuloendothelial system blockage and immunosuppression during parenteral administration [38–40]. The use of tailor-made lipid molecules of varying lengths may obviate this immunosuppression while providing a well-tolerated alternate fuel source [41].

The essential fatty acid requirements in TPN patients can be met by the infusion of 500 ml of a 10% lipid emulsion made from soybean or safflower oil two to three times per week. In addition to replacing essential fatty acids, lipid emulsions may be used to supply a portion of the nonprotein calories on a daily basis, as lipid can be oxidized as an energy substrate by most tissues. In the catabolic, critically ill patient, glucose may be a poorly tolerated energy source, while fat is a particularly valuable energy source as the rate of oxidation of exogenous lipids is increased in stress and sepsis. This increased fat oxidation is accompanied by increases in fat mobilization and turnover [42]. Triglyceride hydrolysis is increased to a much greater extent than fat oxidation, thus accounting for a net increase in lipolysis in the face of injury, sepsis, or burns. In contrast, ketone synthesis is decreased with severe illness or injury [27]. Despite the increased utilization of fat, the provision of fat calories does not decrease gluconeogenesis as significantly as in the normal individual.

Protein

The normal requirement for protein is 0.8 g/kg/day (60–70 g protein/day) and between 1.2 to 2.2 g/kg/day for infants. Protein requirements are increased in severe illness to 1.5 to 2.0 g/kg/day, levels comparable to the requirements of rapidly growing infants and children. During stress both protein catabolism and protein synthesis are increased. However, there is an imbalance of protein breakdown relative to synthesis, resulting in a rapid decrease in lean body mass and overall nitrogen loss [43]. It has been hypothesized that there is a plasma factor that is capable of inducing muscle proteolysis in the face of trauma and sepsis [44].

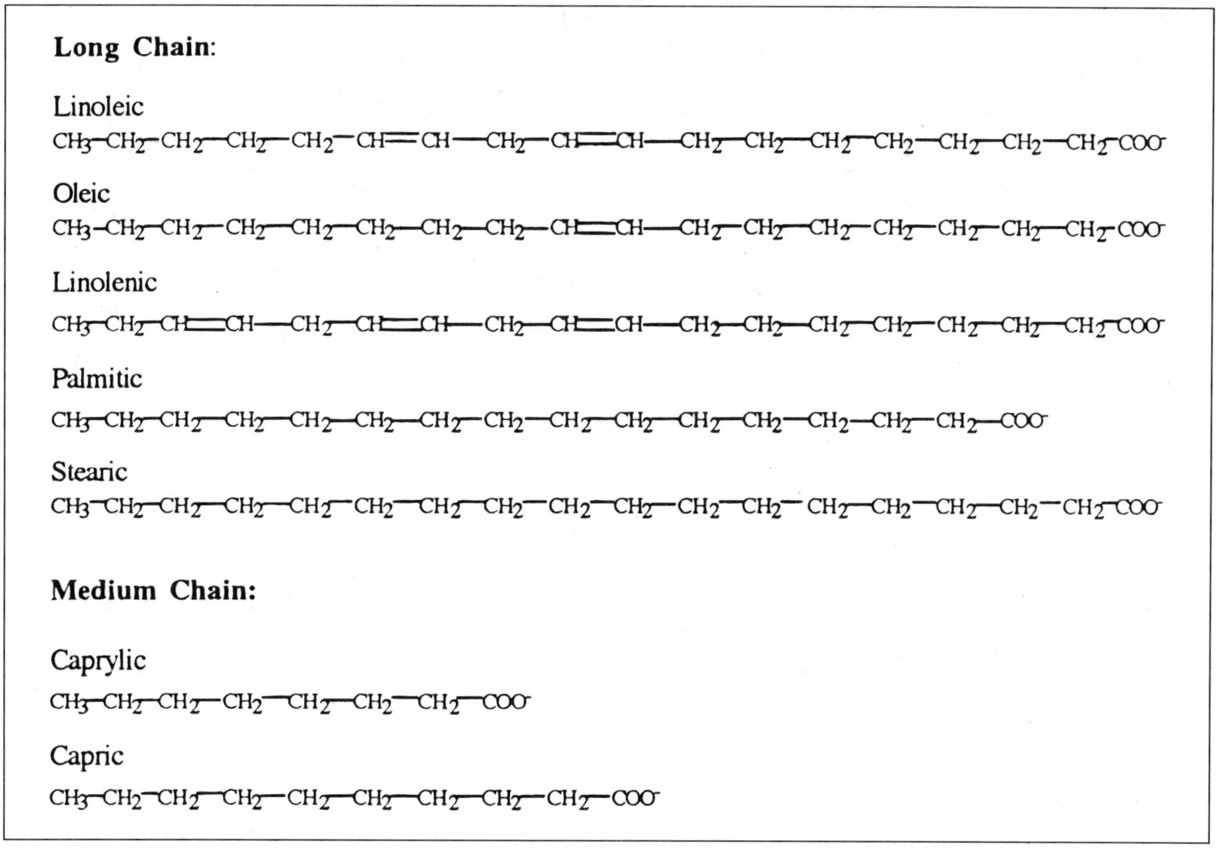

Figure 28-3. Chemical structure of long- and medium-chain fatty acids.

Amino acids mobilized from skeletal muscle, connective tissue, and unstimulated intestine are used to support wound healing, inflammation, acute phase response, and gluconeogenesis. Ideally, one would prefer to provide these substrates via TPN, however, it is not certain whether these changes in protein metabolism are influenced by the specific admixture of TPN provided.

Because part of the response to injury includes increased lipolysis and decreased glucose oxidation, TPN with a mixture of glucose, lipid, and nitrogen would be expected to reduce lipolysis and increase glucose oxidation. Furthermore, such feeding would be expected to increase protein synthesis yet many patients remain in a state of net protein catabolism [45]. While nitrogen balance can be improved, tissue catabolism may not be reversed [46]. Thus, as the degree of illness increases, or when sepsis supervenes, the achievement of net protein synthesis becomes increasingly difficult and may not be attainable. The specific types of fuel sources used in parenterally feeding such patients does not appreciably alter these protein dynamics [32,47–50].

In the hypermetabolic or septic patient, carbohydrate should constitute 60% to 70% of nonprotein calories to avoid the complications of excess glucose infusion [32,33]. In the face of a limited capacity to oxidize glucose, fat should be provided not only to prevent essential fatty acid deficiency (2% to 5% of total calories 1 to 2 times weekly) but as a substantial portion of the nonprotein calories. As a general rule, lipid should be provided on a daily basis and should constitute 25% to 30% of the calories in the hypermetabolic patient. The maximum rate of lipid infusion is 1 g/kg/day to avoid complications of excess lipid infusion. While protein catabolism is unresponsive to protein, glucose, or lipid administration, protein synthesis is responsive to amino acid infusion, and nitrogen balance can be attained through support of protein synthesis [51–53]. Nitrogen balance is an endpoint in the metabolic support of patients. Conventional TPN formulas have a nonprotein calorie-nitrogen ratio of 150 : 1. The stressed, hypermetabolic patient with increased protein requirements and decreased calorie needs requires a calorie-nitrogen ratio that is less (80 to 100 : 1) than that found in standard formulations. Administration of conventional TPN in this setting will result in excessive calorie infusion and insufficient protein delivery. To determine if an adequate quantity and composition of protein is being provided, nitrogen balance should be calculated and followed at least weekly and whenever it appears that the patient is not responding to the current parenteral regimen. In addition, the determination of short turnover proteins including transferrin, retinol binding protein, and thyroxine binding prealbumin will give some indication as to the adequacy of protein and calories provided.

Alternate Parenteral Components

Arginine

Dietary protein content, route of delivery, and composition have all been shown to affect protein utilization. In addition, certain amino acids seem to have functions in addition to serving as substrates for protein synthesis. Arginine is a semi-essential amino acid necessary for growth and for the response to hypermetabolic and septic states [54]. Nitrogen derived from arginine is not only used for protein synthesis but also in the biosynthesis of creatinine, polyamines, and urea. Not only does it support protein synthesis necessary for healing but also promotes T-cell mitogenesis and decreases T-cell dysfunction associated with the post-injury state.

In addition to immunomodulatory effects, arginine has also demonstrated nutritional benefit beyond that of serving as a synthetic substrate. Arginine-enriched parenteral solutions used in tumor-bearing laboratory animals have demonstrated selective host nitrogen balance and body cell mass gain without increased tumor growth [55]. The exact mechanism for this is unclear, but it has been hypothesized that arginine-induced branched-chain amino acid (BCAA) utilization by host tissues may be responsible for this effect.

Arginine has also been shown to inhibit tumor induction, growth, and metastatic spread [56]. These effects may be the result of enhanced tumor surveillance and macrophage phagocytic function. However, T-cell blastogenesis and increased IL-2 production are also noted with parenteral arginine supplementation, and these responses may contribute to the observed effect.

Glutamine

Glutamine is the most abundant circulating and intracellular free amino acid [57]. It serves as a precursor for synthesis of amino acids and proteins. In all dividing cells, it donates nitrogen atoms for the synthesis of purines, pyrimidines, and ultimately deoxyribonucleic and ribonucleic acids [58]. Glutamine is the most important precursor for ammoniagenesis in the kidney and ammonia trapping in the perivenous hepatocytes.

In addition to multiple intracellular functions, glutamine also plays an important role in intertissue physiology. Skeletal muscle, which contains more than half of the free amino acid pool, comprises 60% glutamine [59]. Glutamine is a precursor and nitrogen donor for many intracellular biosynthetic reactions and serves as a transport vehicle for nitrogen and carbon atoms between body tissues [60]. In septic states, skeletal muscle glutamine is mobilized and used for substrate by the liver, kidney, lung, and intestine. Animal studies indicate that glutamine may also play a regulatory role in protein homeostasis. It has been shown to both stimulate protein synthesis [61,62] and inhibit protein degradation [63,64]. In the liver, glutamine stimulates glycogen synthesis [65] and, in rapidly dividing cells such as intestinal mucosa and lymphocytes, glutamine serves as a primary oxidative fuel [66].

The two principal enzymes involved in glutamine metabolism are glutamine synthetase, which catalyzes the synthesis of glutamine from glutamate and ammonia, and glutaminase, which deamidates glutamine resulting in glutamate and ammonia (Figure 28-4) [67]. The gastrointestinal tract is the principal organ of glutamine utilization [68], where it is a key mucosal substrate essential for intestinal structure and function [69]. Glutamine oxidation provides the major energy source for the intestinal mucosa and processes nitrogen and carbon into precursors for hepatic ureagenesis and gluconeogenesis. The entire gastrointestinal tract extracts approximately 20% of circulating glutamine in the postabsorptive state [70], and more than 90% of this extraction is by the enterocytes. Transport from the intestinal lumen and basal membrane is via the system N, sodium-dependent transporter. This high-affinity system is inducible by enteral glutamine but can be inhibited by histidine [71]. Despite avid uptake, the intracellular concentration of glutamine is low. This is because of high affinity glutaminase present within the mitochondria of enterocytes, which rapidly breaks down glutamine [72]. The enterocyte either uses glutamine for fuel substrate via the Kreb's cycle and releases ammonia into the portal venous system or metabolizes glutamine via pyrroline-5-carboxylate and releases proline, ornithine, or citrulline into the portal venous system (Figure 28-5) [73].

In the liver, the periportal hepatocytes, replete with glutaminase, metabolize glutamine to gluta-

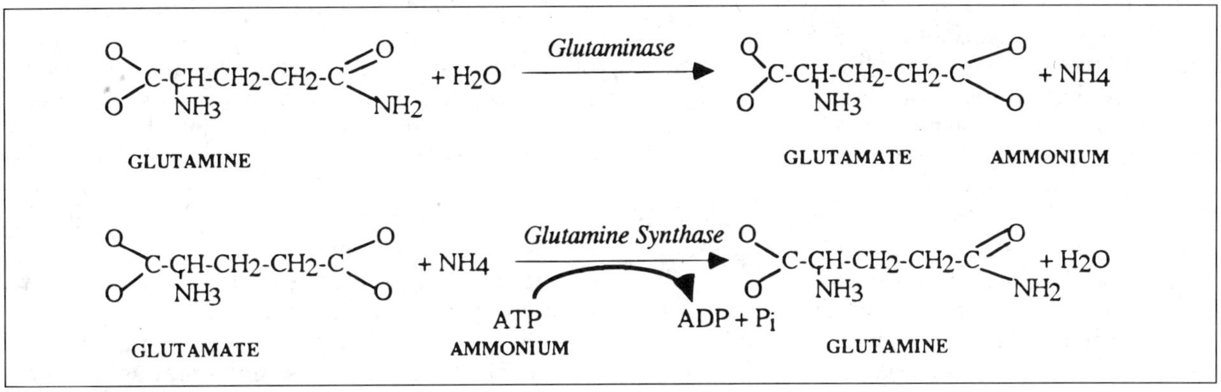

Figure 28-4. Glutamine metabolism.

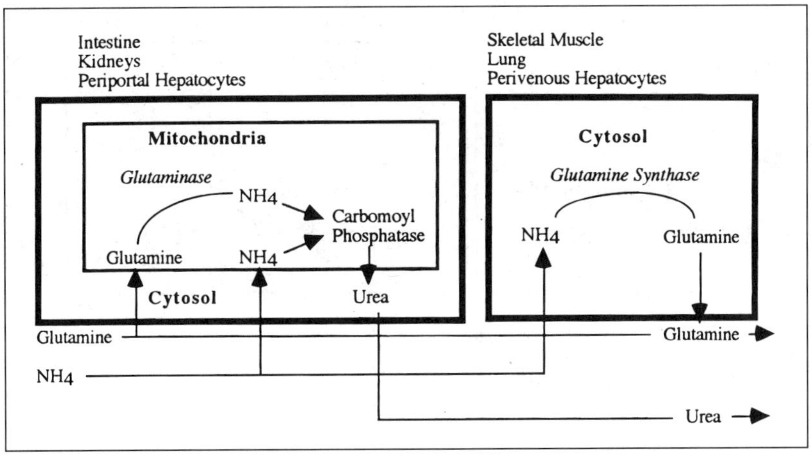

Figure 28-5. Glutamine metabolism in various cell types.

mate and ammonia. In the periportal, hepatocyte carbamoyl phosphatase then combines ammonia with bicarbonate to produce urea. The blood that traverses the hepatic lobule from the portal to the central vein bathes the perivenous hepatocytes, which possess little glutaminase but contain high levels of glutamine synthase [74]. Because of this, the perivenous hepatocytes are able to serve as scavengers of the ammonia produced by the enterocytes and periportal hepatocytes and produce glutamine by combining glutamate and ammonia. This arrangement of glutamine utilization and ammonia release by the enterocytes and periportal hepatocytes and ammonia scavenging by the perivenous hepatocytes theoretically prevents systemic ammonia toxicity. During states of acidosis, when urea production is inhibited, ammonia detoxification is accomplished mainly via glutamine production by the perivenous hepatocyte. The development of hyperammonemia in chronic liver disease has been ascribed to portosystemic shunting and loss of urea cycle enzyme activity. However, in cases of hyperammonemia, perivenous glutamine synthase activity must also be significantly affected. Ammonia flux through glutaminase has been shown to be inversely related with urea synthesis. Furthermore, the capacity of this ammonia detoxifying system is significant and is not likely to be overwhelmed without underlying hepatic dysfunction (Figure 28-6) [75].

Current parenteral nutrition formulations are glutamine free, which may explain some of the mucosal atrophy, impaired intestinal barrier, and diminished immune function observed in patients receiving parenteral nutrition. Numerous studies have attempted to address this issue. Hwang [76], Grant [77], Jacobs [78], and others [79–81] have demonstrated improved villous height and enterocyte protein content when parenteral nutrition is supplemented with glutamine. [*Editor's Note:* While all agree that enteral glutamine increases villous height and enterocyte protein count, not all studies are unanimous in confirming this effect with parenteral glutamine [82]. In addition, glutamine-enriched parenteral nutrition may promote intestinal adaptation after massive small bowel resection [83] and small bowel transplantation [84]. Glutamine has been shown to be stimulatory for intestinal epithelial cell protein synthesis, an effect that occurs for both secreted and nonsecreted proteins [73].

Glutamine supplementation has been shown to provide protective effects in the management of physiologic stress, injury, sepsis, malignant disease, and radiation injury in both animal models and human studies. When glutamine is added to cultured lymphocytes, marked mitogenesis occurs while other amino acids (arginine, asparagine, aspartate, glutamate, glycine, histidine, proline, and serine) only stimulated mitogenesis to 10% to 20% of the stimulation seen with glutamine [85]. Rats treated with parenteral nutrition supplemented with glutamine show improved survival after *Escherichia coli* peritonitis [86]. This phenomenon appears to be independent of nutritional status, as groups were similar in this regard, and is likely to be the result of improved mucosal immune function and possibly enhanced secretory IgA production. Parenteral nutrition supplemented with glutamine has been shown to decrease [*Editor's Note:* or *increase*] bacterial translocation from the intestinal lumen in experimental animals [87]. This decrease in translocation is associated with a normalization of secretory IgA levels and decreased bacterial adherence to enterocytes [88]. When glutamine is added to parenteral nutrition formulations, significant improvement in gastrointestinal immune function

Figure 28-6. Ammonia detoxification.

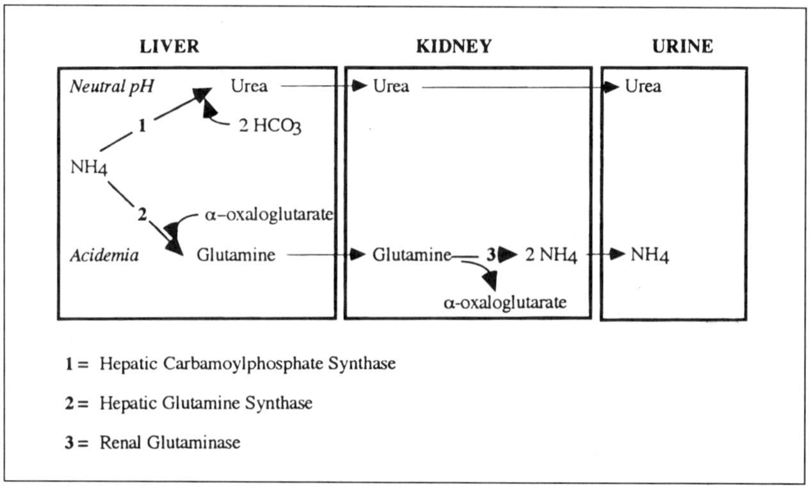

occurs [88]. In patients undergoing bone marrow transplantation for hematologic malignancies, a beneficial effect of glutamine-supplemented TPN has been demonstrated and is associated with a decreased hospital stay [89,90]. In addition to the physiologic effect of glutamine supplementation, administration of glutamine-containing TPN is associated with an improvement in patients' psychosocial status as measured by psychometric testing [91]. The authors hypothesize that glutamine may influence patients' mood either directly by affecting central nervous system neurotransmitters or indirectly through its effects on overall protein status [91].

Dipeptides

Dipeptides may be the solution to stability problems with free amino acids in parenteral formulations. The central feature of a dipeptide is the planar bond that joins two amino acids. Although intermittent cyclization occurs, this arrangement makes a molecule with unique physical properties (Figure 28-7). Because glutamine is considered nonessential and is unstable in solution, it has been excluded from modern parenteral solutions. Glutamine forms cyclic pyroglutamic acid or breaks down to glutamate and ammonia when in solution. However, it can be combined with alanine or glycine to form a stable dipeptide. In light of recent information revealing glutamine's central role in metabolic and immunologic function, its exclusion from parenteral solutions is problematic. [*Editor's Note:* While this view is commonly held, the two studies available concerning use of glutamine-enriched solutions in "normal" perioperative use revealed only a statistical but not likely biologic advantage to the glutamine-containing solution [92,93]. There may be a greater advantage in sicker patients, such as bone marrow transplant patients [90].]

A similar situation exists for tyrosine. Tyrosine is relatively insoluble in aqueous parenteral nutrition solutions at neutral pH. Because of this, physiologic levels of tyrosine in parenteral formulations are not possible. The inability to provide adequate tyrosine is particularly troublesome for low-birth-weight infants. Because tyrosine is critical for optimal growth and development, infants who must be sustained parenterally suffer developmental delays. The parenteral administration of γ-L-glutamyl-L-tyrosine dipeptide has been shown to supply adequate tyrosine for growth and development in laboratory animals [94,95] and may be useful in low-birth-weight infants who do not have adequate enteral function.

The plasma half-life and metabolic fate of dipeptides are affected by both ends of the molecule, but appear to be most dependent on the N-terminal residue [96]. Studies involving dipeptide kinetics have demonstrated rapid disappearance of dipeptides from serum, with little urinary excretion of intact dipeptides and concomitant increase in serum concentrations of the respective amino acids [97]. Although dipeptides infused intravenously may serve as substrate for circulating plasma peptidases, intravascular hydrolysis seems to be relatively unimportant in the metabolic handling of these molecules [98–100]. In general, the liver and kidneys perform the majority of dipeptide processing. The particular organ involved in dipeptide breakdown depends on the specific dipeptide. For L-glycyl-L-glutamine, tissue breakdown, in decreasing order of importance, occurs in the kidneys, splanchnic organs, and skeletal muscle. However, for L-alanyl-L-glutamine, skeletal muscle and the splanchnic bed share responsibility for breakdown equally, with a minor contribution from the kidneys [101,102].

In addition to providing an adequate amino acid complement, parenteral dipeptide formulations may have additional benefits. With current formulations and advancements in the metabolic management of patients on parenteral nutrition, the majority of complications are due to mechanical and septic difficulties related to the central venous catheter. The ability to reduce the osmolarity of parenteral solutions by use of dipeptides may allow administration of nutritionally complete formulations peripherally, thus obviating the

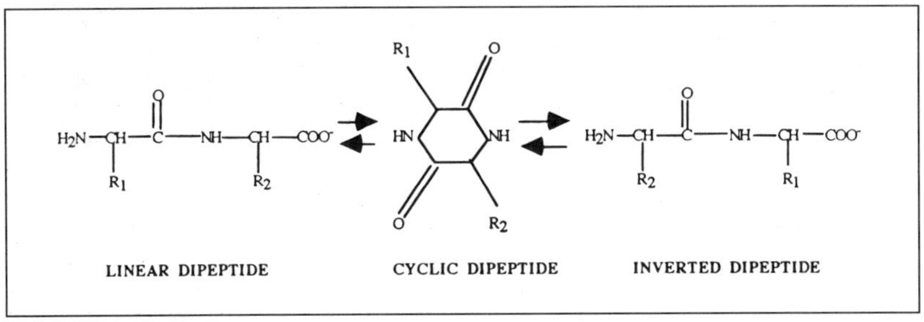

Figure 28-7. Linear and cyclic dipeptides.

need for central venous access. However, in the immediate future, it is unlikely that dipeptides will replace crystalline amino acids as the protein source in parenteral nutrition. Currently dipeptides have limited availability and are expensive to produce. However, combinations of free amino acids and dipeptides may alleviate deficiencies in current parenteral formulations.

Nucleosides and Nucleotides

Rapidly replicating intestinal mucosal cells may require an external source of purines and pyrimidines for optimal growth. Nucleosides are purines or pyrimidines linked to a pentose sugar, either D-ribose or 2-deoxyribose (Figure 28-8). When the phosphate ester of a nucleoside is formed, the result is a nucleotide (Table 28-2). Nucleotides participate, in one way or another, in nearly all biochemical processes. They are the activated precursors of DNA and RNA; they are part of the universal energy carrier ATP; they are part of the coenzymes NAD, FAD, and CoA; and they act as metabolic regulators and second messengers such as cyclic AMP and GMP. Because of this, nutritional supplementation with nucleosides and nucleotides may be beneficial in fully supporting cell growth and division. However, current parenteral formulations are devoid of these molecules. [*Editor's Note:* One wonders whether nucleotides are transported into cells intact.]

Iijima [103] studied rats given standard parenteral nutrition with and without glutamine supplementation. Then, to determine whether an effect on mucosal proliferation could be observed, the experiments were repeated with the addition of a parenteral nucleoside-nucleotide mixture. Significantly less mucosal atrophy was found in the nucleoside-nucleotide mixture group in comparison with the glutamine group. Additionally, the group receiving the nucleoside-nucleotide supplemented solution had significantly greater total and mucosal wet weights, mucosal DNA content, protein content, villous height, and cellular proliferating activity [103]. Whether parenteral supplementation with nucleosides and nucleotides, which appear to improve intestinal structure, will translate into improved physiologic and immune mucosal function remains to be determined. However, these molecules are readily available and easily added to parenteral solutions.

Omega-3 Fatty Acids

The most commonly used lipid emulsion solutions contain a mixture of long-chain fatty acids (LCFAs), with the largest component being the ω-6 linoleic acid. Arachidonic acid is derived from the ω-6 family of fatty acids and gives rise to specific inflammatory eicosanoids (prostaglandins and thromboxanes in the "2" series and leukotrienes in the "4" series), which appear to play a crucial role in the pathogenesis of endotoxic shock. Eicosapentaenoic acid (EPA), found in high concentrations in fish oils, is derived from the ω-3 family of fatty acids and is a competitive inhibitor of arachidonic acid during eicosanoid metabolism. The biologic activities of the eicosanoids derived from EPA differ greatly from those derived from arachidonic acid. Increasing the availability of ω-3 versus ω-

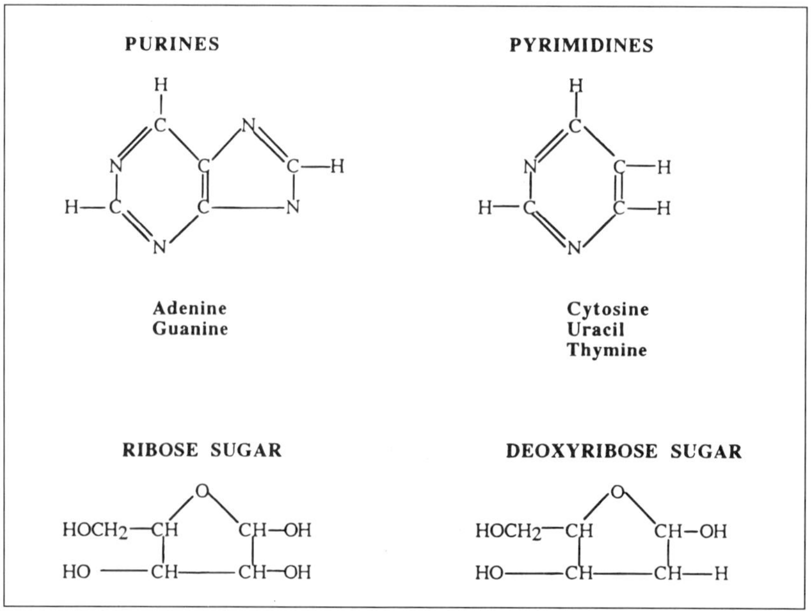

Figure 28-8. Purine and pyrimidine structure.

Table 28-2. Base Nomenclature

Purine Ribonucleoside	5′-Monophosphate Purine Ribonucleoside
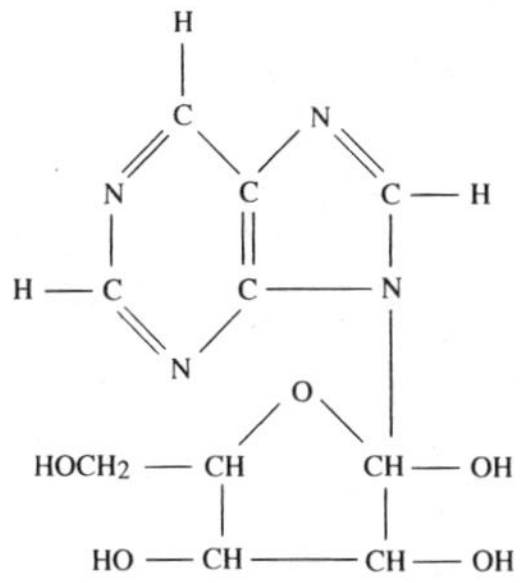	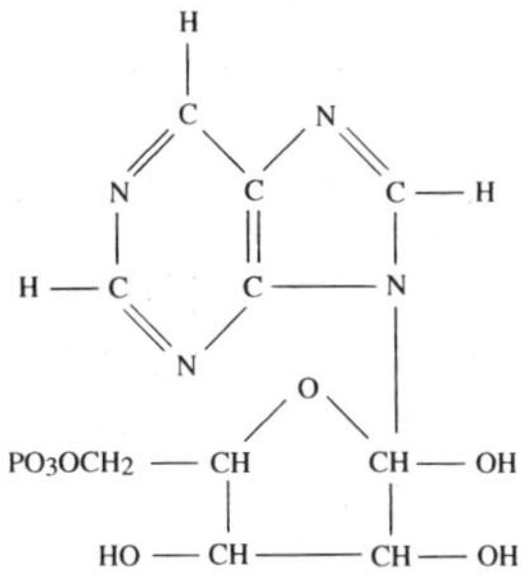

Base	Ribonucleoside	5′-Monophosphate Ribonucleotide
Adenine	Adenosine	Adenylate (AMP)
Guanine	Guanosine	Guanylate (GMP)
Uracil	Uridine	Uridylate (UMP)
Cytosine	Cytidine	Cytidylate (CMP)

Pyrimidine Deoxyribonucleoside	5′-Monophosphate Pyrimidine Deoxyribonucleoside
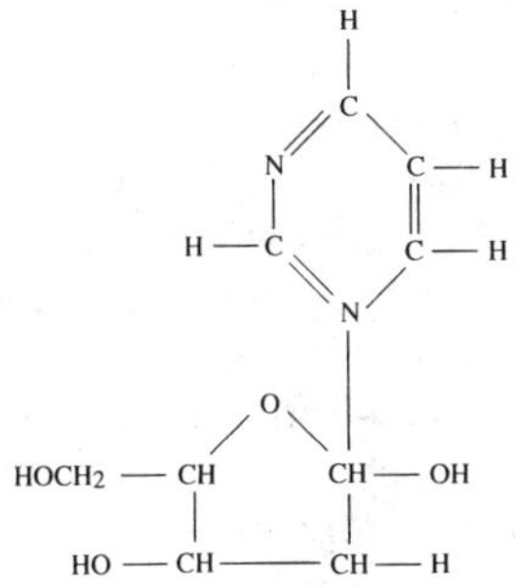	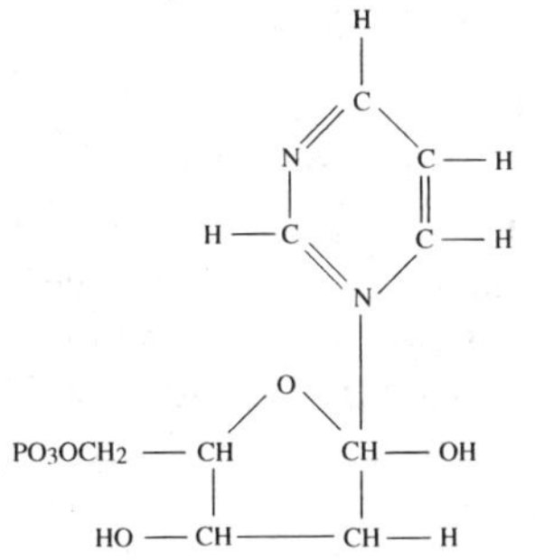

Base	Deoxyribonucleoside	5′-Monophosphate Deoxyribonucleotide
Adenine	Deoxyadenosine	Deoxyadenylate (dAMP)
Guanine	Deoxyguanosine	Deoxyguanylate (dGMP)
Thymine	Deoxythymidine	Deoxythymidylate (dTMP)
Cytosine	Deoxycytidine	Deoxycytidylate (dCMP)

6 precursors for eicosanoid metabolism has been shown to significantly ameliorate the inflammatory response and improve survival in burn injury [41] and endotoxemia [104,105]. However, these same anti-inflammatory effects that are beneficial in certain clinical situations may also be detrimental by altering the normal healing response [106].

Medium-Chain Triglycerides

Fat emulsions are a valuable parenteral energy source, particularly in injured and septic patients. However, in such individuals, long-chain triglycerides (LCTs) may not be completely oxidized, leading to reesterification of some LCFAs to triglycerides in the liver. Medium-chain triglyceride (MCT) emulsions, with esterified monocarboxylic acids containing mainly 8 and 10 carbon atoms, have been shown to be a viable parenteral source of calories when administered in varying proportions in combination with LCTs (see Figures 28-2 and 28-3) [107]. MCTs have different physical properties than LCTs: They are metabolized by separate pathways, are more water soluble, do not require chylomicron formation, and can be transported directly to the liver bound to serum albumin [108,109]. Partial replacement of LCTs with MCTs in parenteral formulas improves reticuloendothelial cell function in the injured animal [39]. In addition, protein sparing is augmented by the use of parenteral MCTs [110,111]. MCTs are directly available to tissues as a fuel source and are more potent stimulants of thermogenesis than LCTs [107]. The most commonly used MCTs contain caprylic (8 : 0) and capric (10 : 0) fatty acids (Figure 28-3).

Structured Fatty Acids

Structured fatty acids are synthesized from glycerol backbones and selected fatty acids (see Fig. 28-2). Interesterification can combine LCTs and MCTs on the same glycerol backbone. In this way, fatty acids can be chosen for superior caloric, immunologic, or structural properties. In addition, MCFAs and LCFAs can be combined to alter chylomicron dynamics.

LCTs rely on carnitine-dependent transport into the mitochondria, have lower plasma clearance rates, lower oxidation rates [37], and less nitrogen-sparing effect than do MCTs. In addition, LCTs accumulate in the reticuloendothelial system causing immunosuppression during parenteral administration [39,40]. However, MCTs also have undefinable side effects. They may be toxic in large doses, do not meet essential fatty acid requirements, and can induce metabolic acidosis. When used in safe concentrations, studies have shown a thermodynamic benefit for MCTs over LCTs [112]. This energy advantage may be due to the energy utilization of triglyceride-free fatty acid cycling that occurs with LCFA but not with MCFA metabolism. Thus, a combination of LCTs and MCTs in quantities sufficient to maximize benefit may have advantages over either individually.

To ascertain the optimal amount of parenteral structured MCT provision, Gollaher et al. [113] administered varying quantities of structured lipids composed of 15% canola oil, 35% menhaden oil, and 50% MCT oil [(final fatty acid composition of 34% caprylic (8 : 0), 18% capric (10 : 0), 13% oleic (18 : 1 ω-9), 7% palmitic (16 : 0), 5% eicosapentaenoic (20 : 5 ω-3), 4% myristic (14 : 0), 4% palmitoleic (16 : 1 ω-7), 4% linoleic (18 : 2 ω-6)], and 11% other to metabolically stressed rats. They found that providing 15% of total calories as structured MCTs maximized whole-body protein synthesis [113]. These findings are in agreement with studies by Trocki [40] and Mochizuki [114] that showed that, in metabolically stressed animals, relatively low fat intake (5%–15% of total calories) optimized protein metabolism. However, albumin synthesis was maximized when fat intake was 30% of total calories. Furthermore, nitrogen excretion was lowest in the group receiving 30% of total calories as MCTs, although this led to markedly elevated serum triglyceride levels. The same parenteral MCTs plus fish oil structured triglyceride has been shown to decrease tumor growth while maintaining host body weight and nitrogen balance in tumor-bearing animals [115].

Sandström et al. [116] randomized 20 patients to receive either 20% Intralipid or structured triglycerides for 5 to 7 days to ascertain safety and tolerance to these lipids. They found rapid clearance of the structured lipid without evidence of intolerance. Resting energy expenditure, carbon dioxide production, oxygen consumption, and nitrogen balance were all comparable between groups, as were serum proteins, liver enzymes, and electrolytes [116].

In summary, lipid emulsions composed of LCTs are currently the standard parenteral lipid sources. However, LCTs may not be the ideal source of parenteral lipid calories. Conversely, MCTs do not require chylomicron formation, can be transported directly to the liver bound to serum albumin [108,109], are directly available to tissues as a fuel source, and are more potent stimulants of thermogenesis than LCTs [107]. However, MCTs may be toxic in large doses, do not meet essential fatty acid requirements, and can induce metabolic acidosis. Therefore, partial replacement of LCTs with MCTs on a glycerol backbone minimizes side effects while providing superior caloric, immunologic, and structural lipid properties. These facts suggest that structured lipids may become the standard lipid therapy in the future.

Dicarboxylic Fatty Acids

Dicarboxylic acids have been found to be a safe parenteral energy source. The citric acid cycle is the final common pathway for the oxidation of amino acids, fatty acids, and carbohydrate. Use of dicarboxylic acids as an energy source, which requires minimal cellular processing, may theoretically offer thermodynamic advantage. Azelaic and sebacic acids are the dicarboxylic acids most commonly studied thus far (Figure 28-9). These molecules are straight-chain, medium-length acids that possess an additional terminal carboxyl group, which accounts for their water solubility. This solubility allows them to remain in simple solution without esterification to a glycerol backbone. They are oxidized to water and carbon dioxide as they pass through acetyl coenzyme A and succinyl coenzyme A formation. During oxidation, they produce calories intermediate to carbohydrate and LCTs [107].

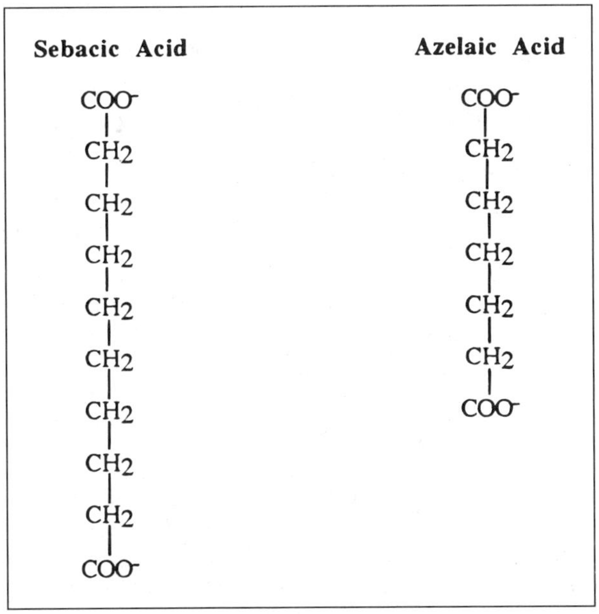

Figure 28-9. Chemical structure of dicarboxylic acids.

The volume of distribution for dicarboxylic acids is the same as that for glycerol esterified MCTs, but their serum half-lives are longer, averaging around 1.5 hours. Unlike parenteral LCT and MCT infusions, these dicarboxylic acids do not increase serum ketone, insulin, or glucose levels, suggesting that their metabolism is insulin-independent. In addition to the possible thermodynamic benefit, the water-soluble azelaic and sebacic acids can be administered in parenteral solutions without emulsification. However, this water solubility also makes the urinary excretion of azelaic acid 70% and sebacic acid 48% [107]. Because of high urinary losses, increased amounts of dicarboxylic acids must be administered to achieve adequate caloric provision.

Phospholipids

Current lipid emulsions contain a considerable amount of phospholipid. In lipid emulsions, phospholipids are in excess and only part of them serve as triglyceride surface emulsifiers. The remainder are present as liposomes, which trap cholesterol and attract apoprotein E. This results in cholesterol- and apoprotein E-rich phospholipids that bind low-density lipoprotein receptors, reducing cellular uptake of endogenous lipoproteins by hepatocytes, fibroblasts, and macrophages. The result is an alteration in cellular membrane lipid content and possible altered cellular function such as decreased platelet aggregation and increased cholesterol flux from macrophages. In addition, plasma cholesterol levels and apoprotein E levels are increased. The adverse effects of these phenomena remain to be elucidated [117].

Growth Hormone

Although current methods of parenteral nutrition support are capable of optimizing whole-body protein synthesis, protein catabolism remains disproportionately high in critically ill patients. This inability to replete body protein in the metabolically stressed individual may be the reason for the limited effectiveness of standard nutritional therapy in most surgical patients [118–120]. Recently there has been a renewed interest in the use of human growth hormone and its potential anabolic effects that enhance protein sparing in critical illness. The effect of pituitary extract on reducing net nitrogen loss during the post-traumatic response was first described by Cuthbertson during his classic studies of stress metabolism [121]. Subsequently, growth hormone and, more recently, recombinant human growth hormone administration has been shown to improve nitrogen retention in a variety of clinical situations. Growth hormone therapy has been studied in postburn injury [122], postoperatively [123–126], in patients with gastrointestinal disease [127,128], and in critically ill patients [129]. In such a heterogeneous population of patients, growth hormone administration given in conjunction with nutrition support enhances whole-body protein synthesis. When administered prior to induction of the catabolic state, growth hormone further enhances the protein-sparing effects of TPN [130]. Growth hormone treatment enhances the efficiency of protein deposition without significantly affecting body fat gain or extracellular water expansion (Figure 28-10) [131]. In addition to its effects on protein deposition, growth hormone therapy was recently shown to enhance immunologic responses, decrease wound infection, and reduce length of hospital stay [132].

Micronutrients

The macronutrients and supplements described above provide the principal energy substrates required by the patient receiving parenteral nutrition. An additional concern is the provision of appropriate amounts of macrominerals, microminerals, and vitamins to deliver a complete diet and to assure proper cellular function.

Macrominerals

The requirements for the major electrolytes (sodium, potassium, chloride, phosphorus, calcium, and magnesium) are dependent on the primary

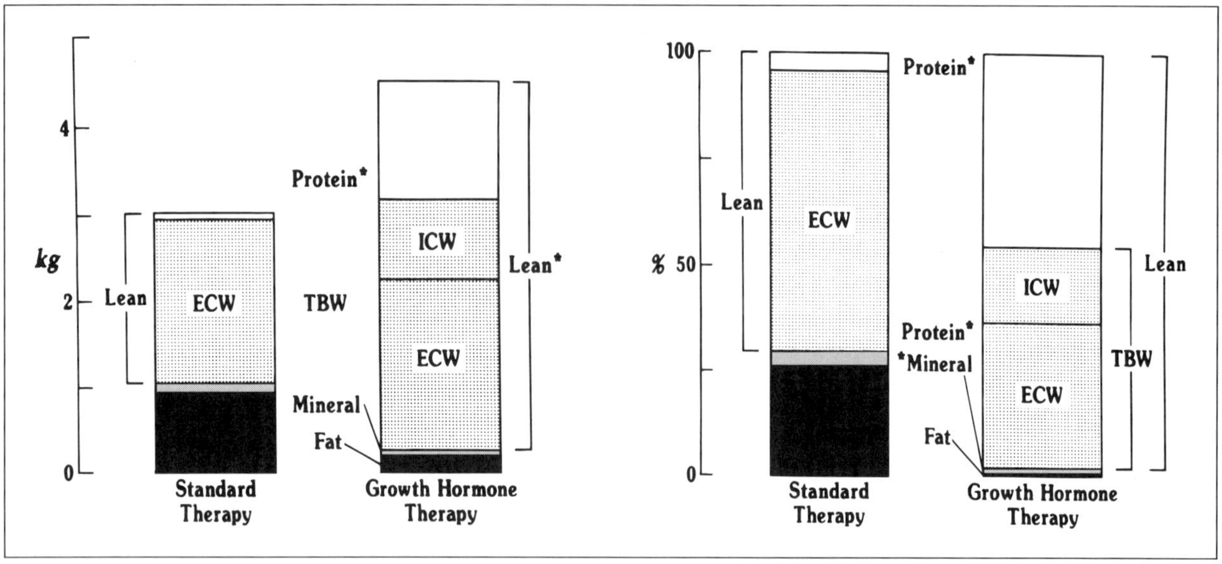

Figure 28-10. *Left:* Gain during 3 weeks of GH therapy. Patients treated with GH gained significantly more lean mass and protein-containing mass ($p < 0.03$) than did patients receiving STD therapy. *Right:* Components of weight change, expressed as a percentage of the change in body weight. Lean* = lean mass; *mineral = mineral mass; protein* = protein-containing mass. (From TA Byrne, et al. Anabolic therapy with growth hormone accelerates protein gain in surgical patients requiring nutritional rehabilitation. *Ann Surg* 218:400, 1993. Reproduced with permission.)

disease state, renal function, hepatic function, nutritional status, medication history, and abnormal losses. The daily provision of the major electrolytes is contingent on measuring serum levels and monitoring excessive losses in the urine or due to fistulas, diarrhea, vomiting, or nasogastric losses. The major intracellular ions (potassium, phosphorus, and magnesium), in particular, require close monitoring during initiation of TPN and once the patient has reached a state of anabolism. It has been demonstrated that nitrogen retention in malnourished patients receiving TPN is only possible when adequate amounts of potassium and phosphorus are included in the TPN solution [133]. Nitrogen, phosphorous, and potassium are retained in the proportions 1 g : 0.08 g : 3.1 mEq respectively.

Microminerals

The trace metals zinc, copper, chromium, selenium, manganese, iodine, and molybdenum are essential nutrients that serve as metabolic cofactors in several enzyme systems. These substances are present in varying amounts as contaminants in a normal diet as well as in infused intravenous fluids, drugs, and blood products. Much of our current understanding about these elements derives from the specific deficiency states described in patients on long-term parenteral nutrition. Because these microminerals are present in small quantities in the normally nourished individual, measurement of serum levels is notoriously inaccurate and difficult to interpret in the determination of specific deficiency states.

Zinc requirements are generally increased in the hypermetabolic patient as there is an increased urinary zinc loss in the face of muscle protein catabolism and aminoaciduria. Significant amounts of zinc may also be lost in the stool in the face of prolonged diarrhea or fistula loss. Zinc deficiency is associated with impaired wound healing, alopecia, disturbances in taste, and a characteristic rash involving the perioral area and in flexion creases [134]. In infants, zinc deficiency may lead to thymic atrophy, immune incompetence, and irritability. Copper deficiency is manifest by a megaloblastic anemia and neutropenia in adults, while infants may develop skeletal demineralization, growth retardation, and central nervous system abnormalities [135–137]. Chromium potentiates the action of insulin in vitro and in vivo [138], and three cases of chromium-responsive glucose intolerance during TPN have been described in which the intravenous administration of chromium chloride almost immediately restored normal insulin sensitivity and glucose tolerance. Manganese plays a role in antioxidant protection and energy metabolism. Although clinical manganese deficiency has never been documented in a patient on long-term TPN, it is considered an essential trace element and should be provided routinely in TPN solutions. The Nutrition Advisory Group of the American Medical Association has provided guidelines for replacement of these four trace elements [139]. Selenium is also an important antioxidant in the protection of the cell from free radical injury [140]. Selenium deficiency in patients undergoing TPN has been reported with clinical findings of cardiomyopathy and myositis [141]. Therefore, selenium should be added daily to the TPN solution along with the other four micronutrients. In particular, selenium stores are depleted in patients with thermal injury [142], acquired immunodeficiency syndrome [143], and liver failure [144]. Zinc, chromium, and selenium are excreted renally while manganese and copper are excreted through the biliary tract. In the face of renal or liver dysfunction, trace element replacement should be adjusted or withheld accordingly. Guidelines for the parenteral replacement of molybdenum, iodine, and the "ultratrace" elements (fluorine, boron, nickel, silicon, and vanadium) have not been established, and their roles as beneficial or essential factors are currently only speculative.

Vitamins

Analogous to the trace elements, vitamins are also essential cofactors necessary for normal metabolism and cellular function and must be provided as a routine component of the TPN solution. Guidelines have been established for the parenteral provision of the 13 essential vitamins in the adult [145] and pediatric [146] populations.

The exact dosages for adequate trace element and vitamin replacement in the critically ill, catabolic patient are unknown. Vitamins C and B complex requirements are increased in the face of hypermetabolism and may be administered in large excesses with impunity. Although the remainder of the vitamins and trace elements can be safely administered in increased amounts, there is little evidence that any benefit would be derived. Therefore, in the majority of patients receiving parenteral nutrition, the standard recommended amounts of trace elements and multivitamins should be provided unless specific losses or deficiencies are identified.

Indications for Initiating Parenteral Nutrition

The length of time an individual can withstand inadequate nutritional intake depends on a number of variables, which include previous state of health and nutrition, the degree of preexisting malnutrition, age, the severity of the illness, the presence of sepsis, and the length of time to the expected return of oral intake. Clinical decisions are based on the presence of malnutrition or the expectation that there will be a significant deterioration in the patient's nutritional status without any intervention. The patient that is malnourished prior to injury or illness will certainly benefit from early, aggressive nutrition support. Similarly, the septic or injured patient in whom a prolonged ICU course is anticipated should also benefit from early nutritional intervention. Techniques of nutrition support are generally better for preservation of lean body mass than for repletion in patients who have lost considerable lean body mass that is difficult to replace once lost. Therefore, it is preferable to initiate nutrition support in appropriate patients as soon as the need is identified [147]. Little definitive data are available regarding specific indications for instituting nutritional support. However, certain guidelines are helpful.

Candidates for parenteral nutrition support include patients who cannot eat, in whom bowel rest is desired, or who are unable to take in sufficient enteral nutrients. If gastrointestinal tract function is present, enteral nutrient administration is the preferred route. As the metabolic rate increases, one has to take into consideration the patient's prior nutritional state in determining a reasonable threshold for instituting appropriate nutrition support (see Figure 28-1). As a general rule, an adult aged 60 or less, with previously normal nutrition, who is moderately catabolic, usually tolerates up to 14 days of starvation without demonstrating a significant nutritional deficit. We do not advocate waiting this prolonged a period of time, but it is usually tolerated. Patients who are 60 to 70 years old tolerate only about 10 days of starvation, and patients who are over 70 years of age tolerate no more than 5 to 7 days of starvation. In critically ill patients, deficits generally occur after 7 to 10 days regardless of age. Thus, nutritional intervention in this latter group should be initiated well before this time to avoid compromises of physiologic function in these catabolic patients.

Acute clinical settings where TPN should be a part of routine care include severely catabolic patients whose gastrointestinal (GI) tracts will be unusable for more than 5 to 7 days, severe malnutrition and a nonfunctional gastrointestinal tract, severe pancreatitis, massive small bowel resection, diseases of the small intestine, radiation enteritis, intractable diarrhea, intractable vomiting, and high-dose chemotherapy, radiation, and/or bone marrow transplantation. TPN is usually helpful in the moderately malnourished patient who requires intensive medical or surgical intervention, in patients in whom adequate enteral nutrition cannot be established within 7 to 10 days, and in the treatment of enterocutaneous fistulas, inflammatory bowel disease, hyperemesis gravidarum, and inflammatory adhesions with small bowel obstruction. Parenteral nutrition is of limited value in a well-nourished patient suffering minimal stress or trauma when the GI tract is expected to be usable within 10 days or in a proven or suspected untreatable disease state. TPN is not indicated when patients have a functional and usable GI tract capable of absorption of adequate nutrients, when the sole dependence on TPN will be less than 5 days, when TPN therapy would delay an urgently needed operation, when aggressive nutrition support is not desired by the patient or legal guardian and when such action is in accordance with hospital policy and existing law, in patients whose prognosis does not warrant aggressive nutrition support, and when the risks of TPN are judged to exceed the benefits [148].

Specific Clinical Situations in Which TPN Provides Primary Therapy

Short-Bowel Syndrome

This condition represents the most dramatic indication for parenteral nutrition because long-term survival on enteral intake may not be possible when there is inadequate absorptive surface available to the individual. In the pediatric population, short-bowel syndrome usually results from congenital loss of a major segment of bowel, necrotizing enterocolitis, or inflammatory bowel disease. Many adult disorders may also lead to short-gut such as vascular accidents secondary to atherosclerotic disease, embolus, thrombotic disease, or volvulus; regional enteritis; radiation enteritis; trauma; and extensive neoplasm. In addition to ensuring adequate nutritional intake for survival, growth, and development, parenteral nutrition promotes the development of adaptive hypertrophy within the gut to allow for enhanced absorption. As a general rule a minimum of approximately 60 cm of intestine beyond the duodenum is required for survival on oral intake alone. Less bowel length may be adequate (as little as 30 cm in length) following an adaptive period on TPN if the pylorus and ileocecal valve are intact and the bowel is allowed to dilate, with villous enlargement and hyperplasia of the intestinal epithelium. It is important to recognize a patient's potential for short-bowel and to begin early aggressive nutrition support. Particular attention must be paid to the likely large losses of fluid and electrolytes as well as particular vitamin deficiencies (B_{12} and fat-soluble vitamins) due to loss of the specialized ileal absorptive region. Additionally, with the loss of the ileum, the enterohepatic circulation is disrupted, leading to an inadequate pool of bile acids and an almost universal development of cholelithiasis. Therefore, cholecystectomy should be considered whenever a massive enterectomy is performed, regardless of the etiology for bowel loss.

Gastrointestinal Fistulas

Despite all of the advances in parenteral nutrition, the overall mortality associated with gastrointestinal fistulas has not been dramatically affected by this nutritional modality [149]. That is not to say that TPN does not play a distinct role in the management of these patients. Malnutrition is common in the setting of a gastric, duodenal, or small-bowel fistula. TPN is therefore indicated in fistula patients who are obviously malnourished or have a high risk for developing malnutrition and have a high fistula output with the need for complete bowel rest. The primary role for parenteral nutrition in fistula management is supportive. By replacing ongoing protein and nutrient losses in conjunction with additional supportive and therapeutic measures (i.e., antibiotics, somatostatin), the likelihood for spontaneous fistula closure is improved [150]. The serum transferrin level has been shown to be predictive of which patients with gastrocutaneous fistulas will close spontaneously, while levels of all of the short-turnover proteins (transferrin, retinol-binding protein, thyroxin-binding prealbumin) are predictive of mortality [151]. If surgical intervention is warranted, then adequate preoperative nutrition improves the patient's tolerance of the intervention as well as decreasing the operative morbidity. Therefore, parenteral nutrition plays a central role in treating the majority of gastrointestinal fistulas.

Bone Marrow Transplantation

At least 50% of patients undergoing bone marrow transplantation have a significant degree of malnutrition [152]. Additionally, most have significant gastrointestinal dysfunction, including mucositis, anorexia, nausea, vomiting, and diarrhea. Thus, enteral nutrition in these patients may be difficult and is often unreliable. Parenteral nutrition, on the other hand, is generally routine in this setting, and its use has been shown to enhance survival, diminish relapse, and shorten the post-transplant hospital stay [153].

Obstetrics

Specialized nutrition support during pregnancy provides supportive therapy for the mother, is crucial for normal fetal growth, and decreases the risk of neonatal death or long-term medical and developmental sequelae [154]. The principal reasons for requiring nutrition support during pregnancy include malnutrition secondary to severe hyperemesis gravidarum or other intercurrent illnesses that affect adequate nutrient intake or absorption. Whenever possible, the enteral route should be utilized with TPN reserved for situations in which gastrointestinal feeding is not tolerated or is contraindicated. Maternal and fetal nutritional status should be closely monitored. Maternal weight gain of at least 1 kg/month in normal weight and 0.5 kg/month in obese women during the second and third trimesters is considered minimal weight gain to assure adequate fetal nutritional status. Ultrasonography is also useful in monitoring the adequacy of the nutritional regimen in providing for adequate fetal growth.

Cardiac Surgery

Protein-calorie deficiency or malnutrition has a definitely deleterious effect on cardiac muscle function and performance [155]. Once depleted, normal cardiac function does not easily return [156]. In the acute setting, the myocardium, like any other muscle, is affected by starvation. Provision of adequate nutrition is essential for efficient cardiac function. In addition, providing adequate calories in the form of glucose and fat (TPN) immediately prior (overnight) to cardiac surgery increases the myocardial glycogen concentration, is associated with the occurrence of fewer severe postoperative ventricular arrhythmias, less pressor dependency, fewer transmural myocardial infarctions, and improved survival [157].

Specific Clinical Situations in Which TPN May Provide Primary Therapy

Acquired Immunodeficiency Syndrome (AIDS)

The combination of malnutrition and gastrointestinal dysfunction is common in patients with AIDS. A component of the disease itself is an increased immunosuppression and the "wasting syndrome," which has been postulated to be secondary to essential fatty acid deficiency. Inhibitors of delta-6-desaturase enzyme activity in the gastrointestinal tract lead to a malabsorption of gamma linoleic acid and/or isopentoic acid [158]. In addition to the nutritional benefits provided by infusion of lipid emulsions, cholesterol extraction may actually decrease the infectivity of the human immunodeficiency virus (HIV) via fluidization of the viral membranes [159]. Once the wasting syndrome begins, nutritional support is considered mandatory [160]. Parenteral nutrition is indicated when intestinal absorption is impaired despite adequate oral or enteral intake. Early institution of TPN has been recommended by some authors to prevent progressive wasting and to retard the progressive immunologic deterioration in AIDS. Ongoing randomized studies are currently under way to define a role for aggressive nutrition support in these complex patients.

Organ Failure

Disease-specific parenteral and enteral formulations have been developed to address specific needs and disorders related to particular organ system dysfunction. As such, these specific solutions have been developed for their potential primary effect on the underlying disease process. These include formulations for patients with liver, kidney, respiratory, and cardiac failure (see Parenteral Nutrition Formulations later in this chapter for discussion of these formulations).

Specific Clinical Situations in Which TPN Provides Supportive Therapy

The nutritional support of TPN is indicated whenever adequate oral or enteral nutrition cannot be provided or tolerated in a patient who is already malnourished or at risk to develop malnutrition without this support. The largest single group of patients in this category are those who require perioperative nutrition support.

Perioperative

A recent study by the Veterans Affairs TPN Cooperative Study Group of patients undergoing elective surgery suggested that, except for severely malnourished patients, the infectious complication rate was higher when TPN was given preoperatively than in the control group [118]. These complications included both catheter-related and noncatheter-related infections, mainly pneumonia and wound infections, suggesting impairment of the immune mechanism in these patients. In cancer patients with moderate malnutrition receiving chemotherapy, McGeer et al. [120] also found that TPN was associated with an increased risk of infection. Other studies have reached similar conclusions. In a recent review of prospective studies that evaluated the use of perioperative nutrition support, Campos and Meguid [119] reached several conclusions: When TPN is given to malnourished patients in adequate amounts for greater than 7 to 15 days preoperatively, significant improvements in both nutritional status and postoperative clinical outcome are likely to occur; perioperative enteral nutrition is as effective as TPN in improving clinical outcome.

Inflammatory Bowel Disease (IBD)

Acute and chronic malnutrition is a significant complicating factor in many patients with IBD [161,162]. Both parenteral and enteral nutritional modalities are well-documented methods for providing metabolic support to the IBD patient to prevent or reverse malnutrition. In Crohn's disease, enteral or parenteral nutrition is likely to facilitate remission in 60% to 80% of patients with acute exacerbations [163]. The enteral route is preferred except in the presence of high-output fistulas, obstruction, or severe diarrhea. TPN is particularly supportive in situations that require intensive medical therapy in combination with bowel rest. In ulcerative colitis, nutrition support does not influence disease activity [164]. However, in acute exacerbations of ulcerative colitis, TPN is beneficial by preserving lean body mass when surgery is being considered.

Pancreatitis

Nutrition support does not improve the course or duration of the disease process in the setting of pancreatitis. Nutritional intervention is of no benefit in the setting of mild, acute, or chronic relapsing pancreatitis [165,166]. Nutrition therapy is indicated for supportive purposes in the presence of severe necrotizing pancreatitis when it is expected that oral intake will not be adequate for a period greater than 7 days [167]. Intestinal feeding should be utilized unless the symptoms of pancreatitis are exacerbated by use of the gastrointestinal tract, in which case parenteral nutrition is indicated. Administration of intravenous lipid emulsions as a calorie source in pancreatitis appears to be safe as long as serum triglyceride levels are monitored and remain below 400 mg/dL [163].

Cancer

Malnutrition commonly complicates the course of malignant disease due to direct effects of the tumor and indirectly as a result of anorexia, chemotherapy, radiation, and surgical intervention. The presence and severity of malnutrition in the cancer patient are inversely related to his or her duration of survival [168,169]. Although nutrition support via the parenteral or enteral route is effective in treating the malnutrition associated with neoplastic disease or antitumor therapy, it is not a treatment for cancer itself. The effect of TPN on tumor growth itself remains a controversial issue. Parenteral nutrition may preferentially stimulate tumor growth [170,171]. However, cytokinetic and immunohistochemical studies in human head and neck cancers have shown no evidence of an effect on tumor growth by TPN [172]. Parenteral nutrition administration does not reduce chemotherapy-associated toxicity, but in malnourished patients who are undergoing chemotherapy TPN does prevent further impairment of nutritional status [173]. In general, if the well-nourished or mildly malnourished cancer patient is capable of tolerating adequate oral intake, specialized nutrition support is not routinely indicated. Additionally, specialized nutrition support is not beneficial and may actually be detrimental in the presence of advanced malignancy that is unresponsive to chemotherapy or radiation [163].

Eating Disorders

Anorexia nervosa and bulimia may be associated with varying degrees of malnutrition depending on the status of the individual's psychological disorder. Primary therapy is directed toward treatment of the underlying psychological, emotional, and cognitive abnormalities. Under certain circumstances, when the patient cannot ingest sufficient calories orally and he or she has significant malnutrition (< 65% of ideal body weight or > 30% recent weight loss), nutritional intervention is required, generally by the enteral route. If the patient is uncooperative or does not tolerate nasoenteric feeding due to emotional or physical reasons, then parenteral nutrition is indicated. It is believed by some clinicians that restoration of a normal nutritional status in this setting may facilitate physical and emotional recovery in select patients. Conversely, forced nutritional therapy may actually worsen the situation because of the emotional trauma associated with the perceived loss of control in this clinical setting. Therefore, a specific role for nutrition support in general and TPN in particular in patients with eating disorders remains controversial and at present is only recommended for replenishment of patients with evidence of severe malnutrition [163].

Critical Illness

The goals of nutrition support in the critically ill patient include the minimization of starvation effects, the attainment of nitrogen balance and reasonable visceral protein levels, the prevention of specific nutrient deficiencies, and the support of the acute phase-inflammatory response until the patient heals and the hypermetabolic response resolves. Premorbid conditions such as malnutrition, organ dysfunction, prior illness, obesity, and pregnancy may further complicate this situation. Enteral delivery of nutrition in this setting has been shown to significantly reduce subsequent septic complications, presumably because of preservation of gastrointestinal barriers and host defenses [163]. If enteral access cannot be obtained, if gastrointestinal feeding is contraindicated, or if enteral feedings do not fully meet the required caloric intake, then parenteral feedings should be administered until a transition to enteral nutrition is possible. A variety of specific nutrients have been proposed for use in the critical care setting and will be discussed later in the chapter (see Parenteral Nutrition Formulations). It is important to recognize that, regardless of the method and specific nutrients administered, as long as the source of infection or stress is present the patient will not be capable of increasing or even maintaining his or her lean body mass. Thus, it is not enough to support these patients nutritionally but is necessary to aggressively seek out and treat the sources for stress hypermetabolism. Because of the complex array of factors that affect these patients' nutritional needs, an accurate assessment of their caloric and nutrient requirements is essential to meet the individual's needs and to avoid the complications of overfeeding (see Determination of Energy Requirements earlier in this chapter; Chapter 19 on Nutritional Assessment).

Parenteral Nutrition Formulations

See Table 28-3 and Figures 28-11 and 28-12.

The traditional TPN formula contains 25% dextrose; 4.25 to 5.0% amino acids; electrolytes, vitamins, and trace elements. In addition, lipid emulsions are provided as a separate infusion to prevent essential fatty acid deficiency. The population of patients who require parenteral nutrition support represent a very heterogeneous group with varied nutritional requirements and metabolic deficits. Therefore, the provision of nutrition support must be individualized to each unique clinical setting and the formulations modified from the traditional formulation (see Table 28-3).

Table 28-3. Total Parenteral Nutrition (TPN) Formulations at the University of Cincinnati Medical Center

	Standard	High Dextrose	Renal[a]	Hepatic	Cardiac[a]	Stress	Peripheral
Caloric substrates[b]							
Dextrose (%)	15	20	46.6	25	35	17.5	5
Amino acids (%)	5[c]	5[c]	1.7[d]	4[e]	5[c]	5.2[f]	3.5[c]
Protein (g)	50	50	17	40	50	52	35
Fat (as TNA) (g)	40	40	—	40	—	40	40
Calorie content							
TNA (Kcal/ml)	1.1	1.3	—	1.3	—	1.0	0.71
Non-TNA (Kcal/ml)	0.71	0.88	1.65	1.0	1.4	0.80	—
Calorie (nonprotein)-nitrogen ratio							
TNA	119:1	141:1	—	208:1	—	114:1	104:1
Non-TNA	67:1	89.1	794:1	142:1	156:1	82:1	—
Electrolytes[g]							
Potassium (K)	18	18	0	12	0	13	10
Sodium (Na)	30	30	2	5	5	23	40
Magnesium (Mg)	5	5	0	8	8	8	8
Calcium (Ca)	4.5	4.5	0	4.7	0	4.7	4.7
Phosphorus (P)	10	10	0	5	5	9	5
Chloride (Cl)	37	37	1	13.5	2	10	40
Acetate (Ac)	55	55	14	31	45	51	52

TNA = Total nutrient admixture.
[a]Renal and cardiac are not formulated as TNA.
[b]All caloric substrate values are expressed per liter of solution.
[c]As balanced amino acid solution (FreAmine III, McGaw).
[d]As essential amino acids (Nephramine, McGaw).
[e]As Hepatamine, McGaw.
[f]As FreAmine HBC, McGaw.
[g]Standard minimum concentrations as mEq/L and phosphorus as mM/L. Maximum total concentrations are: K = 80, Na = 154, Mg = 12, Ca = 9.4, P = 15, Cl = (limited by cation), Ac = 80.

ORDNUT

UNIVERSITY OF CINCINNATI HOSPITAL

PARENTERAL NUTRITION ORDER FORM

Deadline for orders at 9:30 A.M.

Date: ______________ Time: ______________

UMC-375, 8/92

STEP 1: SELECT BASE FORMULA:

Total Nutrient Admixture (TNA) contains: Fat emulsion, Dextrose, & Amino acids.
Non-TNA contains: Dextrose & Amino acids.

Standard Formula:

	❑ TNA	❑ NON-TNA
Each Liter contains:		
Non-Protein Calorie: N	119	67
Total kcal/ml	1.1	0.71
Dextrose (15%)	150 gm	
Amino Acids (5%)	50 gm	
Fat Emulsion (4%)	40 gm (as TNA)	

MVI-12 (10 ml) & Trace elements-5 (3 ml) daily
Vit K 5 mg weekly

Standard Electrolytes (mEq/L)

Na	K	Ca	Mg	P(mM)	Cl	Acetate
30	18	4.5	5	10	37	55

High Dextrose Formula:

	❑ TNA	❑ NON-TNA
Each Liter contains:		
Non-Protein Calorie: N	141	89
Total kcal/ml	1.3	0.88
Dextrose (20%)	200 gm	
Amino Acids (5%)	50 gm	
Fat Emulsion (4%)	40 gm (as TNA)	

MVI-12 (10 ml) & Trace elements-5 (3 ml) daily
Vit K 5 mg weekly

Standard Electrolytes (mEq/L)

Na	K	Ca	Mg	P(mM)	Cl	Acetate
30	18	4.5	5	10	37	55

STEP 2: ORDER <u>TOTAL</u> ADDITIVES IF DIFFERENT FROM ABOVE:

Total Na __________ mEq/L
Total K __________ mEq/L
Total Ca __________ mEq/L
Total Mg __________ mEq/L
Total Phos __________ mM/L
Reg. Insulin __________ units/L

Other per Liter:
____
____
____
____
____

MAXIMUM TOTAL CONC/LITER

K+	80 mEq
Ca	9.4 mEq
Mg	12 mEq
Phos	15 mM
Ac	80 mEq

DAILY TRACE ELEMENTS

Zn	3.0 mg
Cu	1.2 mg
Cr	12 mcg
Mn	0.3 mg
Se	60 mcg

STEP 3: SELECT INFUSION RATE:

INFUSE AT __________ ml/hr or Cycle: __________ ml Total Volume

PHYSICIAN SIGNATURE ______________________ PAGER #: __________

WHITE—CHART YELLOW—PHARMACY

Figure 28-11. Physician's order form for standard and high dextrose parenteral nutrition formulations at the University of Cincinnati Medical Center. (From the Department of Parenteral and Enteral Nutrition, University of Cincinnati Medical Center. Reproduced with permission.)

ORDNUT

UNIVERSITY OF CINCINNATI HOSPITAL

SPECIALTY PARENTERAL NUTRITION ORDER FORM

Deadline for orders at 9:30 A.M.

Date: ______________ Time: ________________

UMC-376, 7/92

STEP 1: SELECT BASE FORMULA:

Total Nutrient Admixture (TNA) contains: Fat emulsion, Dextrose, & Amino acids.
Non-TNA contains: Dextrose & Amino acids.

Hepatic Formula:

❑ TNA ❑ NON-TNA

Each Liter contains:

	TNA	NON-TNA
Non-Protein Calorie: N	208	142
Total kcal/ml	1.3	1.0
Dextrose (25%)	250 gm	
Amino Acids (4%)	40 gm	
Fat Emulsion (4%)	40 gm (as TNA)	

MVI-12 (10 ml) & Trace elements-5 (3 ml) daily
Vit K 5 mg weekly

Standard Electrolytes (mEq/L)

Na	K	Ca	Mg	P(mM)	Cl	Acetate
5	12	4.7	8	5	13.5	31

Renal Formula:

❑ NON-TNA (see step 4) *

Each Liter contains:

Non-Protein Calorie: N	794
Total kcal/ml	1.65
Dextrose (46.7%)	467 gm
Amino Acids (1.7%)	17 gm

MVI-12 (10 ml) & Trace elements-5 (3 ml) daily
Vit K 5 mg weekly

Standard Electrolytes (mEq/L)

Na	K	Ca	Mg	P(mM)	Cl	Acetate
2	0	0	0	0	1	14

Cardiac Formula:

❑ NON-TNA (see step 4) *

Each Liter contains:

Non-Protein Calorie: N	156
Total kcal/ml	1.4
Dextrose (35%)	350 gm
Amino Acid (5%)	50 gm

MVI-12 (10 ml) & Trace elements-5 (3 ml) daily
Vit K 5 mg weekly

Standard Electrolytes (mEq/L)

Na	K	Ca	Mg	P(mM)	Cl	Acetate
5	0	0	8	5	2	45

Peripheral Formula:

❑ TNA

Each Liter contains:

Non-Protein Calorie: N	104
Total kcal/ml	0.71
Dextrose (5%)	50 gm
Amino Acids (3.5%)	35 gm
Fat emulsion (4%)	40 gm

MVI-12 (10 ml) & Trace elements-5 (3 ml) daily
Vit K 5 mg weekly

Standard Electrolytes (mEq/L)

Na	K	Ca	Mg	P(mM)	Cl	Acetate
40	10	4.7	8	5	40	52

STEP 2: ORDER TOTAL ADDITIVES IF DIFFERENT FROM ABOVE:

Total Na ____________ mEq/L
Total K ____________ mEq/L
Total Ca ____________ mEq/L
Total Mg ____________ mEq/L
Total Phos ____________ mM/L
Reg. Insulin ____________ units/L

Other per Liter:
____
____
____
____
____

MAXIMUM TOTAL CONC/LITER	
K+	80 mEq
Ca	9.4 mEq
Mg	12 mEq
Phos	15 mM
Ac	80 mEq

DAILY TRACE ELEMENTS	
Zn	3.0 mg
Cu	1.2 mg
Cr	12 mcg
Mn	0.3 mg
Se	60 mcg

STEP 3: SELECT INFUSION RATE:

Infuse Base Formula at ____________ ml/hr

* STEP 4: SELECT IF NON-TNA FAT EMULSION DESIRED:

❑ 20% FAT EMULSION (250 ML) INFUSE OVER 10 HOURS.

PHYSICIAN SIGNATURE ______________________________ PAGER #: ______________

WHITE—CHART YELLOW—PHARMACY

Figure 28-12. Physician's order form for hepatic, renal, cardiac, and peripheral parenteral nutrition formulations at the University of Cincinnati Medical Center. (From the Department of Parenteral and Enteral Nutrition, University of Cincinnati Medical Center. Reproduced with permission.)

Total Nutrient Admixture

A recent advance in the delivery of parenteral nutrition has been the widespread use of total nutrient admixtures (TNA) in which all components, including lipid, are mixed in a single bag for continuous infusion. This technology allows for the daily administration of a mixed substrate solution and avoids the transient hyperlipidemia seen with separate lipid infusion. This also allows for provision of the required calories while at the same time delivering less glucose calories. It is not clear what the ideal energy substrates are and whether altering this fuel source might affect whole-body protein metabolism in various clinical situations [48]. While provision of glucose calories is known to have a beneficial protein-sparing effect [31,174], this may be countered by various metabolic complications [32,33]. Provision of calories in a mixed substrate of glucose and fat is as effective as pure glucose in achieving anabolism [32,47–50]. Several studies have suggested that injured and/or septic patients may have an obligatory need for fat oxidation [27,45,175], while others have not been able to conclusively demonstrate a benefit in protein sparing with the use of a combination of lipid and glucose [176,177]. It is clear that as the degree of critical illness increases, it becomes increasingly difficult to attain protein synthesis regardless of the energy source. However, delivery of 30% to 50% of the patient's estimated caloric needs as lipid appears equally effective while decreasing the metabolic complications inherent in the use of high concentrations of glucose in the TPN formulations [48], provided the patient is not severely septic or catabolic, in which case lipid may not be as effective in sparing lean body mass [174]. Overfeeding with excessive glucose or lipid may be detrimental and should be avoided. If administering a mixed substrate, the respiratory quotient (RQ) should be in the 0.8 to 0.9 range. If this value is higher, it generally indicates overfeeding, especially with glucose, and the calories provided should be reduced. Serum glucose must be closely monitored and may be regulated over the short term with subcutaneous regular insulin administration and over the long term by insulin infusion or adding regular insulin to the TPN formulation. Serum lipids should also be monitored and if consistently elevated (triglyceride levels > 500 mg/dl), the amount of lipid calories provided should be reduced.

Disease-Specific Formulations

Patients often require further modification of the standard TPN or TNA formulation due to alterations in the function of one or several vital organ systems. Specific formulations can be tailored to better meet the nutritional requirements of patients with renal failure, hepatic failure, pulmonary failure, cardiac insufficiency, and severe metabolic stress (see Table 28-3). Frequently one is presented with a patient suffering from multisystem organ failure that demands a clear understanding of the benefits of each of the specialized formulas and may require the use of a combination of specific nutrients.

Acute Renal Failure

The patient with renal failure may have a wide spectrum of metabolic abnormalities. This includes an increased protein catabolism with an inability to excrete the products of nitrogen metabolism (urea) leading to a rapid rise in blood urea nitrogen (BUN). The anuric and oliguric patient will also have increased fluid retention, acidemia, and elevated serum electrolytes including potassium, magnesium, and phosphate. In addition to the catabolic effect of critical illness, renal failure alone increases the catabolic response and may further impair wound healing and resistance to infection. The goal of nutritional management in these patients is to improve the metabolic state while avoiding the accumulation of excess urea, fluid, acids, and electrolytes. Hemodialysis is very effective in managing fluid retention and controlling azotemia and electrolyte abnormalities. However, hemodialysis itself causes an increased catabolism and negative nitrogen balance [178] due to loss of amino acids across the dialysis membrane [179] and release of granulocyte proteinases after contact of the blood with the membrane [180].

Patients with acute renal failure who are not anuric, are able to handle a modest fluid load, and have no life-threatening electrolyte abnormalities may be managed with a modified renal failure TPN formulation. This solution may contain either essential amino acids [181] or a modest dose of standard amino acids [182] in a high concentration (50%–70%) dextrose solution. The former have been formulated to prevent the development of hyperuremia. Essential amino acids provide protein equivalent of high biologic value and may allow recycling of urea for protein synthesis [181]. An increased survival has been demonstrated in one classic study; however, the number of patients in this study is too small to demonstrate efficacy [181]. Therefore, despite the theoretical advantages offered by solutions high in essential amino acids, the clinical efficacy of these solutions in acute renal failure has not been conclusively proven [183,184]. Survival of patients with acute renal failure is more closely associated with the ability to attain positive energy balance rather than with the formulation of amino acids utilized.

Glucose is the primary energy source utilized in acute renal failure because of its protein-sparing effect in the catabolic patient [174] and because it can be delivered in high concentrations when fluid requirements are limited. Fat may also be utilized as an energy source in moderate amounts (30% of caloric requirements), particularly if the patient is consistently glucose-intolerant. However, fat does not provide as much protein-sparing effect as carbohydrate [170]. Additionally, the lipid emulsion contains 15 mmol/L of phosphate, which may be contraindicated if the patient is already hyperphosphatemic due to renal failure. Serum electrolytes should be closely monitored, especially when initiating TPN because the potassium, phosphate, and magnesium levels may decline rapidly in the face of hypertonic dextrose infusion. In such a formulation, caloric requirements may be administered along with amino acids and electrolytes in a minimal amount of excess volume.

Close attention must be paid to the micronutrients in the renal failure patient. Iron, vitamin D, and the water-soluble vitamins may all be deficient in the patient with chronic renal failure and require supplementation. Conversely, the trace elements (chromium, zinc, and selenium) and electrolytes (magnesium and phosphate), which are primarily excreted via the kidneys, may accumulate and should be administered with caution.

If the patient requires hemodialysis for maintenance of fluid and electrolyte balance or for control of BUN, the TPN regimen may be liberalized to a more standard mixture of nonessential and essential amino acids, carbohydrate, and lipid. It is not necessary to reduce nutrient or volume intake because any excess can be dialyzed off. In certain circumstances, the anuric patient may not be able to tolerate the dialysis regimen due to hemodynamic instability. More recent methods of continuous fluid removal are now available and may be particularly useful in patients with hemodynamic instability. These methods include slow continuous ultrafiltration (SCUF), continuous arteriovenous hemofiltration (CAVH), and continuous arteriovenous hemodialysis (CAVHD). Each of these methods requires a different approach to the parenteral nutrition regimen utilized.

SCUF uses hydrostatic pressure across a membrane to produce ultrafiltration rates of up to 5 ml/min [185]. No dialysis fluid is used, so there is minimal solute removal, thus necessitating intermittent hemodialysis therapy. In this regimen, a "renal formulation" containing minimal fluid, high-concentration dextrose, and essential amino acids might decrease the need for intermittent hemodialysis when control of volume excess is the primary concern. Approximately 90% of the nutrients provided are retained by the patient [186].

CAVH also relies on hydrostatic pressure generated by cardiac output across a membrane that is more permeable than those used for hemodialysis [187]. This allows for an increased rate of hemofiltration of 10 ml/min, which effects removal of solute by convection and may be adequate to maintain acceptable levels of BUN, creatinine, and electrolytes without supplemental hemodialysis. Because of the large volume of fluid removed by this technique, volume restriction is not a concern and, in fact, the majority of patients on CAVH will require supplemental intravenous fluids in addition to the TPN. CAVH allows the administration of a more balanced, standard TPN solution with up to 150 g/day of balanced amino acids with good control of fluid balance and nitrogen accumulation [188,189].

The third method, CAVHD is a continuous therapy that utilizes a reduced flow rate of standard dialysate fluid [190–192]. At such low flow rates, nutrients may be added to the dialysate and are taken up by the patient. This may reduce the efficiency of the dialysis but may obviate the need for separate administration of TPN. Using this technique of "nutritional hemodialysis" with a dialysate containing 5% dextrose and 0.4% amino acids and a flow rate of 27 ml/min, Feinstein et al. [190] demonstrated that 49 g/hr of glucose and 4 g/hr of amino acids were absorbed by the patients.

Hepatic Failure

Many seriously ill patients may have some degree of hepatic dysfunction when their illness is complicated by intra-abdominal sepsis. Such dysfunction does not usually warrant any protein restriction or modification in the TPN solution provided. In contrast, patients with acute fulminant hepatic failure secondary to acute viral or alcoholic hepatitis or patients with acute-on-chronic liver disease may have their clinical course complicated by development of hepatic encephalopathy. These patients have low serum levels of branched-chain amino acids (BCAAs) (leucine, isoleucine, valine) and elevated levels of methionine aromatic amino acids (phenylalanine, tyrosine, tryptophan) [193]. In hepatic dysfunction, BCAAs may supply up to 30% of total energy needs in contrast to the 6% to 7% of calories derived from BCAAs in normal patients. The increased aromatic amino acids are thought to contribute to encephalopathy by effectively competing with the reduced BCAAs at the blood-brain barrier, providing precursors for the synthesis of false neurotransmitters within the brain. A modified hepatic formulation containing 35% BCAAs and decreased amounts of the aromatic amino acids and methionine have been shown to allow positive nitrogen balance with increased protein synthesis and improved ammonia metabolism in muscle while correcting the plasma amino acid profile and ameliorating encephalopathy [194]. Those patients with acute-on-chronic liver disease who have either mild (grade I) or no encephalopathy may tolerate a limited amount (50 to 60 g) of protein in a standard amino acid mixture. If these patients do not tolerate a standard formula or if they present with grade II or greater encephalopathy, then a modified hepatic solution as described above is indicated. Meta-analysis of prospective randomized trials utilizing modified (high BCAAs, low aromatic) and normal mixtures reveals improvement in encephalopathy [195] and in some cases increased survival [196].

Some patients with hepatic dysfunction and ascites may require fluid and sodium restriction to regulate the intra-abdominal accumulation of fluid. Patients with liver disease frequently have micronutrient (thiamine, pyridoxine, riboflavin, folic acid, zinc, and vitamins A, D, E, and K) deficiencies due to abnormalities in nutrient intake, absorption, metabolism, and/or storage. In addition to standard micronutrient supplementation, additional multivitamins, thiamine, folate, and zinc may be provided for these patients. Jaundiced patients may develop excess levels of copper and manganese because these trace elements are excreted primarily via the biliary system. Thus, copper and manganese replacement should be limited, and trace element solutions without copper and manganese may be appropriate to use in such patients. In patients with multiple organ failure, with both hepatic and renal failure, one may have to choose between higher BUN and less encephalopathy (modified high BCAAs, low aromatic) and a lower BUN and a greater degree of encephalopathy (essential amino acids).

Pulmonary Failure

Acute respiratory failure requiring mechanical ventilation results in increased catabolism and hypermetabolism [197]. This is further amplified in the patient with preexisting chronic lung disease in whom weight loss and malnutrition are common [198]. Protein-calorie malnutrition in the mechanically ventilated patient leads to further derangements in pulmonary function and structure [199], reduction in respiratory muscle strength and contractility [199–202], abnormal ventilatory drive [203], decreased production of surfactant [204,205], and altered pulmonary defense mechanisms [199]. Early aggressive nutrition support is essential to avoid these complications of protein-calorie malnutrition in the mechanically ventilated patient. Refeeding malnourished patients with respiratory failure may lead to large shifts of sodium and water from the intracellular into the extracellular compartment. This may further compromise ventilatory function due to development of pulmonary edema. Thus, it is often necessary to restrict sodium and volume administration to these patients.

In addition to serving as substrates for nutrition, the caloric components (amino acids, carbohydrate, and lipid) in parenteral nutrition solutions have important direct effects on pulmonary mechanics and ventilatory function that must be considered. Amino acids have been shown to increase minute ventilation, oxygen consumption, and ventilatory response to hypoxia and hypercarbia [203,206,207]. Specifically, the BCAAs appear to stimulate ventilatory drive [208]. Therefore, in addition to their nutritional value, administration of amino acids appears to also provide a beneficial effect on ventilatory efficiency by stimulating respiratory function.

The administration of glucose in the clinical setting of respiratory failure may lead to an increased carbon dioxide production (VCO_2) [209] and increased ventilatory response to hypoxia [207]. Under rare circumstances, overfeeding with large quantities of carbohydrate in a malnourished, septic patient with inadequate respiratory reserve secondary to chronic obstructive pulmonary disease may lead to excess VCO_2 and difficulty weaning from the ventilator [210,211]. Administration of a mixed substrate glucose/lipid solution should prevent the potential complications of carbohydrate overfeeding in these patients. It is emphasized that despite all of the publicity that this complication has received, it occurs only rarely. In the original publication, excessive VCO_2 and difficulty in weaning only occurred when depleted septic patients suddenly had large loads of glucose administered without adaptation [210]. In a recent clinical trial studying TPN in mechanically ventilated patients, increasing the caloric intake increased the VCO_2 while increasing the proportion of carbohydrate calories had no effect on VCO_2 [212]. Thus, avoiding overfeeding in these patients appears to be more important than the specific composition of the formulation.

Despite the concern that fat emulsions might cause further impairment of pulmonary function, intravenous administration of lipids are usually well tolerated in the clinical setting of pulmonary failure. Furthermore, lipid emulsions have been shown to improve pulmonary mechanical properties and surfactant production in an animal model [213] and, as previously noted, may be a preferred fuel source for the injured and septic patient [27,214]. It is clear that, in the face of respiratory failure and ongoing wasting of skeletal muscle, overall outcome is improved with careful assessment and provision of a mixed substrate fuel formulation. Indirect calorimetry with determination of the patient's REE and RQ allows for accurate determination of the patient's caloric and substrate needs. Lipid calories, with their lower RQ, may be used to provide up to 50% of energy needs while decreasing overall VCO_2. This may become important when one is attempting to wean such patients from mechanical ventilation. In addition to monitoring nutritional parameters, respiratory rate, vital capacity, minute ventilation, and arterial blood gases must be continually assessed as nutrition support is instituted and advanced. Substrate manipulation should be instituted to keep RQ less than 0.9, which reduces minute ventilation and may promote weaning. When proper initial assessment and interval follow-up is applied early in the course of the illness and appropriate amounts of mixed substrate fuel are provided as a total nutrient admixture, excessive VCO_2 and a need for major changes in the nutritional formulation during weaning should be a rare occurrence in such patients.

Cardiac Failure

For some six decades the standing dictum that the heart is spared the ravages of starvation was unquestioned, until the deleterious effects of protein-calorie malnutrition on cardiac muscle were demonstrated [155]. It was further demonstrated that once depleted, normal cardiac function did not easily return [156]. In the acute setting, the myocardium, like any other muscle, is affected by starvation. Provision of adequate nutrition is essential for efficient cardiac function. In general, the myocardium utilizes fatty acids primarily under resting conditions and carbohydrate in the face of ischemia and increased energy demands. Provision of amino acids affects protein turnover in ischemic and septic cardiac muscle. In particular, BCAA-enriched solutions have been shown to improve cardiac function in isolated rat-heart preparations [156]. In addition to serving as nutritional substrate, hypertonic glucose [215], amino acids [216], and, secondarily, insulin and glucagon provide positive inotropic effects in the face of cardiac dysfunction [217–219]. Thus, the nutritional needs of the patient with cardiac failure can be met by utilizing a mixed substrate solution containing glucose, a balanced amino acid solution, and lipid emulsion.

The challenge in providing parenteral nutrition for this population of patients is to provide an adequate amount of calories in a sodium- and volume-restricted solution. By utilizing more concentrated solutions of amino acids (10%), dextrose (70%), and lipid emulsion (20%) while limiting sodium to approximately 1.5 g/day, one can generally meet the cardiac patient's needs in a limited volume of approximately 1500 ml/day. Because of the high density of carbohydrate calories utilized in this setting, blood glucose should be monitored closely. Insulin should be added to the formulation in amounts necessary to control hyperglycemia. An additional consideration in this subset of critically ill patients is that diuretic therapy is often required to maintain an optimal volume status. Vigorous diuresis may lead to substantial losses of potassium, magnesium, and zinc. These losses should be anticipated and, when indicated, additional supplementation of these elements should be provided.

Stressed/Septic Patient

The serum amino acid profile in stressed and septic patients is similar to the profile seen in hepatic failure with the exception that the sulfur-containing amino acids are more prominent in the septic patient [220]. In this setting, the BCAAs are used for fuel preferentially by skeletal muscle and may therefore become depleted. Provision of BCAAs may stimulate protein synthesis while inhibiting protein degradation. Infusion of a conventional TPN solution is also associated with intestinal atrophy. Parenteral nutrition solutions enriched with glutamine have been found to partially reverse gut atrophy [221], although this has not been universally confirmed [82]. The potential benefit of such solutions in stressed patients theoretically is to prevent translocation of potentially pathogenic bacteria and their products across the intestinal wall and into the systemic circulation [222]. However, glutamine is excluded from conventional TPN solutions because it is unstable at room temperature. Infusion of BCAA-enriched solutions increase synthesis and release of glutamine from skeletal muscle [223–225] and may be as effective as glutamine in limiting gut atrophy [223].

TPN formulations containing adequate amounts of essential and nonessential amino acids and enriched with 45% BCAAs theoretically may be beneficial in stressed and septic patients by improving nitrogen retention, increasing visceral protein synthesis, preserving intestinal integrity, improving immune status, and normalizing the plasma amino acid profile [227]. Clinical studies comparing BCAA-enriched with conventional solutions have only shown marginal improvement in nitrogen balance, decreased ureagenesis, and improved plasma levels of short turnover proteins. However, despite the apparently more efficient source of protein provided by BCAA solutions, little major effect on outcome has been demonstrated [228–231]. Because of the increased cost, this formulation should only be reserved for the rare circumstance when severely stressed patients fail to respond to conventional TPN solutions.

Peripheral Parenteral Nutrition (PPN)

This formulation has a low caloric density because it must be isotonic or slightly hypertonic to be infused via a peripheral vein. The solution contains a final concentration of 5% dextrose and, to provide an adequate calorie-nitrogen ratio, 200 ml of 20% lipid emulsion should be administered along with the PPN. This can be compounded as a total nutrient admixture with a caloric density of 0.71 kcal/ml and a calorie-nitrogen ratio of 104 : 1. Because the insertion and placement of central venous catheters remain the main causes of TPN-related complications (see Catheter-Related Complications later in this chapter), parenteral nutrition administration could be made safer by infusion of the nutrient solution via a peripheral vein. The major objection to PPN has been due to the high rate of peripheral vein thrombophlebitis previously associated with this modality. However, changes in the method of parenteral nutrition infusion and attention to catheter composition and care have increased the feasibility of this technique in many patients who may require short-term parenteral nutrition support.

The recognition of the complications of overfeeding and a more accurate assessment of caloric needs have led to an overall reduction in caloric load provided to most hospitalized patients requiring TPN. Very few patients, except for the hypermetabolic critically ill individual, will require more than 30 kcal/kg/day or between 1800 and 2000 kcal per day [16]. The use of total nutrient admixtures allows for infusion of a satisfactory caloric load as PPN while reducing the osmolality of the solution. Administration of growth hormone in this setting has been shown to be an effective adjuvant, with enhanced nitrogen retention and visceral protein synthesis in the presence of hypocaloric peripheral nutrition support [232]. The use of fine-bore (23-gauge) polyurethane or silicone elastomer cannulas in a large vein, with meticulous attention paid to insertion, fixation, and care should minimize the risk of peripheral vein thrombophlebitis. Several adjunctive measures have been advocated to further reduce this complication. These include the use of a 5-μm inline filter to reduce the particulate matter infused [233] and application of transdermal glyceryl trinitrate [234] and topical nonsteroidal anti-inflammatory drug gel [235] adjacent to the cannula site.

PPN is not indicated in the hypercatabolic patient or when long-term TPN is anticipated. However, PPN may be useful when patients have no central venous access or when central venous catheterization is contraindicated. When a patient without central access is unable to tolerate full enteral nutrition or is unable to take in adequate oral nutrients but is expected to improve within a short period of time (5–7 days), PPN infusion may be appropriate to provide supplemental calories and protein and to avoid delays in the initiation of nutrition support.

Venous Access for Parenteral Nutrition Delivery

The optimal method for delivering the required calories in an acceptable volume of solution is to provide the formulation in a hypertonic mixture that is infused into a central vein. It is preferable, but not always possible, to access the central venous system with a single lumen catheter placed percutaneously via the subclavian vein. This should be a new catheter that has not been used for other infusions or monitoring before the initiation of parenteral nutrition and is used solely for its administration.

Before placement of the central line, whenever possible, the patient should be prepared physiologically. Adequate restoration of intravascular volume is of primary importance. Patients who require nutrition support can be markedly hypovolemic early in the course of their illness or injury. At least two to three liters of a balanced intravenous salt solution should be administered to patients who are volume-depleted before central venous cannulation. In addition, coagulation abnormalities as indicated by a prolonged bleeding time or thrombocytopenia (platelet count below 50,000/mm^3) in the multiply transfused and/or septic patient must be considered and, when identified, should be corrected with specific component transfusion prior to attempted line placement. Adequate explanation of the indications and risks of the procedure, sedation, and proper positioning of the patient is of equal importance once the patient is physiologically prepared.

The nature of the procedure is explained in detail with special attention given to describing the position of the patient during the procedure and to teaching the Valsalva maneuver. The physician informs the patient of the risks of the procedure, including possible misdirection of the catheter tip (requiring replacement or redirection of the catheter using fluoroscopy) and the risk of pneumothorax or hemothorax. Adequate documentation of patient teaching, discussion of procedural risks, and a signed consent should be available in the patient's medical record. Once consent has been obtained, the patient should be sedated with small doses of an intravenous benzodiazepine administered slowly via a peripheral intravenous line. The patient should be sedated and relaxed but still able to respond to commands. A rolled blanket is placed from the base of the patient's neck to the small of the back beneath the thoracic spine. This roll allows the patient's shoulders to extend back against the mattress when the patient is in a supine position. An analogy is the position of a "soldier at attention" with his head and shoulders dropped back and his arms at his side, a position that enables a horizontal approach to the subclavian vein. The patient's bed is placed in Trendelenberg position to distend the subclavian vein. The patient's head is turned slightly away from the side of insertion.

Central venous access for parenteral nutrition administration is best administered via subclavian vein cannulation using the Seldinger technique (Figure 28-13). The side of choice is a matter of personal preference and experience but, at times, may be dictated by other concurrent factors. The left subclavian vein is generally easier to cannulate and follows a gentler curve than the right; however, there is a small but finite risk of thoracic duct injury during cannulation on this side. If there has been extensive injury to the subclavian region or known anatomic abnormalities on one side, then the contralateral side should be used. In a situation where a tube thoracostomy is already in place and all other factors are equal, the catheter should be placed on the same side as the chest tube to protect against the development of a pneumothorax and avoid the need for contralateral tube thoracostomy.

Central line insertion is a surgical procedure and mandates the use of strict aseptic technique. Surgical caps and masks should be worn by all personnel in attendance, and sterile drapes are used to drape the field and to shield the patient's face. The operator puts on a sterile gown and sterile gloves. Items present on the subclavian catheter insertion tray should be prepared and laid out in an orderly fashion prior to preparation of the patient's skin. Preparation of the skin is done in three steps. Initially, the skin is cleansed with gauze sponges soaked in alcohol (the area of preparation is bounded laterally by the anterior axillary line and shoulder, superiorly by a line from the shoulder to the angle of the mandible, anteriorly along the mandible, medially by the midline, and inferiorly by a horizontal line through the nipple). Next, the area is cleansed three times with a povidone-iodine solution that should remain in contact with the skin for two minutes. Finally, the povidone-iodine is removed with alcohol. The three small towels or drapes should border the lateral, superior, and medial edges of the field, and a large drape should border the inferior edge of the field and extend over the patient's lower chest and abdomen to provide a work surface.

The point of insertion of the catheter is chosen

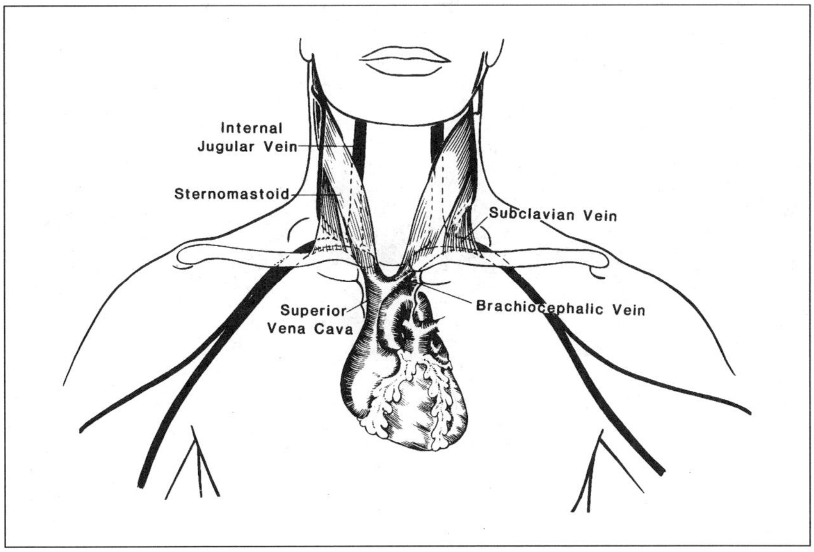

Figure 28-13. Venous anatomy of the thoracic inlet. (From TC Koutlas [ed]. *The Mont Reid Surgical Handbook* [3rd ed]. St. Louis: Mosby-Year Book, 1993. Reproduced with permission.)

at a spot near the junction of the proximal and middle third of the clavicle (Figure 28-14). This point is often found 1 cm inferior to and 1 cm medial to the bend of the clavicle. Using a 25-gauge needle and syringe filled with lidocaine, a skin weal is made at the point of insertion by injecting 1% lidocaine. A 22-gauge needle and lidocaine syringe is then advanced from the point of insertion toward an area below the fingertip of the operator's contralateral hand (placed in the sternal notch). The needle is passed in a horizontal position (not more than 10° off the horizontal). As the needle is advanced, negative pressure is maintained by pulling on the plunger until the needle enters the subclavian vein and there is a return of blood into the syringe. The entire track is then anesthetized by injecting 1% lidocaine while slowly withdrawing the needle. A syringe with an 18-gauge thin-walled Seldinger needle is then inserted along the same track immediately following removal of the small needle. The 18-gauge needle should be advanced slowly with negative pressure applied to the syringe barrel until a "pop" is felt as the vein is entered and the syringe fills with dark (venous) blood. When good intravascular position is attained there will be free aspiration of blood into the syringe. In the absence of free aspiration of blood, threading of the guidewire is unlikely. The patient is then asked to perform a Valsalva maneuver and a soft J-tipped intravascular guidewire is passed through the needle into the superior vena cava. The needle is withdrawn and the central venous catheter is carefully passed over the wire into the superior vena cava. If the patient is being mechanically ventilated, positive pressure ventilation should be temporarily stopped during the time of venipuncture and insertion of the guidewire. The catheter should be anchored to the skin using a single 3-0 silk suture placed at the insertion site. A 5 to 10mm bite of skin should be taken medial to the point of catheter insertion and the knot tied loosely to avoid pressure necrosis of skin. The free ends of the suture are then passed around the catheter and tied securely.

Several points of precaution need to be mentioned. The wire should never be withdrawn through the needle because shearing may result and the wire may migrate, requiring fluoroscopic retrieval. Similarly, when the catheter is being threaded over the guidewire the operator should always hold the guidewire either at the skin level or at the hub end of the catheter to prevent loss of the guidewire through the puncture site. Finally, suturing of the catheter should take place while the wire is still in the catheter lumen to avoid occluding the catheter with the suture and to prevent spillage of blood, leakage of air, or development of thrombus in the catheter. A single suture should be used to anchor the catheter. No additional sutures need to be placed in the catheter hub or along the catheter. The placement of multiple sutures usually results in catheter problems and provides difficulty in cleansing the entire subclavian region during subsequent dressing changes.

The catheter is now ready to be attached to the infusion system. The operator asks the patient to perform a Valsalva maneuver while the guidewire is removed, and a 500-ml bag of 5% dextrose in water is attached to the catheter via sterile intravenous tubing. Opening the roller clamp of the dextrose infusion establishes free flow through the catheter. Lowering the infusion bag below the

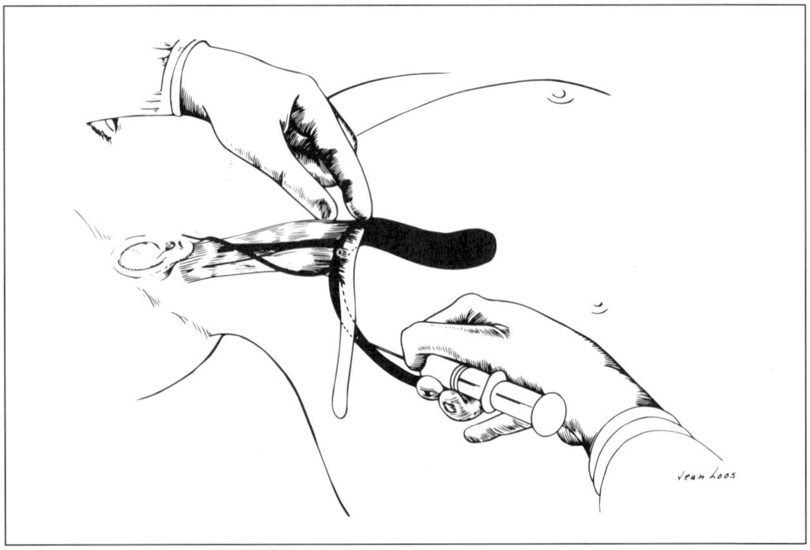

Figure 28-14. Infraclavicular subclavian venipuncture. (From TC Koutlas [ed]. *The Mont Reid Surgical Handbook* [3rd ed]. St. Louis: Mosby-Year Book, 1993. Reproduced with permission.)

level of the patient should result in a reflux of blood into the administration tubing to confirm the intravascular tip position of the catheter. The bag is then raised to its original height to flow. The infusion should be given via an infusion device and run at a rate of 40 ml/hour until proper catheter tip position is confirmed. The rolled sheet is removed from beneath the patient, the bed is taken out of the Trendelenberg position, and a sterile occlusive dressing is applied.

Proper positioning of the catheter must be immediately confirmed by a portable chest roentgenogram. Acceptable positions of the catheter tip include the superior vena cava or the junction of the innominate vein and vena cava. A retrograde location of the catheter tip in the internal jugular or location in the contralateral subclavian vein is unacceptable and can predispose the patient to thrombosis. Such misdirected catheters should be manipulated using aseptic technique under fluoroscopic guidance until they are in an acceptable position. Similarly, location of the catheter tip in the right atrium or ventricle is unacceptable because the stiffness of percutaneous catheters can cause endocardial lesions, which subsequently become a nidus for bacterial or fungal infection. Erosion and perforation of the right atrium have been reported. The procedure has not been completed until the chest x-ray is seen and proper catheter position assured.

At the conclusion of the procedure the operator should write a procedure note documenting the site of insertion, type and dosage of sedative drug and local anesthetic, the type and size of catheter used, the number of needle passes, any complications encountered, and the position of the catheter tip on chest x-ray as well as any roentgenographic abnormalities that are seen on the postinsertion x-ray.

Occasionally the subclavian veins are not available or cannot be cannulated. In this situation central venous access for parenteral nutrition administration should be obtained via internal jugular venous cannulation (see Figure 28-13). The same preparation and precautions are necessary when accessing the internal jugular vein. However, the maintenance of a sterile occlusive dressing on the neck is more difficult than is the subclavian site, thus making these catheters more susceptible to contamination and subsequent catheter sepsis. Hence the subclavian site is preferred whenever possible.

To insert the internal jugular vein catheter, a point of insertion is selected approximately 5 cm above the clavicle along the posterior edge of the sternocleidomastoid muscle or between the two heads of the sternocleidomastoid muscle. Local anesthesia is used to infiltrate the skin, subcutaneous tissue and the catheter insertion track from the point of insertion aiming toward the suprasternal notch or slightly toward the ipsilateral nipple. After localization of the vein with a 22-gauge needle, an 18-gauge Seldinger needle is used for catheter insertion over a guidewire in the same fashion as described above for the subclavian vein.

On rare occasions, the only route for central access is via the femoral veins or a peripherally inserted 24-inch-long central line. Neither of these options is very optimal, and often the risks inherent with these methods outweigh any benefit that can be obtained. Femoral lines are associated with much higher complication rates due to the high density of skin pathogens in the region. Strict care of the entrance site along with frequent (every 48 hours) replacement of the catheter is required to decrease the incidence of complications. The peripherally inserted central lines also are associated with high infection rates and should be removed after 5 days. A much better approach to the patient with limited venous access is to utilize multiple lumen catheters placed via the subclavian or internal jugular veins [236].

Complications of Parenteral Nutrition

Parenteral nutrition can clearly provide an influential effect in many clinical situations where no other route of alimentation is feasible. Many complications associated with malnutrition are obviated, and at times TPN can be a truly life-saving modality. An understanding of essential macronutrient and micronutrient requirements and potential complications associated with parenteral nutrition administration has made this treatment modality quite safe and available in the majority of clinical settings. Multidisciplinary nutrition support teams composed of physicians, nurses, dietitians, and pharmacists have had a marked impact on reducing TPN-related complications [237]. These teams may assist in the delivery of parenteral nutrition as well as developing protocols and standing orders (Figure 28-15) to minimize the risk and sequelae associated with common complications. Despite these advances, there remains a small but finite incidence of catheter (mechanical and sepsis-related) and metabolic morbidity associated with parenteral nutrition administration.

Catheter-Related Complications

Mechanical Complications

Mechanical complications can be divided into those associated with insertion of the central cath-

ORDCHK

UNIVERSITY OF CINCINNATI HOSPITAL

PHYSICIAN'S CHECKLIST/ORDER SHEET

All applicable orders have been checked. A line has been placed through orders that have been voided. ORDERS NOT CHECKED ARE NOT TO BE FOLLOWED. Orders have been modified according to the medical condition of the patient. These orders have been dated, timed and signed by a physician. As an order is filled, the individual doing so must date/time and initial in the space provided. Further orders will be added as needed.

UMC-44 Rev. 8/92

ALLERGIES: ❑ None Known ❑ Yes, Drug/Reaction:______________________

PAGE ________ OF ________

ORDER NUMBER	✔	PARENTERAL NUTRITION (PN) STANDING ORDERS			ORDER NOTED (DATE/TIME)	(INITIAL)
1.	√	Obtain confirmation of appropriate position of central				
		venous access device prior to initiating PN.				
2.	√	Initial and subsequent dressings per nursing procedure.				
3.	√	Phlebotomy by peripheral venipuncture unless peripheral				
		access is exhausted.				
4.	√	Vital signs q8h.				
5.	√	I & O q8h.				
6.	√	Measure initial height and weight. Record weight q				
		Monday, Wednesday, Friday.				
7.	√	If PN is temporarily interrupted, infuse D_5W at PN				
		infusion rate.				
8.	√	Do not infuse IVPB into PN.				
9.	√	Finger stick blood sugar b.i.d. x 3 days unless patient is				
		diabetic, then FSBS q _____. Call MD for >250 mg/dl.				
10.	√	Laboratory studies (use low volume tubes when possible).				
		PRIOR TO STARTING PN	EVERY MONDAY	EVERY THURSDAY		
		Renal (4203)	Renal (4203)	Renal (4203)		
		Bone (4041)	Bone (4041)	Bone (4041)		
		Hepatic (4162)	Hepatic (4162)			
		Transferrin (4706)	Transferrin (4706)			
		Prealbumin (4705)	Prealbumin (4705)			
		Retinol Binding	Retinol Binding			
		Protein (4707)	Protein (4707)			
		Magnesium (4229)	Magnesium (4229)			
		CBC (4032)	CBC (4032)			
		Triglyceride (4726)				
		Prothrombin Time (4204)				
		(See, also, Nursing Procedures)				

White–Chart Yellow–UD Copy
Pink–IV Copy Goldenrod–Floor Copy

Physician signature ______________________

Date ___________ Time ___________

Developed by Robert H. Bower, M.D. Date 1/94 Review Date ___________

Figure 28-15. Physician's standing order form for patients on parenteral nutrition at the University of Cincinnati Medical Center. (From the Department of Parenteral and Enteral Nutrition, University of Cincinnati Medical Center. Reproduced with permission.)

eter and those related to long-term catheterization of a central vein. Insertion-related problems are generally technical in nature and are directly related to the skill and experience of the person inserting the catheter. A detailed knowledge of the anatomy of the central veins and the thoracic inlet as well as strict adherence to the basic surgical principles outlined above (see Venous Access for Parenteral Nutrition Delivery) are key factors in maintaining a low complication rate. An awareness and early recognition of the array of potential insertion-related problems is also important to minimize the extent and severity of these complications. The incidence of complications secondary to insertion of central lines has been reported to be from 2% to 7%. The most commonly reported complications are pneumothorax (approximately 6% incidence) and great vessel injury. Other, less common injuries include cardiac, mediastinal, tracheal, nerve, and lymphatic injury. Additional complications are cardiac arrhythmias, catheter misdirection, and embolism of air or the catheter itself. Prevention of insertion-related complications requires operator skill as well as appropriate preparation of the patient. Placement of a central line for parenteral nutrition is never an emergency, thus the procedure should be delayed until the patient is well hydrated and any coagulopathies or other complicating factors have been corrected or optimized. At the time of insertion, proper positioning and patient cooperation are key factors, and this usually requires the administration of a parenteral short-acting sedative to the patient. Strict sterile technique during the procedure must be followed to minimize the incidence of later septic sequelae. At the completion of the insertion, a chest roentgenogram is imperative to confirm proper placement of the catheter within the superior vena cava and to promptly recognize any insertion-related complications. The procedure should not be considered complete until the chest x-ray is reviewed.

Mechanical complications related to long-term central vein cannulation include venous thrombosis; caval and myocardial perforation secondary to malposition of the catheter; air embolism during tubing changes or due to inadvertent disconnection of the infusion tubing; catheter embolism due to breakage of the catheter; and chronic arterial stenosis, arteriovenous fistula, or pseudoaneurysm formation secondary to an unrecognized arterial injury. Incidences of these mechanical complications are best diminished by using the smallest catheter that will be adequate for delivery of the required solution(s), assuring that the catheter is properly positioned in the superior vena cava, using locking devices at all tubing connections, following strict protocols during tubing changes, and restraining patients who are likely to pull out their catheters. Venous thrombus formation around the catheter is the most common long-term mechanical complication, occurring in approximately 5% to 10% of patients with central lines, and often leads to catheter-related infection due to trapping of organisms within the thrombus. The role of catheter composition in the development of venous thrombus formation and subsequent development of catheter-related infection is well recognized. Rigid catheters such as those composed of polyethylene or Teflon are more often responsible for thromboses than soft silicone or polyurethane catheters [238,239]. In a study comparing a variety of catheter materials for thrombogenicity in an animal model, Borrow and Crowley [240] demonstrated that polyurethane coated with hydromer was least thrombogenic, silicone was the next least, and plain polyurethane was the most thrombogenic. Newer catheter materials containing elastomeric hydrogel change composition to become softer on insertion and may prove to be even less thrombogenic than the materials currently available [241]. The addition of heparin to the TPN solution has been advocated by some as a deterrent to the development of thrombosis. However, this has not been proven to be of any benefit in this situation and is not routinely recommended.

Infectious Complications

Catheter-related sepsis is one of the most common and potentially serious complications associated with TPN infusion. It is defined as either culture documented catheter infection or resolution of fever and signs of sepsis within 24 hours after removal of the line in a patient with no other identifiable source of infection. The most predominant offending organisms are gram-positive skin contaminants (i.e., staphylococcal species). The incidence of TPN line sepsis has been reported in two large clinical series to be between 6.5% and 7% [242,243], but clearly can be minimized by meticulous catheter care [244]. Careful attention to aseptic technique during line placement and subsequent dressing changes are key factors in preventing catheter-related sepsis. Protocols for the careful surveillance of all catheters and meticulous dressing care of these sites should be established by the nutrition support team or a team of specially trained nursing personnel to minimize bacterial colonization of the skin with subsequent progression along the subcutaneous tract of the catheter. When catheter infection is suspected, blood cultures should be obtained through the line as well as via a peripheral site, the catheter should be exchanged over a guidewire, and the catheter tip should be cultured. Preliminary culture results should be available within 24 to 48 hours. If either the central line blood or tip cultures are positive, if the peripheral culture is positive without any other obvious source, or if symptoms of sepsis persist despite negative cultures, the catheter should be removed and a new site chosen if central venous access is still required.

In the patient with limited venous access, it is often necessary to infuse TPN through a multilumen catheter or through the venous infusion port of a pulmonary artery catheter. The use of these catheters allows for the efficient care of the patient and management of multiple infusions while decreasing the risks of individual central line insertions. However, it is controversial as to whether infusion of TPN via these devices will increase the risk of catheter-related sepsis. It is crucial to limit the use of multilumen catheters for TPN infusion to instances in which incompatible solutions are being continuously infused in a patient with limited venous access. The least possible number of lumens should be utilized, and breaks in the continuity of the line for intermittent infusions and blood drawing should be discouraged. Since the use of the 7 French triple-lumen catheter was first introduced into clinical practice in 1983, there have been numerous reports and studies comparing infection rates of these versus single-lumen catheters. The literature on this topic has yielded conflicting results. Some studies have demonstrated markedly increased catheter sepsis rates [245,246], while others have not been able to demonstrate a significant difference in the infection rate [247–251]. In one of the latter studies, Lee et al. [251] hypothesize that the equivalent infection rate may be due to greater attention to skin preparation before insertion and during subsequent dressing changes. The incidence of multilumen catheter-related sepsis appears to increase with the duration of catheter placement and suggests that this begins at approximately 7 to 10 days for triple-lumen catheters [251]. Guidewire exchange of central catheters has long been an accepted method for replacing existing lines with no increased incidence of infection [252,253] unless the catheter and the subcutaneous tunnel has already been colonized by infectious organisms [252,254–256]. Routine exchange of triple-lumen catheters over a guidewire every three to four days has been shown to decrease the incidence of catheter-related sepsis to a rate equivalent to single-lumen catheters, which are not routinely exchanged [257].

In our routine at the University of Cincinnati we require that all multilumen catheters that have TPN infusing through one of the ports be exchanged over a guidewire every 3 days. If there is suspected catheter-related sepsis, both the patient's blood and the catheter tip are cultured and when catheter sepsis is documented or strongly suspected, the line is removed and a new line is inserted at a different site. Occasionally, the only central venous access that an ICU patient has is a pulmonary artery catheter. Horowitz et al. [248] have shown that the use of a pulmonary artery catheter for TPN infusion is a viable alternative to the use of the triple-lumen catheter, with no difference in the rate of catheter-related sepsis as long as the catheter was changed every 3 days. It is the policy at our institution that the pulmonary artery catheter and introducer are exchanged over a guidewire at 3 days and is removed at 6 days and placed at a different site. By adhering to these guidelines, we have been able to maintain an acceptable catheter-related sepsis rate. Between July 1989 and June 1992, 2114 central lines were placed for the administration of TPN with an overall catheter-related sepsis rate of 4.5%, and no difference in sepsis rates between groups was detected (Table 28-4). We define catheter-related sepsis very liberally as either culture-documented catheter infection or resolution of fever and signs

Table 28-4. Central Venous Catheter Sepsis Rates,[a] University of Cincinnati Medical Center, July 1989 to June 1992

Type of Catheter	Number of Catheters	Number of Catheter Sepsis Cases[b]	Catheter Sepsis (%)
Single-lumen	477	20	4.2
Triple-lumen	1562	69	4.4
Pulmonary artery	75	6	8.0
Total	2114	95	4.5

[a]Catheter-related sepsis defined as either culture-documented catheter infection or resolution of fever and signs of sepsis within 24 hr after removal of the line in a patient with no other identifiable source of infection.
[b]No significant difference between groups by analysis of variance (ANOVA).

of sepsis within 24 hours after removal of the line in a patient with no other identifiable source of infection. Between 1989 and 1991, the rate of colonization of the central lines, with or without positive blood cultures, was 3.6% (single-lumen = 2.5%, triple-lumen = 4.2%, pulmonary artery = 1.9%). While the incidence of sepsis is higher than one would like to see, the patient population has changed significantly with many patients who are severely traumatized and immunocompromised.

A variety of antibiotics and antiseptic agents have been bonded to central venous catheters or catheter cuffs and have been associated with significantly lower bacterial colonization and sepsis rates [258–261]. A recent study that evaluated the use of implanting a biodegradable silver impregnated collagen cuff subcutaneously in a triple-lumen catheter site prolonged the time of catheter site use in nonseptic critically ill patients. However, it was of no benefit in reducing infection in septic patients and appeared to predispose these patients to fungal colonization and fungemia [262]. As new technologies introduce more effective materials for the manufacture of central venous catheters along with antibiotic bonding to the catheters and catheter cuffs, catheter-related thrombosis and sepsis should continue to decline. Further studies are required to determine the long-term effectiveness and safety of antibiotic bonded catheters and cuffs. These newer devices may allow for less frequent catheter exchanges. However, these will not replace the need for careful surveillance of all catheters and meticulous dressing care of these sites. Safe and efficient central venous access for delivery of parenteral nutrition is crucial. The risks of mechanical and infectious complications can be minimized by adhering to the guidelines outlined above.

Metabolic Complications

The majority of metabolic complications associated with TPN infusion are related to an excess or deficit of fluid, electrolytes, macronutrients, or micronutrients and are potentially avoidable. Despite an increased understanding of the appropriate composition of these solutions, metabolic complications occur in 5% to 10% of patients receiving parenteral nutrition [243].

Fluid, Electrolytes, and Micronutrients

Fluid and electrolyte abnormalities may be due to increased losses followed by inadequate replacement, excessive administration of certain substances, or the inability to excrete those substances (Table 28-5). With a better understanding of the long-term requirements of essential fatty acids, vitamins, and trace elements and the routine infusion of appropriate amounts of these substances, many of the complications of omission are readily avoidable by following standard regimens for replacing these nutrients. Similarly, identification of clinical situations in which certain trace elements and vitamins (i.e., renal or hepatic failure) or lipids (i.e., hyperlipidemia) may accumulate and reach toxic levels are well recognized and readily avoidable by tailoring the parenteral nutrition solutions to meet specific requirements and deficiencies.

Carbohydrate

One of the most common metabolic complications associated with TPN infusion is hyperglycemia, which occurs in up to 25% of patients at some point during the course of treatment. This may be due to excessive administration of glucose to a patient with underlying diabetes mellitus or as a result of glucose intolerance secondary to "insulin resistance" in the setting of stress and/or sepsis. Ongoing hyperglycemia, if unchecked, can lead to a hyperosmolar state with associated osmotic diuresis, hypovolemia, intracellular dehydration, and acidosis. In rare instances this may progress to coma and death (hyperosmolar hyperglycemic nonketotic coma) [263]. Treatment includes decreasing the dextrose concentration in the TPN solution, frequent monitoring of serum glucose levels with administration of subcutaneous insulin, and addition of insulin to the TPN solution as the daily insulin needs are established. Occasionally it is necessary to utilize an insulin drip to control hyperglycemia in particularly resistant cases. It is essential in this setting to establish a stable dosage of insulin and to control the blood sugar prior to advancing the rate of TPN. In the setting of ongoing stress or sepsis, hyperglycemia will be difficult to treat until the underlying cause of glucose intolerance is addressed. In contrast to hyperglycemia, the sudden withdrawal of a hypertonic dextrose TPN solution after prolonged infusion may lead to hypoglycemia. This is most commonly reported in children and can be prevented or treated by avoiding sudden withdrawal of the infusion and by administering a 5% or 10% dextrose solution intravenously whenever the TPN infusion is suddenly withdrawn or interrupted while monitoring the serum glucose level.

Hepatic Toxicity

One of the more significant metabolic complications is hepatic dysfunction [264], which can be a vexing problem in modern surgical practice. In 1971, Peden first described a pattern of centrilobu-

Table 28-5. Fluid and Electrolyte Complications Associated with Parenteral Nutrition Administration

Complication	Etiology	Therapy/Prevention
Volume overload	Administration of required calories in volume not tolerated due to cardiac or renal insufficiency	Increase caloric density of the solution by increasing dextrose and/or lipid concentration
Dehydration	Excessive fluid losses due to vomiting, diarrhea, drain, or fistula output	Accurate replacement of abnormal fluid losses
Hypernatremia	Administration of hyperosmolar solution to patient unable to increase oral intake of free water	Identify patient at risk and provide an adequate amount of free water in the TPN solution
Hyponatremia	Free water overload	Accurate replacement of free water
Hyperkalemia	Excessive administration; renal failure; acidosis	Reduce potassium dosage; correct acidosis
Hypokalemia	GI losses (vomiting, diarrhea, fistula); renal losses (diuretics); alkalosis; increased insulin levels; hypomagnesemia	Monitor levels frequently and replace deficit and ongoing losses; replace Mg if low
Hypochloremia	Excessive vomiting or sustained gastric suction	Monitor and replace
Hypercalcemia	Excessive administration of calcium and/or vitamin D	Reduce amount administered
Hypocalcemia	Osteomalacia; excessive phosphate administration; severe pancreatitis	Monitor ionized calcium levels and replace
Hypermagnesemia	Renal failure	Reduce Mg administration
Hypomagnesemia	Excessive GI losses; anabolism	Monitor and replace
Hyperphosphatemia	Excessive administration; renal failure	Reduce amount administered (lipid emulsions have high phosphorus concentrations)
Hypophosphatemia	Initial refeeding in malnourished; increased renal excretion (alkalosis, hypokalemia, hypomagnesemia, diabetes, steroid and diuretic treatment)	Monitor and replace; with the institution of TPN in malnourished, give 10–15 mmol/L; replace K and Mg if low
Hyperglycemia*	Excessive glucose administration; diabetes mellitus; glucose intolerance due to "insulin resistance" in stress or sepsis	Decrease dextrose concentration in TPN; frequent monitoring and administration of insulin

Key: GI = gastrointestinal; TPN = total parenteral nutrition.
*Occurs in up to 25% of patients at some point during the course of TPN treatment.

lar cholestasis and early cirrhosis in an infant on TPN [265]. Since that time biochemical and morphologic derangements in liver function and structure have been reported in increasing numbers. These abnormalities may include elevations in alkaline phosphatase and transaminases [266], hyperammonemia [267], intracanalicular or intracellular cholestasis [268], and hepatomegaly, usually as a result of fatty infiltration [269]. In some cases, but mostly in children, these abnormalities have progressed to fibrosis, cirrhosis, liver failure, and death [270,271].

The pathogenesis of these hepatic derangements is not clear, although several theories that have been advanced include toxicity of certain free amino acids (i.e., methionine) [272], amino acid imbalance [264], excessive dextrose administration [273], excessive protein administration [274], toxic products in the infusate [266], exposure of TPN solutions to light with photo-oxidation of amino acids [275], route of administration [276], nutrient deficiency [277–281], the relative immaturity of the neonatal biliary excretory system [282], altered gut hormone secretion [283], and lack of intestinal stimulation with gut mucosal atrophy and translocation of bacteria and/or endotoxin across the gut wall [284–288]. None of these theories have gained prominence as the accepted etiology, and it has not been established that one abnormality inevitably progresses to the next [289]. The hepatic toxicity of TPN that is seen clinically appears to be multifactorial in origin. Most patients develop a combination of hepatic steatosis with evidence of cholestasis and abnormalities in liver function. However, hepatic steatosis appears to be the earliest and most frequent histologic change noted. In a rat model of pure hepatic steatosis, it has been demonstrated that insulin and glucagon appear to play a critical role in the development of TPN-associated hepatic steatosis. The development of hepatic steatosis appears to be directly related to increased synthesis of fatty acid and impaired hepatic release of triglyceride, which may be due to an altered ratio of insulin to glucagon. Specifically, an elevated portal venous insulin-glucagon molar ratio appears to be the primary stimulus, and any treatment that lowers this ratio should diminish hepatic steatosis. The infusion of lipid-free TPN in a hypertonic dextrose base leads to an elevated portal venous insulin-glucagon molar ratio and hepatic steatosis in rats [290]. Parenteral administration of a low dose of glucagon prevents and reverses TPN-related hepatic steatosis by lowering the portal insulin-glucagon molar ratio in these animals while not affecting overall glucose metabolism [291,292]. Additionally, in this model parenteral administration of TPN supplemented with L-glutamine or lipid also lowers the insulin-glucagon ratio and prevents hepatic steatosis [82,293]. Because of the uncertain and probable multifactorial etiology of hepatic toxicity, there has been no consistent therapeutic modality accepted for the treatment of hepatic dysfunction except the forced discontinuance of TPN. However, it appears that the clinical treatment of hepatic steatosis during TPN can be safely performed using any one, or a combination, of modalities, without having to discontinue the TPN infusions. Continued clinical corroboration is required to further knowledge of this particularly vexing complication of TPN.

Immunologic Complications

There is a strong association between nutritional depletion and weakening of various measurable immune responses [294–296]. While it is apparent that severely malnourished patients fare better perioperatively when nutritionally repleted, it is less clear whether the added expense and potential morbidity of TPN can be justified in many moderately malnourished patients. Specifically, the effect of parenterally administered protein and energy substrates on immune function in patients who have undergone surgery is unclear. In a study of early TPN in acute pancreatitis, Sax et al. [166] reported a significantly higher rate of catheter-related sepsis than contemporaneous patients without pancreatitis who received TPN. This is similar to a previous study of TPN in pancreatitis in another teaching institution [297]. The authors of these articles speculated that this was related to an immunosuppressive effect of pancreatitis. However, recent reports have implied that parenteral nutrition itself may have an immunosuppressive effect on patients. In the multicenter Veterans Affairs cooperative trial of perioperative TPN [118], there was a higher overall noncatheter-related infection rate in TPN-treated patients. Furthermore, in the moderately malnourished group, this negated any benefit derived from a decrease in noninfectious complications, and no overall benefit is observed in the group receiving parenteral nutrition [118]. Recent animal studies have suggested that lipid-free TPN may adversely affect the cellular immune system. Administration of lipid-free TPN to rats may have immunosuppressive effects via an elevation of splenic macrophage production of PGE_2 in response to endotoxin [298]. High levels of PGE_2 suppress the immune system and increase the activity of T-suppressor cells [299].

Certain nutrients affect the immunocompetence of the host in various ways. For example, certain essential fatty acids (EFAs) are required in minimal amounts for normal immune function, although excessive intake of these EFAs is associated with impaired immune responses [38,111,300]. Small dietary amounts of the ω-6 EFA linoleic acid are required for the normal propagation and maturation of cell-mediated immune response. However, provision of large amounts of linoleic acid can lead to increased synthesis of PGE_2 by the macrophage. In contrast, lipids of the ω-3 series appear to be immunostimulatory [41,301,302]. Other nutrient additives such as glutamine, arginine, and purines appear to improve immune function when administered parenterally and/or enterally [38,56,87,303].

Metabolic Bone Disease

This is a syndrome associated with long-term parenteral nutrition that may present with pathologic fractures or, more commonly, as lower back and extremity pain. The cause is thought to be due to the abnormal metabolism of vitamin D, aluminum, calcium, protein, and glucose [304]. Symptoms related to metabolic bone disease usually subside if vitamin D is withheld or once TPN can be discontinued. However, it may take from months to years for bone remineralization to occur, depending on the duration of TPN and the extent of demineralization.

Hypersensitivity

Although rare, hypersensitivity reactions have been described secondary to TPN infusion. Because of the multicomponent nature of TPN, no single substance can be singled out as causative. In the majority of cases, the multivitamin component of the solution was implicated [305]. All of the components of TPN, including the lipid emulsions [306], dextrose [307], amino acids, electrolytes, and trace elements [308] have been associated with anaphylactoid reactions. In addition, there are multiple trace substances added to the various components that serve as emulsifiers, solubilizers, wetting agents, and antioxidants that are all potential allergens [308,309]. It is obvious that identification of the offending agent can be quite difficult. The best approach in this situation is to obtain expert consultation from an allergist and to begin with a base solution of dextrose only, adding components one by one until the reaction recurs. Once the specific component of the solution is identified, further specification may be required through the use of epicutaneous allergy testing.

References

1. Wilkinson AW. Historical background of intravenous feeding. *Nutr Diets* 5:295, 1963.
2. Rhode CM, et al. Method for continuous intravenous administration of nutritive solutions suitable for prolonged metabolic studies in dogs. *Am J Physiol* 159:409, 1949.
3. Rhoads JE. Diuretics as an adjuvant in disposing of extra water employed as a vehicle in parenteral hyperalimentation. *Fed Proc* 21:389, 1962.
4. Aubaniac R. L'injection intraveineuse sous-claviculaire: Avantages et technique. *Presse Med* 60:1456, 1952.
5. Dudrick SJ, et al. Long-term total parenteral nutrition with growth, development and positive nitrogen balance. *Surgery* 64:134, 1968.
6. Kudsk K, et al. Enteral versus parenteral feeding: Effects on septic morbidity after blunt and penetrating abdominal trauma. *Ann Surg* 215:503, 1992.
7. Cardona MA, et al. Bacterial translocation through intact ileal mucosa in vitro: An active metabolic process. Presented at Surgical Infection Society, Fort Lauderdale, Florida, April 8–10, 1991.
8. Abernathy GB, et al. Efficacy of tube feeding in supplying energy requirements of hospitalized patients. *JPEN* 13:387, 1989.
9. Cataldi-Betcher EL, et al. Complications occuring during enteral nutrition support: A prospective study. *JPEN* 7:546, 1983.
10. Kemper M, Weissman C, Hyman AI. Caloric requirements and supply in critically ill surgical patients. *Crit Care Med* 20:344, 1992.
11. Wagner DR, Elmore MF, Tate JT. Combined parenteral and enteral nutrition in severe trauma. *Nutr Clin Pract* 7:113, 1992.
12. Bower RH, et al. Postoperative enteral vs. parenteral nutrition. *Arch Surg* 121:1040, 1986.
13. Harris JA, Benedict FG. Biometric studies of basal metabolism in man. Carnegie Institute of Washington, Publication #279, 1979.
14. Long CL, et al. Metabolic response to injury and illness: Estimation of energy and protein needs from indirect calorimetry and nitrogen balance. *JPEN* 3:452, 1979.
15. Makk LJK, et al. Clinical application of the metabolic cart to the delivery of total parenteral nutrition. *Crit Care Med* 18:1320, 1990.
16. Weissman C, et al. Resting metabolic rate of critically ill patients: Measured vs. predicted. *Anesthesiology* 64:673, 1986.
17. Hess D, et al. A comparison of four methods of determining caloric requirements of mechanically ventilated patients. *Respir Care* 86:1197, 1986.
18. Branson RD, et al. Measured versus predicted energy expenditure in mechanically ventilated patients with chronic obstructive pulmonary disease. *Respir Care* 32:748, 1987.
19. Bursztein S, et al. *Energy Metabolism, Indirect Calorimetry and Nutrition.* Baltimore: Williams & Wilkins, 1989.
20. Steinhorn DM, et al. Modular indirect calorimeter suitable for long-term measurements in multipatient intensive care units. *Crit Care Med* 19:963, 1991.
21. Westenskow DR, Roberts SE, Pace NL. Evaluation of a replenishment type oxygen consumption monitor. *Crit Care Med* 17:798, 1989.
22. Bower RH, et al. *Protocol for Nutrition Support* (2nd ed). Cincinnati: University of Cincinnati, 1992.
23. Hankeln KB, et al. Use of continuous noninvasive measurement of oxygen consumption in patients with adult respiratory distress syndrome following shock of various etiologies. *Crit Care Med* 19:642, 1991.
24. Nelson LD, Anderson HB, Garcia H. Clinical validation of a new metabolic monitor suitable for use in critically ill patients. *Crit Care Med* 15:951, 1987.
25. Skootsky SA, Abraham E. Continuous oxygen consumption measurement during initial emergency department resuscitation of critically ill patients. *Crit Care Med* 16:706, 1988.
26. Wolfe RR, Allsop J, Burke JF. Glucose metabolism in man: Responses to intravenous glucose infusion. *Metabolism* 28:210, 1979.
27. Askanazi J, et al. Influence of TPN on fuel utilization in injury and sepsis. *Ann Surg* 191:40, 1980.
28. Shangraw RE, et al. Differentiation between septic and postburn insulin resistance. *Metabolism* 38:983, 1989.
29. Jahoor F, et al. Role of insulin and glucose oxidation in mediating the protein catabolism of burns and sepsis. *Am J Physiol* 257:E323, 1989.
30. Long JM III, et al. Fat-carbohydrate interaction: Effects on nitrogen sparing in total intravenous feeding. *Surg Forum* 25:61, 1974.
31. Woolfson AMJ, Healey RV, Allison SP. Insulin to inhibit protein catabolism after injury. *N Engl J Med* 300:14, 1979.
32. Meguid M, et al. Amelioration of metabolic complications of conventional total parenteral nutrition. *Arch Surg* 119:1294, 1984.
33. Nanni G, Siegel JH, Coleman B. Increased lipid fuel dependence in the critically ill septic patient. *J Trauma* 24:14, 1984.
34. Wretlind A. Recollections of pioneers in nutrition: Landmarks in the development of parenteral nutrition. *J Am Coll Nutr* 11:366, 1992.
35. Harvel RJ, Kane JP, Kashyap ML. Interchange of apolipoproteins between chylomicrons and high density lipoproteins during alimentation lipemia in man. *J Clin Invest* 52:32, 1973.
36. Carlsson LA. Studies on the fat emulsion intralipid. I. Association with serum proteins to intralipid trigyceride particles (ITP). *Scand Lab Invest* 40:139, 1980.
37. Kaufmann RL, et al. Defective lipid disposal mechanisms during bacterial infections in rhesus monkeys. *Metabolism* 25:615, 1976.
38. Fischer GW, et al. Diminished bacterial defenses with Intralipid. *Lancet* 2:819, 1980.

39. Hamawy KJ, et al. The effect of lipid emulsions on reticulo-endothelial system function in the injured animal. *JPEN* 9:559, 1985.

40. Trocki O, et al. Effects of fish oil on postburn metabolism and immunity. *JPEN* 11:521, 1987.

41. Alexander JW, et al. The importance of lipid type in the diet after burn injury. *Ann Surg* 204:1, 1986.

42. Nordenstrom J, et al. Metabolic utilization of intravenous fat emulsion during total parenteral nutrition. *Ann Surg* 196:221, 1982.

43. O'Keefe SJ, Sender PM, James WPT. Catabolic loss of body nitrogen in response to surgery. *Lancet* 2:1035, 1974.

44. Clowes GHA, et al. Muscle proteolysis induced by a circulating peptide in patients with sepsis or trauma. *N Engl J Med* 308:545, 1983.

45. Shaw JHF, Wolfe RR. An integrated analysis of glucose, fat and protein metabolism in severely traumatized patients: Studies in the basal state and the response to total parenteral nutrition. *Ann Surg* 209:63, 1989.

46. Larsson J, et al. Nitrogen requirements in severely injured patients. *Br J Surg* 77:413, 1990.

47. Baker JP, et al. Randomized trial of TPN in critically ill patients: Metabolic effects of varying glucose-lipid ratios as the energy source. *Gastroenterology* 87:53, 1984.

48. DeChalain TMB, et al. The effect of fuel source on amino acid metabolism in critically ill patients. *J Surg Res* 52:167, 1992.

49. Paluzzi M, Meguid MA. A prospective, randomized study of the optimal source of nonprotein calories in TPN. *Surgery* 98:717, 1987.

50. Tracey KJ, et al. Protein and substrate metabolism during starvation and parenteral refeeding. *Clin Sci* 74:123, 1988.

51. Cerra FB, et al. Septic autocannibalism, a failure of exogenous nutritional support. *Ann Surg* 192:570, 1980.

52. Long CL, Jeevanaudan M, Kinney JM. Whole body protein synthesis and catabolism in septic man. *Am J Clin Nutr* 30:1340, 1977.

53. Shaw JHF, Wildbore M, Wolfe RR. Whole body protein kinetics in severely septic patients. *Ann Surg* 205:288, 1987.

54. Bower RH. Nutrition and immune function. *Nutr Clin Pract* 5:189, 1990.

55. Oka T, et al. Effect of arginine-enriched total parenteral nutrition on the host-tumor interaction in cancer-bearing rats. *JPEN* 17:375, 1993.

56. Barbul A. Arginine and immune function. *Nutrition* 6:53, 1990.

57. Smith RJ. Glutamine metabolism and its physiologic importance. *JPEN* 14:40, 1990.

58. Krebs H. Glutamine metabolism in the animal body. In J Mora, R Palacios (eds), *Glutamine Metabolism, Enzymology, and Regulation.* New York: Academic, 1980.

59. Bergstrom J, et al. Intracellular free amino acid concentration in human skeletal muscle tissue. *J Appl Physiol* 36:693, 1974.

60. Marliss EB, et al. Muscle and sphlanchnic glutamine and glutamine metabolism in postabsorptive and starved man. *J Clin Invest* 50:814, 1971.

61. Jepson MM, et al. Relationship between glutamine concentration and protein synthesis in rat skeletal muscle. *Am J Physiol* 255:E166, 1988.

62. Rennie MJ, et al. Characteristics of a glutamine carrier in skeletal muscle have important consequences for nitrogen loss in injury, infection, and chronic disease. *Lancet* 2:1008, 1986.

63. MacLennan PA, Brown RA, Rennie MJ. A positive relationship between protein synthetic rate and intracellular glutamine concentration in perfused rat skeletal muscle. *FEBS Lett* 215:187, 1987.

64. Smith RJ. Regulation of protein degradation in differentiated skeletal muscle cell in monolayer culture. In EA Khairallah, SJ Bond, JWC Bird (eds), *Intracellular Protein Catabolism: Progress in Clinical and Biochemical Research.* New York: Liss, 1984.

65. Katz J, Golden S, Wals PA. Stimulation of hepatic glycogen synthesis by amino acids. *Proc Natl Acad Sci USA* 73:3433, 1976.

66. Newsholme EA, Crabtree B, Ardawi MSM. Glutamine metabolism in lymphocytes: its biochemical, physiological, and clinical importance. *Quart J Exp Physiol* 70:473, 1985.

67. Bode B, et al. Characteristics and regulation of hepatic glutamine transport. *JPEN* 14:51, 1990.

68. Souba WW, et al. Gut glutamine metabolism. *JPEN* 14:45, 1990.

69. Inoue Y, et al. Effect of total parenteral nutrition on amino acid and glucose transport by the human small intestine. *Ann Surg* 217:604, 1993.

70. Klimberg VS, et al. Glutamine-enriched total parenteral nutrition supports gut metabolism. *Surg Forum* 40:175, 1989.

71. Salloum RM, et al. Selective stimulation of brush border glutamine transport in the tumor-bearing rat. *J Surg Res* 50:391, 1991.

72. Pinkus LM, Windmueller HG. Phosphate-dependent glutaminase of small intestine and localization and role in intestinal glutamine metabolism. *Arch Biochem Biophys* 182:506, 1977.

73. Higashiguchi T, et al. Effect of glutamine on protein synthesis in isolated intestinal epithelial cells. *JPEN* 17:307, 1993.

74. Hèussinger D. Liver glutamine metabolism. *JPEN* 14:56, 1990.

75. Kaiser S, Gerok W, Hèussinger D. Ammonia and glutamine metabolism in human liver slices: New aspects of the pathogenesis of hyperammonemia in chronic liver disease. *Eur J Clin Invest* 18:535, 1988.

76. Hwang TL, et al. Preservation of small bowel mucosa using glutamine-enriched parenteral nutrition. *Surg Forum* 38:56, 1987.

77. Grant J. Use of L-glutamine in total parenteral nutrition. *J Surg Res* 44:506, 1988.

78. Jacobs DO, et al. Combined effects of glutamine and epidermal growth factors (EGF) on GI mucosal cellularity. *Surgery* 104:358, 1988.

79. Inoue Y, Grant JP, Snyder PJ. Effect of glutamine-supplemented total parenteral nutrition on recovery of the small intestine after starvation atrophy. *JPEN* 17:165, 1993.

80. Platell C, et al. The influence of parenteral glutamine and branched chain amino acids on total parenteral nutrition-induced atrophy of the gut. *JPEN* 17:348, 1993.

81. van der Hulst RW, et al. Glutamine and the preservation of gut integrity. *Lancet* 341:1363, 1993.

82. Li S, et al. Addition of L-glutamine to total parenteral nutrition (TPN) and its effect on portal insulin and glucagon and the development of hepatic steatosis in rats. *J Surg Res* 48:421, 1990.

83. Tamada H, et al. Alanyl glutamine-enriched total parenteral nutrition restores intestinal adaptation after either

proximal or distal massive resection in rats. *JPEN* 17:236, 1993.

84. Frankel WL, et al. Glutamine enhancement of structure and function in transplanted small intestine in the rat. *JPEN* 17:47, 1993.
85. Ardawi MM, Newsholme EA. Glutamine metabolism in lymphocytes of the rat. *Biochem J* 212:835, 1983.
86. Inoue Y, Grant JP, Snyder PJ. Effect of glutamine-supplemented intravenous nutrition on survival after *Escherichia coli*-induced peritonitis. *JPEN* 17:41, 1993.
87. Burke D, et al. Glutamine-supplemented TPN improved gutimmune function. *Arch Surg* 124:1396, 1989.
88. Alverdy JC. Effects of glutamine-supplemented diets on immunology of the gut. *JPEN* 14:109, 1990.
89. Schloerb PR, Amare M. Total parenteral nutrition with glutamine in bone marrow transplantation and other clinical applications (a randomized, double-blind study). *JPEN* 17:407, 1993.
90. Ziegler TR, et al. Clinical and metabolic efficiency of glutamine-supplemented parenteral nutrition after bone marrow transplantation: A randomized, double-blind, controlled study. *Ann Intern Med* 116:821, 1992.
91. Young LS, et al. Patients receiving glutamine-supplemented intravenous feedings report an improvement in mood. *JPEN* 17:422, 1993.
92. Stehle P, et al. Effect of parenteral glutamine peptide supplements on muscle glutamine loss and nitrogen balance after major surgery. *Lancet* 1:231, 1989.
93. Hammarqvist F, Wernerman et al. Addition of glutamine to total parenteral nutrition after elective surgery spares free glutamine in muscle, counteracts the fall in muscle protein synthesis, and improves nitrogen balance. *Ann Surg* 209:455, 1989.
94. Hilton MA, et al. Use of stable peptide gamma-L-glutamyl-L-tyrosine as an intravenous source of tyrosine in mice. *Metab Clin Exp* 40:634, 1991.
95. Radmacher PG, et al. Use of soluble peptide gamma-L-glutamyl-L-tyrosine to provide tyrosine in total parenteral nutrition in rats. *JPEN* 17:337, 1993.
96. Vazquez JA, Daniel H, Adibi SA. Dipeptides in parenteral nutrition: From basic science to clinical applications. *Nutr Clin Pract* 8:95, 1993.
97. Albers S, et al. Availability of amino acids supplied intravenously in healthy humans as synthetic dipeptides: Kinetic evaluation of L-alanyl-L-glutamine and glycyl-L-tyrosine. *Clin Sci* 75:463, 1988.
98. Abumrad NN, et al. Possible sources of glutamine for parenteral nutrition: Impact on glutamine metabolism. *Am J Physiol* 257:E228, 1989.
99. Hübl W, et al. Influence of molecular structure and plasma hydrolysis on the metabolism of glutamine containing dipeptides in humans. *Metabolism* 38:9, 1989.
100. Krzysik BA, Adibi SA. Cytoplasmic dipeptidase activities of kidney, ileum, liver, muscle, and blood. *Am J Physiol* 233:E450, 1977.
101. Lochs H, et al. Glycylglutamine: Metabolism and effects on organ balances of amino acids in postabsorptive and starved subjects. *Am J Physiol* 262:E155, 1992.
102. Lochs H, et al. Splanchnic, renal, and muscle clearance of alanyl-glutamine in humans and organ fluxes of alanine and glutamine when infused in free peptide forms. *Metabolism* 39:833, 1990.
103. Iijima S, et al. Intravenous administration of nucleosides and a nucleotide mixture diminishes intestinal mucosal atrophy induced by total parenteral nutrition. *JPEN* 17:265, 1993.
104. Mascioli EA, et al. Enhanced survival to endotoxin in guinea pigs fed IV fish oil emulsion. *Lipids* 23:623, 1988.
105. Pomposelli JJ, et al. Short-term TPN containing ω-3 fatty acids ameliorate lactic acidosis induced by endotoxin in guinea pigs. *Am J Clin Nutr* 52:548, 1990.
106. Albina JE, Gladden P, Walsh WR. Detrimental effects of an ω-3 fatty acid-enriched diet on wound healing. *JPEN* 17:519, 1993
107. Mingrone G, et al. Kinetics and thermogenesis of medium-chain monocarboxylic and dicarboxylic acids in man: Sebacate and medium-chain triglycerides. *JPEN* 17:257, 1993.
108. Bach AC, Babyan UK. Medium-chain triglycerides: An update. *Am J Clin Nutr* 36:950, 1982.
109. Senior JR. *Medium-Chain Triglycerides.* Philadelphia: University of Pennsylvania Press, 1968.
110. Jiang ZM, et al. A comparison of medium-chain and long-chain triglycerides in surgical patients. *Ann Surg* 217:175, 1993.
111. Sobrado J, et al. Lipid emulsions and reticuloendothelial system function in healthy and burned guinea pigs. *Am J Clin Nutr* 42:855, 1985.
112. Drews D, Schluter MD, Stein TP. Glycerol kinetics with parenteral lipid emulsions (long-chain triglycerides, medium-chain triglycerides, and structured lipids) in rats. *Metabolism* 42: 743, 1993.
113. Gollaher CJ, et al. The effect of increasing levels of fish oil-containing structured triglycerides on protein metabolism in parenterally fed rats stressed by burn plus endotoxin. *JPEN* 17:247, 1993.
114. Mochizuki H, et al. Optimal content for enteral diets following thermal injury. *JPEN* 8:638, 1984.
115. Ling PR, et al. Structured lipid made from fish oil and medium-chain triglycerides alters tumor and host metabolism in Yoshida-sarcoma-bearing rats. *Am J Clin Nutr* 53:1177, 1991.
116. Sandström R, et al. Structured triglycerides to postoperative patients: A safety and tolerance study. *JPEN* 17:153, 1993.
117. Roulet M, et al. Effects of intravenously infused egg phospholipids on lipid and lipoprotein metabolism in postoperative trauma. *JPEN* 17:107, 1993.
118. Buzby GP, et al (The Veterans Affairs Total Parenteral Nutrition Cooperative Study Group). Perioperative total parenteral nutrition in surgical patients. *N Engl J Med* 325:525, 1991.
119. Campos ACL, Meguid MM. A critical appraisal of the usefulness of perioperative nutritional support. *Am J Clin Nutr* 55:117, 1992.
120. McGeer AJ, Detsky AS, O'Rourke K. Parenteral nutrition in cancer patients undergoing chemotherapy: A meta-analysis. *Nutrition* 6:233, 1990.
121. Cuthbertson DP, Shaw GB, Young FG. The anterior pituitary gland and protein metabolism. II. The influence of anterior pituitary extracts on the metabolic response of the rat to injury. *J Endocrinol* 2:468, 1941.
122. Wilmore DW, et al. Anabolic effects of human growth hormone and high caloric feeding following thermal injury. *Surg Gynecol Obstet* 138:875, 1974.
123. Hammarqvist F, et al. Biosynthetic human growth hormone preserves both muscle protein synthesis and the decrease in muscle-free glutamine, and improves whole body nitrogen economy after operation. *Ann Surg* 216:184, 1992.
124. Jiang Z-M, et al. Low-dose growth hormone and hypocalo-

ric nutrition attenuate the protein-catabolic response after major operation. *Ann Surg* 210:513, 1989.

125. Ponting GA, et al. Postoperative positive nitrogen balance with intravenous hyponutrition and growth hormone. *Lancet* 2:438, 1988.

126. Ward HC, et al. Protein and energy metabolism with biosynthetic human growth hormone after gastrointestinal surgery. *Ann Surg* 206:56, 1987.

127. Ponting GA, et al. Protein and energy metabolism with biosynthetic human growth hormone in patients on full intravenous nutritional support. *JPEN* 14:437, 1990.

128. Ziegler TR, et al. Recombinant human growth hormone enhances the metabolic efficacy of parenteral nutrition: A double-blind, randomized controlled study. *J Clin Endocrinol Metab* 74:865, 1992.

129. Ziegler TR, et al. Use of growth hormone combined with nutritional support in a critical care unit. *JPEN* 14:574, 1990.

130. Koea JB, et al. Growth hormone therapy initiated before starvation ameliorates the catabolic state and enhances the protein-sparing effect of total parenteral nutrition. *Br J Surg* 80:740, 1993.

131. Byrne TA, et al. Anabolic therapy with growth hormone accelerates protein gain in surgical patients requiring nutritional rehabilitation. *Ann Surg* 218:400, 1993.

132. Vara-Thorbeck R, et al. Exogenous growth hormone: Effects on the catabolic response to surgically produced acute stress and on postoperative immune function. *World J Surg* 17:530, 1993.

133. Rudman D, et al. Elemental balances during intravenous hyperalimentation of underweight adult subject. *J Clin Invest* 55:94, 1975.

134. Kay RG, et al. A syndrome of acute zinc deficiency during total parenteral hyperalimentation in man. *Ann Surg* 183:331, 1976.

135. Karpel JT, Peden VH. Copper deficiency in long-term parenteral nutrition. *J Pediatr* 80:32, 1972.

136. Pulmissano DJ. Nutrient deficiencies after intensive parenteral alimentation. *N Engl J Med* 291:799, 1974.

137. Vilter RW, et al. Manifestations of copper deficiency in a patient with systemic sclerosis on intravenous hyperalimentation. *N Engl J Med* 291:188, 1974.

138. Mertz W. Chromium in human nutrition: A review. *J Nutr* 123:626, 1993.

139. Guidelines for essential trace element preparations for parenteral use: A statement by the Nutrition Advisory Group. *JPEN* 8:263, 1979.

140. Burk RF. Protection against free radical injury by selenoenzymes. *Pharmacol Ther* 45:383, 1990.

141. Kien C, Ganther HE. Manifestations of chronic selenium deficiency in a child receiving total parenteral nutrition. *Am J Clin Nutr* 37:319, 1983.

142. Hunt DR, et al. Selenium depletion in burn patients. *JPEN* 8:695, 1984.

143. Dworkin BM, et al. Selenium deficiency in the acquired immunodeficiency syndrome. *JPEN* 10:405, 1986.

144. Dworkin BM, et al. Low blood selenium levels in alcoholics with and without advanced liver disease. *Dig Dis Sci* 30:838, 1985.

145. Multivitamin preparations for parenteral use: A statement by the Nutrition Advisory Group. *JPEN* 3:258, 1979.

146. Green HL, et al. Guidelines for the use of vitamins, trace elements, calcium, magnesium, and phosphorus in infants and children receiving total parenteral nutrition: Report of the Subcommittee on Pediatric Parenteral Nutrient Requirements from the Committee on Clinical Practice Issues of the American Society for Clinical Nutrition. *Am J Clin Nutr* 48:1324, 1988.

147. Bower RH. Nutrition for critically ill patients. In JL Cameron (ed), *Current Surgical Therapy.* St. Louis: Mosby, 1992.

148. American Society for Parenteral and Enteral Nutrition (ASPEN). Guidelines for use of total parenteral nutrition in the hospitalized adult patient. *JPEN* 10:441, 1986.

149. Soeters PB, Ebeid AM, Fischer JE. Review of 404 patients with gastrointestinal fistulas: Impact of parenteral nutrition. *Ann Surg* 190:189, 1979.

150. Fischer JE. The management of gastrointestinal fistulae. *Contemp Surg* 29:104, 1981.

151. Kuvshinoff BW, et al. Serum transferrin as a prognostic indicator of spontaneous closure and mortality in gastrointestinal cutaneous fistulas. *Ann Surg* 217:615, 1993.

152. Donaldson SS, Lenon RA. Alterations of nutritional status: Impact of chemotherapy and radiation therapy. *Cancer* 43:2036, 1979.

153. Weisdorf SA, et al. Positive effect of prophylactic total parenteral nutrition on long-term outcome of bone marrow transplantation. *Transplantation* 43:833, 1987.

154. Institute of Medicine. *Nutrition During Pregnancy.* Washington, DC: National Academy Press, 1990.

155. Abel RM, et al. Adverse hemodynamic and ultrastructural changes in dog hearts subjected to protein-calorie malnutrition. *Am Heart J* 97:733, 1979.

156. Freund HR, et al. The effect of branched chain amino acids on systolic properties of the normal and septic isolated rat heart. *Arch Surg* 120:483, 1985.

157. Lolley DM, et al. Reduction of intraoperative myocardial infarction by means of exogenous anaerobic substrate enhancement: Prospective randomized study. *Ann Thorac Surg* 26:515, 1978.

158. Meguid MM, Muscaritoli M. Current uses of total parenteral nutrition. *Am Fam Phys* 47:383, 1993.

159. Begin ME, Das UN. A deficiency in dietary gamma-linoleic and/or eicosapantaenoic acids may determine individual susceptibility to AIDS. *Med Hypoth* 20:1, 1986.

160. Task Force on Nutritional Support in AIDS: Guidelines for nutritional support in AIDS. *Nutrition* 5:39, 1989.

161. Mullen JL, et al. Ten years experience with intravenous hyperalimentation and inflammatory bowel disease. *Ann Surg* 187:523, 1978.

162. Reilly J, et al. Hyperalimentation in inflammatory bowel disease. *Am J Surg* 131:192, 1976.

163. ASPEN Board of Directors. Guidelines for the use of parenteral and enteral nutrition in adult and pediatric patients: Nutrition support for adults with specific diseases and conditions. *JPEN* 17:12, 1993.

164. McIntyre PB, et al. Controlled trial of bowel rest in the treatment of severe acute colitis. *Gut* 27:481, 1986.

165. Kirby DF, Craig RM. The value of intensive nutritional support in pancreatitis. *JPEN* 9:353, 1985.

166. Sax HC, et al. Early total parenteral nutrition in acute pancreatitis: Lack of beneficial effects. *Am J Surg* 153:117, 1987.

167. Kalfarentzos FE, et al. Total parenteral nutrition in severe acute pancreatitis. *J Am Coll Nutr* 10:156, 1991.

168. Daly JM, Dudrick SJ, Copeland EM. Evaluation of nutritional indices as prognostic indicators in the cancer patient. *Cancer* 43:925, 1979.

169. DeWys WE, et al. Prognostic effect of weight loss prior to chemotherapy in cancer patients. *Am J Med* 69:491, 1980.

170. Heys SD, et al. Stimulation of protein synthesis in human tumours by parenteral nutrition: Evidence for modulation of tumour growth. *Br J Surg* 78:483, 1991.

171. Rossi-Fanelli F, et al. Effect of energy substrate manipulation on tumor cell proliferation in parenterally fed cancer patients. *Clin Nutr* 10:228, 1991.

172. Westin T, et al. Tumor cytokinetic response to total parenteral nutrition in patients with head and neck cancers. *Am J Clin Nutr* 53:764, 1991.

173. De Cicco M, et al. Parenteral nutrition in cancer patients receiving chemotherapy: effects on toxicity and nutritional status. *JPEN* 17:513, 1993.

174. Long JM III, et al. Effect of carbohydrate and fat intake on nitrogen excretion during total intravenous feeding. *Ann Surg* 185:417, 1977.

175. Burke JF, et al. Glucose requirements following burn injury: Parameters of optimal glucose infusion and possible hepatic and respiratory abnormalities following excessive glucose uptake. *Ann Surg* 190:274, 1979.

176. Douglas RG, Shaw JHF. Metabolic response to sepsis and trauma. *Br J Surg* 76:115, 1989.

177. Long CL. Fuel preferences in the septic patient; glucose or lipid. *JPEN* 11:333, 1987.

178. Borah MF, et al. Nitrogen balance during intermittent dialysis therapy of uremia. *Kidney Int* 14:491, 1978.

179. Wolfson M, Jones MR, Kopple JD. Amino acid losses during hemodialysis with infusion of amino acids and glucose. *Kidney Int* 21:500, 1982.

180. Horl WH, Heidland A. Evidence for the participation of granulocyte proteinases on intradialytic catabolism. *Clin Nephrol* 21:314, 1984.

181. Abel RM, et al. Improved survival from acute renal failure after treatment with intravenous essential L-amino acids and glucose: Results of a prospective double-blind study. *N Engl J Med* 288:695, 1973.

182. Abel RM, et al. Amino acid metabolism in acute renal failure: Influence of intravenous essential L-amino acid hyperalimentation therapy. *Ann Surg* 180:350, 1974.

183. Feinstein EI, et al. Clinical and metabolic responses to parenteral nutrition in acute renal failure. A controlled double-blind study. *Medicine* 60:124, 1981.

184. Mirtallo J, et al. A comparison of essential and general amino acid infusions in the nutritional support of patients with compromised renal function. *JPEN* 5:109, 1982.

185. Paganini EP. Continuous replacement modalities in acute renal dysfunction. In EP Paganini (ed), *Acute Continuous Renal Replacement Therapy*. Boston: Martinus Nijhoff, 1986.

186. Paganini EP, et al. Amino acid balance in patients with oliguric acute renal failure undergoing slow continuous ultrafiltration (SCUF). *Trans Am Soc Artif Intern Organs* 28:615, 1982.

187. Kramer P, et al. Arteriovenous hemofiltration: A new simple method for treatment of overhydrated patients resistant to diuretics. *Klin Wochenschr* 55:121, 1977.

188. Kaplan AA, Longnecker RE, Folkert VW. Continuous arteriovenous hemofiltration: A report of six months experience. *Ann Intern Med* 310:358, 1984.

189. Kramer P, et al. Intensive potential of continuous arteriovenous hemofiltration. *Trans Am Soc Artif Intern Organs* 28:28, 1982.

190. Feinstein EI, et al. Nutritional hemodialysis. In K Atsumi, M, Maekawa, K Ota (eds), *Progress in Artificial Organs*. Cleveland: ISAO Press, 1984.

191. Geronemus R, Schneider N. Continuous arteriovenous hemodialysis: A new modality for treatment of acute renal failure. *Trans Am Soc Artif Intern Organs* 30:610, 1984.

192. Sigler M, Teehan BP. Solute transport in continuous hemodialysis: A new treatment for acute renal failure. *Kidney Int* 32:562, 1987.

193. James JH, et al. Hyperammonemia, plasma amino acid imbalance, and blood-brain amino acid transport: A unified theory of portal-systemic encephalopathy. *Lancet* 2:772, 1979.

194. Fischer JE, et al. The effect of normalization of plasma amino acids on hepatic encephalopathy in man. *Surgery* 80:77, 1976.

195. Naylor CD, et al. Parenteral nutrition with branched-chain amino acids in hepatic encephalopathy: A meta-analysis. *Gastroenterology* 97:1033, 1989.

196. Cerra FB, et al. Disease-specific amino acid infusion (FO80) in hepatic encephalopathy: A prospective, randomized, double-blind, controlled trial. *JPEN* 9:288, 1985.

197. Driver AG, LeBrun M. Iatrogenic malnutrition in patients receiving ventilatory support. *JAMA* 244:2195, 1980.

198. Hunter AMB, Carey MA, Larsh HN. The nutritional status of patients with chronic obstructive pulmonary disease. *Am Rev Respir Dis* 124:376, 1981.

199. Edelman NH, Rucker RB, Peavy HH. Nutrition and the respiratory system. *Am Rev Respir Dis* 134:347, 1986.

200. Gertz I, et al. Muscle metabolism in patients with chronic obstructive lung disease and acute respiratory failure. *Clin Sci Mol Med* 52:395, 1977.

201. Rochester DF. Body weight and respiratory muscle function in chronic obstructive pulmonary disease. *Am Rev Respir Dis* 134:646, 1986.

202. Thurlbeck WM. Diaphragm and body weight emphysema. *Thorax* 33:483, 1978.

203. Wilson DO, Rogers RM, Hoffman RM. Nutrition and chronic lung disease. *Am Rev Respir Dis* 132:1347, 1985.

204. Faridy EE. Effect of food and water deprivation on surface activity of lungs of rats. *J Appl Physiol* 29:493, 1970.

205. Sahebjami H, Vassallo CL, Wirman JA. Lung mechanics and ultrastructure in prolonged starvation. *Am Rev Respir Dis* 117:77, 1978.

206. Askanazi J, et al. Effect of protein intake on ventilatory drive. *Anesthesiology* 60:106, 1984.

207. Zwillich CW, Sahn SA, Weil JV. Effects of hypermetabolism upon respiratory gas exchange in normal man. *J Clin Invest* 66:900, 1977.

208. Takala J. Branched chain amino acids and respiratory function in man. In JM Kinney, PR Borum (eds), *Perspectives in Clinical Nutrition*. Baltimore/Munich: Urban & Schwarzenberg, 1989.

209. Rodriguez JL, et al. Ventilatory and metabolic effects of glucose infusions. *Chest* 88:512, 1985.

210. Askanazi J, et al. Respiratory changes induced by large glucose loads of total parenteral nutrition. *JAMA* 243:1444, 1980.

211. Freund HR. Nutritional support in cardiac and pulmonary diseases. In JE Fischer (ed): *Total Parenteral Nutrition* (2nd ed). Boston: Little, Brown, 1991.

212. Talpers SS, et al. Nutritionally associated increased carbon dioxide production: Excess total calories vs. high proportion of carbohydrate calories. *Chest* 102:551, 1992.

213. Bahrami S, et al. Mechanical properties of the lungs of post-traumatic rats are improved by including fat in total parenteral nutrition. *JPEN* 11:560, 1987.

214. Robin AP, et al. Influence of parenteral carbohydrate on fat oxidation in surgical patients. *Surgery* 95:608, 1984.

215. Ko KK, Paradise RR. The effects of substrate on contractility of rat atria depressed with halothane. *Anesthesiology* 31:532, 1969.

216. Abel RM, Subramaniam VA, Gay WA Jr. Effects of an intravenous amino acid nutrient solution on left ventricular contractility in dogs. *J Surg Res* 23:201, 1977.

217. Farah AE, Alousi AA. The actions of insulin on cardiac contractility. *Life Sci* 29:975, 1981.

218. Kao RL, et al. The effect of insulin and anoxia on the metabolism of isolated mature rat cardiac myocytes. *Arch Biochem Biophys* 203:587, 1980.

219. Markovitz LJ, Hasin Y, Freund HR. The effect of insulin and glucagon on systolic properties of the normal and septic isolated rat heart. *Basic Res Cardiol* 80:377, 1985.

220. Freund HR, Ryan JA, Fischer JE. Amino acid derangements in patients with sepsis. *Ann Surg* 188:423, 1978.

221. O'Dwyer ST, et al Maintenance of small bowel mucosa with glutamine-enriched parenteral nutrition. *JPEN* 13:579, 1989.

222. Deitch EA, et al. The gut as a portal of entry for bacteremia. *Ann Surg* 205:681, 1987.

223. Bower RH, Kern K, Fischer JE. Use of branched chain amino acid enriched solutions in patients under metabolic stress. *Am J Surg* 149:266, 1985.

224. Johnson DJ, et al. Branched chain amino acid uptake and muscle free amino acid concentrations predict postoperative muscle nitrogen balance. *Ann Surg* 204:513, 1986.

225. McCauley R, et al. The influence of branched chain amino acid infusions on wound healing. *Aust NZ J Surg* 60:471, 1990.

226. Platell C, et al. Influence of glutamine and branched chain amino acids on the jejunal atrophy associated with parenteral nutrition. *J Gastroenterol Hepatol* 6:345, 1991.

227. Teasley KM, Buss RL. Do parenteral nutrition solutions enriched with high concentrations of branched chain amino acids offer significant benefits to stressed patients? *Ann Pharmacol* 23:411, 1989.

228. Bower RH, et al. Branched chain amino acid-enriched solutions in the septic patient: A randomized, prospective trial. *Ann Surg* 203:13, 1986.

229. Cerra FB, et al. The effect of stress level, amino acid formula, and nitrogen dose on nitrogen retention in traumatic and septic stress. *Ann Surg* 205:282, 1987.

230. Sandstedt S, Jorfeldt L, Larsson J. Randomized, controlled study evaluating effects of branched chain amino acids and alpha-ketoisocaproate on protein metabolism after surgery. *Br J Surg* 79:217, 1992.

231. von Meyenfeldt MF, et al. Effect of branched chain amino acid enrichment of total parenteral nutrition on nitrogen sparing and clinical outcome of sepsis and trauma: A prospective randomized double blind trial. *Br J Surg* 77:924, 1990.

232. Lehmann SL, et al. Growth hormone enables effective nutrition by peripheral vein in postoperative patients: A pilot study. *J Am Coll Nutr* 9:610, 1990.

233. Payne-James JJ, Khawaja HT. First choice for total parenteral nutrition: The peripheral route. *JPEN* 17:468, 1993.

234. Khawaja HT, Williams JD, Weaver PC. Transdermal glyceryl trinitrate to allow peripheral total parenteral nutrition: A double-blind placebo controlled feasibility study. *J Royal Soc Med* 84:69, 1991.

235. Payne-James JJ, et al. Topical nonsteroidal anti-inflammatory gel for the prevention of peripheral vein thrombophlebitis. *Anaesthesia* 47:324, 1992.

236. Rombeau J, Rolandelli R, Wilmore DW. Nutritional support. In DW Wilmore, et al (eds). *Care of the Surgical Patient.* New York: Scientific American, 1989.

237. Nehme AE. Nutritional support of the hospitalized patient: The team concept. *JAMA* 243:1906, 1980.

238. DiConstanzo J, et al. Mechanism of thrombogenesis during total parenteral nutrition: Role of catheter composition. *JPEN* 12:190, 1988.

239. Linder LE, et al. Material thrombogenicity in central venous catheterization: A comparison between soft, antebrachial catheters of silicone elastomer and polyurethane. *JPEN* 8:399, 1984.

240. Borrow M, Crowley JG. Evaluation of central venous catheter thrombogenicity. *Acta Anesth Scand* 81:59, 1985.

241. Crocker KS, et al. Clinical evaluation of elastomeric hydrogel peripheral catheters during home infusion therapy. *J Intraven Nursing* 13:89, 1990.

242. Goldmann DA, Maki DG. Infection control in total parenteral nutrition. *JAMA* 223:1360, 1973.

243. Wolfe BM, et al. Complications of parenteral nutrition. *Am J Surg* 152:93, 1986.

244. Ryan JA Jr, et al. Catheter complications in total parenteral nutrition: A prospective study of 200 consecutive patients. *N Engl J Med* 290:757, 1974.

245. McCarthy MC, et al. Prospective evaluation of single and triple lumen catheters in total parenteral nutrition. *JPEN* 11:259, 1987.

246. Pemberton LB, et al. Sepsis from triple- vs. single-lumen catheters during total parenteral nutrition in surgical or critically ill patients. *Arch Surg* 121:591, 1986.

247. Gil RT, et al. Triple- vs. single-lumen central venous catheters. *Arch Int Med* 149:1139, 1989.

248. Horowitz HW, et al. Central catheter-related infections: Comparison of pulmonary artery catheters and triple lumen catheters for the delivery of hyperalimentation in a critical care setting. *JPEN* 14:588, 1990.

249. Johnson BH, Rypins EB. Single-lumen vs. double-lumen catheters for total parenteral nutrition. *Arch Surg* 125:990, 1990.

250. Kelly CS, et al. Sepsis due to triple lumen central venous catheters. *Surg Gynecol Obstet* 163:14, 1986.

251. Lee RB, Buckner M, Sharp KW. Do multi-lumen catheters increase central venous catheter sepsis compared to single-lumen catheters? *J Trauma* 28:1472, 1988.

252. Armstrong CW, et al. Prospective study of catheter replacement and other risk factors for infection of hyperalimentation catheters. *J Infect Dis* 154:808, 1986.

253. Newsome HHJ, et al. Mechanical complications from insertion of subclavian venous feeding catheters: Comparison of de novo percutaneous venipuncture to change of catheter over guidewire. *JPEN* 8:560, 1984.

254. Graeve AH, Carpenter CM, Schiller WR. Management of central venous catheters using a wire introducer. *Am J Surg* 142:752, 1981.

255. Olson ME, et al. Evaluation of strategies for central catheter replacement. *Crit Care Med* 20:797, 1992.

256. Pettigrew RA, et al. Catheter-related sepsis in patients on intravenous nutrition: A prospective study of quantitative catheter cultures and guidewire changes for suspected sepsis. *Br J Surg* 72:52, 1985.

257. Pomp A, et al. Catheter-related sepsis: Single lumen catheters vs. triple lumen catheters [Abstract]. *JPEN* 12:23, 1988.

258. Kamal GD, Pfaller MA, Rempe LE, et al. Reduced intravascular catheter infection by antibiotic bonding: A prospective, randomized, controlled trial. *JAMA* 265:2364, 1991.

259. Maki DG, et al. An attachable silver-impregnated cuff for prevention of infection with central venous catheters: A prospective randomized multicenter trial. *Am J Med* 85:307, 1988.

260. Trooskin SZ, et al. Prevention of catheter sepsis by antibiotic bonding. *Surgery* 97:547, 1985.

261. Bach A, et al. Prevention of catheter-related infections by antiseptic bonding. *J Surg Res* 55:640, 1993.

262. Norwood S, Hajjar G, Jenkins L. The influence of an attachable subcutaneous cuff for preventing triple lumen catheter infections in critically ill surgical and trauma patients. *Surg Gynecol Obstet* 175:33, 1992.

263. McCurdy DK. Hyperosmolar hyperglycemic nonketotic diabetic coma. *Med Clin N Am* 54:683, 1970.

264. Sheldon GF, Petersen SR, Sanders R. Hepatic dysfunction during hyperalimentation. *Arch Surg* 113:504, 1978.

265. Peden VH, Witzelben CL, Skelton MA. Total parenteral nutrition [Letter]. *J Pediatr* 78:180, 1971.

266. Grant JP, et al. Serum hepatic enzyme and bilirubin elevations during parenteral nutrition. *Surg Gynecol Obstet* 145:573, 1977.

267. Touloukian RG, Seashore JH. Hepatic secretory obstruction with total parenteral nutrition in the infant. *J Pediatr Surg* 10:353, 1975.

268. Postuma R, Trevenen CL. Liver disease in infants receiving total parenteral nutrition. *Pediatrics* 63:110, 1979.

269. Tulikoura I, Huikuri K. Morphological fatty changes and function of the liver, serum free fatty acids and triglycerides during parenteral nutrition. *Scand J Gastroenterol* 17:177, 1982.

270. Cohen C, Olsen MM. Pediatric total parenteral nutrition: Liver histopathology. *Arch Pathol Lab Med* 105:152, 1981.

271. Dahms BB, Halpin TC. Serial liver biopsies in parenteral nutrition-associated cholestasis of early infancy. *Gastroenterology* 81:136, 1981.

272. Moss RL, et al. Hepatobiliary dysfunction during total parenteral nutrition is caused by infusate, not the route of administration. *J Ped Surg* 28:391, 1993.

273. Burke JF, et al. Glucose requirements following burn injury. *Ann Surg* 190:274, 1979.

274. Messing B, et al. Chronic cholestasis and macronutrient excess in patients treated with prolonged parenteral nutrition. *Nutrition* 8:30, 1992.

275. Bhatia J, Rivera et al. Hepatic function during short-term total parenteral nutrition: Effect of exposure of parenteral nutrients to light. *Res Commum Chem Pathol Pharmacol* 78:321, 1992.

276. King WWK, et al. Nutritional efficacy and hepatic changes during intragastric, intravenous, and prehepatic feeding in rats. *JPEN* 7:443, 1983.

277. Buchman AL, et al. Lecithin increases plasma free choline and decreases hepatic steatosis in long-term total parenteral nutrition patients. *Gastroenterology* 102:1363, 1992.

278. Cooper A, et al. Taurine deficiency in the severe hepatic deficiency complicating total parenteral nutrition. *J Pediatr Surg* 19:462, 1984.

279. Keim NL, Mares-Perlman JA. Development of hepatic steatosis and essential fatty acid deficiency in rats with hypercaloric, fat-free parenteral nutrition. *J Nutr* 114: 1807, 1984.

280. Lombardi B, Ugazio G, Raick AN. Choline deficiency fatty liver: Relation of plasma phospholipids to liver triglycerides. *Am J Physiol* 210:31, 1966.

281. Sidransky H, Clark S. Chemical pathology of acute amino acid deficiencies. *Arch Pathol* 72:468, 1961.

282. Quigley EMM, et al. Hepatobiliary complications of total parenteral nutrition. *Gastroenterology* 104:286, 1993.

283. Doty JE, et al. Cholecystokinin prophylaxis of parenteral nutrition-induced gallbladder disease. *Ann Surg* 201:76, 1985.

284. Alverdy JC, Aoys E, Moss GS. Total parenteral nutrition promotes bacterial translocation from the gut. *Surgery* 104:185, 1988.

285. Capron JP, et al. Metronidazole in prevention of cholestasis associated with total parenteral nutrition. *Lancet* 1:446, 1983.

286. Drenick EJ, Fisler J, Johnson D. Hepatic steatosis after intestinal bypass: Prevention and reversal by metronidazole, irrespective of protein calorie malnutrition. *Gastroenterology* 82:535, 1982.

287. Freund HR, et al. A possible beneficial effect of metronidazole in reducing TPN-associated liver function derangements. *J Surg Res* 38:356, 1985.

288. Latham PS, et al. Hyperalimentation-associated jaundice: An example of a serum factor inducing cholestasis in rats. *Am J Clin Nutr* 41:61, 1985.

289. Sax HC, et al. Hepatic steatosis in total parenteral nutrition: Failure of fatty infiltration to correlate with abnormal serum hepatic enzyme levels. *Surgery* 100:697, 1986.

290. Li S, et al. Increasing dextrose concentrations in total parenteral nutrition (TPN) causes alterations in hepatic morphology and plasma levels of insulin and glucagon in rats. *J Surg Res* 44:639, 1988.

291. Li S, et al. Addition of glucagon to total parenteral nutrition (TPN) prevents hepatic steatosis in rats. *Surgery* 104:350, 1988.

292. Li S, et al. Reversal of hepatic steatosis in rats by addition of glucagon to total parenteral nutrition (TPN). *J Surg Res* 46:557, 1989.

293. Nussbaum MS, et al. Addition of lipid to total parenteral nutrition prevents hepatic steatosis in rats by lowering the portal venous insulin/glucagon ratio. *JPEN* 16:106, 1992.

294. Daly JM, Dudrick SJ, Copeland EM. Effects of protein depletion and repletion on cell mediated immunity in experimental animals. *Ann Surg* 188:791, 1978.

295. Dempsey DT, Mullen JL, Buzby GP. The link between nutritional status and clinical outcome: Can nutritional intervention modify it? *Am J Clin Nutr* 47:352, 1988.

296. Haffejee AA, Angorn IB. Nutritional status and the non-specific cellular and humoral immune response in esophageal carcinoma. *Ann Surg* 189:475, 1979.

297. Goodgame JT, Fischer JE. Parenteral nutrition in the treatment of acute pancreatitis: effect on complications and mortality. *Ann Surg* 186:651, 1977.

298. Nussbaum MS, et al. Lipid-free total parenteral nutrition and macrophage function in rats. *Arch Surg* 126:84, 1991.

299. Goodwin JS, Webb DR. Regulation of the immune response by prostaglandins. *Clin Immunol Immunopathol* 15:106, 1980.

300. Jarstrand C, Berghem H, Lahnborg S. Human granulocyte and reticuloendothelial system function during intralipid infusion. *JPEN* 2:663, 1978.

301. Beisel WR, et al. Single-nutrient effects on immunologic functions. *JAMA* 245:53, 1981.

302. Kinsella JE, et al. Dietary polyunsaturated fatty acids and eicosanoids: Potential effects on the modulation of inflammatory and immune cells: an overview. *Nutrition* 6:24, 1990.

303. Rudolph FB, et al. Role of RNA as a dietary source of pyrimidines and purines in immune function. *Nutrition* 6:45, 1990.

304. McCullough ML, Hsu N. Metabolic bone disease in home parenteral nutrition. *J Am Diet Assoc* 87:915, 1987.

305. Nagata MJ. Hypersensitivity reactions associated with parenteral nutrition: Case report and review of the literature. *Ann Pharmacol* 27:174, 1993.

306. Kamath KR, Berry A, Cummins G. Acute hypersensitivity reaction to Intralipid [Letter]. *N Engl J Med* 304:360, 1981.

307. Bower RH, Orr ME, Nussbaum MS. Hypersensitivity reactions to dextrose during home parenteral nutrition (HPN). *JPEN* 15:33, 1991.

308. Pomeranz S, et al. Parenteral nutrition-induced anaphylaxis. *JPEN* 11:314, 1987.

309. Levy M, Dupuis LL. Parenteral nutrition hypersensitivity. *JPEN* 14:213, 1990.

Selected Readings

Buzby GP, et al. (The Veterans Affairs Total Parenteral Nutrition Cooperative Study Group). Perioperative total parenteral nutrition in surgical patients. *N Engl J Med* 325:525, 1991.

This important study of the effects of perioperative TPN screened 3259 patients and studied 1982 patients in which 459 received TPN. There was no difference in short-term or long-term mortality among groups. Noninfectious complications were lower in severely malnourished patients treated with TPN. However, there was a higher rate of infectious complications in all TPN-treated patients. In the moderately malnourished group, this negated any benefit derived from a decrease in noninfectious complications, and no overall benefit was observed in the group receiving parenteral nutrition.

Byrne TA, Morrissey TB, Gatzen C. Anabolic therapy with growth hormone accelerates protein gain in surgical patients requiring nutritional rehabilitation. *Ann Surg* 218:400, 1993.

This prospective randomized clinical trial compared standard nutritional therapy with growth hormone-supplemented nutritional therapy in 14 patients with significant gastrointestinal dysfunction. The results demonstrated that growth hormone administration enhanced protein gain without a significant increase in body fat or the extracellular water compartment leading to an overall acceleration of nutritional repletion in this population.

Dudrick SJ, et al. Long-term parenteral nutrition with growth and development and positive nitrogen balance. *Surgery* 64:134, 1968.

This classic study marked the beginning of the modern era of parenteral nutrition therapy. The authors adapted the technique of subclavian venipuncture and demonstrated that total caloric needs in solutions containing hypertonic dextrose and amino acid could be safely administered to humans for a prolonged time in a reasonable volume with minimal complications.

Harvel RJ, Kane JP, Kashyap ML. Interchange of apolipoproteins between chylomicrons and high density lipoproteins during alimentation lipemia in man. *J Clin Invest* 52:32, 1973.

An early study that revealed parenteral lipid kinetics and documented the body's ability to clear parenterally administered lipids.

Krebs H. Glutamine metabolism in the animal body. In J Mora, R Palacious (eds), *Glutamine Metabolism, Enzymology, and Regulation.* New York: Academic, 1980. P 319.

A comprehensive summation of metabolic pathways of glutamine metabolism and their importance to the intact organism.

29

Enteral Nutrition

Robert H. Bower
Scott M. Berry

Because of its accessibility and voluminous absorptive surface, the gastrointestinal tract represents one of the most significant interfaces between an organism's internal milieu and its environment. As such, it is the ideal portal for internalization of substances capable of altering the organism's physiology [1]. As our understanding of gastrointestinal physiology has expanded, it has become apparent that nutrient assimilation is not the only function performed by the gastrointestinal tract. Modulation of hepatic and skeletal muscle nitrogen processing, the processing of foreign antigens, and regulation of immune response are only a few of its additional functions. Hence, the ability of the gastrointestinal tract to influence a remote organ system's response to external insult or injury has become an exciting field of inquiry [2].

Although enteral nutrition therapies are inexpensive when compared to other forms of medical therapy, their low cost belies their potency. Standard hospital meals cost $10 to $20 a day. Tube feeding costs $30 to $50 a day when administered by gravity or bolus and $40 to $60 a day when administered using a pump [3].

Both the types of nutrients provided and the route of nutrient administration appear to affect the patient's response to nutritional therapy. Studies have shown improved immune function, decreased infection rates, and decreased hospital stays with the use of enteral formulas supplemented with arginine, nucleotides (RNA), and ω-3 fatty acids [2,3]. In addition, the route of nutrient delivery seems to be an important determinant of patient response. Enterally fed patients appear to have improved immune function and a reduced incidence of infectious complications when compared to patients fed parenterally, especially in the post-traumatic setting [4–9]. Considering the lower cost and physiologic superiority of enteral nutrition, an adequate trial of enteral feeding should be attempted in all patients in need of specialized nutrition care. [*Editor's Note:* It is fair to say that whereas previously the knee-jerk response to nutritional support was to place a central line, at present TPN is used only in patients whose needs cannot be met by enteral nutrition.]

History of Enteral Nutrition

Enteral nutrition likely began when multicellular organisms first formed rudimentary gastrointestinal tracts to extract nutrients from the aqueous environment in which they existed. Humans have always been nourished enterally. Intestinal failure led to progressive malnutrition and, unless corrected, was uniformly fatal. Specialized forms of enteral therapy were attempted to save such unfortunate individuals [10]. With the exception of conventional eating and drinking, documentation of specialized enteral nutrition begins with the ancient Egyptian use of rectal feeding (Table 29-1) [11]. Milk, whey, chicken, beef and grain broths, raw eggs, blood, and liquor have all been administered rectally [12]. In the early 1900s the inadequacies of rectal feeding and the availability of rubber tubes made access to the gastrointestinal tract via the nasal route the preferred method [13]. Tubes placed operatively are a relatively recent development. Sites of placement include the pharynx, esophagus, duodenum, stomach, and jejunum. Percutaneous endoscopic or radiographic placement of tubes, with or without laparoscopic assistance, have gained favor as the methods of choice for establishing long-term enteral access for feeding in the past decade.

Defined formula diets were developed in the 1940s. Their development was followed by long-term studies of enteral formulas in the 1960s. Although enteral therapies had long been in use, it was parenteral nutrition research and development that nurtured an understanding of nutrition's benefit to patient care [2–4,14,15]. Before the widespread clinical implementation of parenteral nutrition in the 1970s, early operative intervention for correctable intestinal problems was the only option to reduce malnutrition-related morbidity and mortality. For uncorrectable intestinal problems, such as short-gut syndrome, there was little to offer. The application of parenteral nutrition technology to many disorders was lifesaving. Initially, parenteral nutrition seemed at least equivalent to enteral nutrition, and applications for it seemed limitless. However, as the mechanical, septic, metabolic, and financial complications of parenteral nutrition administration became manifest, proof of benefit was demanded and indiscriminate use discouraged.

Attitudes shifted away from use of parenteral therapies in the 1980s, spawning multiple studies comparing enteral and parenteral nutrition during that decade. Muggia-Sullam et al. [16] showed that in unselected patients parenteral and enteral nutrition regimens were equivalent to promote nitrogen balance, preserve body weight, and promote protein synthesis. However, other studies showed parenteral nutrition superior in achievement of caloric needs, early positive nitrogen balance, and weight gain, although markers of protein synthesis such as albumin and short-turnover proteins were virtually always equivalent [7,8,17–20]. Thus, in unselected general surgery patients in whom complication rates were low [21–24], the route of nutrient delivery assumed

Table 29-1. History of Enteral Nutrition

Ancient Egypt	Nutrient enemas for patients with intestinal failure
1900	Abandonment of nutrient enemas; nasointestinal access
1940	Defined formula diets for pediatric patients with malabsorption
1960	Long-term studies of enteral feeding formulas by NASA for the manned space program
1970	Parenteral nutrition research and development
1980	Realization that enteral and parenteral therapies were not equivalent
1990	Specialized forms of enteral therapy, immunomodulatory enteral nutrition, cost-effectiveness of enteral therapies proven

less importance. This assumption was substantiated by a meta-analysis done by Moore et al. [17] in which, after combining eight prospective randomized trials comparing septic complications between enterally and parenterally fed patients, the incidence of septic complications was not significantly reduced in the elective surgery (9% vs. 21%, NS) and penetrating trauma groups (16% vs. 27.5%, NS). However, in groups of patients in whom septic complications were common, enteral therapy appeared to be superior to parenteral therapy with regard to length of hospital stay and septic complication rates [7,19]. Enterally fed blunt trauma patients had the most significant reduction in sepsis rates (21% vs. 50%, $p < 0.05$) [17]. Enteral nutrition reduced the septic complication rate in blunt trauma patients to that observed in elective surgery patient populations, presumably by removing the combined immunosuppressive effects of blunt trauma and parenteral nutrition. Although enteral nutritional therapy may be superior to parenteral therapy, proof of decreased complication rates in nonselected surgical and penetrating trauma patients will require exceedingly large studies because their rate of infectious complications is so low. Realistically, studies large enough to show superior outcome may never be completed.

Finally, a study in surgical patients by Hamaoui et al. [8] in 1990 showed that the mean daily costs for enteral nutrition were considerably lower than for parenteral ($44.36 ± 8.50 vs. $102.10 ± 11.77, $p < 0.01$). They point out that although the cost of nutrients was similar between groups, the cost of non-nutrient supplies added considerably to the total cost of parenteral nutrition administration (43% for parenteral vs. 13% for enteral). In addition, when the cost of treating complications is divided by the entire group at risk, the costs for enterally fed patients are virtually always lower than for parenterally fed patients because complications are less frequent with enteral nutrition therapies [25,26]. These and other studies suggest that enteral nutrition is less expensive to administer and monitor than parenteral nutrition [27–29]. [*Editor's Note:* While complication rates in enteral nutrition may be lower, there may be more fatalities. The reason is that aspiration is usually a major source of complications in enteral nutrition and may be fatal. In parenteral nutrition, line sepsis is the most common complication and is rarely fatal in a well-run program.]

Macronutrients

The urgency of initiating nutrition support should be evaluated in the context of the patient's care problems. Airway, breathing, circulation, tissue oxygenation, acid-base neutrality, normal electrolyte concentrations, and volume repletion must all be accomplished before nutritional management can proceed. Optimal nutrient metabolism will not occur if any of these patient care issues are neglected. Thus, these problems must be addressed prior to institution of nutrition support. After stabilization, prompt initiation of nutrition support will then ensure maximal nutrition benefit.

Protein

The breakdown of lean body mass is rapid and relentless after five or six days of simple starvation and greater for starvation in the face of the physiologic stress of major illness or operation. Significant protein deficits accumulate each day the patient is without nutrition support. Weight gain, which is usually reflective of fluid retention more than building of body cell mass, should not be a priority in the acute care setting. The goal of nutritional therapy in this setting should be nitrogen equilibrium with maintenance or restoration of structural and functional protein synthesis. If protein intake is inadequate, body tissues may not be replaced.

Generally, healthy individuals require 0.8 to 1.0 g protein/kg/day (Table 29-2). Minimal protein requirements in normal individuals are 0.55 g/kg/

Table 29-2. Components of Nutrient Provision

Component	Usual Requirement	Requirement During Stress
Protein	0.8–1 g/kg/d	1.2–2.5 g/kg/d
Calories		
Carbohydrate	25–35 kcal/kg/d	35–50 kcal/kg/d
Fat	30%–35% of total calories	30%–35% of total calories*

*Fat may be increased to 50% of total enteral calories if serum glucose is uncontrollable or if abdominal distention and pain or osmotic diarrhea develop.

day; the values of 0.8 to 1.0 will support normal activity. Because sepsis leads to mobilization of muscle protein stores, dietary protein requirements are increased 1.2 to 2.5 times during systemic infection. This amount of protein should be administered along with adequate calories (as much as 1.3 to 1.5 times the calculated BEE) to allow protein synthesis.

Dietary proteins are the largest source of amino acids and peptides in humans. However, most of the ingested nitrogen is in the form of intact protein with only a small portion of the ingested protein in the form of free amino acids or peptides. In general, plant protein is difficult to assimilate. Animal protein is more readily digested and assimilated. In addition to ingested protein, the sloughed gastrointestinal tract mucosa, secreted digestive enzymes, and secreted immunoglobulins contribute to the protein pool. Under normal circumstances, almost all secreted protein is reabsorbed as peptides and free amino acids, which then enter the free amino acid pool and are reused for protein synthesis. The 75 g of desquamated cells together with 75 g of secreted digestive enzymes make up the source of half of the 300 g free amino acid pool present in normal individuals. In patients who have excessive intestinal losses, such as can occur with diarrhea or high-output fistulas, much, if not all, of this protein-rich material is lost to the total body economy. Therefore, protein depletion, with its attendant morbidity, is common in these clinical situations.

Protein digestion begins in the stomach where secreted zymogens are acted on by gastric acid to produce a family of proteases. These proteases then cleave the intact proteins into mixtures of mainly peptides with a few free amino acids. However, the importance of these proteases in overall protein assimilation is limited, as positive nitrogen balance may be attained easily after total gastrectomy.

The pancreas releases many proenzymes into the small bowel lumen in response to hormonal and vagal stimulation. The brush-border enzyme enterokinase is released in response to the luminal presence of bile acids. The pancreatic proenzyme trypsinogen cleaves the amino terminus of the trypsinogen peptide protease to produce trypsin. Trypsin is then capable of activating itself and the other pancreatic proteases. These pancreatic proteases are divided broadly in endo- and exopeptidases. The endopeptidases trypsin, chymotrypsin, and elastase and the exopeptidases carboxypeptidase A and carboxypeptidase B digest intact proteins to short peptides 2 to 6 amino acids in length (70%) and free amino acids (30%). As the protein moves aborally, brush-border peptidases cleave the peptides further so that, by the time they reach the jejunum, 50% of the intraluminal nitrogen is in the form of free amino acids.

A number of brush-border proteases cleave protein molecules that are greater than three amino acids in length. These proteases cleave one amino acid at a time from the NH terminus of the peptide. The resulting free amino acids and dipeptides are then absorbed across the luminal membrane and into the enterocyte cytoplasm, where further degradation may occur.

Under normal circumstances, colonic bacterial proteases play no role in protein digestion and assimilation. Because the colon cannot absorb the protein breakdown products, these peptides and amino acids (3%–5% of the total protein ingested) are lost in the feces.

The products of this intraluminal and brush-border protein digestion are assimilated into the cellular cytosol via a variety of amino acid transport systems. System A, system L, system ASC, and system Ly are amino acid transport systems that have different amino acid specificities and transport their respective amino acids via differing mechanisms. Although these systems are present in cells not involved in secretion or nutrient absorption, there are certainly more systems in cells whose primary function is absorption of protein. The transport systems for peptides are different than those for free amino acids, but, like the amino acid transporters, the cellular peptide transporters are incompletely characterized. As much as 70% of dietary protein may be assimilated into the enterocyte as peptides.

Elemental tube feeding formulas arose from the realization that unabsorbed nutrients that remained within the bowel lumen were unavailable for nutritional repletion. It was postulated that predigested nutrients would require less digestive system participation for assimilation and, therefore, be absorbed more readily. However, providing protein in the form of free amino acids confers little, if any, advantage and is probably unnecessary because di- and tripeptides in the bowel lumen are transported into the mucosal cell and then hydrolyzed to free amino acids. In addition, free amino acids have the disadvantage of increased osmolarity when present in tube feedings; this leads to decreased tolerance due to distention, cramping, and diarrhea. Oligopeptides from protein hydrolysates are absorbed and tolerated better than free amino acids and, therefore, should be the major protein source of an enteral formula [30–34]. [*Editor's Note:* This view, commonly held for the past decade, is no longer universally accepted.]

Calories

Calories are provided as a source of fuel for cellular synthetic, degradative, protective, and support functions. When nonprotein calories are provided in sufficient quantities, protein is spared from use as an energy source. In general, a ratio of nonprotein calories to nitrogen of 100 to 125:1 is probably most beneficial to the surgical patient (see Table 29-2). As stated, when external gastrointestinal or renal protein losses are significant, the calorie to nitrogen ratio should be adjusted accordingly. Conversely, when renal clearance of nitrogenous waste products is inadequate or when increased intestinal protein load leads to encephalopathy, the calorie to nitrogen ration may need to be adjusted upward.

The administration of adequate calories for energy and amino acids for protein replacement leads to improved cellular and organ function. Carbohydrate generally makes up 50% to 80% of administered enteral calories. By supplying 20% to 50% of the patient's caloric requirement as lipid, carbohydrate calories can be lessened, and, therefore, the complications associated with carbohydrate overfeeding are reduced. In addition, the provision of 2% to 6% of calories as long-chain fatty acids will prevent essential fatty acid deficiency.

Carbohydrate

In the human diet, starch accounts for most of the carbohydrate present. Starch is composed of the straight-chain glucose polymer amylose and the branched-chain polymer amylopectin. The remainder is made up of the disaccharides sucrose and lactose. A variable portion of dietary carbohydrate is in the form of plant fiber and is unavailable for digestion and absorption.

Salivary and pancreatic amylase cleave the α-1,4 glucose polymer linkage to yield maltose and maltotriose. The 1,6 linkage at the glucose polymer branch points are not hydrolyzed by amylase. As the carbohydrate enters the stomach, it will not be altered to any significant extent until entering the small intestine because no appreciable additional carbohydrate digestion occurs in the stomach.

In the intestinal lumen, pancreatic α-amylase is the only active carbohydrate splitting enzyme. The major products are maltose, maltotriose, and α-limit dextrins. Because α-amylase has little activity against the α-1,4 bonds near the 1,6 branch points, as much as one-third of the starch present cannot be further hydrolyzed by intraluminal enzymes. These α-limit dextrins are, however, rapidly hydrolyzed to usable forms by intestinal brush-border enzymes.

The brush-border enzymes lactase, sucrase, isomaltase, α-limit dextrinase, glucoamylase sucrase, and trehalase play differing roles in carbohydrate digestion because of their differing abilities to cleave specific glycosidic linkages. The activity of these carbohydrases exceeds the intestinal capacity for absorption of the monosaccharides except for lactase. As people age, their ability to break down lactose decreases, leading to lactose intolerance. Once cleaved, hexose sugars are transported across the luminal enterocyte membrane via at least one, and possibly more, transport systems. The glucose absorbed can then be released into the portal venous system. After hepatic extraction the glucose enters the systemic circulation; in the presence of insulin it is used as a fuel source without further modification by most tissues.

The colon plays an important salvage role for malabsorbed sugars and fiber. Although the colon does not absorb monosaccharides directly, it does absorb the short-chain fatty acids that result from bacterial monosaccharide digestion in the colon. Fiber present in the colonic lumen is extensively degraded, with short-chain fatty acids being the main product of polysaccharide digestion. For each gram of dietary fiber, 5 mEq of fatty acids are produced. Twenty percent of these short-chain fatty acids are excreted, while the remainder are absorbed or used by the colonic bacteria.

Most commercially available tube feeding formulas use nonlactose forms of carbohydrate, which are easily degraded and absorbed. Tolerance of enteral formulas may be related to the osmolarity of the formula. Osmolarity reflects the number of osmotically active protein and carbohydrate molecules. The size and length of the molecules do not influence osmolarity. Thus, formulas that utilize peptides and oligosaccharides tend to be better tolerated, provided brush-border enzymatic function is intact.

Fats

The most important dietary lipids are triglycerides, phospholipids, and cholesterol. The steroid hormones and fat-soluble vitamins are also considered in this class of nutrients. Glycerol is the three-carbon backbone to which fatty acids are esterified. When one fatty acid is esterified to the hydroxyl group of glycerol, monoacylglycerol (monoglyceride) is formed; esterification of two fatty acids forms diacylglycerol (diglyceride); and esterification of three fatty acids forms triacylglycerol (triglyceride). Fatty acids are the most abundant constituents of lipid. The saturated fatty acids have a general structure of

$CH_3(CH_2)_nCOOH$. The short-chain fatty acids have an n less than 6 and are polar (soluble in water). The medium-chain fatty acids have an n between 6 and 12 and are also polar. Those fatty acids with an n greater than 12 are considered long-chain and are not polar. Unsaturated fatty acids occur in each of the three categories and are characterized by the presence of one or more double bonds.

Phospholipids are the major component of cell membranes. They have a three-carbon backbone, much like glycerol, with the addition of an esterified phosphorus group. Most phospholipid delivered to the intestinal lumen is derived from endogenous biliary secretions and sloughed intestinal epithelium.

There are different phospholipases capable of hydrolyzing phospholipids. The most important one is pancreatic phospholipase A_2. This enzyme releases fatty acids from the number two position on the glycerol backbone forming free fatty acids and lysophospholipids. Both of these moieties are readily absorbed from the intestinal lumen into the intestinal epithelial cytosol. There they are reesterified by lysolecithin acyltransferase. These reesterified phospholipids are then used as surface coats for lipoproteins, which transport triglycerides from intestinal cells into the lymphatic channels. Eventually, phospholipids are reintegrated into cellular membranes after lipoprotein-cell membrane fusion. The contents of the circulating lipoproteins are internalized into cells and used as metabolic precursors.

Cholesterol consists of three six-carbon rings and 1 five-carbon ring adjoined in a particular stereotopic arrangement. Cholesterol is derived from both plant and animal dietary sources. In addition, biliary secretions and sloughed intestinal epithelium provide a considerable amount, up to 50%, of the intraluminal cholesterol present. When a fatty acid is esterified to one of the six-membered rings, cholesterol ester is formed. Female and male hormones, adrenocortical hormones, and bile acids are all formed from this cyclopentanophenanthrene structure. Approximately 85% of dietary cholesterol is present in the free form, the remainder is present in the intestinal lumen as cholesterol ester. The esters are nonpolar and thus do not interact with the aqueous phase of intraluminal contents. To be absorbed, they must first be cleaved to free cholesterol by pancreatic cholesterol esterase. Micellar solubilization by bile salts is necessary for cholesterol absorption.

Because of its caloric density (9 kcal/g), lipid emulsions provide calories in a relatively small volume. They may, therefore, be useful in patients with volume restrictions to increase the number of calories provided. Most fat absorption occurs in the proximal jejunum. Under normal circumstances, the ileum is exposed to little intraluminal fat. When enteral fat load is increased, the jejunal absorption does not change, but ileal absorption is induced. Patients with diseased distal intestine or enterocutaneous fistulas who are considered candidates for enteral nutrition are often intolerant of the osmotic load of glucose-based enteral formulas. Lipid-based enteral formulas present a lower osmotic load than isocaloric carbohydrate-based formulas, and therefore may be absorbed from the lumen better. In addition, lipid does not exacerbate hyperglycemia and may be used in increased concentration as an alternate source of calories in patients in whom serum glucose management is difficult. When hypertriglyceridemia is present, the amount of lipid that can be safely provided to a patient is limited. Because of dietary requirements for the essential fatty acids, linoleic and linolenic acid, at least 2% to 6% of total calories should be provided as long-chain fatty acids.

Glucose or oligosaccharides, which usually constitute the majority of calories in commercially available enteral formulas, may be tolerated poorly in patients with diseased bowel. Distention, crampy pain, and diarrhea may result from the osmotic load of glucose-based formulas. Therefore, in patients with malabsorption we favor lipid-based formulations that use increased amounts of medium-chain triglycerides, protein as di- and tripeptides, and limited oligosaccharides to minimize osmolarity. Medium-chain fatty acids are absorbed unchanged into the portal system and can be used as a fuel source; however, they provide no essential fatty acids.

Vitamins

Vitamins are organic substances found in minute quantities in foodstuffs that are essential to various metabolic processes. They are chemically dissimilar and have a wide range of functions, usually serving as cofactors to enzymatically driven cellular metabolic reactions (Table 29-3).

Vitamin C is active in the metabolism of aromatic amino acids, regulation of cellular respiration, and structural collagen synthesis. Small amounts of ascorbic acid are absorbed in the ileum by a slow passive diffusion mechanism. The majority is absorbed by a rapid, sodium-dependent, active transport mechanism. Absorption by the carrier mechanism is saturated at relatively low luminal ascorbic acid concentrations. Thus, large enteral doses of vitamin C saturate the protein transporter quickly, with the majority of the re-

Table 29-3. Vitamins

Vitamin	Absorption	Daily Requirement
Ascorbic acid	Ileum; active transport	60 mg/d
Biotin	Jejunum; facilitated diffusion	150–300 μg/d
Folic acid	Small intestine; facilitated diffusion	0.4–0.8 mg/d
Niacin	Small intestine; facilitated diffusion	14–18 mg/d
Pantothenic acid	Small intestine; active transport	4–7 mg/d
Riboflavin	Jejunum and colon; facilitated diffusion	1.2–1.7 mg/d
Thiamine	Jejunum; active transport	0.4–1.2 mg/d
Vitamin B_6	Jejunum; passive diffusion	2.2 mg/d
Vitamin A	Small intestine; saturable, passive carrier-mediated transport, bile-dependent	800–1000 μg/d retinol; or 4200–6000 μg/d β-carotene
Vitamin D	Small intestine; saturable, passive carrier-mediated transport, bile-dependent, transported in lymph	5–10 μg/d (200–400 IU/d)
Vitamin E	Small intestine; passive mechanism, transported in lymph	10–15 mg/d (10–15 IU/day)
Vitamin K	Dietary: small intestine; active transport, bile-dependent, transported in lymph Bacterial: colon; passive, transported in lymph	1 mg/d

maining intraluminal ascorbic acid not assimilated. The ascorbic acid that is transported ultimately accumulates inside the cell against a concentration gradient. The RDA for vitamin C is 60 mg/day.

Biotin is involved as a cofactor in many cellular reactions. Its uptake from the intestinal lumen occurs mainly in the jejunum along the brush-border membrane. The absorption of biotin from the intestinal lumen seems to bear no relationship to an animal's need for biotin, thus it is not an inducible transporter. Normal daily requirements for biotin are 150 to 300 μg/day. Because biotin deficiency is essentially unknown (one anecdotal case has been reported), no RDA exists.

Folic acid functions to transfer single carbon atoms within the cell for purine and serine metabolism. In addition, it is a necessary cofactor for hemopoiesis. Whether intestinal transport of folic acid is by an active or passive mechanism is still argued. Most now feel that it is transported via facilitated diffusion followed by metabolism that is then trapped intracellularly. The RDA for folic acid is 0.4 to 0.8 mg/day.

Niacin functions in the body as a component of glycolytic pathways and cellular respiration. It is easily absorbed from the entire small intestine because it is water soluble and very stable under the wide range of gastrointestinal conditions. Niacin is formed from the precursor tryptophan and RDAs are expressed as both niacin and tryptophan-niacin equivalents (1 mg niacin equals 60 mg tryptophan). The RDA is 14 to 18 mg niacin/day.

Pantothenic acid is part of coenzyme A and acts to release energy from carbohydrate metabolism. It is also necessary for the synthesis and degradation of cholesterol, fatty acids, and steroid hormones. It is absorbed from the small intestinal lumen unchanged, by a sodium-dependent, saturable process. Deficiency is rare due to widespread presence in foodstuffs. The RDA is 4 to 7 mg/day.

Riboflavin acts as a cofactor in tissue oxidation and respiration and plays an important role in protein metabolism. It is water soluble and easily absorbed from the proximal gastrointestinal tract. In addition, riboflavin may also be absorbed from the colonic lumen in quantities sufficient to prevent clinical deficiency. The RDA is 1.2 to 1.7 mg/day.

Thiamine consists of a pyrimidine ring joined to a thiazole nucleus. The bond between the rings is weak and is easily broken by temperature and alkaline environment. It serves as a coenzyme in carbohydrate metabolism. It is highly water soluble and thus easily absorbed from the proximal gastrointestinal tract by an active transport mechanism. The body is unable to store thiamine to any significant extent; when the body is saturated, urinary excretion increases. Thiamine is found in both animal and plant sources. Thiamine deficiency may be precipitated by the administration of large glucose loads to previously malnourished patients. Thiamine deficiency is usually the first vitamin deficiency to manifest itself and should be considered in patients who have otherwise unexplained lactic acidosis. The RDA for thiamine is 0.4 to 1.2 mg/1000 kcal.

Vitamin B_6 refers to three different pyridine derivatives that are all present in foodstuffs and interconverted readily within the body. Vitamin B_6 is involved in amino acid and glycogen metabolism. It is easily absorbed from the proximal small intestine by a passive diffusion mechanism. Even when malabsorption of xylose, fat, and folic acid is severe, vitamin B_6 absorption is unaffected. The RDA is 2.2 mg/day.

Vitamins A, D, E, and K are fat-soluble vitamins, each of which possesses its own unique physiologic function. Vitamin A is necessary for growth and differentiation of epithelial tissues, protein synthesis, and maintenance of vision. Vitamin D is central to calcium homeostasis. It regulates calcium retention in the kidneys and absorption from the intestinal lumen. Vitamin E is an antioxidant that may be critical to cellular surveillance and prevention of neoplastic growth. Vitamin K is critical for the production of clotting factors and is central to hemostasis. The absorptive mechanisms for fat-soluble vitamins are not well defined. Vitamin A is thought to be absorbed by a passive, saturable, carrier-mediated transport that occurs in the small intestine. It is dependent on bile salt concentrations. Vitamin D absorption is thought to be similar to that of vitamin A. Most of the absorbed vitamin D is transported via the lymphatics and a small fraction by the portal system. Vitamin E is absorbed by a passive mechanism. Like vitamin A, most of vitamin E is transported in the small intestinal lymphatics, with a small portion transported via the portal system. Vitamin K is derived from dietary and colonic bacterial sources. Dietary vitamin K differs from bacterial vitamin K at its side chain. Dietary vitamin K is absorbed by an energy-requiring saturable mechanism. Bacterial vitamin K is absorbed via a concentration-dependent passive process. It is also absorbed into the lymphatics and is transported bound to lipoproteins.

Vitamins and trace elements may be rapidly depleted when adequate nutrition is provided to malnourished patients. Patients with high metabolic rates should receive approximately twice the RDA for water-soluble vitamins. If the patient has large wounds, such that extensive tissue repair will be occurring, vitamin C should be provided at 5 to 10 times the RDA. In addition to disturbances in the commonly monitored electrolytes, patients with malabsorption due to diarrhea or fistulas can lose considerable amounts of copper, zinc, and magnesium. We find it useful to monitor serum magnesium levels biweekly and supplement the patient as necessary by providing parenteral magnesium. We do not routinely check serum copper or zinc levels in patients with large gastrointestinal volume losses. However, the amount of copper contained in two ampules of commercially prepared vitamin and trace element preparations given parenterally twice a week usually suffices.

Nutrient Utilization

The route of nutrient delivery can affect the patient's response to nutrients during illness. The benefits of using enteral nutrition nearly always outweigh the risks and favor the use of enteral nutrition when the functional gut is accessible and nutritional therapy is delivered with skill. Currently, there are many fewer contraindications to enteral therapy. Most should be considered relative contraindications (Table 29-4).

Studies of patients who have been given enteral or parenteral nutrition containing equivalent amounts of calories and nitrogen have shown that the enterally fed patients have stimulation of gut trophic hormones, improved systemic immunity, reduced incidence of infection following trauma and burns, and better tolerance of septic insult than parenterally fed patients [6–9]. The reason for this is not completely understood. Unfortunately, it is common to experience difficulty in administering all of a patient's nutritional needs enterally because of feeding intolerance. Mucosal brush-border atrophy and hypoalbuminemia may result in enteral nutrition being poorly absorbed leading to diarrhea and continued nutritional depletion [35]. Tube feeding intolerance may make it impossible to administer all the patient's nutritional needs by the enteral route. However, if the GI tract retains adequate absorptive surface and functions sufficiently to absorb nutrients, then it should be used as soon as possible to provide at least a portion of the patient's nutritional needs. Because it generally takes four to five days to attain target caloric provision with enteral therapy, a period of concurrent enteral and parenteral nu-

Table 29-4. Possible Contraindications to Enteral Feeding

Inability to safely establish enteral access
Intestinal obstruction
High-output fistula
Intractable vomiting
Intractable severe diarrhea
Ischemic bowel
Known intolerance to enteral feeding
Malabsorption
Patient refusal

trition may be necessary to restore mucosal function [35,36].

Many nutrients can be utilized in the periphery with minimal hepatic processing. When significant liver failure occurs, full nutritional resuscitation may be impossible. In addition, peripheral nutrient processing may be affected by the sequelae of surgical disease. The most common severe forms of peripheral cellular dysfunction occur with the systemic inflammatory response associated with burns, blunt trauma, and sepsis. These three inciting events affect cells in the periphery in similar ways and may result in the syndrome of multiple organ failure.

The multiple organ failure syndrome (MOFS) now accounts for over half of all intensive care unit (ICU) deaths [37–39]. As the science of critical care has improved, more patients are surviving their initial insult only later to develop MOFS. The fundamental characteristic of the syndrome is involvement of organs or systems remote from the site of primary pathology. Involvement of these systems may range from subclinical to fulminant failure. Once the cascade of events known as MOFS develops, supportive care is all that is available at present. The best treatment is prevention. However, the prediction of which patients will progress to MOFS after their initial insult can be exceedingly difficult. Infection, inadequate tissue perfusion, and a persistent inflammatory state are the most important risk factors for the development of MOFS [39]. Early recognition and prompt treatment of these states may avert the development of MOFS.

The mortality of MOFS is related to the number of systems involved, even more than to the primary process that initiated the MOFS. This mortality is approximately 25% per organ system involved. Although uncontrolled infection is the inciting event for MOFS in about 50% of cases, in the remainder it occurs without any identifiable source [39].

The role of enteral nutrition support in the management of MOFS has received increasing attention in recent years. The metabolic picture of MOFS is that of a progressively hyperglycemic, hypercatabolic, immunocompromised patient with structural, visceral, and enzymatic protein wasting resulting in organ failure. [*Editor's Note:* It is entirely possible that proteolysis of functional and structural organ proteins may contribute to the dysfunction and ultimately to organ failure.] Controversy still exists over the most appropriate nutrient mix for the patient with MOFS. It is clear, however, that such patients have markedly elevated nutrient requirements and that these nutrients are best provided enterally. Although requirements for both calories and protein are increased, relatively more protein is required than calories. In general, 1.5 to 2.5 g/kg/day of protein should be provided to these patients along with adequate calories to support its utilization [37–39]. Optimal calorie to nitrogen ratio is closer to 100:1 in these critically ill patients than the 150:1 in healthy individuals [38]. With progressively severe organ system failure, it may become necessary to use a formula designed to minimize the metabolic derangements associated with failure of a specific organ system.

Disease-specific enteral and parenteral formulas have been useful in the management of isolated hepatic or renal failure patients and may be efficacious in the management of the patient with MOFS who has particularly severe involvement of these organs. In addition, immune-enhancing enteral feedings enriched with arginine, RNA, and ω-3 fatty acids have been shown to decrease septic complications, speed recovery from infectious complications, and decrease length of ICU stay in critically ill patients [40].

Pharmaconutrients

At present, studies have shown improved immune function, decreased infection rates, and decreased hospital stays with use of a supplemented immunomodulatory enteral formula (Table 29-5) [40,41]. The nutritionally complete formula contains supplemental arginine and nucleotides (RNA) with a fat source, primarily as fish oil, which is rich in ω-3 polyunsaturated fatty acids.

Arginine

Arginine is a semiessential amino acid necessary for growth and the response to hypermetabolic and septic states [37]. Not only does it support protein synthesis necessary for healing, but it promotes T-cell mitogenesis and decreases T-cell dysfunction associated with the post-injury state. In animal models, arginine has been shown to inhibit tumor induction, growth, and metastatic spread [42]. In addition, arginine is the metabolic precursor of nitric oxide, which has widespread functions and a role as a mediator.

Fatty Acids

The lipid composition of the immune cells reflects that of the diet. Because linoleic (ω-6) and linolenic (ω-3) are the precursors to the potent immunomodulators arachidonic, eicosapentaenoic, and docosahexanoic acids, it is not surprising that dietary manipulation of these lipids leads to altered immune function. Diets high in ω-3 fish oils cause

Table 29-5. Pharmaconutrients

Component	Action
Arginine	T-cell mitogen Decreases T-cell dysfunction in post-injury state Augments macrophage phagocytic function Promotes IL-2 production Inhibits tumor induction, growth, and metastatic spread
ω-3 fatty acids	Decreased cyclooxygenase pathway-produced prostanoids Increased lipoxygenase pathway leukotriene production Precursors to the immunomodulators: arachadonic, eicosapentaenoic, and docosahexanoic acids
Ribonucleic acid (RNA)	Enhances delayed cutaneous hypersensitivity Increases mitogen-stimulated lymphocyte proliferation Enhances IL-2 production Enhances T-helper cell and macrophage function

Source: Data from references 15, 64–68.

increased lipoxygenase-pathway utilization resulting in increased amounts of immunostimulatory leukotrienes and decreased amounts of immunodepressive prostanoids from the cyclooxygenase pathway [43,44].

Nucleotides

Delayed cutaneous hypersensitivity, mitogen-stimulated lymphocyte proliferation, graft rejection, and graft-versus-host disease are all suppressed by diets lacking nucleotides. Provision of uracil restores these functions by enhancing T-helper cell and macrophage populations [45,46]. Because of cell mediated-immunity augmentation, these formulas should not be used in the transplant population or in patients in whom immunosuppression is desirable. The greatest benefit of this disease-specific formula over conventional formulas has been observed in patients who have an infection at the time of initiation of feeding, are elderly, or are more acutely ill. Due to improvements in the outcome of critically ill patients as demonstrated by decreased infectious complications and decreased hospital stays [15,41], such a disease-specific formula is currently our choice for enteral nutrition support in most ICU patients.

Because of improvement in immune indices, decreased infectious complications, and decreased hospital stays [40,41], we believe that pharmaconutrients should be the first choice for enteral nutrition support in all except transplant patients.

Clinical Enteral Nutrition

Enteral Access

Critical illness and comorbid conditions may complicate aspiration and enteral tolerance issues considerably. After Einhorn described the inadequacies of rectal feeding in 1910, tubes that were passed through the nose became the preferred vehicle for enteral access [20]. For short-term feeding (weeks), this is still the preferred form of enteral access. Tubes surgically placed in the pharynx, esophagus, duodenum, stomach, and jejunum have been used in the past. More recently, percutaneous endoscopic and laparoscopic methods are usually reserved for those patients requiring intermediate and long-term (months) enteral nutrition support (Table 29-6).

The proper method and location of enteral nutrition delivery is not altogether clear. Intragastric feeding may pose an undue aspiration risk in patients with gastroesophageal reflux or altered mental status (Table 29-7). Patients who have a documented episode of pulmonary aspiration, patients with diabetic neuropathy, hypothyroidism, depressed sensorium, advanced age, and patients ventilated with positive-end expiratory pressure may have an increased aspiration risk [47]. Furthermore, medications such as theophylline, anticholinergics, calcium channel blockers, beta-agonists, and alpha-antagonists cause reduction

Table 29-6. Cost and Success Rates for Postpyloric Tube Placement by Method

Method	Cost ($)	Success (%)
Endoscopic	704	90
Fluoroscopic, in Radiology	297	87
Fluoroscopic, portable	325	85
Blind passage with one x-ray	106	50
Blind passage with metoclopramide	142	85
pH-sensing tube with one x-ray	131	81

Source: Data from references 48–64.

Table 29-7. Factors That May Increase Aspiration or Intolerance

Aspiration	Intolerance
Previous episode of aspiration	Hypertonic formulations
Diabetic neuropathy	Myocardial infarction
Hypothyroidism	Pneumonia
Depressed sensorium	Renal failure
Advanced age	Urinary tract infection
Positive-end expiratory pressure	Intra-abdominal infections
Theophylline	Burns
Beta-agonists	Diabetes
Calcium channel blockers	Abdominal surgery
Alpha-antagonists	Hypoalbuminemia
Anticholinergics	Malnutrition

in lower esophageal sphincter pressure. All of these factors can contribute to an increased incidence of life-threatening pulmonary aspiration. Unfortunately, the question of whether postpyloric feeding reduces aspiration risk is still not adequately answered.

There are conflicting reports about the risk of aspiration with nasogastric versus nasojejunal feedings [48–52]. Studies have included heterogenous groups of patients, some with a preexisting aspiration tendency and some without. In addition, studies in head-injured patients often show no benefit to postpyloric feeding. Diminished gag reflex and impaired oropharyngeal transfer are commonly present in such individuals and may predispose to aspiration of oral contents irrespective of gastroesophageal reflux or regurgitation. Therefore, aspiration in this group may not represent true tube feeding aspiration but aspiration of oral contents.

There is also the separate issue of tube feeding tolerance. While aspiration risk may not be decreased by postpyloric access, enteral tolerance is improved. Patients who have myocardial infarctions, pneumonias, urinary tract infections, acute renal failure, intra-abdominal infections, burns, diabetes, or who are critically ill from other causes often have gastric atony that precludes intragastric enteral nutrition therapy. This failure to tolerate intragastric feeding should not be considered failure of enteral therapy. Exhaustive efforts should be made to ensure successful enteral feeding via duodenal or jejunal access. However, establishing such access can be difficult.

For intermediate-term (weeks to months) enteral nutrition administration, percutaneous endoscopic, radiologic, or laparoscopic methods of enteral access are preferred. Conventional operative placement is reserved for patients with contraindications to, or failure of, the above techniques. For short-term (weeks) access, the transnasal route of intestinal access is preferred. Using this route, intragastric placement is generally easy; however, postpyloric access can be troublesome. In general, the more successful forms of establishing postpyloric access require specialized expertise and equipment in addition to being more expensive to use.

Spontaneous intestinal passage of tubes placed in the stomach is associated with a low immediate success rate and often requires multiple radiographs [53–66]. The administration of metoclopramide may improve the chance of transpyloric passage [54]; however, this, along with additional radiographs, increases the cost of enteral nutrition support considerably. Endoscopic or fluoroscopic placement of tubes is expensive because appropriate expertise and specialized equipment are required [50,51,66].

Bedside clinical indicators of feeding tube placement such as insufflation of air or aspiration of gastric contents are notoriously poor and can lead to fatal complications [62–67]. Radiograph is the most reliable commonly used method to confirm tube position; however, even this can be misinterpreted [67]. Fluoroscopic contrast study through the tube is the gold standard for establishing tube position. However, due to its expense and inconvenience, it is not routinely performed but is reserved for special cases where position confirmation is particularly troublesome. The exception is when a tube is placed primarily under fluoroscopic guidance. Under such circumstances, completion contrast study is generally performed. Even when postpyloric access is attained using endoscopy, tube displacement on removal of the endoscope is not rare and, therefore, generally requires a radiograph after completion of endoscopic placement.

Tubes manufactured with a pH sensor at their

tip may assist in nasointestinal placement by providing continuous pH readings during placement. The rapid change from an acidic gastric pH to that of an alkaline duodenal pH signals passage of the tube into the proximal intestine [68,69]. Our initial experience with these tubes has been favorable, with over an 80% success rate for postpyloric tube placement. Although not 100% successful, most tubes can be placed by this method, obviating the need for more expensive and involved placement methods.

Use of Tube Feeding

Administration of appropriate protein and adequate calories, without over-or underfeeding, is crucial for optimal patient outcome. Illness requiring hospitalization is often accompanied by a hypermetabolic state that, when coupled with any preexisting nutritional depletion, places patients at high risk for nutritional complications such as poor wound healing, depressed immunity, and increased susceptibility to nosocomial infections [1–3,5–9,14,15,38]. However, overfeeding of carbohydrate calories may lead to elevated blood sugars, osmotic diuresis, hyperosmotic nonketotic coma, increased carbon dioxide production, and hepatic steatosis.

To use enteral nutrition support in patients with intestinal dysfunction, there must be at least four feet of functional bowel. Even when enterocutaneous fistulas exist, enteral nutritional therapy may be possible. One may, for example, place the feeding tube in the fistula, provided there are four feet distal to the fistula that are intact. Respectable rates of fistula closure have been achieved using enteral support, although slightly less than those achieved with parenteral nutrition [70–72].

Clinical indicators classically used to determine tube feeding tolerance, such as bowel sounds or nasogastric output, are of questionable value for predicting tube feeding tolerance. We have found little correlation between bowel sounds and enteral feeding tolerance. The only truly reliable test of tube feeding tolerance is a trial of tube feeding. To optimize the chances for a successful trial, tube feeding should be administered through an appropriate tube whose position is confirmed radiographically unless a specific contraindication to the use of the GI tract exists.

The functioning GI tract should be used for nutrition provision. It has been shown that enteral therapies promote nitrogen retention, restore body cell mass, restore cell-mediated immunity, accelerate wound healing, and improve overall nutritional status, in addition to being less costly than equivalent parenteral therapies [5,7,8,17,73–78]. In addition to the use of enteral therapy being more cost-effective than use of parenteral therapy, there are also cost considerations within enteral therapy categories. Because there is little government regulation of food products and most physicians are uninitiated in the basics of nutritional provision, many companies that market enteral feeding products have seized the opportunity to market unproven and expensive "disease-specific formulas." When benefit is unproven, use is suspect and often cost cannot be justified. Most offer no advantage over adequate calories and protein provided by a standard formula, and therefore their use should be curtailed. Efficacy has been established in only a few of these specialty formulas.

The most widely accepted disease-specific enteral formulas are those designed for use in patients with hepatic failure and protein-limiting encephalopathy [79,80] and for patients with renal failure who are not yet dialysis candidates but need protein or volume restriction. While hepatic formulas enriched with branched-chain amino acids and limited aromatic amino acids have been shown effective in limiting encephalopathy in a number of trials, proof of efficacy of renal formulations with decreased amino acids is elusive. Probably the use of a concentrated solution (2 kcal/ml) with a limited amount of balanced amino acids are as effective at limiting the metabolic disturbances associated with renal failure as are those with specialized protein sources [81]. In addition to enteral formulas designed for patients with hepatic failure, enteral formulas that are immunomodulatory are being studied and also seem to be effective at reducing malnutrition-associated costs.

Bower et al. [40] conducted a prospective randomized study in 326 ICU patients comparing a modified enteral formula containing arginine, ω-3 lipids, and ribonucleic acids (RNA) (IMPACT, Sandoz, Minneapolis, MN) to a standard tube feeding (Osmolite HN, Ross, Columbus, OH). In patients who received at least 821 ml/day of formula, they found a reduction in median length of stay of 8 days ($p < 0.05$) in the group treated with the modified formula. In patients who were stratified as septic, the median length of hospital stay was reduced 10 days ($p < 0.05$) along with a major reduction in the incidence of acquired infections ($p < 0.01$) in the patients who received the modified formula. In a similar study done with cancer patients using the same formula, Daly et al. [41] were able to show a decrease in infectious and wound complications (11% vs. 37%, $p = 0.02$) in postoperative patients treated with the modified formula. In addition, mean length of stay (15.8 ± 5.1 vs. 20.2 ± 9.4 days, $p = 0.01$) was also decreased in the group receiving the modified enteral formula. The modest cost of using immunomodulatory enteral formulas compared to the cost savings in decreased complications and decreased length of stay is attractive from a cost-effectiveness standpoint.

Although often overlooked, elemental formulas also fall within the specialized formula class of enteral nutrition. Elemental tube feedings arose from the realization that dietary nutrients contained within the bowel lumen have not been assimilated into the body proper in critical illness and are, therefore, ineffective in nutritional repletion. It was postulated that predigested nutrients would be absorbed more readily and, therefore, would require less digestive system participation for assimilation. [*Editor's Note:* This assumption may be correct because, in the absorption of protein, oligopeptides rather than single amino acids may be the preferred configuration for absorption.] In addition to increased preparation costs, free amino acids increase tube feeding osmolarity, which may lead to decreased tolerance. Measures to evaluate diarrhea or improve tolerance can add considerably to the costs of enteral therapies, diminishing their cost benefit. Furthermore, gastrointestinal intolerance may necessitate more costly parenteral therapy.

Hamaoui et al. [8] were able to show that enteral formulas containing di- and tripeptides were well-tolerated and cost-effective in the immediate postoperative period. Because di- and tripeptides in the bowel lumen are transported into the mucosal cell and then hydrolyzed to free amino acids, providing nitrogen in the form of free amino acids does not confer any advantage and probably adds unnecessary expense. Oligopeptides from protein hydrolysates are better tolerated, absorbed, and less costly to produce than free amino acids and, therefore, should be the major protein source of formulas designed for enhanced absorption [42–46].

The costs of monitoring for complications and treating them when they arise are additional; the cost of providing nutrition therapies is sometimes overlooked (Table 29-8). In a prospective study of 253 hospitalized tube-fed patients, Cataldi-Betcher et al. [26] showed an 11.7% total complication rate. All patients were fed by continuous pump-controlled infusion. Ninety-one percent were fed by nasogastric tube, 4% by gastrostomy, 2% by jejunostomy, 2% by cervical esophagostomy, and 0.5% by nasoduodenal tube. Seventy-nine percent of patients were fed with standard tube feeding formulas (Isocal, Ensure, Compleat B) following a special protocol designed by the nutrition support department. All patients were monitored daily by the nutrition support team. Diarrhea (2.3%), gastric atony (1.6%), vomiting (1.5%), tube dislodgement or obstruction (1.5%), and aspiration pneumonia (0.8%) were the most common gastrointestinal and mechanical complications. Hyperkalemia (0.8%), azotemia (0.4%), and hypokalemia (0.4%) were the most common metabolic complications of enteral therapies. When the total number of patients receiving enteral therapy are considered, the cost of treating these complications is approximately $18.78 per patient day [25]. However, this figure includes the costs of parenteral nutrition for those 9 patients who failed enteral therapy. When the costs of providing parenteral nutrition are excluded, the cost of treating the complications associated with enteral therapy adds only $0.99 to each patient's nutrition care costs. The complication rate in this study was lower than most reported series and was probably the result of standardized protocols and careful daily monitoring by the nutrition support team [82]. With such meticulous monitoring enteral therapy complications are infrequent, and the costs of treating these complications changes total costs of enteral nutrition administration little.

Table 29-8. Complications of Enteral Nutrition

Complication	Patients Suffering Complication (%)
Mechanical	
Diarrhea	2.3
Gastric atony	1.6
Tube dislodgement	1.5
Emesis	1.5
Aspiration	0.8
Metabolic	
Hyperkalemia	0.8
Azotemia	0.4
Hypokalemia	0.4

When the cost of treating all complications is divided by the total number of patient days on enteral therapy, the cost is $0.99/patient day.
Source: From EL Cataldi-Betcher, et al. Complications occurring during enteral nutrition support: A prospective study. *JPEN* 7:546, 1983.

Isosmolar polymeric tube feedings are started at 20 to 40 ml/hr and advanced 20 ml/hr every 12 to 24 hours to target rate as patient tolerance allows. If a hyperosmotic formulation is used for intragastric feeding it can be started at full strength and at a slow rate that is advanced as tolerance is established. If the patient is being fed into the intestine or the patient has had a drainage procedure (antrectomy, pyloroplasty, pyloromyotomy, or gastrojejunostomy), there is no functioning pylorus to protect the small intestine from the hyperosmotic or volumetric load. For these situations, it is usually recommended to begin with a hyposmolar or diluted tube feeding formula, first advancing the rate, then the concentration after tolerance is established. Alternatively, some clinicians will elect to use full strength formula infused at a slow rate of 10 to 20 ml/hr. Enteric tube feeding intolerance is manifested as nausea, vomiting, crampy abdominal pain, abdominal distention, high aspirates, and diarrhea.

During gastric feeding, aspirates should be checked every four hours. If an aspirate is greater than 50% of the volume fed over the previous four hours, the aspirate should be returned, the tube feeding stopped, the tube flushed with 30 ml of water, and the aspirate rechecked after four hours. If it is less than half the original aspirate, the tube feeding should be resumed at a rate that is 20 to 40 ml/hr less than the original rate. The rate can then be advanced 20 ml/hr/day up to target.

During intestinal feeding if evidence of tube feeding intolerance occurs or an aspirate greater than 100 ml is found, the tube feeding should be stopped. Flush the feeding tube with 30 ml of water and check aspirates in 4 hours. Once clinical symptoms of intolerance subside, resume the tube feeding at a slower rate and then advance 20 ml/hr/day to target rate. If the gastric or small intestine aspirates remain high, IV metoclopramide may be useful. If maximal metoclopramide therapy is unsuccessful, erythromycin's prokinetic activity may be helpful. The usual starting dose is 250 mg IV every 6 hours. For patients at high aspiration risk, methylene blue can be added to the tube feeding. If pulmonary suctioning reveals blue-tinged secretions, aspiration into the tracheobronchial tree is occurring and the tube feeding should be stopped. Tube position should be checked by radiograph. If the tube is not in the small intestine, it should be advanced to that point. If it is already in the small intestine and has not been displaced, advancing the tube distal to the ligament of Treitz may improve tolerance.

Diarrhea may become a problem for the tube-fed patient. Usually bowel misbehavior is not due to the tube feeding but rather administration of hyperosmolar medicines, sorbitol-containing elixirs, infections, or compromise in gut integrity (Tables 29-9 and 29-10). It is useful to divide diarrhea pathophysiology into osmotic and secretory. By checking the osmotic gap of the diarrhea (osmotic gap = measured osmolality − 2(sodium + potassium), etiology is suggested. When diarrhea is due to the enteral feeding, it is usually osmotic in nature.

Unfortunately, it is common in critically ill patients to encounter intolerance to gastric feedings. However, because the jejunum functions sufficiently to absorb nutrients even in the presence of gastric and colonic ileus, it should be used as soon as possible to provide at least a portion of the patient's nutritional needs. Mucosal brush-border atrophy and hypoalbuminemia present in critically ill patients may lead to diarrhea and continued nutritional depletion [46]. Because it may take 4 to 5 days to attain target caloric provision with enteral therapy, a period of concurrent enteral and parenteral nutrition may be necessary to sustain the patient while restoring mucosal function [46].

Clinical indicators such as bowel sounds, nonspecific radiographic findings, abdominal girth, or nasogastric output are of little value in predicting intestinal tube feeding tolerance. We have found little correlation between these indicators and enteral feeding tolerance, and consequently believe that the only truly reliable test of tube feeding tolerance is a trial of postpyloric tube feeding.

When intolerance is due to the tube feeding, it may be related to rate of administration, osmolality, or the composition of the formula. These three variables should be altered one at a time until tolerance is established. One option is to simply decrease the rate of tube feeding. Another is to dilute the tube feeding to half strength before a new formula is tried. If after these interventions the patient does not tolerate one-half strength tube feeding at 30 ml/hr, kaolin-pectin, 30 ml every 3 to 4 hours, can be started and appropriate stool studies sent. The exact mechanism of action of kaolin-pectin is unknown; however, it possesses no known side effects, may bind luminal toxins, may aid in intestinal bacteria recolonization, and may stimulate intestinal trophism. The use of antimotility agents should be reserved for patients whose diarrhea is persistent and whose work-up is negative for infectious or toxin-related diarrhea (Tables 29-9 and 29-10).

Adequate calories provided by a standard tube feeding formula will suffice for most patients.

Table 29-9. Laboratory Evaluation of Tube-Feeding-Associated Diarrhea

Stool osmolality
Stool for fecal leukocytes
Clostridium difficile toxin assay
Clostridium difficile culture
Stool culture for enteric pathogens
Stool for ova and parasites (only if patient was admitted with preexisting diarrhea and has a history suggesting exposure)
Malabsorptive studies

Table 29-10. Common Etiologic Agents in Osmotic and Secretory Diarrhea

Osmotic	Secretory
Sorbitol	Lactulose
Antibiotics	*Clostridium difficile*
Antacids	Intestinal motility disorder
Laxatives	Enteric pathogens
H_2 antagonists	Villous adenoma
Stool softeners	HIV-associated
Mucosal atrophy from malnutrition	Neuroendocrine tumors

Fiber-enriched formulas in general provide the same calories and nutrients as low-residue formulas. The addition of fiber may assist in the maintenance of regular bowel activity. The previous statement notwithstanding, patients may exhibit either diarrhea or constipation with the use of fiber-containing formulas, presumably secondary to fiber intolerance. In those cases, a lower fiber content formula or a standard low-residue formula should be used.

Most tube feeding formulas are balanced with regard to the RDA of vitamins and minerals. However, hospitalized patients often receive multiple medications, some of which may affect the absorption of these micronutrients. In addition, it is usually necessary to administer 1500 to 2000 ml of tube feedings daily for the patient's vitamin and trace element needs to be met. If the patient's target rate is less than that, additional supplementation, in the form of a multivitamin, should be given.

The patient receiving enteral nutritional support should have physiologic and metabolic parameters determined at appropriate intervals. This is necessary to ensure that adequate support is being provided and that metabolic derangements can be detected in a timely fashion. In addition, the commonly referred-to short-turnover proteins transferrin, prealbumin (transthyretin), and retinol-binding protein should be checked weekly to assist with nutritional management by gauging protein synthesis. Additional fluids or electrolytes that are necessary can be separately infused in the tube, added to the tube feeding, or be supplemented parenterally.

Transition Therapy

Transition feeding is a directed change in and facilitation of one feeding modality for another [83,84]. Modalities of transition feeding include parenteral nutrition to tube feeding, parenteral nutrition to oral feeding, and tube feeding to oral feeding. Listed below are guidelines used at the University of Cincinnati for transition feeding.

Parenteral Nutrition to Tube Feeding

Initiate full-strength tube feeding at 20 to 40 ml/hr through an appropriate tube. When enteral tolerance is established, parenteral nutrition should be decreased by the amount of calories provided enterally. Peripheral parenteral nutrition can be tapered in a similar fashion, but this is not necessary. Peripheral formulas can be stopped when enteral calorie provision is adequate, so long as volume requirements are being met. We often continue full parenteral support until one-third to one-half of the patient's caloric needs are being met enterally, then we begin tapering. When we achieve 75% to 80% of the patient's needs enterally, we will often discontinue parenteral therapy. "Topping a patient off" with small amounts of parenteral nutrition (<1 liter/day) subjects the patient to the risks of parenteral therapy with minimal benefit; therefore, we do not support this practice. The tube feeding rate can be advanced by 20 ml/hr every 12 to 24 hours until target calories are attained. Feeding can be changed from continuous to intermittent as need and tolerance allow.

Parenteral Nutrition to Oral Diet

Initiate oral diet (usually clear liquids) when patient tolerance will be likely. If the patient demonstrates tolerance, advance to solid food as is appropriate (for most patients, a full liquid diet consisting of high-fat, high-lactose foods is inappropriate after prolonged NPO status). In general, the rate of administration of parenteral nutrition may be decreased once the patient is consuming 500 or more calories daily. Parenteral nutrition may have a blunting effect on appetite in some patients. Consequently, parenteral nutrition may need to be weaned or discontinued to allow appetite to return. Parenteral nutrition should be stopped once the patient is consuming two-thirds of nutritional requirements without difficulty.

Tube Feeding to Oral Intake

Allowing a patient access to oral diets does not preclude use of tube feeding. Often it is necessary to combine these modalities to meet a patient's needs. Once an oral diet of liquids or solid food is initiated, a simple approach is to convert tube feeding from continuous to nocturnal feeding at the same rate and follow oral intake with calorie counts. This allows at least one-half of needs to be met by tube feedings, while the patient is allowed oral intake at mealtimes during the day. We discontinue tube feedings when the patient is consuming two-thirds of caloric needs. Patients who continue to meet less than their documented caloric needs may try a variety of nutritional supplements. The transition from parenteral or enteral nutrition to oral diet implies that patients assume active involvement in their nutritional care. More patient encouragement may be necessary with this phase of transitional feeding.

Disease-Specific Formulas

While the disease-specific concept has certain limitations, the impetus is to tailor the nutrition to meet the altered needs of patients with specific ailments.

Enteral nutrition formulas can be balanced formulas, which are nutritionally complete, or disease-specific formulas, which are adjusted to the altered needs of the patient with certain diseases. There are now many tube feeding formulas produced that claim to aid in the management of patients with specific diseases. Efficacy has been established in only a few of these specialty formulas. Most of the disease-specific enteral formulas available have altered protein composition to correct the metabolic disturbances in protein metabolism encountered with the specific organ failure, while some formulas have altered carbohydrate-lipid ratios. The most widely accepted disease-specific enteral formulas are those designed for use in patients with hepatic failure and protein-limiting encephalopathy and those with renal failure who are not yet dialysis candidates but need protein restriction.

Approximately 50% of patients with hepatic failure will develop grade 2 or greater encephalopathy when attempts to provide adequate dietary protein are made [85]. Limiting their protein intake can have grave nutritional implications. These patients have been shown to benefit from formulas high in branched-chain amino acids and low in aromatic amino acids. It is possible, using these formulas, to provide 70 to 80 g protein/day to most of these patients without inducing encephalopathy [86]. This amount of protein daily is sufficient to support structural and functional protein synthesis. Additionally, the electrolyte composition of these formulas is altered to help limit the electrolyte disturbances that are often present with hepatic failure.

Renal failure patients who are not being dialyzed tolerate protein and volume loads poorly. Therefore, renal formulas attempt to limit protein infusion by providing limited amounts of amino acids of high biologic quality. The protein composition consists of the essential amino acids plus histidine, which is thought to be conditionally essential in renal failure. Theoretically, these formulas provide a high-quality protein source without nonessential protein load that would elevate the patient's BUN to a level requiring dialysis. In addition to protein alterations, renal formulas also use increased dextrose concentrations to limit volume. Magnesium, phosphorus, potassium, and sodium are likewise limited to assist in managing the electrolyte disturbances commonly found in these patients. Once the patient begins dialysis, protein, volume, and electrolyte restrictions are lessened, and they should be switched to a standard enteral formula with balanced amino acids and standard dextrose and lipid concentrations [87].

The last category of enteral formula that has been proven efficacious is the immunomodulatory class. Studies to date have shown improved immune function, decreased infection rates, and decreased hospital stays with use of this class of formulas. They are nutritionally complete and contain increased amounts of the ω-3 fatty acids, arginine, and RNA. Because of the nucleic acid load, blood urea nitrogen may rise, but this is usually not significant.

Conclusion

Early and aggressive nutrition support is requisite to achieving enteral nutrition's benefits on patient outcome. Overfeeding, as well as underfeeding, will negate some of these positive effects. Therefore, the patient should be given micro- and macronutrients in amounts sufficient to support their metabolic state.

Although it is unclear whether intragastric feeding predisposes to pulmonary aspiration, tolerance is clearly improved by postpyloric nutrient provision. Most enteral "specialty" formulas are unproven and probably unnecessary with the exception of hepatic and possibly renal formulations. Elemental diets composed of free amino acids with oligosaccharides as the major calorie source are poorly tolerated and also probably unnecessary. Immunomodulatory nutrients have proven efficacy in both trauma and cancer patients and should be used liberally when enteral nutrition support is deemed necessary.

Nutrition therapies should be transitioned to

enteral (tube feedings, then oral diets) as soon as feasible. This not only improves the patient's response to nutritional therapy but also provides an additional sense of well-being.

References

1. Berry SM, Bower RH. Nutrition in the ICU. *Pract Gastroenterol* 5(7):35, 1993.
2. Chandra RK. Nutrition, immunity, and infection: present knowledge and future directions. *Lancet* 1:688, 1983.
3. Christou NV, et al. Estimating mortality risk in preoperative patients using immunologic, nutritional, and acute phase response variables. *Ann Surg* 210:69, 1989.
4. Bower RH. Nutrition and immune function. *Nutr Clin Pract* 5:189, 1990.
5. Randall HT. Efficacy, feasibility, safety, and cost comparisons of enteral and parenteral elemental nutrition. *Contemp Surg* 28:4, 1986.
6. Alverdy JC, Aoys E, Moss GS. Total parenteral nutrition promotes bacterial translocation from the gut. *Surgery* 104:185, 1988.
7. Moore FA, et al. TEN versus TPN following major abdominal trauma: Reduced septic morbidity. *J Trauma* 29:916, 1989.
8. Hamaoui E, et al. Enteral nutrition in the early postoperative period: A new semi-elemental formula versus total parenteral nutrition. *JPEN* 14:501, 1990.
9. Shukla HS, et al. Enteral hyperalimentation in malnourished surgical patients. *Indian J Med Res* 80:339, 1984.
10. Fagerman K, Lysen LK. Enteral feeding tubes: A comparison and history. *Nutr Supp Serv* 7:10, 1987.
11. Randall HT. Enteral nutrition: tube feeding in acute and chronic illness. *JPEN* 8:113, 1984.
12. Randall HT. History of enteral nutrition. In JL Rombeau, MD Caldwell (eds), *Enteral and Tube Feeding* (1st ed). Philadelphia: Saunders, 1984. P 1.
13. Einhorn M. Duodenal alimentation. *Med Record* 78:92, 1910.
14. Reilly JJ, et al. Economic impact of malnutrition: A model system for hospitalized patients. *JPEN* 12:371, 1988.
15. Smythe PM, et al. Thymolymphatic deficiency and depression of cell mediated immunity in protein-calorie malnutrition. *Lancet* 2:939, 1971.
16. Muggia-Sullam M, et al. Postoperative enteral versus parenteral nutritional support in gastrointestinal surgery. *Am J Surg* 149:106, 1985.
17. Moore FA, et al. Early enteral feeding, compared with parenteral, reduces postoperative septic complications. *Ann Surg* 216:172, 1992.
18. Bower RH, et al. Postoperative enteral vs. parenteral nutrition. *Arch Surg* 121:1040, 1986.
19. Kudsk KA, et al. Enteral versus parenteral feeding. *Ann Surg* 215:503, 1992.
20. Lim STK, et al. Total parenteral nutrition versus gastrostomy in the preoperative preparation of patients with carcinoma of the esophagus. *Br J Surg* 68:69, 1981.
21. Mughal MM, Meguid MM. The effect of nutritional status on morbidity after elective surgery for benign gastrointestinal disease. *JPEN* 11:140, 1987.
22. Detsky AS, et al. Evaluating the accuracy of nutritional assessment techniques applied to hospitalized patients: Methodology and comparisons. *JPEN* 8:153, 1984.
23. Buzby GP, et al. Prognostic nutritional index in gastrointestinal surgery. *Am J Surg* 139:160, 1986.
24. Detsky AS, et al. Predicting nutrition associated complications for patients undergoing gastrointestinal surgery. *JPEN* 11:446, 1987.
25. Twomey PL, Patching SC. Cost-effectiveness of nutrition support. *JPEN* 9:3, 1985.
26. Cataldi-Betcher EL, et al. Complications occurring during enteral nutrition support: A prospective study. *JPEN* 7:546, 1983.
27. Roberts D, Thelen D, Weinstein S. Parenteral and enteral nutrition: A cost-benefit audit. *Minn Med* 65:707, 1982.
28. Meguid MM, Muscaritoli M. Current uses of total parenteral nutrition. *Am Fam Phys* 47:383, 1993.
29. Wolfe BM, Phillips GJ, Hodges RE. Evaluation and management of nutritional status before surgery. *Med Clin North Am* 63:1257, 1979.
30. Adibi SA. Intestinal transport of dipeptides in man: Relative importance of hydrolysis and intact absorption. *J Clin Invest* 50:2266, 1971.
31. Adibi SA. Intestinal phase of protein assimilation in man. *Am J Clin Nutr* 29:205, 1976.
32. Keohane P, et al. Influence of protein composition and hydrolysis method on intestinal absorption of protein in man. *Gut* 26:907, 1985.
33. Matthews DM. Intestinal absorption of peptides. *Physiol Rev* 55:537, 1975.
34. Matthews DM, Adibi SA. Peptide absorption. *Gastroenterology* 71:151, 1976.
35. Adibi SA, Allen ER. Impaired jejunal absorption rates of essential amino acids induced by either dietary caloric or protein deprivation in man. *Gastroenterology* 59:404, 1970.
36. Berry SM, Lacy JA, Nussbaum MS. Basic concepts of enteral and parenteral nutrition. In M Torosian (ed), *Hospital Based Nutrition.* New York: Marcel-Dekker, 1994.
37. Bower RH. Nutrition for critically ill patients. In J Cameron (ed), *Current Surgical Therapy* (4th ed.) St. Louis: BC Decker, 1992. P 1051.
38. Rombeau JL, Rolandelli RH, Wilmore DW. Nutritional support. In D Wilmore, et al (eds), *Care of the Surgical Patient* (1st ed.) New York: Scientific American, 1988. P 1.
39. Deitch EA. Multiple organ failure. *Ann Surg* 216:117, 1992.
40. Bower RH, et al. Early enteral administration of a formula supplemented with arginine, nucleotides and fish oil in intensive care unit patients: Results of a randomized prospective clinical trial. *Crit Care Med* 23(3):430, 1995.
41. Daly JM, et al. Enteral nutrition with supplemental arginine, RNA, and omega-3 fatty acids in patients after operation: Immunologic, metabolic, and clinical outcome. *Surgery* 112:56, 1992.
42. Barbul A. Arginine and immune function. *Nutrition* 6:53, 1990.
43. Kinsella JE, Lokesh B. Dietary lipids, eicosanoids, and the immune system. *Crit Care Med* 18:S94, 1989.
44. Johnson PV, Marshall LA. Dietary fat, the prostaglandins and the immune response. *Prog Food Nutr Sci* 8:3, 1984.
45. Kulkarni AD, et al. Modulation of delayed hypersensitivity in mice by dietary nucleotide restriction. *Transplantation* 44:847, 1987.
46. Kulkarni SS, et al. Functional impairment of T lymphocytes in mouse radiation chimeras by a nucleotide-free diet. *Exp Hematol* 12:694, 1984.
47. Raper S, Maynard N. Feeding the critically ill. *Br J Nurs* 1:273, 1992.

48. Kiver KF, et al. Pre- and postpyloric enteral feeding: Analysis of safety and complications [Abstract]. *JPEN* 8:95, 1984.

49. Burtch GD, Shatney CH. Feeding jejunostomy (versus gastrostomy) passes the test of time. *Am J Surg* 53:54, 1987.

50. Ponsky JL, et al. Percutaneous approaches to enteral alimentation. *Am J Surg* 149:102, 1985.

51. Payne-James J. Enteral nutrition: Accessing patients. *Nutrition* 8:223, 1992.

52. Strong RM, et al. Equal aspiration rates from postpylorus and intragastric-placed small-bore nasoenteric feeding tubes: A randomized, prospective study. *JPEN* 16:59, 1992.

53. Caulfield KA, Page CP, Pestana C. Technique for intraduodenal placement of transnasal enteral feeding catheters. *Nutr Clin Pract* 6:23, 1991.

54. Lord LM, et al. Comparison of weighted vs. unweighted enteral feeding tubes for efficacy of transpyloric intubation. *JPEN* 17:271, 1993.

55. Cardoza JD, Jeffrey RB. Nasojejunal feeding tube placement in immobile patients. *Radiology* 166:893, 1988.

56. Rees RGP, et al. Spontaneous transpyloric passage and performance of "fine bore" polyurethane feeding tubes: A controlled clinical trial. *JPEN* 12:469, 1988.

57. Thurlow PM. Bedside enteral feeding tube placement into duodenun and jejunum. *JPEN* 10:104, 1986.

58. Ugo PJ, Mohler PA, Wilson GL. Bedside postpyloric placement of weighted feeding tubes. *Nutr Clin Pract* 7:284, 1992.

59. Ramos SM, Lindine P. Inexpensive, safe and simple nasoenteral intubation: An alternative for the cost conscious. *JPEN* 10:78, 1986.

60. Boyes RJ, Kruse JA. Nasogastric and nasoenteric intubation. *Crit Care Clin* 8:865, 1992.

61. Rives DA, et al. Endoscopically assisted nasojejunal feeding tube placement. *Am Surg* 55:88, 1989.

62. Metheny N, Spies MA, Eisenberg P. Measures to test placement of nasoenteral feeding tubes. *West J Nurs Res* 10:367, 1988.

63. Metheny N. Measures to test placement of nasogastric and nasointestinal feeding tubes: A review. *Nurs Res* 37:224, 1988.

64. Chang J, et al. Inadvertent endobronchial intubation with nasogastric tube. *Arch Otol* 108:528, 1982.

65. Muthuswamy P, Patel K, Ragendren R. Isocal pneumonia with respiratory failure. *Chest* 81:390, 1982.

66. Torrington K, Bowman M. Fatal hydrothorax empyema complicating a malpositioned nasogastric tube. *Chest* 79:240, 1981.

67. Ghahremani GG, Gould RJ. Nasoenteric feeding tubes, radiographic detection of complications. *Dig Dis Sci* 31:574, 1986.

68. Strong RM, et al. Enteral tube feedings utilizing a pH sensor enteral feeding tube. *Nutr Supp Serv* 8:11, 1988.

69. Dimand R. Cannulation of the small bowel using a pH guided feeding tube in critically ill infants and children [Abstract]. *JPEN* 15:24S, 1991.

70. Smith DW, Lee RM. Nutritional management in duodenal fistula. *Surg Gynecol Obstet* 103:666, 1956.

71. Meguid MM, Campos AC, Hammond WG. Nutrition support in surgical practice. *Am J Surg* 159:427, 1990.

72. Rombeau JL, Rolandelli RH. Enteral and parenteral nutrition in patients with enteric fistulas and short bowel syndrome. *Surg Clin North Am* 67:551, 1987.

73. Stephens RV, Randall HT. Use of concentrated balanced liquid elemental diet for nutritional management of catabolic states. *Ann Surg* 170:642, 1969.

74. Raminski MV. Enteral hyperalimentation. *Surg Gynecol Obstet* 143:12, 1976.

75. Shils ME. Enteral nutrition by tube. *Cancer Res* 37:2432, 1977.

76. Bethel RA, et al. Nasogastric hyperalimentation through a polyethylene catheter: An alternative to central venous hyperalimentation. *Am J Clin Nutr* 32:1112, 1979.

77. Chernoff R. Nutritional support: Formulas and delivery of enteral feeding. *J Am Diet Assoc* 79:426, 1981.

78. Heymsfield SB, et al. Enteral hyperalimentation: An alternative to central venous hyperalimentation. *Ann Int Med* 90:63, 1979.

79. Kearns PJ, et al. Accelerated improvement of alcoholic liver disease with enteral nutrition. *Gastroenterology* 102:200, 1992.

80. Greenberger NJ, et al. Effect of vegetable and animal protein diets in chronic active encephalopathy. *Dig Dis Sci* 22:845, 1977.

81. A.S.P.E.N. Board of Directors. Guidelines for the use of parenteral and enteral nutrition in adult and pediatric patients. *JPEN* 17:1SA, 1993.

82. Brown RO, et al. Enteral nutrition support management in a university teaching hospital: Team versus non-team. *JPEN* 11:52, 1987.

83. Krey SH, Murray RL. Modular and transitional feedings. In JL Rombeau, MD Caldwell (eds), *Enteral and Tube Feeding* (2nd ed). Philadelphia: Saunders, 1990. P 127.

84. Zibrida M, Carlson SJ. Transitional feeding. In MM Gottschlich, LE Matarese, EP Shronts (eds), *Nutrition Support Dietetics Core Curriculum* (2nd ed). Silver Spring, MD: American Society of Parenteral and Enteral Nutrition, 1993. P 459.

85. Shanbhogue RL, et al. Increased protein catabolism without hypermetabolism after human orthotopic liver transplantation. *Surgery* 101:146, 1987.

86. Hehir DJ, et al. Nutrition in patients undergoing orthotopic liver transplant. *JPEN* 9:695, 1985.

87. Fischer JE, Bower RH. Nutritional support in liver disease. *Surg Clin North Am* 61:653, 1981.

Selected Readings

ASPEN Board of Directors. Guidelines for the use of parenteral and enteral nutrition in adult and pediatric patients. *JPEN* 17:1SA, 1993.

General guidelines for the use of both parenteral and enteral nutrition therapies.

Bower RH, et al. Early enteral administration of a formula supplemented with arginine, nucleotides and fish oil in intensive care unit patients: Results of a multicenter prospective, randomized, clinical trial. *Crit Care Med* 23(3):436, 1995. In press.

Documentation of the efficacy of pharmaconutrients in septic and/or critically ill ICU patients.

Daly JM, et al. Enteral nutrition with supplemental arginine, RNA, and omega-3 fatty acids in patients after operation: Immunologic, metabolic, and clinical outcome. *Surgery* 112:56, 1992.

Documentation of the efficacy of pharmaconutrients in postoperative cancer patients.

Moore FA, et al. Early enteral feeding, compared with parenteral, reduces postoperative septic complications. *Ann Surg* 216:172, 1992.

A meta-analysis collating eight studies comparing complication rates between enterally and parenterally fed patients.

30

Critical Evaluation of Results: Cost and Benefit of Nutrition Support

Scott M. Berry
Joseph A. Lacy

In the American health care system we have enjoyed the best that technology has to offer, with little regard for cost. It is what our patient advocates have always demanded, and it is how we are trained to practice medicine. The most technically advanced forms of therapy are usually also the most expensive, primarily due to research and development costs, unfavorable economic scale, and limited availability. We have been willing to escalate care costs for the sake of providing the "best" care. However, "most technically advanced" and "best" are not necessarily synonymous. With a few notable exceptions, the most basic and least expensive nutritional therapies often are the best.

Because of the indolent nature of many nutritional problems, the immediate benefit of nutrition intervention in all but the most severely depleted patients is difficult to demonstrate. Although specialized forms of nutritional therapy can be expensive, when compared to other forms of medical therapy most nutritional therapies are relatively inexpensive. This is especially true for enteral forms of therapy. Therefore, benefit need only be modest to justify cost.

Nutrition is considered so basic to life that to withhold it requires special and profound circumstances. Withholding a medical therapy may allow an established disease to progress; withholding nutrition can create fertile ground for disease occurrence and progression. A patient who can eat should be allowed to do so. If nutritional status is normal and the patient is unable or unwilling to take adequate nutrition by mouth for more than a week, enteral therapy through a tube should be used. If the patient is malnourished, the time interval between decreased oral intake and commencement of enteral therapy is shortened. Few would question the appropriateness or the cost-to-benefit ratio of these measures because most acknowledge that to sustain life, all people require nutrition. However, the use of more expensive specialized enteral formulas and parenteral nutrition is not as straightforward. Specialized enteral and parenteral nutrition formulas have proven benefit in only selected patient populations; therefore, cost-effective use of these therapies requires discrimination.

Morbidity and mortality have been the most commonly used end points in clinical studies. Therapies that lower morbidity and/or mortality are considered effective by the clinician, quite correctly, regardless of cost. Thus, disregard for cost issues is promulgated. Ideally, the terms "effective" and "cost-effective" would be interchangeable; however, such is not always the case. For example, should a $1000 therapy be 10 times more effective than a $100 therapy? Similarly, to justify their existence, should it be required that all therapies save more money in decreased morbidity and mortality than it costs to provide them? Recently, length of stay (LOS), which is a crude measure of hospital costs, has been increasingly used as an end point in clinical studies. Using LOS as an end point in clinical studies serves to focus clinicians on cost issues, albeit indirectly.

There seems to be something distasteful, almost anti-Hippocratic, about applying cost-benefit analysis to health care expenditure. However, the issue is not one of limiting medical therapies to patients in need of them, but rather of the discriminate use of available therapies. Stated in another way, the cost of many technologically advanced therapies mandates use only where medical benefit is proven. In the past, use of medical technology was ultimately dictated by the clinician's interpretation of studies showing diagnostic or therapeutic benefit. While the same principle remains true, "reimbursability" is now an additional environmental pressure shaping the evolution of medical practice. Now, more than ever, it is imperative that the clinician know and understand the applicability and limitations of specific medical therapies. While the inappropriate use of many therapies may not be detrimental to the patient, unless use is clearly indicated and beneficial the patient will not only receive inferior care, but in our new environment reimbursement may be denied. The intelligent use of medical resources is requisite as treatment decisions are more closely scrutinized. Although most of us would choose to be sheltered from cost issues, economic isolation in medicine is truly a thing of the past.

Many tools are available to help resolve the issue of "Is it worth it?" As defined by Twomey and Patching [1], *risk-benefit* analysis compares the morbidity and mortality of medical intervention with the morbidity and mortality of the untreated disease process (Table 30-1). This is the end point most commonly used in clinical studies and is done without regard for cost issues. As advanced and expensive treatments for previously poorly treated or untreatable conditions have developed, demand for these therapies continues to increase. However, supply is often limited by availability and, ultimately, cost constraints. To improve use of resources limited by monetary scarcity, *cost-benefit* analysis—which relates the monetary cost of a therapy to the benefit produced—is often employed. This requires that cost and benefit be in the same units, most commonly dollars. However, assigning a dollar value to pain, loss of function, quality of life, and ultimately life itself requires judgment determinations few would agree on. *Cost-effective* analysis allows comparisons of competing therapies without relying purely on clinical or monetary guidelines. It can compare number of lives saved or diseases prevented per dollar spent, and allows conclusions to be drawn about the most effective use of monetary resources.

Table 30-1. Definitions

Risk-Benefit	Compares the morbidity and mortality of a medical intervention with the morbidity and mortality of the untreated disease process. The end point most commonly used in clinical studies. Done without regard for cost issues.
Cost-Benefit	Relates the monetary cost of a therapy to the benefit produced. Requires that cost and benefit be in the same units, most commonly dollars. Difficult to assign dollar values to pain, loss of function, quality of life, and loss of life. Requires judgment determinations few can agree on.
Cost-Effective	Comparisons of competing therapies without relying purely on clinical or monetary issues. Compares number of lives saved per dollar spent and allows conclusions to be drawn about the most effective use of monetary resources.

Source: Twomey PL and Patching SC. Cost-effectiveness of nutrition support. *JPEN* 9:3, 1985.

Proven benefit is the mainstay of cost-effective medical therapy in general, and cost-effective nutrition support in particular. Medical practice fashioned by the use of medical technology only where patient benefit is proven constitutes good medicine, and good medicine is always cost-effective.

Prevalence and Costs of Malnutrition

It is estimated that more than 5 million patients in the United States receive oral, enteral, or parenteral nutrition therapies annually in hospitals, long-term care facilities, and at home [2]. The total annual costs for this care exceed $3 billion [3]. Malnutrition has many causes and manifestations and represents a clinical continuum from imperceptible to gross structural and functional changes. Total starvation for 3 days in normal adults results primarily in glycogen and water losses, but by day 15 in normally nourished individuals and by day 7 in people with interceding illnesses, functional deficits become increasingly evident [4,5]. Unintended weight loss greater than 10% of normal body weight in hospitalized patients results in more complications, higher mortality rates, longer hospital stays, and, therefore, greater health care resource use [3–14]. In addition, patients with a serum albumin less than 3.0 g/dL, a poor nutritional status by Subjective Global Assessment [15–17], or a Prognostic Nutritional Index [18] of $\geq$ 60 are 3.5 to 4.5 times more likely to experience postoperative complications than those with normal nutritional indices [19].

On admission, as many as 50% of hospitalized patients have moderate malnutrition, while 5% to 10% are severely malnourished (Table 30-2) [8,20–31]. One may quibble over the percentages, but overall the situation demonstrates that a significant number of hospital patients enter malnourished. Further, serial evaluations have shown

Table 30-2. Prevalence of Hospital Malnutrition

Study	Population	Malnutrition Criteria & Incidence
Mullen (1979) [30]	64 nonselected surgical patients	albumin—16% transferrin—50% total protein—5% creatinine-height index—65% triceps skinfold—33% midarm circumference—36% T-lymphocyte rosette formation—36% lymphocyte migration—68% total lymphocyte count—25% delayed hypersensitivity—62%
Forse (1980) [136]	216 nonselected surgical patients	body composition—37%
Buzby (1986) [18]	100 intestinal surgical patients	prognostic nutritional index (PNI): intermediate-risk—23% high-risk—39%
O'Leary (1982) [31]	1225 nonselected VA patients	ideal body weight—13% midarm circumference—16% triceps skinfold—49% arm muscle circumference—8% arm muscle area—27% anergy—35% total lymphocyte count—37% albumin—14%
Baker (1982) [16]	59 nonselected surgical patients	subjective clinical assessment: mild malnutrition—12% severe malnutrition—27%
Kamath (1986) [23]	3047 nonselected patients	albumin—12% hemoglobin—29% total lymphocyte count—46%
Reilly (1988) [9]	771 nonselected patients	likelihood of malnutrition (LOM) score: medical patients—59% surgical patients—48%
Coates (1989) [22]	228 nonselected medical patients	likelihood of malnutrition (LOM) score—46%

Note: Bracketed numbers correspond with references.

that nutritional status worsens over the length of hospitalization in both medical and surgical patients [32–40]. In addition, up to 70% of patients transferred from hospitals to long-term care facilities have evidence of malnutrition [41]. With few exceptions, for patients with the same diagnosis, hospitals receive the same Diagnosis Related Group (DRG) mandated payment whether hospital stay is short and inexpensive or long and expensive. Therefore, shortening hospital stay by speeding convalescence and decreasing complications is paramount from the perspectives of both a patient's well-being and fiscal responsibility. Alternatively, there are specific ways to improve DRG reimbursement, the major determinants of which are (1) principal diagnosis, (2) comorbid conditions (present on admission), (3) complications (nosocomially acquired), (4) procedures performed, and (5) the patient's age and sex. Documentation of comorbid conditions and complications are the two areas of DRG reimbursement documentation that are commonly neglected. Patients are not usually admitted to the hospital for malnutrition per se but may be admitted with a diagnosis that is directly related to poor nutritional status. Although malnutrition may be the antecedent event, it is not the primary diagnosis. Nonetheless, malnutrition is present in a major percentage of hospitalized patients on admission and often increases with length of stay [8,20–40]. In spite of this fact, malnutrition is listed as a comorbid condition or complication in only 5% to 10% of discharge summaries. In the absence of proper documentation, hospitals must absorb the increased expenditure associated with these conditions. Proper documentation of malnutrition as a comorbid condition or as a complication may more than justify the use of nutrition support and the presence of nutrition support departments.

Malnourished patients have excess hospital costs of $1738 and incur $3557 in additional charges when compared to their normally nourished counterparts, according to a 1987 study (Table 30-3) [9]. When complications occur in malnourished patients, those figures increase to $2996 and $6157, respectively [9]. In a study of burn patients, Weinsier et al. [42] showed significantly decreased hospital stay (29 ± 15 vs. 36 ± 19 days , $p < 0.01$) and hospital costs ($17,800 ± $11,300 vs. $24,200 ± $20,000, $p < 0.02$) in patients treated with aggressive nutrition support. Christensen et al. [27,43] showed that, in a community hospital, 32% of the patients were malnourished but consumed 45% of total health care expenditures, costing nearly twice as much to care for than their well-nourished counterparts. Robinson et al. [44] found that in an urban teaching hospital, the incidence of malnutrition was higher than in community hospitals (56%), as was the percentage of expenditure (73%) for the malnourished group.

Studies done by Shaw-Stiffel et al. [45] in general surgical patients and by Anderson et al. [46] in general medical patients have shown that malnutrition increases length of hospital stay by up to 50%. Studies by Robinson et al. [44] and Linn et al. [47] have confirmed this 50% increase in length of stay for malnourished patients, although DRG reimbursement was similar to that for normally nourished individuals. The actual hospital costs for malnourished patients admitted to a general medical ward were $16,791 compared to $5124 for well-nourished patients [46], leaving hospitals to absorb the difference. The institution of DRGs has also led to decreased preoperative time in hospitals for malnourished patients: from 22 days to 6 days [47]. Coinciding with DRG institution and decreased preoperative hospital time has been a 250% increase in mechanical complication rates, a 60% increase in infectious complication rates, and a 10% increase in readmission rates following surgery for head and neck cancers, reiterating that the cost of treating the consequences of malnutrition are far greater than the cost of treatment for malnutrition [47]. These findings are supported by Linn [48], who found that malnourished hospitalized patients had an increased risk of health problems up to one year after discharge. Based on these studies, reduction in morbidity and mortality associated with comorbid and nosocomially acquired malnutrition would seem to justify use of nutrition support in malnourished patients, and early admission for preoperative nutritional repletion for severely malnourished patients.

Enteral Versus Parenteral Trials

Before parenteral nutrition development and clinical implementation in the 1970s, early operative intervention for correctable intestinal problems was the only option to reduce malnutrition-related morbidity and mortality. For uncorrectable intestinal problems, such as short-gut syndrome, there was little to offer. The application of parenteral nutrition technology to certain disorders was truly life-saving. Initially, parenteral nutrition seemed equivalent to enteral nutrition, and applications for this technology seemed limitless. However, as the mechanical, metabolic, septic, and monetary issues surrounding parenteral nutrition administration became manifest, proof of benefit was demanded and indiscriminate use discouraged.

Muggia-Sullam et al. [49] showed that in non-

Table 30-3. Effects of Malnutrition

Study	Population	Findings
Mullen (1979) [30]	64 surgical patients	albumin < 30 g/L: 2.5× complications transferrin < 220 mg/dL: 5× complications anergy to 1 of 3 antigens: 2.5× complications
Buzby (1986) [18]	100 surgical patients	sepsis death PNI < 40%: 3%–8% 3% PNI 40%–49%: 9%–22% 4% PNI ≥ 50%: 26%–28% 33%
Anderson (1984) [137]	74 gynecologic and urologic patients	LOS > 10 days in 48% of patients when albumin, prealbumin, retinol-binding protein, or protein intake was low; when normal, only 20% had > 10-day LOS
Anderson (1985) [46]	135 general medical patients	inability to eat and albumin < 35 g/L predicted LOS > 8 d
Detsky (1987) [19]	202 surgical patients	severe malnutrition by SGA: 4.44× complications albumin < 30 g/L: 4.02× complications admission PNI ≥ 60: 3.61× complications
Reilly (1988) [9]	771 hospital admissions	2.6× minor complications 3.4× major complications 3.8× death rate increased LOS (1.1–12.8 d) increased hospital costs ($1738) increased patient charges ($3557) increased complication costs ($2996) increased complication charges ($6157)
Linn (1988) [47]	120 head and neck cancer patients: malnourished (M) vs. normally nourished (N)	M N postop. stay 17–23 d 10 d complications 3× — infections 32% 19% readmissions 20%–30% 50%–60%
Shaw-Stiffel (1993) [45]	245 surgical patients	LOS 16.5 ± 10.7 days when normally nourished, 23.5 ± 16.5 d when malnourished

LOS = length of stay, PNI = prognostic nutritional index, SGA = subjective global assessment.
Note: Bracketed numbers correspond with references.

selected patients, parenteral and enteral nutrition regimens were equivalent in promoting nitrogen balance, preserving body weight, and promoting protein synthesis. However, other studies show parenteral nutrition superior in achieving caloric needs, early positive nitrogen balance, and weight gain; protein synthetic markers, such as albumin and short-turnover proteins, were virtually always equivalent (Table 30-4) [50–55].

Moore et al. [53] performed a prospective randomized study in trauma patients comparing complication rates between enterally and parenterally fed groups. They found a decreased incidence of abdominal abscesses and pneumonias (3% vs. 20%, $p = 0.003$) in the enterally fed group. In a similar study, Kudsk et al. [54] also showed a decreased incidence of infections per patient (0.4 ± 0.2 vs. 1.2 ± 0.3, $p = 0.03$), intraabdominal abscess (1.9% vs. 13.3%, $p < 0.04$), and pneumonias (11.8% vs. 31%, $p < 0.02$) in the enterally fed group.

However, Bower et al. [52] showed no difference in outcome between groups of nonselected general surgery patients. The results are probably due in part to the low incidence of septic complications that occur in nonselected groups of patients undergoing elective abdominal procedures [10, 15,18,19]. This seems to be substantiated by a meta-analysis done by Moore et al. [51] where, after combining eight prospective randomized trials comparing septic complications between enterally and parenterally fed patients, the incidence of septic complications was not significantly reduced in the elective-surgery (9% vs. 21%, NS) and penetrating-trauma groups (16% vs. 27.5%, NS). Enterally fed blunt trauma patients had the most significant reduction in sepsis rates (21% vs. 50%, $p < 0.05$). Enteral nutrition reduced the sep-

Table 30-4. Enteral Versus Parenteral Trials

Study	Population	Findings
Lim (1981) [55]	24 esophageal cancer patients	PN: superior nitrogen balance, superior weight gain, greater calories received EN: superior albumin gain, superior morale
Muggia-Sullam (1985) [49]	19 general surgical patients	Equivalent body weight maintenance, glucagon, insulin, gastrin, and pancreatic polypeptide levels PN: slightly earlier nitrogen balance, superior prealbumin and retinol-binding protein between days 2 and 6, vasoactive intestinal peptide levels decreased
Bower (1986) [52]	20 general surgical patients	PN: superior nitrogen intake, albumin decreased, cost: \$330.37/d EN: albumin maintained, cost: \$121.34/d
Moore (1989) [53]	59 trauma patients	Equivalent nitrogen balance EN: superior albumin, transferrin, and retinol-binding protein restoration, fewer septic complications (17% vs. 37%), decreased major sepsis (3% vs. 20%)
Hamaoui (1990) [50]	19 surgical patients	Equivalent albumin, prealbumin, transferrin levels PN: superior nitrogen balance, greater calories received, cost: \$102.10/d EN: cost: \$44.36/d
Moore (1992) [51]	230 patient meta-analysis	PN: superior nitrogen balance, superior weight gain, less gastrointestinal discomfort EN: fewer total (38% vs. 59%) and septic (17% vs. 44%) complications, superior glucose control, lower SGOT and LDH, superior total protein, albumin, and transferrin levels, decreased LOS (17 vs. 22 days) and SICU/LOS (4.4 vs. 7.3 d) in penetrating trauma group
Kudsk (1992) [54]	98 trauma patients	Equivalent nitrogen balance PN: higher bilirubin (2.2 vs. 0.3 mg/dL), superior caloric provision, less diarrhea (21% vs. 15%) EN: fewer infections per patient (0.25 vs. 0.71), fewer pneumonias (11.8% vs. 31%), intraabdominal abscesses (1.9% vs. 13.3%), and central line infections (1.9% vs. 13.3%)

EN = enteral nutrition, LDH = lactate dehydrogenase, LOS = length of stay, PN = parenteral nutrition, SGOT = serum glutamic-oxaloucetic transaminase, SICU = surgical intensive care unit.

Note: Bracketed numbers correspond with references.

tic complication rate in blunt trauma patients to that observed in elective surgery patient populations, seemingly removing the combined immunosuppressive effects of blunt trauma and parenteral nutrition. Because the septic potential in nonselected surgical and penetrating trauma patients are low, although enteral nutritional therapy may be superior to parenteral therapy, proof of decreased complication rates in these two groups will require exceedingly large samples. Realistically, studies large enough to show superior outcome may never be done. Finally, a study in surgical patients by Hamaoui et al. [50] in 1990 showed that the mean daily costs for enteral nutrition were considerably lower than for parenteral (\$44.36 ± 8.50 vs. \$102.10 ± 11.77, $p < 0.01$). They point out that although the cost of nutrients was similar between groups, the cost of nonnutrient supplies added considerably to the cost of parenteral nutrition provision (parenteral: 43% vs. enteral: 13% of total costs). In addition, because complications are less frequent with enteral nutrition therapies, when the cost of treating complications is divided by the entire group at risk, enterally fed patient costs are virtually always lower than the costs for parenterally fed patients [1,56]. These and other studies suggest that enteral nutrition is virtually always less expensive to administer and monitor than parenteral nutrition [57–59]. In addition, enteral therapy may give superior nutritional (and immunologic?) response despite inferior nitrogen balance and caloric provision.

Cost-Effective Enteral Nutrition

The functioning gastrointestinal tract should be used for provision of nutrition. It has been shown that enteral therapies promote nitrogen retention, restore body cell mass, restore cell-mediated immunity, accelerate wound healing, and improve overall nutritional status in addition to being less costly than equivalent parenteral therapies [14,50,51,53,60–65]. In addition to the use of enteral therapy being more cost-effective than use of parenteral therapy, there are also cost considerations within enteral therapy categories. Because there is little government regulation of food products and most physicians are uninitiated in the basics of nutritional provision, many companies that market enteral feeding products have seized the opportunity to market unproven and expensive "disease-specific" formulas. When benefit is unproven, use is suspect, and often cost cannot be justified. Most offer no advantage over adequate calories and protein provided by a standard formula and, therefore, their use should be curtailed. Efficacy has been established in only a few of these specialty formulas.

The most widely accepted disease-specific enteral formulas are those designed for use in patients with hepatic failure and protein-limiting encephalopathy [66,67], and for patients with renal failure who are not yet dialysis candidates but need protein or volume restriction. While hepatic formulas enriched with branched-chain amino acids and limited aromatic amino acids have been shown effective in limiting encephalopathy in a number of trials, proof of efficacy of renal formulations with decreased amino acids is elusive. Probably the use of a concentrated solution (2 kcal/ml) with a limited amount of balanced amino acids is as effective at limiting the metabolic disturbances associated with renal failure as are those with specialized protein sources [2], although one study showed much poorer outcome in the nonessential amino acid group [68]. In addition to enteral formulas designed for patients with hepatic failure, enteral formulas that are immunomodulatory are being studied and also seem to be effective at reducing malnutrition-associated costs.

Bower et al. [69] conducted a prospective randomized study in trauma patients comparing a modified enteral formula containing arginine, ω-3 lipids, and ribonucleic acids (Impact, Sandoz, Minneapolis, MN) to a standard tube feeding (Osmolite HN, Ross, Columbus, OH). In this study of 326 patients, they found a 27% decrease in length of stay (22 vs. 30 days, $p = 0.05$) in the group treated with the modified formula. Although the incidence of most infectious complications was lower in the modified formula group, this difference attained significance only for urinary tract infections ($p = 0.05$). Finally, the modified formula group also had a decreased length of stay from the onset of infectious complications to discharge. This decrease was most pronounced for the group of patients who developed pneumonias (19 vs. 27 days, $p = 0.01$). In a similar study done with cancer patients using the same formula, Daly et al. [13] were able to show a decrease in infectious and wound complications (11% vs. 37%, $p = 0.02$) in postoperative patients treated with the modified formula. In addition, mean length of stay (15.8 ± 5.1 vs. 20.2 ± 9.4 days, $p = 0.01$) was also decreased in the group receiving the modified enteral formula. The modest cost of using immunomodulatory enteral formulas when compared to the cost savings in decreased complications and decreased length of stay is attractive from a cost-effectiveness standpoint (Table 30-5).

Table 30-5. Enteral Nutrition Support

Study	Population	Findings
Bower (1993) [69]	326 hospital patients randomized to study or standard enteral formulas	Equivalent mortality and tolerance Study group: decreased LOS (22 vs. 30 d), fewer septic complications, decreased LOS after onset of infectious complication
Daly (1992) [13]	85 GI cancer surgical patients randomized to study or standard enteral formulas	Equivalent calories received, nitrogen received, and nitrogen balance Study group: improved lymphocyte mitogenesis, increased arginine and ornithine levels, fewer infectious and wound complications (11% vs. 37%), decreased LOS (15.8 vs. 20.2 d)
Cataldi-Betcher (1983) [56]	253 hospitalized enterally fed patients	6.2% GI, 3.5% mechanical, and 2.0% metabolic complication rates, 29% specialty formula usage

LOS = length of stay

Note: Bracketed numbers correspond with references.

Although often overlooked, elemental formulas also fall within the specialized formula class of enteral nutrition. Elemental tube feedings arose from the realization that dietary nutrients contained within the bowel lumen have not been assimilated into the body proper in critical illness and are therefore ineffective in nutritional repletion. It was postulated that predigested nutrients would be absorbed more readily and thus required less digestive system participation for assimilation. In addition to increased preparation costs, free amino acids increase tube feeding osmolarity, which may lead to decreased tolerance. Measures to evaluate diarrhea or improve tolerance can add considerably to the costs of enteral therapies, diminishing their cost-benefit ratio. Furthermore, gastrointestinal intolerance may necessitate more costly parenteral therapy. Hamaoui et al. [50] were able to show that enteral formulas containing di- and tripeptides were well tolerated and cost-effective in the immediate postoperative period. Because di- and tripeptides in the bowel lumen are the preferred means of transport into the mucosal cell and then hydrolyzed to free amino acids, providing nitrogen in the form of free amino acids does not confer any advantage, may actually be disadvantageous, and probably adds unnecessary expense. Because oligopeptides from protein hydrolysates are better tolerated and absorbed and are less costly to produce than free amino acids, they should be the major protein source of formulas designed for enhanced absorption [70–74].

The cost of monitoring for complications and treating them when they arise are additional, sometimes overlooked, costs of providing nutrition therapies. In a prospective study of 253 hospitalized tube-fed patients, Cataldi-Betcher et al. [56] showed a 11.7% total complication rate. All patients were fed by continuous pump-controlled infusion; 91% were fed by nasogastric tube, 4% by gastrostomy, 2% by jejunostomy, 2% by cervical esophagostomy, and 0.5% by nasoduodenal tube. Seventy-nine percent of patients were fed with standard tube feeding formulas (Isocal, Ensure, Compleat B) following a special protocol designed by the nutrition support department. All patients were monitored daily by the nutrition support team. Diarrhea (2.3%), gastric atony (1.6%), emesis (1.5%), tube dislodgement or obstruction (1.5%), and aspiration pneumonia (0.8%) were the most common gastrointestinal and mechanical complications. Hyperkalemia (0.8%), azotemia (0.4%), and hypokalemia (0.4%) were the most common metabolic complications of enteral therapies. When the total number of patients receiving enteral therapy are considered, the cost of treating these complications is approximately $18.78 per patient day [1]. However, this figure includes the costs of parenteral nutrition for those 9 patients who failed enteral therapy. When the costs of providing parenteral nutrition are excluded, the cost of treating the complications associated with enteral therapy adds only $0.99 to each patient's nutrition care costs.

Twenty-nine percent of patients in the Cataldi-Betcher study [56] were treated with a more expensive, specialized enteral formula (Vivonex, Vital, HepaticAid, AminAid). Although their published rate of specialty formulation usage was 5.5%, only patients who required HepaticAid or AminAid were considered. However, elemental diets designed for gastrointestinal failure, because of special preparation and increased expense, should also be considered specialized formulas, making their specialty formula usage 29%. In summary, enteral therapy was well tolerated by most patients and was economical to administer [56]. The complication rate was lower than most reported series and was probably the result of standardized protocols and careful daily monitoring by the nutrition support team [74]. With such meticulous monitoring, enteral therapy complications are infrequent, and the costs of treating these complications changes the total costs of enteral nutrition administration only slightly. With major changes in the health care arena rapidly occurring, a caveat exists in that complications may become more problematic secondary to decreased staffing and less education/in-servicing that may occur in a cost-containment environment.

Cost-Effective Parenteral Nutrition

There is little question regarding the cost-benefit ratio of enteral therapies. For the most part, they are relatively inexpensive, have low complication rates, and maximize the potential positive effects of nutrition support [13,14,50,51,53,56,60–65,69]. Because parenteral nutrition is usually more expensive than enteral nutrition [50], often has a higher risk of complications than enteral nutrition, and provides benefit to only certain groups of patients [50,51,53,76–78], its use has been increasingly scrutinized. With the advent of specialized nutrition support teams and improvements in pharmacy technology, the expense and incidence of complications associated with parenteral nutrition use have decreased dramatically in the past 10 years, improving effectiveness of parenteral nutrition. With current technology, the limiting factor to the cost-effective use of parenteral nutrition may be the ability to prospectively recognize groups proven to benefit from the various parenteral nutrition formulations [79].

A meta-analysis published in 1987 by Detsky et al. [76] showed that the routine perioperative use of parenteral nutrition in nonselected patients having major surgery does not decrease the postoperative complication rates to any appreciable extent. More recently, Eisenberg et al. [77] subjected perioperative parenteral nutrition to a cost-benefit analysis and showed similar results. For those patients at low risk for postoperative complications, namely well-nourished individuals, there is neither decreased complication rates nor improved cost-benefit ratio for the perioperative use of parenteral nutrition. However, decreased complication rates did occur in those patients who were malnourished, making the cost of perioperative parenteral nutrition well justified in that group [76,77]. Mullen et al. [80] also showed that for all surgical patients, one week of preoperative parenteral nutrition significantly decreased postoperative complications (18% vs. 39%, $p < 0.01$), major postoperative septic events (4% vs. 21%, $p < 0.01$), and mortality (4% vs. 28%, $p < 0.005$). Of these patients, 50% to 55% had malignancies, with the remainder having nonmalignant conditions requiring major abdominal surgery. When patients were stratified by prognostic nutritional index (PNI) into low-, intermediate-, and high-risk groups, the decrease in complications, major septic complications, and death was significant only in the high-risk group (PNI $\geq$ 50); this study, however, has not been generally accepted because it is retrospective and selected. Similarly, Smale et al. [81] found that patients with intraabdominal, thoracic, or head and neck malignancies who were considered at high nutritional risk (PNI $\geq$ 40), complications (31% vs. 66%, $p < 0.001$), major septic complications (15% vs. 43%, $p < 0.005$), and death (15% vs. 40%, $p < 0.025$) were significantly decreased by preoperative parenteral nutrition. Similar results were found by Sandström et al. [78] and Müller et al. [82] in patients undergoing major surgery. The basic theme underlying all of these studies is that regardless of the patient's primary disease process, malnutrition, which can be at least partially corrected with parenteral nutrition, is a risk factor for complications and death. The great majority of mechanical postoperative complications are influenced by inadequate protein synthesis (wound dehiscence, anastomotic breakdown, fistula formation) [83]. In addition, infectious complications (urinary tract infections, wound infections, pneumonias, intraabdominal abscess), functional disturbances, and the need for additional medical support can be decreased in malnourished patients solely by appropriate nutrient provision (Table 30-6) [11,12,78].

Nevertheless, preoperative parenteral nutrition is expensive. Ten days of preoperative parenteral nutrition adds $3500 to $4500 to a patient's care costs. Despite the fact that parenteral nutrition is expensive, the cost-effectiveness ratios are favorable for those groups of patients where the overall incidence of nutrition-related complications is around 20%. For high-risk groups, incremental cost per complication avoided is approximately $11,515, making the use of preoperative parenteral nutrition cost-effective [84]. However, in low-risk groups, the cost of providing parenteral nutrition is greater than the cost of treating avoided complications. Intrinsic to these data are the ability to recognize high-risk patients, a truth substantiated by parenteral nutrition trials that show no benefit or cost savings for nonselected groups of patients [1,76–79,81,82,84,85]. These data suggest that the use of standard parenteral nutrition formulations should be limited to malnourished patients unable to tolerate enteral therapy. Because inadequate nutrition in a stressed patient for greater than 7 days can lead to significant nutritional deficit, the indications for parenteral nutrition are extended to normally nourished patients without nutrient intake for more than 7 days [32–38]. Probably the most dramatic demonstration of differential cost-benefit ratio was achieved by Buzby et al. [86] in the prospective Veterans Affairs Cooperative Study, where it was demonstrated that only patients with significant severe malnutrition (weight loss of 10% to 15%, albumin of less than 3.0 g/dl) benefited from perioperative parenteral nutrition. In those patients with mild or moderate malnutrition, improvement in mechanical complications (disrupted anastomoses) and the like were outweighed by an increase in noncatheter-related nosocomial infections [86].

When organs specifically involved in total body metabolic activities are dysfunctional and enteral nutrition is not possible, use of specialized formulations may be considered. Efficacy is proven for hepatic formulations, but remains questionable for others. Liver disease is associated with malnutrition and increased operative risk in the majority of chronic liver failure patients [87–89]. Except for glucose, macronutrients are usually well tolerated. However, in the perioperative period, attempts to provide adequate protein intake may lead to hepatic encephalopathy in up to 50% of patients [90,91]. The protein intolerance that is seen in liver failure is particularly trou-

Table 30-6. Parenteral Nutrition Support

Study	Population	Findings		
Heatley (1979) [138]	74 gastric and esophageal cancer patients given nutrition support (NS) or none (N)		NS	N
		wound infection	8%	31%
		major complication	29%	53%
		death	16%	22%
Smale (1981) [81]	159 cancer surgical patients given nutrition support (NS) or none (N)		NS	N
		complications	26%	37%
		deaths	11%	20%
		no nutrition support with a PNI > 40: 2× complications, 3× major sepsis, 3× mortality		
Müller (1982) [82]	125 GI carcinoma patients given nutrition support (NS) or none (N)		NS	N
		wound infection	21%	25%
		major complication	17%	32%
		death	5%	19%
Twomey (1985) [1]	analysis of complications prevented by preoperative nutrition support	wound infections decreased by 11% @ $2000/ea: $22,000 savings; complications decreased by 19% @ $50,000/ea: $950,000 savings; nutrition support costs $800,000: net savings $1720/patient		
Detsky (1987) [76]	analysis of savings by expected incidence of complications when parenteral nutrition support is used	<5% expected complication rate: no benefit to nutrition support use; 20% expected complication rate: $11,515 savings with nutrition support use; 60% expected complication rate: $1031 savings with nutrition support use		
Sandström (1993) [78]	300 surgery patients given nutrition support (NS) or none (N)	no benefit in low nutritional risk patients; nonfed patients had lower energy expenditure, less nitrogen excretion, lower heart rates, lower body temperature; increased cardiac complication in the PN group		
Eisenberg (1993) [77]	incremental costs of providing periop. parenteral nutrition for 16 d; benefit analysis in low, moderate, and high nutritional risk patients	low nutritional risk PN costs $3921, no benefit; moderate nutritional risk PN costs $3195, no benefit; high nutritional risk PN costs $3071, in the high-risk group, 22% decrease in complications was observed with PN therapy, a cost savings of $13,959/patient treated		

PN = parenteral nutrition, PNI = prognostic nutritional index.
Note: Bracketed numbers correspond with references.

bling because amino acids are central to tissue repair, host defense, and enzymatic function [91]. Depressed serum branched-chain amino acid (BCAA) concentrations and elevated serum aromatic amino acid (AAA) concentrations may be causal in this encephalopathy. The inability of the failing liver to clear aromatic amino acids from the blood results in a BCAA-AAA ratio that approaches 1:1 [90,92–96]. Fischer [96] and others [68,97] have shown that 70 to 80 g/day of critical protein equivalent is well tolerated if BCAA-enriched solutions are used.

Nutrition-associated complications, particularly infection and poor wound healing, are common causes of morbidity and mortality among adults with chronic liver disease referred for operation [90]. Given sufficient time, adequate preoperative nutrition can reduce the morbidity and mortality that is associated with malnutrition [87,88]. Prospective randomized trials also indicate that, when given with adequate carbohydrate, BCAA-enriched solutions are more effective than placebo and equal to or more effective than conventional treatment with enterally administered lactulose and/or neomycin in reversing hepatic encephalopathy [68,97,98]. Further evidence suggests improved mortality for patients treated with BCAA-enriched parenteral nutrition support compared with patients given intravenous glucose and conventional hepatic encephalopathy treatment with lactulose and/or neomycin [97].

Renal dysfunction leads to elevated blood urea nitrogen, creatinine, and ammonia levels. Currently used parenteral renal formulations that contain limited amino acid provision composed of essential amino acids usually improves these parameters [99]. However, lowering these laboratory parameters may be at considerable metabolic and monetary expense to the patient and therefore may not be beneficial [100–103]. Because renal formulation may function by limiting protein metabolism or by rendering the urea cycle ineffective, questions regarding possible deleterious effects on protein metabolism have been raised [100,104]. In the absence of clear benefit, some have suggested that acute renal failure patients in need of protein restriction should be supported with less expensive balanced amino acid formulations of limited concentrations [2]. One should not forget, however, that the only study showing efficacy in the treatment of patients with renal failure was carried out with an essential amino acid, high-glucose, low-volume formulation [99]. No other study has been as carefully done or as detailed and, given the expense, is not likely to be repeated. One could argue for utilization of essential amino acid solutions in patients with renal failure.

When the total number of patients who receive parenteral nutrition are considered and the cost of treating complications is divided by the entire group at risk, estimated costs of treating the complications associated with parenteral nutrition (sepsis 0.5%, pneumothorax 4%, subclavian vein thrombosis 0.1%) is approximately $12.50 per patient day [1]. The decreased cost of parenteral nutrition administration that has occurred over the past decade in combination with acceptably low complication rates associated with this form of therapy have tipped the cost-effectiveness scales in favor of parenteral nutrition use. However, the low cost per patient day of treating these complications depends heavily on a low incidence of occurrence, which in turn is a direct result of the presence of multidisciplinary nutrition support teams [105–116].

Nutrition Support Teams

As hospitals grapple with health care reimbursement issues, costly therapies and cost-containment strategies are closely scrutinized. Many of the changes are a direct result of the shift toward prospective payment systems (for example, Medicare's use of DRGs) and the impetus to stem rising health care costs. At the time of this writing, hospitals do not receive higher reimbursement on the basis of the need for parenteral or enteral nutrition except for supplemental payment for malnutrition as a comorbidity [117]. As cost pressures continue to mount, the need to achieve cost-effectiveness in clinical nutrition therapy is more important than ever.

The inception of nutrition support teams was facilitated by the recognition that nutrition support can be complex and optimally requires a multidisciplinary approach. Many institutions have assembled a multidisciplinary team to handle nutrition support functions while team members administratively answer to their respective departments (for example, pharmacy, nursing, dietetics, medicine, and surgery). Other institutions have nutrition support teams organized as free-standing departments, although this appears to be the exception [118]. Nutrition support teams are not immune to the roving eye of fiscal accountability and therefore can be a prime target for budgetary cuts. Specialized nutrition support teams often generate little or no outside revenue while assuming the financial cost of highly trained personnel.

Nutrition support services receive justification by improving quality of care, reducing associated complications of nutritional therapies, ensuring appropriate use of expensive specialized forms of nutritional therapies, and by performing research and attracting funding (Table 30-7). When comparing quality of parenteral and specialized enteral nutrition provision, the establishment of a multidisciplinary team often results in improved nutritional care [119–121] but does not necessarily guarantee optimum therapy [122].

Nutrition support teams are committed to bringing clinical nutrition benefits to patients and to the attention of colleagues, the community, and, increasingly, to administrators. Indeed, a heightened awareness of service activities and attributes for improved patient care (and outcome) is imperative to sequester administrative support.

It is fallacious to assume that because we all eat, we must all have some expertise in nutrition. Nutritional therapies can be extremely complex and expensive. Physicians, nurses, and pharmacists receive little formal nutritional education, whereas most health care givers, including dietitians and pharmacists, receive little formal training in parenteral and specialized enteral nutrition. Leaving the decision-making process regarding nutrition therapy to groups who have not received specialized training or who have not received appropriate experience can foster inefficient and ineffective use of these therapies. Nonetheless, balancing actual cost savings and time required to provide nutrition support is profoundly difficult.

Roberts and Levine [117] quantified potential cost savings of greater than $100,000 per annum regarding nutrition support recommendations in-

Table 30-7. Nutrition Support Teams

Study	Population	Findings		
Sanders (1976) [107]	318 hospital patients treated before NST, 1st NST yr, and after 1 yr with NST	catheter sepsis before NST 28.6%, during 1st yr of NST 12%, and after 1 yr of NST 4.7%		
Nehme (1980) [108]	164 patients without NST, 211 patients with NST	Complication	with NST	without NST
		catheter	3%	33%
		metabolic	11%	93%
		PN deaths	0%	6%
Weinsier (1985) [42]	70 burn patients given nutrition support (NS) or no nutrition support (N)		NS	N
		weight loss	3 ± 5%	13 ± 8%
		hospital stay	29 ± 15 d	36 ± 19 d
		hospital cost	$18,000 ± $11,000	$24,000 ± $20,000
O'Brien (1986) [106]	31 hospital patients	45% were treated differently than NST recommendations with total excess costs: $70,270 ($5000/patient)		
Owens (1989) [111]	248 patients managed by NST	quality assurance program resulted in 60% improvement in metabolic complications and 2.8% wastage rate vs. 13.6% wastage rate before NST		
Powers (1991) [113]	181 patients managed by NST	nutritional goals met in 96%, 10% catheter complication rate, 4% catheter sepsis rate		

NST = nutrition support team, PN = parenteral nutrition.
Note: Bracketed numbers correspond with references.

volving parenteral nutrition. A portion of cost savings are realized by minimizing waste—including waste generated from orders changed after a solution is prepared and/or orders discontinued after a solution is prepared. In a retrospective study, Gianino and co-workers [109] looked at cost-effectiveness of central venous catheter care in patients receiving total parenteral nutrition. Those patients with catheters maintained by a member of the nutrition support team utilizing a specifically designed monitoring protocol sustained a 0.5% catheter-related sepsis rate (compared to a reported 5% incidence and cost average of $20,200) [109].

Powers and co-workers [123] found in a prospective study of 100 patients that team-managed enteral nutrition therapy resulted in improved nutritional care when compared with a nonteam approach. Team-managed patients had more frequent documentation of nutrition assessment, attained estimated energy needs for a significantly greater time period, and had more frequent monitoring parameters performed than nonteam managed care [123]. In a follow-up study, Brown et al. [75] found that nutrition support team management of enteral nutrition reduced associated morbidity and optimized nutrient delivery compared to nonteam therapy.

In conclusion, the benefits of improved nutritional status [8,124], possible reduced morbidity and mortality [125,126], the potential for reduced length of stay [1,13,69], reduced patient and hospital costs [20], as well as reduced liability [127] can be facilitated under the direction of nutrition support teams. Nutrition support teams also enable prompt and effective response to patients who are at high nutrition risk.

Home Nutrition Support

There are approximately 40,000 home parenteral nutrition and 160,000 home enteral nutrition patients in the United States. Total dollars paid for home parenteral therapy in 1992 was $156 million, and for enteral therapy was $137 million [128]. Social and economic climates coupled with technologic advances spell a continued growth in the expansion of the home health care industry, of which nutrition support is a part.

The most common usage for home enteral therapy is malignancy (42%) followed by neurologic swallowing disorders (30%). The remaining 28% of patients on home enteral therapy have various disorders, none of which comprise more than 3% to 4% of the total group (Table 30-8).

During the early years of parenteral nutrition, patients in need of such therapy were hospitalized for many months at a time. The rationale for home parenteral nutrition was, and still remains, to remove patients from expensive institutional care by permitting less costly self-care or assisted-care at home. Approximately two weeks of in-hospital training are required to prepare a motivated patient with adequate support for home parenteral

Table 30-8. Home Nutrition Support

Therapy	Disease	Percent	Mortality	Rehabilitation
Parenteral therapy:	malignancy	35%	70%	<50% minimal
40,000 patients/yr;	Crohn's disease	14%	4%	70% full
$156 million/yr	AIDS enteropathy	4%	80%	<50% minimal
	ischemic bowel	9%	6%–20%	50% full
	motility disorder	8%	"	"
	radiation enteritis	4%	"	"
	congenital defect	3.5%	"	"
	obstruction	2.5%	"	"
	miscellaneous	20%	"	"
Enteral therapy:	malignancy	42%		
160,000 patients/yr;	neurologic deficit	30%		
$137 million/yr	miscellaneous	28%		

Source: North American Home Parenteral and Enteral Nutrition Patient Registry. *Annual Report with Outcome Profiles: First Report Using Longitudinal Data.* Albany, NY: The Oley Foundation; Silver Spring, MD: American Society for Parenteral and Enteral Nutrition, 1992.

nutrition self-care. In general, any stable patient with a probable need for 30 or more days of inpatient parenteral nutrition support is a home parenteral nutrition candidate. Because of the initial training expense necessary to prepare a patient for home care, individuals who will require less than 30 days of home parenteral nutrition are probably not cost-effective candidates. The most common indications for home parenteral nutrition use include malignancy (35%), Crohn's disease (14%), ischemic bowel (9%), motility disorders (8%), acquired immunodeficiency syndrome (AIDS) (4%), associated enteropathy (4%), radiation enteritis (4%), congenital bowel defect (3.5%), and chronic obstruction (2.5%), with the remaining 20% being made up of various disorders [128]. Because nutritional therapy is truly lifesaving in nonterminal disease states such as congenital loss of bowel, chronic obstruction, motility disorders, ischemic bowel, and radiation enteritis, cost-benefit analysis seems unnecessary.

The mortality rate for home parenteral nutrition patients within the above-mentioned group of disorders is 6% to 20%. Of these patients, 20% to 45% resume oral nutrition and 20% to 50% experience complete rehabilitation [128]. With regard to Crohn's disease, home parenteral nutrition has never been shown to prolong life or improve outcome, although hospitalizations may be reduced [129,130]. Trials have shown enteral nutrition therapy to be as effective as parenteral in acute exacerbations of Crohn's disease [131]. The exception may be Crohn's-associated bowel obstruction, where nonoperative resolution is improved by parenteral nutrition [131,132]. However, patients with Crohn's-associated obstructions usually require hospitalization, making the issue of home parenteral therapy moot. The mortality for home parenteral nutrition in Crohn's disease is 4%, with 70% of patients resuming full oral nutrition within 1 year, and 70% percent achieving full rehabilitation (able to carry out normal age-appropriate activities) [128].

When home parenteral nutrition is used in terminal conditions, such as AIDS and cancer, clearly defined end points are requisite. Because parenteral nutrition may reduce hospital stay but will not affect ultimate outcome in these disease states, the decision to institute home care must be weighed by life expectancy and quality of life measures. Many home parenteral nutrition programs sanction the use of parenteral nutrition in these disease states only for those patients under active treatment or those with viable treatment options [133]. The mortality for home parenteral nutrition patients with AIDS and cancer are 80% and 70%, respectively. Only 15% to 25% will ever resume oral intake, and minimal rehabilitation will be achieved in less than 50% [128]. Our own policy in Cincinnati is to rarely, if ever, utilize home parenteral nutrition in patients with cancer. In addition, there is a legitimate question as to accelerated tumor growth in patients given parenteral nutrition.

The cost of home parenteral nutrition therapy is considerable, usually more than that of in-patient parenteral nutrition, and usually must be borne by third-party payers. However, if parenteral nutrition therapy is the sole reason for hospitalization, hospital room and nursing care costs must be weighed against the cost of home therapy and, in this instance, home therapy is virtually always cost-effective [133–135].

References

1. Twomey PL, Patching SC. Cost-effectiveness of nutrition support. *JPENutr* 9:3, 1985.
2. A.S.P.E.N. Board of Directors. Guidelines for the use of parenteral and enteral nutrition in adult and pediatric patients. *JPEN* 17(Suppl 4):1SA, 1993.
3. Rombeau JL, Rolandelli RH, Wilmore DW. Nutritional support. In D Wilmore, et al (eds). *Care of the Surgical Patient* (1st ed). New York: Scientific American, 1988. P 1.
4. Leiter LA, Marliss EB. Survival during fasting may depend on fat as well as protein stores. *JAMA* 248:2306, 1982.
5. Allison SP. Review: The uses and limitations of nutritional support. *Clin Nutr* 11:319, 1992.
6. Studley HO. Percentage of weight loss: A basic indicator of surgical risk in patients with chronic peptic ulcer disease. *JAMA* 106:458, 1936.
7. Windsor JA, Hill G. Weight loss with physiologic impairment: A basic indicator of surgical risk. *Ann Surg* 207:290, 1988.
8. Seltzer MH, et al. Instant nutritional assessment: Absolute weight loss and surgical mortality. *JPEN* 6:218, 1982.
9. Reilly JJ, et al. Economic impact of malnutrition: A model system for hospitalized patients. *JPE Nutr* 12:371, 1988.
10. Mughal MM, Meguid MM. The effect of nutritional status on morbidity after elective surgery for benign gastrointestinal disease. *JPEN* 11:140, 1987.
11. Chandra RK. Nutrition, immunity, and infection: Present knowledge and future directions. *Lancet* 1:688, 1983.
12. Smythe PM, et al. Thymolymphatic deficiency and depression of cell mediated immunity in protein-calorie malnutrition. *Lancet* 2:939, 1971.
13. Daly JM, et al. Enteral nutrition with supplemental arginine, RNA, and omega-3 fatty acids in patients after operation: Immunologic, metabolic, and clinical outcome. *Surgery* 112:56, 1992.
14. Randall HT. Efficacy, feasibility, safety, and cost comparisons of enteral and parenteral elemental nutrition. *Contemp Surg* 28:4, 1986.
15. Detsky AS, et al. Evaluating the accuracy of nutritional assessment techniques applied to hospitalized patients: Methodology and comparisons. *JPEN* 8:153, 1984.
16. Baker JP, et al. Nutritional assessment: A comparison of clinical judgement and objective measures. *N Engl J Med* 306:969, 1982.
17. Baker JP, et al. A comparison of predictive value of nutritional assessment techniques. *Human Nutr Clin Nutr* 36c:233, 1982.
18. Buzby GP, et al. Prognostic nutritional index in gastrointestinal surgery. *Am J Surg* 139:160, 1986.
19. Detsky AS, et al. Predicting nutrition-associated complications for patients undergoing gastrointestinal surgery. *JPEN* 11:446, 1987.
20. Bistrian BR, et al. Protein status of general surgical patients. *JAMA* 230:858, 1974.
21. Bistrian BR, et al. Prevalence of malnutrition in general medical patients. *JAMA* 235:1567, 1976.
22. Coates KG, et al. Hospital-associated malnutrition: A reevaluation 12 years later. *J Am Diet Assoc* 93:27, 1989.
23. Kamath SK, et al. Hospital malnutrition: A 33-hospital screening study. *Research* 86:203, 1986.
24. Willard MD, Gilsdorf RB, Price RA. Protein-calorie malnutrition in a community hospital. *JAMA* 243:1720, 1980.
25. Nelson S, Bottsford JE, Long JM. Finding malnourished patients in a community hospital: Development of a nutritional assessment service. *J S C Med Assoc* 79:9, 1983.
26. Hunt DR, et al. A simple nutrition screening procedure for hospitalized patients. *J Am Diet Assoc* 85:332, 1985.
27. Christensen KS, Gstundter KM. Hospital-wide screening improved the basis for nutrition intervention. *J Am Diet Assoc* 85:704, 1985.
28. Maillet JO. Evaluating your assessment program. *Nutr Supp Serv* 4:19, 1982.
29. Thompson JS, et al. Hospital evaluation of malnutrition. *J Am Diet Assoc* 84:337, 1984.
30. Mullen JL, et al. Implications of malnutrition in the surgical patient. *Arch Surg* 114:121, 1979.
31. O'Leary JP, et al. Incidence of malnutrition among patients admitted to a VA hospital. *South Med J* 75:1095, 1982.
32. Hill GL, et al. Malnutrition in surgical patients: An unrecognized problem. *Lancet* 1:689, 1977.
33. Weisner RL, et al. Hospital malnutrition: A prospective evaluation of general medical patients during the course of hospitalization. *Am J Clin Nutr* 32:418, 1979.
34. Warnold I, Lundholm K. Clinical significance of preoperative nutritional status in 215 non-cancer patients. *Ann Surg* 199:299, 1984.
35. Agradi E, et al. Hospital malnutrition: Incidence and prospective evaluation of general medical patients during hospitalization. *Acta Vitaminol Enzymol* 6:235, 1984.
36. Pinchcofsky GD, Kaminski MV. Increasing malnutrition during hospitalization: Documentation by a nutritional screening program. *J Am Coll Nutr* 4:471, 1985.
37. Hospital nutrition still abounds. *Nutr Rev* 46:315, 1988.
38. Hill GL, et al. Protein status and metabolic expenditure determine the response to intravenous nutrition: A new classification of malnutrition. *Br J Surg* 78:109, 1991.
39. Willcutts HD. Nutritional assessment in 1000 surgical patients in an affluent suburban community hospital [Abstract]. *JPEN* 1:25A, 1977.
40. Kwong C, Wirth J, Avera E. Improved quality assurance through admission screening. *Nutr Supp Serv* 4:48, 1984.
41. Federer JG, Rane-Szos AK, Blanford G. Evidence of malnutrition and prolonged recuperation in an extended care facility [Abstract]. *Abstr Am Diet Assoc,* 69th Annual Meeting, 1986. P 68.
42. Weinsier RL, et al. Cost containment: A contribution of aggressive nutritional support in burn patients. *J Burn Care Rehab* 6:436, 1985.
43. Christensen KS. Hospital-wide screening increases revenue under prospective payment system. *J Am Diet Assoc* 86:1234, 1986.
44. Robinson G, Goldstein M, Levine GM. Impact of nutritional status on DRG length of stay. *JPEN* 11:49, 1987.
45. Shaw-Stiffel TA, et al. Effect of nutrition status and other factors on length of hospital stay after major gastrointestinal surgery. *Nutrition* 9:140, 1993.
46. Anderson MD, et al. Malnutrition and length of stay: A relationship? *Henry Ford Hosp Med J* 33:190, 1985.

47. Linn BS, Robinson DS. The possible impact of DRGs on nutritional status of patients having surgery for cancer of the head and neck. *JAMA* 260:514, 1988.

48. Linn BS. Outcomes of older and younger malnourished and well-nourished patients one year after hospitalization. *Am J Clin Nutr* 39:66, 1984.

49. Muggia-Sullam M, et al. Postoperative enteral versus parenteral nutritional support in gastrointestinal surgery. *Am J Surg* 149:106, 1985.

50. Hamaoui E, et al. Enteral nutrition in the early postoperative period: A new semi-elemental formula versus total parenteral nutrition. *JPEN* 14:501, 1990.

51. Moore FA, et al. Early enteral feeding, compared with parenteral, reduces postoperative septic complications. *Ann Surg* 216:172, 1992.

52. Bower RH, et al. Postoperative enteral vs. parenteral nutrition. *Arch Surg* 121:1040, 1986.

53. Moore FA, et al. TEN versus TPN following major abdominal trauma: Reduced septic morbidity. *J Trauma* 29:916, 1989.

54. Kudsk KA, et al. Enteral versus parenteral feeding. *Ann Surg* 215:503, 1992.

55. Lim STK, et al. Total parenteral nutrition versus gastrostomy in the preoperative preparation of patients with carcinoma of the esophagus. *Br J Surg* 68:69, 1981.

56. Cataldi-Betcher EL, et al. Complications occurring during enteral nutrition support: A prospective study. *JPEN* 7:546, 1983.

57. Roberts D, Thelen D, Weinstein S. Parenteral and enteral nutrition: A cost-benefit audit. *Minn Med* 65:707, 1982.

58. Meguid MM, Muscaritoli M. Current uses of total parenteral nutrition. *Am Family Phys* 47:383, 1993.

59. Wolfe BM, Phillips GJ, Hodges RE. Evaluation and management of nutritional status before surgery. *Med Clin North Am* 63:1257, 1979.

60. Stephens RV, Randall HT. Use of concentrated balanced liquid elemental diet for nutritional management of catabolic states. *Ann Surg* 170:642, 1969.

61. Kaminski MV. Enteral hyperalimentation. *Surg Gynecol Obstet* 143:12, 1976.

62. Shils ME. Enteral nutrition by tube. *Cancer Res* 37:2432, 1977.

63. Bethel RA, et al. Nasogastric hyperalimentation through a polyethylene catheter: An alternative to central venous hyperalimentation. *Am J Clin Nutr* 32:1112, 1979.

64. Chernoff R. Nutritional support: Formulas and delivery of enteral feeding. *J Am Diet Assoc* 79:426, 1981.

65. Heymsfield SB, et al. Enteral hyperalimentation: An alternative to central venous hyperalimentation. *Ann Int Med* 90:63, 1979.

66. Kearns PJ, et al. Accelerated improvement of alcoholic liver disease with enteral nutrition. *Gastroenterology* 102:200, 1992.

67. Greenberger NJ, et al. Effect of vegetable and animal protein diets in chronic active encephalopathy. *Dig Dis Sci* 22:845, 1977.

68. Freund HR, et al. Infusion of branched chain amino acid solutions in patients with hepatic encephalopathy. *Ann Surg* 196:209, 1982.

69. Bower RH, et al. A modified enteral formula reduces hospital length of stay in patients in intensive care units [Abstract]. *Crit Care Med* 21:S275, 1993.

70. Adibi SA. Intestinal transport of dipeptides in man: Relative importance of hydrolysis and intact absorption. *J Clin Invest* 50:2266, 1971.

71. Adibi SA. Intestinal phase of protein assimilation in man. *Am J Clin Nutr* 29:205, 1976.

72. Keohane P, et al. Influence of protein composition and hydrolysis method on intestinal absorption of protein in man. *Gut* 26:907, 1985.

73. Matthews DM. Intestinal absorption of peptides. *Physiol Rev* 55:537, 1975.

74. Matthews DM, Adibi SA. Peptide absorption. *Gastroenterology* 71:151, 1976.

75. Brown RO, et al. Enteral nutrition support management in a university teaching hospital: Team versus non-team. *JPEN* 11:52, 1987.

76. Detsky AS, et al. Perioperative parenteral nutrition: A meta-analysis. *Ann Int Med* 107:195, 1987.

77. Eisenberg JM, et al. Does perioperative total parenteral nutrition reduce medical care costs? *JPEN* 17:201, 1993.

78. Sandström R, et al. The effect of postoperative intravenous feeding (TPN) on outcome following major surgery evaluated in a randomized study. *Ann Surg* 217:195, 1993.

79. Detsky AS, et al. The choice to treat all, some, or no patients undergoing gastrointestinal surgery with nutritional support: A decision analysis approach. *JPEN* 8:245, 1984.

80. Mullen JL, et al. Reduction of operative morbidity and mortality by combined preoperative and postoperative nutritional support. *Ann Surg* 192:604, 1980.

81. Smale BF, et al. The efficacy of nutritional assessment and support in cancer surgery. *Cancer* 47:2375, 1981.

82. Müller JM, et al. Preoperative parenteral feeding in patients with gastrointestinal carcinoma. *Lancet* 1:68, 1982.

83. Christou NV, et al. Estimating mortality risk in preoperative patients using immunologic, nutritional, and acute phase response variables. *Ann Surg* 210:69, 1977.

84. Detsky AS, Jeejeebhoy KN. Cost-effectiveness of preoperative parenteral nutrition in patients undergoing major abdominal surgery. *JPEN* 8:632, 1984.

85. Anderson GF, Steinberg EP. Implications of Medicare's prospective payment system for specialized nutrition services. *Nutr Clin Pract* 1:12, 1986.

86. Buzby GP, et al. (The Veterans Affairs Total Parenteral Nutrition Cooperative Study Group). Perioperative total parenteral nutrition in surgical patients. *N Engl J Med* 325:525, 1991.

87. DiCecco SR, et al. Assessment of nutritional status of patients with end-stage liver disease undergoing liver transplantation. *Mayo Clinic Proc* 64:95, 1989.

88. Shaw BJ, et al. Influence of selected patient variables and operative blood loss on six-month survival following liver transplantation. *Semin Liver Dis* 5:385, 1985.

89. Mendenhall LL, et al. Protein-calorie malnutrition associated with alcoholic hepatitis. *Am J Med* 76:211, 1984.

90. Johnson PJ, et al. Nutritional management and assessment. In R Calne (ed), *Liver Transplantation* (2nd ed). New York: Harcourt Brace Jovanovich, 1987. P 103.

91. Fischer JE, Bower RH. Nutritional support in liver disease. *Surg Clin North Am* 61:653, 1981.

92. Clowes GA. Amino acid clearance in liver disease: Indicator of hepatocyte function, prognosis, and selection of treatment. In WV McDermott (ed), *Surgery of the Liver.* Boston: Blackwell, 1985. P 39.

93. Shanbhogue RL, et al. Nutritional support in surgery of the liver. In WV McDermott (ed), *Surgery of the Liver.* Boston: Blackwell, 1985. P 497.

94. Sherlock S. Liver function. In WV McDermott (ed), *Surgery of the Liver.* Boston: Blackwell, 1985. P 25.

95. Carithers RL, et al. Postoperative care. In WC Maddrey (ed), *Transplantation of the Liver.* New York: Elsevier, 1989. P 111.

96. Fischer J, et al. The effect of normalization of plasma amino acids on hepatic encephalopathy in man. *Surgery* 80:77, 1976.

97. Cerra FB, et al. Disease-specific amino acid infusion (F080) in hepatic encephalopathy: A prospective, randomized, double blind controlled trial. *JPEN* 9:288, 1985.

98. Naylor CD, et al. Parenteral nutrition with branched chain amino acids in hepatic encephalopathy: A meta-analysis. *Gastroenterology* 97:1003, 1989.

99. Abel RM, et al. Improved survival from acute renal failure after treatment with intravenous essential L-amino acids and glucose. *N Engl J Med* 288:695, 1973.

100. Mirtallo J, et al. A comparison of essential and general amino acid infusions in the nutritional support of patients with compromised renal function. *JPEN* 5:109, 1982.

101. Rainford DJ. Nutritional management of acute renal failure. *Acta Chir Scand Suppl* 507:327, 1981.

102. Asbach HW, et al. The treatment of hypercatabolic acute renal failure by adequate nutrition and haemodialysis. *Acta Anaesthesiol Scand* 18:255, 1974.

103. Feinstein EL, et al. Clinical and metabolic responses to parenteral nutrition in acute renal failure: A controlled double-blind study. *Medicine* 60:124, 1981.

104. Flanigan RC, et al. Nutritional assessment and therapy in advanced urothelial cancer. *Urol Clin North Am* 11:671, 1984.

105. Padberg FT, et al. Central venous catheterization for parenteral nutrition. *Ann Surg* 193:264, 1981.

106. O'Brien DD, et al. Recommendations of nutrition support team promote cost containment. *JPEN* 10:300, 1986.

107. Sanders RA, Sheldon GF. Septic complications of total parenteral nutrition. *Am J Surg* 132:214, 1976.

108. Nehme AE. Nutritional support of the hospitalized patient. *JAMA* 243:1906, 1980.

109. Gianino MS, Brunt M, Eisenberg PG. The impact of a nutritional support team on the cost and management of multilumen catheters. *J Int Nurs* 15:327, 1992.

110. Mitchell KA, et al. Standardized TPN order form reduces staff time and potential error. *Nutrition* 6:457, 1990.

111. Owens JP, Geibig CB, Mirtallo JM. Concurrent quality assurance for a nutrition-support service. *Am J Hosp Pharm* 46:2469, 1989.

112. Geibig CB, Mirtallo JM, Owens JP. Quality assurance for a nutritional support service. *Nutr Clin Pract* 6:147, 1991.

113. Powers T, et al. A nutrition support team quality assurance plan. *Nutr Clin Pract* 6:151, 1991.

114. Harper PH, et al. Total parenteral nutrition: Value of a standard feeding regimen. *Br Med J* 286:1323, 1983.

115. MacDonald HL, et al. Parenteral nutrition. *J Royal Coll Surg Edin* 26:173, 1981.

116. Maswoswe JJ, Newcomer DR, Quandt CM. Achieving parenteral nutrition cost savings through prescribing guidelines and formulary restrictions. *Am J Hosp Pharm* 44:1376, 1987.

117. Roberts MF, Levine GM. Nutrition support team recommendations can reduce hospital costs. *Nutr Clin Pract* 7:227, 1992.

118. Finn SC, Zola EM, Sheridan JF. Issues facing nutrition support teams. *Drug Intell Clin Pharm* 18:826, 1984.

119. Traeger SM, et al. Total parenteral nutrition by a nutrition support team: Improved quality of care. *JPEN* 10:408, 1986.

120. Faubion WC, et al. Total parenteral nutrition catheter sepsis: Impact of the team approach. *JPEN* 10:642, 1986.

121. Jacobs DO, et al. Impact of a nutritional support service on VA surgical patients. *J Am Coll Nutr* 3:311, 1984.

122. Dalton MJ, Schepers G, Gee JP. Consultative total parenteral nutrition teams: The effect on the incidence of total parenteral nutrition-related complications. *JPEN* 8:146, 1984.

123. Powers DA, et al. Nutritional support team versus non-team management of enteral nutritional support in a Veterans Administration medical center teaching hospital. *JPEN* 10:635, 1986.

124. Alexander JW, et al. Beneficial effects of aggressive protein feeding in severely burned children. *Ann Surg* 192:505, 1980.

125. Dempsey DT, Mullen JL, Busby GP. The link between nutritional status and clinical outcome: Can nutrition intervention modify it? *Am J Clin Nutr* 47:352, 1988.

126. Lyman B, Pendleton SH, Pemberton LB. The role of the nutritional support team in preventing and identifying complications of parenteral and enteral nutrition. *Qual Rev Bull* 13:232, 1987.

127. Spencer RA, Palmisano DJ. Specialized nutritional support of patients: A hospital's legal duty? *Qual Rev Bull* 11:160, 1985.

128. North American Home Parenteral and Enteral Nutrition Patient Registry. *Annual Report with Outcome Profiles: First Report Using Longitudinal Data.* Albany, NY: The Oley Foundation; Silver Spring, MD: American Society for Parenteral and Enteral Nutrition, 1992.

129. Fleming RC, McGill DB, Berkner S. Home parenteral nutrition as a primary therapy in patients with extensive Crohn's disease of the small bowel and malnutrition. *Gastroenterology* 73:1077, 1977.

130. Rault RMJ, Scribner BH. Treatment of Crohn's disease with home parenteral nutrition. *Gastroenterology* 72: 1249, 1977.

131. Cravo M, Camillo ME, Correia JP. Nutritional support in Crohn's disease: Which route? *Am J Gastroenterol* 86:317, 1991.

132. Russell RI. Review article: Dietary and nutritional management of Crohn's disease. *Aliment Pharmacol Ther* 5:211, 1991.

133. Wesley JR. Home parenteral nutrition: Indications, principles and cost-effectiveness. *Comp Ther* 9:29, 1983.

134. Wateska LP, Sattler LL, Steiger E. Cost of home parenteral nutrition program. *JAMA* 244:2303, 1980.

135. Howard L, et al. Four years of North American registry home parenteral nutrition outcome data and their implications for patient management. *JPEN* 15:384, 1991.

136. Forse RA, Shizgal HM. The assessment of malnutrition. *Surgery* 88:17, 1980.

137. Anderson CF, et al. The sensitivity and specificity of nutrition-related variables in relationship to the duration of hospital stay and the rate of complications. *Mayo Clin Proc* 59:477, 1984.

138. Heatley RV, Williams RHP, Lewis MH. Preoperative intravenous feeding: A controlled trial. *Postgrad Med J* 55:541, 1979.

Selected Readings

Detsky AS, et al. Perioperative parenteral nutrition: A meta-analysis. *Ann Int Med* 107:195, 1987.

This meta-analysis helped to define the role of perioperative parenteral nutrition by revealing benefit only in select groups of patients. The results were used to help define current parenteral nutrition use standards.

Linn BS. Outcomes of older and younger malnourished and well-nourished patients one year after hospitalization. *Am J Clin Nutr* 39:66, 1984.

This paper documents the detrimental long-term effects of ignored hospital malnutrition on convalescence, disease relapse, and hospital readmission rates.

Moore FA, et al. Early enteral feeding, compared with parenteral, reduces postoperative septic complications. *Ann Surg* 216:172, 1992.

This meta-analysis, which combined eight studies, revealed decreased septic complications overall, and in blunt trauma patients in particular. In addition, it reveals how well surgical patients tolerate early enteral therapy.

O'Leary JP, et al. Incidence of malnutrition among patients admitted to a VA hospital. *South Med J* 75:1095, 1982.

The largest series to document the incidence of malnutrition in patients admitted to the hospital.

Weisner RL, et al. Hospital malnutrition: A prospective evaluation of general medical patients during the course of hospitalization. *Am J Clin Nutr* 32:418, 1979.

The first paper to call our attention to nutritional neglect and the progressive nature of malnutrition in hospitalized patients.

Index

Index